Modern Therapeutics in Rheumatic Diseases

Section Editors

Steffen Gay, MD

University Hospital of Zurich, Switzerland

Gary M. Kammer, MD

Wake Forest University School of Medicine, Winston-Salem, NC

Johanne Martel-Pelletier, PhD

Hôpital Notre-Dame, Université de Montréal, Montréal, PQ, Canada

Larry W. Moreland, MD

University of Alabama, Birmingham, AL

Jean-Pierre Pelletier, MD

Hôpital Notre-Dame, Université de Montréal, Montréal, PQ, Canada

George C. Tsokos, MD

Uniformed Services University of the Health Sciences, Bethesda; and Walter Reed Army Institute of Research, Silver Spring, MD

Modern Therapeutics in Rheumatic Diseases

Edited by

George C. Tsokos, MD

Uniformed Services University of the Health Sciences, Bethesda;
and Walter Reed Army Institute of Research, Silver Spring, MD

Humana Press ✴ Totowa, New Jersey

© 2002 Humana Press Inc.
999 Riverview Drive, Suite 208
Totowa, New Jersey 07512

www.humanapress.com

The content and opinions expressed in this book are the sole work of the authors and editors, who have warranted due diligence in the creation and issuance of their work. The publisher, editors, and authors are not responsible for errors or omissions or for any consequences arising from the information or opinions presented in this book and make no warranty, express or implied, with respect to its contents.

This publication is printed on acid-free paper. ∞
ANSI Z39.48-1984 (American National Standards Institute) Permanence of Paper for Printed Library Materials.

Cover illustration: Figure 1A from Chapter 14, "Promoting Articular Cartilage Repair," by Joseph A. Buckwalter and James A. Martin. Adapted from ref. *16*.

Production Editor: Jessica Jannicelli.
Cover design by Patricia F. Cleary.

For additional copies, pricing for bulk purchases, and/or information about other Humana titles, contact Humana at the above address or at any of the following numbers: Tel.: 973-256-1699; Fax: 973-256-8341; E-mail: humana@humanapr.com or visit our Web site: http://humanapress.com

Printed in the United States of America.   10 9 8 7 6 5 4 3 2 1

Library of Congress Cataloging in Publication Data

Modern therapeutics in rheumatic diseases/edited by George C. Tsokos...[et al.]
    p. cm.
  Includes bibliographical references and index.
  ISBN 0-89603-916-1 (alk. paper)
  1. Rheumatism.   I. Tsokos, George, C.

  RC927 .M545 2001
  616.7'2306—dc21

                                        00-053529

Preface

Rheumatic diseases, in general, are of unknown pathogenic origin. Until recently the mainstay in their treatment has been the use of general measures without specificity. Such drugs as prednisone were used in the treatment of most of the diseases to suppress the inflammatory process and a usually overactive immune system. The effect was nonspecific and the side effects were often life-threatening. In the field of such degenerative rheumatic diseases as osteoarthritis, nonspecific anti-inflammatory drugs have been used with minimal benefit and numerous side effects.

During the last two decades, enormous progress has been made in the understanding of the molecular and cellular processes that lead to disease pathology. Several biochemical steps have been identified in most of the systemic diseases and the involved cells have been characterized. The complexities of the immune system have been better understood and the aberrations that lead to autoimmunity have been clarified significantly.

During the last decade rheumatologists have capitalized on the knowledge gained and have begun to develop new treatment modalities designed to interrupt particular pathologic processes in the hope that, by reversing the aberration, clinical improvement will ensue. This approach has enjoyed frequent success. As a consequence, a number of novel biologics and drugs have recently been introduced in the treatment of rheumatic diseases and many more are in clinical trials. These new therapeutic modalities have already changed the way we think about rheumatic diseases and have markedly increased our ability to help suffering patients. The pace of development of these novel drugs is also increasing and a continuous surge of new biologics and drugs that will claim better clinical efficacy, more specificity, and less toxicity seems likely.

Modern Therapeutics in Rheumatic Diseases aims to synthesize this developing knowledge and present it concisely to all those treating rheumatic patients. Without ignoring what is currently standard treatment, it will present, in practical detail, novel treatments and will discuss those that are in clinical trials and about to be introduced in the rheumatology practice. *Modern*

Therapeutics in Rheumatic Diseases provides a single volume, compiled by experts, where this important information can be accessed.

The editors wish to thank Elyse O'Grady for making this book possible and Jessica Jannicelli for her wonderful editing skills.

Steffen Gay
Gary M. Kammer
Johanne Martel-Pelletier
Larry W. Moreland
Jean-Pierre Pelletier
George C. Tsokos

Contents

II. OSTEOARTHRITIS

Jean-Pierre Pelletier and Johanne Martel-Pelletier, Section Editors

III. SYSTEMIC AUTOIMMUNE DISEASES

Gary M. Kammer and George C. Tsokos, Section Editors

Contributors

ROY D. ALTMAN, MD • *University of Miami School of Medicine and Miami Veterans Affairs Medical Center, University of Miami, Miami, FL*

ALEXANDER E. ANNENKOV, PhD • *Bone and Joint Research Unit, St. Bartholomew's and Royal London School of Medicine and Dentistry, Queen Mary, University of London, Charterhouse Square, London, UK*

JOAN M. BATHON, MD • *Division of Rheumatology, Johns Hopkins University School of Medicine, Baltimore, MD*

DIMITRIOS T. BOUMPAS, MD, FACP • *Division of Rheumatology, Clinical Immunology and Allergy, University of Crete Medical School, Heraklion, Greece*

JÜRGEN BRAUN, MD • *Section on Rheumatology, Benjamin Franklin University, Free University Berlin, Berlin, Germany*

BARRY BRESNIHAN, MD • *Department of Rheumatology, St. Vincent's University Hospital, Dublin, Ireland*

S. LOUIS BRIDGES, JR., MD, PhD • *Division of Clinical Immunology and Rheumatology, University of Alabama at Birmingham, Birmingham, AL*

JOSEPH A. BUCKWALTER, MD • *Department of Orthopaedic Surgery, University of Iowa College of Medicine, Iowa City, IA*

RICHARD K. BURT, MD • *Department of Medicine, Division of Immune Therapy and Autoimmune Diseases, Northwestern University Medical Center, Chicago, IL*

LEONARD H. CALABRESE, DO • *R. J. Fasenmeyer Chair of Clinical Immunology, Department of Rheumatic and Immunologic Diseases, The Cleveland Clinic Foundation, Cleveland, OH*

MAURIZIO CEPPI, PhD • *Institut de Biochimie, Universite de Fribourg, Fribourg, Switzerland*

YUTI CHERNAJOVSKY, PhD • *Bone and Joint Research Unit, St. Bartholomew's and Royal London School of Medicine and Dentistry, Queen Mary, University of London, Charterhouse Square, London, UK*

GINA L. COSTA, PhD • *Department of Cellular and Molecular Biology, SurroMed, Mountain View, CA*

DAVID I. DAIKH, MD, PhD • *Department of Veterans Affairs Medical Center and Department of Medicine, University of California, San Francisco, CA*

PAUL EMERY, MD • *Department of Rheumatology, University of Leeds School of Medicine, United Leeds Teaching Hospital, Leeds, UK*

CHRISTOPHER H. EVANS, PhD • *Center for Molecular Orthopaedics, Harvard Medical School, Boston, MA*

C. GARRISON FATHMAN, MD • *Department of Medicine, Division of Immunology and Rheumatology, Stanford University School of Medicine, Stanford, CA*

GARY S. FIRESTEIN, MD • *Division of Rheumatology, Allergy and Immunology, UCSD School of Medicine, La Jolla, CA*

SHERRY D. FLEMING, MD • *Division of Immunology/Rheumatology, Department of Medicine, Uniformed Services University of the Health Sciences, Bethesda; and Walter Reed Army Institute of Research, Silver Spring, MD*

RENATE E. GAY, MD • *WHO Collaborating Center for Molecular Biology and Novel Therapeutic Strategies for Rheumatic Diseases, Department of Rheumatology, University Hospital of Zurich, Zurich, Switzerland*

STEFFEN GAY, MD • *WHO Collaborating Center for Molecular Biology and Novel Therapeutic Strategies for Rheumatic Diseases, Department of Rheumatology, University Hospital of Zurich, Zurich, Switzerland*

MARK C. GENOVESE, MD • *Division of Immunology and Rheumatology, Department of Medicine, Stanford University School of Medicine, Stanford, CA*

STEVEN C. GHIVIZZANI, PhD • *Center for Molecular Orthopaedics, Harvard Medical School, Boston, MA*

WILLIAM R. GILLILAND, MD • *Division of Immunology/Rheumatology, Department of Medicine, Uniformed Services University of Health Sciences, Bethesda, MD*

ERIC L. GREIDINGER, MD • *Division of Immunology and Rheumatology, University of Missouri and Department of Veterans Affairs Medical Center, Columbia, MO*

BOULOS HARAOUI, MD • *Department of Rheumatology, Hôpital Notre-Dame, Centre Hospitalier de l'Université de Montréal, Montréal, Québec, Canada*

JAMES H. HERNDON, MD • *Center for Molecular Orthopaedics, Harvard Medical School, Boston, MA*

ROBERT W. HOFFMAN, DO • *Division of Immunology and Rheumatology, University of Missouri and Department of Veterans Affairs Medical Center, Columbia, MO*

M. ELAINE HUSNI, MD, MPH • *Beth Israel Deaconess Medical Center, Harvard Medical School, Boston, MA*

GABOR G. ILLEI, MD • *Arthritis and Rheumatism Branch, NIAMS, NIH, Bethesda, MD*

KANYAKORN JAOVISIDHA, MD • *Division of Rheumatology, Department of Medicine, Medical College of Wisconsin, Milwaukee, WI*

KENNETH C. KALUNIAN, MD • *Division of Rheumatology, UCLA School of Medicine, Los Angeles, CA*

GARY M. KAMMER, MD • *Section on Rheumatology and Clinical Immunology, Department of Internal Medicine, Wake Forest University School of Medicine, Winston-Salem, NC*

ILDY M. KATONA, MD • *Departments of Pediatrics and Medicine, Uniformed Services University of the Health Sciences, Bethesda, MD*

MUHAMMAD A. KHAN, MD, FRCP, FACP • *Division of Rheumatology, Department of Medicine, Case Western Reserve University, Cleveland, OH*

ROBERT P. KIMBERLY, MD • *Division of Clinical Immunology and Rheumatology, University of Alabama at Birmingham, Birmingham, AL*

JOHN R. KIRWAN, BSC, MD, FRCP (UK) • *Rheumatology Unit, University of Bristol Division of Medicine, Bristol Royal Infirmary, Bristol, UK*

TETSUYA KOBAYASHI, PhD • *Rheumatology, Immunology, and Genetics Program, Institute of Medical Science, St. Marianna University, Kanagawa, Japan*

CLARENCE W. LEGERTON III, MD • *Division of Rheumatology and Immunology, Medical University of South Carolina, Charleston, SC*

PAMELA MANNING, PhD • *Molecular Pharmacology, Monsanto Company, St. Louis, MO*

JOHANNE MARTEL-PELLETIER, PhD • *Osteoarthritis Research Unit, Centre Hospitalier de l'Université de Montréal, Hôpital Notre-Dame, Montréal, PQ, Canada*

JAMES A. MARTIN, PhD • *Department of Orthopaedics, University of Iowa College of Medicine, Iowa City, IA*

ALAN K. MATSUMOTO, MD • *Johns Hopkins University School of Medicine, Baltimore, MD*

JOAN T. MERRILL, MD • *Department of Clinical Pharmacology, Oklahoma Medical Research Foundation, Oklahoma City, OK*

LAURA J. MIRKINSON, MD • *Department of Critical Care, Children's National Medical Center, George Washington University School of Medicine, Washington, DC*

LARRY W. MORELAND, MD • *Division of Clinical Immunology and Rheumatology, University of Alabama at Birmingham, Birmingham, AL*

ULF MÜLLER-LADNER, MD • *WHO Collaborating Center for Molecular Biology and Novel Therapeutic Strategies for Rheumatic Diseases, Department of Rheumatology, Zurich, Switzerland*

KUSUKI NISHIOKA, MD, PhD • *Rheumatology, Immunology, and Genetics Program, Institute of Medical Science, St. Marianna University, Kanagawa, Japan*

JAMES R. O'DELL, MD • *Section of Rheumatology and Immunology, Department of Internal Medicine, University of Nebraska Medical Center, Omaha, NE*

IVAN G. OTTERNESS, PhD • *Department of Pharmacology, Emil Fisher Center, University of Erlangen-Nurenberg, Erlangen, Germany; Current address: 241 Monument St., Groton, CT*

THOMAS PAP, MD • *WHO Collaborating Center for Molecular Biology and Novel Therapeutic Strategies for Rheumatic Diseases, Department of Rheumatology, University Hospital of Zurich, Zurich, Switzerland*

JEAN-PIERRE PELLETIER, MD • *Osteoarthritis Research Unit, Centre Hospitalier de l'Université de Montréal, Hôpital Notre-Dame, Montréal, Quebec, Canada*

JEAN-PIERRE RAYNAULD, MD • *Department of Rheumatology, Hopital Notre-Dame, Centre Hospitalier de l'Université de Montréal, Montréal, Québec, Canada*

JEAN-YVES REGINSTER, MD, PhD • *Head Bone and Cartilage Metabolism Unit, University of Liege, Liege, Belgium*

PAUL D. ROBBINS, PhD • *Department of Molecular Genetics and Biochemistry, University of Pittsburgh School of Medicine, Pittsburgh, PA*

WILLIAM H. ROBINSON, MD, PhD • *Division of Immunology and Rheumatology, Department of Medicine, Stanford University School of Medicine, Stanford, CA*

ANN K. ROSENTHAL, MD • *Division of Rheumatology, Department of Medicine, Medical College of Milwaukee, Milwaukee, WI*

SANDRO RUSCONI, PhD • *Département de Médecine, Institut de Biochimie, Université de Fribourg, Fribourg, Switzerland*

KENNETH G. SAAG, MD, MSC • *Division of Clinical Immunology and Rheumatology, Department of Medicine, University of Alabama at Birmingham, Birmingham, AL*

MARY J. SALTARELLI, PhD • *Clinical Biochemical Measurements, Pfizer Global Research and Development, Groton, CT*

JÖRG SCHEDEL, MD • *WHO Collaborating Center for Molecular Biology and Novel Therapeutic Strategies for Rheumatic Diseases, Department of Rheumatology, University Hospital of Zurich, Zurich, Switzerland*

PETER H. SCHUR, MD • *Division of Rheumatology, Immunology, and Allergy, Brigham and Women's Hospital and Harvard Medical School, Boston, MA*

DAVID L. SCOTT, MD • *Rheumatology Unit, King's College Hospital, London, UK*

JOACHIM SIEPER, MD • *Section on Rheumatology, Benjamin Franklin University, Free University Berlin, Berlin, Germany*

RICHARD M. SILVER, MD • *Division of Rheumatology and Immunology, Medical University of South Carolina, Charleston, SC*

LEE S. SIMON, MD • *Department of Medicine, Beth Isreal Deaconess Medical Center, Harvard Medical School, Boston, MA*

VIBEKE STRAND, MD • *Division of Immunology, Stanford University School of Medicine, Palo Alto, CA*

JOHN S. SUNDY, MD, PhD • *Division of Rheumatology, Allergy and Clinical Immunology, Department of Medicine, Duke University Medical Center, Durham, NC*

PAUL P. TAK, MD, PhD • *Division of Clinical Immunology and Rheumatology, Academic Medical Center, Amsterdam, The Netherlands; and Division of Rheumatology, Allergy and Immunology, UCSD School of Medicine, La Jolla, CA*

ANN E. TRAYNOR, MD • *Division of Immune Therapy and Autoimmune Disease, Department of Medicine, Northwestern University Medical Center, Chicago, IL*

GEORGE C. TSOKOS, MD • *Division of Immunology/Rheumatology, Department of Medicine, Uniformed Services University of the Health Sciences, Bethesda; and Walter Reed Army Institute of Research, Silver Spring, MD*

FONS A. J. VAN DE LOO, PhD • *Rheumatology Research Laboratory, University Medical Center, Nijmegen, The Netherlands*

WIM B. VAN DEN BERG, PhD • *Rheumatology Research Laboratory, University Medical Center, Nijmegen, The Netherlands*

DIMITRIOS VASSILOPOULOS, MD • *Academic Department of Medicine, Hippokration General Hospital, Athens University School of Medicine, Athens, Greece*

MARY C. WASKO, MD, MSC • *Division of Rheumatology, Department of Medicine, University of Pittsburgh Medical Center, Pittsburgh, PA*

ARTHUR WEINSTEIN, MD • *Section of Rheumatology, Washington Hospital Center, Washington, DC*

SEAN J. WOLLASTON, MD • *Division of Rheumatology, UCLA School of Medicine, Los Angeles, CA*

DAVID WOFSY, MD • *Arthritis Unit , Department of Veterans Affairs Medical Center and Department of Medicine, University of California, San Francisco, CA*

I RHEUMATOID ARTHRITIS

1

New Treatment Opportunities for Rheumatoid Arthritis

Larry W. Moreland

In this introductory chapter, it is the intent to point out the tremendous new advances that have been made within the past two years for treating rheumatoid arthritis (RA). The past decade has been marked by a remarkable increase in our knowledge in the pathogenesis of RA. This basic scientific knowledge has translated now into opportunities to target specifically the mediators that are now known to be players in this disease. These new therapies include potentially safer (although not more effective with pain control) cyclooxygenase-2 specific nonsteroidal anti-inflammatory drugs (NSAIDs); leflunomide; and two tumor necrosis factor (TNF) inhibitors, etanercept and infliximab. A device, the Prosorba column has also received approval by the US Food and Drug Administration (FOA) for use with RA patients. Moreover, it is anticipated in the near future that interleukin 1 (IL-1) inhibitors will soon be available. Although these new therapeutic options have shown significant clinical responses in RA patients, these advances will require further analysis with long-term follow-up to determine their true potential to modify the disease and to be safer than currently available therapies.

The ultimate goal of RA management is to restore the patient to normal non-RA status with normal physical, social, and emotional function and capacity to work, and with structurally and anatomically normal joints. Although this goal may be unrealistic in many patients, we can now at least have these goals in our sights. Never before have so many drugs been available to use as treatments for RA, and these new therapies have resulted in the paradigms for treating RA.

Profound clinical improvements have been demonstrated with these new disease-modifying, anti-rheumatic drugs (DMARDs) (leflunomide, etanercept, and infliximab) in placebo-controlled trials. Thus, the challenges we will face as clinicians include how to administer these new therapies either alone or in combination with our currently available DMARDs such as methotoxate, sulfasalazine, hydroxychloroquine, cycyclosporine, gold salts, corticosteroids, and so forth.

There is a growing consensus that we should treat RA patients earlier with our "best" DMARDs. This is based on evidence that up to three-fourths of RA patients have developed evidence of permanent damage (erosion of bone and cartilage) within three years of disease duration. This consensus has been further solidified with the recent evidence that several of our DMARDs (methotrexate, etanercept,

From: *Modern Therapeutics in Rheumatic Diseases*
Edited by: G. C. Tsokos, et al. © Humana Press, Inc., Totowa, NJ

leflunomide, sulfasalazine, infliximab) can slow the disease progression, as measured radiographically.

These new advances in our treatment options are met with several new challenges including when these therapeutic agents should be used in the current treatment paradigms by physicians who see these patients. Decisions that will be important in this regard will need to take into account the comparable efficacy and safety profile as well as the cost-effectiveness of these new therapies. What is becoming increasing clear in the most recent years is that combinations of currently available disease-modifying drugs with each other, or in combination with these new therapies, provides in most cases a better therapeutic result than when each of the agents is used alone. These new therapies will require additional studies in patients to determine which options will provide the most beneficial long-term outcomes.

In Chapter 10, use of combination of our current disease modifying drugs is reviewed *(1–6)*. Methotrexate remains the DMARD used most often and remains the cornerstone for the combination of DMARDs. This chapter reviews in detail each of the treatment approaches with combination therapy published to date. In particular, discussion of therapeutic options for early disease or initial therapy for RA, which may differ from treatment given to patients with more established disease, who have been treated with methotrexate and have failed to have an optimal response (i.e., complete remission). These pivotal studies have provided the basis with which to compare future studies with regards to study design, outcome measures, and so on. Numerous questions are unanswered at this time concerning the appropriateness of combination therapy for specific patients with mild vs more aggressive disease, as well as which specific combination would be the most effective. Further studies might include large clinical trials where patients with certain specific types of mild vs aggressive disease are randomized to specific protocols. Alternatively, we may also see large databases with long-term follow-ups in which therapies given to patients are carefully documented, along with the outcomes of such therapies.

In Chapter 6, there is a review of the current data regarding TNF inhibitors as new therapeutic options for the treatment of RA *(7–19)*. TNF inhibitors have been truly a "bench to bedside" approach in which the lessons learned from both animal models of disease, and an understanding of molecular events gained by several investigators, have represented the first target based treatment for RA. There are currently two TNF inhibitors commercially available for the treatment of RA: etanercept and infliximab. The efficacy of TNF inhibitors in patients with refractory disease has been remarkable; in fact, the percentage of patients that respond to such therapies is in the range of 50–70%. It will be important to predict or understand why some patients have such good clinical responses as we move forward with other targeted therapies, such as IL-1 inhibitors *(20–23)*. Therefore, much research is needed to understand why some patients do not respond to TNF inhibitors; better understanding of the disease in these patients can lead to new therapeutic options. Likewise understanding the mechanisms through which patients have dramatic responses to these TNF inhibitors is important, because as this will ultimately shed light on identifying patients who might be more likely to respond to such targeted therapies. Potential areas of investigation in this regard would involve the analysis of genetic factors that might be predictive of efficacy and/or adverse events. Chapter 2 gives an up-to-date review of the current understanding of the genetics of RA.

One area of investigation has now led to the approval of drugs that will not only improve the signs and symptoms of RA, but also potentially slow the disease, as measured radiographically. Therapies that have been shown to slow the disease radiographically represent a new challenge as we move forward in developing new paradigms in the treatment of RA. Although the short-term (1-yr studies) clearly suggests that drugs such as leflunomide (reviewed in Chapter 8) and the TNF inhibitors (reviewed in Chapter 6), as well as methotrexate and sulfasalazine, can slow the disease, several question remain to be answered, such as whether a radiographic measurement of 1 yr of change will translate into long-term benefits such as improved function and survival. In addition, it is now important to understand if indeed these radiographic changes are truly important and whether these therapies (alone or in combination) should be used in early disease to prevent irreversible damage. This information will require significant further investigation especially regarding what types of combinations of these agents should be used and in what types of patients (i.e., more aggressive vs less aggressive disease).

Another molecular target for potential therapy is IL-1, which has many of the same proinflammatory activities of TNF. The current state of research in IL-1 inhibitors is reviewed in Chapter 7. Specifically, IL-1 receptor antagonists (IL-1ra) have been shown in controlled trials to produce statistically significant improvements in controlling the signs and symptoms of RA, as well as slowing the disease process, as measured radiographically *(20–23)*. The efficacy of IL-1ra might be enhanced potentially with preparations that would increase the half-life or ability to block all IL-1 receptors. In fact, in animal models of arthritis, it has been shown that there is a clear dose response of the amount of IL-1ra given with regards to the efficacy. Therefore, perhaps improved formulations or delivery systems of IL-1ra and/or other mechanisms such as inhibitors of IL-1 converting enzyme *(24)* potentially might be future ways of inhibiting IL-1. In addition, agents that inhibit P38 mitogen activating protein (MAP) kinase *(25–27)*, which would theoretically inhibit the production of both TNF and IL-1, represent another target that is worthy of RA therapy exploration (reviewed in Chapter 11).

Although often thought to be an adjunctive therapy for RA, corticosteroids have been shown to demonstrate remarkable anti-inflammatory effects in a variety of diseases. However, the significant adverse events associated with long-term, high-dose cortisone use (reviewed in Chapter 5) clearly have limited the usefulness of this particular agent as a long-term drug for the treatment of RA. As illustrated in Chapter 5, systemic steroid use in RA remains a highly debated area. The most intriguing aspect that remains to be clearly defined is whether corticosteroids can modify the disease by slowing damage as measured radiographically *(28)*. The mechanisms by which corticosteroids are effective, such as inhibiting proinflammatory cytokines (such as TNF, IL-6, IL-1) would support the role that they might be able to alter disease manifestations. This is of particular importance now that both TNF and IL-1 inhibitors have been able to demonstrate true disease modification in this same manner. However, the long-term side effects, such as steroid-induced osteoporosis, as well as other untoward effects, would argue that the benefit-risk ratio would be unfavorable in using these as long-term disease-modifying drugs.

The increased mortality reported in studies of patients with RA is multifactoral. However, a probable cause of the long-term outcome of many RA patients might relate to many of the medications used to treat the signs and symptoms of this disease. This has been of particular interest with regards to NSAIDs, which have significant toxicities such as peptic ulcer disease with perforations and bleeds. Recent advances in the discovery of the COX-2 isoenzyme and specific inhibitors of COX-2 have led to a new class of drugs, the COX-2-selective NSAID *(29–31)*. These new anti-inflammatory drugs are reviewed in Chapter 3. Although these new agents do not have increased efficacy when compared to the traditional COX-1/COX-2 NSAIDs, the benefit of COX-2 agents relates to their safety profile. Indeed, studies completed to date of patients with RA using upper-endoscopy and the presence of ulcerations as a surrogate marker for severity of toxicity would strongly support the improved safety profile with COX-2-specific NSAIDs. However, longer term trials appropriately powered to determine the true clinical significance, i.e., perforations and bleeds, will more clearly define the safety efficacy profile of these therapies. NSAIDs, either nonselective or selective COX-2 inhibitors, are not disease modifying anti-rheumatic drugs. They do not slow the disease as measured radiographically. Their clinical benefit relates in inhibiting prostaglandin production and thus serving as analgesic and anti-inflammatory agents that improve the signs and symptoms of the disease, allowing patients to be more functional. These new selective COX-2 inhibitors should then offer increased safety as a means of improving pain in patients with this debilitating and crippling form of arthritis.

Another interesting line of investigation in providing new therapeutic targets and potentially significant disease modification involves the use of agents that inhibit the destructive enzymes that destroy cartilage and bone. In this regard, there has been a significant interest in the past several years with the evaluation of drugs such as tetracyclines, in particular minocycline, as agents that could modify the disease *(32–36)*. The recent advances in this field are reviewed in Chapter 9. Although not approved by the FDA for use in RA, tetracyclines are an option that many physicians might consider in patients in combination therapy with other disease modifying drugs.

This line of investigation in inhibitors of matrix metalloproteinases (MMPs) remains an active area of interest. However, a major hurdle is to identify the specific MMPs that are involved in the destructive process in RA, but that are not essential for normal processes in the other areas of the body. MMPs have numerous activities and inhibition of them might result in significant untoward events such as increased fibrosis, or alterations in the immune surveillance with regards to malignancies.

Leflunomide, a pyrimidine-synthesis inhibitor, has also shown significant improvement in signs and symptoms of disease, as well as slowing radiographic progression *(37–43)* in RA patients. Emery, et al. in Chapter 8, have reviewed the clinical data regarding the development of this agent. An area of interest at this time is whether the combination of leflunomide with other drugs such as methotrexate, etanercept, infliximab, and so on will enhance the efficacy of each of these drugs when used in combination.

Although recent advances in new therapies that have been outlined have markedly enhanced our ability potentially to slow the devastating manifestation of RA, the fact is that very few, if any, patients have developed true remissions. In Chapter 11, Genovese outlines other areas of investigation regarding molecular targets that might contribute to improving our therapeutic options over the next few years. In particular in this regard, the ability to inhibit the T cells either with T-cell receptor peptide vaccine *(44)*, or with agents that inhibit the costimulatory pathways *(45–47)*, might potentially lead to combinations of therapies that inhibit not only macrophage molecules (such as IL-1 and TNF) but also T-cell function. In addition, an area of investigation that requires further exploration are agents that inhibit B cells. Rheumatoid factor production is one of the hallmarks of RA, and yet the exact role rheumatoid factors play in the destructive process remain elusive even after several decades of investigation in this area.

In summary, remarkable advances have occurred in the treatment options of RA. Several areas of investigation remain that will be crucial to our understanding of the long-term benefits of these new therapeutic options. Specifically, all of these agents have been studied in relatively short-term clinical trials and our understanding of the long-term benefits and/or toxicity of these new therapies remain elusive. In this regard, it is crucial that the long-term benefits and toxicities of these agents, when used either alone or in combination, are clearly defined as we embark on additional therapies for RA. It is clear that the agents in use now to inhibit targeted areas in human disease also have the potential of interfering with targets that are involved with normal physiological processes. We clearly do not understand the long-term benefits of these new therapies at this time.

The bar for achievable clinical improvement has been substantially raised with these new treatment developments. With further definition of the genetic and nongenetic factors that contribute to the disease, we as rheumatologists can now realistically strive for remission as a goal for our patients with RA. With the human genome project completed, clinical and basic researchers have the opportunity to define which molecular mechanisms are likely operative in the initiation, perpetuation, and ultimate destructive phases of RA. Moreover, with new targets currently being investigated such as inhibitors of IL-1—agents that block costimulatory molecules that block the signaling between T and B cells—the potential of inducing tolerance in RA is now closer to reality. With continued advances in our understanding of cytokine biology, new ways of blocking TNF and IL-1 are likely to evolve.

There is general agreement that the inflammation of RA should be controlled as soon as possible, as completely as possible, and for as long as possible, consistent with patient safety. The risk of RA management has decreased as rheumatologists have gained more experience using combinations of DMARDs, and as increasingly specific and less toxic agents to modify inflammation (e.g., TNF and COX-2 inhibitors) have become available. Potential benefit has increased with the documentation of prevention of structural damage. This improved therapeutic risk/benefit and progressive, irreversible nature of RA joint damage justifies immediate initiation of DMARD treatment of newly diagnosed RA, and this is rapidly becoming the expected standard of care.

In summary, this work on RA therapies succinctly reviews the recent advances in our treatment options for RA and provides a glimpse to the future of other therapies that are currently under investigation for RA. As clinical researchers, the opportunity to take the basic research findings from the bench and to clinical practice provides a remarkable opportunity to improve the quality of life for our patients. Not since the development of cortisone as a therapy for RA has such progress been made in the treatment of RA.

REFERENCES

1. Boers, M., A.C. Verhoeven, H.M. Markusse, et al. 1997. Randomized comparison of combined step-down prednisolone, methotrexate and sulphasalazine with sulphasalazine alone in early rheumatoid arthritis. *Lancet* 350:309–318.

2. Mottonen, T., P. Hannonsen, M. Leirasale-Repo, et al. 1999. Comparison of combination therapy with single-drug therapy in early rheumatoid arthritis: a randomized trial. *Lancet* 353:1568–1573.

3. Tugwell, P., T. Pincus, D. Yocum, et al. 1995. Combination therapy with cyclosporine and methotrexate in severe rheumatoid arthritis. *N. Engl. J. Med.* 333:137–141.

4. Kremer, J.M. 1998. Combination therapy with biologic agents in rheumatoid arthritis: perils and promise. *Arthritis Rheum.* 41:1548–1551.

5. Tsakonas, E, A.A. Fitzgeral, M.A. Fitazcharles, et al. 2000. Consequences of delayed therapy with second-line agents in rheumatoid arthritis: a 3 year followup on the hydroxychloroquine in early rheumatoid arthritis (HERA) study. *J. Rheumatol.* 27:623-929.

6. O'Dell, J.R., C.E. Haire, N. Erikson, et al. 1996. Treatment of rheumatoid arthritis with methotrexate alone, sulfasalazine, and hydroxychloroquine, or a combination of all three medications. *N. Engl. J. Med.* 334:1287–1291.

7. Elliott, M.J., R.N. Maini, M. Feldmann, J.R. Kalden, C. Antoni, J.S. Smolen, et al. 1994. Randomised double-blind comparison of chimeric monoclonal antibody to tumour necrosis factor α (cA2) versus placebo in rheumatoid arthritis. *Lancet* 344:1105–1110.

8. Elliott, M.J, R.N. Maini, M. Feldmann, A. Long-Fox, P. Charles, H. Bijl, and J.N. Woody. 1994. Repeated therapy with nonoclonal antibody to tumour necrosis factor a (cA2) in patients with rheumatoid arthrisis. *Lancet* 344:1125–1127.

9. Lovell, D.J., E.H. Giannini, A. Reiff, G.D. Cawkwell, E.D. Silverman, J.J. Noton, et al. 2000. Etanercept in children with polyarticular juvenile rheumatoid arthritis. *New Engl J Med* 342:763–769, 2000.

10. Maini, R.N., F.C. Breedveld, J.R. Kalden, J.S. Smolen, D. Davis, J.D. MacFarlane, et al. 1998. Therapeutic efficacy of multiple intravenous infusions of anti-tumor necrosis factor a monoclonal antibody combined with low-dose weekly methotrexate in rheumatoid arthritis. *Arthritis Rheum.* 41(9):1552–1563.

11. Maini, RN, F.C. Breedveld, J.R. Kalden, J.S. Smolen, D. Davis, J.D. MacFarlane, et al. 1998. Therapeutic efficacy of multiple intravenous infusions of anti-tumor necrosis factor a monoclonal antibody combined with low-dose weekly methotrexate in rheumatoid arthritis. *Arthritis Rheum.* 41:1552–1563.

12. Moreland, L.W., S.W. Baumgartner, M.H. Schiff, E.A. Tindall, R.M. Fleischmann, A.L. Weaver, et al. 1997. Treatment of rheumatoid arthritis with a recombinant human tumor necrosis factor receptor (p75)-Fc fusion protein. *N. Engl. J. Med.* 337:141–147.

13. Moreland, L.W., G. Margolies, L.W. Heck Jr, A. Saway, C. Blosch, R. Hanna, and W.J. Koopman. 1996. Recombinant soluble tumor necrosis factor receptor (p80) fusion protein: toxicity and dose finding trial in refractory rheumatoid arthritis. *J. Rheumatol.* 23:1849–1855.

14. Moreland, L.W., M.H. Schiff, S.W. Baumgartner, E.A. Tindall, R.M. Fleischmann, K.J. Bulpitt, et al. 1999. Etanercept therapy in rheumatoid arthritis. A randomized, controlled trial. *Ann. Intern. Med.* 130:478–486, 1999.

15. Van de Putte, L.B.A, R. Rau, F.C. Breedfeld, J.R. Kalden, M.G. Malaise, M. Schattekirchner, et al. 1999. Efficacy of the fully human anti-TNF antibody D2E7 in rheumatoid arthritis. *Arthritis Rheum.* 42(Suppl):S1977.

16. Weinblatt, M.E., J.M. Kremer, A.D. Bankhurst, D.J. Bulpitt, R.M. Fleischmann, R.I. Fox, et al. 1999. A trial of etanercept, a recombinant tumor necrosis factor receptor:Fc fusion protein, in patients with rheumatoid arthritis receiving methotrexate. *New Engl. J. Med.* 340:253–259.

17. Maini, R., E.W. St. Clair, F. Breedveld, et al. 1999. Infliximab (chimeric anti-tumour necrosis factor-α monoclonal antibody) versus placebo in rheumatoid arthritis patients receiving concomitant methotrexate: a randomized phase III trial. *Lancet* 354:1932-1939.

18. Moreland, L., M. Schiff, S.W. Baumgartner, et al. 1999. Etanercept therapy in rheumatoid arthritis. *Ann. Int. Med.* 130:478–486.

19. Bathon, J.M., R.W. Martin, R.M. Fleishmann, et al. 2000. A comparison of etanercept and methotrexate in patients with early rheumatoid arthritis. *N. Engl. J. Med.* 343:1583–1586.

20. Arend, W.P., M. Malyak, C.J. Guthridge, and C. Gabay. 1998. Interluikin-1 receptor antagonist: Role in biology. *Annu. Rev. Immunol.* 16:27–55.

21. Bresnihan, B., J.M. Alvaro-Gracia, M. Cobby, M. Doherty, Z. Domljan, P. Emery, et al. 1998. Treatment of rheumatoid arthritis with recombinant human interleukin-1 receptor antagonist. *Arthritis Rheum.* 41:2196–2204.

22. Campion, G.V., M.E. Lebsack, J. Lookbaugh, et al. 1996. Dose-range and dose-frequency study of recombinant human interleukin-1 receptor antagonist in patients with rheumatoid arthritis. *Arthritis Rheum.* 39:1092–1101.

23. Drevlow, B.E., R. Lovis, M.A. Haag, J.M. Sinacore, C. Jacobs, C. Blosche, et al. 1996. Recombinant human interleukin-1 receptor type 1 in the treatment of patients with active rheumatoid arthritis. *Arthritis Rheum.* 39:257–265.

24. Miller, B.E., P.A. Krasney, D.M. Gauvin, K.B. Holbrook, et al. 1995. Inhibition of matue IL-1 beta production in murine macrophanes and a murine model of inflammation by WIN 67694, an inhibitor of IL-1 beta converting enzyme. *J. Immunol.* 154:1331–1338.

25. Jackson, J.R., B. Bolognese, L. Hillegass, et al. 1998. Pharmacological effects of SB 220025, a selective inhibitor of P38 mitogen-activated protein kinase, in angiogenesis and chronic inflammatory disease models. *J. Pharmacol. Exp. Ther.* 284:687–692.

26. Badger, A.M., D.E. Griswold, R. Kapadia, S. Blake, et al. 2000. Disease-modifying activity of SB 242235, a selective inhibitor of p38 mitogen-activated protein kinase, in rat adjuvant-induced arthritis. *Arthritis Rheum.* 43:175-183.

27. Wadsworth, S.A., D.E. Vavender, S.A. Beers, P. Lalan, P.H. Schafer, E.A. Malloy, et al. 1999. RWJ67657, a potent, orally active inhibitor of p38 mitogen-activated protein kinase. *J. Pharmacol. Exp. Ther.* 291:680–687.

28. Kirwan, J.R. and the Arthritis and Rheumatism Council Low-Dose Glucocorticoid Study Group. The effect of glucocorticoids on joint destruction in rheumatoid arthritis. *N. Engl. J. Med.* 333:142–146.

29. Emery, P., H. Zeidler, T.K. Kvien, M. Guslandi, R. Naudin, H. Stead, et al. 1999. Celecoxib versus diclofenac in long-term management of rheumatoid arthritis: randomised double-blind comparison. *Lancet* 354:2106-2111.

30. Schnitzer, T.J., K. Truitt, R. Fleischmann, P. Dalgin, J. Block, Q. Zeng, et al. 1999. The safety profile, tolerability, and effective dose range of rofecoxib in the treatment of rheumatoid arthritis. Phase II Rofecoxib Rheumatoid Arthritis Study Group. *Clin. Ther.* 21:1688–1702.

31. Simon, L.S., A.L. Weaver, D.Y. Graham, A.J. Kivitz, P.E. Lipsky, R.C. Hubbard, et al. 1999. Anti-inflammatory and upper gastrointestinal effects of celecoxib in rheumatoid arthritis: a randomized controlled trial. *JAMA* 282:1921–1928.

32. O'Dell, J.R., G. Paulsen, C.E. Haire, et al. 1999. Treatment of early seropositive rheumatoid arthritis with minocycline: four-year followup of a double-blind, placebo controlled trial. *Arthritis Rheum.* 42:1691–1695.

33. Kloppenburg, M., F.C. Breedveld, J.P. Terwiel, C. Mallee, and B.A. Dijkmans. 1994. Minocycline in active rheumatoid arthritis. *Arthritis Rheum.* 37:629–636.

34. Tilley, B.C., G.S. Alarcon, S.P. Heyse, et al. 1995. for the MIRA Trial Group. Minocycline in rheumatoid arthritis: results of a 48-week double blinded placebo controlled trial. *Ann. Intern. Med.* 122:81–89.

35. O'Dell, J.R., C.E. Haire, W. Palmer, et al. 1997. Treatment of early rheumatoid arthritis with minocycline or placebo: results of a randomized, double-blind, placebo-controlled trial. *Arthritis Rheum.* 40:842–848.

36. Breedveld, F.C., B.A. Dikjmas and H. Mattie. 1990. Minocycline in the treatment for rheumatoid arthritis: an open dose finding study. *J. Rheumatol.* 17:43-46, 1990.

37. Tugwell, P, G. Wells, V. Strand, A. Maetzel, C. Bombardier, B. Crawford, et al. 2000. Clinical improvement as reflected in measures of function and health-related quality of life following treatment with leflunomide compared with methotrexate in patients with rheumatoid arthritis: sensitivity and relative efficiency to detect a treatment effect in a twelve-month, placebo-controlled trial. Leflunomide Rheumatoid Arthritis Investigators Group. *Arthritis. Rheum.* 43:506–514.

38. Sharp, J.T., V. Strand, H. Leung, F. Hurley, and I. Loew-Friedrich. 2000. Treatment with leflunomide slows radiographic progression of rheumatoid arthritis: results from three randomized controlled trials of

leflunomide in patients with active rheumatoid arthritis. Leflunomide Rheumatoid Arthritis Investigators Group. *Arthritis Rheum.* 43:495–505.

39. Strand, V., P. Tugwell, C. Bombardier, A. Maetzel, B. Crawford, C. Dorrier, et al. 1999. Function and health-related quality of life: results from a randomized controlled trial of leflunomide versus methotrexate or placebo in patients with active rheumatoid arthritis. Leflunomide Rheumatoid Arthritis Investigators Group. *Arthritis Rheum.* 42:1870–1878.

40. Smolen, J.S., J.R. Kalden, D.L. Scott, B. Rozman, T.K. Kvien, A. Larsen, et al. 1999. Efficacy and safety of leflunomide compared with placebo and sulphasalazine in active rheumatoid arthritis: a double-blind, randomized, multicentre trial. European Leflunomide Study Group. Lancet 353:259–266.

41. Kremer, J.M. 1999. Methotrexate and leflunomide: biochemical basis for combination therapy in the treatment of rheumatoid arthritis. *Sem. Arthritis Rheum.* 29:14–26.

42. Strand, V., S. Cohen, M. Schiff, A. Weaver, R. Fleischmann, G. Cannon, et al. 1999. Treatment of active rheumatoid arthritis with leflunomide compared with placebo and methotrexate. Leflunomide Rheumatoid Arthritis Investigators Group. *Arch. Int. Med.* 159:2542–2550.

43. Weinblatt, M.E., J.M. Kremer, J.S. Coblyn, A.L. Maier, S.M. Helfgott, M. Morrell, et al. 1999. Pharmacokinetics, safety, and efficacy of combination treatment with methotrexate and leflunomide in patients with active rheumatoid arthritis. *Arthritis Rheum.* 42:1322–1328.

44. Moreland, L.W., E.E. Morgan, T.C. Adamson III, Z. Fronek, L.H. Calabrese, J.M. Cash, et al. 1998. T cell receptor peptide vaccination in rheumatoid arthritis: a placebo-controlled trial using a combination of Vβ3, Vβ14, and Vβ17 peptides. *Arthritis Rheum.* 41:1919–1929.

45. Abrams, J.R., M.G. Lebwohl, C.A. Guzzo, B.V. Jegasothy, M.T. Goldfarb, B.S. Goffe, et al. 1999. CTLA4Ig-mediated blockade of T-cell costimulation in patients with psoriasis vulgaris. *J. Clin. Invest.* 103:1243–1252.

46. Finck, B.K., P.S. Linsley, and D. Wofsy. 1994. Treatment of murine lupus with CTLA-4-Ig. *Science* 265:1225–1227.

47. Kitagawa, M., H. Mitsui, H. Nakamura, S. Yoshino, et al. Differential regulation of rheumatoid synovial cell interleukin-12 production by tumor necrosis factor alpha and CD40 signals. *Arthritis Rheum.* 42:1917–1926.

2

Genetic Influences on Treatment Response in Rheumatoid Arthritis

S. Louis Bridges, Jr. and Robert P. Kimberly

1. INTRODUCTION

The lack of clinical and laboratory markers that reliably predict response, side effects, or toxicity to therapeutic intervention poses a significant challenge in therapeutic decision-making. Consequently, rheumatologists and other physicians treating patients with rheumatoid arthritis (RA) must choose treatment regimens based on their own experience and assessment of the literature which usually consists of clinical trials of heterogeneous patient populations. With the US Food and Drug Administration's (FDA) approval of tumor necrosis factor (TNF) inhibitors such as etanercept (1) and infliximab (2), the era of targeted biological agents for the treatment of RA has begun. Biologic agents differ from traditional medications used for RA in their capacity to target specific pathophysiological pathways not previously accessible to focused therapeutic intervention. However, the expense of these medications (>$10,000/yr), their lack of universally positive clinical responses, and the risk of immunosuppression with regard to infections make the identification of markers for clinically significant responses both clinically and practically important.

Although the mechanism of action of biologic agents may be through molecular events "downstream" from those being directly inhibited, there is rationale for searching for genetic markers of disease within the targeted molecules or their ligands. By identifying genetic markers of treatment response (either positive or negative), rheumatologists hope to be able to stratify patients according to genetic determinants of likelihood of

From: *Modern Therapeutics in Rheumatic Diseases*
Edited by: G. C. Tsokos, et al. © Humana Press, Inc., Totowa, NJ

response or toxicity. Genetic markers that can stratify patients based on their likelihood of response or toxicity may have an impact on clinical trials. For example, incorporation of pharmacogenetic analyses into clinical trials may reduce the number of patients required in phase III trials, but may increase the number of patients to be studied in postmarketing studies. Thus, an understanding of the genetics of clinical responsiveness has the potential to improve safety, cost-effectiveness, and clinical response rates by allowing treatment regimens to be individualized *(3,4)*. It should be noted that although genetic tests may provide guidelines for pharmacologic management, they should not be used by medical insurers to disallow reimbursement for treatments with a particular drug.

GENETIC INFLUENCES ON TREATMENT RESPONSE AND TOXICITY IN HUMAN DISEASES

In the treatment of any disease, there are many factors that can influence response to drugs, including the severity and chronicity of the illness, liver and kidney function, patient age, concomitant treatment with other drugs, coexistent illnesses, and nutritional status *(5)*. Genetic influences on response to drugs have been documented since the 1950s. For example, it was noted that inherited levels of erythrocyte glucose 6-phosphate dehydrogenase (G6PD) activity affected the likelihood of hemolysis after taking antimalarial medications *(6)*. The explosive increase in human genetic information has influenced the field of pharmacology, fostering the burgeoning of pharmacogenetics and pharmacogenomics. For the purposes of this chapter, pharmacogenetics will be used in reference to the study of genetic variation underlying differential response to drugs; pharmacogenomics refers to the systematic application of genomics to discovery of drug-response markers *(7)*.

Genetic markers useful in predicting treatment response or toxicity may lie in genes whose proteins are the target of the drug, are directly involved in the pathogenesis of the disease itself, or are enzymes that influence the metabolic or pharmacokinetic pathways of the drug *(7)*. An example of a genetic marker in the drug target is the presence of coding and promoter polymorphisms in the serotonin receptor *5-HT$_{2A}$* gene, which influence response rates to the antipsychotic drug clozapine *(8)*. For example, there is a polymorphism at position 452 of the 5-HT$_{2A}$ receptor in which either His or Tyr is encoded, based on the allele. In a sample of 153 schizophrenic patients, an association was found between the presence of the Tyr452 allele and poor clinical response to clozapine. A further analysis of multiple polymorphisms in the genes encoding adrenergic receptors, dopamine receptors, serotonin receptors, serotonin transporters, and histamine was performed. Genotypes at six polymorphisms (four in genes for serotonin receptors, one in a gene for serotonin transporter, and one in a histamine gene) yielded a sensitivity of 95% for predicting positive clinical response of schizophrenia to clozapine *(9)*. In Alzheimer's disease, the apolipoprotein E (*apoE*) gene is associated with neurofibrillary tangles and β-amyloid protein in the senile plaques. The presence of particular alleles of the *apoE* gene are associated with response of Alzheimer's to treatment with tacrine *(10)*. There are polymorphic variations in virtually all genes that encode enzymes involved in drug metabolism through modification of functional groups or through conjugation with endogenous substrates (reviewed in ref. 5).

There are many associations between drug response and genetic variations in the metabolic or pharmacokinetic pathways of the drug. The best studied of these associations is that of the cytochrome P450 system. Six cytochrome P450 enzymes (CYP1A2, CYP2C9, CYP2C19, CYP2D6, CYP2E1, and CYP3A4) mediate the oxidative metabolism of most drugs in common use (reviewed in ref. *11*), including some of those used in the treatment of RA, such as nonsteroidal anti-inflammatory drugs *(12,13)* and cyclosporin *(14)*. Some of these enzyme systems (e.g., CYP2C19, CYP2D6) are polymorphic, with specific alleles that are associated with altered (i.e., reduced, deficient, or increased) enzyme activity, which may influence the likelihood of drug toxicity or therapeutic failure *(11)*. A comprehensive discussion of the influence of cytochrome P450 genetic variations is beyond the review of this text, but is reviewed in ref. *15*. In addition, a list of drugs metabolized through this system is available at the Cytochrome P450 Drug Interaction Table on the website of the Georgetown University Medical Center Pharmacology Department <http://dml.georgetown.edu/depts/pharmacology/davetab.html>.

Another example of genetic variations in enzymatic pathways affecting toxicity of drugs is the case of alleles in the thiopurine *S*-methyltransferase *(TPMT)* gene. This enzyme metabolizes the immunosuppressive drug azathioprine (as well as mercaptopurine and thioguanine), and genetic variants in its gene predict hematologic toxicity with use of the drug *(16,17)*. Mutations TPMT*3A or TPMT*2 are found in 80–95% of Caucasians with intermediate or low enzyme activity. In a study from two rheumatology units, 6 of 67 patients (9%) treated with azathioprine for rheumatic diseases were found to be heterozygous for mutant thiopurine methyltransferase alleles. Of note, 5 of the 6 heterozygous patients discontinued therapy within 1 mo of starting treatment because of low leukocyte counts; the sixth patient did not adhere to treatment. In contrast, patients with wild-type *TPMT* alleles received therapy for a median duration of therapy of 39 wk (range 6–180 wk). None of 61 patients with homozygous for the wild-type *TPMT* allele discontinued therapy *(17)*. Genotyping of the *TPMT* gene is now routinely performed on all patients with acute lymphoblastic leukemia (ALL) at the Mayo Clinic; patients with genotypes associated with low TPMT are treated successfully with lower doses of thiopurines *(18–20)*. Perhaps rheumatologists should be using a similar strategy to identify patients with RA and systemic lupus erythematosus (SLE) who require lower doses of azathioprine to avoid toxicity.

Several requirements must be fulfilled for a pharmacogenetic assay to be useful for practicing clinicians *(21)*. First, the test must discriminate between significantly different clinical responses. In RA, a pharmacogenetic assay for efficacy should be able to stratify patients according to improvement in the number of swollen and tender joints, e.g., those meeting American College of Rheumatology (ACR) 50% response criteria vs those failing to meet ACR 20% response criteria. Second, the test must be adequately sensitive. In an assay for toxicity, for example, a sensitivity approaching 100% is desirable whereas in a test of efficacy, identification of 60–80% of responders is clinically useful. The number of false positives (specificity of the test) is also a parameter that influences clinical utility. Finally, the test must be relatively inexpensive, rapid, and yield clear results that are interpretable by practicing physicians. An ideal pharmacogenetic test would require a small blood sample, provide fast and reliable genotype analysis, and accurately predict the treatment response or toxicity to one or more treatment alternatives *(22)*.

GENETIC INFLUENCES ON SUSCEPTIBILITY TO RA
AND ITS SEVERITY

Genes important in susceptibility or severity of RA may also influence treatment response. There is a genetic component to susceptibility to RA, as there is with virtually every form of arthritis, including familial osteoarthritis *(23)*, ankylosing spondylitis *(24)*, SLE *(25)*, and gout *(26)*. Because of the complexity and redundancy of the human immune system and the large number of cell types and molecules involved in its pathogenesis, there are a multitude of genes that may influence RA susceptibility. In addition to contributing to susceptibility, genetic factors may have an effect on disease phenotype as defined by particular clinical manifestations (e.g., erosions or extra-articular manifestations), or may influence response to particular treatments. Potentially relevant genes include those that encode proteins involved in antigen recognition, cell-cell interactions, intracellular signaling, inflammation, apoptosis, cell trafficking, hormonal interactions, and others (reviewed in ref. *27)* A genome-wide screen of 257 multiplex RA families by the North American Rheumatoid Arthritis Consortium (NARAC), revealed evidence for linkage to a number of non-HLA loci on chromosomes 1, 4, 12, 16, and 17 *(27a)*.

Class II MHC Alleles

RA susceptibility is known to be associated with genes in the class II major histocompatibility complex (MHC) *(28,29)*. An association between HLA DR alleles and RA was first reported in 1978 *(30)* and has been confirmed in multiple studies (reviewed in ref. *31)*. It is now generally accepted that particular class II MHC alleles (DR4 subtypes Dw4 [*DRB*0401*], Dw14 [*DRB*0404*], and Dw15 [*DRB*0405*], and some DR1 alleles) are associated with susceptibility to RA in Caucasians. Nucleotide sequence analysis led to the hypothesis that these alleles confer susceptibility to RA based on shared homology at amino acid residues 70–74 of the third hypervariable region of the DRB1 chain, the so-called shared epitope *(32)*. The predisposition to and severity of RA in African-Americans appears to be independent of the presence and dose of the shared epitope in class II MHC alleles *(33)* *(see* below).

In addition to having a role in susceptibility to RA, MHC class II DR4 alleles have been reported to have an affect on disease severity (such as more erosions on radiographs) *(34,35)*. Rheumatoid factor (RF)-positive Caucasians with RA who bear two susceptibility alleles have been shown to be more likely to have severe disease and extra-articular manifestations than heterozygous individuals, suggesting a gene dosing affect *(36)*.

TNF Polymorphisms

In RA, there may be enrichment for genetic polymorphisms that lead to higher levels of cytokines with predominantly proinflammatory effects or lower levels of predominantly anti-inflammatory cytokines. Tumor necrosis factor (TNF), for example, plays a substantial role in the pathogenesis of RA *(37,38)*. There are conflicting reports of the roles of TNF genetic variations in RA, possibly as a result of population admixture and multiple-hypothesis testing *(39)*. Some studies have shown no association between RA susceptibility and the TNF locus *(40–43)*. One study reported an association between the genotypes at the promoter polymorphisms at –238 and –308 and the mean age at disease onset and the presence of rheumatoid nodules, respectively *(43)*. The TNF –238 G/A heterozygous genotype has been reported to be associated, independent of the presence of HLA DR4 alleles, with a paucity of erosions early in the course of the disease *(44)* and with a lower rate of joint damage on hand radiographs as the disease progresses *(45)*. However, functional assays revealed no significant differences in the level of inducible reporter-gene expression between the TNF –238 A and G alleles.

Microsatellite markers in the TNF locus (TNFa, b, c, d, and e) have also been studied with regard to RA susceptibility and severity. Studies have shown an association of TNF microsatellite alleles with RA independent of the MHC locus *(46,47)*, and an association with RA with possible synergy with the MHC locus *(48)*. Criswell and colleagues studied the effect of TNF microsatellite polymorphisms on likelihood of severe RA (defined by rheumatologists' assessments of disease course, joint replacement, hospitalization for RA other than for joint replacement, and severity of erosions on hand/wrist radiographs). Allele 11 of the TNF microsatellite polymorphism TNFa (TNFa11) appeared to be associated with RA severity through an interaction with the MHC shared epitope *(48)*. Most of the severe outcomes were observed among individuals who had inherited both TNFa11 and the shared epitope, whereas individuals who had inherited TNFa11 in the absence of the shared epitope had the best outcomes. Although the mechanism for this interaction remains unclear, both the MHC shared epitope and the TNF-LTα locus appear to be important determinants in RA severity.

DNA MICROARRAYS IN MOLECULAR GENOTYPING AND PHENOTYPING

One of the most exciting biotechnologies to impact on genetics is the development of DNA microarrays, which allow analysis of thousands of genes simultaneously *(49)*. DNA chip technology has facilitated discovery of single nucleotide polymorphisms (SNPs) as well as genotyping of a large number of SNPs in a rapid, accurate fashion *(50,51)*. In addition to SNP discovery and genotyping, DNA microarrays can be used to characterize which of thousands of genes are preferentially expressed in particular tissues (expression profiling) *(52)*. This is a powerful technique that allows molecular comparison of diseased cells or tissues to their normal counterparts and to detect changes in gene expression in response to cytokines, growth factors, and drugs. Thus, DNA microarrays are likely to have a substantial impact on identification of new molecular targets and drug discovery *(53)*. Among the most important potential applications of gene chips is to identify molecular classification of diseases, which may ultimately allow optimization of treatment strategies. For example, Golub et al. used DNA microarrays to profile expression of 6817 genes in bone marrow aspirates of patients with acute myeloid leukemia (AML) and ALL *(54)*. Using 50 informative genes, classification into AML vs ALL, as well as identification of subclasses, was possible. One of the informative genes was topoisomerase II, the target for the anti-leukemia drug etoposide, which illustrates the potential usefulness of molecular classification in pharmacogenetics.

Because RA is a heterogenous disease, molecular phenotyping may someday be useful for determining optimal treatment. Synovial tissue may be obtained through arthroscopic or percutaneous biopsy and expression profiling performed. For results to be interpretable and clinically meaningful, artifacts owing to varying proportions of different cell types must be avoided. There are many ways to exclude this problem, including histologic examination of synovial samples to ensure comparability, or purification of cells of a particular lineage (e.g., T cells, B cells, monocytes, or fibroblasts) by flow sorting or laser-capture microdissection *(54)*.

PHARMACOGENETIC STUDIES IN RA

In approaching pharmacogenetic studies in RA, there are some genetic associations for which the mechanism of side effects or toxicity is unknown. For others, the genetic association may influence drug metabolism or pharmacokinetics. For still others, responsiveness may associate with variations in specific pathophysiologic pathways or with the underlying severity of disease.

Gold salts have been used in the treatment of RA for many years, and can cause side effects such as bone marrow suppression, proteinuria, and mucocutaneous lesions. HLA DR3 may be associated with gold toxicity in RA *(55)*. Further studies indicate that HLA-DQA region genes *(56)* or HLA-B8 and DR3 antigens *(57)* may play an important role in susceptibility to gold-induced nephropathy and that HLA-DR1 *(58)* or HLA-DR5 *(57)* may be involved in susceptibility to mucocutaneous side effects. Although the mechanisms and genes involved remain unknown, such studies helped to set the stage for pharmacogenetics in understanding drug effects in RA. Affecting drug-metabolism genetic variability in the *G6PD* and *TPMT* genes may influence toxicity of antimalarials or azathioprine, respectively, in the treatment of RA. Susceptibility to sulfasalazine-induced agranulocytosis may be influenced by polymorphisms of NAT2 *(59)*.

With the use of immunoglobulin-based biologics, naturally occurring polymorphisms in receptors for immunoglobulins may influence pharmacokinetics and side effects. The efficacy of some of these immunoglobulin-based therapeutics in model systems is Fcγ receptor dependent *(60,61)*. Similarly, the cytokine-release syndrome induced by at least some humanized monoclonal antibodies (MAbs) is also Fcγ receptor-dependent *(62)* (Fig. 1). Tax and colleagues *(63,64)* have shown that in organ transplant recipients, the cell depletion induced by the anti-CD3 MAb, WT31, varies predictably with Fcγ receptor genotype (Fig. 2). Although the effect of naturally occurring polymorphisms in Fcγ receptors on the efficacy of current therapeutic agents in RA has not been explored in depth, an influence on minor infections as an adverse events in both treated and control subjects has been demonstrated *(65)*. Such observations suggest that the genetics of the study population may influence adverse events and impact on formulation strategies as well as affect responsiveness of pathophysiological pathways. Because of the role of TNF in RA and the availability of anti-TNF therapy, TNF and TNF-receptor loci may yield useful pharmacogenetic markers as an example of the latter *(27)*.

The MHC class II shared epitope, which can influence disease severity, may also affect the clinical response of RA to treatment *(66)*. In a study by O'Dell and investigators in the Rheumatoid Arthritis Investigational Network (RAIN), patients were randomized to receive three disease modifying anti-rheumatic drugs (DMARDs) (methotrexate [MTX], hydroxychloroquine, and sulfasalazine), MTX alone, or hydroxychloroquine plus sulfasalazine *(67)*. The three drug regimen was found to be superior to the other two. In a follow-up analysis, all patients were genotyped for the presence of DRB1 *0401, *0404/*0408, *0405, *0101, *1001, and *1402 alleles to determine if there was an influence of the shared epitope on treatment response. Patients with the shared epitope were more likely to achieve ACR 50% response criteria to triple DMARD therapy than

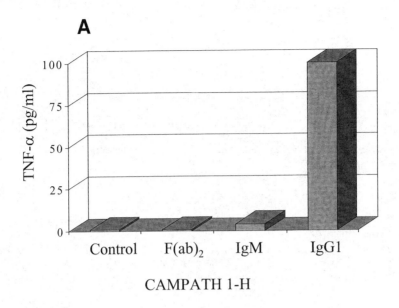

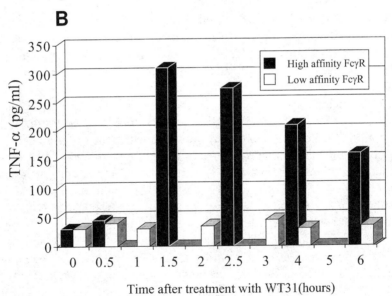

Fig. 1. Role of FcγR in cytokine release syndrome. **(A)** Ex vivo whole-blood cultures demonstrate the central role of Fcγ receptors in TNF-α release by the anti-CD52 MAb, CAMPATH 1-H. Adapted with permission from Wing et al. *(62)*. **(B)** Fcγ receptor-binding affinity for MAb varies with receptor genotype and influences TNF-α production in patients receiving MAb WT31. Adapted from Tax et al. *(64)*.

to MTX alone (94% responders vs 32%, $p < 0.0001$) *(66)*. In contrast, patients without the shared epitope did equally well regardless of treatment (88% responders to triple DMARD therapy vs 83% for MTX alone). Although the number of patients was small, this study suggests that knowing whether or not the patient has alleles containing the shared epitope may be useful in selecting among treatment options.

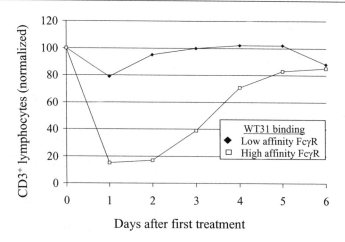

Fig. 2. Percentage of circulating CD3⁺ lymphocytes during anti-CD3 treatment with MAb WT31. The donor with the FcγRIIA genotype which binds WT31 with high affinity showed a more pronounced decrease in circulating CD3⁺ lymphocytes. Adapted from Tax et al. *(64)*.

There are likely to be important racial differences in allele frequencies of genes important in the pathogenesis of RA. As mentioned earlier, MHC class II shared epitope appears to have less of an influence on susceptibility to RA in African-Americans than it does in Caucasians *(33)*. In addition, there are marked differences between African-Americans and Caucasians with regard to the prevalence of an SNP in the *IL-6* gene that appears to play a role in susceptibility to juvenile RA *(68–70)*. Among Spaniards *(71)* and Israeli Jews *(72)*, DR10 alleles appear to be the most important MHC susceptibility genes. Although there are no known racial differences in the overall frequency of mutant TPMT alleles compared to wild-type alleles, it has recently been reported that Caucasians mutant alleles are usually TPMT*3A, whereas Kenyans have the TPMT*3C allele *(73)*. Thus, race should be considered an important variable in genetic analyses of susceptibility, severity, and treatment response in RA.

When pharmacogenetics will be translated to the bedside in the treatment of RA remains to be established, but the future of molecular medicine, and its potential to enhance the management of our patients, appears bright. New agents, including those directed against IL-1 *(74,75)*, and other biologic targets such as costimulatory molecules (e.g., CD40/CD40L, and CTLA4), are being developed, and identification of genetic markers of clinical response or toxicity may provide more efficient and cost-effective therapies.

CONCLUSIONS

There has been an explosion of knowledge of genetic variations among different populations and the influences of genetics on complex autoimmune and inflammatory diseases such as RA. Although class II MHC alleles are important contributors, there are likely to be multiple other genes that modulate the disease phenotype. In addition, genetic markers may allow determination of treatment response, especially in light of the growing number of biologic agents undergoing clinical trials.

REFERENCES

1. Moreland, L.W., S.W. Baumgartner, M.H. Schiff, et al. 1997. Treatment of rheumatoid arthritis with a recombinant human tumor necrosis factor receptor (p75)-Fc fusion protein. *N. Engl. J. Med.* 337:141–147.

2. Maini, R., E.W. St. Clair, F. Breedveld, et al. 1999. Infliximab (chimeric anti-tumour necrosis factor a monoclonal antibody) versus placebo in rheumatoid arthritis patients receiving concomitant methotrexate: a randomised phase III trial. *Lancet* 354:1932–1939.

3. Krynetski, E.Y. and W.E. Evans. 1998. Pharmacogenetics of cancer therapy: getting personal. *Am. J. Human Genet.* 63:11–16.

4. Stix, G. 1998. Personal pills. Genetic differences may dictate how drugs are prescribed (news). *Sci. Am.* 279:17–18.

5. Evans, W.E. and M.V. Relling. 1999. Pharmacogenomics: translating functional genomics into rational therapeutics. *Science* 286:487–491.

6. Carson, P.E., C.L. Flanagan, C.E. Ickes, and A.S. Alving. 1956. Enzymatic deficiency in primaquine-sensitive erythrocytes. *Science* 1956;124:484–485.

7. Kleyn, P.W. and E.S. Vesell. 1998. Genetic variation as a guide to drug development. *Science* 281:1820–1821.

8. Arranz, M.J., D.A. Collier, J. Munro, et al. 1996. Analysis of a structural polymorphism in the 5-HT2A receptor and clinical response to clozapine. *Neurosci. Lett.* 217:177–178.

9. Arranz, M.J., J. Munro, J. Birkett, A. Bolonna, D. Mancam, M. Sodhi, et al. 2000. Pharmacogenetic prediction of clozapine response. *Lancet* 355:1615–1616.

10. Poirier, J., J. Davignon, D. Bouthillier, S. Kogan, P. Bertrand, and S. Gauthier. 1993. Apolipoprotein E polymorphism and Alzheimer's disease. *Lance* 342:697–699.

11. Caraco, Y. 1998. Genetic determinants of drug responsiveness and drug interactions. *Ther. Drug Monit.* 20:517–524.

12. Miners, J.O., S. Coulter, R.H. Tukey, M.E. Veronese, and D.J. Birkett. 1996. Cytochromes P450, 1A2, and 2C9 are responsible for the human hepatic O-demethylation of R- and S-naproxen. *Biochem. Pharmacol.* 51:1003–1008.

13. Mancy, A., M. Antignac, C. Minoletti, et al. 1999. Diclofenac and its derivatives as tools for studying human cytochromes P450 active sites: particular efficiency and regioselectivity of P450 2Cs. *Biochemistry* 38:14,264–14,270.

14. Watkins, P.B. 1990. The role of cytochromes P-450 in cyclosporine metabolism. *J. Am. Acad. Dermatol.* 23:1301–1309.

15. Hasler, J.A. 1999. Pharmacogenetics of cytochromes P450. *Mol. Aspects Med.* 20:12–37.

16. Yates, C.R., E.Y. Krynetski, T. Loennechen, et al. 1997. Molecular diagnosis of thiopurine S-methyltransferase deficiency: genetic basis for azathioprine and mercaptopurine intolerance. *Ann. Intern. Med.* 126:608–614.

17. Black, A.J., H.L. McLeod, H.A. Capell, et al. 1998. Thiopurine methyltransferase genotype predicts therapy-limiting severe toxicity from azathioprine. *Ann. Intern. Med.* 129:716–718.

18. Relling, M.V., M.L. Hancock, G.K. Rivera, et al. 1999. Mercaptopurine therapy intolerance and heterozygosity at the thiopurine S-methyltransferase gene locus. *J. Natl. Cancer Instit.* 91:2001–2008.

19. Balis, F.M. and P.C. Adamson. 1999. Application of pharmacogenetics to optimization of mercaptopurine dosing. *J. Natl. Cancer Instit.* 91:1983–1985.

20. Nelson, N.J. 1999. Genetic profiling for cancer surfaces slowly in the clinic (news). *Natl. Cancer Instit.* 91:1990–1992.

21. Spear, B.B. Clinical applications of pharmacogenomics. Presented at Keystone 2000: Fulfilling the Promises of Genomics Research. March 12–17, 2000, Taos, New Mexico.

22. Schneider, I. 1999. Prescriptions with a personal touch. *Scientist* 6:99.

23. Bleasel J.F., D. Holderbaum, T.M. Haqqi, R.W. Moskowitz. Clinical correlations of osteoarthritis associated with single base mutations in the type II procollagen gene. *J. Rheumatol. Suppl.* 1995;43:34–36.

24. Schlosstein, L., P.I. Terasaki, R. Bluestone, and C.M. Pearson. 1973. High association of an HL-A antigen, W27, with ankylosing spondylitis. *New. Engl. J. Med.* 288:704–706.

25. Criswell, L.A. and C.I. Amos. Update on genetic risk factors for systemic lupus erythematosus and rheumatoid arthritis. *Curr. Opin. Rheumatol.* 2000;12:85–90.

26. Davidson, B.L., M. Pashmforoush, W.N. Kelley, and T.D. Palella. 1989. Human hypoxanthine-guanine phosphoribosyltransferase deficiency. The molecular defect in a patient with gout (HPRTAshville). *J. Biol. Chem.* 264:520–525.

27. Bridges, S.L., Jr. 1999. The genetics of rheumatoid arthritis: Influences on susceptibility, severity, and treatment response. *Cur. Rheumatol. Reports* 1:164–171.

27a. Jawaheer, D., M.F. Seldin, C.I. Amos, W.V. Chen, R. Shigeta, J. Monteiro, et al. for NARAC. 2001. A genome-wide screen in multiplex rheumatoid arthritis families suggests genetic overlap with other autoimmune diseases. *Am. J. Human Genetics* 68:927–936.

28. Rigby, A.S., A.J. Silman, L. Voelm, et al. 1991. Investigating the HLA component in rheumatoid arthritis: an additive (dominant) mode of inheritance is rejected, a recessive mode is preferred. *Genet. Epidemiol.* 8:153–175.

29. Rigby, A.S., L. Voelm, and A.J. Silman. 1993. Epistatic modeling in rheumatoid arthritis: an application of the Risch theory. *Genet. Epidemiol.* 10:311–320.

30. Stastny, P. 1978. Association of the B-cell alloantigen DRw4 with rheumatoid arthritis. *New Engl. J. Med.* 298:869–871.

31. Ollier, W. and W. Thomson. 1992. Population genetics of rheumatoid arthritis. *Rheum. Dis. Clin. N. Am.* 18:741–759.

32. Gregersen, P.K., J. Silver, and R. Winchester. 1987. The shared epitope hypothesis: An approach to understanding the molecular genetics of susceptibility to rheumatoid arthritis. *Arthritis Rheum.* 30:1205–1213.

33. McDaniel, D.O., G.S. Alarcón, P.W. Pratt, and J.D. Reveille. Most African-American patients with rheumatoid arthritis do not have the rheumatoid antigenic determinant (epitope). *Ann. Intern. Med.* 1995;123:181–187.

34. MacGregor, A., W. Ollier, W. Thomson, D. Jawaheer, and A. Silman. 1995. HLA-DRB1*0401/0404 genotype and rheumatoid arthritis: increased association in men, young age at onset, and disease severity. *J. Rheumatol.* 22:1032–1036.

35. Plant, M.J., P.W. Jones, J. Saklatvala, W.E. Ollier, and P.T. Dawes. 1998. Patterns of radiological progression in early rheumatoid arthritis: results of an 8 year prospective study. *J. Rheumatol.* 25:417–426.

36. Weyand, C.M, K.C. Hicok, D.L. Conn, and J.J. Goronzy. 1992. The influence of HLA-DRB1 genes on disease severity in rheumatoid arthritis. *Ann. Intern. Med.* 117:801–806.

37. Chu, C.Q., M. Field, M. Feldmann, and R.N. Maini. 1991. Localization of tumor necrosis factor alpha in synovial tissues and at the cartilage-pannus junction in patients with rheumatoid arthritis. *Arthritis Rheum.* 34:1125–1132.

38. Brennan, F.M., R.N. Maini, and M. Feldmann. 1998. Role of pro-inflammatory cytokines in rheumatoid arthritis. *Springer Semin. Immunopathol.* 20:133–147.

39. Altshuler, D., L. Kruglyak, and E. Lander. 1998. Genetic polymorphisms and disease. *New Engl. J. Med.* 338:1626.

40. Wilson, A.G., N. de Vries, L.B. van de Putte, and G.W. Duff. 1995. A tumour necrosis factor alpha polymorphism is not associated with rheumatoid arthritis. *Ann. Rheum. Dis.* 54:601–603.

41. Campbell, D.A., S. Nelson, R. Madhok, M. Field, and G. Gallagher. 1994. TNF Nco-I RFLP is not an independent risk factor in rheumatoid arthritis. *Eur. J. Immunogenet.* 21:461–467.

42. Field, M., G. Gallagher, J. Eskdale, et al. Tumor necrosis factor locus polymorphisms in rheumatoid arthritis. *Tissue Antigens* 1997;50:303–307.

43. Vinasco, J., Y. Beraun, A. Nieto, et al. 1997. Polymorphism at the TNF loci in rheumatoid arthritis. *Tissue Antigens* 49:74–78.

44. Brinkman, B.M., T.W. Huizinga, S.S. Kurban, et al. 1997. Tumour necrosis factor alpha gene polymorphisms in rheumatoid arthritis: association with susceptibility to, or severity of, disease? *Br. J. Rheumatol.* 36:516–521.

45. Kaijzel, E.L., M.V. van Krugten, B.M. Brinkman, et al. 1998. Functional analysis of a human tumor necrosis factor alpha (TNF-alpha) promoter polymorphism related to joint damage in rheumatoid arthritis. *Mol. Med.* 4:724–733.

46. Mulcahy, B., F. Waldron-Lynch, M.F. McDermott, et al. 1996. Genetic variability in the tumor necrosis factor-lymphotoxin region influences susceptibility to rheumatoid arthritis. *Am. J. Hum. Genet.* 59:676–683.

47. Hajeer, A.H., J. Worthington, A.J. Silman, and W.E. Ollier. 1996. Association of tumor necrosis factor microsatellite polymorphisms with HLA-DRB1*04-bearing haplotypes in rheumatoid arthritis patients. *Arthritis Rheum.* 39:1109–1114.

48. Mu, H., J.J. Chen, Y. Jiang, M-C King, G. Thomson, and L.A. Criswell. 1999. Tumor necrosis factor a microsatellite polymorphism is associated with rheumatoid arthritis severity through an interaction with the HLA-DRB1 shared epitope. *Arthritis Rheum.* 42:438–442.

49. Lipshutz, R.J., S.P. Fodor, T.R. Gingeras, and D.J. Lockhart. 1999. High density synthetic oligonucleotide arrays. *Nature Genet.* 21:20–24.

50. Wang, D.G., J.B. Fan, C.J. Siao, et al. 1998. Large-scale identification, mapping, and genotyping of single-nucleotide polymorphisms in the human genome. *Science* 280:1077–1082.

51. Cargill, M., D. Altshuler, J. Ireland, et al. 1999. Characterization of single-nucleotide polymorphisms in coding regions of human genes. *Nature Genet.* 22:231–238.

52. Duggan, D.J., M. Bittner, Y. Chen, P. Meltzer, and J.M. Trent. 1999. Expression profiling using cDNA microarrays. *Nature Genet.* 21:10–14.

53. Debouck, C. and P.N. Goodfellow. 1999. DNA microarrays in drug discovery and development. *Nature Genet.* 21:48–50.

54. Golub, T.R., D.K. Slonim, P. Tamayo, et al. 1999. Molecular classification of cancer: class discovery and class prediction by gene expression monitoring. *Science.* 286:531–537.

55. Bensen, W.G, N. Moore, P. Tugwell, M. D'Souza, and D.P. Singal DP. 1984. HLA antigens and toxic reactions to sodium aurothiomalate in patients with rheumatoid arthritis. *J. Rheumatol.* 11: 358–361.

56. Sakkas, L.I., I.C. Chikanza, R.W. Vaughan, K.I. Welsh, and G.S. Panayi. 1993. Gold induced nephropathy in rheumatoid arthritis and HLA class II genes. *Ann. Rheum. Dis.* 52:300–301.

57. Rodriguez-Perez, M., J. Gonzalez-Dominguez, L. Mataran, S. Garcia-Perez, and D. Salvatierra. 1994. Association of HLA-DR5 with mucocutaneous lesions in patients with rheumatoid arthritis receiving gold sodium thiomalate. *J. Rheumatol.* 21:41–43.

58. Pickl, W.F., G.F. Fischer, I. Fae, G. Kolarz, and O. Scherak. 1993. HLA-DR1-positive patients suffering from rheumatoid arthritis are at high risk for developing mucocutaneous side effects upon gold therapy. *Human Immunol.* 38:127–131.

59. Wadelius, M., E. Stjerbern, B.-E. Wiholm, and A. Rane. 2000. Polymorphisms of NAT2 in relation to sulphasalazine-induced agranulocytosis. *Pharmacogenetics* 10:43.

60. Clynes, R.A., T.L. Towers, L.G. Presta, and J.V. Ravetch. 2000. Inhibitory Fc receptors modulate in vivo cytotoxicity against tumor targets. *Nature Med.* 6:443–446.

61. Houghton, A.N. and D.A. Scheinberg. 2000. Monoclonal antibody therapies: a 'constant' threat to cancer. *Nature Med.* 6:373–374.

62. Wing, M.G., T. Moreau, J. Greenwood, et al. 1996. Mechanism of first-dose cytokine-release syndrome by CAMPATH 1-H: involvement of CD16 (FcgammaRIII) and CD11a/CD18 (LFA-1) on NK cells. *J. Clin. Invest.* 98:2819–2826.

63. Tax, W.J., L.A. Frenken, C.A. Glaudemans, W.P. Tamboer, and R.A. Koene. 1995. Polymorphism of Fc receptor (Fc gamma RII) is reflected in cytokine release and adverse effects of mIgG1 anti-CD3/TCR antibody during rejection treatment after renal transplantation. *Transplant. Proc.* 27: 867–868.

64. Tax, W.J., W.P. Tamboer, C.W. Jacobs, L.A. Frenken, and R.A. Koene. 1997. Role of polymorphic Fc receptor Fc gammaRIIa in cytokine release and adverse effects of murine IgG1 anti-CD3/T cell receptor antibody (WT31). *Transplantation* 63:106–112.

65. Kimberly, R.P., L.W. Moreland, J. Wu, J.C. Edberg, M.E. Weinblatt, and C. Blosch. 1998. Occurrence of infection varies with Fc receptor genotype. *Arthritis Rheum.* 41:S273 (Abstract).

66. O'Dell, J.R., B.S. Nepom, C. Haire, et al. 1998. HLA-DRB1 typing in rheumatoid arthritis: predicting response to specific treatments. *Ann. Rheum. Dis.* 57:209–213.

67. O'Dell, J.R., C.E. Haire, and N. Erikson, et al. 1996. Treatment of rheumatoid arthritis with methotrexate alone, sulfasalazine and hydroxychloroquine, or a combination of all three medications. *New. Engl. J. Med.* 334:1287–1291.

68. Fishman, D., G. Faulds, R. Jeffery, et al. 1998. The effect of novel polymorphisms in the interleukin-6 (IL-6) gene on IL-6 transcription and plasma IL-6 levels, and an association with systemic-onset juvenile chronic arthritis. *J. Clin. Invest.* 102:1369–1376.

69. Osiri, M., W. Whitworth, J. McNicholl, B. Jonas, L.W. Moreland, and S.L. Bridges, Jr. 1999. A novel single nucleotide polymorphism and five haplotypes in the 5' flanking region of the IL-6 gene: Differences between Caucasians and African-Americans. *Arthritis Rheum.* 42 (Suppl.):S196 (Abstract).

70. Osiri, M., J. McNicholl, L.W. Moreland, and S.L. Bridges, Jr. 1999. A novel single nucleotide polymorphism and five probable haplotypes in the 5' flanking region of the IL-6 gene in African-Americans. *Genes Immun.* 1:166–716.

71. Sanchez, B., I. Moreno, R. Magarino, et al. 1990. HLA-DRw10 confers the highest susceptibility to rheumatoid arthritis in a Spanish population. *Tissue Antigens* 36:174–176.

72. Gao, X., E. Gazit, A. Livneh, and P. Stastny. 1991. Rheumatoid arthritis in Israeli Jews: shared sequences in the third hypervariable region of DRB1 alleles are associated with susceptibility. *J. Rheumatol.* 18:801–803.

73. McLeod, H.L., S.C. Pritchard, J. Githang'a, et al. 1999. Ethnic differences in thiopurine methyltransferase pharmacogenetics: evidence for allele specificity in Caucasian and Kenyan individuals. *Pharmacogenetics* 9:773–776.

74. Koopman, W.J. and L.W. Moreland. 1998. Rheumatoid arthritis: anticytokine therapies on the horizon. *Ann. Intern. Med.* 128:231–233.

75. Gabay, C. and W.P. Arend. 1998. Treatment of rheumatoid arthritis with IL-1 inhibitors. *Springer Semin. Immunopathol.* 20:229–246.

3

Nonsteroidal Anti-Inflammatory Drugs in the Treatment of Rheumatoid Arthritis

John S. Sundy

CONTENTS

INTRODUCTION

Nonsteroidal anti-inflammatory drugs (NSAIDs) continue to be a mainstay of rheumatoid arthritis (RA) management despite exciting recent advances in the therapy of RA (Table 1). Before the era of modern medicine, willow bark, which contains salicylates, was used to treat fever and pain *(1)*. In 1860, salicylic acid was introduced for the treatment of rheumatic diseases, followed by the introduction of acetylsalicylic acid (aspirin) in 1899 *(1)*. Salicylates remained the principle pharmacologic therapy of RA until the introduction of glucocorticoids in the 1940s. In the current era of early, aggressive management of RA with disease modifying anti-rheumatic drugs, the NSAIDs have assumed an adjunctive role in reducing the symptoms of RA.

From: *Modern Therapeutics in Rheumatic Diseases*
Edited by: G. C. Tsokos, et al. © Humana Press, Inc., Totowa, NJ

Table 1
Nonsteroidal Anti-Inflammatory Drugs
in Rheumatoid Arthritis: Important Milestones

Date	Milestone
Pre-modern	Salicylates from botanical sources
1860	Salicylic acid introduced
1949	First nonsalicylate NSAID, phenylbutazone
1971	Mechanism of action of aspirin elucidated
1991	COX-2 discovered
1999	First selective COX-2 inhibitors approved

In 1971, Sir John Vane discovered that aspirin, sodium salicylate, and indomethacin inhibited prostaglandin synthesis *(2)*. Cyclooxygenase was identified in 1976 as the critical enzymatic step in prostaglandin synthesis *(3)*. By the late 1970s, clinicians began to appreciate the significant spectrum of NSAID toxicity. These drugs were shown to cause significant morbidity and mortality primarily owing to gastroduodenal ulcer formation and renal toxicity. The focus of clinical research shifted toward reducing NSAID-induced toxicity. Methods were developed to modify the gastrointestinal (GI) toxicity of NSAIDs through coadministration of gastroprotective drugs. The identification of a second isoform of cyclooxygenase (COX-2) led to the discovery of selective COX-2 inhibitors that exhibit markedly improved GI safety; albeit at greater economic cost. These developments have ushered in the latest era in the evolving history of NSAID therapy of RA.

This chapter reviews the pathogenic mechanisms that support the rationale for NSAID therapy in RA. Evidence for the efficacy of NSAIDs in RA will be presented with particular emphasis on the selective COX-2 inhibitors. NSAID toxicity remains an important issue. Accordingly, this chapter will review the risk factors for NSAID toxicity, methods for minimizing toxicity and the relative safety of selective COX-2 inhibitors vs nonselective COX inhibitors. This review concludes with a discussion of the role of NSAIDs in the modern management of RA.

PATHOGENIC MECHANISMS THAT RATIONALIZE USE OF NSAIDS

The primary molecular target of all NSAIDs is cyclooxygenase (COX), which converts arachidonic acid to prostaglandin G2 (PGG2) and prostaglandin H2 (PGH2) *(4)*. PGH2 is enzymatically converted by prostaglandin synthases to the active forms of PGE2, PGD2, PGI2, and thromboxane A2. Two isoforms of COX have been identified; designated COX-1 and COX-2 *(4)*. COX-1 is constitutively expressed in most tissues and produces prostaglandins important for normal tissue homeostasis. COX-2 is an inducible enzyme that is rapidly upregulated at sites of inflammation and tissue injury. With the exception of sites within the kidney and brain, there is very little constitutive expression of COX-2. Accordingly, COX-2 is the primary source of prostaglandin synthesis in inflamed tissue. Inducers of COX-2 expression in inflamed or injured tissue include: proinflammatory cytokines, immune complexes, lipopolysaccharide, immunoglobulin Fc receptor crosslinking, bradykinin, thrombin, and phospholipase A2 *(4–6)*.

Prostaglandin synthesis is upregulated in virtually all forms of inflammation including RA. Prostaglandins are produced on demand and are not stored in cells. The key regulatory step in the production of prostaglandins is the conversion of membrane phospholipids to arachidonic acid by the phospholipase A2 (PLA2) family of enzymes. A variety of stimuli upregulate PLA2, including proinflammatory cytokines, lipopolysaccharide, oxidized low-density lipoproteins, and small peptide growth factors (7–12).

The biologic effects of prostaglandins are numerous. Their role in regulating inflammatory responses includes the induction of fever, pain, swelling, and the regulation of leukocyte function. Fever is induced, in part, by local production of PGE2 in the brain. PGE2 raises the body temperature set point through interaction with neurons in the hypothalamus (13,14). Prostaglandins do not directly stimulate pain responses. Instead, they contribute to pain responses by inducing a state of hyperalgesia. PGE2 and PGI2 cause sensitization of peripheral nerve terminals and modulate pain processing at a central level in the spinal cord (15). Finally, the role of prostaglandins in swelling is somewhat indirect. Prostaglandins increase blood flow through arteriolar dilation. Edema results from prostaglandin-induced increases in blood flow in conjunction with stimuli that promote endothelial permeability (leukotrienes, bradykinins, platelet-activating factor) (4).

Prostaglandins have a seemingly paradoxical anti-inflammatory effect on leukocytes. Neutrophil chemotaxis and superoxide production are inhibited in vitro by prostaglandins (16). PGE2 inhibits expression of the neutrophil activation marker CD66 (17). PGE2 was also shown to inhibit TNF-α production by monocytes. In fact, administration of NSAIDs to humans and mice enhances lipopolysaccharide-induced TNF-α production, and renders mice more susceptible to the lethal effects of endotoxin (18,19). Enhanced TNF-α production in response to NSAIDs in mice causes alterations in cartilage metabolism that have led to concerns about the role of NSAIDs in accelerating cartilage degradation (20,21). PGE2 has also been shown to downregulate T-lymphocyte proliferation, migration, and cytokine production (22–25). The clinical relevance of these findings is unclear because RA patients who responded to NSAIDs exhibited increased density of T-cell surface markers coincident with reductions in erythrocyte sedimentation rate, c-reactive protein, IgM rheumatoid factor, and clinical parameters of RA activity (26,27). These findings illustrate the importance of differentiating the isolated effects of prostaglandins in vitro from those observed in intact tissue or whole organisms.

Numerous studies provide evidence for the role of prostaglandins in the pathogenesis of RA (28). Prostaglandin E2 can be detected in the synovial fluid of RA patients at a level significantly higher than that seen in synovial fluid from osteoarthritis (OA) patients (29). Accordingly, RA patients express higher levels of COX in synovial tissue than do healthy subjects or patients with OA (30). Clinical responses to NSAIDs in RA patients correlated with reduced PGE2 levels in synovial fluid (31).

The cellular source of prostaglandins in the inflamed joint has not been definitively identified. However, in vitro studies demonstrated upregulated prostaglandin synthesis in macrophages, neutrophils, mast cells, and type I and type II synovial lining cells (32–36). Finally, cytokines important in the pathogenesis of RA, such as Interleukin-1 (IL-1) and TNF-α, are known to upregulate PLA2 and/or COX-2 expression in cultured synovial-tissue fibroblasts (37–40).

NSAIDs may have pharmacologic properties unrelated to inhibition of COX. For instance, anti-inflammatory doses of nonacetylated salicylates (which are weak COX inhibitors) were comparable to other NSAIDs in decreasing pain, joint tenderness, and swelling in RA *(41)*. These data indicate that pharmacologic properties of NSAIDs that are distinct from COX inhibition may have clinical relevance in RA. Numerous molecular pathways related to inflammation but distinct from COX inhibition are modified by NSAIDs. Salicylates were shown to inhibit IL-1 induced COX gene expression in cultured human endothelial cells *(42)*. Aspirin inhibits translocation of the transcription factor NFκB to the nucleus, which can inhibit a variety of inflammatory and immune responses *(43)*. Other mechanisms of action include the accumulation of adenosine, which possesses anti-inflammatory activity *(43)*. The preferential COX-2 inhibitor, nimesulide, induced glucocorticoid-receptor phosphorylation and transcription in cultured human synovial fibroblasts; an action which increases the anti-inflammatory activity of endogenous or exogenous corticosteroids *(44)*. Tenidap, ibuprofen, and naproxen inhibited in vitro T-cell proliferative responses to IL-2 when added to cultures at therapeutic concentrations, whereas indomethacin, piroxicam, and sulindac did not *(45)*. All of these findings suggest that NSAIDs may have anti-inflammatory activities separate from their ability to inhibit COX. The relevance of these findings to the efficacy of NSAIDs in RA has not been determined. It is likely that in the near future, NSAIDs will be developed that have primary activities unrelated to COX inhibition.

NSAIDS IN ANIMAL MODELS OF RA

Two animal model systems are relevant to the role of NSAIDs in RA. The first involves rodent models of RA such as adjuvant-induced arthritis. Remarkably few studies of the activity of NSAIDs have been reported in these systems. A second model system utilizes carrageenan injection and is widely used to assess the anti-inflammatory activity of NSAIDs. Carrageenan, a seaweed extract, induces pain and intense inflammatory responses when administered parenterally in laboratory animals *(46)*. The adjuvant arthritis model and the carrageenan model have been used recently to investigate the effectiveness of selective COX-2 inhibitors. Representative data from this line of research are presented in this section.

Selective COX-2 Inhibition in Carrageenan-Induced Inflammation

The carrageenan model is the classic animal model used to assess the activity of anti-inflammatory agents. Carrageenan injection induces marked increases in prostaglandin synthesis. Most NSAIDs in clinical use were developed for clinical studies based on their ability to reduce the proinflammatory effects of carrageenan in rodents.

The carrageenan model has provided an important tool for dissecting the mechanism by which various inflammatory mediators induce the cardinal manifestations of inflammation. Of particular interest, the carrageenan model helped to support the hypothesis that COX-2 was the critical mediator of inflammation and pain; and provided the in vivo system for initial studies of selective COX-2 inhibitors.

Smith and coworkers undertook a study of the pharmacologic effects of specific COX-1 and COX-2 inhibitors on the production of PGE2, swelling and pain in rats administered carrageenan parenterally (Table 2) *(47)*. Carrageenan injected into the footpad of rats induced inflammatory pain and swelling in association with a four to

Table 2
Analgesic and Anti-Inflammatory Actions of Selective Cyclooxygense Inhibitors

Response parameter	Nonselective COX inhibitor*	Selective COX-1 inhibitor	Selective COX-2 inhibitor
Prevention of footpad edema	+	-	+
Prevention of footpad pain	+	-	+
Prevention of footpad PG production	+	+	+
Therapy of footpad edema	+	-	-
Therapy of footpad pain	+	-	+
Therapeutic reduction in footpad PG levels	+	+	+
Prevention of CSF PGE2 production		-	+
Therapy of CSF PGE2 production		-	+

*PG, prostaglandin; CSF, cerebrospinal fluid; COX, cyclooxygenase. Adapted from ref. *48*.

five-fold increase in local PG production. This inflammatory response was ameliorated by nonselective COX inhibitors *(48)*. In the study by Smith et al., the selective COX-2 inhibitor, celecoxib, but not the selective COX-1 inhibitor, SC-560, prevented increased pain and swelling associated with carrageenan injection *(47)*. Interestingly, the selective COX-1 and COX-2 inhibitors each prevented or treated upregulated PG production in the footpad in response to carrageenan injection. This paradoxical finding indicates that inhibition of local pain and edema at sites of inflammation may be mediated by prostaglandin production at distant sites, such as the central nervous system (CNS). To investigate this possibility, cerebrospinal fluid (CSF) levels of PGE2 were measured after footpad injection of carrageenan. Peripheral inflammation induced by carrageenan footpad injection resulted in markedly upregulated PGE2 production in CSF. Celecoxib, but not the COX-1 selective, SC560 prevented and treated upregulated CSF PGE2 levels in response to footpad injection of carrageenan. These data support the hypothesis that COX-2 is critical for production of PG important in inflammation. Furthermore, these data suggest that the analgesic effect of COX-2 inhibition in response to peripheral inflammation may be mediated in the CNS.

Selective COX-2 Inhibition in Adjuvant Arthritis Models

Adjuvant arthritis is a polyarthritis syndrome induced in rats after immunization with crude mycobacterial-cell wall preparations *(49)*. Selective COX-2 inhibition with celecoxib or rofecoxib reduced the swelling associated with adjuvant arthritis *(50,51)*. Administration of celecoxib to rats with adjuvant arthritis resulted in reduction in serum and paw IL-6 levels and reduced the expression of COX-2 mRNA and protein in affected paws. These effects were comparable to those achieved by the nonselective COX inhibitor, indomethacin. Rofecoxib has also been shown to reduce bone and cartilage damage in the adjuvant arthritis model *(50)*.

CLINICAL TRIALS OF NSAIDS IN RA

Hundreds of clinical trials have been performed using NSAIDs in RA. One of the first such trials in 1965 demonstrated that aspirin was effective in the treatment of RA *(52)*. Numerous trials over the last 40 years have confirmed the effectiveness of NSAIDs in the treatment of RA. However, the interpretation of these clinical trial data is complicated by several factors, which include the introduction of disease-modifying therapy, and changes in accepted measures of clinical outcome. Gotzsche performed a comparative analysis of 196 double-blind trials of NSAIDs in RA and identified three findings: important differences in the variables used to assess efficacy, important errors in statistical methods, and evidence of publication bias *(53)*. Nevertheless, several conclusions may be drawn from these clinical trial data: (1) often patients must try two or more NSAIDs before identifying one that is effective and well-tolerated *(54,55)*; (2) NSAIDs are not disease-modifying drugs in RA *(56)*; (3) although safety and tolerability profiles vary between NSAIDs *(57,58)*, their efficacy is comparable *(58–62)*.

It is difficult to explain the paradox between the comparable efficacy of NSAIDs and the marked variation in individual responses to various NSAIDs. In hundreds of clinical trials assessing over 100 NSAIDs, no one drug or class of NSAID has demonstrated superior efficacy. Yet, it is common for physicians and patients to note marked variation in clinical response. RA patients receiving fixed, blinded doses of ibuprofen, fenoprofen, ketoprofen, and naproxen demonstrated no significant clinical differences as a group. However, there were striking differences in individual responses and clear patient preferences for particular medications *(63)*. This observation led to efforts to identify patients who are responders and nonresponders in clinical trials. In a small trial comparing clinical responses of RA and OA patients to ketoprofen or piroxicam, it was possible to identify "responders" to one or more medications *(64)*. Despite these observations, clinical response or nonresponse has not been correlated with pharmacokinetic parameters; leading some authors to question the concept of nonresponders *(65)*. At present it is not possible to explain the mechanism of differences in clinical responsiveness of individual patients to the various NSAIDs.

Despite reports of hundreds of clinical trials of NSAIDs in RA, study design varies significantly in these trials, making it difficult to summarize clinical findings. Modern RA response criteria have recently been used to compare the efficacy of the new highly selective COX-2 inhibitors with nonselective COX inhibitors *(66)*. These studies have provided the most thorough assessment of the responses of RA patients to therapy with selective COX-2 inhibitors and nonselective COX inhibitors.

In the first such study, celecoxib, was compared with naproxen and placebo in a 12-wk, multi-center, double-blind, randomized controlled trial of 1149 RA patients *(67)*. Participants discontinued NSAIDs or analgesics and were allowed to have a RA flare. Upon experiencing increased RA symptoms, patients were randomized to receive celecoxib at 100, 200, or 400 mg twice daily; naproxen 500 mg twice daily; or placebo. Response rates American College of Rheumatology ([ACR] 20) were 36% in the naproxen group and 39–44% in the celecoxib groups; compared to 29% in the

Table 3
Efficacy and Safety of Celecoxib vs Naproxen vs Placebo in Rheumatoid Arthritis

	Celecoxib (all doses)	Naproxen	Placebo
ACR20 (% responder)	39–44	36	29
Withdrawal owing to treatment failure (%)	21–28	29	45
Patient's global assessment (% improved)	22–30	19	16
Physician's global assessment (% improved)	21–30	20	15
Reduction in number of tender joints	11.6–12.4	9.5	7.6
Reduction in number of swollen joints	7.0–9.1	6.9	5.5
Reduction in arthritis pain VAS (mm)	16.9–20.7	16.9	9.3
Change in AM stiffness (duration-min)	Decr. 98–153	Decr. 90	Incr. 9
Withdrawal due to adverse events (%)	5–7	5	5
Incidence of gastroduodenal ulcer (%)	4–6	26	4
Combined GI adverse events	25–28	31	19
GI adverse events causing withdrawal (%)	1–3	5	1

Adapted from ref. *67.*

placebo group (Table 3). Response rates were comparable in the naproxen and celecoxib groups and both drugs were significantly superior to placebo. Responses to approved doses of active treatments across individual components of the ACR responder index were all superior to placebo except for reduction in C-reactive protein. On average, patients in active treatment groups had 10–12 fewer tender joints, 7–9 fewer swollen joints, and morning stiffness was reduced by 90–120 min. Maximal clinical responses were achieved by 2 wk and were sustained for the duration of the study.

Several important conclusions may be drawn from this study. First, the efficacy of celecoxib in RA arthritis was better than placebo and was comparable to naproxen, a nonselective COX inhibitor that is widely used in RA. Clinical responses to naproxen in this study were comparable to those reported in prior clinical trials in RA *(68,69)*. Second, the active therapies were well-tolerated. The incidence of endoscopically detected ulcers in patients receiving celecoxib was comparable to placebo and significantly lower than patients in patients taking naproxen (*see* Side Effects) *(67)*. Third, despite efficacy of celecoxib and naproxen in most patients, over 25% withdrew from the study because of treatment failure *(67)*. Most withdrawals occurred within 6 wk of initiating treatment. Lack of response in a significant number of patients receiving celecoxib or naproxen may reflect the significant individual to individual variability in clinical responses to NSAIDs.

A second randomized controlled trial performed in Europe compared celecoxib 200 mg twice daily with diclofenac SR 75 mg twice daily in 655 RA patients *(70)*. At 24 wk the efficacy of celecoxib was comparable to that of diclofenac. ACR 20 response rates of 25 and 22% were achieved with celecoxib and diclofenac, respectively. Withdrawal owing to treatment failure occurred in 8% of patients receiving celecoxib and 7% of patients receiving diclofenac.

Finally, a short-term, placebo-controlled trial of rofecoxib, a highly selective COX-2 inhibitor, was performed in 658 RA patients. ACR20 response rates of 44–50% were seen in the rofecoxib group vs 32% in the placebo group *(71)*. Results of large-scale clinical trials in RA using the preferential COX-2 inhibitors nimesulide and meloxicam are not yet available.

SIDE EFFECTS AND PRECAUTIONS

Without question, NSAIDs are effective in treating the signs and symptoms of RA. However, medication-related adverse events ultimately drive clinical decision-making with regard to NSAID use. Up to one-third of patients using conventional NSAIDs develop persistent adverse events, and 10% ultimately discontinue treatment because of adverse events *(72)*. Despite widespread prescribing of over 70 million prescriptions each year, NSAIDs increase the risk of hospitalization and death *(73–75)*. Therefore, considerable attention should be given to identifying patient risk factors for NSAID-related adverse events. In fact, observations of patient-physician encounters indicate that inadequate attention is given to identifying risk factors for NSAID toxicity prior to prescribing *(76)*. Common adverse events associated with NSAID use are detailed below. Differences in rates of adverse events between selective COX-2 inhibitors and nonselective COX inhibitors are highlighted in this section.

Gastrointestinal

The most important adverse event associated with NSAIDs is gastroduodenal ulceration, which is a significant cause of morbidity and mortality worldwide. Clinically relevant gastroduodenal ulceration occurs in up to 6% of patients on long-term NSAID therapy *(77)*. Given the widespread use of NSAIDs this translates into over 100,000 hospitalizations annually; resulting in an estimated 16,000 deaths *(77)*. The direct medical costs in treating these complications exceeded $1.3 billion annually *(77)*. Approximately 40% of the morbidity and mortality is seen in patients with RA *(77)*.

PATHOGENESIS OF NSAID-INDUCED GASTROINTESTINAL TOXICITY

The pathogenesis of NSAID-induced gastrointestinal toxicity results from a combination of local injury to the gastroduodenal mucosa in association with systemic inhibition of normal prostaglandin synthesis, which is important for mucosal homeostasis. Normal gastroduodenal prostaglandin synthesis is mediated almost entirely by COX-1 (reviewed in ref. *78*). Mucosal effects of decreased prostaglandin synthesis include impaired bicarbonate formation, decreased mucus production, reduced mucosal blood flow, and loss of normal epithelial cell proliferation *(78,79)*. Most NSAIDs are weak acids that also mediate local injury to the gastroduodenal mucosa *(72)*. Weak acids are nonionized in the acidic environment of the stomach and can penetrate the protective mucosal layer. In the neutral environment beneath the mucus layer, weak acids release hydrogen ions, which become locally concentrated. The combination of local acid-mediated injury, coupled with systemic loss of prostaglandin-mediated mucosal protection results in the gastroduodenal injury associated with COX-1 inhibitor activity.

RISK FACTORS FOR NSAID-INDUCED GASTROINTESTINAL TOXICITY

Several well-designed epidemiologic studies have characterized risk factors gastro-duodenal ulceration (Table 4). A thorough assessment of each patient's risk factors is necessary to facilitate rational decision-making regarding selection of appropriate

Table 4
Risk Factors for NSAID-Induced Gastroduodenal Ulcers

Established risk factors
>   Advanced age
>   History of gastroduodenal ulcer
>   Concomitant use of corticosteroids
>   High dose NSAIDs/combination of NSAIDs
>   Concomitant anticoagulants
>   Serious systemic disorder

Possible risk factors
>   Concomitant infection with *H. pylori*
>   Cigarette smoking
>   Alcohol consumption

Adapted from ref. *145* with permission.

NSAIDs and concomitant use of gastroprotective medications (*see* below). It is important to appreciate that the risk of NSAID-associated ulcers is greatest in the first month of therapy *(75)*. In fact, most instances of GI bleeding occur in patients taking nonprescription NSAIDs for short periods of time *(80)*. Increasing age is associated with risk of ulceration in a linear fashion. The relative risk of ulceration rises from 1.6 in the sixth decade to 5.6 in the eighth decade of life *(81)*. Other risk factors for gastroduodenal ulceration are shown in Table 4; each of which confers at least a fivefold increased risk of ulceration. The importance of *Helicobacter pylori* in the pathogenesis of NSAID-induced gastropathy is uncertain. *H. pylori* is an independent risk factor for endoscopic and clinically significant ulcers *(82)* Eradication of *H. pylori* prior to instituting NSAID therapy may prevent ulcer recurrence or onset of symptomatic ulcer in chronic NSAID users *(83,84)*. Paradoxically, the presence of *H. pylori* protected against recurrent gastroduodenal ulcerations in arthritis patients using NSAIDs *(85,86)*. Further study is needed to define the role of *H. pylori* in the pathogenesis of NSAID-related gastroduodenal injury.

PREVENTING NSAID-INDUCED GASTROINTESTINAL TOXICITY USING SELECTIVE COX-2 INHIBITORS

Several trials have been performed that demonstrate reduction in the incidence of endoscopic ulcers in patients receiving highly-selective COX-2 inhibitors in comparison to a control population receiving standard NSAIDs. In a 6-mo European trial of celecoxib vs diclofenac in 655 patients with RA, ulcers were detected in 4% of the patients receiving celecoxib and 15% of the patients receiving diclofenac *(70)*. A similar US trial compared celecoxib and naproxen in 1149 RA patients. At 12 wk the cumulative incidence of endoscopic ulcer was 26% in the naproxen group and 4% in the celecoxib groups *(67)*. In a 24-week trial of rofecoxib vs ibuprofen in patients with OA, the cumulative ulcer risk was 10% in patients receiving 25 mg of rofecoxib daily vs 46% in patients receiving ibuprofen 800 mg t.i.d. *(87)*. Finally, the incidence of symptomatic adverse gastrointestinal events was compiled from eight clinical trials of rofecoxib in comparison to ibuprofen, diclofenac, or nabumetone for the treatment of OA *(88)*. In over 5000 patients receiving therapy for 6–52 wk, the incidence of GI-tract perforation, symptomatic gastroduodenal ulcers or upper GI bleeding was 1.3% in the rofecoxib-treated patients vs 1.8% in patients receiving standard NSAIDs. This translated into a relative risk of a clinically significant GI event of 0.51 in patients receiving rofecoxib.

MEDICATIONS USED TO PREVENT NSAID-INDUCED GASTROINTESTINAL TOXICITY

Another important strategy for reducing gastrointestinal complications with NSAIDs is the concomitant use of gastroprotective medications. Clinical trials aimed at reducing NSAID-induced ulcers have been undertaken using sucralfate, type 2 histamine receptor antagonists, proton pump inhibitors and the prostaglandin analog, misoprostol. Sucralfate is not effective (89). The H2-receptor antagonist, ranitidine, given at 150 mg twice daily for 8 wk, reduced duodenal but not gastric ulcers in the setting of nonselective COX-inhibitor use (90,91). However, high-dose famotidine (40 mg b.i.d.) reduced both gastric and duodenal ulcers in a 24-wk study of arthritis patients taking nonselective COX inhibitors (92).

The prostaglandin analog, misoprostol, reduced the incidence of endoscopic ulcers and ulcer complications. Patients taking NSAIDs for OA had a 15-fold reduction in gastric-ulcer risk with concomitant use of misoprostol 200 mcg. q.i.d. (93). A subsequent trial confirmed these findings and extended them to include duodenal ulcers as well (94). More importantly, the reduction in complicated ulcers was studied in the MUCOSA trial, which enrolled 8843 RA patients using NSAIDs (95). Patients were randomized to receive misoprostol 200 mcg. q.i.d. vs placebo for 6 mo. The misoprostol group experienced a 40% reduction in serious upper-GI complications. Consequently, misoprostol is the only drug approved for prophylaxis against NSAID-related gastroduodenal ulcers. Barriers to widespread use of misoprostol prophylaxis include dyspepsia and diarrhea. Lower doses of misoprostol are better tolerated but do not provide the same protection as dosing the drug four times daily (96).

Two large trials demonstrated that proton-pump inhibitors reduce the incidence of NSAID-related gastroduodenal ulcers. The first trial compared omeprazole with ranitidine in the prevention of recurrent ulcers in arthritis patients requiring NSAID therapy (86). About 40–50% of the subjects had RA. Patients with endoscopically diagnosed gastroduodenal ulcers or >10 erosions were treated with omeprazole or ranitidine. Patients who healed completely were randomized to receive concurrent therapy with omeprazole 20 mg daily or ranitidine 150 mg twice daily as prophylaxis against recurrent ulcer or erosions. After 6 mo, 72% of patients receiving omeprazole remained in remission, and 59% of patients receiving ranitidine remained in remission. The difference in relapse rates between omeprazole and ranitidine were statistically significant. The second trial compared omeprazole 20 mg daily with misoprostol 200 mcg. twice daily in the prevention of recurrent gastroduodenal ulcers (85). A placebo arm was also included in this study. Remission was sustained in 61% of patients taking omeprazole, 48% of patients taking misoprostol, and 27% of patients taking placebo. Omeprazole was significantly more effective than misoprostol at the doses used. Both drugs were significantly more effective than placebo. Fewer patients discontinued therapy because of adverse events or lack of efficacy. It is possible that the effectiveness of misoprostol would have been greater if higher doses had been used in this study (96). However, any gain may have been offset by increased adverse events (96).

OTHER GASTROINTESTINAL COMPLICATIONS OF NSAIDs

Although most attention is appropriately given to gastroduodenal ulceration, several other gastrointestinal toxicities occur with NSAID use. Dyspepsia is a common symptom in RA patients using NSAIDs *(97)*. The presence of dyspepsia does not necessarily correlate with endoscopic evidence of mucosal injury. Less than half of patients with dyspepsia have abnormal gastroduodenal mucosa, and up to 40% of patients with gastritis are asymptomatic *(97)*. In studies of ulcer healing or prevention, both histamine-receptor antagonists and proton-pump inhibitors were shown to relieve dyspepsia symptoms *(85,86)*. Other gastrointestinal complications associated with NSAID use include strictures of the esophagus, small bowel, and colon (reviewed in ref. *98)*. Frank ulceration of the small bowel and colon has also been associated with NSAID and may be present in up to 4% of chronic NSAID users *(98,99)*. The pathogenesis of small and large bowel ulcerations is thought to involve the same mechanisms known to occur in the stomach and duodenum.

Nephrotoxicity

There are several manifestations of NSAID-induced nephrotoxicity: hyperkalemia, acute reduction in renal function, nephrotic syndrome with interstitial nephritis, and papillary necrosis (reviewed in ref. *100)*. Reduced renal production of prostaglandins contributes to the pathogenesis of each of these syndromes.

HYPERKALEMIA

NSAIDs contribute to hyperkalemia by indirectly inhibiting aldosterone-induced potassium excretion, and by interfering with normal sodium-potassium exchange in the distal nephron *(100)*. Risk factors for NSAID-induced hyperkalemia include renal insufficiency, diabetes, heart failure, and multiple myeloma *(100)*. Concurrent use of potassium supplements, angiotensin-converting enzyme (ACE) inhibitors, and potassium-sparing diuretics also contributes to the risk of hyperkalemia *(100)*. Hyperkalemia is reversed by discontinuing NSAIDs.

ACUTE REDUCTION IN RENAL FUNCTION

Prostaglandins maintain normal renal blood flow in hypovolemic or low-perfusion states. Inhibition of prostaglandin production in these situations can cause ischemia with acute loss of renal function. Comorbidities that predispose to reduced renal function include congestive heart failure, nephrotic syndrome, dehydration, cirrhosis, chronic renal disease, and advanced age *(100,101)*. Early diagnosis with discontinuation of NSAIDs will usually lead to resolution over several days; whereas continued use may lead to irreversible loss of renal function and even need for dialysis. Indomethacin has been most commonly associated with this adverse effect; whereas naproxen, diclofenac, ibuprofen, and piroxicam have intermediate effects *(100)*. Long-acting NSAIDs may pose greater risk than short-acting NSAIDs *(101)*. COX-2 is constitutively expressed in the kidney and contributes to autoregulation of renal blood flow. Therefore, the same caution must be extended to use of COX-2 inhibitors in high-risk settings.

NEPHROTIC SYNDROME AND INTERSTITIAL NEPHRITIS

A rare complication of NSAIDs is interstitial nephritis with nephrotic syndrome *(100)*. This adverse event is characterized by edema and occasionally reduced urine output. Urinalysis reveals nephrotic range proteinuria with epithelial cell casts and microscopic hematuria. Renal biopsy demonstrates interstitial nephritis in association with minimal change glomerulonephritis. This constellation of pathologic findings and the absence of eosinophilia and urine eosinophils distinguishes this condition from typical drug-induced interstitial nephritis. Proteinuria usually remits within a month of discontinuing NSAIDs. A trial of corticosteroids is recommended for patients who show no reduction in proteinuria within 2 wk *(102)*.

RENAL PAPILLARY NECROSIS

Acute renal papillary necrosis is associated with excessive NSAID doses combined with a volume depleted state *(100)*. Necrosis results from infarction of the distal segment of the renal pyramid. The underlying conditions resulting in papillary necrosis resolve with discontinuation of NSAIDs. However, patients may have permanent defects in maximally concentrating urine. Chronic renal papillary necrosis results from long-standing, excessive ingestion of analgesic combinations containing phenacetin.

Cardiovascular

HYPERTENSION

Elevated blood pressure is perhaps the most common cardiovascular side effect of NSAID use. In a study of over 19,000 Medicare patients, the prescribing of NSAIDs doubled the risk of requiring anti-hypertensive therapy within the first year of treatment *(103)*. Two large meta-analyses of clinical trial data revealed in increase in mean arterial pressure of 3–6 mm Hg depending on the particular NSAID studied *(104,105)*. Although this effect seems modest, it is known that increased diastolic blood pressure of 5 mm Hg sustained over several years is associated with a 15% increased risk of coronary artery disease and a 67% increased risk of stroke *(106)*. No single NSAID has been associated with consistently significant increases in blood pressure. However, aspirin and sulindac were shown in both meta-analyses to have negligible impact on blood pressure. Patients with hypertension at the time of initiating NSAID therapy demonstrated the greatest rise in blood pressure *(104,105)*. NSAIDs diminish the effectiveness of anti-hypertensives; an effect that is most pronounced for β-blockers *(100)*. Because the renal effects of selective COX-2 inhibitors are similar to those of nonselective COX inhibitors, careful monitoring of blood pressure is also required. Given the lengthy duration of NSAID therapy for many RA patients, the clinician should regard modest elevations in blood pressure as a significant risk factor for cardiovascular disease and treat patients accordingly.

CONGESTIVE HEART FAILURE

NSAIDs induce clinically insignificant sodium and fluid retention in many patients. Symptomatic edema occurs in 3–5% of patients and is usually not associated with clinical impairment in cardiac or renal function *(102)*. However, concurrent use of NSAIDs and diuretics in a patient population aged 55 or greater was associated with a doubling in the risk for hospitalization for congestive heart failure (CHF) *(107)*. NSAIDs may lead to sodium and fluid retention with subsequent exacerbation of CHF through a variety of mechanisms (reviewed in ref. *108*). The most important effect is through inhibition of prostaglandin synthesis. Compensated CHF is dependent on the vasodilatory effect of prostaglandins on renal afferent arterioles. Prostaglandins also counteract the actions of angiotensin II on the systemic vasculature. NSAIDs can also attenuate the pharmacologic effects of diuretics and ACE inhibitors (109,110). NSAIDs do not directly impair myocardial function. Exacerbation of CHF has been reported with both selective COX-2 inhibitors and nonselective COX inhibitors. Exacerbations of CHF in patients treated with NSAIDs are commonly associated with impairment in renal function, which may magnify the harmful effects of NSAIDs used in this setting. NSAIDs should be initiated with extreme caution in patients with compensated CHF, and only in situations in which the benefits outweigh potential risks.

Hepatotoxicity

Liver injury as a result of NSAID therapy is rare, occurring in less than 0.1% of patients (111). Toxic reactions are generally idiosyncratic or immune-mediated and are unpredictable (111,112). One exception is aspirin, which is an intrinsic hepatotoxin and will cause liver injury in all persons exposed to sufficient concentrations of the drug (113). Risk factors for NSAID induced liver injury are thought to be the same as those for drug-induced liver injury in general and include: age > 40, female gender, polypharmacy, chronic ethanol ingestion, over- or under-nutrition, and genetic polymorphisms in the cytochrome P-450 system (111).

Hepatoxicity is viewed as a class effect of NSAIDs (111). Spontaneous reports of adverse events to the US Food and Drug Administration (FDA) indicate that hepatotoxicity may be more common for diclofenac than other commonly used NSAIDs such as nabumetone, naproxen, and piroxicam (114). However, these findings have not been borne out in epidemiologic studies, which have detected no significant differences in rates of hepatotoxicity for commonly prescribed NSAIDs (115). In studies of approved COX-2 inhibitors in the United States, elevations in liver aminotransferases occurred at rates similar to those of comparator drugs. No reports of severe hepatic injury have been reported for rofecoxib or celecoxib at this time.

Patterns of liver toxicity include both hepatocellular and cholestatic injury. Patients may present with new onset of constitutional symptoms, elevated aminotransferase levels, and/or cholestatic jaundice. Rarely patients may present with fulminant hepatic failure (116–118). The most common manifestation of liver injury is elevated aminotransferase levels. This presents a diagnostic challenge because patients with RA often have transient elevations in aminotransferases unrelated to NSAID use (119). NSAID-induced liver injury is usually reversible but may progress to irreversible injury with continued use of offending drugs (111,120). Therefore, the clinician must maintain a high index of suspicion for NSAID-induced liver injury in RA patients. Periodic monitoring of liver function studies should be undertaken in all patients using NSAIDs regularly (121). A trial withdrawal of an NSAID is appropriate in patients with persistently abnormal laboratory studies.

NSAID Hypersensitivity Syndromes

A small subset of patients demonstrate heightened sensitivity to aspirin and all nonselective COX inhibitors. The rheumatologist should be aware of the manifestations and management of these syndromes because severe and sometimes fatal attacks of asthma may be precipitated by ingestion of NSAIDs. Two syndromes are generally recognized. The first is the "aspirin triad," which comprises aspirin-sensitivity, asthma, and nasal polyposis *(122)*. Approximately 10% of asthmatics experience NSAID-induced exacerbation of symptoms *(123)*. The syndrome is slightly more common in women *(123)*. A second syndrome of NSAID-induced urticaria and/or angiodema occurs in a subset of patients who virtually always have underlying chronic urticaria *(124)*. About 20–30% of patients with chronic urticaria exhibit exacerbations of urticaria and angioedema upon exposure to NSAIDs *(124)*.

Although these syndromes are typically associated with aspirin, it is important to note that all drugs that demonstrate COX-1 inhibition have been associated with NSAID-hypersensitivity syndromes. Patients who experience respiratory symptoms with ingestion of NSAIDs should be carefully educated as to the generic and trade names of NSAIDs and instructed to avoid them. Particular attention should be given to over-the-counter medications that may contain aspirin or other NSAIDs. In addition, patients should ask about the contents of medications prescribed by other practitioners who may not be aware of the extensive crossreactivity of most NSAIDs in hypersensitivity syndromes.

Some NSAIDs are safe to use in the setting of NSAID sensitivity. Patients can usually safely take sodium salicylate, salicylamide, and choline magnesium trisalicylate *(125)*. Nimesulide and meloxicam, which have preferential COX-2 selectivity, may be administered in lower doses to patients with NSAID sensitivity *(126–128)*. In theory, the highly selective COX-2 inhibitors, rofecoxib and celecoxib, should be safe to use in NSAID-sensitive patients *(125)*. As of yet, no studies have been reported to confirm this hypothesis. Current medication labeling cautions against using these drugs in NSAID-sensitive patients.

Aspirin desensitization may be undertaken to reduce the respiratory symptoms of NSAID sensitivity. Typically nasal congestion responds to desensitization better than asthma symptoms *(125)*. Desensitization is not effective for urticaria or angioedema. Desensitization can reduce symptoms of nasal congestion, slow further formation of polyps, and allow the patient with RA to safely take NSAIDs.

Acute urticaria or anaphylaxis may occur as an immunologic hypersensitivity reaction to the parent drug or a metabolite. In this setting, hypersensitivity is confined to the parent drug and does not require avoidance of all NSAIDs. Patients are usually able to tolerate an alternate NSAID, especially if it is of a chemically distinct class.

Hematologic

The most important hematologic toxicity of NSAIDs is also one of the most important therapeutic effects (reviewed in ref. *129*). NSAIDs impair platelet function through inhibition of TBXA2 synthesis by COX-1. Aspirin irreversibly inhibits COX-1 through acetylation, whereas nonaspirin COX inhibitors reversibly inhibit COX-1. The highly selective COX-2 inhibitors have no effect on platelets at therapeutic doses. Aspirin reduces mortality in the primary and secondary prevention of coronary artery disease. Inhibition of platelet function can lead to complications such as ulcer bleeding or intracranial hemorrhage. Fortunately, the latter is quite rare. Excessive use of alcohol may impair platelet function further, thus contributing to the risk for bleeding complications. The duration of impaired platelet function in the setting of aspirin use is 4–7 d. The nonaspirin NSAIDs inhibit platelet function for a variable period based upon half-life.

Miscellaneous Side Effects

PULMONARY

Pulmonary infiltrates and eosinophilia are rarely reported as a complication of NSAID therapy *(130)*. Patients have typically presented with fever, shortness of breath, cough, and infiltrates on chest X-ray. Leukocyte differential demonstrates an absolute eosinophilia. Biopsy of affected lung tissue demonstrates granulomas with eosinophilic infiltrates. This syndrome has been associated with naproxen, ibuprofen, fenoprofen, and sulindac. This complication is usually self-limited and resolves with discontinuation of the NSAID.

CENTRAL NERVOUS SYSTEM

Aseptic meningitis is a rare complication of NSAID therapy *(131)*. This complication has typically been associated with naproxen but may occur with any NSAID. There have been no reports of aseptic meningitis with use of the selective COX-2 inhibitors, rofecoxib and celecoxib. Patients present with meningeal signs and headache. Fever was present in over 90% of reported cases of NSAID-related aseptic meningitis. Analysis of cerebrospinal fluid (CSF) demonstrates a pleocytosis with a median of 280 cells that are predominantly neutrophils. Aseptic meningitis probably represents a hypersensitivity reaction. Some reports indicate that patients tolerated challenge with the same NSAID after resolution of aseptic meningitis. However, given the number of available NSAIDs it is reasonable to avoid exposing patients to the same drug if NSAIDs are required. Finally, transient cognitive dysfunction has been reported in elderly patients taking NSAIDs *(132)*.

SKIN

The most common adverse event involving the skin is an urticarial drug eruption. Pseudoporphyria has been reported rarely *(133,134)*.

SALICYLATE TOXICITY

Salicylates cause dose-related adverse events involving the ears, (CNS), and liver *(135)*. In therapeutic doses, patients may experience tinnitus and/or hearing loss that is reversible with discontinuation of the drug. Excessive doses may lead to coma and liver injury. Salicylate levels should be monitored periodically in patients using high therapeutic doses.

PREGNANCY

NSAIDs may be continued if necessary during the first half of pregnancy. A single case-control study described aspirin and NSAID use in early pregnancy as a risk factor for persistent pulmonary hypertension of the newborn pregnancy *(136)*. Low doses of aspirin are frequently used during the second half of pregnancy to treat preeclampsia *(137)*. High doses of NSAIDs in the second half of pregnancy may cause constriction of the ductus arteriosis and oligohydramnios *(138)*. NSAIDs should only be continued in late pregnancy if absolutely necessary and in close association with an experienced high-risk obstetrician. Usually it is possible to substitute alternative analgesic and anti-inflammatory medications in this setting.

CURRENT RECOMMENDATIONS ON NSAID USE IN RA

Over the last 20 years, the role of NSAIDs in RA therapy has shifted to one of symptom modification when used in association with disease-modifying drugs. Preventing NSAID toxicity has become a critical aspect of the appropriate use of these medications. The following recommendations on the use of NSAIDs in RA are derived from the data reviewed previously:

Use of NSAIDs in RA

It is appropriate to offer NSAID therapy to any patient with RA who does not have an underlying condition that would prohibit safe use. NSAIDs have been proven to relieve the signs and symptoms of RA using current response criteria (67,70). Furthermore, patients prefer NSAIDs over other analgesic medications, and are willing to accept additional risks of adverse events in order to achieve better symptom control (139,140). Given that NSAIDs are not believed to be disease-modifying, it is appropriate for patients to use NSAIDs on an as needed basis if desired. However, patients should be aware that the analgesic effects of NSAIDs have rapid onset, whereas it may take 1–2 wk to achieve maximal anti-inflammatory benefit (141).

Assessment of Risk Factors for NSAID Toxicity

Risk factors for NSAID toxicity should be assessed for every patient initiating therapy. Particular emphasis should be placed on assessing risks for GI and renal toxicity. Elderly patients and those with a history of peptic ulcer disease, renal disease, CHF, and asthma represent a high-risk population. System review should focus on eliciting symptoms that may indicate one or more of these diseases are present. Risk-factor assessment should not be delayed as toxicity occurs early in the course of NSAID therapy (75,121). The American College of Rheumatology recommends a baseline laboratory evaluation that includes a complete blood count, creatinine, and liver aminotransferases (121). Concurrent medication use must be considered as important drug-drug interactions influence toxicity (see below). Patients should be educated about potential toxicity and should be informed of warning signs of toxicity (e.g., edema, dark/tarry stools, persistent abdominal discomfort, rash, etc.).

Monitoring for NSAID toxicity

Symptoms of potential NSAID toxicity should be elicited periodically—at least yearly. The American College of Rheumatology recommends that a complete blood count, serum creatinine, and serum aminotransferases be monitored yearly (121). Decreasing hemoglobin, and increased creatinine or aminotransferases should all be considered signs of NSAID toxicity. Weekly monitoring of serum creatinine for the first 3 wk of therapy is recommended for NSAID users taking diuretics or ACE inhibitors (121). Patients using diclofenac should have liver-function studies repeated within the first 8 wk of therapy (package insert).

Selection of NSAIDs

Efficacy of the various NSAIDs in RA is comparable among groups of patients (141). Therefore, selection of an NSAID should focus on patient factors such as risk of complications, cost, and convenience. Individual patients may show marked variability

Table 5
Important Interactions of NSAIDs with Commonly Prescribed Drugs

Drug	Interaction	Action necessary	Reference
Lithium	Reduced clearance	Monitor lithium levels	(147)
Methotrexate	Reduced clearance	Careful methotrexate toxicity monitoring	(121)
Warfarin	Bleeding ulcer; hemorrhage	Avoid COX-1 inhibitors	(148)
Diuretics	Hyperkalemia	Monitor potassium	(121)
ACE Inhibitors	Hyperkalemia	Monitor potassium	(109)

in clinical responses. In this setting, changing to an alternate NSAID is appropriate in order to identify an effective and well-tolerated therapy. Maximal clinical responses are usually achieved within 2–3 wk. There is no data supporting improved efficacy with combination NSAID therapy (142). Patients who are anti-coagulated should not receive NSAIDs that inhibit COX-1. In this setting highly selective COX-2 inhibitors (celecoxib, rofecoxib) appear to be safe as long as the prothrombin time is carefully followed.

Prevention of NSAID-Related Gastroduodenal Ulceration

Decision-making on selection of NSAIDs or the concomitant use of gastroprotective medications should be driven by analysis of individual patient risk factors (Table 4). Inevitably, an individual patient's financial means and risk tolerance will influence prescribing as well. Patients with RA and no risk factors for NSAID-induced ulcer have a 0.4% risk of a serious GI event over 6 mo (95), whereas 10% of patients with four or more risk factors will experience a serious GI event within 6 mo (95). Some studies suggest that nabumetone and etodolac may have lower rates of GI toxicity; suggesting that these drugs may be preferable to other nonselective COX inhibitors (143,144). Patients with one or more risk factors for NSAID-related gastroduodenal ulceration should be treated with a selective COX-2 inhibitor, or concomitant use of a proton-pump inhibitor (20 mg omeprazole, 20 mg lansoprazole, 20 mg rabeprazole, or 40 mg pantoprazole daily) or misoprostol (200 mcg b.i.d.-q.i.d.) (141,145).

Patients with symptoms of dyspepsia may be treated with H_2-receptor antagonists or proton-pump inhibitors for symptom relief. Despite the poor correlation of dyspepsia with gastroduodenal ulceration, persistent symptoms of dyspepsia warrant additional investigation to rule out gastroduodenal ulcer.

The role of *H. pylori* infection in NSAID-related ulcers is unclear. Therefore, current recommendations are to identify and treat *H. pylori* in patients diagnosed with gastroduodenal ulcer (145). Routine screening for *H. pylori* in asymptomatic patients taking NSAIDs is not recommended (145).

Important Drug-Drug Interactions

Many drug interactions have been described with NSAIDs (146). A selected listing of important interactions of NSAIDs with commonly prescribed drugs is shown (Table 5).

CONCLUSIONS

The NSAIDs continue to be important in the management of RA. The primary objective of NSAID use is to reduce symptoms of RA rather than to modify the disease course. Given the comparable efficacy of NSAIDs, decisions regarding NSAID selection are driven predominantly by the need to minimize the risks of therapy. In this regard, the selective COX-2 inhibitors represent an important step forward in reducing the incidence of GI toxicity. Progress anticipated in the future includes the introduction of more selective COX-2 inhibitors, the development of irreversible COX-2 inhibitors, and NSAIDs that inhibit alternate pathways of inflammatory mediator production in RA.

REFERENCES

1. Vane, J.R. and R.M. Botting. 1998. Mechanism of action of nonsteroidal anti-inflammatory drugs. *Am. J. Med.* 104:2S–8S; discussion 21S–22S.

2. Vane, J.R. 1971. Inhibition of prostaglandin synthesis as a mechanism of action for aspirin-like drugs. *Nat New Biol.* 231:232–235.

3. Hemler, M. and W.E. Lands. 1976. Purification of the cyclooxygenase that forms prostaglandins. Demonstration of two forms of iron in the holoenzyme. *J. Biol. Chem.* 251:5575–5579.

4. Griffiths, R. 1999. Prostaglandins and inflammation. *In* Inflammation: Basic Principles and Clinical Correlates. J.I. Gallin, and R. Snyderman, editors. Lippincott Williams & Wilkins, Philadelphia. 349–360.

5. O'Neill, G.P. and A.W. Ford-Hutchinson. 1993. Expression of mRNA for cyclooxygenase-1 and cyclooxygenase-2 in human tissues. *FEBS Lett.* 330:156–160.

6. Balsinde, J., H. Shinohara, L.J. Lefkowitz, C.A. Johnson, M.A. Balboa, and E.A. Dennis. 1999. Group V phospholipase A(2)-dependent induction of cyclooxygenase-2 in macrophages. *J. Biol. Chem.* 274:25,967–25,970.

7. Couturier, C., A. Brouillet, C. Couriaud, K. Koumanov, G. Bereziat, and M. Andreani. 1999. Interleukin 1beta induces type II-secreted phospholipase A(2) gene in vascular smooth muscle cells by a nuclear factor kappaB and peroxisome proliferator-activated receptor-mediated process. *J. Biol. Chem.* 274:23,085–23,093.

8. Ozaki, M., Y. Yamada, K. Matoba, H. Otani, M. Mune, S. Yukawa, and W. Sakamoto. 1999. Phospholipase A2 activity in ox-LDL-stimulated mesangial cells and modulation by alpha-tocopherol. *Kidney Int. Suppl.* 71:S171–S173.

9. Terry, C.M., J.A. Clikeman, J.R. Hoidal, and K.S. Callahan. 1999. TNF-alpha and IL-1alpha induce heme oxygenase-1 via protein kinase C, Ca2+, and phospholipase A2 in endothelial cells. *Am. J. Physiol.* 276:H1493–H1501.

10. Shankavaram, U.T., D.L. DeWitt, and L.M. Wahl. 1998. Lipopolysaccharide induction of monocyte matrix metalloproteinases is regulated by the tyrosine phosphorylation of cytosolic phospholipase A2. *J. Leukoc. Biol.* 64:221–227.

11. Pruzanski, W., E. Stefanski, P. Vadas, B.P. Kennedy, and H. van den Bosch. 1998. Regulation of the cellular expression of secretory and cytosolic phospholipases A2, and cyclooxygenase-2 by peptide growth factors. *Biochim. Biophys. Acta.* 1403:47–56.

12. Lyons-Giordano, B., G.L. Davis, W. Galbraith, M.A. Pratta, and E.C. Arner. 1989. Interleukin-1 beta stimulates phospholipase A2 mRNA synthesis in rabbit articular chondrocytes. *Biochem. Biophys. Res. Commun.* 164:488–495.

13. Ushikubi, F., E. Segi, Y. Sugimoto, T. Murata, T. Matsuoka, T. Kobayashi, et al. 1998. Impaired febrile response in mice lacking the prostaglandin E receptor subtype EP3. *Nature* 395:281–284.

14. Stitt, J.T. 1986. Prostaglandin E as the neural mediator of the febrile response. *Yale J. Biol. Med.* 59:137–149.

15. Ferreira, S.H., M. Nakamura, and M.S. de Abreu Castro. 1978. The hyperalgesic effects of prostacyclin and prostaglandin E2. *Prostaglandins.* 16:31–37.

16. Wheeldon, A. and C.J. Vardey. 1993. Characterization of the inhibitory prostanoid receptors on human neutrophils. *Br. J. Pharmacol.* 108:1051–1054.

17. Honig, M., H.H. Peter, P. Jantscheff, and F. Grunert. 1999. Synovial PMN show a coordinated up-regulation of CD66 molecules. *J. Leukoc. Biol.* 66:429–436.

18. Pettipher, E.R., and D.J. Wimberly. 1994. Cyclooxygenase inhibitors enhance tumour necrosis factor production and mortality in murine endotoxic shock. *Cytokine* 6:500–503.

19. Martich, G.D., R.L. Danner, M. Ceska, and A.F. Suffredini. 1991. Detection of interleukin 8 and tumor necrosis factor in normal humans after intravenous endotoxin: the effect of antiinflammatory agents. *J. Exp. Med.* 173:1021–1024.

20. Bottomley, K.M., R.J. Griffiths, T.J. Rising, and A. Steward. 1988. A modified mouse air pouch model for evaluating the effects of compounds on granuloma induced cartilage degradation. *Br. J. Pharmacol.* 93:627–635.

21. Pettipher, E.R., B. Henderson, J.C. Edwards, and G.A. Higgs. 1989. Effect of indomethacin on swelling, lymphocyte influx, and cartilage proteoglycan depletion in experimental arthritis. *Ann. Rheum. Dis.* 48:623–627.

22. Goodwin, J.S., A.D. Bankhurst, and R.P. Messner. 1977. Suppression of human T-cell mitogenesis by prostaglandin. Existence of a prostaglandin-producing suppressor cell. *J. Exp. Med.* 146: 1719–1734.

23. Snijdewint, F.G., P. Kalinski, E.A. Wierenga, J.D. Bos, and M.L. Kapsenberg. 1993. Prostaglandin E2 differentially modulates cytokine secretion profiles of human T helper lymphocytes. *J. Immunol.* 150:5321–5329.

24. van der Pouw Kraan, T.C., L.C. Boeije, R.J. Smeenk, J. Wijdenes, and L.A. Aarden. 1995. Prostaglandin-E2 is a potent inhibitor of human interleukin 12 production. *J. Exp. Med.* 181:775–779.

25. Oppenheimer-Marks, N., A.F. Kavanaugh, and P.E. Lipsky. 1994. Inhibition of the transendothelial migration of human T lymphocytes by prostaglandin E2. *J. Immunol.* 152:5703–5713.

26. Cush, J.J., P.E. Lipsky, A.E. Postlethwaite, R.E. Schrohenloher, A. Saway, and W.J. Koopman. 1990. Correlation of serologic indicators of inflammation with effectiveness of nonsteroidal antiinflammatory drug therapy in rheumatoid arthritis. *Arthritis Rheum.* 33:19–28.

27. Cush, J.J., H.E. Jasin, R. Johnson, and P.E. Lipsky. 1990. Relationship between clinical efficacy and laboratory correlates of inflammatory and immunologic activity in rheumatoid arthritis patients treated with nonsteroidal antiinflammatory drugs. *Arthritis Rheum.* 33:623–633.

28. Sundy, J.S. and B.F. Haynes. 1998. Rheumatoid arthritis. *In* The Autoimmune Diseases. N.R. Rose, and I.R. Mackay, editors. Academic Press, Boston. 343–380.

29. Hishinuma, T., H. Nakamura, T. Sawai, M. Uzuki, Y. Itabash, and M. Mizugaki. 1999. Microdetermination of prostaglandin E2 in joint fluid in rheumatoid arthritis patients using gas chromatography/selected ion monitoring. *Prostaglandins Other Lipid Mediat.* 58:179–186.

30. Sano, H., T. Hla, J.A. Maier, L.J. Crofford, J.P. Case, T. Maciag, and R.L. Wilder. 1992. In vivo cyclooxygenase expression in synovial tissues of patients with rheumatoid arthritis and osteoarthritis and rats with adjuvant and streptococcal cell wall arthritis. *J. Clin. Invest.* 89:97–108.

31. Seppala, E., M. Nissila, H. Isomaki, H. Wuorela, and H. Vapaatalo. 1990. Effects of non-steroidal anti-inflammatory drugs and prednisolone on synovial fluid white cells, prostaglandin E2, leukotriene B4 and cyclic AMP in patients with rheumatoid arthritis. *Scand. J. Rheumatol.* 19:71–75.

32. Loetscher, P., B. Dewald, M. Baggiolini, and M. Seitz. 1994. Monocyte chemoattractant protein 1 and interleukin 8 production by rheumatoid synoviocytes. Effects of anti-rheumatic drugs. *Cytokine* 6:162–170.

33. Moilanen, E., J. Alanko, M. Nissila, M. Hamalainen, H. Isomaki, and H. Vapaatalo. 1989. Eicosanoid production in rheumatoid synovitis. *Agents Actions* 28:290–297.

34. Weissmann, G., C. Serhan, H.M. Korchak, and J.E. Smolen. 1984. Mechanisms of mediator release from neutrophils. Adv. Exp. Med. Biol. 172:527–552.

35. Tetlow, L.C., N. Harper, T. Dunningham, M.A. Morris, H. Bertfield, and D.E. Woolley. 1998. Effects of induced mast cell activation on prostaglandin E and metalloproteinase production by rheumatoid synovial tissue in vitro. *Ann. Rheum. Dis.* 57:25–32.

36. Bomalaski, J.S., C.S. Goldstein, A.T. Dailey, S.D. Douglas, and R.B. Zurier. 1986. Uptake of fatty acids and their mobilization from phospholipids in cultured monocyte-macrophages from rheumatoid arthritis patients. *Clin. Immunol. Immunopathol.* 39:198–212.

37. Crofford, L.J., R.L. Wilder, A.P. Ristimaki, H. Sano, E.F. Remmers, H.R. Epps, and T. Hla. 1994. Cyclooxygenase-1 and -2 expression in rheumatoid synovial tissues. Effects of interleukin-1 beta, phorbol ester, and corticosteroids. *J. Clin. Invest.* 93:1095–1101.

38. Szczepanski, A., T. Moatter, W.W. Carley, and M.E. Gerritsen. 1994. Induction of cyclooxygenase II in human synovial microvessel endothelial cells by interleukin-1. Inhibition by glucocorticoids. *Arthritis Rheum.* 37:495–503.

39. Mino, T., E. Sugiyama, H. Taki, A. Kuroda, N. Yamashita, M. Maruyama, and M. Kobayashi. 1998. Interleukin-1alpha and tumor necrosis factor alpha synergistically stimulate prostaglandin E2-dependent production of interleukin-11 in rheumatoid synovial fibroblasts. *Arthritis Rheum.* 41:2004–2013.

40. Butler, D.M., M. Feldmann, F. Di Padova, and F.M. Brennan. 1994. p55 and p75 tumor necrosis factor receptors are expressed and mediate common functions in synovial fibroblasts and other fibroblasts. *Eur. Cytokine Netw.* 5:441–448.

41. Preston, S.J., M.H. Arnold, E.M. Beller, P.M. Brooks, and W.W. Buchanan. 1989. Comparative analgesic and anti-inflammatory properties of sodium salicylate and acetylsalicylic acid (aspirin) in rheumatoid arthritis. *Br. J. Clin. Pharmacol.* 27:607–611.

42. Xu, X.M., L. Sansores-Garcia, X.M. Chen, N. Matijevic-Aleksic, M. Du, and K.K. Wu. 1999. Suppression of inducible cyclooxygenase 2 gene transcription by aspirin and sodium salicylate. *Proc. Natl. Acad. Sci. USA* 96:5292–5297.

43. Cronstein, B.N., M.C. Montesinos, and G. Weissmann. 1999. Sites of action for future therapy: an adenosine-dependent mechanism by which aspirin retains its antiinflammatory activity in cyclooxygenase-2 and NFkappaB knockout mice. *Osteoarthritis Cartilage.* 7:361–363.

44. Di Battista, J.A., M. Zhang, J. Martel-Pelletier, J. Fernandes, N. Alaaeddine, and J.P. Pelletier. 1999. Enhancement of phosphorylation and transcriptional activity of the glucocorticoid receptor in human synovial fibroblasts by nimesulide, a preferential cyclooxygenase 2 inhibitor. *Arthritis Rheum.* 42:157–166.

45. Hall, V.C. and R.E. Wolf. 1997. Effects of tenidap and nonsteroidal antiinflammatory drugs on the response of cultured human T cells to interleukin 2 in rheumatoid arthritis. *J. Rheumatol.* 24:1467–1470.

46. Di Rosa, M. 1972. Biological properties of carrageenan. *J. Pharm. Pharmacol.* 24:89–102.

47. Smith, C.J., Y. Zhang, C.M. Koboldt, J. Muhammad, B.S. Zweifel, A. Shaffer, et al. 1998. Pharmacological analysis of cyclooxygenase-1 in inflammation. *Proc. Natl. Acad. Sci. USA* 95:13,313–13,318.

48. Zhang, Y., A. Shaffer, J. Portanova, K. Seibert, and P.C. Isakson. 1997. Inhibition of cyclooxygenase-2 rapidly reverses inflammatory hyperalgesia and prostaglandin E2 production. *J. Pharmacol. Exp. Ther.* 283:1069–1075.

49. Wooley, P.H. 1991. Animal models of rheumatoid arthritis. *Curr. Opin. Rheumatol.* 3:407–420.

50. Chan, C.C., S. Boyce, C. Brideau, S. Charleson, W. Cromlish, D. Ethier, et al. 1999. Rofecoxib [Vioxx, MK-0966; 4-(4'-methylsulfonylphenyl)-3-phenyl-2-(5H)-furanone]: a potent and orally active cyclooxygenase-2 inhibitor. Pharmacological and biochemical profiles. *J. Pharmacol. Exp. Ther.* 290:551–560.

51. Anderson, G.D., S.D. Hauser, K.L. McGarity, M.E. Bremer, P.C. Isakson, and S.A. Gregory. 1996. Selective inhibition of cyclooxygenase (COX)-2 reverses inflammation and expression of COX-2 and interleukin 6 in rat adjuvant arthritis. *J. Clin. Invest.* 97:2672–2679.

52. Fremont-Smith, K. and T. Bayles. 1965. Salicylate therapy in rheumatoid arthritis. *JAMA* 192:1133.

53. Gotzsche, P.C. 1990. Sensitivity of effect variables in rheumatoid arthritis: a meta-analysis of 130 placebo controlled NSAID trials. *J. Clin. Epidemiol.* 43:1313–1318.

54. Dukes, M.N. and I. Lunde. 1981. The regulatory control of non-steroidal anti-inflammatory agents. *Eur. J. Clin. Pharmacol.* 19:3–10.

55. Pincus, T. and L.F. Callahan. 1993. Variability in individual responses of 532 patients with rheumatoid arthritis to first-line and second-line drugs. *Agents Actions Suppl.* 44:67–75.

56. Borg, A.A., P.D. Fowler, M.F. Shadforth, and P.T. Dawes. 1993. Use of the Stoke Index to differentiate between disease-modifying agents and non-steroidal anti-inflammatory drugs in rheumatoid arthritis. *Clin. Exp. Rheumatol.* 11:469–472.

57. Fries, J.F., D.R. Ramey, G. Singh, D. Morfeld, D.A. Bloch, and J.P. Raynauld. 1993. A reevaluation of aspirin therapy in rheumatoid arthritis. *Arch. Intern. Med.* 153:2465–2471.

58. Wijnands, M., P. van Riel, M. van 't Hof, F. Gribnau, and L. van de Putte. 1991. Longterm treatment with nonsteroidal antiinflammatory drugs in rheumatoid arthritis: a prospective drug survival study. *J. Rheumatol.* 18:184–187.

59. Rochon, P.A., J.H. Gurwitz, R.W. Simms, P.R. Fortin, D.T. Felson, K.L. Minaker, and T.C. Chalmers. 1994. A study of manufacturer-supported trials of nonsteroidal anti-inflammatory drugs in the treatment of arthritis. *Arch. Intern. Med.* 154:157–163.

60. Gotzsche, P.C. 1993. Meta-analysis of NSAIDs: contribution of drugs, doses, trial designs, and meta-analytic techniques. *Scand. J. Rheumatol.* 22:255–260.

61. Luggen, M.E., P.S. Gartside, and E.V. Hess. 1989. Nonsteroidal antiinflammatory drugs in rheumatoid arthritis: duration of use as a measure of relative value. *J. Rheumatol.* 16:1565–1569.

62. Pincus, T., S.B. Marcum, L.F. Callahan, R.F. Adams, J. Barber, W.F. Barth, et al. 1992. Longterm drug therapy for rheumatoid arthritis in seven rheumatology private practices: I. Nonsteroidal antiinflammatory drugs. *J. Rheumatol.* 19:1874–1884.

63. Huskisson, E.C., D.L. Woolf, H.W. Balme, J. Scott, and S. Franklin. 1976. Four new anti-inflammatory drugs: responses and variations. *Br. Medical J.* 1:1048–1049.

64. Walker, J.S., R.B. Sheather-Reid, J.J. Carmody, J.H. Vial, and R.O. Day. 1997. Nonsteroidal antiinflammatory drugs in rheumatoid arthritis and osteoarthritis: support for the concept of "responders" and "nonresponders." *Arthritis Rheum.* 40:1944–1954.

65. Brooks, P.M. and R.O. Day. 1991. Nonsteroidal antiinflammatory drugs—differences and similarities. *N. Engl. J. Med.* 324:1716–25.

66. Felson, D.T., J.J. Anderson, M. Boers, C. Bombardier, M. Chernoff, B. Fried, et al. 1993. The American College of Rheumatology preliminary core set of disease activity measures for rheumatoid arthritis clinical trials. The Committee on Outcome Measures in Rheumatoid Arthritis Clinical Trials. *Arthritis Rheum.* 36:729–740.

67. Simon, L.S., A.L. Weaver, D.Y. Graham, A.J. Kivitz, P.E. Lipsky, R.C. Hubbard, et al. 1999. Anti-inflammatory and upper gastrointestinal effects of celecoxib in rheumatoid arthritis: a randomized controlled trial. *JAMA* 282:1921–1928.

68. Day, R.O., D.E. Furst, S.H. Dromgoole, B. Kamm, R. Roe, and H.E. Paulus. 1982. Relationship of serum naproxen concentration to efficacy in rheumatoid arthritis. *Clin. Pharmacol. Ther.* 31:733–740.

69. Gall, E.P., E.M. Caperton, J.E. McComb, R. Messner, C.V. Multz, M. O'Hanlan, and R.F. Willkens. 1982. Clinical comparison of ibuprofen, fenoprofen calcium, naproxen and tolmetin sodium in rheumatoid arthritis. *J. Rheumatol.* 9:402–407.

70. Emery, P., H. Zeidler, T.K. Kvien, M. Guslandi, R. Naudin, H. Stead, et al. 1999. Celecoxib versus diclofenac in long-term management of rheumatoid arthritis: randomised double-blind comparison. *Lancet* 354:2106–2111.

71. Schnitzer, T.J., K. Truitt, R. Fleischmann, P. Dalgin, J. Block, Q. Zeng, et al. 1999. The safety profile, tolerability, and effective dose range of rofecoxib in the treatment of rheumatoid arthritis. Phase II Rofecoxib Rheumatoid Arthritis Study Group. *Clin. Ther.* 21:1688–1702.

72. Schoen, R.T., and R.J. Vender. 1989. Mechanisms of nonsteroidal anti-inflammatory drug-induced gastric damage. *Am. J. Med.* 86:449–458.

73. Gabriel, S.E., R.L. Jaakkimainen, and C. Bombardier. 1993. The cost-effectiveness of misoprostol for nonsteroidal antiinflammatory drug-associated adverse gastrointestinal events. *Arthritis Rheum.* 36:447–459.

74. Hochberg, M.C. 1992. Association of nonsteroidal antiinflammatory drugs with upper gastrointestinal disease: epidemiologic and economic considerations. *J Rheumatol.* 19 Suppl 36:63–67.

75. Gabriel, S.E., L. Jaakkimainen, and C. Bombardier. 1991. Risk for serious gastrointestinal complications related to use of nonsteroidal anti-inflammatory drugs. A meta-analysis. *Ann. Intern. Med.* 115:787–796.

76. Tamblyn, R., L. Berkson, W.D. Dauphinee, D. Gayton, R. Grad, A. Huang, et al. 1997. Unnecessary prescribing of NSAIDs and the management of NSAID-related gastropathy in medical practice. *Ann. Intern. Med.* 127:429–438.

77. Singh, G. 1998. Recent considerations in nonsteroidal anti-inflammatory drug gastropathy. *Am. J. Med.* 105:31S–38S.

78. Wolfe, M.M. and A.H. Soll. 1988. The physiology of gastric acid secretion. *N. Engl. J. Med.* 319:1707–1715.

79. Whittle, B.J. 1977. Mechanisms underlying gastric mucosal damage induced by indomethacin and bile-salts, and the actions of prostaglandins. *Br. J. Pharmacol.* 60:455–460.

80. Peura, D.A., F.L. Lanza, C.J. Gostout, and P.G. Foutch. 1997. The American College of Gastroenterology Bleeding Registry: preliminary findings. *Am. J. Gastroenterol.* 92:924–928.

81. Garcia Rodriguez, L.A. and H. Jick. 1994. Risk of upper gastrointestinal bleeding and perforation associated with individual non-steroidal anti-inflammatory drugs. *Lancet* 343:769–772.

82. Kim, J.G. and D.Y. Graham. 1994. Helicobacter pylori infection and development of gastric or duodenal ulcer in arthritic patients receiving chronic NSAID therapy. The Misoprostol Study Group. *Am. J. Gastroenterol.* 89:203–207.

83. Bianchi Porro, G., F. Parente, V. Imbesi, F. Montrone, and I. Caruso. 1996. Role of Helicobacter pylori in ulcer healing and recurrence of gastric and duodenal ulcers in longterm NSAID users. Response to omeprazole dual therapy. *Gut* 39:22–26.

84. Chan, F.K., J.J. Sung, S.C. Chung, K.F. To, M.Y. Yung, V.K. Leung, et al. 1997. Randomised trial of eradication of Helicobacter pylori before non-steroidal anti-inflammatory drug therapy to prevent peptic ulcers. *Lancet* 350:975–979.

85. Hawkey, C.J., J.A. Karrasch, L. Szczepanski, D.G. Walker, A. Barkun, A.J. Swannell, and N.D. Yeomans. 1998. Omeprazole compared with misoprostol for ulcers associated with nonsteroidal antiinflammatory drugs. Omeprazole versus Misoprostol for NSAID-induced Ulcer Management (OMNIUM) Study Group. *N. Engl. J. Med.* 338:727–734.

86. Yeomans, N.D., Z. Tulassay, L. Juhasz, I. Racz, J.M. Howard, C.J. van Rensburg, et al. 1998. A comparison of omeprazole with ranitidine for ulcers associated with nonsteroidal antiinflammatory drugs. Acid Suppression Trial: Ranitidine versus Omeprazole for NSAID-associated Ulcer Treatment (ASTRONAUT) Study Group. *N. Engl. J. Med.* 338:719–726.

87. Laine, L., S. Harper, T. Simon, R. Bath, J. Johanson, H. Schwartz, et al. 1999. A randomized trial comparing the effect of rofecoxib, a cyclooxygenase 2-specific inhibitor, with that of ibuprofen on the gastroduodenal mucosa of patients with osteoarthritis.Rofecoxib Osteoarthritis Endoscopy Study Group. *Gastroenterology* 117:776–783.

88. Langman, M.J., D.M. Jensen, D.J. Watson, S.E. Harper, P.L. Zhao, H. Quan, et al. 1999. Adverse upper gastrointestinal effects of rofecoxib compared with NSAIDs. *JAMA* 282:1929–1933.

89. Agrawal, N.M., S. Roth, D.Y. Graham, R.H. White, B. Germain, J.A. Brown, and S.C. Stromatt. 1991. Misoprostol compared with sucralfate in the prevention of nonsteroidal anti-inflammatory drug-induced gastric ulcer. A randomized, controlled trial. *Ann. Intern. Med.* 115:195–200.

90. Robinson, M.G., J.W. Griffin, Jr., J. Bowers, F.J. Kogan, D.G. Kogut, F.L. Lanza, and C.W. Warner. 1989. Effect of ranitidine on gastroduodenal mucosal damage induced by nonsteroidal antiinflammatory drugs. *Dig. Dis. Sci.* 34:424–428.

91. Ehsanullah, R.S., M.C. Page, G. Tildesley, and J.R. Wood. 1988. Prevention of gastroduodenal damage induced by non-steroidal anti-inflammatory drugs: controlled trial of ranitidine. *BMJ* 297:1017–1021.

92. Taha, A.S., N. Hudson, C.J. Hawkey, A.J. Swannell, P.N. Trye, J. Cottrell, et al. 1996. Famotidine for the prevention of gastric and duodenal ulcers caused by nonsteroidal antiinflammatory drugs. *N. Engl. J. Med.* 334:1435–1439.

93. Graham, D.Y., N.M. Agrawal, and S.H. Roth. 1988. Prevention of NSAID-induced gastric ulcer with misoprostol: multicentre, double-blind, placebo-controlled trial. *Lancet* 2:1277–1280.

94. Graham, D.Y., R.H. White, L.W. Moreland, T.T. Schubert, R. Katz, R. Jaszewski, et al. 1993. Duodenal and gastric ulcer prevention with misoprostol in arthritis patients taking NSAIDs. Misoprostol Study Group. *Ann. Intern. Med.* 119:257–262.

95. Silverstein, F.E., D.Y. Graham, J.R. Senior, H.W. Davies, B.J. Struthers, R.M. Bittman, and G.S. Geis. 1995. Misoprostol reduces serious gastrointestinal complications in patients with rheumatoid arthritis receiving nonsteroidal anti-inflammatory drugs. A randomized, double-blind, placebo-controlled trial. *Ann. Intern. Med.* 123:241–249.

96. Raskin, J.B., R.H. White, J.E. Jackson, A.L. Weaver, E.A. Tindall, R.B. Lies, and D.S. Stanton. 1995. Misoprostol dosage in the prevention of nonsteroidal anti-inflammatory drug-induced gastric and duodenal ulcers: a comparison of three regimens. *Ann. Intern. Med.* 123:344–350.

97. Singh, G., D.R. Ramey, D. Morfeld, H. Shi, H.T. Hatoum, and J.F. Fries. 1996. Gastrointestinal tract complications of nonsteroidal anti-inflammatory drug treatment in rheumatoid arthritis. A prospective observational cohort study. *Arch. Intern. Med.* 156:1530–1536.

98. Bjorkman, D. 1998. Nonsteroidal anti-inflammatory drug-associated toxicity of the liver, lower gastrointestinal tract, and esophagus. *Am. J. Med.* 105:17S–21S.

99. Kessler, W.F., G.T. Shires, 3rd, and T.J. Fahey, 3rd. 1997. Surgical complications of nonsteroidal antiinflammatory drug-induced small bowel ulceration. *J. Am. Coll. Surg.* 185:250–254.

100. Whelton, A. 1999. Nephrotoxicity of nonsteroidal anti-inflammatory drugs: physiologic foundations and clinical implications. *Am. J. Med.* 106:13S–24S.

101. Henry, D., J. Page, I. Whyte, R. Nanra, and C. Hall. 1997. Consumption of non-steroidal anti-inflammatory drugs and the development of functional renal impairment in elderly subjects. Results of a case-control study. *Br. J. Clin. Pharmacol.* 44:85–90.

102. Whelton, A. and C.W. Hamilton. 1991. Nonsteroidal anti-inflammatory drugs: effects on kidney function. *J. Clin. Pharmacol.* 31:588–598.

103. Gurwitz, J.H., J. Avorn, R.L. Bohn, R.J. Glynn, M. Monane, and H. Mogun. 1994. Initiation of antihypertensive treatment during nonsteroidal anti-inflammatory drug therapy. *JAMA* 272:781–786.

104. Pope, J.E., J.J. Anderson, and D.T. Felson. 1993. A meta-analysis of the effects of nonsteroidal anti-inflammatory drugs on blood pressure. *Arch. Intern. Med.* 153:477–484.

105. Johnson, A.G., T.V. Nguyen, and R.O. Day. 1994. Do nonsteroidal anti-inflammatory drugs affect blood pressure? A meta-analysis. *Ann. Intern. Med.* 121:289–300.

106. Collins, R., R. Peto, S. MacMahon, P. Hebert, N.H. Fiebach, K.A. Eberlein, et al. 1990. Blood pressure, stroke, and coronary heart disease. Part 2, Short-term reductions in blood pressure: overview of randomised drug trials in their epidemiological context. *Lancet* 335:827–838.

107. Heerdink, E.R., H.G. Leufkens, R.M. Herings, J.P. Ottervanger, B.H. Stricker, and A. Bakker. 1998. NSAIDs associated with increased risk of congestive heart failure in elderly patients taking diuretics. *Arch. Intern. Med.* 158:1108–1112.

108. Feenstra, J., D.E. Grobbee, W.J. Remme, and B.H. Stricker. 1999. Drug-induced heart failure. *J. Am. Coll. Cardiol.* 33:1152–1162.

109. Sturrock, N.D. and A.D. Struthers. 1993. Non-steroidal anti-inflammatory drugs and angiotensin converting enzyme inhibitors: a commonly prescribed combination with variable effects on renal function. *Br. J. Clin. Pharmacol.* 35:343–348.

110. Laiwah, A.C. and R.A. Mactier. 1981. Antagonistic effect of non-steroidal anti-inflammatory drugs on frusemide-induced diuresis in cardiac failure. *Br. Medical J. (Clin. Res. Ed.).* 283:714.

111. Tolman, K.G. 1998. Hepatotoxicity of non-narcotic analgesics. *Am. J. Med.* 105:13S–19S.

112. Scully, L.J., D. Clarke, and R.J. Barr. 1993. Diclofenac induced hepatitis. 3 cases with features of autoimmune chronic active hepatitis. *Dig. Dis. Sci.* 38:744–751.

113. Zimmerman, H.J. 1981. Effects of aspirin and acetaminophen on the liver. *Arch. Intern. Med.* 141:333–342.

114. Miwa, L.J., J.K. Jones, A. Pathiyal, and H. Hatoum. 1997. Value of epidemiologic studies in determining the true incidence of adverse events. The nonsteroidal anti-inflammatory drug story. *Arch. Intern. Med.* 157:2129–2136.

115. Carson, J.L., B.L. Strom, A. Duff, A. Gupta, and K. Das. 1993. Safety of nonsteroidal anti-inflammatory drugs with respect to acute liver disease. *Arch. Intern. Med.* 153:1331–1336.

116. Rabkin, J.M., M.J. Smith, S.L. Orloff, C.L. Corless, P. Stenzel, and A.J. Olyaei. 1999. Fatal fulminant hepatitis associated with bromfenac use. *Ann. Pharmacother.* 33:945–947.

117. Lewis, J.H. 1984. Hepatic toxicity of nonsteroidal anti-inflammatory drugs. *Clin. Pharm.* 3:128–138.

118. Paulus, H.E. 1982. FDA Arthritis Advisory Committee meeting. *Arthritis Rheum.* 25:1124–1125.

119. Weinblatt, M.E., J.R. Tesser, and J.H.D. Gilliam. 1982. The liver in rheumatic diseases. *Semin. Arthritis Rheum.* 11:399–405.

120. Aithal, P.G. and C.P. Day. 1999. The natural history of histologically proved drug induced liver disease. *Gut* 44:731–735.

121. American College of Rheumatology Ad Hoc Committee on Clinical Guidelines. 1996. Guidelines for monitoring drug therapy in rheumatoid arthritis. 1996. *Arthritis Rheum.* 39:723–731.

122. Samter, M. and R.F. Beers, Jr. 1968. Intolerance to aspirin. Clinical studies and consideration of its pathogenesis. *Ann. Intern. Med.* 68:975–983.

123. Szczeklik, A. and M. Sanak. 2000. Genetic mechanisms in aspirin-induced asthma. *Am. J. Respir. Crit. Care Med.* 161:S142–S146.

124. Stevenson, D.D. and R.A. Simon. 1998. Sensitivity to aspirin and nonsteroidal antiinflammatory drugs. In Allergy: Principles and Practice. vol. 2. J. E. Middleton, C.E. Reed, E.F. Ellis, N.F. Adkinson, J.W. Yunginger, and W.W. Busse, editors. Mosby, Philadelphia. 1225–1234.

125. Szczeklik, A. and D.D. Stevenson. 1999. Aspirin-induced asthma: advances in pathogenesis and management. *J. Allergy Clin. Immunol.* 104:5–13.

126. Bianco, S., M. Robuschi, G. Petrigni, M. Scuri, M.G. Pieroni, R.M. Refini, et al. 1993. Efficacy and tolerability of nimesulide in asthmatic patients intolerant to aspirin. *Drugs* 46:115–120.

127. Kosnik, M., E. Music, F. Matjaz, and S. Suskovic. 1998. Relative safety of meloxicam in NSAID-intolerant patients. *Allergy* 53:1231–1233.

128. Andri, L., G. Senna, C. Betteli, S. Givanni, I. Scaricabarozzi, P. Mezzelani, and G. Andri. 1994. Tolerability of nimesulide in aspirin-sensitive patients. *Ann. Allergy* 72:29–32.

129. Schafer, A.I. 1999. Effects of nonsteroidal anti-inflammatory therapy on platelets. *Am. J. Med.* 106:25S–36S.

130. Goodwin, S.D. and R.W. Glenny. 1992. Nonsteroidal anti-inflammatory drug-associated pulmonary infiltrates with eosinophilia. Review of the literature and Food and Drug Administration Adverse Drug Reaction reports. Arch. Intern. Med. 152:1521–1524.

131. Moris, G. and J.C. Garcia-Monco. 1999. The challenge of drug-induced aseptic meningitis. *Arch. Intern Med.* 159:1185–1194.

132. Goodwin, J.S. and M. Regan. 1982. Cognitive dysfunction associated with naproxen and ibuprofen in the elderly. *Arthritis Rheum.* 25:1013–1015.

133. Checketts, S.R., K.A. Morrison, and R.D. Baughman. 1999. Nonsteroidal anti-inflammatory-induced pseudoporphyria: is there an alternative drug? *Cutis* 63:223–225.

134. Checketts, S.R. and G.J. Morgan, Jr. 1999. Two cases of nabumetone induced pseudoporphyria. *J. Rheumatol.* 26:2703–2705.

135. Yip, L., R.C. Dart, and P.A. Gabow. 1994. Concepts and controversies in salicylate toxicity. *Emerg. Med. Clin. North Am.* 12:351–364.

136. Van Marter, L.J., A. Leviton, E.N. Allred, M. Pagano, K.F. Sullivan, A. Cohen, and M.F. Epstein. 1996. Persistent pulmonary hypertension of the newborn and smoking and aspirin and nonsteroidal antiinflammatory drug consumption during pregnancy. *Pediatrics* 97:658–663.

137. CLASP Collaborative Group. 1995. Low dose aspirin in pregnancy and early childhood development: follow up of the collaborative low dose aspirin study in pregnancy. *Br. J. Obstet. Gynaecol.* 102:861–868.

138. Theis, J.G. 1996. Acetylsalicylic acid (ASA) and nonsteroidal anti-inflammatory drugs (NSAIDs) during pregnancy. Are they safe? *Can. Fam. Physician.* 42:2347–2349.

139. Wolfe, F., S. Zhao, and N. Lane. 2000. Preference for nonsteroidal antiinflammatory drugs over acetaminophen by rheumatic disease patients: a survey of 1,799 patients with osteoarthritis, rheumatoid arthritis, and fibromyalgia. *Arthritis Rheum.* 43:378–385.

140. Bagge, E., M. Traub, M. Crotty, P.G. Conaghan, E. Oh, and P.M. Brooks. 1997. Are rheumatoid arthritis patients more willing to accept non-steroidal anti-inflammatory drug treatment risks than osteoarthritis patients? *Br. J. Rheumatol.* 36:470–472.

141. American College of Rheumatology Ad Hoc Committee on Clinical Guidelines. 1996. Guidelines for the management of rheumatoid arthritis. *Arthritis Rheum.* 39:713–722.

142. Furst, D.E., K. Blocka, S. Cassell, E.R. Harris, J.M. Hirschberg, N. Josephson, et al. 1987. A controlled study of concurrent therapy with a nonacetylated salicylate and naproxen in rheumatoid arthritis. *Arthritis Rheum.* 30:146–154.

143. Roth, S.H., E.A. Tindall, A.K. Jain, F.G. McMahon, P.A. April, B.I. Bockow, et al. 1993. A controlled study comparing the effects of nabumetone, ibuprofen, and ibuprofen plus misoprostol on the upper gastrointestinal tract mucosa. *Arch. Intern. Med.* 153:2565–2571.

144. Schattenkirchner, M. 1990. An updated safety profile of etodolac in several thousand patients. *Eur. J. Rheumatol. Inflamm.* 10:56–65.

145. Wolfe, M.M., D.R. Lichtenstein, and G. Singh. 1999. Gastrointestinal toxicity of nonsteroidal antiinflammatory drugs. *N. Engl. J. Med.* 340:1888–1899.

146. Verbeeck, R.K. 1990. Pharmacokinetic drug interactions with nonsteroidal anti-inflammatory drugs. *Clin. Pharmacokinet.* 19:44–66.

147. Stein, G., M. Robertson, and J. Nadarajah. 1988. Toxic interactions between lithium and non-steroidal anti-inflammatory drugs. *Psychol. Med.* 18:535–543.

148. Chan, T.Y. 1995. Adverse interactions between warfarin and nonsteroidal antiinflammatory drugs: mechanisms, clinical significance, and avoidance. *Ann. Pharmacother.* 29:1274–1283.

4

Additional Considerations on the Use of Nonsteroidal Anti-Inflammatory Drugs

M. Elaine Husni and Lee S. Simon

CONTENTS

INTRODUCTION

Physicians have the capacity to attenuate most types of pain, but the effectiveness of the presently available medications is typically limited by their toxic effects. One such class of analgesic medications is the nonsteroidal anti-inflammatory drugs (NSAIDs), which have been shown to be anti-inflammatory, analgesic, and antipyretic. NSAIDs represent one of the most commonly used classes of drugs in the world, with more than 17,000,000 Americans using various NSAIDs on a daily basis.

The following chapter describes how NSAIDs exert their effect on pain and inflammation, details the associated toxicities including serious gastrointestinal (GI) events, and reviews the newest available drugs, the cyclooxygenase-2 (COX-2) inhibitors. These new medications have been proven to be as efficacious as traditional NSAIDs while inducing substantially less risk of GI toxicity.

From: *Modern Therapeutics in Rheumatic Diseases*
Edited by: G. C. Tsokos, et al. © Humana Press, Inc., Totowa, NJ

With the aging of the US population, the Centers for Disease Control predicts a significant increase in the prevalence of painful degenerative and inflammatory rheumatic conditions, leading to a probable parallel increase in the use of NSAIDs *(1–2)*. They are widely used to reduce pain, decrease gel phenomenon and improve function in patients with osteoarthritis (OA), rheumatoid arthritis (RA), and treatment of pain including headache, dysmenorrhea, and postoperative pain.

Approximately 60 million NSAID prescriptions are written each year in the United States, with the number for elderly patients exceeding those for younger patients by approx 3.6-fold *(2–3)*. Some of these NSAIDs are also available over the counter such as aspirin (ASA), ibuprofen, naproxen, and ketoprofen. At equipotent doses, the clinical efficacy and tolerability of the various NSAIDs are similar; however, individual responses are highly variable *(4–6)*. Anecdotally, although it is believed that if a patient fails to respond to one NSAID of one class that it is reasonable to try another NSAID from a different class, however, no one has studied this in a prospective controlled manner.

The origin of NSAIDs dates back to 1763, at which time sodium salicylic acid was discovered. Various impure forms of salicylates had been used as analgesics and antipyretics throughout the previous century. Once purified and synthesized the acetyl derivative of salicylate, acetylsalicylic acid (ASA), was found to provide more anti-inflammatory activity than salicylate alone. However, GI toxicity (particularly dyspepsia) associated with the use of ASA led to the introduction of phenylbutazone, an indoleacetic acid derivative, in the early 1950s. This was the first nonsalicylate NSAID developed for use in patients with painful and inflammatory conditions. Phenylbutazone is a weak prostaglandin synthase inhibitor that also induces uricosuria, and was rapidly shown to be useful in patients diagnosed with ankylosing spondylitis and gout. However, adverse events such as bone marrow toxicity, particularly in women over the age of 60, have essentially eliminated the use of this drug.

Indomethacin, another indoleacetic acid derivative, was subsequently developed in the 1960s as a substitute for phenylbutazone. Although this medication was safer, it had significant toxicity as well and the search for safer and at least equally effective NSAIDs ensued. Other clinical issues have driven the development of newer agents, such as once a day (QD) or twice a day (BID) dosing to help improve compliance. Today, there are at least 20 different NSAIDs currently available in the United States. In addition, COX-2 specific inhibitors have been introduced (e.g., celecoxib and rofecoxib) with similar efficacy to traditional NSAIDs but significantly decreased effects on the GI tract and on platelet effects *(7–11)*.

PHARMACOLOGY

Bioavailability

In experimental situations, all NSAIDs are completely absorbed after oral administration. However absorption rates may vary in patients with altered GI blood flow or motility and, with certain NSAIDs when taken with food. For example, taking naproxen with food may decrease absorption by 16% although this is likely not clinically important. Enteric coating may reduce direct effects of NSAIDs on the gastric mucosa but may also reduce the rate of absorption of active drug.

Table 1
Diseases That Can Affect
Glomerular Filtration Rate

Congestive heart failure
Established renal disease
Diabetes
Hypertension
Dehydration
Significant hypoalbuminemia

Most NSAIDs are weak organic acids; once absorbed they are >95% bound to serum albumin. This is a saturable process. Clinically significant decreases in serum albumin levels or institution of other highly protein-bound medications may lead to an increase in the free component of NSAID in serum. This may be important in patients who are elderly or are chronically ill especially with associated hypoalbuminemic states. Importantly, owing to increased vascular permeability in localized sites of inflammation, this high degree of protein binding may result in delivery of higher levels of NSAIDs.

In general, the pharmacology of NSAIDs is characterized by a negligible first-pass hepatic metabolism, high protein binding with small volumes of distribution, and poor dialysis potential. NSAIDs may also be detrimental to renal function. Anti-inflammatory agents are inhibitors of prostaglandin synthesis and in a variety of diseases (i.e., congestive heart failure, liver disease, chronic renal failure, systemic lupus erythematosis (SLE) with renal involvement, or clinically important dehydration) prostaglandins appear to be important in maintaining renal blood flow (Table 1) *(12)*. Therefore, treating such patients with NSAIDs can have an incremental worsening of their renal function. The kinetics of NSAIDs can also differ in various clinical conditions. In the elderly population or those with hepatic cirrhosis, naproxen clearance, for example, is reduced by 50%. On the other hand, renal disease does not have an important effect, because urinary excretion of unchanged drug is negligible for most NSAIDs, except for indomethacin, aclofenac, azapropazone, and tiaprofenic acid (10–60% of which is excreted in the urine) *(12)*.

Mechanism of Action

There is a clear individual variation in response to NSAID therapy; some patients seem to respond better to one drug than to others *(6,13–15)*. Adverse events also seem to be variable among individual drugs and patients. Some of the variability in clinical effects may be explained as certain NSAIDs appear to be more potent inhibitors of prostaglandin synthesis, whereas others may more prominently affect nonprostaglandin mediated biologic events. Differential effects have also been attributed to variations in the enantiomeric state of the agent, as well as its pharmacokinetics, pharmacodynamics, and metabolism *(6,14,16)*. The theoretical and real differences between NSAIDs have been reviewed by Brooks and Day and Furst *(6,17)*. Although variability can be explained in part by absorption, distribution, and metabolism, potential differences in mechanism of action must be considered as an important explanation for their variable effects.

The primary effect of NSAIDs is to inhibit COX enzyme (prostaglandin synthetase), thereby blocking the transformation of arachidonic acid to prostaglandins, prostacyclin, and thromboxanes. These drugs are primarily anti-inflammatory and analgesic by decreasing production of these prostaglandins, specifically of the E series. Prostanoic acids are proinflammatory, increasing both vascular permeability, as well as sensitivity to the release of bradykinins. By inhibiting prostaglandin synthesis, NSAIDs have also been shown to inhibit the formation of prostacyclin and thromboxane; thus, resulting in complex effects on vascular permeability and platelet aggregation undoubtedly contributing to the overall clinical effects of these compounds.

Polyunsaturated fatty acids include arachidonic acid, constituents of all cell membranes, exist in ester linkage in the glycerols of phospholipids and are subsequently converted first through the action of phospholipase A_2 or phospholipase C ultimately to prostaglandins or leukotrienes. Free arachidonic acid, released by the phospholipase acts as a substrate for the PGH synthase complex or COX, which includes both an oxygenase and peroxidase step. These enzymes catalyze the conversion of arachidonic acid to the unstable cyclic-endoperoxide intermediates, PGG_2 and PGH_2. These arachidonic acid metabolites are then converted to the more stable PGE_2 and PGF_2 compounds by specific tissue prostaglandin synthases. NSAIDs inhibit COX activity by blocking the capacity of arachidonate from binding into the active site and thereby reducing the conversion of arachidonic acid to PGG_2.

THE COX ENZYME

At least two isoforms of the COX enzymes have been identified: COX-1 and COX-2. Although they share 60% homology in the amino acid sequences considered important for catalysis of arachidonic acid, they are products of two different genes. They differ most importantly in their regulation and expression of the enzymes in various tissues (18–19).

COX-1 or prostaglandin synthase H_1 (PGHS-1) is a "housekeeping enzyme" that regulates normal cellular processes and is stimulated by hormones or growth factors. It is constitutively expressed in most tissues, and is inhibited by all NSAIDs to varying degrees depending on the applied experimental model system used to measure their drug effects (20). COX-1 is important in maintaining the integrity of the gastric and duodenal mucosa and many of the toxic effects of the NSAIDs on the GI tract are attributed to its inhibition. It is also important in the activity leading to platelet aggregation.

The other isoform, COX-2 or prostaglandin synthase H_2 (PGHS-2) is an inducible enzyme and is usually undetectable, or is at very low levels in most tissues. Its expression is increased during states of inflammation or experimentally in response to mitogenic stimuli. For example, in the monocyte/macrophage systems, endotoxin stimulates COX-2 expression; in fibroblasts various growth factors, phorbol esters, and interleukin-1 (IL-1) also upregulate the enzyme. This isoform is also constitutively expressed in the brain, specifically cortex and hippocampus; in the female reproductive tract, such as the ovum and associated with implantation of the fertilized ovum, in the male vas deferens, in bone, and at least in some models in human kidney specifically, in the macula densa and associated with the thick ascending limb of henle. The expression of COX-2 is inhibited by glucocorticoids. COX-2 is also inhibited by all of the presently available

NSAIDs to a greater or lesser degree. Thus, differences in the effectiveness with which a particular NSAID inhibits an isoform of cyclooxygenase may affect both its activity and its potential toxicity. It has been proposed that the ideal NSAID would inhibit the inducible COX-2 isoform (thereby decreasing inflammation) without having any effect on the constitutive COX-1 isoform (thereby minimizing toxicity) at any efficacious therapeutic dose.

The in vitro systems used to define the actions on the COX enzymes of the available NSAIDs are based on using either cell-free systems, pure enzyme, or whole cells (20). Each drug studied to date has demonstrated different measurable effects within each system. As an example: it appears that nonacetylated salicylates inhibit the activity of COX-1 and COX-2 in whole cell systems but are not active against either COX-1 or COX-2 in recombinant enzyme or cell-membrane systems. This evidence suggests that salicylates act early in the arachidonic acid cascade, perhaps by inhibiting enzyme expression rather than direct inhibition of COX.

Recently evidence has accumulated that several NSAIDs are selective for COX-2 enzyme effects over COX-1. For example, in vitro effects of etodolac demonstrate an approx a 10-fold inhibition of COX-2 compared to COX-1, at low doses. However, at higher anti-inflammatory doses this specificity appears to be mitigated, as both enzymes are affected. However, two highly selective or specific COX-2 inhibitors, celecoxib (Celebrex) and rofecoxib (Vioxx) have been approved from the US Food and Drug Administration (FDA). Both of these specific COX-2 inhibitors are at least 300 times more effective at inhibiting COX-2 activity than COX-1, and have no measurable effect on COX-1 mediated events at any therapeutic doses. Both COX-2 specific inhibitors (or CSI's) have been shown as effective at inhibiting osteoarthritis pain, dental pain, and the pain and inflammation associated with RA as naproxen at 500 mg BID, ibuprofen 800 mg TID (3×/d), diclofenac 50 mg TID or 75 mg BID, without endoscopic evidence of gastroduodenal damage and without affecting platelet aggregation (8–10,21–24). Unfortunately, owing to the design of the randomized controlled clinical trials used for many investigations, the important questions regarding the renal effects of the specific COX-2 inhibitors remain unanswered.

Arachidonic acid can also serve as a substrate for 5- or 12-lipoxygenase. The 5-lipoxygenase enzyme catalyzes the conversion of arachidonic acid to biologically active leukotriene and hydroxyeicosatetraenoic acids (HETEs) products. None of the presently available NSAIDs used to treat arthritis inhibit 5-lipoxygenase directly, although several compounds presently under development may have inhibitory effects on both cyclooxygenase and lipoxygenase. It remains to be seen whether these will be clinically useful.

Biologic and Other Effects of the NSAIDs

NSAIDs are lipophilic and become incorporated in the lipid bilayer of cell membranes and thereby may interrupt protein-protein interactions important for signal transduction. For example, stimulus response coupling, which is critical for recruitment of phagocytic cells to sites of inflammation has been demonstrated in vitro to be inhibited by some NSAIDs (24–27). There are data suggesting that NSAIDs inhibit activation and chemotaxis of neutrophils as well as reducing toxic oxygen radical production in stimulated neutrophils. There is also evidence that several NSAIDs scavenge superoxide radicals (24).

Salicylates have been demonstrated to inhibit phospholipase C activity in macrophages. Some NSAIDs have been shown to affect T-lymphocyte function experimentally by inhibiting rheumatoid factor production in vitro (25). Another newly described action not directly related to prostaglandin synthesis inhibition, is a decrease in the expression of L-selectin thus affecting a critical step in the migration of granulocytes to sites of inflammation (26). NSAIDs have been demonstrated in vitro to inhibit NF-κB (nitric oxide [NO] transcription factor)-dependent transcription thereby inhibiting inducible nitric-oxide synthetase [NOS] which has been associated with increasing inflammation (27). Anti-inflammatory levels of ASA have been shown to inhibit expression of inducible NOS and subsequent production of nitrite in vitro. At pharmacologic doses, sodium salicylate, indomethacin, and acetaminophen have been studied and had no effect; however, at suprapharmacologic dosages, sodium salicylate inhibited nitrite production.

Recently it has been described that prostaglandins inhibit apoptosis (programmed cell death) and that NSAIDs, via inhibition of prostaglandin synthesis may reestablish more normal cell cycle responses (20). There is also evidence suggesting that some NSAIDs may reduce PGH synthase gene expression thereby supporting the clinical evidence of differences in activity in NSAIDs in sites of active inflammation.

The importance of these prostaglandin and nonprostaglandin mediated processes in reducing clinical inflammation is not entirely clear. Although nonacetylated salicylates have been shown in vitro to inhibit neutrophil function and to have equal efficacy in patients with rheumatoid arthritis (RA), clinically there is no substantial evidence to suggest that biologic effects other than prostaglandin-synthase inhibition are more important for anti-inflammatory and/or analgesic effects (28).

Metabolism

Nonsteroidal anti-inflammatory agents are metabolized predominantly in the liver by the cytochrome P450 system, the 2C9 isoform, and subsequently excreted in the urine. This must be taken into consideration when prescribing NSAIDs for patients with hepatic and/or renal dysfunction. Some NSAIDs such as oxyprozin have two metabolic pathways, whereby some portion is directly secreted into the bile and another part is further metabolized and excreted in the urine. Others have a prominent enterohepatic circulation, resulting in a prolonged half-life and should be used with caution in the elderly (i.e., Indomethacin, sulindac, and piroxicam). In patients with renal insufficiency, some inactive metabolites may be resynthesized in vivo to the active compound. Diclofenac, flurbiprofen, celecoxib, and rofecoxib are metabolized in the liver, and should be used with care and at lowest possible doses in patients with clinically significant liver disease. This would mean patients with significant liver dysfunction such as patients with cirrhosis with or without ascites, prolonged prothrombin times, falling serum albumin levels, or important elevations in liver transaminases in blood.

Salicylates are the least highly protein bound NSAID: approx 68%. Zero order kinetics is dominant in salicylate metabolism. Thus, increasing the dose of salicylates is effective over a narrow range but once the metabolic systems are saturated, then incremental dose increases may lead to very high serum salicylate levels. Thus, changes in salicylate doses need to be carefully considered at chronic steady state levels particularly in patients with altered renal or hepatic function.

Table 2
The Nonsteroidal Anti-Inflammatory Drugs and Cox-2 Inhibitors

NSAID	Trade name	Daily recommended adult doses (mgs/24 h)	Plasma half-life (h)
Carboxylic acids			
Aspirin (acetylsalicylic acid)	Multiple	1300–5000	4–15
Buffered aspirin	Multiple	Same	Same
Enteric-coated salicylates	Multiple	Same	Same
Salsalate	Disalcid	1500–3000	Same
Choline magnesium trisalicylate	Trilisate	Same	Same
Diflunisal	Dolobid	500–1500	7–15
Proprionic acids			
Ibuprofen	Motrin, Rufen	1600–3200	2
Naproxen	Naprolan, Anaprox	500–1000	13
Fenoprofen	Nalfon	1200–3200	3
Ketoprofen	Orudis	150–300	2
Flurbiprofen	Ansaid	200–300	3–9
Oxaprozin	Daypro	600–1800	40–50
Acetic acid derivatives			
Indomethacin	Indocin, Indocin SR	75–200	3–11
Tolmetin	Tolectin	800–1600	1
Sulindac	Clinoril	300–400	16
Diclofenac	Voltaren, Arthrotec	100–200	1–2
Etodolac	Lodine	600–1200	2–4
Ketorolac	Toradol	20–40	2
Fenamates			
Meclofenamate	Meclomen	200–400	2–3
Mefenamic acid	Ponstel	500–1000	2
Enolic acids			
Piroxicam	Feldene	10–20	30–86
Phenylbutazone	Butazolidin	200–600	40–80
Meloxicam	Mobic	7.5	20
Naphthylkanones			
Nabumetone	Relafen	500–1000	19–30
COX-2 inhibitors			
Celecoxib	Celebrex	100–400	11
Rofecoxib	Vioxx	12.5–50	17

Plasma Half-Life

Significant differences in plasma half-lives of the NSAIDs may be important in explaining their diverse clinical effects (Table 2). Those with long half-lives typically do not attain maximum plasma concentrations quickly and clinical responses, such as acute analgesia, may be delayed. Plasma concentrations can vary widely owing to differences in renal clearance and metabolism. Piroxicam has the longest serum half-life of currently marketed NSAIDs: 57 ± 22 h. In comparison, diclofenac has one of the shortest: 1.1 ± 0.2 h. Although drugs have been developed with very long half-lives to improve patient compliance, the fact that piroxicam has such a long half-life is less attractive for the elderly patient at risk for specific NSAID-induced toxic effects. In the older patient, it is sometimes preferable to use drugs with a shorter half-life so that when the drug is discontinued the unwanted effects may be more rapidly eliminated.

Sulindac and nabumetone are "prodrugs," in which the active compound is produced after first pass metabolism through the liver. Theoretically, prodrugs were developed to decrease the exposure of the gastrointestinal mucosa to the local effects of the NSAIDs. Unfortunately, as was noted, with adequate systemic inhibition of COX-1 the patient is placed at substantial risk of an NSAID-induced upper GI event as long as COX-1 activity remains inhibited. This is true for drugs such as ketorolac given as an injection or by these prodrugs when given at adequate therapeutic doses (29). Once steady state has been achieved, synovial-fluid concentrations of NSAIDs, do not vary much. Although theoretically important for clinical effect, this has not been shown in vivo (30). Thus, choices to prescribe specific NSAIDs are largely based on issues of safety and convenience/compliance.

Miscellaneous

Other pharmacologic properties may be important clinically. NSAIDs, which are highly lipid soluble in serum will penetrate the central nervous system (CNS) more effectively and occasionally may produce striking changes in mentation, perception, and mood. Indomethacin has been associated with many of these side effects, even after a single dose, particularly in the elderly.

ADVERSE EFFECTS

Hepatotoxicity

Elevation in hepatic transaminase levels is not uncommon, although it occurs more often in patients with juvenile RA or systemic lupus erythematosus (SLE). Unless elevations exceed 2–3× upper limit of normal (ULN) or serum albumin and/or prothrombin times are altered, these effects are usually not considered clinically significant (31).

Nonetheless, overt liver failure has been reported following use of many NSAIDs: including diclofenac, flurbiprofen, and sulindac (31). Garcia-Rodriguez et al. preformed a retrospective study of 625,000 patients who received more than 2 million prescriptions for NSAIDs and evaluated for newly diagnosed acute liver injury. The incidence of acute liver injury was 3.7/100,000 NSAID users and none of these had a fatal outcome (33).

Of all NSAIDs, sulindac has been associated with the highest incidence of cholestasis in certain countries, whereas there is evidence that diclofenac not uncommonly varies transaminases serum levels (31). Therefore it is recommended that patients at risk for liver toxicity be followed very carefully. When initiating NSAID treatment, all patients should be evaluated again within 8–12 wk and serious consideration given to performing a blood analysis evaluating for serum transaminase changes. In addition, a drop in serum albumin (suggestive of a synthetic defect induced by the drug) or a prolonged prothrombin time should warrant the cessation of NSAID therapy.

PULMONARY EFFECTS

Many adverse reactions attributed to NSAIDs are owing to inhibition of prostaglandin synthesis in local tissues. The broadest example are patients with allergic rhinitis, nasal polyposis, and/or a history of asthma, in whom all NSAIDs effectively inhibit prostaglandin synthetase and increase their risk for anaphylaxis. In high doses, even nonacetylated salicylates may sufficiently decrease prostaglandin synthesis to induce an anaphylactic reaction (33). Although the exact mechanism for this effect remains unclear, it is known that E prostaglandins serve as bronchodilators. When COX activity is inhibited in patients at risk, a decrease in synthesis of prostaglandins that contributes to bronchodilation results (33).

Another explanation implicates the alternate pathway of arachidonate metabolism, whereby shunting of arachidonate into the leukotriene pathway occurs when COX is inhibited (34). This explanation implies that large stores of arachidonate released in certain inflammatory situations lead to excess substrate for leukotriene metabolism when cyclooxygenase is inhibited. This results in release of products that are highly reactive and may stimulate anaphylaxis (34).

HEMATOLOGIC EFFECTS

Platelet Effects/Neutropenia

Platelet aggregation and thus the ability to clot is primarily induced through stimulating thromboxane production with activation of platelet COX-1. There is no COX-2 enzyme activity in the platelet. NSAIDs and aspirin inhibit the activity of COX-1, but the COX-2 specific inhibitors have no effect on COX-1 at clinically effective therapeutic doses (10). We also have little information about the use of the COX-2 specific inhibitors and the risk of thrombosis because there is no effect of these drugs on platelet function. However, Leese et al has recently published a double-blind randomized placebo-controlled study to compare the effects on platelet function of supratherpeutic doses of celecoxib (600 mg BID, which is 2–3× the treating doses) with a standard dose of naproxen (500 mg BID). The study results indicate that even at supratherapeutic doses, celecoxib will not interfere with normal mechanisms of platelet aggregation and hemostasis, thus supporting the premise that celecoxib is COX-1 sparing relative to traditional NSAIDs (10). Only aspirin has been studied prospectively to determine inhibition of potential for thrombosis and low-dose aspirin should be given concomitantly with either NSAIDs or specific COX-2 inhibitors in patients at risk. Given the additive ulcerogenic potential associated with the use of multiple NSAIDs, it is advisable to use specific COX-2 inhibitors with aspirin when considering combination cardioprotective/anti-inflammatory therapies.

The effect of the nonsalicylate NSAIDs on platelet function is reversible and related to the half-life of the drug; whereas the effect of aspirin (ASA), which is acetylsalicylic acid and acetylates the COX-1 enzyme serving to permanently inactivate it. The individual platelet cannot synthesize new COX enzyme so for the life span of the platelet exposed to ASA the platelet does not function appropriately. Therefore, the effect of ASA on the platelet does not wear off as the drug is metabolized as with the nonsalicylate NSAIDs. Thus, patients awaiting surgery should be able to stop their NSAIDs at a time determined by 4–5 times their serum half-life, whereas ASA needs to be discontinued

1–2 wk before the planned procedure to allow the platelet population to reestablish itself with platelets unexposed to ASA.

GI TOLERABILITY

The most clinically significant adverse effects following use of NSAIDs occurs in the GI mucosa and appears to be owing to local effects of the drug, or more importantly, owing to systemic inhibition of prostaglandin synthesis. NSAIDs cause a wide range of GI problems including esophagitis, esophageal stricture, gastritis, mucosal erosions, hemorrhage, peptic ulceration and/or perforation, obstruction, and death *(35)*.

NSAIDs can interfere with multiple components of GI tract homeostasis. It can disrupt the local milieu by the process of ion trapping. NSAIDs are weak organic anions that, at the pH of the stomach lumen, remain unchanged and can penetrate the thick gastric mucous barrier and then the mucosal-cell layers accumulate at high levels within cells causing direct cellular toxicity. Effects secondary to prostaglandin depletion include increased acid production, decreased mucin and bicarbonate production, and decreased epithelial-cell proliferation, and decreased mucosal blood flow. Endothelial effects include microvascular injury by causing stasis within the small blood vessels within GI mucosa leading to ischemia and ulceration.

In addition, to the known effects on gastric and duodenal mucosa, there is increasing evidence that the mucosa of the large bowel as well as the small bowel can be affected. These agents may also induce stricture formation *(36)*. These strictures may manifest as diaphragms that precipitate small or large bowel obstruction, and may be very difficult to detect on contrast radiographic studies. Additionally, there is evidence to suggest that NSAIDs induce dysfunction in GI mucosal permeability. The magnitude of risk for GI adverse events is controversial. The FDA reports an overall risk of 2–4% for NSAID-induced gastroduodenal ulcer and its complications, whereas the point prevalence of gastroduodenal ulcer determined by endoscopy is 15–31% *(35,37,38)*.

In general, the relative risk as summarized in multiple clinical trials, ranges from 4.0–5.0 for development of gastric ulcer, from 1.1 and 1.6 for development of duodenal ulcer, and a relative risk of 4.5–5.0 for development of clinically significant gastric ulcer with hemorrhage, perforation, obstruction, or death. Although there have been many epidemiological studies attempting to prove causal associations, most have had inherent design flaws that complicate estimation of true risk. There are data which suggest that the risk of hospitalization for adverse GI effects may be 7–10-fold greater in patients with RA treated with NSAIDs compared with those who are not receiving these agents.

Epidemiologic studies suggest that the safest NSAIDs are nonacetylated salicylates (salsalate, magnesium choline trisalicylate, and diflunisal). Other drugs such as nabumetone, lower doses of ibuprofen, and etodolac are usually listed together with similar effects. Those NSAIDs with prominent enterohepatic circulation and significantly prolonged half-lives such as sulindac and piroxicam have been linked to increased GI toxicity owing to increased reexposure of gastric and duodenal mucosa to bile reflux and thus the active moiety of the drug.

As noted, other sites in the GI tract including the esophagus and small and large bowel may also be affected. Exposure to NSAIDs is probably a major factor in the development of esophagitis and subsequent stricture formation. Effects on small and

Table 3
Risk Factors for NSAID-Induced
Gastoduodenal Toxic Effects

Age over 65
Past history of peptic ulcer disease (including GI bleeding)
Concomitant use of NSAIDs with glucocorticoid therapy
Use of combination or maximum dose of the NSAIDs
History of GI toxicity due to to other NSAIDs

large bowel have increasingly been reported. An autopsy study of 713 patients showed that small bowel ulceration defined as ulcers >3 mm in diameter were observed in 8.4% of patients exposed to NSAIDs compared to 0.6% of nonusers of *(39)*. Ulcerations of stomach and duodenum were observed in 22% of NSAID users compared with 12% of nonusers.

Endoscopic studies have clearly demonstrated that NSAID administration results in shallow erosions or submucosal hemorrhage which, although occurring at any site in the GI tract are more commonly observed in the stomach near the prepyloric area and the antrum. Typically, these lesions are asymptomatic making prevalence data very difficult to determine. Nor do we know the number of lesions that spontaneously heal or that progress to ulceration, frank perforation, gastric or duodenal obstruction, serious GI hemorrhage, and/or subsequent death. Risk factors for the development of important GI ulcer complications in patients receiving NSAIDs include: age > 60, prior history of peptic ulcer disease or GI bleeding, prior use of anti-ulcer therapies for any reason, concomitant use of glucocorticoids particularly in patients with RA, comorbidities such as significant cardiovascular disease, or patients with severe RA as determined by a disability index (Table 3) *(8,37,38,41)*. Other risk factors include increasing dose of specific and individual NSAIDs, or combination NSAIDs at full dose *(41)*.

Endoscopic data from large numbers of patients treated with COX-2 specific inhibitors demonstrate that ulcers are induced at the same rate as in patients who received placebo; whereas the active comparators may induce ulcers (as documented by endoscopy) from 15% (diclofenac 75 mg BID, ibuprofen 800 mg TID) to 19% (naproxen 500 mg BID) following 1 wk of treatment in healthy volunteers. In addition, after 12 wk of treatment, 26% (naproxen 500 mg BID) of patients with OA and RA demonstrate ulcers. A meta-analysis of the randomized controlled trials (RCTs) regarding rofecoxib demonstrated the bleeding complication rate to be 50%, whereas a similar study with celecoxib demonstrated about 77% decrease in bleeding with active comparators in both the RCT and open-label trials *(42)*. Patients treated with low dose aspirin for cardiovascular prophylaxis or who are infected with *Helicobacter pylori* are considered independent risk factor for ulcer formation. A large outcome trial (intention to treat cohort), which compared the effects of celecoxib 400 mg bid (2–4 times the treating dose for OA and RA), compared with ibuprofen 800 mg TID and diclofenac 75 mg BID for 6 mo demonstrated a 65% reduction of complications including bleeds, perforations and obstructions in the non-ASA-treated cohort *(8)*. It will be important for long-term outcomes to address issues of a delay in healing of ulcers induced by ASA or *H. pylori* in order to fully elucidate the magnitude of this individual risk, which currently is based on theoretical data.

APPROACH TO THE PATIENT AT RISK
FOR NSAID-INDUCED GI ADVERSE EVENTS

The approach to the patient with arthritis who requires chronic NSAID treatment and has developed or is at risk for an NSAID-induced GI event is straightforward but is complicated by the issue of cost of therapy. Many patients with dyspepsia or upper GI distress typically manifest superficial erosions by endoscopy, which often heal spontaneously without change in therapy. Even more difficult to evaluate is whether agents documented as cytoprotective actually alter NSAID-induced symptoms which may or may not predict significant GI events. One clinical study demonstrated that >80% of patients who developed significant NSAID-induced endoscopic abnormalities were asymptomatic *(43)*.

However, prospective observational trials have demonstrated that patients are surprisingly more symptomatic when they develop NSAID-induced toxicities than previously thought *(44)*. The patient who develops a gastric or duodenal ulcer while taking NSAIDs should have treatment discontinued and therapy for ulcer disease, either H_2-antagonist or proton pump inhibitors instituted. If NSAIDs must be continued concomitantly then the patient will be required to receive therapy for longer periods of time. Typically most patients with uncomplicated gastric or duodenal ulcers will heal within 8 wk of initiating H_2-antagonists. If NSAID treatment is continued then perhaps 16 wk of therapy may be necessary for adequate healing. Diagnostic tests to determine if the patient is *H. pylori* positive should be performed and if the patient has measurable antibodies, then specific antibiotic therapy to eradicate the infection should be administered. Prophylaxis to prevent NSAID-induced gastric and/or duodenal ulcers is more complicated. To date, there has been no evidence that agents other than misoprostol therapy will prevent NSAID-induced gastric ulceration and its complications *(40,45,46)*.

Although H_2-antagonists or proton pump inhibitors have been demonstrated to prevent NSAID-induced duodenal ulcers, prevention of gastric ulcerations has not been clearly shown. Endoscopy has shown that famotidine at twice the approved dose (40 mg BID) significantly decreased the incidence of both gastric and duodenal ulcers *(47)*. Similarly, endoscopy demonstrated that treatment with omeprazole decreased gastroduodenal ulcers *(48)*.

Although both H_2-antagonist and proton pump inhibitors (PPIs) decrease dyspeptic symptoms quite effectively, neither has been studied to determine if they decrease the incidence of ulcer complications. Misoprostol is a prostaglandin analog, which locally replaces the prostaglandins normally synthesized in the gastric mucosa but whose synthesis is inhibited by NSAIDs. A large prospective trial evaluated 8843 patients with RA to determine whether misoprostol would decrease the incidence of ulcers but also their complications *(41,46)*. Patients received various NSAIDs and were followed for 6 mo either on misoprostol co-therapy or placebo. The study was powered based on endoscopic observations of an 80% decrease with concomitant misoprostol therapy in endoscopically proven ulcers >0.3–0.5 cm in diameter with obvious depth in the gastric and duodenal mucosa *(40,46)*. Misoprostol successfully inhibited development of ulcer complications such as bleeding, perforation, and obstruction. There was a 40% reduction in patients treated with misoprostol as opposed to those receiving placebo. Further analysis demonstrated that patients with health-assessment questionnaire (HAQ) scores

> 1.5 (thus worse disease) had an 87% reduction in risk for an NSAID-induced toxic event if concomitantly treated with misoprostol *(45)*.

These data suggest that high-risk patients may benefit from concomitant misoprostol therapy if NSAID treatment is indicated. Unfortunately, the major adverse event causing withdrawal in approx 10% of patients was diarrhea. Therefore medications such as stool softeners and cathartics should be stopped. There are data suggesting that concomitant treatment with misoprostol once an ulcer develops will allow healing *(48)*. These data are preliminary, at best. The use of COX-2 specific inhibitors in high risk patients may clearly be cost-effective; further studies in the general population are warranted.

RENAL ADVERSE EFFECTS

The effects of NSAIDs on renal function include retention of sodium, changes in tubular function, interstitial nephritis, and reversible renal failure owing to alterations in filtration rate and renal plasma flow. Prostaglandins and prostacyclins are important for maintenance of intrarenal blood flow and tubular transport *(49)*. All NSAIDs except nonacetylated salicylates have the potential to induce reversible impairment of glomerular-filtration rate; this effect occurs more frequently in patients with congestive heart failure; established renal disease with altered intrarenal plasma flow including diabetes, hypertension, or atherosclerosis; and with induced hypovolemia: dehydration, salt depletion, or significant hypoalbuminemia *(12)*. Triamterene-containing diuretics, which increase plasma renin levels, may predispose patients receiving NSAIDs to develop precipitously acute renal failure. NSAIDs have been implicated in the development of acute and chronic renal insufficiency, owing to inhibition of vasodilating prostaglandins, thereby reducing renal blood flow, as has been observed infrequently in patients with lupus nephritis.

NSAID-associated intersitial nephritis is typically manifested as nephrotic syndrome, characterized by edema or anasarca, proteinuria, hematuria, and pyuria. The usual stigmata of drug-induced allergic nephritis such as eosinophilia, eosinophiluria, and fever are not typically present. Interstitial infiltrates of mononuclear cells are seen histologically with relative sparing of the glomeruli. Phenylproprionic acid derivatives such as fenoprofen, naproxen, and tolmetin along with the indoleacetic acid derivative indomethacin are most commonly associated with the development of interstitial nephritis. Inhibition of prostaglandin synthesis intrarenally by NSAIDs decreases renin release and thus produces a state of hyporeninemic hypoaldosteronism with resulting hyperkalemia. Physiologically, this effect may be amplified in patients taking potassium sparing diuretics. Salt retention precipitated by some NSAIDs which may lead to peripheral edema, is likely owing to both inhibition of intrarenal prostaglandin production, which decreases renal medullary blood flow and increases tubular reabsorption of sodium chloride as well as direct tubular effects. NSAIDs have also been reported to increase anti-diuretic hormone effect, thereby reducing excretion of free water, resulting in hyponatremia. Thiazide diuretics may produce an added effect on the NSAID-induced hyponatremia. All NSAIDs have been demonstrated to interfere with medical management of hypertension and heart failure and indomethacin appears to be the prescribed NSAID most commonly associated with this adverse reaction.

All NSAIDs with the exception of the nonacetylated salicylates have been associated with increases in mean blood pressure. Patients receiving antihypertensive agents including beta blockers, ACE inhibitors, thiazide and loop diuretics must be checked regularly when initiating therapy with a new NSAID to insure that there are no significant continued and sustained rises in blood pressure. Because these patients have elevated levels of angiotensin II and norepinephrine, their kidneys increase the release of vasodilator prostaglandins, which act locally to minimize the degree of renal ischemia (50). NSAIDs can interfere with this compensatory response and the increase in renal and systemic vascular resistance can cause an elevation in blood pressure.

The mechanism of acute renal failure induced in the "at risk" patient treated with NSAIDs is believed to be prostaglandin mediated. However, the role of COX-2 in maintenance of renal homeostasis in the human remains unclear. COX-2 activity is notably present in the macula densa and tubules in animals and humans, and is upregulated in salt depleted animals. In humans COX-1 is an important enzyme for control of intrarenal blood flow. There is sufficient evidence to indicate the new COX-2-specific inhibitors are not safer than traditional NSAIDs in terms of renal function. Any patient at high risk for renal complications should be monitored very carefully. No patient with a creatinine clearance of <30 cc/min should be treated with either a NSAID or a COX-2-specific inhibitor. The COX-2 inhibitors at normal approved treating doses in OA (celecoxib 100 mg BID and 200 mg QD and rofecoxib 12.5 mg and 25 mg QD) and RA seem to be a cause of edema and hypertension at the same rate as the traditional NSAIDs (2–3%).

IDIOSYNCRATIC ADVERSE EFFECTS

Many of the untoward effects of NSAIDs are related to their mechanism of action, via prostaglandin inhibition; but they also have important idiosyncratic effects. A typical nonspecific reaction includes skin rash and photosensitivity, associated with all currently available NSAIDs and particularly the phenylproprionic acid derivatives. The phenylproprionic acid derivatives may also induce aseptic meningitis especially in patients with SLE. The underlying mechanism of action remains unknown. This class of NSAIDs has also been associated with a reversible toxic amblyopia.

The CNS side effects of NSAIDs include aseptic meningitis, psychosis, and cognitive dysfunction. The latter changes are more commonly seen in elderly patients treated with indomethacin, whereas the phenylproprionic acid derivatives are more commonly associated with the development of aseptic meningitis and toxic amblyopia. Patients at the extremes of age may not manifest this side effect. Unfortunately, there is conflicting data about the effects of NSAIDs on cognitive function, particularly in the elderly (51).

Tinnitus is a common problem with higher doses of salicylates as well as the nonsalicylate NSAIDs. The mechanism is unknown. Interestingly, the young and the elderly may not complain of tinnitus but only of hearing loss. Decreasing the dose usually alleviates the effect. In all circumstances tinnitus is reversible with discontinuation of medication.

Owing to the antiplatelet effects of all NSAIDs except the nonacetylated salicylates and COX-2 specific inhibitors, concomitant therapy with coumadin puts patients at great risk for bleeding. Because concomitant NSAID therapy would displace coumadin from its albumin-binding sites, the prothrombin time may be prolonged; in addition, given the increased relative risk for NSAID-induced gastroduodenal ulcers and bleeding, there is an increased risk for bleeding when the NSAIDs are used concomitantly with warfarin. In that the COX-2 specific inhibitors rarely induce ulcers of the GI tract and do not alter platelet function, the patient on warfarin would have less risk for a significant GI bleed when treated with these drugs than traditional NSAIDs. However, both rofecoxib and celecoxib have been shown to prolong the international normal ratio (INR) in patients concomitantly treated with the anti-inflammatory and coumadin. Thus, the INR should be monitored at a 2 wk interval after initiation of therapy. Effects such as these may also be seen with Dilantin or other highly protein-bound drugs such as antibiotics. The NSAIDs inhibit the renal excretion of lithium and should be used with caution in patients taking this drug. Cholysteramine, an anion-exchange resin reduces the rate of NSAID absorption and its bioavailability.

There are little data documenting the effects of the NSAIDs on pregnancy or the fetus. In animal models, the NSAIDs have been shown to increase the incidence of dystocia, post-implantation loss as well as delay of parturition. The effect of prostaglandin inhibition may result in premature closure of the ductus arteriosus. Thus, the drug is usually stopped at least 6–8 wk before delivery. ASA has been associated with smaller babies and neonatal bruising; however, it has been used for many years in the treatment of patients who require NSAIDs while pregnant. In animals there is no evidence that ASA is a teratogen. The NSAIDs are excreted in breast milk. It is believed that salicylates in normally recommended doses are not considered dangerous to nursing infants. Although there are a few case reports of reversible infertility associated with the use of NSAIDs, given the large numbers of patients who regularly use NSAIDs, there does not appear to be a generalized epidemic of infertility *(52)*.

SUMMARY AND CONCLUSIONS

NSAIDs are important in treating patients with arthritis and effectively relieving the pain, inflammation, and stiffness. In the past, potential GI and or renal toxicity was the major reason for not prescribing NSAIDs as first-line therapy for OA given the age of the typical patient who suffers such a clinical problem. With the availability of the COX-2 specific inhibitors, the search for efficacious analgesic and anti-inflammatory drugs with decreased toxicity, namely reduced deleterious GI side effects and no platelet effects has questioned the use of the traditional NSAIDs in such a patient population. Thus it is logical that the COX-2 inhibitors may play a larger role in the repertoire of treatment for OA. As more individuals are exposed to COX-2 inhibitors, a different adverse-event profile may emerge. Of greatest concern, there are pending questions regarding the unwanted effects on renal function with chronic use, the possible increased risk of thromboembolic events in at risk patients, and/or the repair process following tissue injury. In addition, COX-2 specific inhibitors may also have important effects on other diseases affecting the same population of patients who suffer from OA, which would give them a distinct advantage relative to traditional NSAIDs. Given the safety profile of the COX-2 inhibitors, these drugs are being studied for use in decreasing the progression of Alzheimer's disease, prevention and treatment of colon cancer, and celecoxib has been recently approved for use in preventing polyps and decreasing polyp size in Familial Adenomatous Polyposis.

Unfortunately, NSAIDs have not been shown to decrease erosions in RA, to retard osteophyte formation in OA, or to protect cartilage from mechanical or inflammatory injury; thus they have not been shown to alter the natural history of any of these destructive tissue processes. Interestingly, in contrast, pretreatment with NSAIDs has repeatedly been demonstrated to decrease heterotopic bone formation after joint replacement *(53)*. In other experimental models, specific NSAIDs have been shown in vitro to inhibit chondrocyte proteoglycan synthesis *(27)*. There are a few case reports that suggest that the chronic use of some NSAIDs accelerated cartilage damage in OA (i.e., indomethacin), and some investigators believe the data to be compelling enough to preclude the use of NSAIDs in standard therapy for OA *(54)*. Amin et al have also presented similar in vitro data regarding the effects of the COX-2-specific inhibitors on cartilage. Although this effect may have profound implications, the evidence is inferential that chronic use of NSAIDs in general or the COX-2-specific inhibitors clearly damage cartilage in humans and/or worsens the clinical course of OA. Until our understanding of biochemical events affecting the articular cartilage and subchondral bone improve, there is still a need to aggressively treat both acute and chronic pain in order to maintain function in patients with OA. Both the NSAIDs and the COX-2 inhibitors have been demonstrated to be equally efficacious in palliating the pain and inflammation of OA and to improve function and quality of life of these patients. The combination of nonpharmacologic interventions with acetaminophen, NSAIDs, and/or COX-2 inhibitors will allow control of pain in patients with OA, and the availability of the COX-2 specific therapies will allow for a safer side-effect profile for those who need chronic therapy.

REFERENCES

1. Morbidity and Mortality Weekly Report, 1994.
2. Morbidity and Mortality Weekly Report, 1995.
3. Simon, L.S., F.L. Lanza, P.E. Lipsky, R.C. Hubbard, S. Talwalker, B.D. Schwartz, et al. 1998. Preliminary study of the safety and efficacy of SC-58635, a novel cyclooxygenase 2 inhibitor: efficacy and safety in two placebo-controlled trials in osteoarthritis and rheumatoid arthritis, and studies of gastrointestinal and platelet effects. *Arthritis Rheum.* 41:1591–1602.
4. Rehman, Q. and N.E. Lane. 1999. Getting control of osteoarthritis pain. An update on treatment options. *Postgrad. Med.* 106:127–134
5. Brooks, P.M. and R.O. Day. 1991. Nonsteroidal antiinflammatory drugs: differences and similarities. *N. Engl. J. Med.* 324:1716–1725.
6. Simon, L.S. and V. Strand. 1997. Clinical response to nonsteroidal antiinflammatory drugs. *Arthritis Rheum.* 40:1940–1943
7. Fosslien, E. 1998. Adverse effects of nonsteroidal anti-inflammatory drugs on the gastrointestinal system. *Ann. Clin. Lab. Sci.* 28:67/81.
8. Silverstein, F.E., G. Faich, J.L. Goldstein, L.S. Simon, T. Pincus, A. Whelton, et al. 2000. The celecoxib long-term safety study (CLASS): a randomized double-blind controlled trial. *JAMA* 284: 1247–1255.
9. Laine, L., S. Harper, T. Simon, et al. 1999. A randomized trial comparing the effect of rofecoxib, a cyclooxygenase-2 specific inhibitor, with that of ibuprofen on gastroduodenal mucosa of patients with osteoarthritis. *Gastroenterology* 117:776–783.
10. Leese, P., R. Hubbard, A. Karim, P. Isakson, S. Yu, and S. Geis. 2000. Effects of celecoxib, a novel cyclooxygenase-2 inhibitor, on platelet function in healthy adults: a randomized, controlled trial. *J. Clin. Pharmacol.* 40:124–132.
11. Brater, C. 2000. Pharmacokinetics. In: *Up to Date*, Rose, B.D. (ed.), Up to Date, Wellesley, MA.
12. Schlondorff, D. 1993. Renal complications of nonsteroidal anti-inflammatory drugs. *Kid. Int.* 44:643–653.

13. Brooks, P.M. and R.O. Day. 1991. Nonsteroidal antiinflammatory drugs: differences and similarities. *N. Engl. J. Med.* 324:1716–1725.

14. Mahmud, T., S.S. Rafi, D.L. Scott, J.M. Wrigglesworth, and I. Bjarnason. 1996. Nonsteroidal antiinflammatory drugs and uncoupling of mitochondrial oxidative phosphorylation. *Arthritis Rheum.* 39:1998–2003.

15. Walker, J.S., R.B. Sheather-Reid, J.J. Carmody, J.H. Vial, and R.O. Day. 1997. Nonsteroidal antiinflammatory drugs in rheumatoid arthritis and osteoarthritis: support for the concept of "responders" and "nonresponders" *Arthritis Rheum.* 40:1944–1954.

16. Furst, D.E. 1994. Are there differences among nonsteroidal antiinflammatory drugs? Comparing acetylated salicylates, nonacetylated salicylates, and nonacetylated nonsteroidal antiinflammatory drugs. *Arthritis Rheum.* 37(1):1–9.

17. Crofford, L.J., P. Lipsky, P. Brooks, S.B. Abramson, L.S. Simon, L.B.A. van de Putte. 2000. Basic biology and clinical application of cyclooxygenase-2. *Arthritis Rheum.* 43:4–13.

18. Dubois, R.N., S.B. Abramson, L. Crofford, R. Gupta, L.S. Simon, L.B. Van De Putte, P.E. Lipsky. 1998. Cyclooxygenase in biology and disease. *FASEB. J.* 12:1063–1073.

19. Mitchell, J.A., P. Akarasereenont, C. Thiemermann, R.J. Flower, and J.R. Vane. 1994. Selectivity of nonsteroidal antiinflammatory drugs as inhibitors of constitutive and inducible cyclooxygenase. Proc. *Natl. Acad. Sci. USA* 90:11,693–11,697.

20. Bensen, W.G., J.J. Fiechtner, J.I. McMillen, W.H. Zhao, S.S. Yu, E.M. Woods, et al. 1999. Treatment of osteoarthritis with celecoxib, a cyclooxygenase-2 inhbitor: A randomized controlled trial *Mayo Clin. Proc.* 1999; 74:1095–1105.

21. Ehrich, E.W., A. Dallob, I. De Lepeleire, A. Van Hecken, D. Riendeau, W. Yuan W, et al. Characterization of rofecoxib as a cyclooxygenase-2 isoform inhibitor and demonstration of analgesia in the dental pain model. *Clin. Pharmacol. Ther.* 1999;65:336–347.

22. Schnitzer, T.J., M. Kamin, and W.H. Olson. 1999. Tramadol allows reduction of naproxen dose among patients with naproxen-responsive osteoarthtis pain: a randomized, double blind, placebo controlled trial. *Arthritis Rheum.* 42:1370–1377.

23. Simon, L.S. 1996. Nonsteroidal antiinflammatory drugs and their effects: the importance of COX selectivity. *J. Clin. Rheum.* 2:135–140.

24. Simchowitz, L., J. Mehta, and I. Spilberg. 1979. Chemotactic factor-induced generation of superoxide radicals by human neutrophils: effect of metabolic inhibitors and antiinflammatory drugs. *Arthritis Rheum.* Jul;22(7):755–763.

25. Goodwin, J.S. 1984. Immunologic effects of nonsteroidal anti-inflammatory drugs. *Am. J. Med.* Oct 15;77(4B):7–15.

26. Díaz-González, F., I. González-Alvero, M.R. Companero, et al. Prevention of in vitro neutrophil-endothelial attachment through shedding of L-selectin by nonsteroidal antiinflammatory drugs. *J. Clin. Invest.* 1995; 95(4):1756–1765.

27. Amin, A.R., P. Vyas, M. Attur, J. Leszczynska-Piziak, I.R. Patel, G. Weissmann, and S.B. Abramson. 1995. The mode of action of aspirin-like drugs: effect on inducible nitric oxide synthase. *Proc. Natl. Acad. Sci. USA* 92:7926–7930.

28. Bombardier, C., P.M. Peloso, and C.H. Goldsmith. 1995. Salsalate, a nonacetylated salicylate, is as efficacious as diclofenac in patients with rheumatoid arthritis. Salsalate-diclofenac study group. *J. Rheumatol.* 22:617–624.

29. Agrawal, N.M., J. Caldwell, A.J. Kivitz, et al. 1999. Comparison of the upper gastrointestinal safety of Arthrotec 7 and nabumetome in osteoarthritis patients at high risk for developing nonsteroidal anti-inflammatory drug-induced gastrointestinal ulcers. *Clin. Ther.* April; 21(4):659–674.

30. Simon, L.S., C. Basch, and D. Robinson. 1991. Naproxen levels in plasma and synovial fluid of patients with rheumatoid arthritis. *Curr. Therapeut.* 13(supp.) 4:35–43.

31. Garcia Rodriguez, L.A., R. Williams, L.E. Derby, A.D. Dean, and H. Jick. 1994. Acute liver injury asociated with nonsteroidal antiinflammatory drugs and the role of risk factors. *Arch. Intern. Med.* 154:311–316.

32. Helfgott, S.M., J. Sandberg-Cook, D. Zakim, and J. Nestler. 1990. Diclofenac-associated hepatotoxicity. *JAMA* 264:2660–2662.

33. Simon, L.S. 1996. Actions and toxicities of the NSAIDs. *Curr. Opin. Rheum.* 8:169–175.

34. Robinson, D.R., M. Skoskiewicz, K.J. Bloch, G. Castorena, et al. 1986. Cyclooxygenase blockade elevates leukotriene E4 production during acute anaphylaxis in sheep. *J. Exp. Med.* Jun 1;163(6):1509–1517.

35. Wolfe, M.M., D.R. Lichtenstein, and G. Singh. 1999. Gastrointestinal toxicity of the nonsteroidal antiinflammatory drugs. *N. Engl. J. Med.* 340:1888–1899.

36. Bjarnson, I., J. Hyllar, A.J. Macpherson, and A.S. Russell. 1993. Side effects of the nonsteroidal anitinflammatory drugs on small and large intestine. *Gastroenterology* 104:1832–1847.

37. Fries, J.P., S.R. Miller, and P.W. Spitz. 1989. Toward an epidemiology of gastropathy associated with nonsteroidal antiinflammatory drug use. *Gastroenterology* 96:647–655.

38. Gabriel, S.E., L. Jaaklimainen, and C. Bombadier. Risk for serious gastrointestinal complications related to use of nonsteroidal antiinflammatory drugs: a meta-analysis. *Ann. Int. Med.* 1991; 115:787–796.

39. Allison, M.C., A.G. Howatson, and C.J. Torance. 1992. Gastrointestinal damage associated with the use of nonsteroidal antiinflammatory drugs. *N. Engl. J. Med.* 327:749–754.

40. Silverstein, F.E., D.Y. Graham, J.R. Senior, et al. 1995. Misoprostol reduces serious gastrointestinal complications in patients with rheumatoid arthritis receiving nonsteroidal anti-inflammatory drugs. *Ann. Intern. Med.* 123:214

41. Griffin, M.R., J.M. Piper, J.R. Daugherty, M. Snowden, and W.A. Ray. 1991. Nonsteroidal antiinflammatory drug use and increased risk for peptic ulcer disease in elderly persons. *Ann. Intern. Med.* 114:257–263.

42. Langman, M.J., D.M. Jensen, D.J. Watson, S.E. Harper, P.L. Zhao, H. Quan, et al. 1999. Adverse upper gastrointestinal effects of rofecoxib compared with NSIADs. *JAMA* 282:1929–1933.

43. Scheiman, J.M. and L. Laine. 1996. Nonsteroidal antiinflammatory drug gastropathy. *Gastrointet. Endosc. Clin. North. Am.* 6:489–504.

44. Singh, G., D.R. Ramey, D. Morfeld, H. Shi, H.T. Hatoum, and J.F. Fries. 1996. Gastrointestinal tract complications of nonsteroidal antiinflammaotry drug treatment in rheumatoid arthritis. A prospective observational study. *Arch. Intern. Med.* 156:1530–1536.

45. Simon, L.S., H.T. Hatoum, R.M. Bittman, W.T. Archambault, and R.P. Polisson. 1996. Risk factors for serious nonsteroidal-induced gastrointestinal complications: regression analysis of the MUCOSA trial. *Fam. Med.* 28:202–208.

46. Graham, D.Y., R.H. White, L.W. Moreland, et al. 1993. Duodenal and gastric ulcer prevention with misoprostol in arthritis patients taking NSAIDs. *Ann. Intern. Med.* 119:257–262.

47. Taha, A., N. Hudson, C.J. Hawkey, A.J. Swannell, P.N. Trye, J. Cottrell, et al. 1996. Famotidine for the prevention of gastric and duodenal ulcers caused by nonsteroidal antiinflammaotry drugs. *N. Engl. J. Med.* 334:1435–1439.

48. Hawkey, C.J., J.A. Karrasch, L. Szczepanski, D.G. Walker, A. Barkun, A.J. Swannell, et al. 1998. Omeprazole compared with misoprostol for ulcers associated with nonsteroidal antiinflammatory drugs. *N. Engl. J. Med.* 338: 727–734.

49. McAdam, B.F., F. Catella-Lawson, I.A. Mardini, S. Kapoor, J.A. Lawson, and G.A. FitzGerald. 1999. Systemic biosynthesis of prostacyclin by cyclooxygenase (COX)-2: the human pharmacology of a selective inhibitor of COX-2. *Proc. Natl. Acad. Sci. USA* May 11;96(10):5890.

50. Patrono, C. and M.J. Dunn. 1987. The clinical significance of inhibition of renal prostaglandin synthesis. *Kid. Int.* 32:1.

51. Saag, K.G., L.M. Rubenstein, E.A. Chrischilles, and R.B. Wallace. 1995. Nonsteroidal antiinflammatory drugs and cognitive decline in the elderly. *J. Rheumatol.* 22: 2142–2147.

52. Simon, L.S. 1998. Biology and toxic effects of nonsteroidal anti-inflammatory drugs. *Curr. Opin. Rheumatol.* May 10(3):153–158.

53. Nilsson, OS and P.E. Persson. 1999. Heterotopic bone formation after joint replacement. *Curr. Opin. Rheumatol.* 11:127–131.

54. Huskisson, E.C., H. Berry, P. Gishen, R.W. Jubb, and J. Whitehead. 1995. Effects of antiinflammatory drugs on the progression of osteoarthritis of the knee. LINK Study Group. Longitudinal investigation of nonsteroidal anti-inflammatory drugs in knee osteoarthritis. *J. Rheumatol.* 22:1941–1946.

55. Amin, A.R., M. Attur, R.N. Patel, G.D. Thakker, P.J. Marshall, et al. 1997. Superinduction of cyclooxygenase-2 activity in human osteoarthritis-affected cartilage. Influence of nitric oxide. *J. Clin. Invest.* Mar 15;99(6):1231–1237.

5

Glucocorticoid Therapy in Rheumatoid Arthritis

Kenneth G. Saag and John R. Kirwan

CONTENTS

INTRODUCTION

Discovered over 50 years ago, synthetic cortisone was first shown to be remarkably effective in relieving the inflammation associated with rheumatoid arthritis (RA) *(1,2)*. This pioneering work by Hench, Kendall, and colleagues subsequently resulted in a Nobel Prize in Medicine. Today, synthetic glucocorticoid use in RA remains one of the most controversial and commonly debated areas of modern arthritis management *(3–8)*. Attitudes towards glucocorticoid use in RA range from disdain *(6,9)* to widespread acceptance *(3,5)*. Despite this contentiousness, it is widely agreed that moderate- or high-dose glucocorticoid therapy is highly effective in controlling acute RA inflammation, but may result in significant serious adverse events. In addition to their recognized short- and medium-term efficacy for disease activity, increasing evidence favors a potential RA disease modifying effect of these agents. Lastly, controversy continues to surround the toxicity of low-dose therapy in RA, particularly its effects on bone.

From: *Modern Therapeutics in Rheumatic Diseases*
Edited by: G. C. Tsokos, et al. © Humana Press, Inc., Totowa, NJ

POTENTIAL MECHANISMS OF GLUCOCORTICOID ACTION

Glucocorticoids act as anti-inflammatory mediators via a number of pathways, which continue to be further elucidated *(10–12)*. Oral steroids in standard doses (<30 mg daily) circulate in the plasma and diffuse through the plasma membrane where they bind to cytosolic glucocorticoid receptors. Two types of effect can then occur. In one, heat-shock protein chaperons this complex to the nucleus where it exerts potent effects on transcription via binding to positive and negative glucocorticoid response elements in the promoter region of target genes. An alternative route is through direct interaction with pathways within the cytosol that control the production of inflammatory mediators. The relative effects of these two mechanisms are not yet fully understood, but in combination they result in the decreased synthesis of proinflammatory cytokines such as interleukin (IL)-1, IL-6, and tumor necrosis factor (TNF)α *(11,12)*. They also influence the production of arachidonic acid metabolites including both prostaglandins and leukotrienes. Specifically, they inhibit phospholipase A2 via upregulation of lipocortin, and glucocorticoids are selective inhibitors of cyclooxygenase 2 (COX-2) *(11,13–17)*. Suppression of endothelial factors and nitric oxide (NO) as well as activation of β-adrenoreceptors, endonucleases, and neutral endopeptidases explains other observed effects *(12,18)*. Glucocorticoids have a direct effect on lymphocytes by decreasing T-cell function and circulating number. New evidence suggests *(10)* that when glucocorticoids are given in high dose (e.g., >200 mg intravenously) all glucocorticoid receptors become saturated and additional therapeutic effects emerge that are mediated by incorporation of glucocorticoid molecules into cell membranes.

PHYSICIAN PERCEPTIONS AND BEHAVIORS RELATED TO DAILY GLUCOCORTICOID TREATMENT

Although the majority of physicians prescribing glucocorticoids are generalists *(19)*, rheumatologists comprise one of the largest group of specialists who commonly prescribe these agents, particularly for the treatment of RA. On a population basis, RA constitutes the most common indication for chronic glucocorticoid use *(20)*. Most US rheumatologists report that they use "low-dose" glucocorticoid therapy in their management of RA *(21)*. Physicians' interest in using glucocorticoids is supported by their perceived efficacy for this therapy. Wolfe found that 30% of rheumatologists considered prednisone to be "good" or "excellent" in efficacy, third only behind methotrexate (65%) and combination therapy (53%) *(22)*. In contrast, European rheumatologists are more inclined to use higher doses of glucocorticoids at the onset of disease, in an effort to induce disease remission *(23)*. The term "low-dose" therapy, however, is not well defined. Some authorities suggest 10 mg/d as the upper threshold *(24)*. In a 1994 survey of 301 practicing US rheumatologists, 43% agreed with this definition but 36% considered a maximum of 7.5 mg/d as low dose *(21)*. Here we adopt the more conservative definition.

There continues to be widespread variation in glucocorticoid use with prescribing dependent on both clinician and patient factors. Criswell and colleagues demonstrated that independent of insurance status and other patient characteristics, physicians were highly variable in glucocorticoid-prescribing patterns even among similar patients *(25)*. Although some rheumatologists report use of glucocorticoids in up to 80%

of their RA patients *(26)*, other practitioners claim that <10% of their patients use glucocorticoids *(6)*. However, in a 1997 survey of American College of Rheumatology (ACR) members by Schlessinger and colleagues, only 7% of respondents reported never using glucocorticoids in RA *(27)*. In the 1994 survey of US rheumatologists, 85% reported use of low-dose glucocorticoids either routinely (33%) or as "bridge" therapy when initiating second-line anti-rheumatic agents (52%). Nearly three-fourths of these rheumatologists estimated that they most often prescribed between 5 and 10 mg/d of prednisone, a proportion only modestly higher than the 63% use of glucocorticoids just recently documented in a 1999 survey of a random sample of over 130 ACR members (Saag and Kirwan, unpublished data). A survey of UK rheumatologists *(28)* found that 63% "never" or "very infrequently" initiated corticosteroid treatment in uncomplicated RA, whereas a survey of current outpatients showed that 24% were actually currently taking glucocorticoids.

The possibility that physicians' perceptions of glucocorticoid treatment may not always reflect their documented practices is further evidenced in a group of 819 RA patients followed for a mean of 14.2 yr by Wolfe and colleagues, 69.1% took prednisone at some point during their disease course *(29)*. In 857 RA outpatients seen at a Midwestern US medical center over a 5-yr period, 34% were taking glucocorticoids, a proportion second only to nonsteroidal anti-inflammatory drugs (NSAIDs) of all RA medications *(30)*. To our knowledge, and owing in part to difficultly with RA case definition in community-based cohorts, there have been no population-based surveys addressing glucocorticoid use by generalists for the treatment of RA. In summary of the available data on physician beliefs and practices, approx 25–40% of RA patients in many US and European practices are receiving glucocorticoids at any given time *(6,25,26,29,31)*.

EVIDENCE FOR EFFICACY OF DAILY GLUCOCORTICOIDS ON SYMPTOM CONTROL

Short- to moderate-term glucocorticoid studies fairly consistently reveal similar or improved disease activity when compared with control therapy *(32)*. In an effort to define improvement in disease activity, interventional studies compare glucocorticoid preparations with placebo, aspirin, other NSAIDs, and less potent second-line anti-rheumatic drugs. Million and colleagues, in a randomized but unblinded study, reported improvements in functional capacity (measured on a 1–5 scale) attributable to low-dose glucocorticoids *(33)*. A Cochrane Library meta-analysis by Gotzche and colleagues confirmed short-term efficacy (outcomes measured closest to 1 wk) with superior improvement in joint tenderness and pain in comparison to NSAIDs *(34,35)*.

Moderate term low-dose glucocorticoid effectiveness (outcomes measured closest to 6 mo) was assessed in a meta-analysis and subsequent Cochrane Review by Saag, Criswell, and colleagues *(36,37)*. Of 32 studies identified, only nine satisfied a relatively modest list of inclusion criteria for the meta-analysis. The remainder of the studies were not randomized, used an excessive dose, were of too short a duration or did not quantitatively define the endpoints. The meta-analysis of satisfactory studies concluded that glucocorticoids were significantly as or more effective than placebo in four out of six outcomes measured (tender joints, swollen joints, pain, and functional status). Compared with alternative therapies such as chloroquine and aspirin, glucocorticoids were as or more effective in improving RA disease activity.

Although the evidence demonstrates that up to several months of reduction in RA disease activity can be achieved with glucocorticoids, documented long-term anti-inflammatory benefits of glucocorticoids are not well-supported by the current literature. In a randomized controlled clinical trial of prednisolone vs placebo in addition to standard therapy *(38)*, anti-inflammatory benefits of glucocorticoids declined considerably after the first year, such that by 18 mo patients receiving prednisolone or placebo had statistically indistinguishable Health Assessment Questionnaire and articular index scores. A randomized controlled trial by Van Gestel and colleagues also indicated little differential benefit in disease activity score between gold/prednisolone vs placebo/gold beyond the 3-mo point *(32)*. In a study of elderly onset RA, Van Schaardenburg and colleagues compared prednisone vs chloroquine over a 2-yr period. Disease activity improved in both groups to a similar extent, whereas there was a heightened need for other DMARDs in those on chloroquine *(39)*. Similarly, neither the Dutch COBRA study nor a second Dutch clinical trial demonstrated protracted anti-inflammatory benefits of glucocorticoids beyond 5 mo *(40,41)*. In contrast to these consistent report from well-designed trials, a preliminary results from the German Low Dose Prednisolone Study Group (discussed further below) suggested that 5 mg of prednisolone resulted in better joint indices and ACR remission criteria than among patients taking placebo at 2 yr *(42)*. In contrast to the accumulating data on disease modification potential (discussed below), the majority of these studies raise concerns about the long-term benefits of glucocorticoids on disease activity. It has been suggested that there may be separate mechanisms responsible for development of RA erosions (regulated by synovial hypertrophy) and those responsible for inflammation (influenced by the degree of synovitis) this might account for this perceived disparity *(43)*.

EVIDENCE FOR CONTROL OF RA RADIOGRAPHIC PROGRESSION WITH DAILY GLUCOCORTICOIDS

In addition to disease activity (as evidenced by synovial inflammation), it is necessary to examine the definitive outcome of continuing joint destruction by radiographic progression. Firm conclusions on the long-term efficacy of glucocorticoid therapy in this respect have been lacking, because only a few studies have exceeded 1 yr in follow-up duration. Studies reporting on the effects of glucocorticoids on radiographic progression are summarized in Table 1.

The early studies of the Empire Rheumatism Council *(44)* and Joint Committee of the Medical Research Council (MRC) and Nuffield Foundation *(45)* failed to observe significant improvements in radiographic progression of patients treated with cortisone compared with aspirin preparations over a 1 yr period. However, a subsequent and less widely quoted MRC study *(46)* compared prednisolone with either aspirin or phenylbutazone and demonstrated that glucocorticoid treatment was associated with significantly less destructive joint changes of hand radiographs (41% progression in prednisolone group and 72% progression in analgesic group at yr 2; $p<0.03$). This later investigation has been criticized for incomplete follow-up of many patients over the full 2-yr study period. Critics also note that one-third of patients in both groups showed further radiographic deterioration in the final year *(6,47)*. When the patients from this second MRC study were followed over a full 4 yr, there was a significantly better radiographic outcome in those who received prednisolone (1.06 erosions per

Table 1
Studies of Oral Glucocorticoids and Radiographic Progression in RA

Study (reference/yr)	Experimental group	Control group	Study type (number of subjects)	Effect on radiologic progression of disease	Comments
MRC (44) 1955	Cortisone (69 mg/d)	ASA	CT (100)	No difference	Trend toward protective effect
MRC (46) 1959	Prednisolone (Initial 20 mg, 12 mg/d by yr 1, 10 mg/d by yr 2)	ASA	CT (77)	Reduction after 2 yr, less after 3 yr	Control patients offered prednisolone in yr 3
Bernsten (51) 1961	Various glucocorticoids, dose not reported	IM Gold, analgesics	Retrospective (388)	Deterioration in all groups	Many patients had already failed other Rx
Harris (50) 1983	Prednisone (5 mg/d) and DMARD	Placebo and DMARD	DB RCT (34)	No significant difference	Trend towards reduction
Million (33) 1984	Prednisolone and DMARD	No prednisolone	RCT (103)	Significant reduction	10-yr study
Kirwan (38) 1995	Prednisolone (7.5 mg/d) and DMARD	Placebo and DMARD	DB RCT (106)	Significant reduction	
Boers (40) 1997	Prednisolone (60 mg/d with taper) and MTX, SSZ	Placebo and SSZ	DB RCT (102)	Significant reduction	
Hansen (41) 1999	Prednisolone (6 mg/d) and DMARD	DMARD	RCT (102)	No significant difference	Trend towards reduction
Wassenberg (56)* 1999	Prednisolone (5 mg/d) and either AU or MTX	Placebo and either AU or MTX	DB RCT (196)	Significant reduction	Relatively new onset RA
Van Everdingen (57)* 1999	Prednisolone (10 mg/d)	Placebo	DB RCT (81)	Significant reduction	Only study since the MRC to not allow background DMARDs. SSA allowed after 6 mo

* Abstract.

MRC, Medical Research Council; R, randomized; CT, controlled trial; DB, double blind; IM intramuscular; ASA, high dose aspirin; MTX, methotrexate; SSZ, sulfasalazine; AU, auranofin; DMARD, disease modifying anti-rheumatic drug.

patient-year on prednisolone vs 3.25 erosions per patient-year on analgesics) *(48)*. Additionally, only half as many glucocorticoid-treated patients developed new erosions (51 vs 94%) *(49)*.

Although limited by the small number of patients, a clinical trial by Harris and colleagues suggested a disease-modifying effect of low-dose glucocorticoid therapy, as evidenced by the finding of erosions in 4 controls vs 1 prednisone- treated patient, although this was not statistically significant *(50)*. Million and colleagues also detected a small but significant reduction in joint erosions in some anatomic areas; however, this study was marred by an only 64% completion rate and a failure to adjust already large *p*-values for multiple comparisons *(33)*. In contrast to these later studies, a retrospective comparison of 183 glucocorticoid-treated RA patients with 205 patients taking either gold or analgesics and found similar levels of radiographic deterioration in both groups *(51)*. These later findings, however, were limited by the use of uncertain glucocorticoid doses and comparison of the glucocorticoid group with historical controls. In contrast to oral use, Hansen-treated RA patients with monthly intravenous methylprednisolone and observed no significant radiographic improvements in comparison to a control group receiving only saline infusions *(52)*.

Several recent studies using randomized controlled designs have provided further insight into this controversy. Kirwan and colleagues evaluated measures of disease activity and examined changes in radiographic severity scores (graded using the Larsen system), over a 2-yr period in patients treated with glucocorticoids in addition to standard therapy *(38)*. For those patients receiving 7.5 mg/d of prednisolone, a statistically significant difference in progression of radiographic erosion was detected at the 2-yr follow-up (0.72 U in the prednisolone group vs 5.37 U in the placebo group, $p = 0.0004$). The results of this large and well-designed study were questioned by some because of the chance occurrence of slightly more severe disease in the placebo group at baseline, ambiguities in the statistical approach to radiographic assessment, and the decision to treat each patient's hand radiograph as an independent outcome *(53)*. However, subsequent "blinded" follow-up of these patient showed that after prednisone was discontinued a significant deterioration in the Larsen index occurred *(54)*. In support of the effects of prednisolone on retardation of radiographic progression, levels of N propeptide of type III procollagen were reduced by 26% ($p < 0.001$), whereas patients were on prednisolone compared to levels when they were withdrawn from glucocorticoids *(55)*.

Results from the Dutch COBRA study showed that patients randomized to high-dose prednisolone (initially 60 mg/d tapered in 6 weekly steps to 7.5 mg/d) in combination with methotrexate and sulphasalazine may have experienced an arrest of radiographic progression after the first 6 mo of active treatment *(40)*. Further, the clinical differences between the subjects receiving the triple combination vs those on sulfasalazine alone were no longer significant once prednisolone was stopped. A second Dutch study of 102 patients with active RA of variable duration detected a nonsignificant trend towards reduction in radiographic progression among those randomized to DMARD plus prednisolone vs prednisolone alone *(41)*.

The preliminary report of a double-blind randomized controlled clinical trial by Wassenberg and colleagues compared 5 mg of prednisolone with placebo in 196 patients with RA of only 2 yr duration. All patients also received comedication with auranofin or methotrexate. Using a modified Sharp method, erosions were significantly fewer

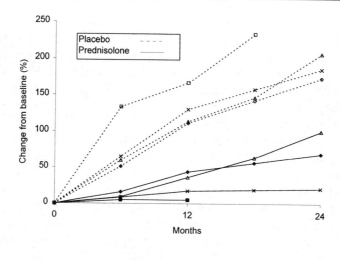

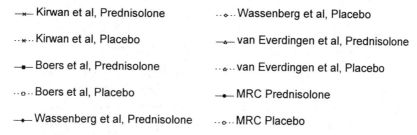

Fig. 1. Proportion change in the erosion score in five trials of prednisolone in RA.

among patients randomized to prednisolone (erosion score 7.6% of maximum at yr 2) vs control (12.7% of maximum) *(56)*.

With the exception of the very early MRC studies, all of the investigations just noted have been accompanied by the concomitant use of disease modifying anti-rheumatic agents. Thus, it has been difficult to discern the independent effects of glucocorticoids in these studies. Only one preliminary report has compared prednisolone alone with placebo in patients with very early RA defined as less than 1 yr and no prior RA treatment *(57)*. For the first 6 mo of this study patients received only the study medications but could later receive sulfasalazine. At 2 yr, a significant ($p = 0.02$) inhibition of radiographic change was seen and less than 65% of patients later required sulfasalazine. As most of these studies included patients of similar severity and disease duration, it is reasonable to directly compare their results. Figure 1 shows such a comparison, based on the proportionate change from baseline. The cumulative magnitude and consistency of these findings supports a protective effect of glucocorticoids on joint destruction.

ALTERNATIVE SYSTEMIC DOSING REGIMENS

The majority of glucocorticoid use in RA appears to be by daily oral dosing. However, alternative dosing regimens have been explored.

Timing of administration of the glucocorticoid dose may influence both efficacy and toxicity. Daily split-dose therapy should be used only for short duration owing to its more profound disruption of the normal hypothalamic-pituitary-adrenal (HPA) axis function. Administration of short acting glucocorticoid very early in the morning (0200 h), in contrast to later in the day, may better complement the normal diurnal variation in endogenous hormones and further block pro-inflammatory cytokine production such as IL-6 *(58)*. In contrast to other rheumatic disease where alternate day therapy may be both effective and less toxic, <50% of RA patients tolerate alternate-day regimens because of increased symptoms on "off" days *(59)*. Some physicians, however, have reported success with these regimens *(60)*.

Pulse therapy administered either intramuscularly or intravenously has been investigated in predominately small studies. Intramuscular pulses was beneficial for disease activity in combination with chrysotherapy *(61)*, but not apparently with sulfasalazine *(62)*. Intravenous pulse therapy has been recently reviewed *(23)*. Of note, intermittent 1 g infusions of solumedrol (as a rapid infusion) have shown modest clinical improvements *(63,64)* but a heightened risk of electrolyte, metabolic, and cardiovascular complications *(65)*. At least one study has touted long-term benefits on disease progression of intermittent pulse therapy *(66)*.

INTRA-ARTICULAR AND OTHER TYPES OF LOCAL GLUCOCORTICOID THERAPY

Intra-articular glucocorticoids are often used successfully in RA to control localized inflammation for periods of up to 3 mo *(67,68)*. When injected, triamcinolone hexacetonide, triamcinolone acetonide, and long-acting methylprednisolone are the preferred preparations with dosing ranging from 10 mg for small joints to 40 mg for larger joints. Local injections of triamcinolone into crioarytenoid joints may be an adjunct to systemic therapy for patients developing stridor or airway obstruction owing to RA involvement in this region *(69,70)*. Although even intra-articular therapy may have systemic spillover leading to blood-sugar effects and decrements in biochemical markers of bone formation *(71)*, this mode of administration is safer with respect to long-term toxicity *(72)*. Local complications have been suspected if injections are administered very frequently. These have included avascular necrosis *(67)*, Charcot-type arthropathy *(73)*, and tendon rupture *(74)*. There has been surprisingly little investigation into the long-term efficacy or disease modification potential of intra-articular therapy.

SPECIAL GLUCOCORTICOID INDICATIONS IN RA

High dose glucocorticoids are the therapeutic mainstay for managing serious visceral manifestations of RA *(75)*. Potential glucocorticoid responsive RA complications and extra-articular manifestations include: interstitial lung disease *(30,76–78)*, bronchiolitis obliterans with organizing pneumonia (BOOP) *(79)*, pericarditis *(80)*, vision-threatening eye involvement *(81,82)*, and vasculitis *(75)*. The vasculitis indication is somewhat controversial because older studies have suggested a potential etiologic role of glucocorticoids in vasculitis pathogenesis *(83,84)*. However, these studies are limited by selection bias or rapid fluctuation of dose leading to vasculitis flares. For Felty's syndrome, glucocorticoids are of questionable benefit. Although glucocorticoids will increase the white blood cell count, the risk for infection may actually be higher. For most of these serious disorders enumerated, glucocorticoids are typically administered in the dose range of 1 mg/kg prednisone equivalent. For life or organ-threatening complications, intravenous pulse therapy is often considered (500–1000 mg of methylprednisolone), although data supporting this regimen are predominately anecdotal *(85)*.

Glucocorticoids are often used in pregnant RA patients to control peri-partum disease activity. Although clearly safer than most other anti-rheumatics during pregnancy, glucocorticoid use has been suggested to cause fetal growth retardation and low birth-weight offspring. It is difficult, however, to discern fully whether these adverse fetal outcomes are owing to the glucocorticoids or the underlying chronic inflammatory disorder *(86,87)*. The American Academy of Pediatrics considers prednisone and its active metabolite prednisolone to be compatible with breast-feeding *(88,89)*. Even at doses above 1 mg/kg, the amount of glucocorticoid secreted into the breast milk is less than 10% of a nursing infant's endogenous cortisol production *(90)*.

Two other indications for glucocorticoid administration in RA are worthy of comment. Some physicians offer glucocorticoids as first-line therapy to patients with elderly-onset RA and predominantly generalized stiffness similar to polymyalgia rheumatica *(91)*. However, heightened concerned about the effects of glucocorticoids on bone in these often already osteoporotic patients, has challenged this traditional approach *(92)*. Finally, some RA patients who are at particular risk for NSAID-induced gastropathy or renal insufficiency may be more safely managed with low-dose glucocorticoids than with NSAIDs.

Evidence for Toxicity

Studies of glucocorticoid toxicity in RA tend to be retrospective and observational. The ability to differentiate bad outcomes attributable to glucocorticoids from those occurring owing to RA or other comorbidities, therefore, confounds the picture. A strong physician selection bias for glucocorticoid use exists as physicians are inclined to treat more severe RA patients with glucocorticoids. The use of glucocorticoids at variable points in the disease course, limited data defining the "threshold" dose for particular adverse events, and toxicity reports covering a heterogeneous group of glucocorticoid-treated diseases (which do not always extrapolate to RA) all further confound interpretation of toxicity data.

Mortality and hospitalization are important discrete outcomes analyzed in several studies of glucocorticoid use. Scott and colleagues noted 35% mortality by 20 yr in a follow-up study of RA patients assigned to a standard regimen that included prednisone *(93)*. The investigators attributed at least some of these deaths to glucocorticoids. Based on an analysis of the large Arthritis Rheumatism and Aging Medical Information System (ARAMIS) database, a 1.5-fold increased risk of mortality for glucocorticoid-treated patients was seen when compared with controls (hazards ratio ranging from 1.3–1.6) *(94)*. In another ARAMIS study, prednisone at an average dose of 6.9 mg/d resulted in a high frequency of attributable hospitalizations, particularly related to fractures and cataracts *(95)*. Although risk estimates in these studies were adjusted for case mix, ARAMIS is limited to self-report for much of its data and, it is not possible to account fully for all comorbidities in such cohorts.

Several large retrospective reviews indicate that long-term, low-dose glucocorticoid use is a significant independent predictor of numerous, potentially serious adverse events *(21,29,96)*. In a recent study, even after statistical adjustment for significant disease severity factors such as the presence of rheumatoid nodules and bony erosions, average

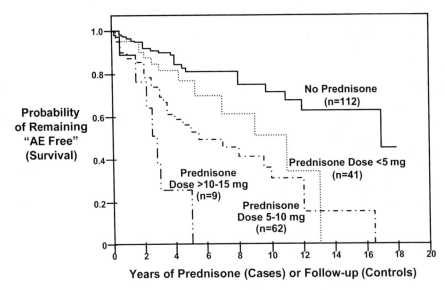

Fig. 2. Probability of remaining free from adverse events (adverse events) over time while on low-dose (<5 mg), intermediate dose (5–10 mg) or high-dose (>10–15 mg) prednisone compared with a control group. Adapted from ref. *21.*

prednisone dose was the strongest predictor of a serious adverse event potentially attributable to glucocorticoid therapy (odds ratio [OR] = 4.5 for 5–10 mg, 95% confidence interval [CI] 2.1–9.6 and OR = 32.3 for 10–15 mg, 95% CI 4.6–220) *(21).* Lending further credibility to causality, a glucocorticoid-adverse event association was both dose- and time-dependent (Fig. 2). This investigation and other studies indicate that both cumulative and mean glucocorticoid dose are independent important adverse-event predictors. Our conclusion is that, over and above the reduced life expectancy owing to RA alone, glucocorticoid toxicity probably does include an element of increased mortality in the long term. The confounding effect of patient selection, physician bias, and comorbidity will continue to make it difficult to estimate the risk precisely.

Interestingly, less serious toxicities (e.g., skin thinning, cushingoid appearance) may be of great concern to patients, whereas more debilitating toxicities, e.g., including vertebral crush deformity, cataracts, and glucocorticoid-induced hypertension, may be initially unrecognized or asymptomatic. Compared with other anti-rheumatic agents, glucocorticoids have a low incidence of short-term symptomatic toxicity and patients uncommonly discontinue therapy for these reasons *(95,97).* What follows is an overview of the most common glucocorticoid toxicities that may occur in RA.

Bone and Muscle

Glucocorticoid-induced osteoporosis (GIOP) is the most potentially devastating complication of protracted glucocorticoid therapy in RA. Lukert and Raisz estimate that over 50% of glucocorticoid users will develop bone loss leading to fracture *(98).* However, there have been no randomized controlled trials in RA large or long enough to clarify the full magnitude of the fracture risk of lower dose therapy in patients followed under optimal clinical trial conditions. The mechanisms of GIOP include:

(1) direct inhibition of osteoblast activity; (2) decreased calcium absorption through the gastrointestinal (GI) tract; (3) increased renal calcium loss (both of which may increase PTH); and (4) diminished sex-hormone production, all of which lead to enhanced osteoclast-mediated bone resorption. Recent findings suggest that a glucocorticoid-induce defect in bone formation may be the predominant pathway of importance *(99)*. Prednisone doses as low as 2.5 mg/d orally or even intra-articular therapy can suppress osteocalcin, a biochemical marker of bone formation *(71,98)*. Steroid-induced osteoporosis initially affects trabecular bone. However, with chronic glucocorticoid use, cortical bone at sites such as the femoral neck is also affected *(100)*. Most studies of GIOP define bone mass as bone mineral density (BMD), commonly measured using dual energy X-ray absorptiometry (DXA). Comparison of studies is made more difficult by the differential timing of glucocorticoid initiation, variable-dosing regimens, use of different bone-mass measurement techniques, and disparities between the sites of measurement. Indeed, bone-mass changes may vary considerably between sites measured *(41)*.

Laan and colleagues reported that changes in spinal BMD, measured by quantitative computerized tomography (QCT), occurred within the initial 5 mo of low-dose therapy (mean dose = 7.5 mg prednisone), but that RA patients had significant (although not complete) reversal of their bone loss once the prednisone was discontinued *(101)*. Although well-designed, this study has been criticized owing to its use of QCT, a technique that may overestimate the effects of glucocorticoid on bone. Additional studies of RA and those with other glucocorticoid-requiring diseases confirm a mean first-year loss of bone of up to 15% at the dose range ≤10 mg/d prednisone *(102–105)*. Few of these studies, however, have been randomized controlled clinical trials and the mean glucocorticoid doses used in individual studies somewhat vary. With continued use beyond a year, bone loss is greater than normal and is estimated at approx 3%/yr in subsequent years *(98,104)*. Although a decline in BMD is strongly correlated with fracture risk and BMD is considered the best overall predictor *(106,107)*, the rate of bone turnover, bone quality, and other factors also play important roles in fracture risk *(108)*. Several studies including a recent meta-analysis have failed to demonstrate an association of low-dose glucocorticoid use with low axial BMD, even in the setting of an increased fracture rate *(102,103,109,110)*. However, one of the studies included in the meta-analysis reported improved BMD at the lumbar spine, but paradoxically showed bone loss at all other locations measured *(111)*.

Some investigators argue that glucocorticoids may prevent bone loss in RA because of their inhibitory effects on proinflammatory cytokines that modulate osteoclast activity as well as their beneficial effects on functional status, which promotes more weight-bearing activities *(112,113)*. Sambrook and colleagues could not demonstrate a statistically significant decline in axial bone mass over a 24-wk period when patients taking a mean dose of 8 mg/d of prednisone were compared with controls *(102)*. However, a trend was present in this small cross-sectional study. A subsequent longitudinal study by the same investigators also failed to associate glucocorticoids with bone loss in RA *(114)*. Gough and colleagues *(115)* reported greater bone loss at a prednisone dose between 1 and 5 mg rather than a dose >5 mg, and hypothesized that the outcome might be related to poorer control of disease activity in the group less aggressively treated. A small set of data collected in a randomized controlled trial of prednisolone *(38)* did not point to any

Table 2
Mean (sd) Changes (%) in Bone Mineral Density in a Subset of Patients[a]
in the ARC Low Dose Glucocorticoid Study *(38)*

Years of treatment	Prednisolone 7.5 mg daily (n = 11)		Placebo (n = 10)	
	Spine	*Hip*	*Spine*	*Hip*
1	−1.6 (5.0)	−2.2 (7.1)	−2.3 (6.5)	−0.6 (5.6)
2	−3.0 (5.6)	−1.2 (3.1)	−1.3 (4.6)	−4.0 (2.5)[b]

[a]Patients were chosen for bone mineral density measurement because they were attending study centers where measurement facilities were readily available at the time of the study. Only those patients for whom measurements at the spine and hip were available after yr 1 and yr 2 are included.

[b]P = 0.04 for difference from the prednisolone group (T-test).

substantial increase in osteoporosis (Table 2). Thus the confounding effects in trying to identify an association between glucocorticoid treatment and osteoporosis in RA relate to two principal issues: the heightened risk of osteoporosis caused by the RA disease process itself *(116–121)* and a higher rate of osteoporosis in postmenopausal women, the demographic group with the highest prevalence of RA.

Given the inconsistencies in BMD studies and the knowledge that fractures in glucocorticoid-treated patients may occur at a higher BMD and may be dependent on other factors *(108,122)*, it is necessary to examine long-term studies that evaluate actual fracture incidence. Michel and colleagues *(123)* reported that 34% of more than 300 women on a mean dose of prednisone of 8.6 mg/d had a self-reported fracture within 5 yr of follow-up. Two case-control studies of hip fractures in patients both with and without RA showed a two-fold increased risk even after adjusting for the presence of RA *(121,124)*. At least two retrospective studies identify fractures as one of the most commonly documented complication of supraphysiologic glucocorticoid use *(21,96)*. As previously noted, observational studies of these types may be prone to confounding by indication, whereby RA patients with more severe and active disease are also more likely to develop a comorbidity independent of glucocorticoid use.

Alternate-day therapy may have some benefits for bone preservation *(125)*, but the cumulative glucocorticoid dose appears most important *(100,116,126,127)*. The presence of biochemical changes with very low oral *(98)*, intra-articular *(71)*, or even inhaled steroids *(128,129)* argues against a "safe" glucocorticoid dose from the standpoint of bone *(114)*.

Osteonecrosis of bone is a significant problem in patients receiving high glucocorticoid doses, particularly for treatment of systemic lupus erythematosus (SLE). However, osteonecrosis can rarely occur in RA patients receiving low-dose therapy. In one retrospective RA cohort, no cases of known osteonecrosis were found, and in another study, osteonecrosis occurred in <3 % of patients given physiologic glucocorticoids for adrenal insufficiency *(21,130)*. Osteonecrosis is seldom noted when the prednisone dose is maintained <20 mg/d *(131)*.

Similar to osteonecrosis, the occurrence of myopathy in patients receiving low-dose glucocorticoids is rare. Based on small studies, fluorinated glucocorticoid preparations, such as triamcinolone, appear to be more closely associated with myopathy than prednisone *(132)*. Of note, myopathy has been reported to occur at a dose as low as 8 mg/d of triamcinolone after only 3 mo of treatment. In general, myopathy attributable to prednisone requires a higher dose and longer duration of treatment.

Cardiovascular

Steroids promote fluid retention *(133)*, a problem of particular concern in patients with underlying heart or kidney disease. Patients with essential hypertension require closer surveillance of blood pressure and may need modification of their anti-hypertensive regimens while on low-dose glucocorticoid therapy. Often, in patients receiving <10 mg/d, age and elevated pre-treatment blood pressure may better explain significant hypertension than the use of glucocorticoids *(134)*.

Another troublesome but difficult-to-study potential toxicity of low-dose glucocorticoids is the development of premature atherosclerotic vascular disease. Increasing attention to the importance of accelerated atherosclerotic disease in RA and other inflammatory conditions has raised interesting questions about the role of chronic inflammation on the vascular endothelium *(135)*. Although atherosclerotic vascular disease is known to be accelerated in patients with Cushing's disease, there are insufficient data to implicate a similar heightened risk in RA patients owing to glucocorticoids. Kalbak *(136)* reported a threefold increase of atherosclerosis in RA patients treated with glucocorticoids compared with nonsteroid-treated patients, although the dose consumed and other confounding factors were not reported. In another report, moderate- to low-dose glucocorticoids (20 mg tapered to 5 mg over 3 mo) had no significant adverse effect on lipoprotein levels if other risk factors were controlled *(137)*.

Dermatologic

Even at the low doses typically used in RA, skin thinning and ecchymoses represent one of the most common glucocorticoid adverse events. It is estimated from ARAMIS data that 32 cases of purpura developed for every 1000 patient-years of follow-up *(95)*. A cushingoid appearance is very troubling to patients, but is uncommon at doses below physiologic range. However, in one study, moon facies did develop in 13% of patients receiving 4–12 mg of triamcinolone for <60 d *(138)*. Alternate-day therapy decreases the incidence of cushingoid appearance. Steroid acne and, to a lesser extent, hirsutism and striadverse event are other undesirable dermatologic side effects that occur even at doses used for RA.

Gastrointestinal

Although most investigators agree that glucocorticoids are considerably less toxic to the upper GI tract than NSAIDs, glucocorticoids may slightly increase the risk of adverse GI events such as gastritis, ulceration, and GI bleeding. Among 477 RA patients treated with varying glucocorticoid doses Bollet and colleagues found a 7.5% prevalence of ulcers *(139)*. If glucocorticoids independently increase GI events, the effect is slight, with estimated relative risks varying from 1.1 (not significant) to 1.5 (marginally significant) *(140,141)*. In addition to reports of upper GI morbidity, there are anecdotal reports of intestinal rupture, diverticular perforation, and pancreatitis believed to be caused by low-dose glucocorticoids *(142–144)*. Glucocorticoids are frequently used concurrently with NSAIDs in RA, and meta-analyses confirm that the combination of glucocorticoids and NSAIDs synergistically result in a higher risk of GI adverse events *(141,145)*. One meta-analysis *(145)* reported that glucocorticoids caused a nearly two-fold increased risk of GI adverse events (OR = 1.8, 95% CI 1.2–2.8) among NSAID users; whereas in another study, combined use of NSAIDs and glucocorticoids resulted in more than a four-fold increased risk of GI adverse events over nonusers (OR = 4.4, 95% CI 2.0–9.7) *(141)*. These meta-analyses were conducted before the availability of COX-2 selective NSAIDs, therefore, the combined GI effects of glucocorticoids with selective COX-2 NSAIDs is unknown.

Infectious Diseases and Immunologic Dysfunction

Moderate- to high-dose glucocorticoid therapy can lead to an increased risk of serious infections requiring hospitalizations, surgery, or both. However, to our knowledge, no studies have explored the risk of infection specifically to RA patients treated with lower dose glucocorticoids. The risk of infection appears to be lessened by initiating alternate-day therapy *(146)*. A meta-analysis by Stuck and colleagues *(147)* showed that the rate of infection was not significantly increased in patients given a mean dose of <10 mg/d of prednisone or a cumulative dose of <700 mg. One investigation of 250 RA patients demonstrated that asymptomatic bacteriuria was almost three-fold more frequent ($p < 0.05$) in those taking less than 7.5 mg/d of prednisolone for more than 6 mo (the minimal or average glucocorticoid dose was not reported) *(148)*.

Herpes zoster has a higher incidence among RA patients treated with immunosuppressive agents. In one analysis, eight glucocorticoid-treated RA patients developed zoster compared with only one control ($p < 0.04$) *(21)*. However, it is difficult to separate the independent effects of glucocorticoid use from those of other commonly used anti-rheumatic agents such as methotrexate. It is anticipated that association of glucocorticoids with infectious sequeladverse event may become an even greater concern if glucocorticoids are used in combination with biological anti-rheumatic agents (i.e., TNF-α inhibitors) that may predisopose to infections. At this time, the independent role of glucocorticoids in this infectious disease outcome of RA patients is uncertain.

Metabolic and Endocrine

RA patients with diabetes mellitus will commonly have higher blood-glucose levels while taking glucocorticoids *(149)*. Moreover, in patients with early diabetes or glucose intolerance new-onset hyperglycemia or, rarely, a nonketotic hyperosmolar state, may develop without warning for the first time. Ketosis in glucocorticoid-associated diabetes is very rare, as the gluconeogenic and glycogenic effects of glucocorticoids offer protection against this complication *(150)*. It is uncommon for frank diabetes to develop *de novo* as a result of glucocorticoid therapy *(151)*.

An additional concern of chronic glucocorticoid use is hypothalamic-pituitary-adrenal (HPA) insufficiency. HPA insufficiency appears to be both dose- and duration-specific. High-dose therapy can result in protracted suppression of adrenocorticotropic hormone release and adrenal hypo-responsiveness in as little as 5 d *(152)*. Spontaneous recovery of the HPA axis is usual in patients on ≤5 mg of prednisone *(153)*; however, subphysiologic doses (<7.5 mg/d) given for long-term periods may lead to HPA blunting *(154)*. HPA suppression is worsened if glucocorticoids are given twice daily. Steroid withdrawal syndrome is not clearly associated with HPA insufficiency but presents as extreme weakness and arthralgias *(155)*; therefore, too rapid a glucocorticoid withdrawal can be confused with an exacerbation of RA disease activity. Van Gestel and colleagues demonstrated that tapering from 20 mg/d by increments of 2.5 mg/d every 2 wk resulted in rebound deterioration in 58% of responders *(32)*. Indeed, difficulty withdrawing patients from glucocorticoids is sometimes cited as a compelling reason for not initiating them *(156)*. Despite these widely held sentiments, with the exception of Kirwan's study where patients were successfully withdrawn form 7.5 mg of prednisolone over 4 wk without a prominent flare, there have been no randomized controlled trials of lower dose withdrawal to specifically address this issue.

Neuropsychiatric

Many RA patients receiving low-dose therapy report a slight increase in their overall sense of well-being, which appears to be independent of improvement in disease activity. Symptoms of akathisia, insomnia, and depression are also occasionally observed in patients taking low-dose therapy. Memory impairment, particularly in older patients, can occur even at low doses *(157)*. Daily split-dose therapy, in particular, tends to be troublesome because the evening dose disrupts normal diurnal variation in endogenous glucocorticoid levels and promotes sleep disturbances. True glucocorticoid psychosis is distinctly uncommon at doses <20 mg/d of prednisone *(158)*.

Ophthalmologic

Posterior subcapsular cataracts are a well-described complication of prolonged corticosteroid use. Although some clinicians believe there is no minimal safe dose with respect to this complication and reports exist of cataract formation even with inhaled glucocorticoid preparations *(159)*. Others note that cataracts rarely occur in patients taking <10 mg/d for <1 yr *(160,161)*. Cataracts were detected in 29% of 112 RA patients taking a mean dose of 8 mg/d for an average of 6.9 yr compared with an 18% incidence in matched controls ($p < 0.05$) *(96)*. In their preliminary analysis of 819 RA patients *(29)*, Wolfe and colleagues reported an almost threefold increased risk of cataracts for >15 mg-yr (i.e., 5 mg/d for 3 yr) of prednisone (OR = 2.7, 95% CI 1.7–4.4).

In addition to cataracts, glucocorticoid-treated patients may develop increased intra-ocular pressure, which can lead to minor visual disturbances *(162)*. The development of frank glaucoma, particularly with low-dose therapy, is rare and tends to appear in patients who are otherwise predisposed to the condition *(163,164)*. Highlighting a potential risk of even low-dose therapy, glaucoma may occur with inhaled glucocorticoids as well *(165)*.

Evidence-Based Treatment Guidelines

Owing to difficulties balancing effectiveness data with toxicity concerns, as well as the advent of numerous other RA specific therapies, there is little consensus about the current place of glucocorticoid in the majority of RA clinical scenarios. Potential indications for glucocorticoid use in RA patients are outlined in Table 3; however, several of these recommendations are debatable. A fixed, low dose of prednisolone for patients with early active disease as an erosion-suppressing treatment may be justified

Table 3
Indications for Possible Use of Glucocorticoids in RA

- "Bridge" therapy for patients who have experienced a severe functional decline with limitations interfering with necessary daily living or vocational activities
- Patients with NSAID contraindications who have acute inflammation unlikely to respond rapidly enough to second-line agents
- Extra-articular manifestations or other serious life-threatening or organ-damaging RA manifestation (i.e., pericarditis, scleromalacia perforans)
- Men or women not at reduced risk of bone loss, for whom chronic glucocorticoids may be reasonable in combination therapy regimens with a single daily dose <10 mg/d
- Pregnant or lactating women
- Suppression of joint destruction in patients with early, active disease

NSAID, nonsteroidal anti-inflammatory drugs; RA, rheumatoid arthritis.

Table 4
Recommendations for Safe and Effective Glucocorticoid Use

- Use the smallest dose possible to accomplish clinical objectives
- Taper dose more rapidly to near a physiologic range (<7.5 mg/d), then taper more slowly to avoid steroid withdrawal flare-ups that may require dosage increases
- Exercise special caution in individuals on concomitant NSAIDs, because of a heightened risk of gastropathy, fluid retention, and other synergistic toxicities
- Monitor blood sugar, blood pressure, and consider periodic ophthalmologic examinations to avoid preventable glucocorticoid toxicity
- Protect the bones
  o Encourage osteoporosis risk factor modification
  o Obtain baseline bonemass determination to assess the need for anti-osteoporotic therapy
  o Supplement all at-risk patients to achieve 1500 mg/d of elemental calcium and add vitamin D
  o Replace gonadal hormone deficiencies if not contra-indicated
  o Strongly consider bisphosphonate therapy

NSAID, nonsteroidal anti-inflammatory drugs.

for the first 2 yr or so, but long-term therapy or "background" treatment for symptom control is not clearly supported based on the evidence available.

Once the decision is made to initiate glucocorticoids, every effort should be made to use these agents as safely and effectively as possible (Table 4). Increasing data argues that more aggressive use of higher dose glucocorticoids earlier rather than later in the course of disease might be best supported by the available evidence. However, practitioners skeptical of the disease-modifying benefits of glucocorticoid therapy and choosing to use these agents long-term should strive to achieve the lowest effective dose. Many rheumatologists report significant difficulties in tapering glucocorticoids for most RA patients and abrupt withdrawal may result in dramatic flares in disease activity *(32,50)*. Thus, more gradual withdrawal regimens are generally necessary to avoid re-exacerbations. However further research on appropriate tapering regimens is greatly needed.

All RA patients with or at risk of glucocorticicoid-induced osteoporosis (GIOP) should receive conservative therapy with calcium and vitamin D *(166,167)* with strong consideration given to the addition of a bisphosphonate *(168–171)*. Hormone-replacement therapy and calcitonin should also be considered in selected individuals, although the data is less conclusive than that seem with the newer bisphosphonates *(172)*. Despite this accumulating data, only a minority of patients on glucocorticoids receive preventative therapy or diagnostic testing for bone loss *(19,20,173–176)*.

ACKNOWLEDGMENTS

Special thanks to Ms. Laurie Tipton for her expert assistance with manuscript preparation.

REFERENCES

1. Hench, P.S., E.C. Kendall, C.H. Slocumb, et al. 1949. Effects of a hormone of the adrenal cortex (17-hydroxy-11 dehydrocorticosterone: compound E) and of pituitary adrenocorticotrophic hormone on rheumatoid arthritis: Preliminary report. *Proc. Staff Meet Mayo Clin.* 24:181–197.

2. Hench, P.S., E.C. Kendal, C.H. Slocumb, et al. 1950. Effects of cortisone acetate and pituitary ACTH on rheumatoid arthritis, rheumatic fever and certain other conditions. *Arch. Intern. Med.* 85:545–666.

3. Weiss, M.M. 1989. Corticosteroids in rheumatoid arthritis. *Semin. Arthritis Rheum.* 19:9–21.

4. George E. and J.R. Kirwan. 1990. Corticosteroid therapy in rheumatoid arthritis. *Bailliere's Clin. Rheumatol.* 4:621–647.

5. Weisman, M.H. 1993. Should steroids be used in the management of rheumatoid arthritis? *Rheum. Dis. Clin. North Am.* 19(1):189–199.

6. Ramos-Remus, C., J. Sibley, A.S. Russell. 1992. Steroid in rheumatoid arthritis: the honeymoon revisited (editorial). *J. Rheumatol.* 19:667–670.

7. Laan, R.F., T.L. Jansen, and P.I. van Riel. 1999. Glucocorticosteroids in the management of rheumatoid arthritis (review). *Rheum. (Oxford).* 38(1):6–12.

8. Kirwan, J.R. and A.S. Russell. 1998. Systemic glucocorticoid treatment in rheumatoid arthritis - a debate. *Scand. J. Rheumatol.* 27:247–251.

9. Fries, J.F. and G. Singh. 1995. Glucocorticoids and joint destruction in rheumatoid arthritis (letter to editor). *N. Engl. J. Med.* 333:142–146.

10. Buttgereit, F., M. Wheling, and G.R. Burmester. 1998. A new hypothesis of modular glucocorticoid actions - Steroid treatment of rheumatic diseases revisited. *Arthitis Rheum.* 41:761–767.

11. Boumpas, D.T., G.P. Chrousos, R.L. Wilder, et al. 1993. Glucocorticoid therapy for immune-mediated diseases: Basic and clinical correlates. *Ann. Intern. Med.* 119:1198–1208.

12. Barnes, P.J., and I. Adcock. 1993. Anti-inflammatory actions of steroids: molecular mechanisms. *TiPS.* 14:436–441.

13. Gustafsson, J-A., J. Carlstedt-Duke, L. Poellinger. et al. 1987. Biochemistry, molecular biology, and physiology of the glucocorticoid receptor. *Endocr. Rev.* 8:185–234.

14. Kern, J.A., R.T. Laumb, J.C. Reed, R.P. Daniel, and P.L. Nowell. 1988. Dexamethasone inhibition of interleukin-1beta production by human monocytes: post-transcriptional mechanisms. *J. Clin. Invest.* 81:237–244.

15. Vishwanath, B.S., F.J. Frey, M.J. Bradtury, M.F. Dallman, and B.M. Frey. 1993. Glucocorticoid deficiency increases phospholipase A2 activity in rats. *J Clin Invest.* 92:1974–1980.

16. Cronstein, B.N., S.C. Kimmel, R.I. Levin, F. Martiniuk, and G. Weissmann. 1992. A mechanism for the anti-inflammatory effects of corticosteroids: the glucocorticoid receptor regulates leukocyte adhesion to endothelial cells and expression of endothelial-leukocyte adhesion molecule-1 and intercellular adhesion molecule 1. *Proc. Natl. Acad. Sci. USA* 89:9991–9995.

17. Szczepanski, A., T. Moatter, W.W. Carley, and M.E. Gerritsen. 1994. Induction of cyclooxygenase II in human synovial microvessel endothelial cells by interleukin-1. Inhibition by glucocorticoids. *Arthritis Rheum.* 37:495–503.

18. Palmer, R.M., L. Bridge, N.A. Foxwell, and S. Moncada. 1992. The role of nitric oxide in endothelial cell damage and its inhibition by glucocorticoids. *Br. J. Pharmacol.* 105:11–12.

19. Mudano, A., J. Allison, J. Hill, T. Rothermel, and K. Saag. 1999. Glucocorticoid-induced osteoporosis: process of care and patient outcomes in a managed care population. *Arthritis Rheum.* 42:S73.

20. Walsh, L.J., C.A. Wong, M. Pringle, and A.E. Tattersfield. 1996. Use of oral corticosteroids in the community and the prevention of secondary osteoporosis: a cross sectional study. *BMJ* 313:344–346.

21. Saag, K.G., R. Koehnke, J.R. Caldwell, et al. 1994. Low dose long-term corticosteroid therapy in rheumatoid arthritis: an analysis of serious adverse events. *Am. J. Med.* 96:115–123.

22. Wolfe, F., D.A. Albert, and T. Pincus. 1998 A survey of United States rheumatologists concerning effectiveness of disease-modifying antirheumatic drugs and prednisone in the treatment of rheumatoid arthritis. *Arthritis Care Res.* 11(5):375–381.

23. Weusten, B.L.A.M., J.W.G. Jacobs, and J.W.J. Bijlsma. 1993. Corticosteroid pulse therapy in active rheumatoid arthritis. *Semin Arthritis Rheum.* 23:183–192.

24. Caldwell, J.R., and D.E. Furst. 1991. The efficacy and safety of low-dose corticosteroids for rheumatoid arthritis. *Semin. Arthritis Rheum.* 21:1–11.

25. Criswell, L.A., and W.J. Redfearn. 1994. Variation among rheumatologists in the use of prednisone and second-line agents for the treatment of rheumatoid arthritis. *Arthritis Rheum.* 37(4):476–480.

26. Pincus, T., R.H. Brooks, and C.M. Stein. 1995. Changing patterns of patient care in rheumatoid arthritis: use of methotrexate or prednisone in > 80% (both in 57%) of patients and frequent combination therapy with minimal evidence of disease in 36% of patients (abstract). *Arthritis Rheum.* 38:S366.

27. Schlesinger, N., K. Farrukh, K. Barrett, B. Hoffman, and R.H. Schumacher. 1997. A survey of corticosteroid use in rheumatoid arthritis. *Arthritis Rheum.* 40:S194.

28. Byron, M.A., and A.G. Mowat. 1985. Corticosteroid prescribing in rheumatoid arthritis: The fiction and the fact. *Br. J. Rheum.* 24:164–166.

29. Wolfe, F., D. Furst, N. Lane, et al. 1995. Substantial increases in important adverse events follow low dose prednisone therapy of rheumatoid arthritis (RA). *Arthritis Rheum.* 38:S312.

30. Saag, K.G., S. Kolluri, R.K. Koehnke, et al. 1996. Rheumatoid arthritis lung disease: Determinants of physiologic and radiographic abnormalities. *Arthritis Rheum.* 39(10):1711–1719.

31. Bird, H. 1985. Conference report. The role of steroids in the treatment of arthritis. *Ann. Rheum. Dis.* 44:642–643.

32. Van Gestel, A.M., R.F.J.M. Laan, C.J. Haagsma, L.B.A. Van de Putte, and P.L.C.M. Van Riel. 1995. Low-dose oral steroids as bridge therapy in rheumatoid arthritis patients starting with parenteral gold. A randomized double-blind placebo-controlled trial. (and personal correspondence). *Br. J. Rheumatol.* 34(4):347–351.

33. Million, R., P. Poole, J.H. Kellgren, and M.I. Jayson. 1984. Long-term study management of rheumatoid arthritis. *Lancet* 1:812–816.

34. Gotzsche, P.C., and H.K. Johansen. 1999. Short-term, low-dose corticosteroids and nonsteroidal anti-inflammatory drugs for rheumatoid arthritis (Cochrane Review). *The Cochrane Library,* Update Software, Oxford.

35. Gotzsche, P.C., and H.K. Johansen. 1998. Meta-analysis of short term low dose prednisolone versus placebo and non-steroidal anti-inflammatory drugs in rheumatoid arthritis. *BMJ* 316:811–818.

36. Saag, K.G., L.A. Criswell, K.M. Sems, M.D., Nettleman, and Kolluri S. Low-dose corticosteroids in rheumatoid arthritis: a meta-analysis of their moderate-term effectiveness. *Arthritis Rheum.* 1996;39(11):1818–1825.

37. Criswell, L.C., K.G. Saag, K.M. Sems, et al. 1999. Rheumatoid Arthritis (RA): Moderate-Term Low Dose Corticosteroids for Rheumatoid Arthritis (Cochrane Review). *The Cochrane Library.* vol. Issue 1. Update Software, Oxford.

38. Kirwan, J.R., Arthritis and Rheumatism Council Low Dose Glucocorticoid Study Group. 1995. The effect of glucocorticoids on joint destruction in rheumatoid arthritis. *N. Engl. J. Med.* 333:142–146.

39. Van Schaardenburg, D., R. Valkema, B.A.C. Dijkmans, et al. 1995. Prednisone for elderly-onset rheumatoid arthritis: Outcome and bone mass in comparison to treatment with chloroquine. *Arthritis Rheum.* 38:334–342.

40. Boers, M., A.C. Verhoven, H.M. Markusse, et al. 1997. Randomised comparison of combined step-down prednisolone, methotrexate and sulphasalazine with sulphasalazine alone in early rheumatoid arthritis. *Lancet* 350(9074):309–318.

41. Hansen, M., J. Podenphant, A., Florescu, et al. 1999. A randomised trial of differentiated prednisolone treatment in active rheumatoid arthritis. Clinical benefits and skeletal side effects. *Ann. Rheum. Dis.* 58:713–718.

42. Zeidler, H., R. Rau, and P. Steinfeld, 1999. Efficacy and safety of low dose prednisolone in early rheumatoid arthritis (RA). *Arthritis Rheum.* 42:9 (Suppl.):S271.

43. Kirwan, J.R. 1997. The relationship between synovitis and erosions in rheumatoid arthritis. *Br. J. Rheum.* 36:225–228.

44. Empire Rheumatism Council Sub-Committee. 1955. Multi-Center controlled trial comparing cortisone acetate and acetyl salicylic acid in the long-term treatment of rheumatoid arthritis. *Ann. Rheum. Dis.* 14:353–363.

45. Joint Committee of the Medical Research Council and Nuffield Foundation on Clinical Trials of Cortisone A, and Other Therapeutic Measures in Chronic Rheumatic Diseases. A comparison of cortisone and aspirin in the treatment of early cases of rheumatoid arthritis. *BMJ* 1954;1:1223–1227.

46. Joint Committee of the Medical Research Council and Nuffield Foundation on Clinical Trials of Cortisone A, and Other Therapeutic Measures in Chronic Rheumatic Diseases. 1959. A comparison of prednisolone with aspirin or other analgesics in the treatment of rheumatoid arthritis. *Ann. Rheum. Dis.* 18:173–187.

47. Joint Committee of the Medical Research Council and Nuffield Foundation on Clinical Trials of Cortisone A, and Other Therapeutic Measures in Chronic Rheumatic Diseases. 1960. A comparison of prednisolone with aspirin or other analgesics in the treatment of rheumatoid arthritis. *Ann. Rheum. Dis.* 19:331–337.

48. West, H.F. 1967. Rheumatoid arthritis: the relevance of clinical knowledge to research activities. *Abstr. World Med.* 41:401–417.

49. Masi, A.T. 1983. Low dose glucocorticoid therapy in rheumatoid arthritis (RA): transitional or selected add-on therapy? (editorial). *J. Rheumatol.* 10:675–678.

50. Harris, E.D., R.D. Emkey, J.E. Nichols, and A. Newberg. 1983. Low dose prednisone therapy in rheumatoid arthritis: A double blind study. *J. Rheumatol.* 10:713–721.

51. Berntsen, C.A. and R.H. Freyberg. 1961. Rheumatoid patients after five or more years of corticosteroid treatment: A comparative analysis of 183 cases. *Ann. Intern. Med.* 54:938–953.

52. Hansen, T.M., P. Kryger, H. Elling, et al. 1990. Double blind placebo controlled trial of pulse treatment with methylprednisolone combined with disease modifying drugs in rheumatoid arthritis. *BMJ* 301:268–270.

53. Porter, D. 1995. Glucocorticoids and joint destruction in rheumatoid arthritis (letter to editor). *N. Engl. J. Med.* 333:1569.

54. Hickling, P., R.K. Jacoby, and J.R. Kirwan. 1998. Joint destruction after glucocorticoids are withdrawn in early rheumatoid arthritis. *Br. J. Rheumatol.* 37:930–936.

55. Sharif, M., C. Salisbury, D.J. Taylor, and J.R. Kirwan. 1998. Changes in biochemical markers of joint tissue metabolism in a randomized controlled trial of glucocorticoid in early rheumatoid arthritis. *Arthritis Rheum.* 41(7):1203–1209.

56. Wassenberg, S., R. Rau, and H. Zeidler. 1999. Low dose prednisolone therapy (LDPT) retards radiographically detectable destruction in early rheumatoid arthritis. *Arthritis Rheum.* 42(9 (Suppl.): S243.

57. van Everdingen, A.A., J.W.G. Jacobs, D.R. van Reesema, and W.J. Bijlsma. 1999. Low dose glucocorticoids in early RA inhibit radiological joint damage. *Arthritis Rheum.* 42(9) (Suppl.):S271.

58. Arvidson, N.G., B. Gudbjornsson, A. Larsson, and R. Hallgren. 1997. The timing of glucocorticoid administration in rheumatoid arthritis. *Ann. Rheum. Dis.* 56:27–31.

59. Fitzcharles, M.A., J. Halsey, and H.L.F. Currey. 1982. Conversion from daily to alternate daily corticosteroids in rheumatoid arthritis. *Ann. Rheum. Dis.* 41:66–68.

60. Neustadt, D.H. 1983. Recent strategies in the use of corticosteroids in rheumatoid arthritis. *Clin. Rheum. Pract.* (5):196-204.

61. Corkhill, M.M., B.W. Jirkham, K. Chikanza, T. Gibson, and G.S. Panayi. 1990. Intramuscular depot methylprednisolone induction of chrysotherapy in rheumatoid arthritis: a 24 week randomised controlled trial. *Br. J. Rheumatol.* 29:274–279.

62. Gough, A., T. Sheeran, V. Arthur, G. Panayi, and P. Emery, 1994. Adverse interaction between intramuscular methylprednisolone and sulphasalazine in patients with early rheumatoid arthritis. *Scand. J. Rheumatol.* 23:46–48.

63. Liebling, M.R., E. Leib, and K. McLaughlin, 1981. Pulse methylprednisolone in rheumatoid arthritis. *Ann. Intern. Med.* 4:21–26.

64. Forster, P.J.G., K.A. Grindulis, and V. Neumann, et al. 1982. High dose intravenous methylprednisolone in rheumatoid arthritis. *Ann. Rheum. Dis.* 41:444–446.

65. Stubbs, S.S., and R.M. Morrell. 1973. Intravenous methylprednisolone sodium succinate: Adverse reactions reported in association with immunosuppressive therapy. *Transplant Proc.* 5:1145–1146.

66. Heytman, M., M.J. Ahern, M.D. Smith, and P.J. Roberts-Thomson. 1994. The long term effect of pulsed corticosteroids on the efficacy and toxicity of chrysotherapy in rheumatoid arthritis. *J. Rheumatol.* 21:435–441.

67. Hollander, J. 1969. Intra-synovial corticosteroid therapy in arthritis. *MD State. Med. J.* 19: 62–66.

68. Gray, R.G., J. Tenenbaum, and N.L. Gottlieb. 1981. Local corticosteroid injection treatment in rheumatic disorders. *Semin. Arthritis Rheum.* 10:231–254.

69. Dockery, K., A. Sismanis, and E. Abedi, 1991. Rheumatoid arthritis of the larynx: the importance of early diagnosis and corticosteroid therapy. *South. Med. J.* 84:95.

70. Habib, M.A. 1977. Intra-articular steroid injection in acute rheumatoid arthritis of the larynx. *J. Laryngol. Otol.* 91:909.

71. Emkey, R.D., R. Lindsay, J. Lyssy, et. al. 1996. The systemic effect of intraarticular administration of corticosteroid on markers on bone formation and bone resorption in patients with rheumatoid arthritis. *Arthritis Rheum.* 39:277–282.

72. Green, M.J., P.G. Conaghan, S. Proudman, et al. 1999. 2 year longitudinal bone densitometry to assess efficacy and toxicity of combination therapy including intra-articular corticosteroid injections in severe early RA. *Arthritis Rheum.* 42(9) (Suppl.):S238.

73. Bentley, G., and J.W. Goodfellow. 1969. Disorganization of the knees following intra-articular hydrocortisone injections. *J. Bone Joint Surg.* 51B:498–502.

74. Noyes, F.R., E.S. Grood, N.L. Nussbaum, et al. 1977. Effect of intraarticular corticosteroids on ligament properties: a biochemical and histologic study in rhesus knees. *Clin. Orthop.* 123:197–209.

75. Matteson, E.L., and D.L. Conn., M.H. Weisman, M.E. Weinblatt, editors. 1995. Extraarticular manifestations of rheumatoid arthritis. In: Treatment of the Rheumatic Diseases: Companion to the Textbook of Rheumatology. Philadelphia: W. B. Saunders; 52–67.

76. Turner-Warwick, M., and R.C. Evans. 1977. Pulmonary manifestations of rheumatoid disease. *Clin. Rheum. Dis.* 3:549.

77. Wallaert, B., P.Y. Hatron, J.M. Grosbois, et al. 1986. Subclinical pulmonary involvement in collagen vascular diseases assessed by bronchoalveolar lavage. *Am. Rev. Respir. Dis.* 133:574.

78. Saag, K.G., J. Kline, G. Hunninghake. 1998. Interstitial Lung Diseases. In: G.L. Baum, J.D. Crapo, B.R. Celli, and J.B. Karlinsky, eds. Textbook of Pulmonary Diseases. 6th ed. Philadelphia: Lippincott-Raven; 341–365.

79. van Thiel, R.J., S. van der Burg, A.D. Groote, G.D. Nossent, and S.H. Wills. 1991. Bronchiolitis obliterans organizing pneumonia and rheumatoid arthritis. *Eur. Respir. J.* 4:905.

80. Franco, A.E., H.D. Levine, and A.P. Hall. 1972. Rheumatoid pericarditis: report of 17 cases diagnosed clinically. *Ann. Intern. Med.* 77:837.

81. Watson, P.G. and S.S. Hayreh. 1976. Scleritis and episcleritis. *Br. J. Ophthalmol.* 60:163.

82. Watson, P. 1980. The diagnosis and management of scleritis. *Ophthalmol.* 87:716.

83. Kemper, J.W., A.H. Baggenstoss, and C.H. Slocumb. 1957. The relationship of therapy with cortisone to the incidence of vascular lesions in rheumatoid arthritis. *Ann. Intern. Med.* 46:831.

84. Conn, D.L., R.B. Tompkins, and W.L. Nichols. 1988. Glucocorticosteroids in the management of vasculitis: a double-edged sword? *J. Rheumatol.* 15:1181.

85. Cash, J.M., and R.L. Wilder. 1995. Treatment-resistant rheumatoid arthritis. *Rheum. Dis. Clin. NA* 21:1–18.

86. Rayburn, W.F. 1992. Glucocorticoid therapy for rheumatic diseases: maternal, fetal, and breast-feeding considerations. *Am. J. Reprod. Immunol.* 28:138–140.

87. Reinisch, J.M., N. Simon, W. Karow, and R. Gandelman. 1978. Prenatal exposure to prednisone in humans and animals retards intrauterine growth. *Science* 202:436–438.

88. Committee on Drugs American Academy of Pediatrics 1989. The transfer of drugs and other chemicals into human breast milk. *Pediatrics* 84:924–936.

89. Katz, F.H., and B.R. Duncan. 1975. Entry of prednisone into human milk. *N. Engl. J. Med.* 293:1154.

90. Ost, L., G. Wettrell, I. Bjorkhem, and A. Rane. 1985. Prednisolone excretion in human milk. *J. Pediatr.* 106:1008–1011.

91. Lockie, L.M., E. Gomez, and D.M. Smith.1983. Low dose adrenocorticosteroids in the management of elderly patients with rheumatoid arthritis: selected examples and summary of efficacy in the long-term treatment of 97 patients. *Sem. Arth. Rheum.* 12(4):373–381.

92. Haugeberg, G., T. Uhlig, J.A. Falch, J.I. Halse, and T.K. Kvien. 2000. Bone mineral density and frequency of osteoporosis in female patients with rheumatoid arthritis. Arthritis Rheum. 43(3): 522–530.

93. Scott, D.L., D.P.M. Symmons, B.L. Coulton, et al. 1987. Long-term outcome of treating rheumatoid arthritis: results after 20 years. *Lancet* 1108–1111.

94. Wolfe, F., D.M. Mitchell, J.T. Sibley, et al. 1994. The mortality of rheumatoid arthritis. *Arthritis Rheum.* 37:481–494.

95. Fries, J.F., C.A. Williams, D. Ramey, et al. 1993. The relative toxicity of disease-modifying antirheumatic drugs. *Arthritis Rheum.* 36:297–306.

96. McDougall, R., J. Sibley, M. Haga, and A. Russell. 1994. Outcome in patients with rheumatoid arthritis receiving prednisone compared to matched controls. *J. Rheum.* 21:1207–1213.

97. Pincus, T., S.B. Marcum, and L.F. Callahan. 1992. Longterm drug therapy for rheumatoid arthritis in seven rheumatology private practices: II. Second line drugs and prednisone. *J. Rheumatol.* 19:1885–1894.

98. Lukert, B.P., and L.G. Raisz. 1990. Glucocorticoid-induced osteoporosis: pathogenesis and management. *Ann. Intern. Med.* 112:352–364.

99. Manolagas, S.C., R.S. Weinstein. 1999. New developments in the pathogenesis and treatment of steroid-induced osteoporosis. *J. Bone Miner Res.* 14:1061–1066.

100. Dykman, T.R., O.S. Gluck, W.A. Murphy, T.J. Hahn, and B.H. Hahn. 1985. Evaluation of factors associated with glucocorticoid-induced osteopenia in patients with rheumatic diseases. *Arthritis Rheum.* 28:361–368.

101. Laan, R.F.J.M., P.L.C.M. van Riel, L.B.A. van de Putte, et al. 1993. Low-dose prednisone induces rapid reversible axial bone loss in patients with rheumatoid arthritis. *Ann. Intern. Med.* 119:963–968.

102. Sambrook, P.N., J.A. Eisman, M.G. Yeates, et. al. 1986. Osteoporosis in rheumatoid arthritis: safety of low dose corticosteroids. *Ann. Rheum. Dis.* 45:950–953.

103. Verstraeten, A., and J. Dequeker, 1986. Vertebral and peripheral bone mineral content and fracture incidence in postmenopausal patients with rheumatoid arthritis: effect of low dose corticosteroids. *Ann. Rheum. Dis.* 45:852–857.

104. Reid, I.R., and A.B. Grey. 1993. Corticosteroid osteoporosis. *Bailliere's Clin. Rheumatol.* 7:573–587.

105. LoCasio, V., E. Bonucci, B. Imbimbo, et al. 1984. Bone loss after glucocorticoid therapy. *Bone Mineral* 8:39–51.

106. Hochberg, M.C., P.D. Ross, D. Black, et al. 1999. Larger increases in bone mineral density during alendronate therapy are associated with a lower risk of new vertebral fractures in women with postmenopausal osteoporosis. *Arthritis Rheum.* 42(6):1246–1254.

107. Wasnick, R.D., and P.D. Miller. 2000. Antifracture efficacy of antiresorptive agents are related to changes in bone density. *J. Clin. Endocrinol. Metab.* 85:231–236.

108. Peel, N.F.A., D.J. Moore, N.A. Barrington, D.E. Bax, and R. Eastell. 1995. Risk of vertebral fracture and relationship to bone mineral density in steroid treated rheumatoid arthritis. *Ann. Rheum. Dis.* 54:801–806.

109. O'Malley, M., A.J. Kenrick, D.J. Sartoris, et al. 1989. Axial bone density in rheumatoid arthritis: comparison of dual-energy projection radiography and dual-photon absorptiometry. *Radiology* 170:501–505.

110. Verhoeven, A.C., and M. Boers. 1997. Limited bone loss due to corticosteroids: a systematic review of prospective studies in rheumatoid arthritis and other diseaes. *J. Rheumatol.* 24:1495–503.

111. Messina, O.D., J.C. Barreira, J.R. Zanchetta, et al. 1992. Effect of low doses of deflazacort vs prednisone on bone mineral content in premenopausal rheumatoid arthritis. *J. Rheumatol.* 19:1520–1526.

112. Poole, A.R., and P. Dieppe. 1994. Biological markers in rheumatoid arthritis. *Semin. Arthritis Rheum.* 23:17–31.

113. Guyatt, G.H., C.E. Webber, A.A. Mewa, et al. 1984. Determining causation-a case study: adrenocorticosteroids and osteoporosis. *J. Chron. Dis.* 37:343–352.

114. Sambrook, P.N., M.L. Cohen, J.A. Eisman, N.A. Pocock, G.D. Champion, and M.G. Yeates. 1989. Effects of low dose corticosteroids on bone mass in rheumatoid arthritis: a longitudinal study. *Ann. Rheum. Dis.* 48:535–538.

115. Gough, K.S., J. Lilley, S. Eyre, R.L. Holder, and P. Emery. 1994. Generalized bone loss in patients with early rheumatoid arthritis. *Lancet* 344:23–27.

116. Hall, G.M., T.D. Spector, J.A. Griffin, A.S.M. Jawad, M.L. Hall, and D.V. Doyle. 1993. The effect of rheumatoid arthritis and steroid therapy on bone density in postmenopausal women. *Arthritis Rheum.* 36:1510–1516.

117. Lane, N.E., A.R. Pressman, V.L. Star, S.R. Cummings, and M.C. Nevitt. 1995. Rheumatoid arthritis and bone mineral density in elderly women. *J. Bone Min. Res.* 10:257–263.

118. Gough, A., P. Sambrook, J. Devlin, et al. 1998. Osteoclastic activation is the principal mechanism leading to secondary osteoporosis in rheumatoid arthritis. *J. Rheumatol.* 25:1282–1289.

119. Towheed, T.E., D. Brouillard, E. Yendt, and T. Anastassiades. 1995. Osteoporosis in rheumatoid arthritis: Findings in the metacarpal, spine, and hip and a study of the determinants of both localized and generalized osteopenia. *J. Rheumatol.* 22:440–443.

120. Spector, T.D., G.M. Hall, E.V. McCloskey, and J.A. Kanis. 1993. Risk of vertebral fracture in women with rheumatoid arthritis. *BMJ* 306:558.

121. Cooper, C., C. Coupland, and M. Mitchell. 1995. Rheumatoid arthritis, corticosteroid therapy and hip fracture. *Ann. Rheum. Dis.* 54:49–52.

122. Luengo, M., C. Picado, L. Del Rio, N. Guanabens, J.M. Montserrat, and J. Setoain. 1991. Vertebral fractures in steroid dependent asthma and involutional osteoporosis: a comparative study. *Thorax* 46:803–806.

123. Michel, B.A., D.A. Bloch, and J.F. Fries. 1991. Predictors of fractures in early rheumatoid arthritis. *J. Rheumatol.* 18:804–808.

124. Baltzan, M.A., S. Suissa, D.C. Bauer, and S.R. Cummings. 1999. Hip fractures attributable to corticosteroid use (research letters). *Lancet* 353(9161):1327.

125. Gluck, O.S., W.A. Murphy, and T.J. Hahn, et al. 1981. Bone loss in adults receiving alternate day glucocorticoid therapy. *Arthritis Rheum.* 24:892–898.

126. Kroger, H., R. Honaken, S. Saarikoski, and E. Alhava. 1994. Decreased axial bone mineral density in perimenopausal women with rheumatoid arthritis-a population based study. *Ann. Rheum. Dis.* 53:18–23.

127. Reid, I.R., and S.W. Heap. 1990. Determinants of vertebral mineral density in patients receiving long-term glucocorticoid therapy. *Arch. Intern. Med.* 150:2545–2548.

128. Teelucksingh, S., P.L. Padfield, L. Tibi, K.L. Gough, and P.R. Holt. 1991. Inhaled corticosteroids, bone formation, and osteocalcin. *Lancet* 338(8758):60–1.

129. Marystone, J.F., E.L. Barrett-Connor, and D.J. Morton. 1995. Inhaled and oral corticosteroids: their effects on bone mineral density in older adults. *Am. J. Public Health* 1995;85:1693–1695.

130. Vreden, S.G.S., A.R.M.M. Hermus, P.A. van Liessum, et al. 1991. Aseptic bone necrosis in patients on glucocorticoid replacement therapy. *Neth. J. Med.* 39:153–157.

131. Zizic, T.M., C. Marcoux, and D.S. Hungerford. 1985. Corticosteroid therapy associated with ischemic necrosis of bone in systemic lupus erythematosus. *Am. J. Med.* 79:596–604.

132. Afifi, A.K., A. Bergman, and J.C. Harvey. 1968. Steroid myopathy: clinical histologic and cytologic observations. *Johns Hopkins Med. J.* 123:158.

133. Lieberman, P., R. Patterso, and R. Kunske. 1972. Complications of long-term steroid therapy for asthma. *J. Allergy Clin. Immunol.* 49:329–336.

134. Jackson, S.H.D., D.G. Beevers, and K. Myers. 1981. Does long-term low-dose corticosteroid therapy cause hypertension? *Clin. Sci.* 61:381s–383s.

135. Pasceri, V., and E.T.H. Yeh. 1999. A tale of two diseases: atherosclerosis and rheumatoid arthritis (editorial). *Circulation* 100(21):2124–2126.

136. Kalbak, K. 1972. Incidence of arteriosclerosis in patients with rheumatoid arthritis receiving long-term corticosteroid therapy. *Ann. Rheum. Dis.* 31:196–200.

137. Svenson, K.L.G., H. Lithell, R. Hällgren, et al. 1987. Serum lipoprotein in active rheumatoid arthritis and other chronic inflammatory arthritides: II. Effects of anti-inflammatory and disease-modifying drug treatment. *Arch. Intern. Med.* 147:1917–1920.

138. Shubin, H. 1965. Long term (five or more years) administration of corticosteroids in pulmonary diseases. *Dis. Chest.* 48:287–290.

139. Bollet, A.J., R. Black, and J.J. Bunim. 1955. Major undesirable side-effects resulting from prednisolone and prednisone. *JAMA* 158:459–463.

140. Messer, J., D. Reitman, H.S. Sacks, H.J. Smith, and T.C. Chalmers. 1983. Association of adrenocorticosteroid therapy and peptic-ulcer disease. *N. Engl. J. Med.* 309:21–24.

141. Piper, J.M., W.A. Ray, J.R. Daugherty, and M.R. Griffin. 1991. Corticosteroid use and peptic ulcer disease: role of noncorticosteroidal anti-inflammatory drugs. *Ann. Intern. Med.* 114:735–740.

142. Canter, J.W., and P.E. Shorb Jr. 1971. Acute perforation of colonic diverticula associated with prolonged adrenocorticosteroid therapy. *Am. J. Surg.* 46–51.

143. Nelp, W.B. 1961. Acute pancreatitis associated with steroid therapy. *Arch. Int. Med.* 108: 702–710.

144. Sterioff, S., M. Orringer, and J. Cameron. 1974. Colon perforations associated with steroid therapy. *Surgery* 75:56–58.

145. Gabriel, S.E., L. Jaakkimainen, and C. Bombardier. 1991. Risk for serious gastrointestinal complications related to use of nonsteroidal anti-inflammatory drugs. *Ann. Intern. Med.* 115:787–796.

146. Fauci, A.S. 1976. Glucocorticosteroid Therapy: Mechanisms of action and clinical considerations. *Ann. Intern. Med.* 1976;84:304–15.

147. Stuck, A.E., C.E. Minder, and F.J. Frey. 1989. Risk of infectious complications in patients taking glucocorticosteroids. *Rev. Infect. Dis.* 11:954–963.

148. Burry, H.C. 1973. Bacteriuria in rheumatoid arthritis. *Ann. Rheum Dis.* 32:208–211.

149. Hoogwerf, B., and R.D. Danese. 1999. Drug selection and the management of corticosteroid-related diabetes mellitus (Review). *Rheum. Dis. Clin. North Am.* 25(3):489–505.

150. Alavi, I.A., B.K. Sharma, and V.K.G. Pillay. 1971. Steroid-induced diabetic ketoacidosis. *Am. J. Med. Sci.* 262:15–23.

151. Olefsky, J.M., and G. Kimmerling. 1976. Effects of glucocorticoids on carbohydrate metabolism. *Am. J. Med. Sci.* 1976;271:202–210.

152. Streck, W.F., and D.H. Lockwood. 1979. Pituitary adrenal recovery following short-term suppression with corticosteroids. *Am. J. Med.* 66:910–914.

153. LaRochelle, G.E.J., A.G. LaRochelle, R.E. Ratner, et al. 1993. Recovery of the hypothalamic-pituitary-adrenal (HPA) axis in patients with rheumatic diseases receiving low-dose prednisone. *Am. J. Med.* 95:258–264.

154. Daly, J.R., A.B. Myles, P.A. Bacon, et al. 1967. Pituitary adrenal function during corticosteroid withdrawal in rheumatoid arthritis. *Ann. Rheum. Dis.* 26:18–24.

155. Dixon, R.B., and N.P. Christy. 1980. On the various forms of corticosteroid withdrawal syndrome. *Am. J. Med.* 68:224–230.

156. Glass, D., M.L. Snaith, A.S. Russell, and J.R. Daly. 1971. Possible unnecessary prolongation of corticosteroid therapy with rheumatoid arthritis. *Lancet* 2:334–337.

157. Keenan, P.A., M.W. Jacobson, R.M. Soleymani, et al. 1996. The effect on memory of chronic prednisone treatment in patients with systemic disease. *Neurology* 47:1396–1402.

158. Kershner, P., and R. Wang-Cheng. 1989. Psychiatric side effects of steroid therapy. *Psychomatics* 30:135–139.

159. Cumming, R.G., P. Mitchell, and S.R. Leeder. 1997. Use of inhaled corticosteroids and the risk of cataracts. *N. Engl. J. Med.* 337:8–14.

160. Skalka, H.W., and J.T. Prchal. 1980. Effect of corticosteroids on cataract formation. *Arch. Ophthalmol.* 98:1773–1777.

161. Berkowitz, J.S, D.S. David, and S. Sakai, et al. 1973. Ocular complications in renal transplant recipients. *Am. J. Med.* 55:492–495.

162. Garbe, E., J. LeLorier, J.-F. Biobin, and S. Suissa. 1997. Risk of ocular hypertension or open-angle glaucoma in elderly patients on oral glucocorticoids. *Lancet* 350:979–82.

163. Francois, J. 1977. Corticosteroid glaucoma. *Ann. Ophthalmol.* 1075–1080.

164. Tripathi, R.C., S.K. Parapuram, B.J. Tripathi, Y. Zhong, and K.V. Chalam. 1999. Corticosteroids and glaucoma risk (review). *Drugs and Aging* 15(6):439–450.

165. Garbe, E., J. LeLorier, J-F. Boivin, and S. Suissa. 1997. Inhaled and nasal glucocorticoids and the risks of ocular hypertension or open-angle glaucoma. *JAMA* 277:722.

166. Sambrook, P., J. Birmingham, P. Kelly, et al. 1993. Prevention of corticosteroid osteoporosis. A comparison of calcium, calcitriol, and calcitonin. *N. Engl. J. Med.* 328:1747–1752.

167. Buckley, L.M., E.S. Leib, K.S. Cartularo, P.M. Vacek, and S.M. Cooper. 1996. Calcium and vitamin D3 supplementation prevents bone loss in the spine secondary to low-dose corticosteroids in patients with rheumatoid arthritis. *Ann. Intern. Med.* 125:961–968.

168. Saag, K.G., R. Emkey, T. Schnitzer, et al. 1998. Alendronate for the treatment and prevention of glucocorticoid-induced osteoporosis. *N. Engl. J. Med.* 339:292–299.

169. Adachi, J.D., W.G. Bensen, J. Brown, D. Hanley, et al. 1997. Intermittent etidronate therapy to prevent corticosteroid-induced osteoporosis. *N. Engl. J. Med.* 337:382–387.

170. Reid, D., C. Cohen, S. Pack, A. Chines, and D. Ethgen. 1998. Risedronate reduces the incidence of vertebral fratures in patients on chronic corticosteroid therapy. *Arthritis Rheum.* 41:S136.

171. Cohen, S., R.M. Levy, Keller M., et al. 1999. Risedronate therapy prevents corticosteroid-induced bone loss: A twelve-month, multicenter, randomized, double-blind, placebo-controlled, parallel-group study. Arthritis Rheum. 42(11):2309–2318.

172. Adachi, J., and G. Ioannidis. 2000. Primer on Corticosteroid-Induced Osteoporosis. Philadelphia: Lippincott-Williams and Wilkins.

173. Peat, I.D., S. Healy, D.M. Reid, et. al. 1995. Steroid induced osteoporosis: an opportunity for prevention? *Ann. Rheum. Dis.* 54:66–68.

174. Buckley, L.M., M. Marquez, R. Feezor, D.M. Ruffin, and L.L. Benson. 1999. Prevention of corticosteroid-induced osteoporosis. *Arthritis Rheum.* 42(8):1736–1739.

175. Aagaard, E., P. Lin, G. Modin, and N.E. Lane. 1999. Prevention of glucocorticoid-induced osteoporosis: Provider practice at an urban county hospital. *Am. J. Med.* 107:456–460.

176. Osiri, M., K.G. Saag, A.M. Ford, and L.W. Moreland. 2000. Practice pattern variation among internal medicine specialists in the prevention of glucocorticoid-induced osteoporosis. *J. Clin. Rheumatol.* 6:117–122.

6

Anti-Tumor Necrosis Factor Agents

Alan K. Matsumoto and Joan M. Bathon

CONTENTS

INTRODUCTION

The development of inhibitors of tumor necrosis factor (TNF) evolved from a targeted bench-to-bedside approach in which lessons learned from basic pathophysiological research were tested in patients with debilitating chronic inflammatory diseases, particularly rheumatoid arthritis (RA) and inflammatory bowel disease. Insofar as all prior treatments for (RA) evolved primarily from serendipitous observations, the TNF inhibitors represent the first "rationally based" treatment, as well as the first Food and Drug Administration (FDA)-approved recombinant proteins ("biologics") for the treatment of RA. This chapter will focus on RA as a paradigm for examining the role of TNF in the pathogenesis and propagation of chronic inflammation, and for evaluating anti-TNF therapy as a strategy for the treatment of chronic inflammatory disease.

RA is a chronic disease with genetic and autoimmune components that is characterized by intense inflammation, resulting in destruction and dysfunction of the joints and, potentially, other organs as well. The characteristic histopathologic findings in the joint are hyperplasia of the synovial lining (or intima), which consists primarily of macrophages and fibroblasts, and an inflammatory influx of lymphocytes, plasma cells, and other cell types in the subintimal area *(1)*. In addition, the joint cavity is invaded by large numbers of activated neutrophils. The destruction of articular cartilage and bone is presumed to occur not only from the direct invasion of contiguous hypertrophied synovium, but also by the synovial fluid neutrophils bathing the cartilage, and by resident chondrocytes, which become activated to degrade their surrounding matrix *(1)*.

From: *Modern Therapeutics in Rheumatic Diseases*
Edited by: G. C. Tsokos, et al. © Humana Press, Inc., Totowa, NJ

Work by Stastny *(2)* and Nepom *(3,4)* more than 15 years ago demonstrated the association of HLA-DR4, a Class II major histocompatibility antigen, with RA. The specificity for this association resides in a conserved five amino acid sequence in the DR-β chain of the associated DR4 alleles (and in several other DR molecules), and is referred to as the "shared epitope" *(5)*. Recent work has suggested that the shared epitope not only conveys disease susceptibility, but is also a marker of disease severity and of extra-articular manifestations, at least in Caucasian patients *(6,7)*. Furthermore, results from epidemiologic and family studies are consistent with the involvement of multiple genes, rather than a single gene, in conveying susceptibility to rheumatoid arthritis. Candidate genes currently under investigation include T-cell receptor, TNF-α, hsp 70, large multifunctional protease (LMP) , and transporter associated with antigen processing (TAP) *(8)*.

RA is also characterized by the presence of several autoantibodies. The most prominent of these is the so-called "rheumatoid factor," an antibody (usually IgM) directed against self-IgG, which occurs in approx 80% of patients with RA. Other autoantibodies described in RA include those directed against keratin, glycoprotein-39, collagen type II, p205, and the G1 domain of aggrecan *(9–12)*. None of these autoantibodies, including rheumatoid factor, is specific to RA, and it is more likely that they play a role in propagating inflammation rather than serving as causative agents.

While the identification of susceptibility genes, and the role of autoantibodies, remain to be clarified in RA it is clear that the sustained inflammatory process, leading to the secretion of matrix-degrading proteases, is ultimately responsible for joint damage and dysfunction in RA. Attention has focused recently, therefore, on strategies that will interrupt this inflammatory cycle. A major advance in this regard is the elucidation of the role of TNF-α in this destructive process.

PATHOGENIC MECHANISMS

The Rheumatoid Synovium

The rheumatoid synovium is hyperplastic with increased numbers of macrophages, fibroblasts, and lymphocytes. Activated T cells and T-cell-derived cytokines have been difficult to identify in the rheumatoid synovium *(13)*, and clinical trials in RA of agents designed to deplete, or inhibit function of, T cells have demonstrated only modest, transient clinical improvement (reviewed in ref. *14*). In contrast, there is an abundance of macrophage and fibroblast-derived cytokines, proteases, and prostanoids in the rheumatoid synovium and synovial fluid *(13,15)*. These observations have led to the suggestion that, although a T-cell mediated, antigen-specific process is undoubtedly critical to the initiation of disease, sustained inflammation is at least equally dependent on cytokine production by synovial macrophages and fibroblasts, which may act on each other in an autocrine or paracrine manner *(16)*. Thus, TNF-α and IL-1, which are primarily products of macrophages, induce the synthesis and secretion from synovial fibroblasts of matrix-degrading proteases, prostanoids, interleukin-6 (IL-6), interleukin-8 (IL-8), and granulocyte-macrophage colony stimulating factor (GM-CSF) *(17,18)* (Fig. 1). Local synthesis of IL-6 promotes the synthesis of immunoglobulins, including rheumatoid factor, by synovial plasma cells; IL-8 induces selective recruitment of neutrophils to the joint cavity; prostaglandin E_2 causes bone resorption; and the

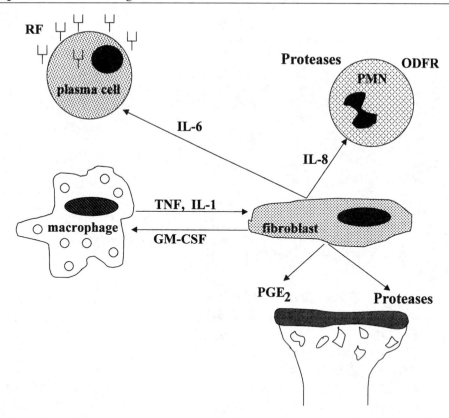

Fig. 1. Simplified scheme of interaction of synovial macrophages and fibroblasts.

matrix metalloproteases degrade the extracellular matrices of bone and cartilage. TNF-α and IL-1 also induce a variety of adhesion molecules, which enables the influx of inflammatory cells to the rheumatoid joint *(19,20)*. GM-CSF produced by the fibroblast may contribute in a positive feedback loop to sustaining macrophage activation, although some have suggested that the fibroblast may become independent of macrophage influence by transformation to an autonomous phenotype *(21)*.

These in vitro observations, suggesting a central of TNF-α and IL-1 in the pathogenesis of RA, prompted a series of studies in animal models and in patients to provide "proof of concept." Two IL-1 inhibitors have been evaluated in patients with longstanding RA: a soluble human type I IL-1 receptor (sHuIL-1R), and a human IL-1 receptor antagonist (IL-1ra). Clinical results were discouraging for both constructs (reviewed in ref. *14*). However, the selection of the sHuIL-1R was premature as subsequent data confirmed a higher affinity of sHuIL-1R for IL-1ra over IL-1 *(22)*; and, in the case of IL-1ra, its only modest performance may be owing to a short half-life. Although IL-1 and TNF-α act alone and synergistically to elicit a nearly identical spectrum of biological responses *(23)*, it has been suggested that a hierarchy exists in which IL-1 acts downstream of TNF-α—for example, blocking TNF-α abolishes IL-1 production and bioactivity in synovial-cell cultures *(24)*. The relative contribution of each cytokine to rheumatoid joint damage remains controversial. Nonetheless, therapeutic attention has predominantly focused on inhibition of TNF-α.

Table 1
Selected Members of the TNF Ligand/Receptor Superfamily[a]

Ligands	Receptors
Lymphotoxin-α	TNF-R1 and -RII
TNF-α	TNF-RI and -RII
Lymphotoxin-β	LT-βR
OX40L	OX40
CD40L	CD40
FasL	Fas
CD27L	CD27
CD30L	CD30
4-1BBL	4-1BB

[a]This is not a complete list. For complete list of TNF ligands and receptors, and updated nomenclature, *see* ref. *81.*

TNF and TNF Receptors

TNF-α was originally named for its ability to trigger necrosis of transplanted tumor cells in mice *(25)*. The purification and cloning of cachectin, a mediator of wasting in chronic diseases, was subsequently found to be identical to TNF-α *(26)*. TNF is produced primarily by macrophages and, to a lesser extent, by lymphocytes *(26)*. It is one of 17 known members of a family of polypeptides that bind to a corresponding family of receptors. The polypeptide ligands are characterized by a common core sequence predicted to contain 10 β-sheet forming sequences, and include TNF-α, lymphotoxin-α and-β, Fas ligand, CD40 ligand, and others *(27)* (Table 1). TNF-α is initially synthesized and expressed as a transmembrane molecule, the extracellular portion of which is subsequently cleaved by TNF-α converting enzyme (TACE) to release the soluble 17 kDa molecule. Soluble TNF-α circulates as a homotrimer and engages its cognate receptors on cell surfaces *(28)*.

In contrast to the relatively restricted synthesis of TNF-α by macrophages and T cells, TNF receptors (TNF-R) are expressed by nearly every mammalian cell. This ubiquitous expression, in conjunction with cell-specific effector molecules that are triggered by the TNF-R, may explain the variety of effects of TNF, which include apoptosis, the synthesis of protein and lipid inflammatory molecules, and transcription factors *(27,28)*. Unlike other ligands of the TNF-R family that bind to a single receptor, TNF and lymphotoxin-α are capable of binding to each of the two TNF-R designated as TNF-RI (or p55) and TNF-RII (or p75) *(28)*. Interaction of TNF with its receptor triggers a conformational change and dimerization or clustering of receptors that, in turns, triggers the cellular response *(29)*. TNF-R, like their ligand, can be cleaved from the cell surface by TACE *(30)* but soluble TNF-R are believed to be present in small amounts relative to membrane-bound TNF-R *(28)*.

The effects of TNF are mediated by its ability to directly or indirectly trigger a variety of signal-transduction pathways including proteases of the caspase family, transcription factors, phospholipases, and protein kinases. TNF-induced activation of the cysteine protease family of caspases leads to apoptotic cell death *(31)*. In contrast, the induction by TNF of cytokine production is mediated, at least in part, by its ability to

Table 2
TNF Inhibitors Currently Approved or in Development

Name	Description	Status
Infliximab	Mouse-human chimeric anti-huTNF MAb	FDA-approved
D2E7	Fully human anti-huTNF MAb	In development
Etanercept	p75sTNF-RII-Fc (dimeric)	FDA-approved
NA	PEG-p55sTNF-RI (monomeric)	In development
Lenercept	p55sTNF-RI-IgG1 (dimeric)	Development terminated

NA, not available.

enhance gene expression and/or increase stability of messenger RNA. Gene expression is upregulated by TNF either via activation of transcription factors such as *NF-κB*, or increased synthesis of transcription factors such as *IRF1*. TNF signaling mechanisms have been reviewed in detail recently *(27)*. An unanswered question is whether the TNF-R have any intrinsic mechanism for downregulating their responses to TNF-α, such as desensitization or internalization, or whether the receptor continues to signal as long as TNF-α is available.

Development of TNF Inhibitors

The two strategies for inhibiting TNF that have been most extensively studied to date consist of monoclonal anti-TNF antibodies and soluble TNF receptors (sTNF-R) (Table 2). Both constructs will theoretically bind to circulating TNF-α, thus limiting its ability to engage cell membrane-bound TNF receptors and activate inflammatory pathways. Soluble TNF-R, but not anti-TNF antibodies, would also be expected to bind lymphotoxin.

With regard to anti-TNF monoclonal antibodies (MAbs), the best studied to date is infliximab (Remicade™), originally referred to as cA2. Infliximab is a chimeric human/mouse anti-TNF-α MAb composed of the constant regions of human (Hu) IgG1κ, coupled to the Fv region of a high-affinity neutralizing murine anti-HuTNFα antibody *(32)*. The antibody exhibits high affinity (K^a 10^{10}/mol) for recombinant and natural huTNF-α, and neutralizes TNF-mediated cytotoxicity and other functions in vitro *(32)*. It has been extensively studied in animal models of arthritis, as well as in patients with RA and inflammatory bowel disease, and is now approved for use in both diseases (*see* below). Because of the potential for an immune reaction to the mouse protein components of a chimeric antibody, an alternate strategy has been to develop a fully human anti-TNF MAb. One such antibody, known as D2E7, was generated by phage- display technology. A high-affinity murine anti-TNF MAb was used as a template for guided selection, which involves complete replacement of the murine heavy and light chains with human counterparts and subsequent optimization of the antigen-binding affinity *(33)*. Although not FDA-approved, early clinical trials with D2E7 are also promising and are discussed briefly below.

In the second approach to TNF inhibition, soluble TNF-R have been engineered as fusion proteins in which the extracellular ligand-binding portion of the huTNF-RI or huTNF-RII is coupled to a human immunoglobulin-like molecule. Although TNF-RI is thought to mediate most of the biological effects of TNF in vivo *(28)*, engineered sTNF-RI and sTNF-RII constructs both appear to be effective in vivo inhibitors of TNF. Although these constructs consist entirely of human protein, the linkage region between the receptor and the immunoglobulin molecule represents an unnatural sequence and, therefore, has the potential for eliciting an anti-drug antibody response. This was the case with lenercept, a fusion protein of two sTNF-RI (p55) with human IgG1-Fc. Pharmacokinetic data indicated enhanced clearance of lenercept with repeated dosing due to the development of anti-lenercept antibodies, and there was an inverse correlation of drug concentration with antibody levels *(34)*. Although the antibodies were non-neutralizing and patients treated with lenercept demonstrated clinical improvement, further development of the drug was terminated in view of concerns about durability of the response and long-term safety.

Etanercept (sTNF-RII:Fc; Enbrel™) is the best studied of the sTNF-R and is approved for the treatment of RA in adults and in children. Like lenercept, it is a dimeric construct in which two sTNF-RII (p75) are linked to the Fc portion of human IgG1 *(35)*. The dimeric receptor has a significantly higher affinity for TNF-α than the monomeric receptor (50–1000-fold higher), and the linkage to the Fc structure significantly prolongs the half-life of the construct in vivo *(35)*. Although it also has an unnatural linkage site, anti-etanercept antibodies have been infrequent. Another mechanism for prolonging the half-life of monomeric receptors is via conjugation with polyethylene glycol. One such construct, PEG-sTNF-RI (p55), has shown efficacy in several animal models of arthritis and is now in early clinical trials (*see* below).

ANIMAL STUDIES

Several lines of evidence exist in animal models that support the importance of TNF-α in the pathogenesis of human RA. Although no animal model of inflammatory arthritis is thought to completely mimic human RA, studies in animals have provided important information on inflammatory mediators and their potential as therapeutic targets in human disease. Most compelling are the findings of elevated levels of TNF-α in the joints of mice with collagen-induced arthritis (CIA), amelioration, or prevention of CIA with anti-TNF blocking antibodies and the spontaneous development of inflammatory arthritis in transgenic mice overexpressing TNF-α.

Collagen-induced arthritis (CIA) in the mouse is induced by immunization of susceptible mice strains with native type II collagen. Macroscopically evident arthritis occurs between d 28–35 after immunization and persists for several months until the joints ankylose *(36)*. CIA shares several histopathologic features with RA including mononuclear-cell infiltration and synovial-cell hyperplasia, resulting in pannus formation with bone and cartilage destruction. In both RA and CIA, disease susceptibility is restricted by MHC class II alleles *(37)* and autoreactive T cells are prominent in the joint with restriction in Vβ T-cell receptor usage *(38)*. Because of these similarities, CIA is a widely used experimental model for RA.

Similar to RA, several studies with CIA mice have demonstrated elevated TNF levels in the arthritic joints *(39–41)*. Recently, to assess the level of cytokine expression during the course of CIA, CIA mice were sacrificed on a weekly basis starting at d 21, before the onset of clinical arthritis. Cytokine mRNA levels in joint tissue were measured by highly quantitative RNA protection assays *(42)*. Levels of TNF-α together with TNF-β, interleukin 11 (IL-11), interleukin 1 receptor antagonist (IL-1Ra), macrophage inhibitory factor 1 α (MIP-1α), and RANTES were elevated early in the CIA disease course and persisted at high levels through the later stages. By contrast, IL-1β, IL-2, MIP-2, and IL-6 rose early in the disease course but rapidly returned to normal levels. Transforming growth factor β1 (TGF-β1), TGF-β2, and TGF-β3 increased slowly, peaking in late disease. Elevated TNF-α mRNA levels were also found in macroscopically and microscopically uninvolved joints. The pattern of persistent elevation TNF-α mRNA throughout the disease course and prior to the onset of arthritis supports the role of TNF-α both in the initiation and maintenance of chronic joint inflammation.

The availability of potent inhibitors of TNF-α have added valuable tools to further elucidate the importance of TNF-α in chronic inflammatory arthritis. CIA mice treated weekly with a neutralizing hamster MAb to TNF-α starting prior to the onset of arthritis, ameliorated the severity of the disease both histologically and clinically although the incidence of arthritis did not change. Antibody treatment starting soon after the onset of arthritis (d 30) had a similar but less pronounced effect on decreasing the severity of the arthritis *(43)*. Anti-TNF had diminishing benefit when used later in the disease course. Treatment of CIA mice with a neutralizing rat anti-TNF-α monoclonal was effective in improving joint scores when given before the onset or 2 d the onset of the arthritis, but was ineffective if given 7 d after onset of arthritis *(44)*. Of interest, use of a polyclonal antibody (PAb) against IL-1α and IL-1β was effective in CIA in both early and late disease. The effectiveness of anti-TNF therapy limited to early disease in murine CIA is in marked contrast to the efficacy of TNF inhibitors in humans with both early and longstanding RA (*see* Clinical Trials below).

Similar results were also obtained using a sTNF-R1- IgG1 fusion protein construct. Administration of the sTNF-R1-IgG1 starting prior to the onset of arthritis decreased severity of arthritis but differed from the MAb studies in decreasing the incidence of arthritis as well. Mice deficient in TNF-R1 by gene targeting were resistant to development of CIA, confirming the importance of TNF-R1 *(45)*, possibly through mediating TNF-induced adhesion-molecule expression and mononuclear-cell infiltration into the joint space *(46)*.

Transgenic mice expressing a modified human TNF-α transgene spontaneously develop a chronic polyarthritis, providing further evidence for the direct involvement of TNF in the pathogenesis of human RA *(47)*. Mice carrying a human TNF transgene with a modified 3′ region from a human globin gene show deregulated human TNF expression with constitutive low-level expression of TNF in a variety of tissues. In contrast, mice carrying a wild-type human TNF transgene show appropriate macrophage-specific inducible TNF expression in response to lipopolysaccharide. Mice with deregulated TNF expression develop a chronic symmetric polyarthritis with histologic features similar to human RA.

Despite the differences with human RA, these animal models support TNF as an important therapeutic target for RA. In addition, the models raise intriguing questions regarding other potential cytokine targets and the utility of inhibiting these targets at different stages of the disease process.

Table 3
Composite Scores for Assessing Clinical Responses in Rheumatoid Arthritis

ACR 20% Response[a]

    Must include: 20% improvement in tender joint count

                   20% improvement in swollen joint count

    And   20% improvement in 3 of 5 of the following criteria:

                   Patient pain assessment

                   Patient global assessment

                   Physician global assessment

                   Patient self-assessed disability

                   Acute phase reactant value (ESR or CRP)

Paulus 20% Response[b]

    Requires improvement in 4 of 6 criteria:

                   Painful joint score by 20%

                   Swollen joint score by 20%

                   Morning stiffness by 20%

                   ESR by 20%

                   Physician global assessment

                   Patient global assessment

[a]*See* ref. 57.
[b]*See* ref. 82.

CLINICAL TRIALS

The clinical efficacy of TNF inhibition has been studied most extensively in RA and, to a lesser extent, in inflammatory bowel disease. Data from clinical trials with etanercept and infliximab have been encouraging, and have resulted in the FDA approval of both agents for the treatment of RA, and of infliximab for inflammatory bowel disease (*see* Current Recommendations).

Because the safety of the TNF inhibitors in humans was unknown, early trials in RA targeted patients with severe, longstanding disease that had failed to respond adequately to conventional treatments such as methotrexate, gold salts, immunosuppressives, and others. More recently, as the safety of these agents unfolded, patients with juvenile RA and adults with early RA have been targeted. An evolution in the selection of study outcomes has also occurred in that earlier trials focused on clinical parameters as endpoints, whereas more recent trials have focused on structural (radiographic) endpoints.

Infliximab in Advanced RA

Favorable results for both safety and efficacy in a small open-label pilot study of infliximab in advanced RA *(32)* prompted a larger double-blind trial comparing infliximab to placebo *(48)*. In the latter study, 73 patients were randomized to a single infusion of infliximab 1 mg/kg or 10 mg kg or placebo, and their fulfillment at wk 4 of the Paulus 20% response criteria (*see* Table 3) was evaluated in an intention-to-treat analysis. The profile of participants in this study is very representative of most of the studies to follow—that is, predominantly women approx 50 yr of age with disease duration of 9–10 yr who had failed an average of three disease-modifying anti-rheumatic

Table 4
Effect of MTX on Frequency of Anti-Chimeric Antibody
Response in Patients Treated with Infliximab[a]

Infliximab, mg/kg	+ MTX	- MTX			+ MTX		
	0	1	3	10	1	3	10
Median duration of Paulus 20 response (wk)	0	2.6	17.2	10.4	16.5	16.5	>18.1
Antibody response, %	N/A	53	21	7	17	7	0

[a]From ref. 50.

drugs (DMARDs). Baseline disease activity was considerable as evidenced by a mean of 28 tender joints, 23 swollen joints, 3 h of morning stiffness, erythrocyte sedimentation rate (ESR) of 63, C-reactive protein (CRP) of 6.2 mg/dL. At wk 4, only 8% of placebo-treated patients fulfilled Paulus 20 and Paulus 50 criteria, whereas response rates in the high-dose infliximab group were 79 and 58% respectively, and in the low-dose group were 44 and 28%, respectively. Comparably dramatic decreases in acute-phase reactants, especially CRP, were observed in conjunction with clinical improvement, often within 2 wk of treatment. This important study provided the first proof-of-concept for a pivotal role for TNF-α in the inflammatory process in the rheumatoid joint. Equally important, the responses to infliximab were robust and rapid, and the treatment was well-tolerated (*see* Side Effects and Precautions).

Interestingly, some decay in the clinical and CRP responses was observed in the low-dose group by wk 4. Furthermore, several patients who were enrolled in a follow-up, multiple-dosing trial developed antichimeric antibodies, and a progressive decrease in the duration of the response to each successive infliximab infusion was noted in several patients (49). These observations raised the possibility that repeated dosing of infliximab may not be feasible in patients with anti-chimeric antibody response owing to a reduction in the half-life of infliximab.

This question was examined in a subsequent study by Maini et al. (50) in which the investigators reasoned that concomitant methotrexate might suppress the antibody response to infliximab. In this protocol, 101 patients with active RA despite methotrexate were randomized to treatment with placebo or one of three doses of infliximab (1, 3, or 10 mg/kg). Low-dose methotrexate (7.5 mg/wk) was continued throughout the study. Infliximab (or placebo) treatments were administered at 0, 2, 6, 10, and 14 wk, and Paulus response criteria were evaluated at 26 wk.

Robust clinical responses to infliximab alone were again observed at all three doses by wk 2 of treatment, but the low-dose (1 mg/kg) group became unresponsive to repeated dosing. Co-administration of infliximab 1 mg/kg with methotrexate significantly prolonged the duration of the 20% Paulus response in >60% of patients from a median of 2.6 wk to 16.5 wk ($p < 0.006$ vs no methotrexate) (Table 4). Approximately 60% of patients receiving infliximab at 3 or 10 mg/kg, with or without methotrexate, achieved the 20% Paulus criteria and these responses were sustained for a median duration of 10.4 to > 18.1 wk ($p < 0.001$ vs placebo). The frequency of antichimeric antibodies was inversely proportional to the dose of infliximab, and significantly reduced by concomitant treatment with methotrexate (Table 4). These data suggest that immunologic tolerance to infliximab was induced with higher doses, and potentiated by

Table 5
Effect of Infliximab Dosing Schedule on ACR 20 Responses

Treatment	Dosing Schedule	Proportion (%) of patients responding	
		30 wk[a]	*54 wk[b]*
Placebo	every 4 wk	20	17
Infliximab 3 mg/kg	every 4 wk	53	48
Infliximab 3 mg/kg	every 8 wk	50	42
Infliximab 10 mg/kg	every 4 wk	58	59
Infliximab 10 mg/kg	every 8 wk	52	59

[a]*See* ref. *51.*
[b]*See* ref. *52.*

the simultaneous administration of methotrexate. Current FDA guidelines advise the use of methotrexate along with infliximab (*see* Current Recommendations below).

In view of the apparent prolongation of the half-life of infliximab when given in conjunction with methotrexate, a long-term study was undertaken to determine whether the frequency of dosing of infliximab could be reduced further without sacrificing efficacy *(51)*. Four hundred twenty-eight patients with RA of 6 mo duration or more who were active despite methotrexate therapy (median dose 15 mg/wk) were randomized to one of five treatment groups: placebo; infliximab 3 mg/kg every 4 or 8 wk; infliximab 10 mg/kg every 4 or 8 wk, intravenously (Table 5). At 30 wk, comparable proportions of patients in all four infliximab treatment groups (50–58%) achieved ACR 20 responses, compared to only 20% in the placebo (methotrexate only) group. There were no statistically significant differences in the percent responding at 4 vs 8 wk of treatment for either dosage, and current FDA guidelines recommend treatment every 8 wk (*see* below). However, at 54 wk of treatment, there was a slight decay in the ACR 20 responses in the 3 mg/kg at both dosing intervals, compared to the higher dose of infliximab (Table 5) *(52)*.

The improvement in the clinical signs of RA observed with TNF inhibitors is likely to reflect a reduction in inflammation and damage to the joint. The accepted surrogate marker for joint damage is the radiographic demonstration of joint space narrowing (cartilage degradation) and joint erosion (bone degradation) in the small joints of the hands and/or feet. There are a number of validated radiographic scoring systems for quantifying the accumulation of erosions and joint space narrowing over time. In the aforementioned study with infliximab *(52)*, the Sharp score with modification by van der Heijde *(53,54)* was utilized. Placebo-treated patients exhibited radiographic progression at a rate of 7.0 Sharp units/yr, whereas the four infliximab groups progressed at rates ranging from –0.7–1.6 *(52)*. These data confirm a significant disease modifying effect of the combination of infliximab/methotrexate compared to methotrexate alone.

Etanercept in Advanced RA

Favorable results have been observed with etanercept for the treatment of longstanding refractory RA also. A preliminary dose-ranging study, in which a small number of patients with refractory RA were treated for 1 mo with increasing doses of etanercept,

Table 6
ACR Responses in Patients Treated with Etanercept

| | Percent of patients responding | | |
| | *Etanercept dose* | | |
Criterion	*0*	*10 mg*	*25 mg*
ACR20			
3 months	23	45	62
6 months	11	51	59
ACR50			
3 months	8	13	41
6 months	5	24	40
ACR70			
3 months	4	8	15
6 months	1	9	15

demonstrated a trend towards clinical improvement *(55)*. Therefore, a larger placebo-controlled, double-blinded trial was undertaken in which 180 patients with active, refractory RA were randomly assigned to twice weekly subcutaneous injections of placebo or one of three doses of etanercept (0.25, 2, or 16 mg/m^2 of body-surface area) *(56)*. Clinical response was defined as the achievement at 3 mo of the ACR20 composite score *(57)* (Table 3).

Robust ACR20 responses were observed in response to etanercept, as follows: 14% response in the placebo group, 33% in the 0.25 mg/m^2 group, 46% in the 2 mg/m^2 group, and 75% in the 16 mg/m^2 group ($p < 0.001$ for all treatment groups compared to placebo). The calculated ACR50 response was also robust at the highest dose of etanercept (57% compared to 7% in the placebo group, $p < .001$). Withdrawal of etanercept led to a rapid rebound in clinical-disease activity, consistent with the relatively short half-life of etanercept (2–3 d). No antibody responses to etanercept were observed. In a subsequent trial, etanercept doses of 10 or 25 mg (rather than dosing by body surface area) were utilized and treatment was continued for a total of 6 mo *(58)*. No significant decay in the clinical response was observed during the longer follow-up, and a dose-dependent reduction in clinical activity was reconfirmed (Table 6).

The treatment of RA has been evolving, like that of cancer, towards simultaneous therapy with multiple drugs. Weinblatt et al. *(59)* evaluated the safety and efficacy of adding etanercept to methotrexate in patients who had had inadequate responses to methotrexate alone. Eighty-nine patients with persistently active RA, despite at least 6 mo of methotrexate therapy at a stable dose of 15–25 mg/wk (or as low as 10 mg/wk if unable to tolerate higher doses), were randomized to receive either etanercept 25 mg or placebo subcutaneously twice weekly for 6 mo in addition to methotrexate. The addition of etanercept to methotrexate resulted in rapid and sustained improvements (*see* Table 7) without potentiating the known toxicities of methotrexate. An unanswered question is whether the combination of etanercept and methotrexate is more efficacious than etanercept alone.

Table 7
ACR Responses at 6 Mo in Patients Receiving Concomitant
Methotrexate and Etanercept (or Placebo)

Clinical response	*Percent of patients responding*	
	Placebo and methotrexate	*Etanercept and methotrexate*
ACR20	27	71
ACR50	3	39
ACR70	0	15

TNF-α Inhibitors in Early RA

Radiographic studies in RA indicate that, in patients who ultimately develop erosions, 40% exhibit their first erosions in the first year of disease, and 90% within the second year *(54,60–62)*. These observations have prompted recommendations for the initiation of disease-modifying treatment early in disease *(63)*. Toward this end, the ability of etanercept to prevent or slow radiographic erosions was evaluated in patients with early disease *(64)*. Six hundred thirty-two patients with an average disease duration of 1 yr were randomized to receive etanercept 25 mg, etanercept 10 mg, or methotrexate (mean dose, 18.3 mg/p wk). Radiographs were evaluated by the modified Sharp score. Robust clinical responses were observed in all three groups. Furthermore, all three treatments dramatically reduced the rate of radiographic progression. Sharp scores at study entry after a mean of 1 yr of disease were 9, 8, and 9 U in the etanercept 25 mg, etanercept 10 mg, and methotrexate groups, respectively; after 1 yr of treatment, Sharp scores had only increased by 0.8, 1.4, and 1.3 U, respectively. These results confirm the ability of this TNF inhibitor, as a single agent, to slow the progression of RA.

TNF Inhibitors in Juvenile RA

Etanercept is the only TNF inhibitor that has been studied in children. In a study by Lovell et al. *(64)*, patients (4–17 yr old) were enrolled in an open-label period in which they received etanercept 0.4 mg/kg of body weight (up to a maximum of 25 mg) twice weekly for 3 mo. Those who met criteria for 30% improvement were invited to continue in a 4-mo double-blind arm of the trial in which they were randomized either to placebo or to continue etanercept. The occurrence of flare of disease, and time to disease flare, were quantified. Of the 64 patients who completed the open-label phase of the study, 51 (75%) met criteria for response. In the double-blind phase of the trial, 21 of the 26 patients (81%) who were randomized to placebo withdrew from the study owing to disease flare, compared to only 7 of the 25 patients (28%) who were randomized to continue etanercept ($p = 0.003$). The median time to disease flare with placebo was 28 d, compared to more than 116 d in the etanercept group ($p < 0.001$). In light of these encouraging results, etanercept has been approved by the FDA for use in patients with polyarticular juvenile RA.

TNF Inhibitors in Inflammatory Bowel Disease

Several small open-label studies *(65–68)*, and one larger double-blind study *(69)*, of anti-TNF inhibitors in patients with inflammatory bowel disease have shown encouraging results. In the last study *(69)*, 108 patients were randomized to receive a single infusion of one of the following: 5 mg/kg infliximab, 10 mg/kg infliximab, or 20 mg/kg infliximab, or placebo. Four weeks after treatment, 81, 50, and 64% of the infliximab groups, respectively, had achieved criteria for clinical response compared to only 17% of patients in the placebo group ($p < 0.001$). In a follow-up study *(70)*, four repeated treatments of these patients with 10 mg/kg infliximab every 8 wk proved safe and efficacious. Infliximab is the only TNF inhibitor approved for use in inflammatory bowel disease (*see* below).

Other TNF Inhibitors in Development

The fully human anti-TNF antibody known as D2E7 was evaluated in a Phase II 3-mo dose finding study in active RA in which a total of 283 patients were randomized to receive placebo, 20, 40, or 80 mg of D2E7 by weekly subcutaneous injection *(69)*. ACR responses in the preliminary report were 10, 49, 57, and 56%, respectively, confirming the clinical efficacy of D2E7. A disease-modifying effect of D2E7 was also suggested by analysis of serial radiographs from a small number of patients participating in a Phase I trial *(70)*.

PEG-p55sTNFR-1, the PEGylated p55-soluble receptor, is earlier in development. It does not appear to be immunogenic *(71)*, but its overall safety and clinical efficacy are currently under investigation in clinical trials.

TNF INHIBITORS: SIDE EFFECTS AND PRECAUTIONS

In controlled clinical trials in RA infliximab and etanercept have been safe and well tolerated with no demonstrable major organ toxicities and no dose-limiting side effects. No significant differences in the incidence of serious adverse events were seen between treatment and placebo groups. Infliximab has also been well-tolerated in clinical trials in Crohn's disease *(70)*. Despite the demonstrated safety in short-term clinical trials, in the absence of long-term treatment data, there remain continued concerns about the potential for increased infections and increased malignancies because of the role TNF may play in these processes. In addition, as these agents are genetically engineered proteins that will be given repeatedly over long periods for the treatment of chronic diseases, issues of immunogenicity and injection reactions require scrutiny. These issues will be briefly addressed.

Injection Reactions

With both etanercept and infliximab, injection reactions represent the most frequent and consistent side effect, although rarely limiting administration of the drugs. Injection site reactions occur in approx 40% of patients treated with etanercept and consist of raised urticarial lesions limited to the injection sites *(58)*. Reactions occur early after initiation of treatment, are generally mild and self-limited, decrease and then resolve completely with repeated dosing. The injection-site reactions are limited to the skin and are not associated with other features of immediate hypersensitivity. No specific therapy is generally required, although topical antihistamines or topical corticosteroids may be tried. Similarly, infusion reactions are the most common side effect of infliximab, manifested most frequently by headache and nausea in approx 20 and 15% of patients, respectively. The infusion reactions are transient and controlled by slowing the rate of infusion or treatment with acetaminophen or antihistamines. The infusion reactions do not increase over time (51).

Infection

Multiple studies in humans and animals demonstrate the importance of TNF-α as a defense against infection with intracellular organisms, raising concerns about the potential for increased infections with chronic TNF inhibition. TNF is increased in the systemic circulation after administration of endotoxin or bacteria, and TNF together with IL-1 are responsible for the physiologic alterations seen in septic shock (28). Mice deficient in TNF-α by gene targeting lack primary B-cell follicles and demonstrate impaired humoral immune responses to both T-dependent and T-independent antigens (74). Mice deficient in TNF-α, TNFR1 (p55), or TNFR2 (p75) are highly susceptible to infection by Listeria monocytogenes (74–76). In a human clinical trial, treatment of septic shock with etanercept resulted in increased mortality in patients with gram positive organisms (77).

Despite these concerns, controlled clinical trials with etanercept alone (58) or in combination with methotrexate (59) did not show an increase in either frequency, type, or severity of infections. This was confirmed in long-term open label experience (78,79). In the infliximab study by Maini et al. (51), patients receiving 10 mg/kg infliximab every 8 wk or every 4 wk had a 64 or 73% incidence of any infection, which was signficantly higher than the 40% seen in the placebo group. However, in patients receiving 3 mg/kg every 8 wk, the incidence of any infection was 53%, which was not statistically different compared with placebo. The incidence of serious infections (those requiring hospitalization and/or intravenous antibiotics) did not differ among the treatment and placebo groups. However investigators reported one patient who died of complications of tuberculosis and one patient who died of coccidiomycosis in the infliximab groups (51). These infliximab results were also confirmed with long-term data (52,80).

Although these studies are reassuring, clinicians should continue to be vigilant for infections. Anti-TNF therapy may suppress the cardinal signs of infection such as fever or malaise, resulting in a delay of appropriate anti-microbial therapy. Both infliximab and etanercept should be used with caution in patients who are prone to frequent infections or who are immunocompromised. The lack of heptotoxicity with these agents make their use appealing in chronic viral hepatitis, but there is no information regarding therapy in these patients. Both agents should be held if an acute infection is present or suspected, keeping in mind the long half-life of the drugs.

Malignancy

The immune system has an important role in surveillance for malignancy, and the role of TNF, in particular, in triggering apoptosis of some tumor-cell types has already been noted. Thus, an increased risk of malignancy is of theoretical concern with chronic long-term TNF inhibition. Unfortunately, short-term clinical trials cannot adequately answer these questions. In the 30 wk infliximab trial (51), representing 445 patient-years of follow-up (359 in the infliximab groups, 86 in the placebo group), 3 patients were reported to have malignancy:1 recurrence of breast cancer, 1 squamous-cell carcinoma and melanoma, and 1 B-cell lymphoma. All three patients were treated with 10 mg/kg infliximab every 4 wk (51). However the incidence of malignancy in the trial was not different than the 2.8 cases expected based on an age and sex matched control population from the Surveillance Epidemiology and End Results (SEER) database of the National Institutes of Health . Similarly in the long-term etanercept data, 9 patients were reported with cancer, not higher than the 9.2 cases expected from the SEER database *(78)*. Definitive answers to the risk of malignancy await long term treatment data in a wider population. Registries have been established to collect these data.

Immunogenicity

As noted earlier, infliximab is a chimeric monoclonal antibody containing 25% mouse sequence at the binding site for TNF. Of concern is the potential of the mouse sequence to elicit an anti-infliximab or human anti-chimeric antibody response that would limit the therapeutic efficacy. In the study of Maini et al. discussed earlier *(51)*, the incidence of anti-chimeric antibodies was significant and inversely correlated with dose of infliximab (Table 4). Concomitant methotrexate reduced the incidence of anti-chimeric antibodies, but improved the rate and duration of clinical response only in the 1 mg/kg infliximab group. In the Crohn's study, patients treated with 10 mg/kg infliximab every 8 wk had an incidence of anti-chimeric antibodies of 15% without an apparent effect on long-term efficacy *(70)*. The effect of these antibodies on limiting therapeutic efficacy remains unclear and they do not increase the risk of infusion reactions.

Although etanercept is composed entirely of human sequence, neoepitopes might be generated at the joining regions of the TNF receptor and the immunoglobulin Fc region, which could elicit an anti-etanercept antibody response. This does not appear to be relevant. In the two published trials, non-blocking anti-etanercept antibodies were found in only two patients and did not have a notable effect on efficacy *(58,59)*.

Of unclear etiology and clinical signficance is the development of low titers of anti-double stranded DNA (anti-ds-DNA) antibodies in patients treated with infliximab and etanercept. Anti-ds-DNA antibodies are specific for systemic lupus erythematosus (SLE), and generally are not found in drug-induced lupus syndromes. In the study by Maini et al *(51)* study, 16% of patients developed anti-ds-DNA antibodies at titers >10 U/mL by the Farr assay, and 4% of patients had titers >25 U/mL. Samples positive by the Farr assay were confirmed by the more specific Crithidia assay. However only one patient developed a drug-induced lupus syndrome characterized by rash and that patient had no detectable antibodies to ds-DNA *(51)*. In the earlier dose-finding study, 8% of patients treated with infliximab developed anti-ds-DNA antibodies with one patient developing a drug-induced clinical syndrome, which resolved after stopping the drug. In trials with etanecept, 4% of patients developed anti-ds-DNA antibodies by radioimmunoassay, but none of the samples were confirmed positive by serial assays with Crithidia. No patient in the etanercept trial developed a lupus syndrome or other connective-tissue disease. Although issues of immunogenicity and autoantibody formation remain, continued efficacy and tolerability of both etanercept and infliximab in long-term trials provides increasingly stronger evidence to alleviate these concerns.

CURRENT RECOMMENDATIONS

Infliximab (Remicade™) is currently FDA-approved, in combination with methotrexate, for the reduction in signs and symptoms and inhibition of the progression of structural damage, in patients with moderate to severely active RA who have had an inadequate response to methotrexate. Remicade is also approved for the reduction in signs and symptoms of moderately to severely active Crohn's disease who have had an inadequate response to conventional therapy, and for the reduction of draining enterocutaneous fistulae in patients with fistulizing Crohn's disease. The safety and efficacy of infliximab beyond a single dose for active Crohn's disease, and beyond three doses for enterocutaneous fistulae owing to Crohn's disease, have not been adequately established.

Etanercept (Enbrel™) is currently FDA-approved for reduction in signs and symptoms and inhibition of progress of structural damage in patients with moderately to severely active RA. Etanercept can be used alone or in combination with methotrexate in patients who do not respond to methotrexate alone. Etanercept is also indicated for reduction in signs and symptoms of moderately to severely active polyarticular-course juvenile RA in patients who have had an inadequate response to one or more disease-modifying drugs.

For both infliximab and etanercept, caution is advised in the use of these agents in patients with a chronic infection or a history of recurrent infection. Neither agent should be given in a patient with a clinically important, active infection. Patients who develop a new infection while undergoing treatment with either agent should be monitored closely. If a patient develops a serious infection or sepsis while on remicade or etanercept, the TNF inhibitor should be discontinued. TNF inhibitors should not be used in patients with multiple sclerosis.

CONCLUSIONS

In vitro studies suggested that TNF is a critical and proximal mediator of the inflammatory pathway in the rheumatoid joint. Proof-of-concept for this hypothesis has now been provided by animal studies and clinical trials. Not only does TNF inhibition dramatically reduce markers of inflammation, but it also slows or halts structural damage, and these effects appear to be as potent in early disease as they are in late disease. In human terms, these efficacies should translate to less functional disability and higher quality of life.

The robust responses to treatment with TNF inhibitors in RA and inflammatory bowel disease are likely to be the tip of the iceberg. Any chronic (noninfectious) inflammatory disease that is primarily macrophage-driven could be a potential target for anti-TNF therapy. For example, pilot trials are now underway to evaluate the efficacy of TNF inhibitors in Wegener's granulomatosis, psoriatic arthritis, congestive heart failure (CHF), and other illnesses.

The potential contribution of IL-1, independent of TNF-α, in chronic inflammatory states remains to be clarified, but it is likely that a combined approach to inhibit both monokines will be even more potent than either solitary approach. Finally, the rebound in disease activity that occurs after cessation of anti-TNF therapy is a sobering reminder that the inflammatory cascade has been interrupted by neutralizing TNF, but that the underlying cause(s) of the disease itself has not been addressed.

REFERENCES

1. Firestein, G.S. 1998. Rheumatoid synovitis and pannus. *In Rheumatology*. J.H. Klippel, and P.A. Dieppe, eds. Mosby International, London, pp. 13.1–13.24.

2. Stastny, P. 1978. Association of the B-cell alloantigen DRw4 with rheumatoid arthritis. *N. Engl. J. Med.* 298:869–871.

3. Nepom, B.S., G.T. Nepom, E. Mickelson, P. Antonelli, and J.A. Hansen. 1983. Electrophoretic analysis of human HLA-DR antigens from HLA-DR4 homo cell lines: correlation between beta-chain diversity and HLA-D. *PNAS* 80:6962–6966.

4. Nepom, G.T., C.E. Seyfried, S.L. Holbeck, K.R. Wilske, and B.S. Nepom. 1986. Identification of HLA-Dw14 genes in DR4+ rheumatoid arthritis. *Lancet* 2:1002–1004.

5. Gregersen, P.K., J. Silver, and R.J. Winchester, 1987. The shared epitope hypothesis. An approach to understanding the molecular genetics of susceptibility to rheumatoid arthritis. *Arthritis Rheum.* 30:1205–1213.

6. Weyand, C.M., K.C. Hicok, K.L. Conn, and J.J. Goronzy. 1992. Influence of HLA-DRB1 genes on disease severity in rheumatoid arthritis. *Ann. Intern. Med.* 117:801–806.

7. Weyand, C.M., T.G. McCarthy, and J.J. Goronzy. 1995. Correlation between disease phenotype and genetic heterogeneity in rheumatoid arthritis. *J. Clin. Invest.* 95:2120–2126.

8. van Jaarsveld, C.H., E.J. ter Borg, J.W. Jacobs, G.A. Schellekens, F.H. Gmelig,-Meyling, C. van Booma-Frankfort, et al. 1999. The prognostic value of the antiperinuclear factor, anti-citrullinated peptide antibodies and rheumatoid factor in early rheumatoid arthritis. *Clin. Exp. Rheumatol.* 17:689–697.

9. Sebbag, M., M. Simon, C. Vincent, C. Masson-Bessiere, E. Girbal, J-J. Durieux, and G. Serre, 1995. The antiperinuclear factor and the so-called antikeratin antibodies are the same rheumatoid arthritis-specific autoantibodies. *J. Clin. Invest.* 95:2672–2679.

10. Verheijden, G.F.M., A.W.M. Rijnders, E. Bos, C.J.J. Coenen-de Roo, C.J. van Staveren, A.M.M. Miltenburg, et al. 1997. Human cartilage clycoprotein-39 as a candidate autoantigen in rheumatoid arthritis. *Arthritis Rheum.* 40:1115–1125.

11. Blass, S., F. Schumann, N.A.K. Hain, J-M. Engel, B. Stuhlmuller, and G.R. Burmester. 1999. p205 is a major target of autoreactive T cells in rheumatoid arthritis. *Arthritis Rheum.* 42:971–980.

12. Guerassismov, A., Y. Zhang, S. Banerjee, A. Cartman, J-Y. Leroux, L.C. Rosenberg et al. 1998. Cellular immunity to the G1 domain of cartilage proteoglycan aggrecan is enhanced in patients with rheumatoid arthritis but only after removal of keratan sulfate. *Arthritis Rheum.* 41:1019–1025.

13. Firestein, G.S., W.D. Xu, K. Townsend, D. Broide, J. Alvaro-Garcia, A. Glasebrook, and N. Zvaifler. 1988. Cytokines in chronic inflammatory arthritis. I. Failure to detect T cell lymphokines (IL-2 and IL-3) and presence of macrophage colony-stimulating factor (CSF-1) and a novel mast cell growth factor in rheumatoid synovitis. *J. Exp. Med.* 168:1573–1586.

14. Moreland, L.W., L.W. Heck Jr., and W.J. Koopman. 1997. Biologic agents for treating rheumatoid arthritis. *Arthritis Rheum.* 40:397–409.

15. Firestein, G.S., J.M. Alvaro-Gracia, R. Maki. 1990. Quantitative analysis of cytokine gene expression in rheumatoid arthritis. *J. Immunol.* 144:3347–3353.

16. Firestein, F.S. and N.J. Zvaifler. 1990. How important are T cells in chronic rheumatoid synovitis. *Arthritis Rheum.* 33:768–773.

17. Saklatvala, J., S.J. Sarsfield, Y. Townsend. 1985. Pig interleukin 1. Purification of two immunologically different leukocyte proteins that cause cartilage resorption, lymphocyte activation, and fever. *J. Exp. Med.* 162:1208–1215.

18. Dayer, J.M., B. Beutler, and A. Cerami. 1985. Cachectin/tumor necrosis factor stimulates collagenase and prostaglandin E2 production by human synovial cells and dermal fibroblasts. *J. Exp. Med.* 162:2163–2168.

19. Cavender, D., Y. Saegusa, and M. Ziff. 1987. Stimulation of endothelial cell binding of lymphocytes by tumor necrosis factor. *J. Immunol.* 139:1855–1860.

20. Gamble, J.R., J.M., Harlan, S.J. Klebanoff, and M.A. Vadas. 1985. Stimulation of the adherence of neutrophils to umbilical vein endothelium y human recombinant tumor necrosis factor. *Proc. Natl. Acad. Sci. USA* 82:8667–8671.

21. Firestein, G.S. 1996. Invasive fibroblast-like synoviocytes in rheumatoid arthritis: passive responders or transformed aggressors? *Arthritis Rheum.* 39:1781–1790.

22. Arend, W.P., M. Malyak, M.F. Smith, Jr., T.D. Whisenend, J.L. Slack, J.E. Sims, et al. 1994. Binding of the IL-1α, IL-1β, and IL-1 receptor antagonist by soluble IL-1 receptors and levels of soluble IL-1 receptors by synovial fluids. *J. Immunol.* 153:4766–4774.

23. Le, J. and J. Vilcek. 1987. Tumor necrosis factor and interleukin-1: cytokines with multiple overlapping biological activities. *Lab. Invest.* 56:234–248.

24. Brennan, F.M., D. Chantry, A. Jackson, R. Maini, and M. Feldmann. 1989. Inhibitors effect of TNF α antibodies on synovial cell interleukin-1 production in rheumatoid arthritis. *Lancet* ii:244–247.

25. Carswell, E.A., L.J. Old, R.L. Kassel, S. Green, N. Fiore, and B. Williamson. 1975. An endotoxin-induced serum factor that causes necrosis of tumors. *Proc. Natl. Acad. Sci. USA* 72:3666–3670.

26. Beutler, B., D. Grenwald, J.D. Hulmes, M. Chang, Y.C. Pan, J. Mathison, R. Ulevitch, and A. Cerami. 1985. Identity of tumour necrosis factor and the macrophage-secreted factor cachectin. *Nature* 316:552–554.

27. Wallach, D., E.E. Varfolomeev, N.L. Malinin, Y.V. Goltsev, A.V. Kovalenko, and M.P. Boldin. 1999. Tumor necrosis factor receptor and Fas signaling mechanisms. *Annu. Rev. Immunol.* 17:331–367.

28. Bazzoni, F. and B. Beutler. 1996. The tumor necrosis factor ligand and receptor families. *N. Engl. J. Med.* 334:1717–1725.

29. Engelmann, H., H. Holtmann, C. Brakebusch, Y.S. Avni, I. Sarov, Y. Nophar, et al. 1990. Antibodies to a soluble form of a tumor necrosis factor (TNF) receptor have TNF-like activity. *J. Biol. Chem.* 265:14,497–14,504.

30. Williams, L.M., D.L. Gibbons, A. Gearing, R.N. Maini, M. Feldmann, and F.M. Brennan. 1996. Paradoxical effects of a synthetic metalloproteinase inhibitor that blocks both p55 and p75 TNF receptor shedding andn TNFα processing in RA synovial membrane cell cultures. *J. Clin. Invest.* 97:2833–2841.

31. Yonehara, S., A. Ishii, and M. Yonehara. 1989. A cell-killing monoclonal antibody (anti-Fas) to a cell surface antigen codownregulated with the receptor of tumor necrosis factor. *J. Exp. Med.* 169:1747–1756.

32. Elliott, M.J., R.N. Maini, M. Feldmann, A. Long-Fox, P. Charles, P. Katsikis, et al. 1993. Treatment of rheumatoid arthritis with chimeric monoclonal antibodies to tumor necrosis factor α. *Arthritis Rheum.* 12:1681–1690.

33. Salfeld, J., Kaymakcalan, A., Tracey, D., Roberts, A., and Kamen, R. 1998. Generation of fully human anti-TNF antibody D2E7. *Arthritis Rheum.* 41(Suppl.):S57.

34. Kneer, J., Luedin, E., Lesslauer, W., Birnboeck, H., Stevens, R.M. 1998. An assessment of the effect of anti-drug antibody formation on the pharmacokinetics and pharmacodyamics of a TNF-r55-IgG (Lenercept) in patients with rheumatoid arthritis. *Arthritis Rheum.* 41(Suppl.):S58.

35. Mohler, K.M., D.S. Torrance, C.A. Smith, R.S. Goodwin, K.E. Stremler, V.P. Fung, et al. 1993. Soluble tumor necrosis factor (TNF) receptors are effective therapeutic agents in lethal endotoxemia and function simultaneously as both TNF carriers and TNF antagonists. *J. Immunol.* 151:1548–1561.

36. Courtnay, J.S., M.J. Dallman, A.D. Dayan, A. Martin, and B. Mosedale. 1980. Immunization against heterologous type II collagen induces arthritis in mice. *Nature* 283:666–668.

37. Holmdahl, R.R., M. Karlsson, M.E. Andersson, L. Rask, and L. Andersson. 1989. Localization of a critical restriction site on the I-Aβ chain that determines susceptibility to collagen induced arthritis in mice. *Proc. Natl. Acad. Sci. USA* 86:9475.

38. Banerjee, S., T.M. Haqqi, H.S. Luthra, J.M. Stuart, and C.S. David. 1988. Possible role of Vβ T cell receptor genes in susceptibility to collagen induced arthritis in mice. *J. Exp. Med.* 167:832.

39. Marinova-Mutafchieva, L., R.O. Williams, L.J. Mason, C. Mauri, M. Feldmann, and R.N. Maini. 1997. Dynamics of proinflammaotry cytokine expression in the joints of mice with collagen induced arthritis (CIA). *Clin. Exp. Immunol.* 107:507–512.

40. Mussener, A., M.J. Litton, E. Lindroos, and L. Klareskog. 1997. Cytokine production in synovial tissue of mice with collagen-induced arthritis (CIA). *Clin. Exp. Immunol.* 107:485–493.

41. Stasiuk, L.M., O. Abehsira-Amar, and C. Fournier. 1996. Collagen-induced arthritis in DBA/1 mice: Cytokine gene activation following immunization with type II collagen. *Cell Immunol.* 173: 269–275.

42. Thorton, S., Duwel, L.E., Boivin, G.P., Ma, Y., and Hirsch, R. 1999. Association of the course of collagen-induced arthritis with distinct patterns of cytokine and chemokine messenger RNA expression. *Arthritis Rheum.* 42:1109–1118.

43. Williams, R.O., Feldmann, M., and Maini, R.N. 1992. Anti-tumor necrosis factor ameliorates joint disease in murine collagen-induced arthritis. *Proc. Natl. Acad. Sci. USA* 89:9784–9788.

44. Joosten, L.A.B., M.M.A. Helsen, F.A.J. van de Loo, and W.B. van den Berg. 1996. Anti-cytokine treatment of established type II collagen induced arthritis in DBA/1 mice. *Arthritis Rheum.* 39:797–809.

45. Mori, L., S. Iselin, G. De Libero, W. and Lesslauer, 1996. Attenuation of collagen-induced arthritis in 55-kDa TNF receptor type 1 (TNFR1)-IgG1 treated and TNFR1 deficient mice. *J. Immunol.* 157:3178–3182.

46. Neumann, B., T. Machleidt, A. Lifka, K. Pfeffer, D. Vestweber, T.W. Mak, et al. 1996. Crucial role of 55 kilodalton TNF receptor in TNF-induced adhesion molecule expression and leukocyte organ infiltration. *J. Immunol.* 156:1587–1593.

47. Keffer, J., L. Probert, H. Cazlaris, S. Georgopoulos, E. Kasalaris, D. Kioussis, and G. Kollias. 1991. Transgenic mice expressing human tumour necrosis factor: a predictive genetic model of arthritis. *EMBO* 10:4025–4031.

48. Elliott, M.J., R.N. Maini, M. Feldmann, J.R. Kalden, C. Antoni, J.S. Smolen, et al. 1994. Randomised double-blind comparison of chimeric monoclonal antibody to tumour necrosis factor α (cA2) versus placebo in rheumatoid arthritis. *Lancet* 344:1105–1110.

49. Elliott, M.J., R.N. Maini, M. Feldmann, A. Long-Fox, P. Charles, H. Bijl, and J.N. Woody. 1994. Repeated therapy with monoclonal antibody to tumour necrosis factor alpha (cA2) in patients with rheumatoid arthritis. *Lancet* 344:1125–1127.

50. Maini, R.N., F.C. Breedveld, J.R. Kalden, J.S. Smolen, D. Davis, J.D. MacFarlane, et al. 1998. Therapeutic efficacy of multiple intravenous infusions of anti-tumor necrosis factor α monoclonal antibody combined with low-dose weekly methotrexate in rheumatoid arthritis. *Arthritis Rheum.* 41:1552–1563.

51. Maini, R., E.W. St. Clair, F. Breedveld, D. Furst, J. Kalden, M. Weisman, et al. 1999. Infliximab (chimeric anti-tumour necrosis factor α monoclonal antibody) versus placebo in rheumatoid arthritis patients receiving concomitant methotrexate: a randomized phase III trial. *Lancet* 354:1932–1939.

52. Lipsky, P.E., D.M.F.M. van der Heijde, E.W. St. Clair, et al. 2000. Infliximab and methotrexate in the treatment of rheumatoid arthritis. *N. Engl. J. Med.* 343:1594–1602.

53. Sharp, J.T. 1989. Radiologic assessment as an outcome measure in rheumatoid arthritis. *Arthritis Rheum.* 32:221–229.

54. Van der Heijde, D.M.F.M., M.A. van Leewen, P.L.C.M. van Riel, et al. 1992. Biannual radiographic assessments of hands and feet in a three-year prospective followup of patients with early rheumatoid arthritis. *Arthritis Rheum.* 35:26–34.

55. Moreland, L.W., G. Margolies, L.W. Heck Jr, A. Saway, C. Blosch, R. Hanna, and W.J. Koopman. 1996. Recombinant soluble tumor necrosis factor receptor (p80) fusion protein: Toxicity and dose finding trial in refractory rheumatoid arthritis. *J. Rheumatol.* 23:1849–1855.

56. Moreland, L.W., S.W. Baumgartner, M.H. Schiff, E.A. Tindall, R.M. Fleischmann, A.L. Weaver, et al. 1997. Treatment of rheumatoid arthritis with a recombinant human tumor necrosis factor receptor (p75)-Fc fusion protein. *N. Engl. J. Med.* 337:141–147.

57. Felsen, D.T., J.J. Anderson, M. Boers, C. Bombardier, M. Chernoff, B. Fried, et al. 1993. The American College of Rheumatology preliminary core set of disease activity measures for rheumatoid arthritis clinical trials. *Arthritis Rheum.* 36:729–740.

58. Moreland, L.W., M.H. Schiff, S.W. Baumgartner, E.A. Tindall, R.M. Fleischmann, K.W. Bulpitt, et al. 1999. Etanercept therapy in rheumatoid arthritis. A randomized, controlled trial. *Ann. Intern. Med.* 130:478–486.

59. Weinblatt, M.E., J.M. Kremer, A.D. Bankhurst, D.J. Bulpitt, R.M. Fleischmann, R.I. Fox, et al. 1999. A trial of etanercept, a recombinant tumor necrosis factor receptor:Fc fusion protein, in patients with rheumatoid arthritis receiving methotrexate. *N. Engl. J. Med.* 340:253–259.

60. Plant, M.J., P.W. Jones, J. Saklatvala, W.E.R. Ollier, P.T. Dawes. 1998. Patterns of radiological progression in early rheumatoid arthritis: Results of an 8 year prospective study. *J. Rheumatol.* 25:416–426.

61. Brook, A. and M. Corbett. 1977. Radiographic changes in early rheumatoid disease. *Ann. Rheum. Dis.* 36:71–73.

62. Fuchs, H.A., J.J. Kaye, L.F. Callahan, E.P. Nance, and T. Pincus. 1989. Evidence of significant radiographic damage in rheumatoid arthritis within the first 2 years of disease. *J. Rheumatol.* 16:585–591.

63. Pincus, T. and L.F. Callahan. 1990. Remodeling the pyramid or remodeling the paradigms concerning rheumatoid arthritis: lessons from Hodgkin's disease and coronary artery disease. *J. Rheumatol.* 17:1582–1585.

64. Bathon, J.M., R.W. Martin, R.M. Fleischmann, J.R. Tesser, M.H. Schiff, E.C. Keystone, et al. 2000. A comparison of etanercept and methotrexate in patients with early rheumatoid arthritis. *N. Eng. J. Med.* 343:1586–1593.

65. Lovell, D.J., E.H. Giannini, A. Reiff, G.D. Cawkwell, E.D. Silverman, J.J. Noton, et al. 2000. Etanercept in children with polyarticular juvenile rheumatoid arthritis. *N. Engl. J. Med.* 342:73–769.

66. Evans, R.C., L. Clarke, P. Heath, S. Stephens, A.I. Morris, and J.M. Rhodes. 1997. Treatment of ulcerative colitis with an engineered human anti-TNFalpha antibody CDP571. *Aliment. Pharmacol. Ther.* 11:1031–1035.

67. Stack, W.A., S.D. Mann, A.J. Roy, P. Heath, M. Sopwith, J. Freeman, et al. 1997. Randomised controlled trial of CDP571 antibody to tumour necrosis factor-alpha in Crohn's disease. *Lancet* 349:521–524.

68. van Dullemen, H.M., S.J. van Deventer, D.W. Hommes, H.A. Bijl, J. Jansen, G.N. Tytgat, and J. Woody. 1995. Gastroenterology. Treatment of Crohn's disease with anti-tumor necrosis factor chimeric monoclonal antibody (cA2). *Gastroenterology* 109:129–135.

69. Targan, S.R., S.B. Hanauer, J.H. Sander, L. Mayer, D.H. Present, T. Braakman, et al. 1997. A short-term study of chimeric monoclonal antibody cA2 to tumor necrosis factor α for Crohn's disease. *N. Engl. J. Med.* 337:1029–1035.

70. Rutgeerts, P., G. D'Haens, S. Targan, E. Vasiliauskas, S.B. Hanauer, D.H. Present, et al. 1999. Efficacy and safety of retreatment with anti-tumor necrosis factor antibody (infliximab) to maintain remission in Crohn's disease. *Gastroenterology* 117:761–769.

71. Van de Putte, L.B.A., R. Rau, F.C. Breedfeld, J.R. Kalden, M.G. Malaise, M. Schattekirchner, et al. 1999. Efficacy of the fully human anti-TNF antibody D2E7 in rheumatoid arthritis. *Arthritis Rheum.* 42(Suppl.):S1977 (Abstract).

72. Rau, R., G. Herborn, O. Sander, L.B.A. van de Putte, P.L.C. van Riel, A. den Broder, et al. 1999. Long-term treatment with the fully human anti-TNF-antibody D2E7 slows radiographic disease progression in rheumatoid arthritis. *Arthritis Rheum.* 42(Suppl.):S1978 (Abstract).

73. Davis, M.W., J.I. Frazier, and S.W. Martin. 1999. Non-immunogenicity of a pegylated soluble tumor necrosis factor receptor type I (PEG sTNF-R1 [p55]). *Arthritis Rheum.* 42(Suppl.):S37 (Abstract).

74. Pasparakis, M., L. Alexopoulou, L., V. Episkopou, and G. Kollias, 1996. Immune and inflammatory responses in TNF-α- deficient mice: a critical requirement for TNF-α in the formation of primary B cell follicles, follicular dendritic cell networks and germinal centers, and in the maturation of the humoral immune response. *J. Exp. Med.* 184:1397–1411.

75. Rothe, J., W. Lesslauer, H. Lotscher, Y. Lang, P. Koebel, F. Kontgen, and A. Althage. 1993. Mice lacking the tumor necrosis factor receptor 1 are resistant to TNF-mediated toxicity but highly susceptible to infection by Listeria monocytogenes. *Nature* 364:798–802.

76. Erickson, S.L., F.J. de Sauvage, K. Kikly, K. Carver-Moore, S. Pitts-Meek, N. Gillett, et al. 1994. Decreased sensitivity to tumour-necrosis factor but normal T-cell development in TNF receptor-2-deficient mice. *Nature* 372:560–563.

77. Fisher, C.J., J.M. Agosti, S.M. Opal, S.F. Lowry, R.A. Balk, J.C. Sadoff, et al. 1996. Treatment of septic shock with the tumor necrosis factor receptor:Fc fusion protein. *N. Engl. J. Med.* 1996;334:1697–702.

78. Moreland, L.M., S.B. Cohen, S. Baumgartner, M. Schiff, E.A. Tindall, and D.J. Burge. 1999. Long-term use of etanercept in patients with DMARD-refractory rheumatoid arthritis. *Arthritis Rheum.* 42(Suppl.):S401.

79. Weinblatt, M.J., J.M. Kremer, M. Lange, and D.J. Burge. 1999. Long-term safety and efficacy of combination therapy with methotrexate and etanercept (Enbrel). *Arthritis Rheum.* 42(Suppl.):S401.

80. Kavanaugh, A., T. Schaible, K. DeWoody, P. Marsters, K. Dittrich, and G. Harriman. 1999. Long-term followup of patients treated with infliximab (anti-TNF antibody) in clinical trials. Arthritis Rheum. 42(Suppl.):S401.

81. Kwon, B., B.-S. Youn, and B.S. Kwon. 1999. Functions of newly identified members of the tumor necrosis factor receptor/ligand superfamilies in lymphocytes. *Curr. Opinions Immunol.* 11:340–345.

82. Paulus, H.E., M.J. Egger, J.R. Ward, and H.J. Williams. 1990. Analysis of improvement in individual rheumatoid arthritis patients treated with disease-modifying antirheumatic drugs, based on the findings in patients treated with placebo. The Cooperative Systematic Studies of Rheumatic Diseases Group. *Arthritis Rheum.* 33:477–484.

7

Interleukin-1 Receptor Antagonist Treatment in Rheumatoid Arthritis

Barry Bresnihan

CONTENTS

1. INTRODUCTION

The pathogenesis of rheumatoid arthritis (RA) is complex. It includes the production of many proinflammatory and destructive mediators by inflamed synovial tissue (1). A widely accepted paradigm suggests that tumor necrosis factor α (TNF-α) and interleukin-1 (IL-1) are critical pathogenetic cytokines (2). The rationale supporting anti-TNFα therapy and the clinical efficacy and safety of two therapeutic compounds, used either in monotherapeutic strategies (3,4) or in combination with methotrexate (MTX) (5,6), have been described. This chapter will highlight the role of IL-1β in the pathogenesis of both synovial inflammation and cartilage matrix degradation in RA. In addition, the effects of inhibiting IL-1β-mediated pathogenetic pathways by targeted therapeutic intervention in experimental arthritis models and in RA will be examined.

The IL-1 gene family includes IL-1α, IL-1β and IL-1 receptor antagonist (IL-1Ra) (7). IL-1α and IL-1β share 26% amino acid homology. Both forms are produced as 31 kDa precursor peptides (pro-IL-1α and pro-IL-1β), which are cleaved to generate either a 17.5 kDa protein for mature IL-1α or a 17.3 kDa protein for mature IL-1β. IL-1α (both the pro- and mature forms) and IL-1β (only the mature form) are agonist molecules that can influence the functions of most cell types. Stimulation of IL-1 gene expression may result from almost any cell perturbation including cell-cell contact, cell contact with extra-cellular matrix elements, soluble factors, some immune complexes, complement fragments, crystals, bacteria, and viruses. TNF-α may also stimulate IL-1 production

From: *Modern Therapeutics in Rheumatic Diseases*
Edited by: G. C. Tsokos, et al. © Humana Press, Inc., Totowa, NJ

(8,9). Moreover, IL-1 production may increase following IL-1 secretion in an autocrine or paracrine regulatory system *(10)*. Activated monocytes and macrophages are the principal source of IL-1α and IL-1β, although almost all cells can produce IL-1 to some extent *(2,7)*. IL-1β is secreted after the cleavage of its proform by IL-1β converting enzyme (ICE). IL-1α is not secreted and may have important functions either as an intracellular cytokine or as a membrane bound protein. The agonist functions of IL-1 result from the interaction between IL-1α or IL-1β and an IL-1 receptor (IL-1R) located on the target cell surface. There are two distinct receptors designated type I (IL-1RI) and type II (IL-1RII). IL-1 binding to IL-1RI results in signal transduction and cell activation. IL-1RII is believed to be a "decoy" receptor that may have a function in scavenging IL-1α and IL-1β, but does not have a role in cell signaling *(11)*. Binding of IL-1β, in particular, to IL-1RI produces many effects that are central to the pathogenesis of RA *(2,7)*. IL-1β may bind to IL-1RI on vascular endothelial cells and result in the upregulation of endothelial adhesion-molecule expression. Similarly, IL-1β may upregulate adhesion molecule expression on circulating lymphocytes and monocytes to initiate or augment infiltration into inflamed tissues. IL-1β also increases chemotaxis of polymorphonuclear leukocytes, lymphocytes, and monocytes. Other IL-1β-mediated agonistic effects include activation of T cells and the stimulation of proteolytic enzyme release by fibroblast-like synoviocytes and tissue macrophages in the synovial lining layer and at the cartilage-pannus junction.

IL-1Ra is the third member of the *IL-1* gene family that binds the IL-1 receptors *(2,7,12,13)*. Four different peptides are derived from the same gene. One isoform is produced as a 177 amino acid protein, including a 25 amino acid hydrophobic leader sequence that is cleaved, resulting in a 152 amino acid protein. This 17 kDa protein, sIL-1Ra, is then glycosylated and secreted with a molecular weight of 22–25 kDa. The three other IL-1Ra isoforms do not possess a leader sequence and therefore remain intracellular (icIL-1Ra). Like IL-1α and IL-1β, sIL-1Ra is produced primarily by activated monocytes and tissue macrophages. icIL-1Ra is constitutively expressed by skin epithelial cells and the gastrointestinal (GI) tract. The agonistic effects of IL-1 are partially blocked by the interaction between IL-1Ra and IL-1RI. When IL-1Ra binds to IL-1RI, it blocks the binding of IL-1α and IL-1β and inhibits signal transduction. The agonistic effects of IL-1 are also partially regulated by IL-1RII *(11)*.

INTERLEUKIN-1 AND ARTHRITIS

Experimental Arthritis

The importance of IL-1 in the pathogenesis of RA is widely accepted *(2)*. Elevated IL-1 levels were observed in the early phase of experimental arthritis *(14,15)*. Intra-articular injection of IL-1 in rabbits induced an initial transient infiltration of neutrophils into the joint space followed by influx of mononuclear cells *(16)*. Proteoglycan loss from articular cartilage was also observed. Repeated intra-articular injection of IL-1 in rats induced synovial-membrane mononuclear cell infiltration but without bone or cartilage destruction *(17)*. However, in the rats whose joints were previously injected with streptococcal cell wall peptidoglycan-polysaccharide complex, intra-articular IL-1 markedly accentuated the inflammatory appearances with pannus formation and cartilage destruction.

Similarly, in a study of antigen-induced arthritis in mice, it was observed that intra-articular methylated bovine serum albumin (mBSA) resulted in mild and transient synovitis without cartilage or bone loss *(18)*. However, when IL-1 was administered it resulted in severe arthritis in the antigen injected knee with pannus formation and extensive cartilage and bone erosion. This predominant role of IL-1 in cartilage and bone destruction has been repeatedly emphasized *(19)*. Moreover, it has been demonstrated that both IL-1α and IL-1β have the potential to cause bone and cartilage damage in antigen-induced arthritis *(20,21)*. The dominance of IL-1β over IL-1α in the development of collagen-induced arthritis has been demonstrated in studies of IL-1β knock-out mice *(22)*. In contrast to the many studies that demonstrated the effects of IL-1 on joint damage, a study of antigen-induced arthritis in rats demonstrated that IL-1 injected into knee joints led to amelioration of arthritis with a reduction in inflammation and joint damage *(23)*. This observation has not been explained but may be owing in part to the induction of IL-1 inhibitors including IL-1Ra.

Rheumatoid Arthritis

The association between IL-1, joint inflammation, and joint damage highlighted in animal studies has also been observed in studies of RA *(2)*. Peripheral blood monocytes from patients with RA produced more IL-1 in vitro than cells from normal subjects or patients with osteoarthritis (OA) *(24,25)*. Synovial fluid levels of IL-1β have been related to some measures of disease activity *(26,27)*. Therapeutic benefit following methotrexate treatment has been associated with reduced in vitro production of IL-1 by circulating mononuclear cells *(28)*, and a decrease in synovial fluid IL-1β concentration *(29)*.

Up to 10% of isolated synovial-tissue cells expressed IL-1β mRNA *(30)*. In immuno-histologic studies of synovial tissue, IL-1α and IL-1β production has been demonstrated in macrophages accumulating at the cartilage-pannus junction and in lining-layer and sublining-layer macrophage populations *(31,32)*. In a study of IL-1β production by synovial tissue explants, it was observed that the highest levels were produced by samples demonstrating lymphoid follicle formation compared to samples that did not demonstrate lymphoid aggregation *(33)*. This suggested that lymphoid-follicle formation, associated with increased IL-1β production, represented a more immunologically active phase of synovitis.

IL-1Ra is also produced in abundance by synovial-tissue macrophages *(34–36)*. In a study udertaken to quantify IL-1Ra and IL-1 gene expression and production by RA synovial membrane, it was observed that IL-1Ra, IL-1α, and IL-1β were present in fresh and cultured synovial cells obtained from patients with RA and OA *(37)*. The IL-1Ra:IL-1 ratios were significantly below the 10–100-fold excess of IL-1Ra required to inhibit IL-1 bioactivity. Moreover, isolated synovial tissue macrophages were demonstrated to produce IL-1Ra, but in amounts that were much less than alveolar- or in vitro-derived macrophages. It was concluded that IL-1Ra production by synovial tissue cells in RA is deficient relative to the total production of IL-1. Similar observations were reported following a study of IL-1Ra and IL-1β production by cultured synovial-tissue samples *(38)*. The IL-1Ra:IL-1β imbalance was reversed to favor an anti-inflammatory effect by the addition of IL-4 and, to a lesser extent, IL-10.

IL-1 RECEPTOR ANTAGONIST TREATMENT
IN ANIMAL MODELS OF ARTHRITIS

IL-1Ra as Monotherapy

IL-1Ra has been administered therapeutically in several in vitro and in vivo experimental models of arthritis with dramatic effects *(19)*. In in vitro studies, IL-1Ra resulted in inhibition of prostaglandin production by chondrocytes and synovial cells, and collagenase production by IL-1-activated synovial cells. The effects of IL-1α and IL-1β in cartilage organ cultures were suppressed in a dose-dependent manner by IL-1Ra *(39)*. IL-1Ra suppressed IL-1-activated matrix metalloproteinase and prostaglandin production by articular chondrocytes. These observations were extended in a further study that demonstrated that intravenous administration of IL-1Ra to rabbits could inhibit leukocyte accumulation and cartilage proteoglycan loss caused by intra-articular injection of IL-1 *(40)*.

In in vivo models, IL-1Ra caused inhibition of joint swelling in rat streptococcal cell wall-induced arthritis reactivated by challenge with peptidoglycan-polysaccharide polymers *(41)*. In another study, IL-1Ra administered intraperitoneally profoundly suppressed the incidence and delayed the onset of immune collagen-induced arthritis *(42)*. In contrast, in the same study IL-1Ra did not affect the pathogenesis of antigen-induced arthritis (AIA) provoked by mBSA. Similarly, in a study of rabbit AIA provoked by ovalbumin, the administration of IL-1Ra had no detectable effect *(43)*. In these studies, IL-1Ra was administered intravenously at 6-h intervals. However, administration of IL-1Ra by continuous intraperitoneal infusion totally prevented the suppression of proteoglycan synthesis *(21)*. Of interest, the effect on proteoglycan synthesis was independent of any effect on joint inflammation. Similar profound effects of continuous intraperitoneal IL-1Ra infusion were observed in murine immune complex-induced arthritis *(44)*. The inhibition of proteoglycan synthesis and cellular influx into the synovium were fully blocked. Intraperitoneal infusion of IL-1Ra also resulted in marked suppression of murine collagen-induced arthritis (CIA): histologic analysis demonstrated markedly reduced cartilage destruction and autoradiography demonstrated full recovery of chondrocyte proteoglycan synthesis *(45)*. In conclusion, IL-Ra is a potent inhibitor of cartilage degradation in several experimental models of arthritis. This effect is maximal following continuous infusion of IL-1Ra and can occur in the absence of a major effect on synovial inflammation. The uncoupling of anti-inflammatory effects and effects on tissue degradation in experimental arthritis may have implications for the treatment of human disease.

Combination Treatment

Combination of IL-1Ra with methotrexate (MTX) in an adjuvant arthritis rat model demonstrated synergistic or additive effects *(46)*. Treatment with IL-1Ra alone resulted in a 6% inhibition of paw swelling, compared to 47% inhibition following MTX alone. The combination of IL-1Ra and MTX resulted in an 84% decrease in swelling. IL-1Ra alone produced 53% decrease in bone resorbtion, compared to 58% inhibition following MTX alone. The combination of IL-1Ra and MTX resulted in a 97% decrease in bone resorbtion. These findings provided experimental support for proceeding to randomized clinical trial protocols combining IL-1Ra and MTX in RA patients.

Gene Therapy

Specific cytokine effects in disease have been successfully modulated by advances in gene therapy, the transfer of genes to patients for therapeutic purposes *(47)*. Using a retroviral vector, the human *IL-1Ra* protein gene was transferred to the knee joints of rabbits with AIA *(48)*. Gene expression was fivefold higher in the inflamed joints than noninflamed joints. Increased gene expression produced a marked reduction in the degree of cartilage damage and a less marked effect on joint inflammation. Moreover, increased *IL-1Ra* gene expression resulted in reduced concentrations of rabbit IL-1β, suggesting inhibition of an autocrine regulatory loop. In a similar study, the human *IL-1Ra* gene was transferred to the synoviocytes of rats with recurrent streptococcal cell wall-induced arthritis *(49)*. Gene transfer in this model significantly reduced the severity of arthritis and partially attenuated erosion of cartilage and bone. In a third experimental model, the effects of human IL-1Ra gene transfer on collagen induced arthritis in mice was studied *(50)*. The onset of CIA was almost completely prevented in the knee joints containing human IL-1Ra-producing cells. Moreover, the onset of CIA in the ipsilateral paws of the human IL-1Ra-producing knee joints was also prevented. In contrast, joints containing nontransfected cells demonstrated severe synovial inflammation and cartilage degradation. These experiments demonstrate the feasibility of gene transfer as a therapeutic approach to arthritis. They also highlight the potential benefits of treatment with IL-1Ra on synovial inflammation and, in particular, on progressive joint degradation.

IL-1 RECEPTOR ANTAGONIST THERAPY IN HUMAN DISEASE

Septic Shock

IL-1β is an important mediator in the pathogenesis of sepsis syndrome and septic shock *(51–53)*. A total of 893 patients with sepsis syndrome were recruited to the first randomized, double-blind, placebo-controlled, multicenter clinical trial of recombinant human IL-Ra in humans *(54)*. The treatment doses used were a 100 mg intravenous loading dose followed by continuous intravenous infusion of 1.0 or 2.0 mg/kg/h for 72 h. The results failed to demonstrate a statistically significant effect of IL-1Ra treatment on survival time compared to placebo. Secondary and retrospective analyses of efficacy did suggest that treatment with IL-1Ra resulted in a dose-related increase in survival time among patients with sepsis and organ dysfunction and/or a predicted risk of mortality of 24% or greater.

Modulation of IL-1 Effects in RA

The first therapeutic attempt to modulate IL-1β-mediated pathogenetic effects in RA employed a recombinant human IL-1 receptor. Twenty-three patients with active RA were enrolled into a randomized, double-blind, placebo-controlled study *(55)*. Treatment or placebo was administered subcutaneously for 28 consecutive days. The rationale for the study was that competitive binding of circulating IL-1 to soluble receptor would inhibit IL-1-mediated inflammatory activity. Soluble IL-1RI had suppressed inflammation in a number of experimental models including arthritis *(56)*. Patients received daily doses of 125, 250, 500, or 1000 mg/m^2. Only one patient in the entire cohort (who had received 1000 mg/m^2/d) demonstrated clinically relevant improvement. Treatment was discontinued prematurely because of dose-limiting rashes in a further two patients who were receiving 1000 mg/m^2/d. No other adverse events prevented continuation to the end of the study. Treatment did result in a reduction of monocyte cell surface IL-1α, which indicated that the dosages administered were functional. In theory, a study employing recombinant human IL-1RII might inhibit IL-1β-mediated clinical effects more efficaciously *(11)*.

Treatment of RA with IL-1Ra

DOSE-RANGE STUDY

One hundred and seventy-five patients with active RA were enrolled in a randomized, double-blind study of recombinant human IL-1Ra administered by subcutaneous injection *(57)*. The rationale for this study was that the administration of IL-1Ra would restore the normal IL-1/IL-1Ra balance and result in suppression of IL-1-mediated pathogenetic events in patients with active RA. Preliminary studies had demonstrated that IL-1Ra was 95% bioavailable with a half-life of 6 h. The dosing schedule in the study was complicated with nine different treatment groups. During the initial 3-wk treatment phase, patients received IL-1Ra 20, 70 or 200 mg once, three times or seven times each week. This was followed by a 4-wk maintenance phase, during which all patients received the initiation phase dose once weekly. Treatment was well-tolerated. Owing to the multiple small treatment groups and the lack of a placebo control group, it was not possible to draw firm conclusions regarding efficacy from this study. However, the results did suggest that daily dosing was more effective than weekly dosing with respect to the number of swollen joints, the investigator and patient assessments of disease activity, pain score, and C-reactive protein (CRP) levels. The findings were considered encouraging and a randomized, placebo-controlled, Phase II clinical trial was designed.

RANDOMIZED CLINICAL TRIAL

In this study 472 patients with active and severe RA were recruited into a 24-wk, double-blind, randomized, placebo-controlled, multicenter study *(58,59)*. Patients were randomized into one of four groups: placebo or IL-1ra 30, 75, or 150 mg/d given by a self-administered subcutaneous injection. Disease duration was >6 mo and <8 yr. Doses of nonsteroidal anti-inflammatory drugs and corticosteroids ($\leq$prednisolone 10 mg/d) remained stable throughout the study. Any disease-modifying anti-rheumatic drugs previously administered (maximum 3) had been discontinued at least 6 wk prior to enrolment. Pretreatment disease severity was similar in the four groups.

The primary therapeutic endpoint was an American College of Rheumatology (ACR) 20% response *(60)*, achieved by 27% of the placebo group compared to 43% of the IL-1Ra 150 mg/d group. The clinical responses in the 150 mg/d group were superior to those observed in the other treatment groups and were statistically better than the placebo group with respect to number of swollen joints, tender joints, Health Assessment Questionnaire (HAQ), erythrocyte sedimentation rate (ESR), and CRP. The clinical responses were observed after 2 wk of therapy and the maximal fall in the acute phase response occurred during the first week of treatment.

Radiologic evaluation of the hands demonstrated a statistically significant slowing in the rate of progressive joint damage following treatment when compared to placebo.

Serial measurements of the Larsen scores *(61)* demonstrated a 41% reduction in the rate of radiologic progression and a 46% reduction in the erosive joint count. A further analysis of radiologic change was performed using a scoring system that distinguishes two aspects of joint damage, articular erosion and joint space narrowing *(62)*. This analysis demonstrated a 58% slowing in the rate of progressive joint space narrowing compared to a 38% slowing in the rate of joint erosion. These findings suggested that the predominant early manifestation of blocking IL-1β-mediated joint damage is a reduction in the rate of cartilage degradation rather than invasion of cartilage and bone by synovial cell proliferation. The observation that IL-1Ra can prevent joint damage is encouraging with positive implications for minimizing the disability that is frequently associated with RA *(1)*.

A small subgroup of patients participating in this trial underwent a synovial biopsy before and after treatment to determine the effects of IL-1Ra on inflamed synovial tissue *(63)*. Twelve paired biopsy specimens were available, three from the placebo group, six from the IL-1Ra 30 mg/d group, none from the IL-1Ra 75 mg/d group, and three from the IL-1Ra 150 mg/d group. There was a notable reduction in intimal layer macrophages and subintimal layer macrophages and lymphocytes following IL-1Ra 150 mg/d. Increased cellular infiltration was observed in all patients receiving placebo and variable changes were observed following IL-1Ra 30 mg/d. Downregulation of the cell adhesion molecules E-selectin, vascular cell adhesion molecule-1, and intercellular adhesion molecule-1 were also associated with the IL-1Ra 150 mg/d dose. Expression of these molecules is regulated by IL-1β *(2,7)*. In addition, the apparent arrest of progressive joint damage seen in four of nine patients studied was significantly associated with the cessation or reversal of intimal layer macrophage accumulation. These observations represent the inhibition by IL-1Ra of biologically relevant IL-1-mediated pathogenetic effects and may help explain some of the critical mechanisms involved.

EXTENSION STUDY

The patients who completed the 24-wk randomized clinical trial had the option of continuing into a further 24-wk extension phase *(64)*. Patients who had received placebo were randomized to one of the three treatment groups and. Three hundred and forty five patients had completed the randomized clinical trial. Of these, 309 (89.9%) entered the extension study. Seventy-six had been receiving placebo and were randomized to one of the three treatment groups. Patients in each of the three treatment groups continued to receive their previous dosages. Seventy-one (93.4%) of the 76 randomized from placebo completed the extension phase. On completion of the extension phase, 55% of the total who had previously received placebo achieved a 20% ACR response. This was maximal at 71% in the group who had been randomized to the highest treatment dose (IL-1Ra 150 mg/d). Significant improvements were also observed in this group for each of individual ACR components. Two hundred and thirty-three patients continued to receive their previous dose of IL-1Ra throughout the extension phase and 223 (95.7%) completed the study. Of this total, 49% maintained an ACR 20% response at 48 wk. Radiologic evaluation of all patients who had completed the extension study was also undertaken *(62)*. The results demonstrated that the reduced rate of progressive joint-space narrowing, or cartilage degradation, observed during the first 24 wk was maintained during the second phase of treatment. However, the rate of joint erosion, reflecting cartilage and bone invasion by proliferating pannus, demonstrated further significant slowing during the extension phase of the study. This suggested that maintaining IL-1Ra treatment resulted in augmentation of the protective effect on joint damage.

IL-1RA COMBINED WITH METHOTREXATE IN RA

MTX is the most widely used disease-modifying therapeutic compound in the treatment of RA. The efficacy of combining IL-1Ra treatment with MTX was evaluated in a randomized, double-blind, placebo-controlled study over 24 wk *(65)*. Four hundred and nineteen patients receiving maintenance doses of 12.5–25 mg MTX weekly for at least 6 mo were recruited. Patients entering the study were required to have manifestations of active disease despite maintenance MTX. The inclusion criteria included six or more swollen joints and at least two of the following: nine or more painful or tender joints, morning stiffness greater than 45 min, and CRP greater than 1.5 mg/d. At entry, the mean MTX dose was 17 mg/wk and mean disease duration was 7 yr. The mean number of swollen joint was 18. There were six treatment groups: placebo, IL-1Ra 0.04, 0.1, 0.4, 1.0, and 2.0 mg/kg/d, administered as a daily subcutaneous injection. IL-1Ra 1.0 mg/kg/d was the optimal dose with 42% demonstrating an ACR 20% response *(41)* at 24 wk compared to 23% of the placebo/MTX group. An ACR 50% response was observed in 24% of this treatment group compared to 4% of the control group, and an ACR 70% response was seen in 10% of the treated patients. These findings indicate that IL-1Ra provides significant additional clinical improvements to patients who are only partially responding to MTX alone.

IL-1RA GENE THERAPY IN RA

Phase I clinical trials of experimental *IL-1Ra* gene therapy in RA have commenced *(47)*. Human IL-1Ra gene was transferred to synovium using a retroviral vector. The preliminary results indicated that the treated synovial tissues successfully expressed IL-1Ra protein *(66)*. The clinical benefits of *IL-1Ra* gene therapy have not yet been evaluated.

Prospects for Future Drug Development

It has been demonstrated in several experimental models that continuous intraperitoneal infusion of IL-1Ra provided considerably better therapeutic results than bolus administration *(21,44,45)*. The maximal efficacy of sustained blood levels of IL-1Ra on inflammation and bone resorbtion was confirmed in rats developing adjuvant arthritis or with established collagen-induced arthritis *(67)*. It was suggested that optimal blood levels of IL-1Ra may not have been achieved by daily subcutaneous injection in human studies to allow continuous saturation of IL-1 receptors. Thus, improvements in human drug delivery systems may result in further increased therapeutic efficacy in patients with RA.

SIDE EFFECTS

IL-1Ra is generally well tolerated. An injection-site reaction was the most frequent adverse event, reported in 25% of patients receiving placebo and 81% of patients receiving maximum dose IL-1Ra in the randomized clinical trial *(58)*. These reactions were usually mild and transient and resulted in premature withdrawal from the study in only 5%. Other adverse events, including infections, were uncommon and encountered as frequently in the placebo group as in the treatment groups. No serious adverse events were observed during the extension study. The adverse events observed during the combination study with methotrexate *(65)* were similar in frequency and severity to those seen in the randomized clinical trial.

CONCLUSIONS

Anticytokine therapy offers new hope to those suffering from RA. The prospect of specifically targeting and modulating the effects of key proinflammatory cytokines or destructive mediators in a complex pathogenetic network may represent a new therapeutic era *(68)*. Anti-TNF-α therapy is already available to many. The symptomatic benefits described, both in monotherapeutic regimes and in combination with MTX, have been impressive *(3–6)*. Anti-TNF-α therapy delayed radiographic progression over 1 yr when administered in combination with MTX *(69,70)*. However, approx 30% of patients failed to respond symptomatically to TNF-α inhibition *(3–6)*. IL-1β is also pivotal in the pathogenesis of synovial inflammation and articular destruction. The inhibition of IL-1β-mediated effects by IL-1Ra, administered as monotherapy to patients with severe RA, resulted in clinical improvements and measureable slowing of progressive joint damage after only 24 wk *(58,59,62)*. Clinical improvements were also observed in patients who were responding suboptimally to stable therapeutic doses of MTX *(65)*. These observations strongly suggest a potential role for IL-1Ra as a novel therapeutic modality in the future management of RA. Further Phase III studies are in progress.

REFERENCES

1. Tak, P.P. and B. Bresnihan. 2000. The pathogenesis and prevention of joint damage in rheumatoid arthritis: Advances from synovial biopsy and tissue analysis. *Arthritis Rheum.* 43:2619–2633.

2. Arend, W.P. and J.-M. Dayer. 1995. Inhibition of the production and effects of interleukin-1 and tumor necrosis factor α in rheumatoid arthritis. *Arthritis Rheum.* 38:151–160.

3. Elliott, M.J., R.M. Maini, M. Feldmann, J.R. Kalden, C. Antoni, J.S. Smolen, et al. 1994. Randomised double-blind comparison of chimeric monoclonal antibody to tumour necrosis factor α (cA2) versus placebo in rheumatoid arthritis. *Lancet* 344:1105–1110.

4. Moreland, L.W., S.W. Baumgartner, M.H. Schiff, E.A. Tindall, R.M. Fleischmann, and A.L. Weaver. 1997. Treatment of rheumatoid arthritis with a recombinant human tumor necrosis factor receptor (p75)-Fc fusion protein. *N. Engl. J. Med.* 337:141–147.

5. Maini, R.N., F.C. Breedveld, J.R. Kalden, J.S. Smolen, D. Davis, J.D. Macfarlane, et al. 1998. Therapeutic efficacy of multiple intravenous infusions of anti-tumor necrosis factor α monoclonal antibody combined with low-dose weekly methotrexate in rheumatoid arthritis. *Arthritis Rheum.* 41:1552–1563.

6. Weinblatt, M.E., J.M. Kremer, A.D. Bankhurst, K.J. Bulpitt, R.M. Fleischmann, R.I. Fox, et al. 1999. A trial of etanercept, a recombinant tumor necrosis factor receptor:Fc fusion protein, in patients with rheumatoid arthritis receiving methotrexate. *N. Engl. J. Med.* 340:253–259.

7. Dinarello, C.A. 1996. Biologic basis for interleukin-1 in disease. *Blood* 87:2095–2147.

8. Philip, R. and L.B. Epstein. 1986. Tumour necrosis factor as immunomodulator and mediator of monocyte cytotoxicity induced by itself, gamma-interferon and interleukin-1. *Nature* 323:86–89.

9. Nawroth, P.P., I. Bank, D. Handley, J. Cassimeris, L. Chess, and D. Stern. 1986. Tumor necrosis factor/cachectin interacts with endothelial cell receptors to induce release of interleukin-1. *J. Exp. Med.* 163:1363–1375.

10. Vannier, E. and C.A. Dinarello. 1993. Histamine enhances interleukin (IL)-1-induced IL-1 gene expression and protein synthesis via H-2 receptors in peripheral blood mononuclear cells: Comparison with IL-1 receptor antagonist. *J. Clin. Invest.* 92:281–287.

11. Colatta, F., S.K. Dower, J.E. Sims, and A. Mantovani. 1994. The type II "decoy" receptor: A novel regulatory pathway for interleukin-1. *Immunol. Today* 15:562–566.

12. Arend, W.P., H.P. Welgus, and R.C. Thompson. 1990. Biological properties of human monocyte-derived interleukin-1 receptor antagonist. *J. Clin. Invest.* 85:1694–1697.

13. Arend, W.P., M. Malyak, C.J. Guthridge, and C. Gabay. 1998. Interleukin-1 receptor antagonist: Role in biology. *Annu. Rev. Immunol.* 16:27–55.

14. Pettipher, E.R., B. Henderson, T. Hardingham and A. Ratcliffe. 1989. Cartilage proteoglycan depletion in acute and chronic antigen-induced arthritis. *Arthritis Rheum.* 32:601–607.

15. Pettipher, E.R., B. Henderson, S. Moncada, and G.A. Higgs. 1988. Leucocyte infiltration and cartilage proteoglycan loss in immune arthritis in the rabbit. *Br. J. Pharmacol.* 95:169–176.

16. Pettipher, E.R, G.A. Higgs, and B. Henderson. 1986. Interleukin-1 induces leukocyte infiltration and cartilage proteoglycan degradation in the synovial joint. *Proc. Natl. Acad. Sci. USA* 83:8749–8753.

17. Stimpson, SA, F.G. Dalldorf, I.G. Otterness, and J.H. Schwab. 1988. Exacerbation of arthritis by IL-1 in rat joints previously injected with peptidoglycan-polysaccharide. *J. Immunol.* 140:2964–2969.

18. Staite, N.D., K.A. Richard, D.G. Aspar, K.A. Franz, L.A. Galinet, and C.J. Dunn. 1990. Induction of acute erosive monarticular arthritis in mice by interleukin-1 and methylated bovine serum albumin. *Arthritis Rheum.* 33:253–260.

19. van den Berg, W.B. 1997. Lessons for joint destruction from animal models. *Curr. Opin. Rheumatol.* 9:221–228.

20. van de Loo, F.A.J., O.J. Arntz, A.C. Bakker, P.L.E.M. van Lent, M.J.M. Jacobs, and W.B. van den Berg. 1995. Role of interleukin-1 in antigen-induced exacerbations of murine arthritis. *Am. J. Pathol.* 146:239–249.

21. van de Loo, F.A.J., L.A.B. Joosten, P.L.E.M. van Lent, O.J. Arntz, and W.B. van den Berg. 1995. Role of interleukin-1, tumor necrosis factor α, and interleukin-6 in cartilage, proteoglycan metabolism and destruction: effect of in situ blocking of murine antigen- and zymosan-induced arthritis. *Arthritis Rheum.* 38:164–172.

22. Fantuzzi, G. and C.A. Dinarello. 1996. The inflammatory response in IL-1β-deficient mice: comparison with other cytokine-related knock-out mice. *J. Leukocyte Biol.* 59:489–493.

23. Jacobs, C., D. Young, and S. Tyler, et al. 1988. In vivo treatment with IL-1 reduces the severity and duration of antigen-induced arthritis in rats. *J. Immunol.* 141:2967–2974.

24. Dulary, B., C.I. Westacott, and C.J. Elson. 1992. IL-1 secreting cell assay and its application to cells from patients with rheumatoid arthritis. *Br. J. Rheumatol.* 31:19–24.

25. Zangerle, P.F., D. DeGroote, M. Lopez, R.J. Meuleman, Y. Vrindts, F. Fauchet, et al. 1992. Direct stimulation of cytokines (IL-1β, TNFα, IL-6, IFNγ and GM-CSF) in whole blood. II. Application to rheumatoid arthritis and osteoarthritis. *Cytokine* 4:568–575.

26. Rooney, M., J.A. Symons, and G.A. Duff. 1990. Interleukin-1 beta in synovial fluid is related to local disease activity in rheumatoid arthritis. *Rheumatol. Int.* 10:217–219.

27. Holt, I., R.G. Cooper, J. Denton, A. Meager, and S.J. Hopkins. 1992. Cytokine inter-relationship and their association with disease activity in arthritis. *Br. J. Rheumatol.* 31:725–733.

28. Chang, D.-M., M.E. Weinblatt, and P.H. Schur. 1992. The effects of methotrexate on IL-1 in patients with rheumatoid arthritis. *J. Rheumatol.* 19:1678–1682.

29. Thomas, R. and G.J. Carroll. 1993. Reduction of leukocyte and interleukin-1 beta concentrations in the synovial fluid of rheumatoid arthritis patients treated with methotrexate. *Arthritis. Rheum.* 36:1244–1252.

30. Firestein, G.S., J.M. Alvaro-Gracia, and R. Maki. 1990. Quantitative analysis of cytokine gene expression in rheumatoid arthritis. *J. Immunol.* 144:3347–3353.

31. Chu, C.Q., M. Field, S.A. Allard, E. Abney, M. Feldmann, and R.N. Maini. 1992. Detection of cytokines at the cartilage/pannus junction in patients with rheumatoid arthritis: implications for the role of cytokines in cartilage destruction and repair. *Br. J. Rheumatol.* 31:653–661.

32. Wood, N.C., E. Dickens, J.A. Symon, and G.W. Duff. 1992. In situ hybridisation of interleukin-1 in CD14 positive cells in rheumatoid arthritis. *Clin. Immunol. Immunopathol.* 62:295–300.

33. Yanni, G., A. Whelan, C. Feighery, and B. Bresnihan. 1993. Contrasting levels of in vitro cytokine production by rheumatoid synovial tissues demonstrating different patterns of mononuclear cell infiltration. *Clin. Exp. Immunol.* 93:387–395.

34. Deleuran, B.W., C.Q. Chu, M. Field, F.M. Brennan, P. Katsikis, M. Feldmann, and R.N. Maini. 1992. Localisation of interleukin-1α, type 1 interleukin-1 receptor and interleukin-1 receptor antagonist in the synovial membrane and cartilage/pannus junction in rheumatoid arthritis. *Br. J. Rheumatol.* 31:801–809.

35. Firestein, G.S., A.E. Berger, D.E. Tracey, J.G. Chosay, D.L. Chapman, M.M. Paine, et al. 1992. IL-1 receptor antagonist protein production and gene expression in rheumatoid arthritis and osteoarthritis synovium. *J. Immunol.* 149:1054–1062.

36. Koch, A.E., S.L. Kunkel, S.W. Chensue, G.K. Haines, and R.M. Strieter. 1992. Expression of interleukin-1 and interleukin-1 receptor antagonist by human rheumatoid synovial tissue macrophages. *Clin. Immunol. Immunopathol.* 65:23–29.

37. Firestein, G.S., D.L. Boyle, C. Yu, M.M. Paine, T.D. Whisenand, N.J. Zvaifler, W.P. Arend. 1994. Synovial interleukin-1 receptor antagonist and interleukin-1 balance in rheumatoid arthritis. *Arthritis Rheum.* 37:644–652.

38. Chomarat, P., E. Vannier, J. Dechanet, M.C. Rissoan, J. Banchereau, C.A. Dinarello, and P. Miossec. 1995. Balance of IL-1 receptor antagonist in rheumatoid synovium and its regulation by IL-4 and IL-10. *J. Immunol.* 154:1432–1439.

39. Smith, R.J., J.E. Chin, L.M. Sam, and J.M. Justen. 1991. Biologic effects of interleukin-1 receptor antagonist protein on interleukin-1 stimulated cartilage erosion and chondrocyte responsiveness. *Arthritis Rheum.* 34:78–83.

40. Henderson, B., R.C. Thompson, T. Hardingham, and J. Lewthwaite. 1991. Inhibition of interleukin-1 induced synovitis and articular cartilage proteoglycan loss in the rabbit knee by recombinant human interleukin-1 receptor antagonist. *Cytokine* 3:246–249.

41. Schwab, J.H., S.K. Anderle, R.R. Brown, F.G. Dalldorf, and R.C. Thompson. 1991. Pro- and anti-inflammatory roles of interleukin-1 in recurrence of bacterial cell wall-induced arthritis in rats. *Infect. Immun.* 59:4436–4442.

42. Woolley, P.H., J.D. Whalen, D.C. Chapman, A.E. Berger, K.A. Richard, D.G. Aspar, and N.D. Staite. 1993. The effect of interleukin-1 receptor antagonist protein on type 11 collagen-induced arthritis and antigen-induced arthritis in mice. *Arthritis Rheum.* 36:1305–1314.

43. Leuthwaite, J., S.M. Blake, T.E. Hardingham, P.J. Warden, and B. Henderson. 1994. The effect of recombinant human interleukin-1 receptor antagonist on the induction phase of antigen induced arthritis in the rabbit. *J. Rheumatol.* 21:467–472.

44. van Lent, P.L.E.M., F.A.J. van de Loo, A.E.M. Holthuysen, et al. 1995. Major role for interleukin-1 but not tumor necrosis factor in early cartilage damage in immune complex arthritis in mice. *J. Rheumatol.* 22:2250–2258.

45. Joosten, L.A.B., M.M.A. Helsen, F.A.J. van de Loo, and W.B. van den Berg. 1996. Anticytokine treatment of established type 11 collagen-induced arthritis in DBA/1 mice. A comparative study using anti-TNFα, anti-IL-1β and IL-1ra. *Arthritis Rheum.* 39:797–809.

46. Bendele, A., G. Sennello, T. McAbee, J. Frazier, E. Chlipala, and B. Rich. 1999. Effects of interleukin-1 receptor antagonist alone or in combination with methotrexate in adjuvant arthritic rats. *J. Rheumatol.* 26:1225–1229.

47. Evans, C.H., S.C. Ghivazzani, R. Kang, T. Muzzonegri, M.C. Wasco, J.H. Herndon, and P.D. Robbins. 1999. Gene therapy for rheumatic diseases. *Arthritis Rheum.* 42:1–16.

48. Otani, K., I. Nita, W. Macaulay, H.I. Georgescu, P.D. Robbins, and C.H. Evans. 1996. Suppression of antigen-induced arthritis by gene therapy. *J. Immunol.* 156:3558–3562.

49. Makarov, S.S., J.C. Olsen, W.N. Johnston, S.K. Anderle, R.R. Brown, A.S. Baldwin, et al. 1996. Suppression of experimental arthritis by gene transfer of interleukin-1 receptor antagonist cDNA. *Proc. Natl. Acad. Sci. USA* 93:402–406.

50. Bakker, A.C., L.A.B. Joosten, O.J. Arntz, M.M.A. Helsen, A.M. Bendele, F.A.J. van de Loo, and W.B. van den Berg. 1997. Gene therapy of murine collagen-induced arthritis: local expression of human IL-1ra protein prevents onset. *Arthritis Rheum.* 40:893–900.

51. Hesse, D.G., K.J. Tracey, Y. Fong, K.R. Manogue, M.A. Palladino Jr., A. Cerami, et al. 1988. Cytokine appearance in human endotoxemia and primate bacteremia. *Surg. Gynecol. Obstet.* 166: 147–153.

52. Waage, A. and T. Espevik T. 1988. Interleukin-1 potentiates the lethal effects of tumor necrosis factor/cachectin in mice. *J. Exp. Med.* 167:1987–1992.

53. Cannon, J.G., R.G. Tompkins, J.A. Gelfand, H.R. Mitchie, G.G. Stanford, J.W.M. van der Meer, et al. 1990. Circulating interleukin-1 and tumor necrosis factor in septic shock and experimental endotoxin fever. *J. Infect. Dis.* 161:79–84.

54. Fisher, C.J., J.-F.A. Dhainaut, S.M. Opal, J.P. Pribble, R.A. Balk, G.J. Slotman, et al. for the Phase 3 rhIL-1ra Sepsis Syndrome Study Group. 1994. Recombinant human interleukin 1 receptor

antagonist in the treatment of patients with sepsis syndrome. Results from a randomized, double-blind, placebo-controlled trial. *JAMA* 271:1836–1843.

55. Drevlow, B.E., R. Lovis, M.A. Haag, J.M. Sinacore, C. Jacobs, C. Blosche, et al. 1996. Recombinant human interleukin-1 receptor type 1 in the treatment of patients with active rheumatoid arthritis. *Arthritis Rheum.* 39:257–265.

56. Schorlemmer, H.U., E.J. Kanzy, K.D. Langner, and R. Kurrle. 1993. Immunomodulatory activity of recombinant IL-1 receptor (IL-1-R) on models of experimental rheumatoid arthritis. *Agents Actions* 39:c113–c116.

57. Campion, G.V., M.E. Lesback, J. Lookabaugh, G. Gordon, M. Catalano, and The IL-1Ra Arthritis Study Group. 1996. Dose-range and dose-frequency study of recombinant human interleukin-1 receptor antagonist in patients with rheumatoid arthritis. *Arthritis Rheum.* 39:1092–1101.

58. Bresnihan, B., J.M. Alvaro-Gracia, M. Cobby, M. Doherty, Z. Domljan, P. Emery, et al. 1998. Treatment of rheumatoid arthritis with recombinant human interleukin-1 receptor antagonist. *Arthritis Rheum.* 41:2196–2204.

59. Bresnihan, B. 1999. Treatment of rheumatoid arthritis with interleukin-1 receptor antagonist. *Ann. Rheum. Dis.* 58(Suppl. I), 96–98.

60. Felson, D.T., J.J. Anderson, M. Boers, C. Bombardier, M. Chernoff, B. Fried, et al. 1993. The American College of Rheumatology preliminary core set of disease activity measures for rheumatoid arthritis clinical trials. *Arthritis Rheum.* 36:729–740.

61. Larsen, A., K. Dale, and M. Eek. 1977. Radiographic evaluation of rheumatoid arthritis and related conditions by standard reference films. *Acta. Radiol. Diagn.* 18:481–491.

62. Jiang, Y., H.K. Genant, I. Watt, M. Cobby, B. Bresnihan, R. Aitchison, and D. McCabe. 2000. A multicenter, double-blind, dose-ranging, randomized and placebo controlled study of recombinant human interleukin-1 receptor antagonist in patients with rheumatoid arthritis: radiologic progression and correlation of Genant and Larsen scoring methods. *Arthritis Rheum.* 43:1001–1009.

63. Cunnane, G., A. Madigan, E. Murphy, O. FitzGerald, and B. Bresnihan. 2000. The effects of treatment with interleukin-1 receptor antagonist on the inflamed synovial membrane in rheumatoid arthritis. *Rheumatology* 40:62–69.

64. Nuki, G., B. Rozman, K. Pavelka, P. Emery, J. Lookabaugh, and P. Musikic. 1997. Interleukin-1 receptor antagonist continues to demonstrate clinical improvement in rheumatoid arthritis. *Arthritis Rheum.* 40:S224.

65. Cohen, S., E. Hurd, J.J. Cush, M.H. Schiff, M.E. Weinblatt, L.W. Moreland, et al. 1999. Treatment of interleukin-1 receptor antagonist in combination with methotrexate in rheumatoid arthritis patients. *Arthritis Rheum.* 42:S273.

66. Evans, C.H., P.D. Robbins, S.C. Ghivizzani, J.H. Herndon, M.C. Wasko, M. Tomaino, et al. 1999. Results from the first human clinical trial of gene therapy for arthritis. *Arthritis Rheum.* 42:S170.

67. Bendele, A., T. McAbee, G. Sennello, J. Frazier, E. Chlipala, and D. McCabe. 1999. Efficacy of sustained blood levels of interleukin-1 receptor antagonist in animal models of arthritis: Comparison of efficacy in animal models with human clinical data. *Arthritis Rheum.* 42:498–506.

68. O'Dell. J.R. 1999. Anticytokine therapy: A new era in the treatment of rheumatoid arthritis? *N. Engl. J. Med.* 340:310–312.

69. Bathon, J.M., R.W. Martin, R.M. Fleischmann, J.R. Tesser, M.H. Schiff, E.C. Keystone, et al. 2000. A comparison of etanercept and methotrexate in patients with early rheumatoid arthritis. *N. Engl. J. Med.* 343:1586–1593.

70. Lipsky, P., D. van der Heijde, E.W. St. Clair, D.E. Furst, F.C. Breedveld, J.R. Kalden, J.S. Smolen, et al. 2000. Infliximab and methotrexate in the treatment of rheumatoid arthritis. *N. Engl. J. Med.* 343:1594:1594–1602.

8 Leflunomide

An Immunomodulatory Drug for the Treatment of Rheumatoid Arthritis

Paul Emery, David L. Scott, and Vibeke Strand

INTRODUCTION

Leflunomide is a new disease-modifying anti-rheumatic drug (DMARD) that is classified as an isoxazol, and is rapidly converted from its prodrug form to its active metabolite, A77 1726, by first-pass metabolism in the gut and liver. At therapeutic doses (20 mg/d) in rheumatoid arthritis (RA) patients, A77 1726 blocks the *de novo* synthesis of pyrimidines by inhibiting dihydroorotate dehydrogenase (DHODH), the rate-limiting enzyme in pyrimidine production *(1–4)* necessary for the clonal expansion of activated T and B lymphocytes. The following overview will address the mode of action and the preclinical and clinical experience with leflunomide in the treatment of RA.

PATHOGENESIS OF RA AND LEFLUNOMIDE MODE OF ACTION

The specific pathogenic events leading to RA remain unknown. It is generally believed, however, that an undefined antigen causes the activation of T cells in a genetically susceptible set of the population, leading to the development of RA *(5–6)*. Proliferation of activated T cells, in turn, stimulate monocytes, dendritic cells, B cells, and fibroblast-like synoviocytes via cytokine release or direct cell-cell contact *(7)*. The

From: *Modern Therapeutics in Rheumatic Diseases*
Edited by: G. C. Tsokos, et al. © Humana Press, Inc., Totowa, NJ

monocytes and synoviocytes, in response to this stimulation, produce pro-inflammatory cytokines, including IL-1 and TNF-α, as well as growth factors that perpetuate the process of inflammation. In addition, they produce matrix metalloproteinases (MMPs) and collagenases involved in the process of degradation *(8–10)*, leading to the permanent structural damage of articular cartilage and bone associated with RA.

In vitro studies indicate that proliferation of mitogen-stimulated CD4+ T cells require an 8- to 16-fold increase of pyrimidine pools in order to support ribonucleic acid (RNA) and deoxyribonucleic acid (DNA) synthesis *(11)*. The blockade of DHODH activity by A77 1726, and the resultant inhibition of pyrimidine biosynthesis, halt T-cell proliferation by arresting the activated cell during the G1/S phase of the cell cycle *(12)*. Other cells that utilize the salvage pathways to collect pyrimidine precursors are less affected by A77 1726 *(13)*. Thus leflunomide specifically inhibits cells such as activated T cells that predominantly use the *de novo* pathway of pyrimidine synthesis and are thought to mediate the development of RA *(14)*.

THE EFFECTIVENESS OF LEFLUNOMIDE IN ANIMAL MODELS OF ARTHRITIS

Preclinical animal studies have demonstrated the effectiveness of leflunomide in both spontaneous and induced arthritis, as well as in other autoimmune disease models *(15–25)*. In a 12-wk study of proteoglycan-induced arthritis in mice *(22)*, leflunomide (35 mg/kg/d) showed improvement in the signs of arthritis by 2 wk of treatment. There was also a reduction in the circulating antibodies to both mouse and human proteoglycan that correlate with the improvement of arthritic signs following treatment with leflunomide. Similar effectiveness has been shown in a rat model of adjuvant-induced arthritis. Oral leflunomide dosed at 5–10 mg/kg/d for 26 d resulted in a significant reduction in both the arthritis score and joint swelling compared to untreated controls *(26)*.

The bone-protective properties of leflunomide have been demonstrated with an in vitro assay modeling osteoclast resorption of bone, where treatment with leflunomide reduced the number of osteoclast resorption pits formed on the surface of ivory plates. The same study showed a reduction of bone resorption in vivo in collagen-induced arthritis in mice *(27)*. Leflunomide treatment was also found to preserve the mechanical properties and matrix integrity of rat bone in an adjuvant-induced model of arthritis *(28)*.

REVIEW OF CLINICAL TRIALS

The efficacy and safety of leflunomide for the treatment of RA has been assessed in one phase II dose-ranging study, two placebo-controlled phase III studies, and a large phase III comparative investigation (Table 1). With study extensions, the phase III clinical trials evaluated the effectiveness of leflunomide for the treatment of RA over 2 yr. The cumulative patient database represents one of the largest groups of RA patients to be studied in a controlled clinical setting. This review will focus on results from the primary trials, but not the extensions.

Phase II Clinical Trial of Leflunomide

The clinical efficacy of leflunomide for the treatment of RA was initially shown in a randomized, double-blind, placebo-controlled phase II clinical trial *(29)*. Four hundred

Table 1
Phase II and III Studies with Leflunomide in Patients with Active RA

Study	YU 203	MN 301	MN 302	US 301 US/Canada
Design	Randomized, double-blind	Randomized, double-blind	Randomized, double-blind	Randomized, double-blind
Duration (mo)	6	6	12	12
Treatment groups	Leflunomide Placebo	Leflunomide Sulfasalazine Placebo	Leflunomide Methotrexate	Leflunomide Methotrexate Placebo
Patients randomized (n)	402	358	999	485
Location	Former Yugoslavia	Europe Australia New Zealand South Africa	Europe South Africa	United States Canada
Extension (mo)	24	6, 12	12	12

and two patients diagnosed with active RA as defined by the American College of Rheumatology (ACR) *(30)*, were randomly selected to receive either placebo or 1 of 3 leflunomide dosing regimens (50 mg on d 1, followed by 5 mg/d, or 100 mg on d 1, followed by either 10 or 25 mg/d) for 24 wk.

The primary measures of clinical effectiveness included tender and swollen joint counts and scores (based on 66–68 joints) and global assessments of disease activity by both the patient and physician. Treatment with leflunomide at 25 mg/d significantly improved all primary and secondary efficacy parameters when compared to placebo. Patients treated with 10 mg/d also showed significant improvement in the primary variables, but there was no statistical difference in tender joint counts compared to placebo.

The data derived from the dose-ranging study were used in a population pharmaco-kinetics model to determine an optimal clinical dose for phase III trials *(31)*.

Clinical success was directly related to the plasma concentration of A77 1726. Eighty percent of the maximum response was achieved by steady-state plasma concentrations of between 10 and 15 mg/L. Based on this analysis the dosing regime for phase III clinical trials, discussed below, was 100 mg/d for 3 d, followed by a maintenance dose of 20 mg/d.

Phase III Clinical Trials of Leflunomide

US301 was a double-blind, placebo-controlled clinical trial conducted in 42 centers in the United States and Canada that randomly assigned 482 patients to either leflunomide, methotrexate, or placebo groups in a ratio of 3:3:2 *(32)*. Methotrexate was initially dosed at 7.5 mg/wk for wk 1–6, with dose titrations to 15 mg/wk after wk 7, in increments of 2.5 mg/wk. The study protocol mandated that all patients receive folate supplementation (1 mg qd or bid).

MN301 was a multicenter trial conducted in Europe, Australia, New Zealand, and South Africa. Thirty-six centers participated in the 6-mo, randomized, double-blind, placebo-controlled trial comparing leflunomide to sulfasalazine. One hundred and thirty patients were assigned to the leflunomide group; an equal number of patients was assigned to the sulfasalazine treatment group and received an initial dose of 0.5 g/d that was titrated at weekly intervals to 2 g/d by wk 4 *(33)*.

A third study, a comparative investigation of the efficacy of leflunomide and methotrexate (MN302), was designed as a multinational, multicenter, double-blind investigation, in which 999 patients were randomly assigned to receive either leflunomide or methotrexate for a 1-yr period of treatment. Methotrexate was provided at an initial dose of 7.5 mg/wk for wk 1–4, increased to 10 mg/wk during wk 5–12, and maintained at 10 or 15 mg/wk for the duration of the study *(34)*. Folate supplementation was not mandated in this comparative investigation.

Leflunomide: Clinical Improvement in Signs and Symptoms of RA

The ACR response criteria *(35)* were used for a summary evaluation of the efficacy measurements *(36)* in the clinical trials evaluating the effect of leflunomide in the treatment of RA. The ACR 20% response rate is defined as a $\geq$ 20% improvement in tender and swollen joint counts in addition to comparable improvement in 3 of 5 clinical parameters, including: patient global assessment of disease activity, physician global assessment of disease activity, functional ability (Health Assessment Questionnaire [HAQ] or the Modified HAQ [MHAQ]), pain intensity, and erythrocyte sedimentation rate (ESR) or C-reactive protein (CRP) levels. The 50 and 70% response rates signify 50 and 70% improvement of the same variables *(35)*.

The ACR 20% response rate in US301 establishes that a significantly higher percentage of patients treated with leflunomide (52%) met the criteria than those receiving placebo (26%); the rate was comparable to that for the methotrexate group (46%) at the study endpoint *(30)*. The ACR 20, 50, and 70% response rates are shown in Fig. 1A. Four to five times more leflunomide patients met the more stringent ACR 50 and 70% criteria than in the placebo-treated group.

In MN301, 55% of the leflunomide patients achieved ACR 20% response rates (Fig. 1B). That percentage proved significantly greater than placebo (29%) and was comparable to sulfasalazine (56%) *(33)*. Twice as many leflunomide and sulfasalazine as placebo patients fulfilled the criteria for ACR 50% response.

Leflunomide showed significantly early onset of action with respect to the efficacy parameters evaluated in this study. At 4 wk, in 8 of 10 outcome measures (tender and swollen joint counts, patient and physician assessments, pain intensity, HAQ, CRP, and rheumatoid factor [RF]), leflunomide showed significant improvement compared to placebo and sulfasalazine *(33)*. The early onset of action may be attributed in part to the initial 100 mg/d loading dose *(33)*.

The large comparative study of leflunomide and methotrexate (MN302) at 1 yr establishes that 51% of the leflunomide-treated patients met the ACR 20% criteria, and significantly more methotrexate patients (65%) met the same level of response *(34,37)* (Fig. 1C). A comparison of the two methotrexate groups showed a disparate ACR 20% response rate to methotrexate treatment (46 vs 65%). An important difference between MN302 and US301 was that concomitant folate administration was not mandated in MN302. Methotrexate treatment without folate supplementation in MN302 was associated with higher clinical efficacy but a higher incidence of hepatotoxicity. With respect to this observation leflunomide is equal in effectiveness to methotrexate when

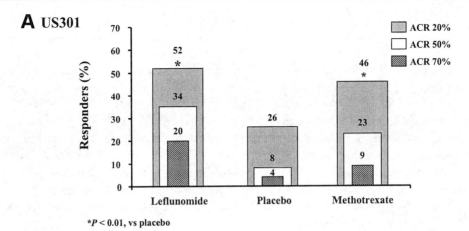

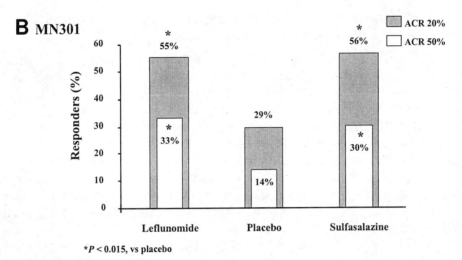

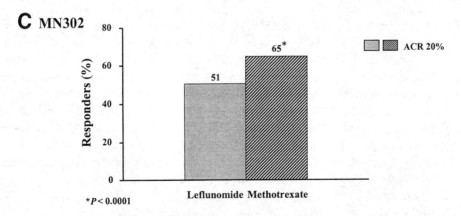

Fig. 1. Comparison of ACR response rates in US301 (A), MN301 (B), and MN302 (C).

administered simultaneously with folate *(38)*. A comparison of the ACR 20% response for leflunomide across the phase III trials indicates a consistent effectiveness at study endpoint (52, 55, and 50.5% in US301, MN301, and MN302, respectively).

An area under the curve (AUC) analysis accounts for the cumulative effects of therapy, by summing the clinical response over the duration of the investigation *(39)*. The AUC analysis of the ACR 20% response adds a temporal component that may offer a better evaluation of clinical effect than can be obtained at a single time-point *(32)*. In US301, the number of weeks leflunomide patients reported ACR 20% response (23.7 wk) was significantly greater than in the placebo group (12.6 wk) and similar to the number in the methotrexate group (22.7 wk) *(32)*. AUC analysis of ACR response in MN302 found equal efficacy for leflunomide and methotrexate in the treatment of RA. The mean duration of clinical effect was 23.0 wk for leflunomide treatment and 25.4 wk for methotrexate therapy, and both treatments were statistically equivalent *(34)*.

Leflunomide: Clinical Improvement of Patient Function and Health-Related Quality of Life

Impairment of physical function resulting from RA disease progression significantly interferes with activities of daily living and adversely affects patient quality of life *(40)*. The three phase III clinical trials evaluated the impact of leflunomide therapy on patient function and health-related quality of life via health assessment instruments, including: HAQ *(41)*, MHAQ *(42)*, the Problem Elicitation Technique (PET) *(43)*, and the Medical Outcomes Study Short Form 36 (SF-36) *(44)*.

Analysis of the correlation between clinical improvement, defined by the ACR response criteria, and patient function and health-related quality of life instruments (HAQ, MHAQ, PET, and SF-36) indicates that the functional assessments were sensitive to the identification of clinical benefits that are of significant importance to patients *(45)*.

The HAQ score comprises patient responses to questions in eight categories related to patient function, including: dressing and grooming, rising, eating, walking, hygiene, reach, grip, and activities of daily living. The average or mean HAQ score is calculated by dividing the sum of the individual sub-scores by the number of questions. A decrease in any of the scores indicates an improvement *(41)*. In US301 leflunomide treatment resulted in significant improvement (Fig. 2) in all categories of the HAQ score compared to placebo. Significant improvement compared to methotrexate was seen in the categories of rising, eating, walking, hygiene, activities of daily living, and the disability index *(46)*. In terms of the MHAQ (representing a shortened form of the HAQ), leflunomide-treated patients showed significant improvement compared to both the placebo and methotrexate groups *(46)*.

Functional assessment via the HAQ score was also significantly improved in leflunomide-treated patients compared to both placebo and sulfasalazine in MN301 (Fig. 3), with statistically significant improvement observed after as little as 1 mo of therapy in the leflunomide group *(33)*.

In both placebo-controlled trials, leflunomide treatment resulted in substantially reduced HAQ scores at study endpoint, –0.45, and –0.50 in US301 and MN302, respectively. The clinical impact of these reductions in HAQ scores are enhanced by the observation that a minimally significant change in HAQ score equals –0.22 *(47)*.

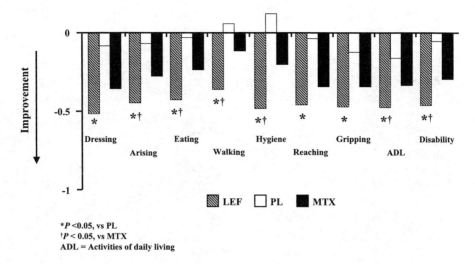

Fig. 2. HAQ scores in US301 comparing leflunomide (LEF) to methotrexate (MTX) and placebo (PL). Reprinted with permission from ref. *46*.

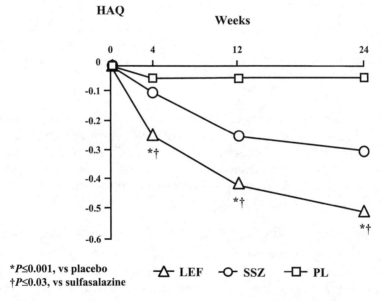

Fig. 3. The change in HAQ score from baseline in MN301. Leflunomide (LEF) shows significant improvement in HAQ scores compared to placebo (PL) and sulfasalazine (SSZ) at 4, 12, and 24 wk of treatment. Reprinted with permission.

Significant improvement in health-related quality of life in US301 was also shown by the SF-36 following leflunomide treatment in comparison with the placebo group. The SF-36 score responses to questions are summarized in eight domains, including: physical functioning, role physical, bodily pain, general health, vitality, social functioning, role emotional, and mental health. Leflunomide treatment resulted in significant improvement in the domains of bodily pain and vitality compared to methotrexate *(46)*.

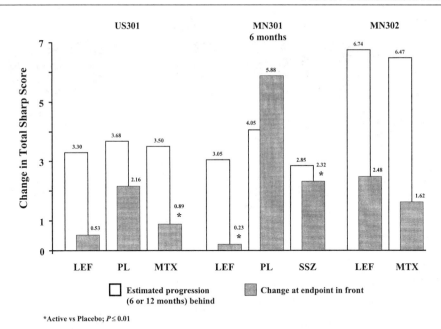

Fig. 4. Change in total Sharp score in phase II clinical trials of leflunomide. Dark bars show the change in Sharp score for each of the treatment groups (foreground). The predicted progression of RA is estimated from the baseline radiographic score divided by the disease duration for each patient, and is shown by the open bars in the background. Reprinted with permission from ref. *48.*

Leflunomide-treated patients in US301 showed significant improvement in the weighted top five scores of the PET compared to both the methotrexate- and placebo-treatment groups *(46)*. The PET assessment allows patients to prioritize the functional assessments, identifying those functional aspects that are of greatest importance to them. They can also indicate where they would like to see the greatest improvement in function and quality of life *(43)*.

Leflunomide: Slowing of Radiographic Disease Progression

After 1 yr of therapy with leflunomide, significantly fewer patients showed radiographically assessed progression of RA in US301 *(32)* compared to placebo, as indicated by changes in total Sharp scores and erosion and joint-space narrowing scores. It was also observed that leflunomide-treated patients had less disease progression than methotrexate-treated patients, but the result was not statistically equivalent ($p \leq 0.05$) *(32)*.

Employing the Larsen method of scoring radiographic progression, leflunomide- and sulfasalazine-treated patients exhibited significantly less disease progression than those receiving placebo in MN301, and both active treatment groups were comparable *(33)*.

Sharp et al. recently presented a comparative analysis of radiographic disease progression across the three phase III clinical trials *(48)*. The objective of the analysis was to determine if treatment with either leflunomide, methotrexate or sulfasalazine retards disease progression. In all cases, active treatment resulted in significantly less disease progression than placebo at 6 and 12 mo of therapy (Fig. 4). In general, leflunomide treatment was equivalent to both methotrexate and sulfasalazine in retarding the advancement of structural damage in RA. These studies represent the first 6- and 12-mo, randomized, placebo- and active-controlled clinical trials to demonstrate slowing of radiographic progression of disease following therapy with a new DMARD *(48)*.

Leflunomide: Combination Therapy with Methotrexate

The clinical safety and pharmacokinetics of leflunomide in combination with methotrexate has been assessed in an open-label, clinical trial of 52 wk duration. Thirty RA patients with active disease despite methotrexate therapy (17 ± 4 mg/wk for 6 mo or greater) were treated with leflunomide (100 mg/d loading dose for 2 d, 10–20 mg/d thereafter) in addition to methotrexate *(49)*. The study found no significant variation in the pharmacokinetic parameters of either drug when the two were administered together, indicating no pharmacokinetic interactions between the drugs *(49)*.

At study endpoint, 53% of the patients fulfilled the ACR 20% criteria for clinical improvement and two patients met the criteria for remission. In general, the combination was well tolerated, with the exception of elevations of liver enzymes. Of the seven patients withdrawn from the study, three were owing to persistent elevation of plasma transaminase levels *(49)*. Because of the potential risk of serious liver damage when methotrexate and leflunomide are used in combination, careful dose titration and patient monitoring are essential *(49)*.

CURRENT RECOMMENDATIONS

Based on the prescribing information *(50)* leflunomide is indicated for adults with active RA to improve the signs and symptoms of the disease and retard structural damage. The recommended dosing includes a 100 mg/d loading dose for 3 d, followed by a maintenance dose of 20 mg/d. Leflunomide may be taken without regard to meals, and in combination with aspirin, nonsteroidal anti-inflammatory drugs (NSAIDs), and corticosteroids. With regard to age, there is no indicated dosage adjustment for patients older than 65 yr, but leflunomide is not recommended for patients under 18 yr of age *(50)*.

Special precautions regarding leflunomide are advised for patients with renal insufficiency, and the drug is not recommended for patients with significantly impaired hepatic function *(50)*. Because preclinical animal studies of leflunomide have shown teratogenic properties, the drug must not be given to women of childbearing potential before testing for pregnancy and obtaining assurances that they are using reliable contraception *(50)*.

Cholestyramine and charcoal are recommended for the accelerated elimination of leflunomide *(50)*. Cholestyramine given orally at a dose of 8 g 3 times daily for 1 d has been shown to reduce levels of A77 1726 by 40% in a 24-h period and by 49–65% in a 48-h period *(50)*. Oral administration of a suspension of activated charcoal (50 g every 6 h for 24 h) has been shown to reduce plasma concentration of A77 1726 by 37% in 24 h and 48% in 48 h *(50)*.

SIDE EFFECTS

The most common adverse events (Table 2) observed during Phase II and Phase III clinical trials of leflunomide were gastrointestinal (G.I.; e.g., diarrhea and nausea), elevated liver enzymes (ALT and AST), reversible alopecia, and skin rash *(29)*. Most of these events were mild to moderate in severity and resolved without further

Table 2
Adverse Events[a] with an Incidence Rate of >5%

| Adverse event | Placebo-controlled | | | Active-controlled | | | All trials |
	Leflunomide (n = 315)	PL (n = 210)	SSZ (n = 133)	MTX (n = 182)	Leflunomide (n = 501)	MTX (n = 486)	Leflunomide (n = 1339)
Gastrointestinal							
Diarrhea	26.7	11.9	9.8	19.2	22.2	10.0	17.0
Nausea	13.0	11.0	18.8	18.1	12.8	18.1	9.3
Dyspepsia	10.2	10.0	9.0	13.2	5.8	7.0	4.9
Abdominal pain	5.7	4.3	8.2	6.8	8.0	7.6	4.6
Vomiting	5.1	4.3	2.7	3.8	3.2	3.4	2.8
Hepatic							
Elevated LFT	10.2	2.4	3.8	10.4	5.8	16.9	4.9
CNS							
Headache	13.3	11.4	12.0	20.9	9.6	7.8	6.8
Dizziness	5.1	3.3	6.0	4.9	7.0	6.2	4.2
Cardiovascular							
Hypertension	8.9	4.3	3.8	2.7	9.8	4.0	10.3
Respiratory							
Respiratory infection	21.0	20.5	20.3	31.9	26.5	24.5	15.1
Bronchitis	5.1	1.9	3.8	6.6	8.0	6.8	6.5
Skin							
Rash	12.4	6.7	10.5	8.8	10.8	9.6	9.9
Alopecia	8.9	1.4	6.0	6.0	16.2	9.8	9.7

[a]Includes all phase II and phase III trials with leflunomide; analyses of phase III trials pertains to 1-yr treatment period. PL, Placebo; SSZ, Sulfasalazine; MTX, Methotrexate; LFT, Liver-function test.

complication. Treatment withdrawals for leflunomide-treated patients were higher than those observed for placebo controls, but were comparable to both sulfasalazine- and methotrexate-treatment groups.

Leflunomide was associated with clinically significant elevations of liver enzymes (ALT and AST), at a rate of 10% in US301 and MN301 and 6% in MN302 (32,33,50). Most of these elevations were mild and ≤2 times the upper limit of normal (ULN). They usually resolved without discontinuation of therapy. Serious elevations of <3 ULN were infrequent and reversed with either dose reduction or withdrawal from therapy.

Rare and potentially serious adverse events in the methotrexate-treated group included five potentially fatal interstitial pneumonitis cases and three cases of reversible renal failure (32). There were no instances of these events in the leflunomide-treated population. Two cases of agranulocytosis requiring hospitalization were reported for sulfasalazine-treated patients; this condition was also not observed in the leflunomide groups (33).

CONCLUSIONS

Preclinical investigations of leflunomide have identified a unique immunomodulatory mode of action. Leflunomide primarily targets activated T cells that use *de novo* synthetic pathways to generate pyrimidines necessary for proliferation, and thus potentially suppress the T-cell-centered pathogenesis of RA. Because of this specific mode of action, leflunomide is believed to function as an immunomodulatory agent.

The results from clinical trials indicate that leflunomide is safe and well tolerated, capable of producing significant improvement in the signs and symptoms of RA placebo, and comparable to both sulfasalazine and methotrexate in effectiveness. Of greater significance to the patient, leflunomide offers substantially significant improvement in patient function and health-related quality of life when compared to placebo, sulfasalazine, and methotrexate in placebo-controlled trials. The active and placebo-controlled trials show that leflunomide can provide significant slowing of radiographically measured disease progression compared to placebo and is at least as effective in slowing RA progression as sulfasalazine and methotrexate.

REFERENCES

1. Cherwinski, H.M., N. Byars, S.J. Ballaron, G.M. Nakano, J.M. Young, and J.T. Ransom. 1995. Leflunomide interferes with pyrimidine nucleotide biosynthesis. *Inflamm. Res.* 44:317–322.

2. Zielinski, T., D. Zeitter, S. Müllner, and R.R. Bartlett. 1995. Leflunomide, a reversible inhibitor of pyrimidine biosynthesis. *Inflamm. Res.* 44(Suppl. 2):207–208.

3. Xu, X., J.W. Williams, H. Gong, and A. Finnegan, and A.S.F. Chong. 1996. Two activities of the immunosuppresive metabolite of leflunomide, A77 1726: inhibition of pyrimidine nucleotide synthesis and protein tyrosine phosphorylation. *Biochem. Pharmacol.* 52:527–534.

4. Rückemann, K., L.D. Fairbanks, E.A. Carrey, C.M. Hawrylowicz, D.F. Richards, B. Kirschbaum, and H.A. Simmonds. 1998. Leflunomide inhibits pyrimidine de novo synthesis in mitogen-stimulated T-lymphocytes from healthy humans. *J. Biol. Chem.* 273:21,682–21,691.

5. Panayi, G.S., J.S. Lanchbury, and G.H. Kingley, 1992. The importance of the T cell in initiating and maintaining the chronic synovitis of rheumatoid arthritis. *Arthritis Rheum.* 35:729–735.

6. Panayi, G.S. 1997. T-cell–dependent pathways in rheumatoid arthritis. *Curr. Opin. Rheumatol.* 9:236–240.

7. Deage, V., D. Burger, and J-M Dayer, 1998. Exposure of T lymphocytes to leflunomide but not to dexamethasone favors the production by monocytic cells of interleukin-1 receptor antagonist and the tissue-inhibitor of metalloproteinases-1 over that of interleukin-1β and metalloproteinases. *Eur. Cytokine News* 9:663–668.

8. Firestein, G.S. 1996. Invasive fibroblast-like synoviocytes in rheumatoid arthritis: passive responders or transformed aggressors? *Arthritis Rheum.* 39:1781–1790.

9. Malik, N., B.W. Greenfield, A.F. Wahl, and P.A. Kiener. 1996. Activation of human monocytes through CD40 induces matrix metalloproteinases. *J. Immunol.* 156:3952–3960.

10. Ivashkiv, L.B. 1996. Cytokine expression and cell activation in inflammatory arthritis. *Advances in Immunol.* 63:337–376.

11. Fairbanks, L.D., M. Bofil, K. Ruckemann, and H.A. Simmonds. 1995. Importance of ribonucleotide availability to proliferating T-lymphocytes from healthy humans. *J. Biol. Chem.* 270:29,682–29,691.

12. Fox, R.I. 1998. Mechanism of action of leflunomide in rheumatoid arthritis. *J. Rheumatol.* 25(Suppl. 53):20–26.

13. Fox, R.I., M.L. Herrmann, C.G. Frangou, G.M. Wahl, R.E. Morris, and B.J. Kirschbaum. 1999. How does leflunomide modulate the immune response in rheumatoid arthritis? *BioDrugs* 12:301–315.

14. Fox, R.I., M.L. Herrman, C.G. Frangou, G.M. Wahl, R.E. Morris, V. Strand, and B.J. Kirschbaum. 1999. Mechanism of action for leflunomide in rheumatoid arthritis. *Clin. Immunol.* 93:1–11.

15. Bartlett, R.R. and R. Schleyerbach. 1985. Disease modifying action of a novel isoxazol derivative, HWA 486, on adjuvant-arthritis of the rat. *Int. J. Immunopharmacol.* 7:1-1. (Abstract)

16. Popovic, S. and R.R. Bartlett. 1986. Disease modifying activity of HWA 486 on the development of SLE in MRL/1-mice. *Agents Actions* 19:313–314.

17. Pasternak, R.D., N.S. Wadopian, R.N. Wright, P. Siminoff, J.A. Gylys, and J.P. Buyniski. 1987. Disease modifying activity of HWA 486 in rat adjuvant-induced arthritis. *Agents Actions* 21: 241–243.

18. Bartlett, R.R., S. Popovic, and R.X. Raiss. 1988. Development of autoimmunity in MRL/lpr mice and the effects of drugs on this murine disease. *Scand. J. Rheumatol.* 75:290–299.

19. Thoenes, G.H., T. Sitter, K.H. Langer, R.R. Bartlett, and R. Schleyerbach. 1988. Testing of the effectiveness of new potential antirheumatic drug, HWA 486 (leflunomide) against acute inflammatory interstitial nephritis in the rat. *Z. Rheumatol.* 47:290 (Abstract)

20. Thoenes, G.H., C. Kuechle, K.H. Langer, R.R. Bartlett, and R. Schleyerbach. 1990. Novel immunosuppressive drug, leflunomide, inhibits acute rejection of kidney transplants in rats. *Kidney Int.* 37:1184 (Abstract).

21. Bartlett, R.R., M. Dimitrijevic, T. Mattar, T. Zielinski, T. Germann, E. Rüde, et al. 1991. Leflunomide (HWA 486), a novel immunomodulating compound for the treatment of autoimmune disorders and reactions leading to transplantation rejection. *Agents Actions* 32:10–21.

22. Glant, T.T., K. Mikecz, R.R. Bartlett, R. Schleyerbach, E.J.M.A. Thonar, J.M. Williams, et al. 1992. Immunomodulation of proteoglycan-induced progressive polyarthritis by leflunomide. *Immunopharmacology* 23:105–116.

23. Glant, T.T., K. Mikecz, F. Brennan, G. Negroiu, and R.R. Bartlett. 1994. Suppression of autoimmune responses and inflammatory events by leflunomide in an animal model for rheumatoid arthritis. *Agents Actions* C267-C270.

24. Robertson, S.M. and L.S. Lang. 1993. Efficacy of topical or oral leflunomide in S-antigen induced autoimmune uveitis. Symposium Leflunomide- Inflammation '93 Vienna:1–1. (Abstract).

25. Thoss, K., S. Henzgen, P.X. Patrow, and R. Braeuer. 1994. Immunomodulation of antigen-induced arthritis by leflunomide in the rat. *Z. Rheumatol.* 53:70 (Abstract).

26. Thoss, K., S. Henzgen, P.K. Petrow, D. Katenkamp, and R. Brauer, R. 1996. Immunomodulation of rat antigen-induced arthritis by leflunomide alone and in combination with cyclosporin A. *Inflamm. Res.* 45:103–107.

27. Arai, U., S. Ueyama, Y. Yoshida, H. Kitagawa, M. Inazu, and M. Yaguchi. 2000. Leflunomide inhibits bone resorption in vitro and the severity of type II collagen-induced arthritis (CIA) in mice. *Ann. Rheum. Dis.* 59:144 (Abstract).

28. Ueyama, S., Y. Arai, Y. Yoshida, H. Kitagawa, M. Inazu, and M. Yaguchi. 2000. Leflunomide inhibits loss of bone mineral density and the reduction of bone mechanical strength in rats with adjuvant-induced arthritis. *Ann. Rheum. Dis.* 59:144 (Abstract).

29. Mladenovic, V., Z. Domljan, B. Rozman, I. Jajic, D. Mihajlovic, J. Dordevic, et al. 1995. Safety and effectiveness of leflunomide in the treatment of patients with active rheumatoid arthritis: Results of a randomized, placebo-controlled, phase II study. *Arthritis Rheum.* 38:1595–1603.

30. Arnett, F.C., S.M. Edworthy, D.A. Bloch, D.J. McShane, J.F. Fries, N.S. Cooper, et. al. 1988. The American Rheumatism Association 1987 revised criteria for the classification of rheumatoid arthritis. *Arthritis Rheum.* 31(3):315–324.

31. Weber, W. and L. Harnisch, L. 1997. Use of a population approach to the development of leflunomide: A new disease-modifying drug in the treatment of rheumatoid arthritis, European cooperation in the field of scientific and technical research. Edited by L.P. Aarons, M. Balant, M. Danhof, U.A. Gex-Fabry, M.O. Gundert-Remy, F. Karlsson, et al. European Commission Directorate-General Science, Research and Development, Brussels. 239.

32. Strand, V., S. Cohen, M. Schiff, A. Weaver, R. Fleischmann, G. Cannon, et al. 1999. Treatment of active rheumatoid arthritis with leflunomide compared to placebo and methotrexate. *Arch. Intern. Med.* 159:2542–2550.

33. Smolen, J.S., J.R. Kalden, D.L. Scott, B. Rozman, T.K. Kvien, I. Loew-Friedrich, et al. European Leflunomide Study Group. 1999. Efficacy and safety of leflunomide compared with placebo and sulphasalazine in active rheumatoid arthritis: a double-blind, randomised, multicentre trial. *Lancet* 353:259–266.

34. Emery, P., F. Breedveld, E.M. Lemmel, J.P. Kaltwasser, P.T. Dawes, B. Gomer, et al. 2000. A comparison of the efficacy and safety of leflunomide and methotrexate for the treatment of rheumatoid arthritis. *Rheumatology* 39:655–665.

35. Felson, D.T., J.J. Anderson, M. Boers, C. Bombardier, M. Chernoff, B. Fried, et al. 1993. The American College of Rheumatology preliminary core set of disease activity measures for rheumatoid arthritis clinical trials. *Arthritis Rheum.* 36:729–740.

36. Felson, D.T., J.J. Anderson, M. Baers, C. Bombardier, D. Furst, C. Goldsmith, et al. 1995. American College of Rheumatology preliminiary definition of improvement in rheumatoid arthritis. *Arthritis Rheum.* 38(6):727–735.

37. Emery, P., F.C. Breedveld, R.W. Jubb, H. Sorensen, C. Oed, and I. Loew-Friedrich. 2000. Efficacy and safety of leflunomide vs methotrexate in rheumatoid arthritis (RA): results of a double-blind, randomized, 2-year trial. *Arthritis Rheum.* 42 (Suppl.):(Abstract).

38. Schiff, M.H. 1999. Leflunomide versus methotrexate: A comparison of the European and American Experience. Scand. *J. Rheumatol.* 28(Suppl.)112:31–35.

39. Pham, B., A. Cranney, M. Boers, A.C. Verhoeven, G. Wells, and P. Tugwell. 1999. Validity of area-under-the-curve analysis to summarize effect in rheumatoid arthritis clinical trials. *J. Rheumatol.* 26:712–716.

40. Scott, D.L. 1999. Leflunomide improves quality of life in rheumatoid arthritis. Scand. *J. Rheumatol.* 28(Suppl.)112:23–29.

41. Fries, J.F., P.W. Spitz, and D.Y. Young. 1982. The dimensions of health outcomes: the health assessment questionnaire, disability and pain scales. *J. Rheumatol.* 9:789–793.

42. Pincus, T., J.A. Summey, S.A. Soraci, Jr., K.A. Wallston, and N.P. Hummon. 1983. Assessment of patient satisfaction in activities of daily living using a modified Stanford health assessment questionnaire. *Arthritis Rheum.* 26:1346–1353.

43. Bakker, C.H. 1998. Health-related utility measurement: concept and application. *Rheumatol. Eur.* 27:5–6.

44. Ware, Jr, J.E. and C.D. Sherbourne. 1992. The MOS 36-item short-form health survey (SF-36). I. Conceptual framework and item selection. *Med. Care* 30:473–483.

45. Tugwell, P., G. Wells, V. Strand, A. Maetzel, C. Bombardier, B. Crawford, et al. 2000. On behalf of the Leflunomide Rheumatoid Arthritis Investigators Group. 43:506–514.

46. Strand, V., P. Tugwell, C. Bombardier, A. Maetzel, B. Crawford, C. Dorrier, et al. 1999. Leflunomide Rheumatoid Arthritis Investigators Group. Function and health-related quality of life. Results from a randomized controlled trial of leflunomide versus methotrexate or placebo in patients with active rheumatoid arthritis. *Arthritis Rheum.* 42:1870–1878.

47. Wells, G.A., P. Tugwell, G.R. Kraag, P.R.A. Baker, J. Groh, and D.A. Redelmeier. 1993. Minimum important difference between patients with rheumatoid arthritis: the patient's perspective. *J. Rheumatol.* 20:557–560.

48. Sharp, J.T., V. Strand, H. Leung, F. Hurley, and I. Loew-Friedrich. 2000. Leflunomide Rheumatoid Arthritis Investigators Group. Treatment with leflunomide slows radiographic progression of rheumatoid arthritis. *Arthritis Rheum.* 43:495–505.

49. Weinblatt, M.E., J.M. Kremer, J.S. Coblyn, A.L. Maier, S. Helfgott, and M. Morrell. 1999. Pharmacokinetics, safety, and efficacy of the combination of methotrexate and leflunomide in patients with active rheumatoid arthritis. *Arthritis Rheum.* 42:1322–1328.

50. Aventis Pharmaceuticals Inc. 1998. Arava™ prescribing information.

9

Matrix Metalloproteinase Inhibitors as Therapies for Rheumatoid Arthritis

Sean J. Wollaston and Kenneth C. Kalunian

CONTENTS

INTRODUCTION
PATHOGENIC MECHANISMS
REVIEW OF ANIMAL DATA
REVIEW OF CLINICAL TRIALS
CURRENT RECOMMENDATIONS
SIDE EFFECTS AND PRECAUTIONS
CONCLUSIONS
REFERENCES

INTRODUCTION

The matrix metalloproteinases (MMPs) are a family of enzymes, that have the capacity to degrade all components of the connective tissue matrix *(1)*. MMPs are felt to play an important role in the irreversible damage of the extracellular matrix in rheumatoid arthritis (RA) *(2)*. Antibiotics, including tetracycline, have been used for many years for RA based on the hypothesis that RA is caused by an infectious agent, particularly a persistent Mycoplasma infection *(3,4)*. In fact, gold and sulfasalazine were initially used in RA based on their antimicrobial properties. This causal association, however, has not been substantiated despite extensive research efforts to do so and tetracycline-derivatives without any antimicrobial activity have proven to be efficacious in rats with adjuvant arthritis *(5,6)*. A small double-blind study comparing tetracycline 250 mg/d with placebo for 1 yr was unable to demonstrate any significant benefit *(7)*.

Tetracycline and its derivatives have recently become more intriguing based on new data that shows multiple immunomodulating and anti-inflammatory effects, as well as the capacity to inhibit MMPs from neutrophils, macrophages, osteoblasts, chondrocytes, epithelial cells, and rheumatoid synoviocytes *(8)*. Minocycline and doxycycline are even more effective than tetracycline in inhibiting MMPs. Oral minocycline at a dose of 100 mg twice daily has been shown to reduce collagenase activity in the synovial tissue of patients with RA *(9)*.

From: *Modern Therapeutics in Rheumatic Diseases*
Edited by: G. C. Tsokos, et al. © Humana Press, Inc., Totowa, NJ

Table 1
Matrix Metalloproteinases

MMP	Protein	Substrate
MMP-1	Collagenase	Fibrillar collagens
MMP-2	Gelatinase A (72 kd)	Type IV and V collagens, fibronectin
MMP-3	Stromelysin	Laminin, fibronectin, nonfibrillar collagen
MMP-7	Matrilysin	Laminin, fibronectin, nonfibrillar collagen
MMP-8	Neutrophil collagenase	Fibrillar collagens
MMP-9	Gelatinase B (92 kd)	Fibrillar collagens
MMP-10	Stromelysin-2	Laminin, fibronectin, nonfibrillar collagen
MMP-11	Stromelysin-3	Serpin
MMP-12	Metalloelastase	Elastin
MMP-13	Collagenase-3	Fibrillar collagens
MMP-14	MT1-MMP	Pro-MMP-2 (gelatinase A)
MMP-15	MT2-MMP	Pro-MMP-2 (gelatinase A)
MMP-16	MT3-MMP	Pro-MMP-2 (gelatinase A)
MMP-17	MT4-MMP	Pro-MMP-2 (gelatinase A)
MMP-18	Collagenase-4	Fibrillar collagens
MMP-19	(no common name)	Gelatin
MMP-20	Enamelysin	Amelogenin
MMP-21	72kd type IV collagenase	Type IV collagen
MMP-23	(no common name)	(unknown)
MMP-24	MT5-MMP	Pro-MMP-2 (gelatinase A)
MMP-25	MT6-MMP	Pro-MMP-2 (gelatinase A)
MMP-26	Macrophase metalloelastase	Gelatin, beta-casein

There are four main groups of MMPs (Table 1): the collagenases, stromelysins, gelatinases, and membrane metalloproteinases (10). The MMPs all contain zinc at the active center of each enzyme; are synthesized as a proenzyme which requires proteolytic cleavage of a propeptide domain for activation; and require calcium to maintain activity (11). The MMPs are carefully regulated at several different points, including synthesis and secretion, activation of the proenzyme, and inhibition of the active enzymes.

There are four collagenases: collagenase-1 (MMP-1), collagenase-3 (MMP-13), neutrophil collagenase (MMP-8), and collagenase-4 (MMP-18). The collagenases cleave fibrillar collagens at a single site and differ in their specificities for different collagens. MMP-1 and MMP-13 are synthesized by fibroblasts and macrophages when these cells are stimulated with inflammatory mediators. Neutrophil collagenase is predominantly synthesized by neutrophils and released upon stimulation of the cell (12). The natural substrates of the stromelysins are probably the proteoglycans, fibronectin, and laminin (13). Stromelysin-1 is not expressed significantly in normal tissues but can be induced by growth factors and cytokines, such as interleukin-1 (IL-1). Stromelysin is also able to activate latent collagenase, which provides a positive feedback signal for matrix destruction. There are two gelatinases, MMP-2 and MMP-9, which cleave denatured collagen, type IV and V collagen, and elastin (14). MMP-9, like MMP-8, is found within the specific granules of the neutrophil, whereas the others are produced by a variety of connective-tissue cells after stimulation by cytokines.

All active MMPS are inhibited by tissue inhibitors of metalloproteinases (TIMPs), which are produced by chondrocytes and synovial fibroblasts. There are at least three members of the TIMP family: TIMP-1, TIMP-2, and TIMP-3. The TIMPs bind specifically with the active matrix metalloproteinases to form 1:1, noncovalent, but tight-binding complexes that inactivate the enzymes *(15,16)*. Interleukin-6 (IL-6) increases TIMP-1 production. These TIMPs are essential in controlling connective tissue damage by blocking the action of the activated MMPs *(17)*.

PATHOGENIC MECHANISMS

Collagenase-1 (MMP-1) and stromelysin-1 (MMP-3) play a critical role in RA *(2)*. Normal fibroblasts produce very low levels of both of these enzymes *(2,18)*. In RA, as well as in osteoarthritis (OA), levels increase markedly in response to cytokines such as interleukin-1α (IL-1α), interleukin-1β (IL-1β), epidermal growth factor, platelet-derived growth factor, and tumor necrosis factor α (TNF–α). The levels of collagenase-1 and stromelysin 1 activity in OA and RA cartilage correlate with lesion severity *(19,20)*. Initial studies on the role of stromelysin in arthritis were performed on the streptococcal cell wall model in Lewis rats, which is a destructive form of arthritis marked by significant matrix degradation. Large amounts of stromelysin mRNA was present in the synovial tissues from these rats with chronic arthritis *(21)*. It has also been shown that there is significantly more stromelysin protein in synovial tissue in patients with RA than with OA *(22)*. Rheumatoid synoviocytes also secrete large amounts of collagenase-1 and *in situ* hybridization studies have demonstrated significantly more collagenase mRNA in RA synovium than from OA synovial tissue *(23,24)*. Although it has been shown that significantly greater amounts of stromelysin-1 and collagenase-1 are present in patients with chronic RA, there is less known about their presence in early disease. A recent synovial biopsy study of patients with early RA (1–3 mo in duration) demonstrated significant collagenase mRNA expression *(24)*.

TIMP gene expression is similar in RA and OA and thus the ratio of TIMP to collagenase is greater in noninflammatory arthritis than it is in RA. This difference has important implications for the pathogenesis of joint damage in RA and suggests that the TIMP system is overwhelmed by the marked increase in MMPs in RA *(23)*. There are important inhibitors other than the TIMPs. Most of the collagenase inhibitory activity in serum is owing to α2-macroglobulin (α2M), which also has the capacity to bind and inactivate MMPs. α2M is inactivated when neutrophils when present in high numbers in synovial fluid owing to the release of elastase and serine proteases, which inactivate the inhibitor *(25,26)*.

REVIEW OF ANIMAL DATA

Breedveld et al. studied the effect of tetracyclines in rats with arthritis (27). They studied 63 rats that were immunized with chick type II collagen and 94 rats that were injected with Freund's adjuvant and gave each group minocycline 125 mg/kg/d or placebo. Minocycline decreased the incidence of arthritis in both groups (collagen: $p = 0.01$; adjuvant: $p = 0.0005$) and decreased the severity, graded by an arthritic index, in both but only only reached significance in the adjuvant model ($p < 0.02$).

Conway et al. identified GI168 as a potent MMP inhibitor with sufficient stability and solubility to allow evaluation in an experimental model of chronic destructive arthritis in rats *(28)*. This model of arthritis is induced by injecting the rats with Freund's adjuvant, which induces acute and chronic synovial inflammation and severe bone and cartilage destruction within 3 wk of the adjuvant injection. GI168 was administered systemically by subcutaneous infusion beginning on d 8 after adjuvant injection and continued thru d 21 at doses of 6, 12, and 25 mg/kg/d. Ankle swelling was reduced in a dose-related fashion and radiological and histological evaluation on d 22 revealed a profound decrease in bone and cartilage destruction in the rats treated with the MMP inhibitor compared to rats treated with placebo. The investigators concluded that the benefit from GI168 supports the role of MMPs in the destructive process in inflammatory arthritis.

Cartilage oligomeric matrix protein (COMP) is a glycoprotein found in articular, tracheal, and nasal cartilage *(29–31)*. COMP turnover is increased in RA and OA, and studies have shown elevated levels of COMP in the serum and synovial fluid of these patients *(32)*. Goldberg et al. showed that the IL-1α stimulation of bovine nasal cartilage resulted in the loss of COMP and that this was partially inhibited by the metalloproteinase inhibitor CGS 27023A, suggesting that the loss of COMP induced by IL-1α involves metalloproteinases *(33)*. Ganu et al. demonstrated in vitro that IL-1α-stimulated articular cartilage generates COMP fragments and that COMP is a substrate for stromelysin-1, collagenase-1, 92-kd gelatinase, and collagenase-3. Ganu et al. showed that the production of these COMP fragments was inhibited by MMP inhibitors CGS 27023A and BB-94 *(34)*.

REVIEW OF CLINICAL TRIALS

Breedveld et al. studied 10 patients with active RA and treated them with oral minocycline for 16 wk in an open study. They reported that half of the outcome measures had improved significantly after 4 wk (morning stiffness, Ritchie Index, erythrocyte sedimentation rate [ESR], and platelet count) and that after 16 wk all variables were improved significantly, including swollen joint count and bilateral grip strength *(35)*. Panayi et al. reported an open study in reactive arthritis that showed some effectiveness of minocycline *(36)*. They reported that morning stiffness improved from baseline of 416 min to 40 min after 3 mo of minocycline, that the number of active joints decreased from baseline of 5 to 2.6 after 3 mo, and that a visual analog scale for pain decreased from a baseline of 56 mm to 44 mm. Lauhio et al. performed a double-blind, placebo controlled trial that showed beneficial results of lymecycline in patients with Chlamydia-induced reactive arthritis, but not reactive arthritis with non-Chlamydial infectious etiologies *(37)*. Of the group with Chlamydia-induced arthritis, the lymecycline treated group had arthralgia for 17.9 wk compared to 32.8 wk in the placebo group ($p = 0.022$). The investigators also showed statistically significant changes in acute phase reactants (duration of elevated ESR was 10.4 wk in lymecycline group vs 23.0 wk in the placebo group; duration of elevated C-reactive protein [CRP] was 4.6 wk in lymecycline group and 23.0 in the placebo group). However, these studies of reactive arthritis were clearly targeting a population of inflammatory arthritis with a well-described infectious link. Langevitz et al. reported the results of a 48-wk open study in which 18 patients with active RA resistant to disease-modifying anti-rheumatic drugs (DMARDs) were given minocycline 100 mg twice daily. Statistically significant changes were demonstrated in patient and physicians' global assessments, tender joint count, swollen joint count, duration of morning stiffness, grip strength, and ESR *(38)*.

In 1994, Kloppenburg et al. were the first to publish results of a double-blind, placebo-controlled trial of minocycline for RA *(39)*. This study randomized 80 patients with mean disease duration of 13 yr, all of whom were required to be taking or to have been previously treated with at least one DMARD. The subjects were characterized as responders if there was 25% or more improvement; subjects were considered failures if there was 25% or greater worsening in two of the following three: Ritchie articular index, number of swollen joints, and CRP level. There were 15 responders in the minocycline group and 7 responders in the placebo group ($p < 0.05$). There were no treatment failures in the minocycline group and 9 in the placebo group ($p < 0.005$). Secondary efficacy measures that revealed statistically significant improvements in the minocycline group included the Ritchie articular index (change from baseline of –0.8 in minocycline group vs 0.6 in placebo), number of swollen joints (change from baseline of –0.8 in minocycline group vs 0.6 in placebo), ESR (change from baseline of –14 in minocycline group vs –4 in placebo), CRP (change from baseline of –1.6 in minocycline vs –0.6 in placebo), hemoglobin (change from baseline of 0.4 in minocycline group vs –0.1 in placebo), and platelet count (change from baseline of –73 in minocycline group vs 12 in placebo). Blinded assessment of hand, wrist, and feet radiographs obtained at baseline and at 6 mo revealed no difference in erosions, joint space narrowing, or number of affected joints between the minocycline and placebo groups.

In 1995, Tilley et al. completed a 48-wk double-blind, placebo-controlled study, known as the Minocycline in Rheumatoid Arthritis (MIRA) Trial *(40)*. Minocycline 100 mg twice daily was added to background nonsteroidal anti-inflammatory drugs (NSAIDs) or low-dose prednisone therapy in patients not receiving concomitant DMARDs. There were 219 patients enrolled with an average disease duration of 8.5 yr. Approximately 50% of the patients enrolled had been treated previously with a DMARD and less than one-third were actively treated with low-dose corticosteroids (≤10 mg of prednisone). There were two prespecified primary outcome measures: improvement in joint swelling and improvement in joint tenderness (assessed at the end of the 48-wk trial). A patient was considered improved if 50% of the affected joints capable of response improved. In the minocycline group, 54% of patients had improvement in joint swelling compared to 39% in the placebo group ($p = 0.023$). Fifty-six percent of patients in the minocycline group and 41% in the placebo group showed improvement in joint tenderness ($p = 0.021$). Secondary outcome measures that demonstrated a statistically significant difference include ESR (change from baseline of –10.8 in minocycline group vs –0.7 in placebo), hematocrit (change from baseline of 0.6 in minocycline group vs –1.1 in placebo), and platelet count (change from baseline of –89.6 in minocycline group vs –10.2 in placebo).

The radiographic data from the MIRA trial demonstrated that patients given placebo tended to develop more radiographic changes than patients given minocycline, but failed to show a statistically significant difference *(41)*. Bluhm et al. calculated the probability of detecting a difference between the two groups in this trial and concluded that there was a low power to detect a 50% difference based on the number of patients in this trial.

In 1997, O'Dell et al. published a double-blind, placebo-controlled study of minocycline in 46 patients with early RA *(42)*. All patients were required to have active disease with disease duration of less than 1 yr. The primary endpoint was successful completion of the 6 mo study while meeting 50% improvement on the modified Paulus criteria at months 3 and 6. Fifteen of the 23 patients (65%) in the minocycline group met the 50% improvement at 3 mo and maintained it through the 6 mo of the trial compared with 3 of the 23 (13%) in the placebo group ($p < 0.001$). Secondary efficacy parameters, which revealed a statistically significant improvement in the minocycline group compared to placebo, include change in morning stiffness and patient and physician global assessments.

In 1999, O'Dell et al. reported on the 4-yr follow-up results of the patients from their prior trial (44). Twenty of the 23 patients in the minocycline group and 18 of the 23 patients in the placebo group were available for follow-up. After the blinded portion of the prior study, the physician was informed of the randomization and was then free to prescribe any combination of prednisone, minocycline, or DMARDs that was deemed appropriate. Of the 15 patients that had a good response to minocycline during the blinded period, all had a subsequent flare and most were put back on minocycline. Ten of the 20 patients originally treated with minocycline never required treatment with DMARDs (other then minocycline) or steroids. Eight of the 20 patients in the minocycline follow-up group and only 1 of 18 in the placebo group were in remission without DMARDs (except minocycline) or steroids. ($p = 0.02$). Thirteen of the 20 patients in the minocyline group and 4 of 18 in the placebo group met ACR 75% response criteria at this long-term follow-up ($p = 0.01$).

In 1998 Nordstrom et al. reported on the clinical response and collagenase activity in 12 RA patients treated with doxycycline for 3 mo (43). The patients were given 150 mg/d of doxycycline and at 3 mo significant reductions were seen in a joint score index ($p < 0.01$) and a pain visual analog scale (VAS) ($p < 0.05$). Also, collagenase activity as measured from saliva by quantitative sodium dodecye sulfate-polyaerylamide gel electrophoresis (SDS-PAGE) electrophoresis was significantly reduced after the 3 mo of treatment ($p < 0.01$).

In 1999, Keyszer et al. showed that MMP-3 plasma levels were markedly elevated in RA compared to healthy controls and OA, but were also markedly elevated in systemic lupus erythematosus (SLE) (45). MMP-1 plasma levels were significantly elevated in RA, OA, psoriatic arthritis, SLE, and mixed connective tissue disease. In contrast, MT complex (MMP-1/TIMP-1 complex) plasma level was elevated in RA only. Plasma TIMP-1 level was no different from controls.

CURRENT RECOMMENDATIONS

Currently the only MMP inhibitors available for clinical use are the tetracyclines and their role in the treatment of RA is not well delineated. The three major clinical trials by Kloppenburg et al., Tilley et al., and O'Dell et al. have proven that minocycline has utility in the treatment of RA (39,40,42). Clearly, the trial by O'Dell et al. demonstrated the most striking results with 15 of 23 patients (65%) in the minocycline group vs 3 of 23 patients (13%) in the placebo group achieving 50% improvement at 3 mo and maintaining it through 6 mo. The 4-yr follow-up of this trial demonstrated that there were a significant number of patients who responded to early treatment with minocycline and continued to do well without needing any other DMARDs or corticosteroids (44). The trial by O'Dell et al. evaluated a markedly different disease population than either the trial by Kloppenburg et al. or the MIRA Trial, which both recruited populations with much longer disease duration. Also, the trial by O'Dell et al. required patients to be DMARD and corticosteroid naïve, whereas the trial by Kloppenburg et al. required patients to have active disease despite concurrent DMARD or past DMARD therapy and the MIRA Trial allowed patients to be on low-dose corticosteroid (prednisone ≤ 10 mg) and only required that any DMARDs have been stopped for at least 4 wk prior to study entry. These two major differences likely account for the disparate degree of improvement seen in the trial by O'Dell et al. compared to the others.

There have not been any studies yet that have sufficiently addressed whether the tetracyclines alter radiographic progression. The study by Kloppenburg et al. did not reveal any radiographic difference between study groups but the number of patients was small (total of 63) and there was only 26 wk between radiographs, making it unlikely that any difference could even be detected *(39)*. The MIRA Trial also was unable to detect a difference in the radiographic progression between groups and Bluhm et al. concluded that the number of patients was insufficient to answer the question *(40,41)*. The trial by O'Dell et al. did not assess radiographic progression *(42,44)*. Despite all theoretical suggestions that MMPs are important in joint destruction and that the inhibition of MMPs may alleviate this damage, studies need to be undertaken in order to conclusively decide whether minocycline or doxycycline are effective in slowing disease progression.

At the current time, minocycline 100 mg twice daily or doxycyline 150–200 mg/d is likely useful for patients with mild to moderate, nonerosive RA. These drugs have a very good adverse effect profile, substantially better than most other DMARDs, and this probably justifies their use in this subset of patients. The benefits of minocycline are certainly better-documented, though doxycycline may be equally effective and associated with less hyperpigmentation than minocycline *(44)*. If a patient responds to a tetracycline, it likely needs to be continued indefinitely. However, if after a reasonable trial it has not produced a good response, then it is probably prudent to either replace or add another DMARD to the therapeutic regimen. The maximum benefit of minocycline may not occur until after 1-yr of therapy *(44)*, but it is probably not justified to wait this length of time in a patient who continues to have active disease, unless it is very mild.

SIDE EFFECTS AND PRECAUTIONS

During the study by Kloppenburg et al., the frequency of reported adverse effects was significantly higher in the minocycline group as compared with placebo group *(39)*. The most common adverse effects were gastrointestinal (GI) (23 in the minocycline group vs 6 in the placebo group), including nausea, vomiting, increased appetite (10 in the minocycline group vs 0 in the placebo group), and change of taste (seven in the minocycline group vs 0 in the placebo group). The only other common adverse effect in this study was dizziness (16 in the minocycline group vs 6 in the placebo group) with two of these patients in the minocycline group sustaining falls that resulted in upper extremity fractures. Four patients in the minocycline group and none in the placebo group withdrew from the study secondary to these GI adverse effects and four patients from the minocycline group and one from the placebo group withdrew from the study secondary to dizziness. There were no clinically relevant alterations in serum tests, including white blood cell (WBC) count, creatinine, albumin, and hepatic enzymes and there were no serious adverse events reported.

O'Dell et al. noted significantly less adverse effects in their trial, especially with regard to dizziness *(42,44)*. The reason for the difference is unclear, but it may be that the study by O'Dell et al. had a younger patient population (mean age at onset: 45 yr) than did the Netherlands trial by Kloppenburg, et al. and the MIRA trial (mean age at onset: 56 and 54 yr, respectively). Subsequent to the blinded phase of the study, three of the minocycline treated patients discontinued the drug secondary to hyperpigmentation and one reported hyperpigmentation but elected to continue therapy. The hyperpigmentation in these four patients occurred at 1, 2.5, 3, and 3.5 yr of therapy. No patients in the 4-yr follow-up reported dizziness that required the drug to be discontinued.

Minocycline is frequently prescribed for acne vulgaris, as well as a few infectious diseases and several side effects have been reported in these patients. Sitbon et al. reported on eight patients that had developed pulmonary infiltrates and eosinophilia that was felt to be secondary to minocyline *(46)*. Several cases of pseudotumor cerebri have been reported that were attributed to minocycline *(47–49)*. One adverse effect that occurs commonly with minocycline but not with other tetracyclines is vestibular dysfunction, which is manifested as dizziness, vertigo, or ataxia *(50–54)*. The incidence of vertigo is reported to be higher in women than men (70% and 28%, respectively). Poliak et al. reported that 4 of 72 adult patients on chronic minocycline developed discoloration of their teeth *(55)*. There have been reports of minocycline-induced hepatic failure, though it is rarer than with tetracycline *(56)*. More than 20 cases of autoimmune hepatitis attributed to minocycline have been reported *(57)*. The signs and symptoms of hepatitis typicallly resolved after discontinuation of the drug. Photosensitivity reactions may be caused by tetracyline and its derivatives, including minocycline. Morrow et al. reported bilateral blue-gray discoloration of the sclera in a patient on chronic minocycline who also had pigmentation of the teeth, hard palate, ears, nail beds, and skin *(58)*. After discontinuation of minocycline, the hyperpigmentation faded except for the sclera and teeth. Hyperpigmentation of the skin generally occurs after chronic exposure to minocycline, usually involves scar tissue or sun exposed skin, and typically fades after discontinuing the drug *(59,60)*. Gough et al. reported 11 patients that had developed drug-induced lupus secondary to minocycline in the United Kingdom through 1994 *(57)*. Drug-induced lupus is considered a late-type of reaction, occurring on average 2 yr after drug onset. It has only been noted with minocycline and not with other tetracyclines.

CONCLUSIONS

There is currently tremendous interest in the role of MMPs in joint destruction in the inflammatory arthritides as well as OA, and speculation about the role of MMP-inhibitors in therapy. The tetracycline-derivatives, minocycline and doxycycline, are probably most useful in patients with mild to moderate, nonerosive RA or in combination with other agents in patients with early disease. Their role as adjunctive agents in combination with other DMARDs along with their ability to decrease radiographic progression needs to be defined. The future holds hope for better-designed MMP-inhibitors that are more specific and potent in their ability to inhibit the most important MMPs. There has been some concern raised that current clinical and laboratory outcome measures are focused on inflammation and that therapies, such as MMP-inhibitors, that are not anti-inflammatory agents may be inappropriately analyzed particularly in short-term trials and may require plasma and/or synovial fluid measures of extracellular matrix turnover. This issue will need to be further addressed when these drugs near clinical trials and it is hoped that by then the appropriate surrogate markers will be better-defined.

REFERENCES

1. Alarcon, G.S. 1998. Minocycline for the treatment of rheumatoid arthritis. *Rheum. Dis. Clin. North. Am.* 24(3):489–499.

2. Harris, E.J. 1990. Rheumatoid arthritis: pathophysiology and implications for therapy. *N. Engl. J. Med.* 322:1277–1289.

3. Alarcon, G.S. and I.S. Mikhail. 1994. Antimicrobials in the treatment of rheumatoid arthritis and other arthritides: a clinical perspective. *Am. J. Med. Sci.* 308:201–209.

4. Ford, D.K and M. Schulzer. 1994. Synovial lymphocytes indicate "bacterial" agents may cause some cases of rheumatoid arthritis. *J. Rheumatol.* 21:1447–1449.

5. Golub, L.M., T.F. McNamara, G. D'Angelo, R.A. Greenwald, and N.S. Ramamurthy. 1987. A nonantibacterial chemically modified tetracycline inhibits mammalian collagenase activity. *J. Dent. Res.* 66:1310–1314.

6. Golub, L.M, K. Soumalainen, and T. Sorsa. 1992. Host modulation with tetracyclines and their chemically modified analogues. *Curr. Opin. Dent.* 2:80–90.

7. Skinner, M., E.S. Cathcart, J.A. Mills, and R.S. Pinals. 1971. Teytracycline in the treatment of rheumatoid arthritis: a double-blind controlled study. *Arthritis Rheum.* 14:727–32.

8. Kloppenburg, M., B.A. Dijkmons, F.C. Breedveld, et al. 1995. Antimicrobial therapy for rheumatoid arthritis. *Baillieres Clin. Rheumatol.* 9:759–769.

9. Greenwald, R.A, L.M. Golub, B. Lavietes, N.S. Ramamurthy, B. Gruber, Laskin, and T.F. McNamara. 1987. Tetracyclines inhibit human synovial collagenase in vivo and in vitro. *J. Rheumatol.* 14:28–32.

10. Woessner, J.F. 1992. Matrix metalloproteinases and their inhibitors in connective tissue remodeling. *FASEB J.* 5:2145–2154.

11. Matrisian, L.M. 1992. The matrix-degrading metalloproteinases. Bioessays 14:455–463.

12. Dioszegi, M., P. Cannon, and H.E. Van Wart. 1995. Vertebrate collagenases. *Methods Enzymol.* 248:413–431.

13. Nagase, H. 1995. Human stromelysin 1 & 2. *Methods Enzymol.* 248:449–470.

14. Murphy, G., T. Crabbe, A. and B. Gelatinases. 1995. *Methods Enzymol.* 248:470–484.

15. Cawston, TE. 1996. Metalloproteinase inhibitors and the prevention of connective tissue breakdown. *Pharm. Ther.* 3:163–182.

16. Murphy, G. and F. Willenbrock. 1995. Tissue inhibitors of matrix metalloendopeptidases. *Methods Enzymol.* 248:496–510.

17. Denhardt, D.T., B. Feng, D.R. Edwards, E.T. Cocuzzi, and U.M. Malyankar. 1993. Tissue inhibitor of metalloproteinases (TIMP, aka EPA): structure, conrol of expression and biological functions. *Pharmacol. Ther.* 59:329–341.

18. Brincekerhoff, C.E. and D.T. Auble. 1990. Regulation of collagenase gene expression in synovial fibroblasts. *Ann. N.Y. Acad. Sci.* 580:355–374.

19. Dean, D.D., J. Martel-Pelletier, J.P. Pelletier, D.S. Howell, and J.F. Woessner Jr. 1989. Evidence for metalloproteinase inhibitor imbalance in human osteoarthritic cartilage. *J. Clin. Invest.* 84:678–685.

20. Martel-Pelletier, J., N. Fujimoto, K. Obata, J.-M. Cloutier, and J.-P. Pelletier. The imbalance between the synthesis level of metalloproteases and TIMPs in osteoarthritic and rheumatoid arthritis cartilage can be enhanced by interleukin-1 (abstract). *Arthritis Rheum.* 1993;36(Suppl. 9):S191.

21. Case, J.P., H. Sano, R. Layfatis, E.F. Remmers, G.K. Kumkumian, and R.L. Wilder. 1989. Transin/stromelysin expression in the synovium of rats with experimental erosive arthritis. In situ localization and kinetics of expression of the transformation-associated metalloproteinase in euthymic and athymic Lewis rats. *J. Clin. Invest.* 84:1731–1740.

22. Hasty, K.A., R.A Reife, A.H. Kang, and J.M. Stuart. 1990. The role of stromelysin in the cartilage destruction that accompanies inflammatory arthritis. *Arthritis Rheum.* 33:388–397.

23. Firestein, G.S., M.M. Paine, and B.H. Littman. 1991. Gene expression (collagenase, tissue inhibitor of metalloproteinases, complement, and HLA-DR) in rheumatoid arthritis and osteoarthritis synovium: Quantitative analysis and effect of intraarticular corticosteroids. *Arthritis Rheum.* 34:1094–1105.

24. McCachren, S.S., B.F. Haynes, and J.E. Niedel. 1990. Localization of collagenase mRNA in rheumatoid arthritis synovium by in situ hybridization histocemistry. *J. Clin. Immunol.* 10:19–27.

25. Zvaifler, N.J., D. Boyle, and G.S. Firestein. 1994. Early synovitis-synoviocytes and mononuclear cells. *Semin. Arthritis Rheum.* 23(Suppl 2):11–16.

26. Zvaifler, N.J. and G.S. Firestein. Pannus and pannocytes. 1994. Alternative models of joint destruction in rheumatoid arthritis. *Arthritis Rheum.* 37(6):783–789.

27. Breedveld, F.C. and D. E. Tentham. 1988. Suppression of collagen and adjuvant arthritis by a tetracycline (abstract). *Arthritis Rheum.* 31(Suppl. 1):R3.

28. Conway, J.G., J.A. Wakefield, R.H. Brown, et al. 1995. Inhibition of cartilage and bone destruction in adjuvant arthritis in the rat by a matrix metalloproteinase inhibitor. *J. Exp. Med.* 182(2):449–457.

29. Hedbom, E., P. Antonsson, A. Hjerpe, et al. 1992. Cartilage matrix poroteins: an acidic oligomeric protein (COMP) detected only in cartilage. *J. Biol. Chem.* 267:6132–6136.

30. DiCesare, P.E., M. Morgelin, K. Mann, and M. Paulsson. 1994. Cartilage oligomeric matrix protein and thrombospondin 1: purification from articular cartilage, electron microscopic structure, and chondrocyte binding. *Eur. J. Biochem.* 223:927–937.

31. DiCesare, P.E., M. Morgelin, C.S. Carlson, S. Pasumati, and M. Paulsson. 1995. Cartilage oligomeric matrix protein: isolation and characterization from human articular cartilage. *J. Orthop. Res.* 13:422–428.

32. Saxne, T. and D. Heingard. 1992. Cartilage oligomerix matrix protein: a novel marker of cartilage turnover detectable in synovial fluid and blood. *Br. J. Rheumatol.* 32:583–591.

33. Goldberg, R.L., S. Spirito, J.R. Doughty, V. Ganu, and D. Heinegard. 1995. Time dependent release of matrix components from bovine cartilage after IL-1alpha treatment and the relative inhibition by matrix metalloproteinase inhibitors [abstract]. *Trans. Orthop. Res. Soc.* 20:125.

34. Ganu, V., R. Goldberg, J. Peppard, et al. 1998. Inhibition of interleukin-1alpha-induced cartilage oligomeric matrix protein degradation in bovine articular cartilage by matrix metalloproteinase inhibitors potential role for matrix metalloproteinases in the generation of cartilage oligomeric matrix protein fragments in arthritic synovial fluid. *Arthritis Rheum.* 41(12):2143–2151.

35. Breedveld, F.C., B.A. Dijkmas, and H. Mattie. 1990. Minocycline in the treatment for rheumatoid arthritis: an open dose finding study. *J. Rheumatol.* 17(1):43–46.

36. Panayi, G.S. and B. Clark. 1989. Minocycline in the treatment of patients with Reiter's syndrome. *Clin. Exp. Rheumatol.* 7(1):100–101.

37. Lauhio, A., M. Leirisalo-Repo, J. Lähdevirta, P. Saikku, and H. Repo. 1991. Double-blind, placebo-controlled study of three-month treatment with reactive arthritis, with special reference to Chlamydia arthritis. *Arthritis Rheum.* 34:6–14.

38. Langevitz, P., D. Zemer, M. Book, and M. Pras. 1992. Treatment of resistant rheumatoid arthritis with minocycline: an open study. *J. Rheumatol.* 19:1502–1504.

39. Kloppenburg, M., F.C. Breedveld, J.P Terwiel, C. Mallee, and B.A. Dijkmans. 1994. Minocycline in active rheumatoid arthritis. *Arthritis Rheum.* 37(5):629–636.

40. Tilley, B.C., G.S. Alarcón, S.P. Heyse, et al. for the MIRA Trial Group. 1995. Minocycline in rheumatoid arthritis: reults of a 48-week double blinded placebo controlled trial. *Ann. Intern. Med.* 122:81–89.

41. Bluhm, A.B., J.T. Shar, B.C. Tilley, et al. 1997. Radiographic reults from the minocycline in rheumatoid arthritis (MIRA) trial. *J. Rheumatol.* 24(7):1295–1302.

42. O'Dell, J.R., C.E. Haire, W. Palmer, et al. 1997. Treatment of early rheumatoid arthritis with minocycline or placebo: results of a randomized, double-blind, placebo-controlled trial. *Arthritis Rheum.* 40(5):842–848.

43. Nordstrom, D., O. Lindy, A. Lauhio, T. Sorsa, S. Santavirta, and Y.T. Konttinen. 1998. Anti-collagenolytic mechanism of action of doxycycline treatment in rheumatoid arthritis. *Rheumatol. Int.* 17(5):175–180.

44. O'Dell, J.R., G. Paulsen, C.E. Haire, et al. 1999. Treatment of early seropositive rheumatoid arthritis with minocycline: four-year followup of a double-blind, placebo controlled trial. *Arthritis Rheum.* 42(8):1691–1695.

45. Keyszer, G., I. Lambiri, R. Nagel, et al. 1999. Circulating levels of matrix metalloproteinases MMP-3 and MMP-1, tissue inhibitor of metalloproteinases 1 (TIMP-1), and MMP-1/TIMP-1 complex in rheumatic disease. Correlation with clinical activity of rheumatoid arthritis versus other surrogate markers. *J. Rheumatol.* 26(2):251–258.

46. Sitbon, O., N. Bidel, C. Dussopt, et al. 1994. Minocycline pneumonitis and eosinophilia. A report on eight patients. *Arch. Intern. Med.* 154(14):1633–1640.

47. Beran, R.G. 1980. Pseudotumor cerebri associated with minocycline therapy for acne. *Med. J. Aust.* 1(7):323–324.

48. Donnet, A., H. Dufour, N. Graziani, and F. Grisoli. 1992. Minocycline and benign intracranial hypertension. *Biomed. Pharmocother.* 46(4):171–172.

49. Moskowitz, Y., E. Leibowitz, M. Ronen, and E. Aviel. 1993. Pseudotumor cerebri induced by vitamin A combined with minocycline. *Ann. Opthalmol.* 25(8):306–308.

50. Jacobson, J.A. and B. Daniel. 1975. Vestibular reactions associated with minocycline. *Antimicrob. Agents Chemother.* 8(4):453–456.

51. Fanning, W.L. and D.W. Gump. 1976. Distressing side-effects of minocycline hydrochloride. *Arch. Intern. Med.* 136(7):761–762.

52. Masterton, G. and C.B. Schofield. 1974. Letter: side-effects of minocycline hydrochloride. *Lancet* 2(7889):1139.

53. Nicol, C.S. and J.D. Oriel. 1974. Letter: minocycline: possible vestibular side-effects. *Lancet* 2(7891):1260.

54. Garnier, R., A. Castot, P. Louboutin, D. Muzard, and F. Conso. 1981. Vestibular-like reactions associated with minocycline. *Therapie* 36(3):313–317.

55. Poliak, S.C., J.J. DiGiovanna, E.G. Gross, G. Gantt, and G.L. Peck. 1985. Minocycline-associated tooth discoloration in young adults. *JAMA* 254(20):2930–2932.

56. Davies, M.G. and P.J. Kersey. 1989. Acute hepatitis and exfoliative dermatitis associated with minocycline. *BMJ* 298(6686):1523–1524.

57. Gough, A., S. Chapman, K. Wagstaff, P. Emery, and E. Elias. 1996. Minocycline induced autoimmune hepatitis and systemic lupus erythematosus-like syndrome. *BMJ* 312(7024):169–172.

58. Morrow, G.L. and R.L. Abbott. 1998. Minocycline-induced scleral, dental, and dermal pigmentation. *Am. J. Opthalmol.* 125(3):396–397.

59. Pepine, M., F.P. Flowers, and F.A. Ramos-Caro. 1993. Extensive cutaneous hyperpigmentation caused by minocycline. *J. Am. Acad. Dermatol.* 28:292–295.

60. Leffell, D.J. 1991. Minocycline hydrochloride hyperpigmentation complicating treatment of venous ectasia of the extremities. *J. Am. Acad. Dermatol.* 24(3):501–502.

10 Combination Disease-Modifying Anti-Rheumatic Drug (DMARD) Therapy

James R. O'Dell

CONTENTS

INTRODUCTION

Over the last decade, there has been a major shift in the way that rheumatologists think about and treat patients with rheumatoid arthritis (RA). Methotrexate remains the gold standard and is most often considered the drug of choice in the treatment of this disease that has the potential to result in progressive disability in the majority of patients. Methotrexate continues to demonstrate superior long-term efficacy compared with other conventional disease-modifying anti-rheumatic drugs (DMARD) *(1,2)*. However, therapy combining methotrexate with other DMARDs is now used for treatment of the growing number of patients with RA who fail to achieve disease control with methotrexate monotherapy *(3)*. A recent survey of US rheumatologists revealed that 99% used combination DMARDs to treat an estimated 24% of all patients. Another recent survey *(4)* has shown that almost half of rheumatologists in the United States are currently using combinations of DMARDs to treat over 30% of their patients; this

From: *Modern Therapeutics in Rheumatic Diseases*
Edited by: G. C. Tsokos, et al. © Humana Press, Inc., Totowa, NJ

number has gone up dramatically from less than 15% just 4 yr ago. Other approaches utilizing combination therapy include methotrexate plus biological agents that decrease tumor necrosis factor (TNF) activity. Clinical studies of such agents (infliximab, etanercept) in patients who had less than optimal responses to methotrexate have shown each of them to be more effective than placebo when added to the baseline methotrexate *(5,6)*. With very few exceptions, all of the clinical trials that have demonstrated the success of combination therapy for RA have included methotrexate as part of the combination. Thus, methotexate is currently the cornerstone of combination therapy *(7)*.

The combination of methotrexate with DMARDs or with biological agents with different mechanisms of action offers the potential for four possible outcomes. One possible outcome is that the efficacy and/or toxicity of the combination therapy will be less favorable than with single-drug therapy. This is of particular concern with regard to toxicity, such as the potential for additive liver blood test abnormalities with methotrexate and leflunomide combination *(8)*. Another possible outcome is that the efficacy and/or toxicity will be no different than with single-drug therapy. Alternatively, efficacy and/or toxicity could be additive; this outcome of additive efficacy could represent either a true additive effect on each individual patient or the sum of two subpopulations of patients, each of which is responsive to one of the two individual drugs. Finally, the outcome of combination therapy may be synergistic for efficacy and/or toxicity.

DESIGN AND INTERPRETATION OF COMBINATION STUDIES

There are several issues central to the design and interpretation of studies of combination therapy in the treatment of RA. First, a sufficiently long duration of therapy ($\geq$1 yr) is essential. This allows sufficient time for dose escalation and for assessment of longer-term efficacy and safety, thereby allowing differences to manifest themselves between/among treatments. Second, dosage is critical to study design; in particular, automatic dose escalation upon failure to achieve a predetermined level of clinical success and, therefore, assuring comparability of dose escalation between treatment arms. Third, patient population characteristics will influence results. Responsiveness to therapy is believed to be affected by previous history of treatment failure with specific DMARDs and by the duration of disease, with late disease being less responsive than early disease. Last, combinations can be evaluated in one of three methods: the step-down approach, the step-up approach, or the parallel approach. The step-down approach is one in which two or more DMARDs are administered initially, then individual agents are removed after symptoms are controlled. The step-up approach has one DMARD administered initially and another added if the first agent is insufficient. The parallel approach evaluates two treatment approaches head-to-head.

WHEN IS COMBINATION THERAPY INDICATED?

The decision of when in the course of RA to use combination therapy is much-debated. Recent studies *(9,10)* suggest that combination therapy may be best utilized as initial therapy for RA. Additional studies clearly demonstrate the benefit of combination DMARD therapy in patients who have not had an optimal response to methotrexate *(5,6,8,11)*. Therefore, studies in both of these two distinct categories of patients will be reviewed. First, patients with early disease who have not previously been treated

Table 1
The Cobra Trial *(9)*

- 155 patients with early RA (<2 yr)
- Double-blind, randomized to receive sulfasalzine (SSA) or a combination of SSA, methotrexate (7.5 mg/wk), and prednisolone
- MTX stop at wk 40 and prednisolone decreased rapidly from 60 mg/d to 7.5 mg/d and stopped by 28 wk
- Significantly fewer withdrawals in combination group (39% vs 8%)
- ACR 20 and 50 better in combination group at 28 wk
- Less erosions in combination group at 54 and 80 wk

with DMARDs, and second, those patients who have been treated with methotrexate and have failed to respond optimally.

TREATMENT OF EARLY DISEASE OR INITIAL THERAPY OF RA

Increasingly, rheumatologists have recognized the benefit of treating patients as early in their disease process as possible. Studies have clearly shown that delays in disease modifying therapy for as little as 8–9 mo may result in less optimal outcomes for patients *(12,13)*. Therefore, it makes sense to consider the most potent therapy right from the beginning. Over a decade ago, Wilske and Healey proposed a step-down bridge approach for the treatment of early RA *(14)*. The central tenet of this approach was to completely control disease as early as possible; to achieve this lofty goal, the authors proposed that multiple therapies be started simultaneously in the beginning of the treatment of RA to assure the quickest possible control of disease and later to taper the patient off a number of these drugs, leaving them on the simplest possible long-term maintenance regimen. This is clearly an attractive hypothesis, but until 1997 there were little or no data to support it.

Researchers in the Netherlands recently reported on such an approach: the COBRA (Combinatietherapie Bij Reumatoide Artritis) Trial *(9)*. In this trial, 155 patients with early disease (less than 2 yr) were randomly assigned to two groups (Table 1). The first group was treated with a combination of prednisolone, methotrexate and sulfasalazine; the second group was treated with sulfasalazine alone. Prednisolone was started at 60 mg/d and was rapidly tapered to 7.5 mg/d over the course of several weeks; it was discontinued completely by wk 28. The dose of methotrexate was 7.5 mg and remained at that level until wk 40, when the patients were tapered off of this medication. The dose of sulfasalazine was the same in both groups and was rapidly accelerated to 2 gm/d. At 28 wk, the combination group was significantly better than the sulfasalazine alone group, with the American College of Rheumatology (ACR) 20s (to review this index *see* ref. *15*) of 72% vs 49% ($p = 0.006$) and ACR 50s of 49% vs 27% ($p = 0.007$). As the prednisolone and methotrexate were tapered, the response rates became more similar in the two groups. However, it is important to note, in terms of a number of important parameters, that significant benefits existed in patients in the combination-treated group at 54 wk, and again at 80 wk. The progression of total sharp score and erosion scores were less in the combination group ($p < 0.01$) than in the sulfasalazine alone group, and

Table 2
FIN-RA Trial *(10)*

- 199 patients, early RA (<2 yr)
- Open, 2-yr, randomized
- SSA ± prednisolone or MTX-SSA-HCQ + prednisolone
- Major endpoint remission, combination 28% remission vs SSA 11% (odds ratio 2.7)

patients in the combination group were more likely to be employed and were working more hours. Importantly, the withdrawal rate was much higher in the sulfasalazine alone group (39 vs 8%), demonstrating that combination therapy was not more toxic, as define by the number of patients who were withdrawn from the protocol by their treating physician for possible toxicity, than mono-DMARD therapy.

Some have discounted the results of the COBRA trial because of the high dose of prednisolone that was used up front. I believe this is a mistake as this study convincingly demonstrates that if an effective induction regimen is used, patients with RA can gain long-term benefits. One way to interpret the results of this study would be to consider this a successful approach for induction therapy in RA patients and to recognize that better ways to maintain control need to be elucidated.

The Fin-RA (Finland Rheumatoid Arthritis) trial group has recently completed another important study in patients with early RA *(10)*. In this study, 199 patients were randomized to receive combination DMARD therapy vs mono-therapy with sulfasalazine (Table 2). The patients had less than 2 yr of disease and had not received previous DMARD therapy. The combination used in this study was methotrexate, sulfasalazine, hydroxychloroquine, and low-dose prednisolone. Patients in the sulfasalazine alone group had the option of receiving prednisolone as well, and also of switching to methotrexate if they had suboptimal responses to sulfasalazine alone. Importantly, the major end-point of this study was remission. Unlike the COBRA trial mentioned earlier, this prospective randomized study was an open trial. At 2 yr, it was determined that the only factor that predicted remission in this group of patients was whether or not they had received combination therapy in the beginning (odds ratio 2.7). Rheumatoid factor status, number of swollen joints, number of tender joints, disease duration and gender had no ability to predict whether patients would be in remission at 2 yr.

Another important observation made in the FIN-RA trial was that if only those patients who were HLA-DR4 shared epitope positive were analyzed, the odds ratio for the ability of combination therapy to predict remission at 2 yr was increased. HLA-DR4 is associated with an increased risk and severity of RA. Again, in this trial, patients on combination therapy tolerated this therapy very well. It is also important to note that secondary endpoints in this trial, including ACR 20 and 50 responses, were numerically better, but not statistically different from those patients who received mono-therapy with sulfasalazine.

With the data provided from the COBRA and Fin-RA trial, a convincing case can be made to treat most patients initially with combination therapy. However, trials to define whether a step-down approach is better than a rapid step-up program have not been done and are clearly needed. Additionally, every clinician knows many patients who have done very well with mono-DMARD therapy. The question remains, do all patients need combinations up front or can we somehow select patients that would benefit the

Table 3
Studies Needed

Early/initial disease	Later established RA

• Step-down vs rapid step-up approach
• MTX + TNF blockade vs MTX
  + prednisone
• Randomization by epitope status
• Attempts to identify predictors of response
	• MTX + TNF blockade vs MTX + HCQ-
	  SSA
	• Infliximab + MTX vs etanercept + MTX
	• Identification of predictors of response

Table 4
Current Recommendations

Early/initial disease	Suboptimal MTX responders

• Rapid acceleration of MTX dose +/– low-dose
  prednisone
• Aggressive step-up to combinations (add HCQ
  and/or SSA)
• Switch to TNF blockers +/– MTX
	• Aggressive step-up to combinations
	• Switch to TNF blockers +/– MTX

most? Until the studies outlined in Table 3 are done, the recommendations for treating this group of patients are as outlined in Table 4.

PATIENTS WITH A SUBOPTIMAL RESPONSE TO METHOTREXATE

Methotrexate has gained almost universal acceptance in the United States as the initial DMARD of choice to treat patients with RA *(3)*. Unfortunately, many patients fail to have a complete response and are characterized as incomplete or suboptimal responders. Usually these patients are defined by the dose of methotrexate that they have received and, currently, patients who have received somewhere between 15 mg and 25 mg of methotrexate have been described as suboptimal responders. The response to parenteral methotrexate is superior to oral methotrexate in some patients because oral absorption is highly variable *(16)*; therefore, it would seem prudent to give most patients a trial of subcutaneous methotrexate before giving up on this form of therapy. Because partial responses to methotrexate are a very common clinical problem, a number of studies have been designed to look at this group of patients *(5,6,8,11)*. Other studies have been designed to compare combination therapy head-to-head with methotrexate therapy *(17)*. These studies have validated the usefulness of all three combination DMARD trial designs: step-up, step-down, and parallel. However, patient characteristics recommending one therapeutic regimen over another remain to be fully clarified and will be the key to optimal treatment in the future.

METHOTREXATE CYCLOSPORINE COMBINATION

The first study to show combination therapy with methotrexate and another disease-modifying drug, compared with continued therapy with methotrexate alone in this group of patients was advantageous was the cyclosporine/methotrexate trial *(11)*. In this trial, 148 patients with active disease despite methotrexate in doses up to 15 mg (mean

Table 5
Triple Therapy: MTX-SSA-HCQ *(17)*

- 102 patients, disease duration mean >6 yr
- Double-blind, randomized, 2-yr trial
- 3 groups: MTX, SSA-HCQ, all 3 drugs
- Triple well-tolerated, fewer withdrawals
- Paulus 50% at 2 yr: MTX 33%, SSA-HCQ 40%, Triple 77% ($p < 0.003$)

dose of methotrexate 10.2 mg) were randomized to receive either cyclosporine in low to moderate doses or placebo in addition to their baseline methotrexate. Forty-eight percent of the patients in the cyclosporine treatment group had achieved an ACR 20 response by 6 mo compared with 16% of the patients in the placebo group ($p = 0.001$). Creatinine elevations did occur in some patients in the cyclosporine group and dosage adjustments were necessary, with creatinines being greater in the cyclosporine-treated group than those treated with placebos at the end of the study ($p = 0.02$). More importantly, long-term use of cyclosporine is associated with a high rate of withdrawal, most commonly because of elevated creatinine levels, hypertension, and/or lack of efficacy. Of the 355 patients enrolled in an open-label extension study, only 22% continued cyclosporine for 3 yr *(18)*.

METHOTREXATE-SULFASALAZINE-HYDROXYCHLOROQUINE (TRIPLE THERAPY)

Long-term methotrexate combination therapy is well-tolerated and superior in efficacy to methotrexate monotherapy in patients with late disease. In a 2-yr, randomized, double-blind, parallel combination strategy study of 102 patients (mean disease duration >6 yr), triple-drug therapy with methotrexate/sulfasalazine/hydroxychloroquine (Table 5) was superior to the combination therapy of hydroxychloroquine/sulfasalazine and monotherapy with methotrexate *(17)*. Seventy-seven percent of patients receiving the triple-drug therapy achieved a 50% Paulus composite response (*see* ref. *19*) compared to 40% of the sulfasalazine-hydroxychloroquine patients and 33% of the methotrexate alone patients ($p = 0.003$). This combination was well tolerated with numerically fewer withdrawals in the combination group compared to the other two groups. This therapy has also been shown to be durable; follow-up of the patients who continued on triple-drug therapy over a 5-yr period revealed that 62% (36/58) tolerated therapy well and continued to maintain a 50% efficacy response *(20)*. A similar long-term response rate (67%) occurred in 15 patients who switched to triple-drug therapy after suboptimal response to monotherapy with methotrexate (17.5 mg/wk) *(21)*. Remissions, as defined by ACR criteria *(22)*, were uncommon in this study (12%) and patients tended to deteriorate when any of the components of the triple therapy were discontinued. This same research group has recently completed enrollment of a new long-term study comparing triple-drug therapy to treatment with methotrexate/sulfasalazine or methotrexate/hydroxychloroquine and preliminary data presented in abstract reveals that the triple combination is more efficacious than either of the two double combinations *(23)*.

OTHER COMBINATIONS WITH METHOTREXATE

The newest DMARD, leflunomide, is comparable in efficacy to other conventional therapies, such as methotrexate *(24)* and sulfasalazine *(25)*. The absence of major hematological, renal and liver toxicity with leflunomide monotherapy suggests that it may assume the position of second-line therapy after or along-side methotrexate. However, only a single, open-label, pilot study has examined the use of leflunomide in combination with methotrexate. Leflunomide (10 mg/d) was added to the treatment regimen of 30 patients with late disease (mean disease duration 13.6 yr) who had suboptimal responses to methotrexate at a dosage of >15 mg/wk *(8)*. The ACR 20% criteria for clinical response were met by 54% of the combination therapy patients after 6 mo of treatment. The combination was generally well-tolerated, but transiently elevated alanine aminotransferase levels occurred in 18 patients and resulted in treatment withdrawal of two patients. Whether these liver blood test abnormalities will prove to be problematic for the clinical use of this combination remains to be seen.

COMBINATIONS INVOLVING BIOLOGICALS

Clearly, one of the most exciting developments in the treatment of RA in the last decade has been the agents that block the action of TNF-α (etanercept and infliximab). Both of these agents have shown substantial efficacy in advanced RA as mono-therapy when compared to placebo *(26,27)*. Additionally, both etanercept and infliximab have been shown to work well when used with methotrexate *(5,6)* in patients who have suboptimal responses to methotrexate (again in comparison to methotrexate plus placebo-treated patients). In the case of infliximab, the combination with methotrexate may be particularly important as a possible way to decrease antibodies, to the mouse component, that may develop to this compound. In this regard, this agent is currently recommended by the FDA as combination (with methotrexate) therapy only. Table 6 shows the percent of ACR 20 and 50 responders in the different trials that have used methotrexate in combination with etanercept or infliximab.

NONCONVENTIONAL "DMARDS"

Steroids are not traditionally considered as DMARDs. However, they clearly fulfill all the criteria for DMARDs, including retarding radiographic erosions *(28–30)*. Few clinicians that care for patients with RA dispute their efficacy. Indeed, they have been used as baseline therapy for approx half of patients included in most of the combination trials discussed above *(5,6,8,11,17)*. This fact, more than any study, attests to their current usefulness, or at least perceived usefulness, in the clinical treatment of RA. Prednisolone was undoubtably a critical component of the success seen in the COBRA protocol *(9)* and may have played a role in the success of the combination group in the FIN-RA trial *(10)*. Steroids clearly deserve further investigation as a component of combination therapy. The COBRA trial has raised the interesting question of whether short courses of high dose steroids could/should be used as a form of induction therapy.

Doxycycline has demonstrated impressive efficacy in animal models of inflammatory and osteoarthritis (OA) *(31,32)*. This efficacy appears to result because of their ability to inhibit metalloproteinases and, presumably in this way, prevent or inhibit joint

Table 6
TNF Inhibition in MTX Failures

Study	Treatment group	% ACR 20 response	% ACR 50 response
Weinblatt *(5)*	Mtx + placebo	27%	3%
Weinblatt *(5)*	Mtx + etanercept	71%	39%
Lipsky *(6)*	Mtx + placebo	20%	8%
Lipsky *(6)*	Mtx + infliximab[a]	42–59%	21–39%

[a]Four different doses regimens of infliximab.

destruction. Studies in patients with RA with the closely related compound minocycline have also demonstrated efficacy *(33–35)*. In two studies in patients with advanced disease (duration 9 and 13 yr), a similar degree of modest but statistically significant benefit was seen *(33,34)*. A much more significant effect was seen in the one double-blind study that has been done in patients with early disease *(35)*. In this study, 65% of minocycline-treated patients achieved an 50% improvement, compared to only 13% of those in the placebo group. This response to minocycline when used in early disease was shown to be durable in a 4-yr follow-up study *(36)*.

THE WAY FORWARD: SELECTING THE RIGHT PATIENTS FOR DIFFERENT THERAPIES

The key to unlocking a brighter future for our patients with RA lies in selecting the correct patients for different therapies. Factors that predict a poor prognosis for patients with RA are well accepted and include rheumatoid factor, elevated erythrocyte sedimentation rate (ESR), the number of joints involved, erosions, the presence of certain genetic markers, and so on. Therefore, some have advocated that patients with certain combinations of these factors should be treated more aggressively. However, unless these factors can be shown to predict response to certain therapies in a differential fashion, their use should not be advocated. For example; it is conceivable that patients in an intermediate or even low-risk group may benefit the most from the early use of certain "aggressive therapies," whereas patients with the worst prognostic marks will do poorly regardless of therapy. Although patient characteristics recommending one therapeutic regimen over another remain to be fully elucidated, genetic differences have been suggested to influence outcomes in a differential fashion. In an attempt to predict response to specific RA treatment regimens, patients with late disease, described previously *(17)*, were tested for the presence of shared HLA-DRB1 epitope alleles *(37)*. Patients who were shared-epitope positive were much more likely to achieve a 50% response if treated with triple therapy (methotrexate-sulfasalazine-hydroxychloroquine) compared with methotrexate alone (94 vs 32% responders, $p < 0.0001$). In contrast, shared-epitope-negative patients did equally well regardless of the treatment provided (88% responders for triple-drug therapy vs 83% for methotrexate monotherapy). This observation has been supported by the FIN-RA trial data that suggests that those patients who were HLA-DR4 positive benefitted the most from combination therapy.

FUTURE RESEARCH

Currently, treatment of RA using methotrexate combinations may be the new gold standard to which future therapies are compared. Many questions remain to be answered (Table 3) regarding the appropriateness of combination therapy and the optimal combinations for specific patients (e.g., differentiated according to clinical and/or genetic features) and for specific clinical situations (e.g., induction, maintenance and/or acute interventional therapy). Other unanswered questions regarding combination therapy involve appropriate monitoring and long-term safety, particularly as they relate to infection, lymphoma, and hepatotoxicity. Furthermore, the cost-benefit implications of long-term combination therapy and any additional monitoring have yet to be addressed. Future research is needed to clarify the role of biological response modifiers, specifically anti-TNF therapies (infliximab, etanercept) and matrix metalloproteinase inhibitors (minocycline, doxycycline), both as components of and alternatives to methotrexate combination regimens.

REFERENCES

1. Pincus, T., S.B. Marcum, and L.F. Callahan. 1992. Long-term drug therapy for rheumatoid arthritis in seven rheumatology private practices: II. Second line drugs and prednisone. *J. Rheumatol.* 19:1885–1894.

2. Wolfe, F. 1995. The epidemiology of drug treatment failure in rheumatoid arthritis. *Baillieres-Clin.-Rheumatol.* 9:619–632.

3. O'Dell, J. 1997. Rheumatoid Arthritis Investigational Network (RAIN). Combination DMARD therapy for rheumatoid arthritis: apparent universal acceptance. *Arthritis Rheum.* 40(Suppl.):S50 (Abstract).

4. Mikuls, T. and J. O'Dell. 1999. The treatment of rheumatoid arthritis: current trends in therapy. *Arthritis Rheum.* 42:S79.

5. Maini, R.N., F.C. Breedveld, J.R. Kalden, et al. 1998. Therapeutic efficacy of multiple intravenous infusions of anti-tumor necrosis factor alpha monoclonal antibody combined with low-dose weekly methotrexate in rheumatoid arthritis. *Arthritis Rheum.* 41:1552–1563.

6. Weinblatt, M.E., J.M. Kremer, A.D. Bankhurst, et al. 1999. A trial of etanercept, a recombinant tumor necrosis factor receptor:Fc fusion protein, in patients with rheumatoid arthritis receiving methotrexate. *N. Engl. J. Med.* 340:253–259.

7. Kremer, J.M. 1998. Combination therapy with biologic agents in rheumatoid arthritis: perils and promise. *Arthritis Rheum.* 41:1548–1551.

8. Weinblatt, M.E., J.M. Kremer, J.S. Coblyn, et al. 1999. Pharmacokinetics, safety, and efficacy of combination treatment with methotrexate and leflunomide in patients with active rheumatoid arthritis. *Arthritis Rheum.* 48(7):1322–1328.

9. Boers, M., A.C. Verhoeven, H.M. Markusse, et al. 1997. Randomized comparison of combined step-down prednisolone, methotrexate and sulphasalazine with sulphasalazine alone in early rheumatoid arthritis. *Lancet* 350:309–318.

10. Mottonen, T., P. Hannonsen, M. Leirasalo-Repo, et al. Comparison of combination therapy with single-drug therapy in early rheumatoid arthritis: a randomised trial. *Lancet* 1999; 353:1568–1573.

11. Tugwell, P., T. Pincus, D. Yocum, et al. 1995. Combination therapy with cyclosporine and methotrexate in severe rheumatoid arthritis. *N. Engl. J. Med.* 333:137–141.

12. Egsmose, C., B. Lung, G. Borg, et al. 1995. Patients with rheumatoid arthritis benefit from early second-line therapy: 5-year follow-up of a prospective double-blind placebo-controlled study. *J. Rheumatol.* 22:2208–2213.

13. Tsakonas, E., A.A. Fitzgerald, M.A. Fitazcharles, et al. 2000. Consequences of delayed therapy with second-line agents in rheumatoid arthritis: a 3 year followup on the hydroxychloroquine in early rheumatoid arthritis (HERA) study. *J. Rheumatol.* 27(3):623–629.

14. Wilske, K.R. and L.A. Healey. 1989. Remodeling the pyramid—a concept whose time has come. *J. Rheumatol.* 16:565–567.

15. Felson, D.T., J.J. Anderson, M. Boers, et al. 1995. American College of Rheumatology preliminary definition of improvement in rheumatoid arthritis. *Arthritis Rheum.* 38:727–735.

16. Herman, R.A., P. Veng-Pedersen, J. Hoffman, et al. 1989. Pharmacokinetics of low-dose methotrexate in rheumatoid arthritis patients. *J. Pharm. Sci.* 78:165.

17. O'Dell, J.R., C.E. Haire, N. Erikson, et al. 1996. Treatment of rheumatoid arthritis with methotrexate alone, sulfasalazine, and hydroxychloroquine, or a combination of all three medications. *N. Engl. J. Med.* 334:1287–1291.

18. Yocum, D.E., M. Stein, and T. Pincus. 1998. Long-term safety of cyclosporin/Sandimmune™ (CsA/SIM) alone and in combination with methotrexate (MTX) in the treatment of active rheumatoid arthritis (RA): analysis of open-label extension studies. *Arthritis Rheum.* 41(Suppl.):S364 (Abstract).

19. Paulus, H.E., M.J. Egger, J.R. Ward, and J.H. William. 1990. Analysis of improvement in individual rheumatoid arthritis patients treated with disease-modifying antirheumatic drugs, based on the findings in patients treated with placebo. *Arthritis Rheum.* 33:477–484.

20. O'Dell, J., G. Paulsen, C. Haire, W. Palmer, S. Wees, J. Eckhoff, L. Klassen, and G. Moore. 1998. Combination DMARD therapy with methotrexate (M) - Sulfasalazine (S) - Hydroxychloroquine (H) in rheumatoid arthritis (RA): continued efficacy with minimal toxicity at 5 years. *Arthritis Rheum.* 41(9; Suppl.):S132.

21. O'Dell, J.R., C. Haire, N. Erikson, W. Drymalski, W. Palmer, P. Maloley, et al. 1996. Efficacy of triple DMARD therapy in patients with RA with suboptimal response to methotrexate. *J. Rheumatol.* 23(Suppl 44):72–74.

22. Pinals, R.S, A.T. Masi, and R.A. Larsen. 1981. Subcommittee for Criteria of Remission in Rheumatoid Arthritis of the American Rheumatism Association Diagnostic and Therapeutic Criteria Committee. Preliminary criteria for clinical remission in rheumatoid arthritis. *Arthritis Rheum.* 24:1308–1315.

23. O'Dell, J., R. Leff, G. Paulsen, C. Haire, J. Mallek, P.J. Eckhoff, et al. 1999. Methotrexate (M)-Hydroxychloroquine(H)-Sulfasalazine(S) versus M-H or M-S for rheumatoid arthritis (RA): Results of a double-blind study. *Arthritis Rheum.* 42:S117.

24. Weaver, A., J. Caldwell, N. Olsen, S. Cohen, et al. 1998. Treatment of active rheumatoid arthritis with leflunomide compared to placebo or methotrexate. *Arthritis Rheum.* 41(Suppl.):S131 (Abstract).

25. Smolen, J.S., J.R. Kalden, B. Rozman, et al. 1998. A double-blind, randomized, phase III trial of leflunomide vs placebo vs sulfasalazine in rheumatoid arthritis. *Arthritis Rheum.* 41(Suppl.):S131 (Abstract).

26. Elliott, M.J., R.N. Maini, M. Reldmann, et al. 1994. Randomised double-blind comparison of chimeric monoclonal antibody to tumor necrosis factor α (eA2) versus placebo in rheumatoid arthritis. *Lancet* 344:1105–1110.

27. Moreland, L.W., S.W. Baumgartner, M.H. Schiff, et al. 1997. Treatment of rheumatoid arthritis with a recombinant human tumor necrosis factor receptor (p75)-Fc fusion protein. *N. Engl. J. Med.* 337:141–147.

28. Kirwan, J.R. and the Arthritis and Rheumatism Council Low-Dose Glucocorticoid Study Group. 1995. The effect of glucocorticoids on joint destruction in rheumatoid arthritis. *N. Engl. J. Med.* 333:142–146.

29. The Joint Committee of the Medical Research Council and Nuffield Foundation on Clinical Trials of Cortisone, ACTH, and Other Therapeutic Measures in Chronic Rheumatic Diseases. 1959. A comparison of prednisolone with aspirin or other analgesics in the treatment of rheumatoid arthritis. *Ann. Rheum. Dis.* 18:173–187.

30. Idem. 1960. A comparison of prednisolone with aspirin or other analgesics in the treatment of rheumatoid arthritis. *Ann. Rheum. Dis.* 19:331–337.

31. Greenwald, R.A., S.A. Moak, N.S. Ramamurthy, and L.M. Golub. 1992. Tetracyclines suppress matrix metalloproteinase activity in adjuvant arthritis and in combination with flurbiprofen ameliorate bone damage. *J. Rheumatol.* 19:927–938.

32. Yu, L.P., G.N. Smith, K. Brandt, et al. 1993. Reduction of the severity of canine osteoarthritis by prophylactic treatment with oral doxycycline. *Arthritis Rheum.* 35:1150–1159.

33. Kloppenburg, M., F.C. Breedveld, J. Terwiel, C. Mallee, B.A.C. Dijkmans. 1994. Minocycline in active rheumatoid arthritis. *Arthritis Rheum.* 37:629–636.

34. Tilley, B.C., G.S. Alarcon, S.P. Heyse, D.E. Trentham, R. Neuner, D.A. Kaplan, et al. 1995. Minocycline in rheumatoid arthritis. *Ann. Int. Med.* 122:81–89.

35. O'Dell, J.R., C.E. Haire, W. Palmer, W. Drymalski, S. Wees, K. Blakely, et al. 1997. Treatment of early rheumatoid arthritis with minocycline or placebo. *Arthritis Rheum.* 40:842–848.

36. O'Dell, J.R., G. Paulsen, C.E. Haire, K. Blakely, W. Palmer, S. Wees, et al. 1999. Treatment of early seropositive rheumatoid arthritis with minocycline: Four-year followup of a double-blind, placebo-controlled trial. *Arthritis Rheum.* 42:1691–1695.

37. O'Dell, J.R., B.S. Nepom, C. Haire, V.H. Gersuk, L. Gaur, G.F. Moore, et al. 1998. HLA-DRB1 typing in rheumatoid arthritis: predicting response to specific treatments. *Ann. Rheum. Dis.* 57:209–213.

11

Experimental Therapeutics for Rheumatoid Arthritis

Mark C. Genovese
and William H. Robinson

CONTENTS

INTRODUCTION

Rheumatoid arthritis (RA) is a disease of complex pathogenesis characterized by chronic inflammatory synovitis. The inflammatory synovitis in RA results in synovial proliferation and the formation of pannus that leads to erosive joint destruction. RA is mediated by T cells, B cells, and macrophages, although the target of the inflammatory response remains elusive. It is likely that an autoimmune T-cell response induces production of TNF-α that drives the inflammatory synovitis and erosive joint

From: *Modern Therapeutics in Rheumatic Diseases*
Edited by: G. C. Tsokos, et al. © Humana Press, Inc., Totowa, NJ

destruction. As discussed in detail in Chapter 6, systemic administration of soluble TNF-α receptor-immunoglobulin fusion proteins and anti-TNF-α antibodies result in clinical improvement in patients with RA and in murine models of RA. However, anti-TNF-α therapy, like methotrexate and other DMARDs, is not curative and active synovitis rapidly returns following discontinuation of therapy. There is tremendous clinical need for other more fundamental therapeutic approaches.

In this chapter we discuss a variety of novel therapeutic approaches for RA directed at terminating the underlying autoimmune process and blocking mediators of joint destruction. We review the evidence for RA being an autoimmune disease and the rationale for the discussed novel therapeutic approaches. We discuss the current status of therapeutic approaches based on inhibition of T-cell activation via costimulatory molecule-blockade, including therapies targeting CD40-CD40L and B7-CD28. Cytokine-based strategies for inducing immune-deviation, including blockade of interleukin-6 (IL-6) and IL-12 as well as counter regulation of proinflammatory cytokines via use of interferon β (IFN-β), are reviewed. Peptide and T-cell receptor (TOR)-based strategies for inactivating or eliminating autoreactive T cells are presented. Additional novel therapeutic strategies involving gene therapy and blockade of mediators of synovitis and joint destruction through the use of molecules such as IL-1-converting enzyme inhibitors, P38 inhibitors, and complement inhibitors are discussed. We will not cover every potential therapy, but instead will concentrate on those that are under current investigation and offer the greatest potential. Although many of these novel therapeutic approaches have tremendous promise based on both theory and animal models, well-designed and rigorous clinical trials are paramount to establish which of these approaches are safe and effective for use in patients with RA. Figure 1 offers a schematic for T-cell-driven erosive arthritis and potential therapeutic targets.

RATIONALE FOR THERAPEUTICS TARGETING T CELLS IN RA

Pathogenic T cells that have evaded mechanisms promoting self-tolerance are felt to play a primary role in initiating and perpetuating the inflammatory response in RA. Evidence that T cells play a critical role in RA includes the: (1) predominance of CD4+ T cells infiltrating the synovium, (2) clinical improvement associated with suppression of T cell function with drugs such as cyclosporine, and (3) the association of RA with certain HLA-DR alleles (1). The HLA-DR (class II MHC) allele polymorphisms associated with RA include a similar sequence of amino acids, termed the "shared epitope" at positions 67–74 in the third hypervariable region of the β chain that are involved in binding and presentation of peptides to T cells (1). The only known function of amino acid residues at this location within the MHC molecule is to bind and present antigenic peptides to T cells, and this is in itself indirect but strong evidence that T cells play an important role in RA.

Adjuvant-induced and collagen-induced (CIA) arthritis are murine models of T-cell-mediated autoimmunity that share many features with RA. The resulting arthritis is characterized by synovitis and erosions that histologically resemble RA (2). Depletion of CD4+ T cell attenuates the incidence and delays onset of both adjuvant-induced arthritis and CIA (3), although such therapy has demonstrated only modest effects in human RA. The failure of this strategy in human RA is likely owing to the entrenched nature

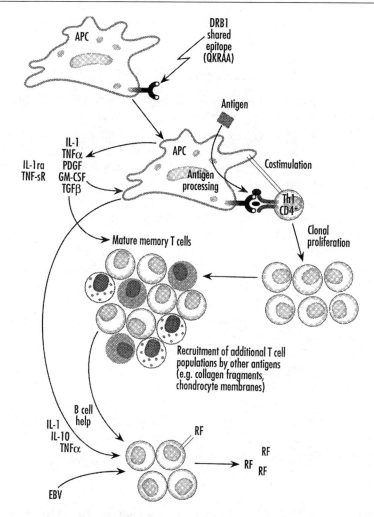

Fig. 1. Pathophysiology of RA: T-cell-driven erosive arthritis and potential targets for therapeutic intervention. The putative autoantigen is taken up by antigen presenting cells (APC), proteolytically processed, and antigen-peptide:MHC complexes formed. These antigen-peptide:MHC complexes are expressed on the surface of the APC, and present the antigenic peptide to potentially autoreactive T cells. The DRB1 shared epitope, a polymorphism in the peptide binding groove of the DRB1 MHC molecule containing the amino acid sequence QKRAA, is associated with increased likelihood of developing RA. MHC molecules containing the shared epitope are believed to more efficiently bind antigenic peptides that activate autoreactive T cells in RA. T-cell activation requires a costimulatory signal (*see* Fig. 2). In RA, T cell activation results in production of cytokines such as TNF-α by macrophages. TNF-α drives a cascade of inflammatory cytokines, including IL-1 and GM-CSF, that cause an inflammatory synovitis and erosive arthritis. Memory T cells are formed and the inflammatory synovitis may be perpetuated by other antigens (e.g., collagen fragments, chondrocyte membranes) and stimuli (e.g., infections and nonspecific joint irritation). As described in the text, potential targets for therapeutic intervention include blocking activation of autoreactive T cells and blocking the mediators of the inflammatory synovitis. Adapted with permission from ref. *1.*

of human autoimmune responses, with a significant burden of autoreactive memory T cells not easily eliminated by anti-CD4 antibody therapies.

CYTOKINE-BASED THERAPEUTIC STRATEGIES

Cytokines play several important roles in the pathophysiology of RA. First, cytokines influence the type of CD4+ helper T cells response generated, e.g., Th1 vs Th2, which can have a large influence on the development of and tissue-damage induced by autoimmune responses. Second, evidence from animal models suggests that proinflammatory cytokines, such as TNF-α, can drive synovitis and erosive joint destruction independent of an ongoing autoimmune response *(4)*.

The CD4+ helper T-cell response plays an important role in regulating autoimmunity in murine models of RA and preliminary evidence suggests that this may also be the case in human RA. Th1 immune responses, characterized by CD4+ T cells that produce IL-2, IL-12, and IFN-γ, are capable of tissue destruction and are associated with autoimmune disease. In contrast, Th2 CD4+ T cells produce IL-4 and IL-5 that mediate phagocyte-independent host defenses involving allergic (IgE) responses and parasite immunity. Th2-mediated immune responses are associated with protection against autoimmunity. The Th1 cytokines IL-12 and IFN-γ promote Th1 responses, while the Th2 cytokine IL-4 promotes Th2 responses.

In murine models of RA, Th1-type CD4+ T-cell responses result in active disease, whereas Th2-type T-cell responses ameliorate disease *(5)*. In human RA patients, there is growing evidence for Th1-like immune responses that may in part drive disease. Thus, a strategy for treatment of human RA would be to induce immune deviation of the autoimmune response towards the nonpathogenic Th2-type response. This can potentially be accomplished by inhibition or blockade of Th1-driving cytokines, or administration of Th2-driving cytokines.

IL-12

Studies in the murine models have demonstrated that the Th1 cytokine IL-12 plays a central role in mediating CIA *(6)*. Mice deficient for expression of IL-12 and wild-type mice treated with anti-IL-12 antibody have reduced severity of arthritis *(6–8)*. Use of a combination of anti-IL-12 plus anti-TNF-α antibodies synergistically suppressed CIA to a significantly greater extent than either antibody alone *(9)*. Furthermore, the combination of anti-IL-12 plus anti-TNF-α antibodies was able to successfully treat CIA following the onset of clinical disease *(9)*.

Increased levels of IL-12 have been detected in the serum and synovial fluid of patients with RA relative to controls with osteoarthritis (OA) *(10)*. There is a case report of a patient with RA who had a severe exacerbation of disease following receiving recombinant IL-12 as an experimental therapy for cervical cancer *(11)*. Thus, there is evidence that the Th1 cytokine IL-12 may contribute to the autoimmune pathogenesis of RA.

In humans, studies are underway looking at mechanisms to interfere with IL-12. It is too early to speculate on their potential utility, however a targeted approach may yield a potentially exciting therapy.

IFN-β

Recombinant human IFN-β has efficacy in and is Food and Drug Administration (FDA)-approved for the treatment of relapsing remitting multiple sclerosis (MS) *(12)*. Although its mechanism of action is poorly understood, IFN-β is thought to antagonize the effects of IFN-γ and other proinflammatory cytokines and to downregulate T-cell activity. IFN-β suppresses mitogen-stimulated production of TNF-α in peripheral blood mononuclear cells, and this effect could be especially beneficial in the treatment of RA. Treatment of CIA by intraperitoneal implantation of syngeneic fibroblasts expressing IFN-β resulted in significant amelioration of arthritis *(13)*.

There is optimism that IFN-β might also be an efficacious therapy for human RA. Eleven patients with active RA were treated with INF-β subcutaneously 3 times/wk for 12 wk with varying dosages, 6 million IU, 12 million IU, and 18 million IU *(14)*. After 3 mo, 4 patients had achieved an ACR 20 response. In addition, all patients underwent synovial biopsies at three time-points: before therapy, 1 mo after initiation of therapy, and 3 mo after initiation of therapy. Based on immunohistologic analysis of the biopsies, there was a significant reduction in CD3+ T cells as well as a reduction in expression of MMP-1 and TIMP-1 at 1 mo, IL-1β at 1 and 3 mo, and CD38+ plasma cells and IL-6 at 3 mo. TNF-α expression also decreased at all time points. The use of regulatory cytokines such as IFN-β that oppose the production and effects of pro-inflammatory cytokines such as TNF-α, IL-1β, and INF-γ, may prove a useful strategy in the future treatment of RA. Phase II clinical trials in RA are now underway.

IL-6

IL-6 has been shown to play an important role in both murine models of RA and in human RA. IL-6 has pleiotrophic effects on a variety of cells, and is involved in the generation of inflammatory responses. TNF-α induces synovial cell proliferation and production of IL-6. IL-6-deficient mice have a dramatic reduction in the severity of adjuvant-induced arthritis, relative to wild type controls *(15)*.

Elevated levels of both IL-6 and soluble IL-6 receptor are observed in the serum and synovial fluid of patients with RA *(16–18)*. An open-label pilot study was conducted to examine use of a mouse anti-IL-6 antibody in five patients with RA *(19)*. These patients were treated with iv injections of anti-IL-6 antibody daily for 10 d. A trend towards clinical improvement was observed for several months following treatment and no adverse events were reported.

Anti-IL-6 receptor antibody is also being studied in human RA patients *(20)*. Treatment with this antibody was associated with a decrease in rheumatoid factor titers and an overall anti-inflammatory effect.

INHIBITION OF T-CELL ACTIVATION BY COSTIMULATORY MOLECULE BLOCKADE

T-cell activation requires two signals (Fig. 2). The first signal is delivered by engagement of the TCR with an antigenic peptide complexed with the major histocompatibility complex (MHC) on the surface of an antigen-presenting cell (APC). Therapies that

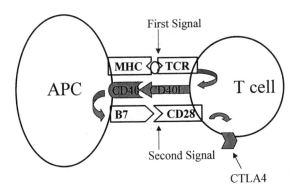

Fig. 2. T-cell activation requires two signals. The first signal, T-cell receptor (TCR) engagement with MHC:antigen-peptide, provides antigen-specificity to the T-cell response. The second signal, CD28 engagement by B7 (CD80 and/or CD86), is an essential costimulatory signal for T-cell activiation. The first signal in the absence of the second signal induces T-cell tolerance (anergy or deletion). Candidate therapeutic agents, including anti-CD40/CD40L, CTLA4-Ig, and anti-CD80/CD86, all block T-cell activation by antagonizing the second signal.

target this first signal include cyclosporin, soluble MHC class II peptides, and altered peptide ligands. A second signal, also known as the costimulatory signal, is required for T cell activation. The costimulatory molecules that interact to mediate the second signal include CD40L-CD40 and CD28-B7(including B7-1 and B7-2, also known as CD80 and CD86). The first signal in the absence of the second signal results in T-cell anergy or deletion (immune tolerance). Antagonizing one or more of the molecules that mediate the second signal results in unopposed signaling through the TCR and T cell tolerance. Thus, therapies that block signaling through the CD40-CD40L and CD28-B7 pathways have the potential to induce immune tolerance and thereby turn off unwanted autoimmune responses.

CD40L

Interference with CD40-CD40L interactions has been shown to reduce the manifestations of autoimmune disease in animal models of systemic lupus erythematosus (SLE), MS, RA, and inflammatory bowel disease. The CD40L-CD40 interaction may be important in the pathogenesis of RA. In the CIA model, treatment with anti-CD40L antibodies at the time of immunization prevents the development of CIA (21). Anti-CD40L antibodies block the development of serum antibodies to collagen, synovial inflammation, and joint erosions. However, treatment with anti-CD40L antibodies did not ameliorate established disease in the CIA model. Administration of anti-CD40L and anti-intracellular adhesion molecule-1 (ICAM-1) antibodies together completely inhibited established CIA, suggesting that other agents combined with anti-CD40L antibodies may be the preferred therapeutic approach for human RA (22).

Anti-CD40L antibodies may prevent engagement of CD40 on macrophages and synoviocytes and inhibit the production of proinflammatory cytokines and other mediators inside the joint, such as nitric oxide (NO) and matrix metalloproteinases (MMPs). The CD40-CD40L interaction appears to be a critical component of CD4+T-cell contact-dependent activation of monocyte IL-1 synthesis (23). Ligation of CD40 also appears to augment proliferation of synovial-membrane fibroblasts and their production of IL-6, (ICAM-1), and vascular adhesion molecule-1 (VCAM-1) *(24)*. Blocking this interaction should decrease IL-6 levels and synovial proliferation. Disruption of the CD40-CD40L interaction may also reduce IL-12 expression, which in turn may reduce the Th1 cellular response in RA *(25)*. CD4+ T-cell depletion and anti-CD40L antibodies reduce IL-12 production by synovial cells. However, IL-12 production by these cells is relatively unaffected by treatment with anti-TNF-α antibodies. On the other hand, anti-TNF-α antibodies but not CD4+ T cell depletion or anti-CD40L antibodies inhibit LPS-stimulated IL-12 production. IL-12 production in RA appears to be controlled through two different pathways, a T cell-dependent CD40-CD40L mechanism and a T-cell-independent process mediated by TNF-α *(26)*. Additional work has shown that ligation of CD40 on synovial tissue from RA patients significantly increases production of TNF-α in a dose-dependent fashion. Moreover, CD40L-induced TNF-α production is enhanced by IFN-γ, IL-4, and IL-13, and decreased by IL-10 *(27)*. These findings suggest that activated T cells drive synovial inflammation in RA via CD40L stimulated production of TNF-α.

Although the CD40-CD40L interactions are important in priming of antigen-specific T cells, the synovial microenvironment in established RA contains a large proportion of memory T cells in which antigen priming has already occurred. Treatment with anti-CD40L antibodies may still have an effect at this point in the disease process in these cell populations. CD40L expression on the surface of T cells is downregulated after CD40 receptor interaction. As well, it appears that in previously activated, but downmodulated T cells, CD40L can be rapidly reexpressed upon subsequent activation or stimulus *(28)*. It is possible that memory T cells or already primed T cells may harbor intracellular stores of preformed CD40L that are available for reexpression. Patients exhibiting CD40L on >10% of CD4+ T cells (CD40L high+) have been shown to have greater disease activity when compared to CD40L low+ groups *(29)*. It may be this group that benefits more substantially from treatment with anti-CD40L antibody therapy.

Anti-CD40L antibody therapy has been utilized in humans for the treatment of other autoimmune diseases including SLE. There have been two antibody preparations used in human clinical trials of this disease, Biogen-9588 and IDEC-131. In the autumn of 1999, the Biogen molecule (BG-9588) was implicated as a potential cause of thrombo-embolic complications after a number of thrombotic adverse events developed in clinical trials. Additional human studies with BG9588 were stopped pending further evaluation of these events and additional preclinical evaluation. The etiology or pathogenesis of these thrombotic complications is not known. However, it is known that CD40L can be expressed by human vascular endothelial cells as well as platelets. CD40L is expressed on activated platelets in thrombus in vivo, and CD40L has also been reported to be responsible for the platelet-mediated activation of endothelial cells in vitro *(30)*. However, different anti-CD40L antibodies recognize distinct epitopes in the CD40L molecule and both side effects and efficacy may depend on these differences. Given this, there is a second molecule, IDEC-131, which is a humanized anti-CD40L monoclonal antibody (MAb) that binds specifically and with high affinity to CD40L. This molecule has been studied extensively in animal models and has completed evaluation in humans in both phase I and II clinical trials for SLE.

It does not appear that therapy with anti-CD40L antibodies results in untoward immunosuppression or an increased risk for infection in animal models or in human trials. There is, however, a theoretical reason for concern. Humoral immunity is impaired in humans with X-linked hyper immunoglobulin M syndrome (HIM), a syndrome associated with severe reduction of thymus-dependent responses and Ig isotype switching that results from point mutations in the gene for CD40L *(31)*. Cell mediated immunity however remains intact. Patients suffering from this disease as well as CD40L knockout animals appear at increased risk for certain opportunistic infections (*Pneumocystis carinii, Cryptosporidia,* and *Leishmania*) and conceivably some viral infections *(31–33)*.

It is anticipated that anti-CD40L antibody could be used in the future for the treatment of RA, and has the potential to result in potent anti-inflammatory and disease modifying effects. The long-term safety of this approach is unclear.

CD40

CD40 is a member of the TNF receptor supergene family and is a potent receptor molecule enabling T cells to regulate a host of immune and inflammatory functions. It is expressed on the surface of APCs, including B cells, activated macrophages, dendritic cells, fibroblasts, synoviocytes, and endothelial cells. Engagement of CD40 by CD40L leads to a host of downstream changes including T-cell costimulation, cytotoxic T-lymphocyte priming, up-regulation of B-cell costimulatory molecules (B7-1 and B7-2), promotion of B-cell differentiation, germinal center formation, B-cell responsiveness to T-cell cytokines, and immunoglobulin class switching. Interference with the CD40L-CD40 interaction as outlined above can prevent the development of a number of autoimmune diseases including CIA, experimental allergic encephalomyelitis, and can prolong allograft survival in transplantation. Overall, less is known regarding the targeting of the CD40 receptor than CD40 ligand.

CD40 is expressed on rheumatoid synovial pannus and fibroblasts. IFN-γ and TNF-α have been found to upregulate CD40 expression on fibroblasts. Additionally, the engagement of fibroblast CD40 with CD40L increases IL-1-induced production of granulocyte macrophage-colony stimulating factor and macrophage inflammatory protein-1 α, suggesting that CD40 may contribute to proliferation of rheumatoid synovium *(34)*. It appears that CD40 is involved in chronic activation of RA synovial monocytes. Interference with ligation of the CD40 receptor through utilization of anti-CD40 antibodies can inhibit secretion of TNF-α from RA synovial monocytes *(35)*. As well, CD40 signaling appears to be important in the production of human RF production. Blockade of the CD40L-CD40 interaction results in deletion of rheumatoid factor producing B cells, while activating antibodies to CD40 can promote the survival of RF precursor cells and stimulate RF synthesis *(36)*.

Interestingly, there is a report of an individual developing seronegative RA in the face of a non-X-linked HIM syndrome *(37)*. The patient was found to express CD40L normally on activated T cells, but CD40-mediated signal transduction in B cells was defective, failing to allow heavy-chain switching. This brings into question whether simple interference with the CD40L-CD40 pathway through targeting of CD40 will be sufficient to result in alteration or prevention of RA, as this patient developed RA despite dysfunction of the CD40 pathway.

Nevertheless, clinical trials in humans utilizing a humanized MAb against CD40 are currently underway. The safety and potential efficacy of this approach remains to be established. Given the constitutive nature of expression of this molecule on the surface of many cell types as opposed to the inducible nature of CD40L, B7, and CTLA-4, this may not be the ideal candidate target. However, in theory this could lead to the induction of tolerance and significant reduction in autoimmune and inflammatory disease.

B7

As outlined earlier, B7-1 and B7-2 (CD80 and CD86, collectively referred to as B7) represent inducible costimulatory molecules expressed on the surface of APC. B7-1 and B7-2 are expressed on activated B cells and bind to CD28 on the surface of T cells. Engagement of B7 with CD28 (second signal), in conjunction with simultaneous signaling through the TCR (first signal), results in T cell activation (Fig. 2). Data from animal models demonstrate that B7-mediated signals through CD28 are essential for the induction of arthritis. Mice deficient for CD28 are highly resistant to induction of CIA *(38)*.

CTLA-4-Ig blocks B7 engagement of CD28, and treatment of mice or rats with CTLA-4-Ig significantly ameliorates development of arthritis *(39,40)*. Use of anti-B7-1 and anti-B7-2 antibodies revealed that simultaneous blockade of both molecules was needed to suppress induction of CIA in mice as well as to decrease disease activity in mice with established CIA *(39)*. Blockade of either B7-1 or B7-2 alone was insufficient *(39)*. Thus, B7 engagement of CD28 plays a critical role in the induction of autoimmune arthritis in rodents and represents an important therapeutic target for human RA.

In humans, the cellular interactions between synovium and infiltrating T cells mediated through the B7/CD28 pathways are associated with the development of exacerbations/inflammation in the synovial cells *(41)*. Both B7-1 and B7-2 can be found expressed within rheumatoid synovium and synovial fluid mononuclear cells *(42,43)*. However, rheumatoid synovium expresses much higher levels of B7-2 than B7-1. B7-2 can be readily detected in rheumatoid synovium, whereas B7-1 positive cells are infrequently found in synovium from both patients with early disease and those with more established disease *(44)*. This data might suggest that interference with B7-CD28 signaling may downmodulate inflammation in patients with RA. As well, it may suggest that B7-2 may be the preferred target over B7-1, although inhibition of both has been necessary for efficacy in animal models of RA *(39)*.

Clinical trials have been designed to utilize anti-B7-1 and anti-B7-2 antibodies both individually and collectively for the treatment of RA in humans. These studies are currently under evaluation for both funding and implementation. It remains to be seen whether one or both molecules will need to be targeted to result in amelioration of disease. In addition, the safety of either single or combination blockade has yet to be established in humans.

CTLA-4

CTLA-4 represents another opportunity to interfere with the costimulatory pathway by which T cells become activated and initiate immune responses. CTLA-4 is a regulatory molecule expressed on the surface of helper T cells following activation. Expression of CTLA-4 blocks excitatory costimulatory signals and delivers inhibitory signals to T cells *(44)*. It is thought that expression of CTLA-4 acts to attenuate T-cell responses following activation, so that overactive T-cell responses do not develop *(45)*.

In mice lacking expression of CTLA-4, activated T cells continue unchecked and a fatal lymphoproliferative disorder develops *(46)*. CTLA-4 has a 100-fold higher affinity, and 500–2500-fold greater avidity, than CD28 for binding to B7 *(47–50)*. When expressed, CTLA-4 preferentially binds B7 thereby preventing B7 from delivering costimulatory signals through CD28. Thus, in addition to delivering inhibitory signals to T cells, CTLA-4 is a natural competitive inhibitor of CD28. Based on these properties, CTLA-4 serves as an inhibitory regulatory check-point during T-cell activation.

One approach to blockade of costimulation has utilized CTLA-4 as a fusion protein, called CTLA-4Ig. This fusion protein consists of the extracellular portion of CTLA-4 joined to the Fc portion of an IgG molecule. In rat models CTLA-4-Ig prevents induction of CIA *(40)*. In studies in mice, not only was CTLA-4-Ig able to block induction of CIA it significantly reduced paw thickness, numbers of joints affected, and joint destruction in established CIA *(39)*. In lupus models use of CTLA-4-Ig in NZB/NZW mice blocked antibody production, and resulted in prolonged life *(51)*. In the MS model, mice treated with CTLA-4-Ig failed to develop EAE *(52)*. In humans, use of CTLA-4-Ig has been reported to significantly improve psoriasis. In a small Phase I study in psoriasis CTLA-4-Ig led to a 50% clinical improvement in disease activity *(53)*. A Phase II study has been completed in humans looking at the safety and efficacy of CTLA-4-Ig in the treatment of RA and results are expected soon. CTLA-4-Ig has the potential to be a very efficacious means of treating autoimmune disease.

T-CELL RECEPTOR-BASED VACCINE STRATEGIES

In susceptible rodent strains, adjuvant-induced arthritis and CIA are mediated by T cells expressing a limited set of TCR V gene segments. In CIA in DBA/1 (H-2^q) mice pathogenic T cells specific for type II collagen utilize a limited number of Vα (Vα8, Vα11, and Vα22) and Vβ (Vβ8, Vβ1, and Vβ6) chains, with almost 60% utilizing Vβ8.2 *(53,54)*. Injection of MAb specific for Vβ8.2 in DBA/1 mice prevents induction of CIA, demonstrating the importance of T cells expressing Vβ8 in induction of CIA *(56,57)*. Although such antibody therapy is effective, anti-TCR antibody works by depleting potentially pathogenic T cells and these populations of T cells reemerge after degradation of the antibody.

Human RA patients expressing DR4 also utilize a limited number of T-cell receptor V gene segments, including Vβ3, Vβ14, and Vβ17. A randomized, placebo-controlled, multicenter, phase II human trial examined use of a TCR peptide vaccine in 99 RA patients *(58)*. This vaccine contained a combination of 3 peptides derived from Vβ3, Vβ14 and Vβ17, and demonstrated a trend towards improvement in the groups receiving the TCR-derived peptides.

A second phase II study was reported in which two different TCR peptide vaccines derived from Vβ3, Vβ14, and Vβ17 were compared in a double-blind randomized placebo controlled study of 6-mo duration. There was a trend toward improvement in those patients receiving vaccination, particularly in those patients with less than 3 yr of disease duration and in those on less than 7.5 mg of prednisone/d. In virtually all the treatment groups improvement was seen following three injections, but waned by wk 20 *(59)*.

Given the heterogeneity of human autoimmune responses in RA, with different patients utilizing different combinations of TCR V gene segments, TCR peptide-based therapeutics are likely to only possess efficacy for a subset of RA patients. Such constraints, combined with their modest efficacy, dampen enthusiasm for wide-scale use of such a strategy.

GENE THERAPY FOR RA

While still in its infancy, gene therapy for the treatment or possibly the prevention of arthritis is a promising field *(60)*. Gene therapy-based strategies offer the potential to deliver proteins, which are not orally active, to selected anatomic sites in a clinical useful manner. Several gene therapy-based therapeutics have demonstrated efficacy in rodent models of RA. Systemic genetic delivery of IL-4, IL-10, IL-13 or TGF-β inhibits arthritis in animal models *(60,61)*. Systemic adenoviral-mediated delivery of a TNF p55 receptor-IgGFc chimeric molecule and IL-1ra suppress CIA *(60,62)*. In CIA and RA synovial cell proliferation and production of degradative enzymes results in pannus formation and joint destruction. These synovial cells, as well as activated T cells, express high levels of Fas. Engagement of Fas causes apoptosis, and intra-articular genetic delivery of Fas-ligand (CD95) results in apoptosis of synovial cells and attenuation of CIA *(63)*.

In the first human clinical trial of gene therapy for arthritis, IL-1ra cDNA was transferred to the metacarpal phalangeal joints (MCP) of patients with RA to express that DNA intra-articularly *(64,65)*. Autologous synovial fibroblasts were stably transduced with a retrovirus carrying IL-1ra cDNA. Nine postmenopausal women received transduced cells or controlled cells in a double-blind dose escalation fashion. One week after gene transfer, the MCP joints were surgically removed and the retrieved tissues were analyzed for evidence of successful gene transfer and gene expression. All joints receiving the transgene showed evidence of gene expression, and curiously a number of joints receiving control cells also showed evidence of gene expression. This finding remains unexplained. No adverse events were reported in any of the patients in this study with follow-up extending beyond 3 yr in several patients. However, the detection of transgene expression in the control joints highlights lack of understanding regarding migration of cells and viruses between joints and just one of the many potential impediments to development and adoption of this field of therapy.

Gene therapy offers tremendous potential for the development of novel effective therapies for RA. Given the recent human deaths associated with adenovirus-based gene therapies *(66)*, careful evaluation of potential therapeutics first in animal models and subsequently in human RA patients is essential.

THERAPEUTIC MODULATION OF MEDIATORS OF INFLAMMATORY ARTHRITIS

P38

Another of the promising pathways being explored for possible therapeutic intervention in RA is that of the stress-activated protein kinases (SAPK) and the mitogen-activated protein kinases (MAPK). Cellular gene expression is modified in response to physical stresses and inflammatory triggers such as cytokines, fever, shock, ischemia, or toxins. These stimuli trigger a cascade starting with cell-membrane receptors that activate kinases leading to expression of cytokines and growth factors. Phosphorylation and activation of these kinases can lead to translocation to the nucleus, activation of transcription factors, and alteration of gene expression *(67)*. The transduction of signals through the kinase pathways allows for mitosis, differentiation, or promotion of growth. Ultimately the response to stress as modulated through one or more of these pathways can result in adaptation through apoptosis, immune activation, and inflammation *(67)*. P38 is one such protein kinase. Activation of P38 is believed to inducibly upregulate TNF-α, IL-1, IL-6, IL-8, NO production, and cyclooxygenase-2 (COX-2) expression. Inhibition of P38 is believe to potentially downregulate these proinflammatory products, but may not result in immune suppression because only inducible production would be affected while constitutive expression of these products would continue unaffected.

The p38 MAPK inhibitors are efficacious in several disease models, including inflammation, septic shock, and animal models of arthritis. SB 203580, a pyridinylimidazole compound, inhibits the catalytic activity of p38 MAPK *(68,69)*. It has been studied in several animal models of cytokine inhibition and inflammatory disease. It was demonstrated to inhibit cytokine production in vivo in both mice and rats, and appears to be effective in preventing the development of CIA as well as adjuvant-induced arthritis. It was also found to reduce mortality in a murine model of endotoxin-induced shock, and block induction of TNF and IL-1β-stimulated IL-6 and IL-8 production in vitro *(70,71)*. Nitric oxide (NO) is an inflammatory mediator and has been implicated in animal models of RA and in vitro models of cartilage degradation. In studies, SB 203850 inhibited IL-1-stimulated p38 MAP kinase activity and NO production *(72)*.

Another molecule, SB 220025, a selective p38 inhibitor, has been shown to reduce angiogenesis and reduce TNF-α production. In murine CIA it was found to prevent the progression of established arthritis *(73)*. A newer and more selective p38 inhibitor, SB 242235, was evaluated in a Lewis rat model of adjuvant-induced arthritis. It inhibited the development of paw edema if given prophylactically during the induction phase of the disease, and effectively treated the disease if given for the treatment of established disease. It was found to inhibit LPS-stimulated TNF-α expression and reduce serum IL-6 levels. It appeared to have disease modifying activity by demonstrating protection of bone, cartilage, and soft tissue histologically *(74)*.

Yet another p38 MAP kinase inhibitor RWJ 67657 appears to inhibit the release of TNF-α in LPS treated human peripheral blood mononuclear cells (PBMCs), as well as the release of TNF-α from PBMCs treated with the superantigen staphylococcal enterotoxin B, suggesting that monocyte and T-cell production and release can be inhibited. This molecule also appears to have very selective effects on p38 without effects on other protein kinases *(75)*.

P38 MAPK appears to be a rationale target for therapeutic intervention in autoimmune and inflammatory disease. There are currently multiple p38 kinase inhibitors under investigation for the treatment of autoimmune-based disease. These agents offer the potential to modulate inducible expression of proinflammatory cytokines as orally bioavailable agents. As such they may be potent disease-modifying agents, and offer an alternative to the currently available biologic-response modifiers directed against TNF-α and IL-1. Human trials with p38 inhibitors are underway.

ICE Inhibition

The inhibition of IL-1β converting enzyme (ICE or caspase-1) offers a potential means to treat autoimmune diseases. Pro-IL-1β is synthesized by activated monocytes and macrophages as a 31 kDa, biologically inactive precursor. ICE is a cysteine protease that catalyzes the conversion of the inactive precursor form of IL-1β to a biologically active mature form that is 17 kDa. IL-1β is involved in mediating inflammatory responses, regulating Fas-mediated apoptosis of lymphoid cells, and believed to be involved in the progression of RA.

In animal models, ICE inhibition has been shown to slow progression of disease, and mouse knockout models for ICE do not develop CIA. VE-13,045 was studied in murine CIA *(76)* Prophylactic treatment with VE-13,045 significantly delayed the onset of inflammation and demonstrated a 60% overall reduction in disease severity. It was also more effective than either indomethacin or methyl prednisolone. When given to mice with established disease, VE-13,045 was also effective in reducing inflammation and progression of arthritis *(76)*.

The ICE inhibitor, SDZ 224-015, was examined in the rat carrageenin paw model of inflammation, and it significantly reduced paw edema *(77)*. In a model of pyrexia induced by lipopolysaccharide (LPS), pyrexia was similarly reduced *(77)*. Another molecule L-709,049, a tetrapeptide inhibitor of ICE, effectively suppressed the production of mature IL-1β in a murine model of endotoxic shock *(78)*. In this LPS model L-709,049 reduced elevations of IL-1β, but had no effect on LPS induced elevations in IL-1 α and IL-6, suggesting ICE inhibitors have relative selectivity for this single proinflammatory cytokine *(78)*. Similarly, WIN 67694, a selective inhibitor of human ICE has been shown to inhibit the release of mature IL-1 without any effect on the release of IL-1 α, IL-6, or TNF-α *(79)*.

The inhibition of ICE poses a potent therapeutic avenue for the treatment of autoimmune diseases. Currently, agents are under investigation in humans for the treatment of arthritis. However, many questions remain as the regulation and mechanisms of activation of ICE are poorly understood, and the degree inhibition of IL-1β that is required to effectively reduce inflammation and slow disease is not clear. Despite this, there may be a future role for synthetic inhibitors of the IL-1β converting enzyme (ICE).

COMPLEMENT INHIBITION

Upon activation of the complement system, C5 is cleaved into its proinflammatory components C5a and C5b-9. These activated terminal complement components have been implicated as pro-inflammatory mediators leading to leukocyte activation, cytokine release, production of matrix metallo-proteases, and upregulation of adhesion molecules. With the use of anti-C5 antibodies it is possible to selectively prevent the cleavage of C5 into its byproducts, yet still preserve the body's normal abilities to generate C3b and maintain normal opsonization and immune complex functions. In murine models of CIA, antibodies to C5 demonstrated the ability to prevent the development of arthritis when given prior to the development of disease, as well as the ability to substantially reduce arthritis in animals with established disease *(80)*.

Antibodies to C5 are under development for the treatment of SLE and RA in humans. The results of a phase I study looking at a humanized antibody against C5 (h5G1.1) in RA showed that with single dose administration the agent was generally well-tolerated without safety or laboratory value abnormalities *(81)*. In the 8 mg/kg cohort there was also a suggestion of improvement in the number of tender and swollen joints as well as a significant reduction in the mean CRP levels. Currently a phase II multi-dose safety and efficacy study of h5G1.1 in RA patients is underway.

NEED FOR RIGOROUS TESTING OF NOVEL THERAPEUTIC AGENTS IN HUMAN CLINICAL TRIALS

Of critical importance is clear demonstration of the safety and efficacy of novel therapeutic agents in human patients with RA. There is frequent discordance between the safety and efficacy of various therapeutic agents in animal models as compared with human patients. In SLE, CD40-CD40L blockade resulted in unexpected thrombotic events in human patients that were not previously observed in animal models. Oral feeding of collagen attenuated arthritis in animal models but failed to show efficacy in human RA *(82,83)*. IL-10 and anti-ICAM-1 therapy ameliorated arthritis in animal models but did not show significant benefit in RA *(84,85)*. IL-1ra cures arthritis in animal models but has only modest efficacy in human RA *(86)*. Clinical experience in another T cell-mediated autoimmune disease, MS further highlights the need to carefully evaluate novel therapeutic agents. IFN-γ and anti-TNF-α each cured experimental autoimmune encephalomyelitis in mice but worsened disease in human MS patients *(87)*. An air of skepticism will be crucial in the interpretation of animal data and its applicability to humans with what are believed to be similar diseases.

SUMMARY: TREMENDOUS PROGRESS, TREMENDOUS POTENTIAL

Over the past decade, tremendous progress has been made towards better understanding the underlying pathophysiology of RA. Based on this knowledge, novel therapeutic agents, such as TNF-α antagonists, have been developed, demonstrated to have efficacy in clinical trials, and implemented in clinical practice. Although such agents have great clinical value, they are in no manner curative. Tremendous potential exists for the development of more fundamental therapies that terminate the autoimmune response and inflammatory synovitis in RA. With the start of the new millennium the next generation of novel biological agents, designed to induce immune tolerance at a fundamental level, are undergoing rigorous evaluation in human clinical trials. These next generation agents include CD40-CD40L and B7-CD28 antagonists, which block costimulatory signals necessary to activate T cells, and offer the potential to terminate the autoimmune response believed to drive the inflammatory synovitis in RA. Beyond global costimulatory blockade, additional novel agents designed to tolerize the autoimmune response and terminate the inflammatory synovitis are currently being evaluated in animal models of RA. Rigorous evaluation in well-designed human clinical trials is essential to demonstrate the safety and efficacy of each novel therapeutic agent in RA as we continue to take molecules and proteins from the bench to the bedside.

REFERENCES

1. Harris, E.D. Ed. 1997. *Rheumatoid Arthritis.* W.B. Saunders, Philadelphia.

2. Courtenay, J.S., M.J. Dallman, A.D. Dayan, A. Martin, and B. Mosedale. 1980. Immunization against heterologous type II collagen induces arthritis in mice. *Nature* 283:666–668.

3. Ranges, G.E., S. Sriram, and S.M. Cooper. 1985. Prevention of type II collagen-induced arthritis by in vivo treatment with anti-L3T4. *J. Exp. Med.* 162:1105–1110.

4. Butler, D.M., A.M. Malfait, L.J. Mason, P.J. Warden, G. Kollias, R.N. Maini, et al. 1997. DBA/1 mice expressing the human TNF-alpha transgene develop a severe, erosive arthritis: characterization of the cytokine cascade and cellular composition. *J. Immunol.* 159:2867–2876.

5. Mauri, C., R.O. Williams, M. Walmsley, and M. Feldmann. 1996. Relationship between Th1/Th2 cytokine patterns and the arithrogenic response in collagen-induced arthritis. *Eur. J. Immunol.* 26:1511–1518.

6. McIntyre, K.W., D.J. Shuster, K.M. Gillooly, R.R. Warrier, S.E. Connaughton, L.B. Hall, et al. 1996. Reduced incidence and severity of collagen-induced arthritis in interleukins-12-deficient mice. *Eur. J. Immunol.* 26:2933–2938.

7. Joosten, L.A.B., E. Lubberts, M.M.A. Helsen, and W.B. van den Berg. Dual role of IL-12 in early and late stages of murine collagen Type II arthritis. *J. Immunol.* 159:4094–4102.

8. Malfait, A.M., D.M. Butler, D.H. Presky, R.N Maini, F.M. Brennan, and M. Feldmann. 1998. Blockade of IL-12 during the induction of collagen-induced arthritis (CIA) markedly attenuates the severity of the arthritis. *Clin. Exp. Immunol.* 111:377–383.

9. Butler, D.M., A.M. Malfait, R.N. Maini, F.M. Brennan, and M. Feldmann. 1999. Anti-IL-12 and anti-TNF antibodies synergistically suppress the progression of murine collagen-induced arthritis. *Eur. J. Immunol.* 29:2205–2212.

10. Kim, W.U., S.Y. Min, M.L. Cho, J. Youn, D.J. Min, S.H. Lee, et al. 2000. The role of IL-12 in inflammatory activity of patients with rheumatoid arthritis (RA). *Clin. Exp. Immunol.* 119(1):175–181.

11. Peeva, E., A.D. Fishman, G. Goddard, S. Wadler, and P. Barland. 2000. Rheumatoid arthritis exacerbation caused by exogenous interleukin-12. *Arthritis Rheum.* 43:461–463.

12. IFNB Multiple Sclerosis Study Group. 1993. Interferon beta-1b is effective in relapsing-remitting multiple sclerosis. I. Clinical results of a multicenter, randomized, double-blind, placebo-controlled trial. The IFNB Multiple Sclerosis Study Group. *Neurology* 43:655–661.

13. Triantaphyllopoulos, K.A., R.O. Williams, H. Tailor, and Y. Chernajovsky. Amelioration of collagen-induced arthritis and suppression of interferon-gamma, interleukin-12, and TNF-α production by interferon-beta gene therapy. *Arthritis Rheum.* 42:90–99.

14. Smeets, T.J., J.M. Dayer, M.C. Kraan, J. Versendaal, R. Chicheportiche, F.C. Breedveld, and P.P. Tak. 2000. The effects of interferon-beta treatment of synovial inflammation and expression of metalloproteinases in patients with rheumatoid arthritis. *Arthritis Rheum.* 43:270–274.

15. Alonzi, T., E. Fattori, D. Lazzaro, P. Costa, L. Probert, G. Kollias, et al., 1998. Interleukin 6 is required for the development of collagen-induced arthritis. *J. Exp. Med.* 187:461–468.

16. Hirano, T., Matsuda, T., Turner, M., Miyasaka, N., Buchan, G., Tang, B., Sato, K., Shimizu, M., Maini, R., Feldmann, M., et al. 1988. Excessive production of interleukin 6/B cell stimulatory factor-2 in rheumatoid arthritis. *Eur. J. Immunol.* 181:797–801.

17. Brozik, M., I. Rosztoczy, K. Meretey, G. Balint, M. Gaal, Z. Balogh, et al., 1992. Interleukin 6 levels in synovial fluids of patients with different arthritides: correlation with local IgM rheumatoid factor and systemic acute phase protein production. *J. Rheumatol.* 19:63–8.

18. Uson, J., A. Balsa, D. Pascual-Salcedo, J.A. Cabezas, J.M. Gonzalez-Tarrio, E. Martin-Mola, and G. Fontan. 1997. Soluble interleukin 6 (IL-6) receptor and IL-6 levels in serum and synovial fluid of patients with different arthropathies. *J. Rheumatol.* 24:2069–2075.

19. Wendling, D., E. Racadot, and J. Wijdenes. 1993. Treatment of severe rheumatoid arthritis by anti-interleukin 6 monoclonal antibody. *J. Rhematol.* 20:259–262.

20. Panayi GS. 1999. Targeting of cells involved in the pathogenesis of rheumatoid arthritis. *Rheumatology* 38(Suppl. 2):8–10.

21. Durie, F.H., R.A. Fava, T.M. Foy, A. Aruffo, J.A. Ledbetter, and R.J. Noelle. 1993. Prevention of collagen-induced arthritis with an antibody to gp39, the ligand for CD40. *Science* 261:1328–1330.

22. Souza, D., E. Raymond, and G. Nabozny. 1999. Synergistic inhibition of established collagen induced arthritis (CIA) through dual inhibition of ICAM-1 and CD40L Pathways. *Arthritis Rheum.* Sept 1999 (Abstract) #320.

23. Wagner, D.H. Jr., R.D. Stout, and J. Suttles. 1994. Role of the CD40-CD40 ligand interaction in CD4+ T cell contact-dependent activation of monocyte interleukin-1 synthesis. *Eur. J. Immunol.* 24:3148–3154.

24. Yellin, M.J., S. Winikoff, S.M. Fortune, D. Baum, et al. 1995. Ligation of CD40 on fibroblasts induces CD54 (ICAM-1) and CD106 (VCAM-1) up-regulation and IL-6 production and proliferation. *J. Leukoc. Biol.* 58:209–216.

25. Kelsall, B.L., E. Stuber, M. Neurath, and W. Strober. 1996. Interleukin-12 production by dendritic cells. The role of CD40-ICD40L interactions in Th 1 T- cell responses. *Ann. NY Acad. Sci.* 795: 116–126.

26. Kitagawa, M., Mitsui, H., Nakamura, H., Yoshino, S, et al. 1999. Differential regulation of rheumatoid synovial cell interleukin-12 production by tumor necrosis factor alpha and CD40 signals. Arthritis Rheum. 42:1917–1926.

27. Harigai, M., M. Hara, S. Nakazawa, C. Fukasawa, et al. 1999. Ligation of CD40 induced tumor necrosis factor-alpha in rheumatoid arthritis: a novel mechanism of activation of synoviocytes. *J. Rheumatol.* 26:1035–1043.

28. MacDonald, K.P., Y. Nishioka, P.E. Lipsky, and R. Thomas. 1997. Functional CD40 Ligand is expressed by T Cells in Rheumatoid Arthritis. *J. Clin. Invest.* 100:2404–2414.

29. Berner, B., G. Wolf, K.M Hummel, G.A. Muller, et al. 2000. Increased expression of CD40 ligand (CD154) on CD4+ T cells as a marker of disease activity in rheumatoid arthritis. *Ann. Rheum. Dis.* 59:190–195.

30. Henn, V., J.R. Slupsky, M. Grafe, I. Anagnostopoulos, et al. 1998. CD40 ligand on activated platelets triggers an inflammatory reaction of endothelial cells. *Nature* 391:591–594.

31. Datta, S.K. and S.L. Kalled. 1997. CD40-CD40 Ligand interaction in autoimmune disease. *Arthritis. Rheum.* 40:1735–1745.

32. Soong, L., J.-C. Xu, I.S. Grewal, P. Kima, J. Sun, B.A. Longley, Jr., et al. 1996. Disruption of CD40-CD40 ligand interactions results in an enhanced susceptibility to leishmania amazonensis infection. *Immunity* 4:263–273.

33. Wiley, J. and A.G. Harmsen. 1995. CD40 ligand is required for resolution of pneumocystis carinii pneumonia in mice. *J. Immunol.* 155:3523–3529.

34. Rissoan, M.C., C. Van Kooten, P. Chomarat, L. Galibert, et al. 1996. The functional CD40 antigen of fibroblasts may contribute to the proliferation of rheumatoid synovium. *Clin. Exp. Immunol.* 106:481–490.

35. Sekine, C., H. Yagita, N. Miyasaka, and K. Okumura. 1998. Expression and function of CD40 in rheumatoid arthritis synovium. *J. Rheumatol.* 25:1048–1053.

36. Kyburz, D., M. Corr, D.C. Brinson, A. Von Damm, et al. 1999. Human rheumatoid factor production is dependent on CD40 signaling and autoantigen. *J. Immunol.* 163:3116–3122.

37. Sibilia, J., A. Durandy, T. Schaeverbeke, and J.P. Fermand. 1996. Hyper-IgM syndrome associated with rheumatoid arthritis: report of RA in a patient with primary impaired CD40 pathway. *Br. J. Rheumatol.* 35:282–284.

38. Tada, Y., K. Nagasawa, A. Ho, F. Morito, O. Ushiyama, N. Suzuki, H. Ohta, and T.W. Mak. 1999. CD28-deficient mice are highly resistant to collagen-induced arthritis. *J. Immunol.* 162:203–208

39. Webb, L.M., M.J. Walmsley, and M. Feldmann. 1996. Prevention and amelioration of collagen-induced arthritis by blockade of the CD39 co-stimulatory pathway: requirement for both B7-1 and B7-2. *Eur. J. Immunol.* 26:2320–2328.

40. Knoerzer, D.B., R.W. Karr, B.D. Schwartz, and L.J. Mengle-Gaw. 1995. Collagen-induced arthritis in the BB rat. Prevention of disease by treatment with CTLA-4-Ig. *J. Clin. Invest.* 96:987–993.

41. Shimoyama, Y., H. Nagafuchi, N. Suzuki, T. Ochi, et al. 1999. Synovium infiltrating T cells induce excessive synovial cell function through CD28/B7 pathway in patients with rheumatoid arthritis. *J. Rheumatol.* 26:2094–2101.

42. Liu, M.F., H. Kohsaka, H. Sakurai, M. Azuma, et al. 1996. The presence of costimulatory molecules CD86 and CD28 in rheumatoid arthritis synovium. *Arthritis Rheum.* 39:110–114.

43. Ranheim, E.A. and T.J. Kipps. 1994. Elevated expression of CD80 (B7/BB1) and other accessory molecules on synovial fluid mononuclear cell subsets in rheumatoid arthritis. *Arthritis Rheum.* 37:1637–1646.

44. Balsa, A., J. Dixey, D.M. Sansom, P.J. Maddison, et al. 1996. Differential expression of the costimulatory molecules B7.1 (CD80) and B7.2 (CD86) in rheumatoid synovial tissue. *Br. J. Rheumatol.* 35:33–37.

45. Schwartz, R.S. 1999. The new immunology—the end of immunosuppressive drug therapy? *N. Engl. J. Med.* 340:1754–1756.

46. Tivol, E.A., F. Borriello, A.N. Schweitzer, W.P. Lynch, J.A. Bluestone, and A.H. Sharpe. 1995. Loss of CTLA-4 leads to massive lymphoproliferation and fatal multiorgan tissue destruction, revealing a critical negative regulatory role of CTLA-4. *Immunity* 3:541–547.

47. Linsley, P.S., W. Brady, L. Grosmaire, J.A. Ledbetter, and N. Damle. 1991. CTLA-4 is a second receptor for B cell activation antigen B7. *J. Exp. Med.* 174:561–569.

48. Linsley, P.S., J.L. Greene, W. Brady, J. Bajorath, J.A. Ledbetter, and R. Peach. 1994. Human B7-1 (CD80) and B7-2 (CD86) bind with similar avidities but distinct kinetics to CD28 and CTLA-4 receptors. *Immunity* 1:793–801.

49. Peach, R.J., J. Bajorath, W. Brady, et al. 1994. Complementarity determining region 1(CDRa)- and CDR3-analogous regions in CTLA-4 and CD28 determine the binding to B7-1. *J. Exp. Med.* 180:2049–2058.

50. Greene, J.L., G.M. Leytze, J. Emswiler, R. Peach, J. Bajorath, W. Cosand, and P.S. Linsley, 1996. Covalent dimerization of CD28/CTLA-4 and oligomerization of CD80/CD86 regulates T cell costimulatory interactions. *J. Biol. Chem.* 271:26,762–26,771.

51. Finck, B.K., P.S. Linsley, and D. Wofsy. 1994. Treatment of murine lupus with CTLA-4-Ig. *Science* 265:1225–1227.

52. Cross, A.H., T.J. Girard, K.S. Giacoletto, R.J. Evans, et al. 1995. Long-term inhibition of murine experimental autoimmune encephalomyelitis using CTLA-4-Fc supports a key role for CD28 costimulation. *J. Clin. Invest.* 95:2783–2789.

53. Abrams, J.R., M.G. Lebwohl, C.A. Guzzo, B.V. Jegasothy, et al. 1999. CTLA-4-Ig-mediated blockade of T-cell costimulation in patients with psoriasis vulgaris. *J. Clin. Invest.* 103:1243–1252.

54. Haqqi, T.M., G.D. Anderson, S. Banerjee, and C.S. David. 1992. Restricted heterogeneity in T-cell antigen receptor Vβ gene usage in the lymph nodes and arthritic joints of mice. *Proc. Natl. Acad. Sci. USA* 89:1253–1255.

55. Osman, G.E., M. Toda, O. Kanagawa, and L.E. Hood. 1993. Characterization of the T cell receptor repertoire causing collagen arthritis in mice. *J. Exp. Med.* 177:387–395.

56. Moder, K.G., H.S. Luthra, M. Griffiths, and C.S. David. 1993. Prevention of collagen-induced arthritis in mice by deletion of T cell receptor Vβ8 bearing T cells with monoclonal antibodies. *Brit. J. Rheum.* 32:26–30.

57. Haqqi, T.M., X.-M. Qu, D. Anthony, J. Ma and M.-S. Sy. 1995. Immunization and T cell receptor Vb chain peptides deletes pathogenic T cells and prevents the induction of collagen-induced arthritis in mice. *J. Clin. Invest.* 97:2849–2858.

58. Moreland, L.W., E.E. Morgan, T.C. Adamson, 3rd, Z. Fronek, L.H. Calabrese, J.M. Cash, et al. T cell receptor peptide vaccination in rheumatoid arthritis: a placebo-controlled trial using a combination of Vbeta3, Vbeta14, and Vbeta17 peptides. *Arthritis Rheum.* 1998 Nov;41(11):1919–1929.

59. Matsumoto, A.K., L.W. Moreland, V. Strand, E. Morgan, C.J. Nardo, S.P. Richieri, and S.W. Brostoff. 1999. Results of phase IIb rheumatoid arthritis clinical trial using T-cell receptor peptides. *Arthritis Rheum.* Sept 1999 (Abstract) #281.

60. Evans, C.H., S.C. Ghivizzani, R. Kang, T. Muzzonigro, M.C. Wasko, J.H. Herndon, and P.D. Robbins. 1999a. Gene therapy for rheumatic diseases. *Arthritis Rheum.* 42:1–16.

61. Song, X.Y., M. Gu, W.W. Jin, M. Klinman, and S.M. Wahl. 1998. Plasmid DNA encoding transforming growth factor-β1 suppresses chronic disease in a streptococcal cell wall-induced arthritis model. *J. Clin. Invest.* 101:1–7.

62. Le, C.H., A.G. Nicolson, A. Morales, and K.L. Sewell. 1997. Suppression of collagen-induced arthritis through adenovirus-mediated transfer of a modified TNF-α receptor gene. *Arthritis Rheum.* 40:1662–1669.

63. Zhang, H., Y. Yang, J.L. Horton, E.B. Samoilova, T.A. Judge, L.A. Turka, J.M. Wu, and Y. Chen, 1997. Amelioration of collagen-induced arthritis by CD95 (Apo-1/FasL) ligand gene transfer. *J. Clin. Invest.* 100:1951–1957.

64. Evans, C.H., P.D. Robbins, S.C. Ghivizzani, J.H. Herndon, R. Kang, A.B. Bahnson, et al. 1996. Clinical trial to assess the safety, feasibility, and efficacy of transferring a potentially anti-arthritic cytokine gene to human joints with rheumatoid arthritis. *Hum. Gene Ther.* 7:1261–1280.

65. Evans, C.H., P.D. Robbins, S.C. Ghivizzani, J.H. Herndon, M.H. Wasko, M. Tomaino, et al. 1999b. Results from the first human clinical trial of gene therapy for arthritis. *Arthritis Rheum.* Sept 1999 (Abstract) #600.

66. Commander, H. 2000. Biotechnology industry responds to gene therapy death. *Nature Med.* 6:118.

67. Tibbles, L.A. and J.R. Woodgett, 1999. The stress-activated protein kinase pathways [In Process Citation] *Cell Mol. Life Sci.* 55:1230–1254.

68. Lee, J.C., S. Kassis, S. Kumar, A. Badger, et al. 1999. p38 mitogen-activated protein kinase inhibitors: mechanisms and therapeutic potentials. *Pharmacol. Ther.* 82:389–397.

69. Wilson, K.P., P.G. McCaffrey, K. Hsiao, S. Pazhanisamy, et al. 1997. The structural basis for the specificity of pyridinylimidazole inhibitors of p38 MAP kinase. *Chem Biol.* 4:423–431.

70. Badger, A.M., J.N. Bradbeer, B. Votta, J.C. Lee, et al. 1996. Pharmacological profile of SB 203580, a selective inhibitor of cytokine suppressive binding protein/p38 kinase, in animal models of arthritis, bone resorption, endotoxin shock and immune function. *J. Pharmacol. Exp. Ther.* 279:1453–1461.

71. Suzuki, M., T. Tetsuka, S. Yoshida, N. Watanabe, et al. 2000. The role of p38 mitogen-activated protein kinase in IL-6 and IL-8 production from the TNF-alpha- or IL-1beta-stimulated rheumatoid synovial fibroblasts. *FEBS Lett.* 465:23–27.

72. Badger, A.M., M.N. Cook, M.W. Lark, T.M. Newman-Tarr, et al. 1998. SB 203580 inhibits p38 mitogen-activated protein kinase, nitric oxide production, and inducible nitric oxide synthase in bovine cartilage- derived chondrocytes. *J. Immunol.* 161:467–473.

73. Jackson, J.R., B. Bolognese, L. Hillegass, S. Kassis, et al. 1998. Pharmacological effects of SB 220025, a selective inhibitor of P38 mitogen-activated protein kinase, in angiogenesis and chronic inflammatory disease models. *J. Pharmacol. Exp. Ther.* 284:687–692.

74. Badger, A.M., D.E. Griswold, R. Kapadia, S. Blake, et al. 2000. Disease-modifying activity of SB 242235, a selective inhibitor of p38 mitogen-activated protein kinase, in rat adjuvant-induced arthritis. *Arthritis Rheum.* 43:175–183.

75. Wadsworth, S.A., D.E. Cavender, S.A. Beers, P. Lalan, P.H. Schafer, E.A. Malloy, et al. 1999. RWJ 67657, a potent, orally active inhibitor of p38 mitogen-activated protein kinase. *J. Pharmacol Exp. Ther.* 291:680–687.

76. Ku, G., T. Faust, L.L. Lauffer, D.J. Livingston, et al. 1996. Interleukin-1 beta converting enzyme inhibition blocks progression of type II collagen-induced arthritis in mice. *Cytokine* 8:377–386.

77. Elford, P.R., R. Heng, L. Revesz, and A.R. MacKenzie. 1995. Reduction of inflammation and pyrexia in the rat by oral administration of SDZ 224-015, an inhibitor of the interleukin-1 beta converting enzyme. Br. J. Pharmacol. 115:601–606.

78. Fletcher, D.S., L. Agarwal, K.T. Chapman, J. Chin, et al. 1995. A synthetic inhibitor of interleukin-1 beta converting enzyme prevents endotoxin-induced interleukin-1 beta production in vitro and in vivo. J. Interferon. *Cytokine Res.* 15:243–248.

79. Miller, B.E., P.A. Krasney, D.M. Gauvin, K.B. Holbrook, et al. 1995. Inhibition of mature IL-1 beta production in murine macrophages and a murine model of inflammation by WIN 67694, an inhibitor of IL-1 beta converting enzyme. *J. Immunol.* 154:1331–1338.

80. Wang, Y., S.A. Rollins, J.A. Madri, and L.A Matis. 1995. Anti-C5 monoclonal antibody therapy prevents collagen-induced arthritis and ameliorates established disease. *Proc. Natl. Acad. Sci.* USA 92:8955–8959.

81. Jain, R.I., L.W. Moreland, J.R. Caldwell, S.A. Rollins, and C.F Mojcik. 1999. A single dose, placebo controlled, double blind, phase I study of the humanized anti-C5 antibody H5g1.1 in patients with rheumatoid arthritis. *Arthritis Rheum.* Sept 1999 (Abstract) #42.

82. Trentham, D.E., R.A. Dynesius-Trentham, E.J. Orav, D. Combitchi, C. Lorenzo, K.L. Sewell, et al. 1993. Effects of oral administration of type II collagen on rheumatoid arthritis. *Science* 261:1727–1730.

83. Sieper, J., S. Kary, H. Sorensen, R. Alten, U. Eggens, W. Huge, et al. 1996. Oral type II collagen treatment in early rheumatoid arthritis. A double-blind, placebo-controlled, randomized trial. *Arthritis Rheum.* 39:41–51.

84. Smeets, T.J., M.C. Kraan, J. Versendaal, F.C. Breedveld, and P.P. Tak. Analysis of serial synovial biopsies in patients with rheumatoid arthritis: description of a control group without clinical improvement after treatment with interleukin 10 or placebo. *J. Rheumatol.* 26:2089–2093.

85. Kavanaugh, A.F., H. Schulze-Koops, L.S. Davis, and P.E. Lipsky. 1997. Repeat treatment of rheumatoid arthritis patients with a murine anti-intercellular adhesion molecule 1 monoclonal antibody. *Arthritis Rheum.* 40:849–853.

86. Bendele, A., T. McAbee, G. Sennello, J. Frazier, E. Chlipala, and D. McCabe. 1999. Efficacy of sustained blood levels of interleukin-1 receptor antagonist in animal models of arthritis: comparison of efficacy in animal models with human clinical data. *Arthritis Rheum.* 42:498–506.

87. Steinman L. 1999. Assessment of animal models for MS and demyelinating disease in the design of rational therapy. *Neuron* 24:511–514.

II   OSTEOARTHRITIS

12

Slow-Acting Drugs for the Treatment of Osteoarthritis

Jean-Yves Reginster and Roy D. Altman

CONTENTS

INTRODUCTION

Potential treatment options in therapy of osteoarthritis (OA) are symptom- or structure (disease)-modifying *(1,2)*. Symptomatic therapies for OA can have a rapid onset of effect, such as nonsteroidal anti-inflammatory drugs (NSAIDs). This effect is appreciated in hours, or in days at the most. Alternatively, some of the present-day therapies may have a slow onset of benefit and symptomatic improvement may not be achieved for weeks after the onset of therapy. There is no therapy of OA that is universally accepted as structure-modifying. However, new data suggests that several agents, including those with a slow onset of symptomatic benefit, may have structure-modifying properties. In this chapter, we review regulatory issues and the information available on a few of the available slow-acting drugs for OA.

REGULATORY ISSUES

Several sets of guidelines, recommendations, or points to consider have been issued by regulatory authorities *(2,3)* or scientific groups *(4)* regarding regulatory requirements for registration of drugs to be used in the treatment of OA.

One of the major issues to be faced by pharmaceutical industries wishing to develop a new chemical entity in this particular area is the inconsistency between Europe and the United States, in the classification of drugs for the treatment of OA and the indication for their use *(4)*.

The European Agency for the Evaluation of Medicinal Products (EMEA) *(2)* in accordance with the European Experts from the scientific community *(4)* recognizes a classification dividing anti-OA drugs into two categories, i.e., symptom-modifying

From: *Modern Therapeutics in Rheumatic Diseases*
Edited by: G. C. Tsokos, et al. © Humana Press, Inc., Totowa, NJ

drugs and structure-modifying drugs. Requirements for registration will be depending on the requested indication.

Symptom-modifying drugs act on symptoms with no detectable effect on the structural changes of the disease. Registration of such drugs would require demonstration of a favorable effect on symptoms with no clinically significant adverse effects on the structural changes of the disease.

Structure-modifying drugs, based on their mechanism of action, are expected to have an effect on the progression of the pathological changes in OA. They may or may not have an independent effect on symptoms.

The claims discussed in the most recent Food and Drug Administration (FDA) draft guidelines *(3)* for the drugs intended for the treatment of OA cover a broader scope of potential indications. Although the claims "treatment of symptoms pain and function" and "delay in structural progression" can be considered rather close, if not similar, to their European counterparts, the FDA has introduced a new concept by proposing a "prevention of OA" claim. However, the FDA acknowledges that demonstration of the prevention at the occurrence of OA in patients with prevalent OA or at risk to develop it, will be challenging. Actually, a prerequisite to the set up of trials with such an objective would be the definition of "new OA" taking into account the highly variable kinetics of apparition of the clinical and radiographic features of OA, respectively *(2)*. Eventually, the FDA recognized that other claims, such as "delay in time to surgery" are also possible, in principle.

For symptom-modifying drugs, US and European agencies request demonstration of a beneficial effect on both pain and function. Measurement of pain requires validated methods using visual analog or Likert scales. Whereas the EMEA wants to see a separate assessment of use-related and rest pain, the FDA request the evaluation of the effect of the tested compound on nonsignal joint (e.g., contralateral knee/hip or hand OA) and a standardization of the effects of confounders (osteophytes, rescue medications, etc.) in the protocol and in the analysis. Studies should be powered to demonstrate an effect on pain and function in separate analysis. For European registration, a compound showing a statistically significant benefit only for pain would be accepted providing no deterioration is shown in functional ability. In the United States, a product that affects much more pain than function (or vice versa) could be approved if the pain relief is large enough to yield overall success. In both continents, a limited effect on one of the two requested endpoints (pain and function) will be reflected in the indication granted.

Self administered instruments (Western Ontario MacMasters Universities Osteoarthritis index [WOMAC] or Lequesne index) are recommended to assess disability arising from OA of the knee or the hip. A patient global assessment is considered an essential endpoint by the US regulators, but the wording and exact objective of the global assessment is not clear.

The requested duration of the pivotal studies evaluating symptom modifying drugs in OA is shorter in the United States (3 mo) compared to the European requirements (6 mo). However, the FDA draft guidelines do state that product- or device-specific considerations may lenghten the duration of the studies. On the other hand, if enough experience already exists for other products in the same class (e.g., NSAIDs), trials could be shortened to 6 wk. In practice, longer trials are recommended.

Both agencies are willing to consider the global risk/benefit assessment of such compounds, including their absence of toxicity on joint structure, even if no structure claim is sought. For EMEA, this absence of deleterious effect on the joint structure should be monitored for at least 1 yr. In agreement with the FDA, X-rays are to be performed when the trial lasts 1 yr or more. Although the FDA does not specifically address the issue of the appropriate comparator for evaluation of symptom-modifying anti-OA drugs, EMEA suggests such studies be performed with the most favorable comparator. A three-arm study, including study drug, placebo, and an active control, are strongly recommended.

For structure-modifying drugs, the situation is slightly more confusing. The major unsolved question remains whether the regulatory agencies are prepared to grant registration to a new chemical entity having shown some benefits on structural endpoints (usually radiological feature of OA hip or knee) without or with only limited evidence of short-term clinical benefit. In other words, the validity of short-term radiologic changes as surrogate for long-term hard clinical endpoint is still not unequivocally accepted. EMEA guidelines acknowledge that epidemiological data support a relation between structural changes and long-term clinical outcomes. However, because the nature and the magnitude of the structural changes that are likely to be clinically relevant in the long-term remains uncertain, clinical endpoints such as the necessity of joint replacement, time to the need for surgery, and long-term clinical evolution (pain and disability) are considered preferable in the assessment of the efficacy of such drugs. Therefore, in any case, clinical signs and symptoms should be monitored in trials assessing the structural effect of anti-OA drugs.

Both agencies recognize the value of standard plain X-rays as presently the best and most standardized method to assess the progression of OA. Joint-space narrowing appears to be the best-characterized measurement for the evaluation of joint preservation. Notwithstanding, measurements of osteophytes or extra-cartilage structure might also be of interest. Magnetic resonance imaging (MRI) may be soon able to replace standard X-rays but remaining technical problems make this technology a tool for tomorrow rather than a currently validated endpoint.

Although the level of clinical benefit requested in Europe for a drug seeking a structure-modifying indication remains rather vague, the US authorities have gone a step further by defining a hierarchy of claims for structural outcomes and clarifying the level of clinical evidence that should be associated to each of them. If the normalization of joint-space narrowing is demonstrated on a plain X-ray, the drug would be granted a "normalization of X-ray" claim that would be considered the most convincing outcome of a positive effect on structural integrity. A level below this, another convincing outcome that would not require parallel demonstration of a symptomatic effect would be the apparition, during the trial, of a reversal in joint-space narrowing reflecting new or regrown cartilage. More ambiguous is the possibility to claim for slowing joint-space narrowing without reducing symptoms. From the FDA point of view, a preliminary contact between the sponsor and the agency would be necessary. In principle, the slowing of joint-space narrowing should be no smaller than 50% than the control population cohort. Both agencies agree that demonstration of structural improvement connotes an element of durability and therefore, that studies evaluating these outcomes should be longer than those performed for symptom modification. United States draft guidelines specify that trials should last at least 1 yr but that imprecision of the joint-space narrowing measurement often results in trials lasting even longer. European guidelines recommend double-blind, placebo-controlled, parallel group design for at least 2 yr for this indication.

Although the position of the United States and European agencies regarding registration of anti-OA drugs has been significantly harmonized during the last years, there are still a certain number of discrepancies that may generate troubles for pharmaceutical companies wishing to develop new chemical entities in this indication or for scientists, aiming at prescription of these drugs to their patients. The common grounds include the recognition of two categories of anti-OA drugs, acting on either symptoms and/or structure. Demonstration of nontoxicity on the joint is also considered a prerequisite, even for compounds that do not seek a structure-modifying claim.

The ideal outcomes currently include pain and function assessment for symptom-modifying drugs and joint-space narrowing assessed by plain X-ray for structure-modifying compounds. Points that remain to be harmonized are application for a structure-modifying drug related to the duration of studies and to the level of evidence of clinical benefit.

MATRIX PRECURSORS

Chondroitin Sulfate

Chondroitin sulfate (CS) is a major component of the extracellular matrix from many connective tissues, such as cartilage, bone, skin, ligaments, and tendons. CS is a sulfated glycosaminoglycan, composed of a long unbranched polysaccharide chain with a repeating disaccharide structure of *N*-acetylgalactosamine and glucuronic acid *(5,6)*. Most of the N-acetylgalactosamine residues are sulfated, particularly in the 4- or 6-position, making CS a strongly charged polyanion with a high water-draining power. In the articular cartilage, the high content of CS in the aggrecan plays a major role in creating a large osmotic swelling pressure, which expands the matrix and places the collagen network under tension *(5)*.

In OA, changes in the structure of CS were reported in different models, with the apparition of a longer chains length and the chains containing more epitopes recognized by specific antibodies *(5,7)*. In a model of human articular chondrocytes, cultivated in clusters, CS (100–1000 µg/mL) increased the production of proteoglycans, with no detectible effects on collagen II synthesis. In the presence of interleukin-1β (IL1β, CS counteracted the effects of the cytokines on proteoglycans, collagen II, and prostaglandins E2 (synthesis) suggesting that, in this particular model, CS can reduce collagenolytic activity and increase matrix-components production *(8)*. In articular chondrocytes isolated from rabbits, CS (100 µg/mL) decreased (average 28%) the number of apopoptic cells, after exposure to nitric oxide (NO) donors (sodium nitroprussite) *(9)*.

In a rabbit model of OA, chymopapain is injected into the knee joint. After 84 d, there was less reduction in proteoglycan content than in those where CS was started 10 d prior to the chymopapain injection *(10)*. This was more effective with the oral administration than the intramuscular administration of CS. This suggests that CS may have a protective effect on the damaged cartilage, assisting resynthesize of proteoglycans.

Several clinical trials have investigated the effects of CS to patients with OA. In 127 patients suffering from uni- or bilateral knee OA (Kellgren-Lawrence radiographic scores grade I to III), CS 400 mg tid or 1200 mg once daily for 3 mo reduced spontaneous joint pain 50% by visual analog scale (VAS), and reduced Lequesne algofunctional index 40–45% *(11)*. This compared favorably to placebo where improvement was 10–15%.

In a similar population (*n* = 146), CS 400 mg three times daily was compared to diclofenac 50 mg three times daily *(12)*. Improvement with diclofenac in Lequesne's index, spontaneous pain, and pain on weight bearing was 30–59% by d 30 and 40–50% at d 90. However, these improvements were lost after the 3-mo treatment when diclofenac was discontinued. With CS, the therapeutic improvement was not realized until d 60, was present in 80–85% of patients by d 90 and lasted in 50–80% for up to 90 d after CS was discontinued.

In a 3-mo dose-ranging study of 140 patients with OA of the knee, CS 200, 800, and 1200 mg daily were compared to placebo *(13)*. CS 200 mg/d was not more effective than placebo. The two higher doses were significantly superior than CS 200 mg/d and placebo in relation to pain (VAS) and Lequesne algofunctional index.

CS 800 mg/d was further tested in two knee OA double-blind, placebo-controlled trials of 85 and 140 patients with similar results *(14,15)*. One of the trials *(14)* also showed significant improvement in the CS group (10%) vs the none in the placebo group in the the time to walk 20 m. In the other study, the CS group demonstrated no change in the width of the medial tibiofemoral joint in 12 mo, with a decrease in the placebo group *(15)*. The surface area minimum width and mean thickness of the medial femorotibial joint were measured by a digitized automatic image analyser.

The structure-modifying properties of CS were also assessed in a double-blind, placebo-controlled trial including 119 patients with interphalangeal OA *(16)*. After 3 yr, the group taking CS 1200 mg daily had a significant decrease in the number of patients with new "erosive" OA finger joints (8.8%) compared to the placebo group (29.4%).

Glucosamine Sulfate

Glucosamine (GS) is an aminosaccharide, acting as a preferred substrate for the biosynthesis of glycosaminoglycan chains. These glycosaminoglycan chains are incorporated into the production of aggrecan and other proteoglycans in cartilage *(17)*. Owing to the essential role of aggrecans in cartilage, compounds enhancing their synthesis might be beneficial in OA.

In human OA chondrocytes, GS sulfate was tested for its ability to regulate the expression of genes, encoding constitutive extracellular matrix macromolecules, GS (50 μ*M*) induced a twofold increase in the steady levels of both perlecan and aggrecan mRNA and caused a modest although consistent decrease in the levels of stromelysin mRNA *(18)*. The same authors later reported that GS not only increased the expression of the aggrecan core protein but also downregulated, in a dose-dependent manner, both matrix metalloproteinases (MMPs) I and Ill expression *(19)*. These studies suggested that GS may exert beneficial effects in OA owing to its effect on the balance between synthesis and degradation of extracellular cartilage and on articular cartilage function.

These transcriptional effects were supported by reports that when using a model of human chondrocytes from OA femoral heads, cultivated in a three-dimensional system for 12 d, GS (10–100 μg/mL) increased proteoglycan synthesis with no effect on their physico-chemical form neither on type II collagen production or on cell proliferation, assessed by quantifying DNA synthesis *(20)*.

GS also inhibited, in a rat chondrosarcoma cell line and bovine cartilage explants, the aggrecan degradation, which was mediated by aggrecanase, a proteinase induced by IL-1 or retinoic acid *(21)*. The inhibition of aggrecanase response was reported to be a consequence of metabolic changes that followed a marked increase in the intracellular GS concentration, the exact mechanisms thereof being not yet fully elucidated. More recently, N-acetylglucosamine was shown to suppress IL1-β and tumor necrosis factor α (TNF-α) induced NO production in human articular chondrocytes, together with an inhibition of inducible nitric oxide synthase (NOS) mRNA and protein expression. In the same experiment, N-acetylglucosamine also suppressed the production of IL-1-β induced cyclooxygenase II (COX II) and IL-6 with no effect on the constitutively expressed COX I *(22)*.

Although identifying novel mechanisms, these results support the anti-inflammatory properties of GS, which were previously described in various classical models, including the carrageenin-induced pleuritis or inflamed paw in the rat *(17)*. On the other hand, OA cartilage is also characterized by a potential defective repair process related to the inability of proliferated cells to migrate in damaged areas. OA fibrilated cartilage was associated with a highly significant decrease in chondrocyte adhesion to extracellular matrix proteins and more specifically to fibronectin *(23)*. In chondrocytes isolated from flbrilated areas of cartilage from OA femoral heads, GS (50–500 μM) restored their decreased adhesion to fibronectin *(24)*. The authors suggested that activation of protein kinase C (PKC), considered to be involved in the physiological phosphorylation of the α-6 A integrin subunit, could be one of the possible mechanisms, through which GS restores fibrilated cartilage chondrocytes adhesion to fibronectin; hence, improving the ability of repair process in osteoarthritic cartilage *(24)*.

Pharmacokinetics studies in man have shown that 90% of GS is absorbed after oral administration. Oral, intravenous, or intramuscular ^{14}C labeled GS is incorporated in the plasma proteins in similar pharmacokinetic patterns *(25)*. However, the area under the curve obtained after oral administration is 26% of that obtained with intravenous or intramuscular administration.

In rabbits with transection of the anterior cruciate ligament, after 8 wk, GS (120 mg/kg/d) significantly reduced the level of chondropathy measured by both an S-grade macroscopic score and an overall assessment using a 100-mm visual analogic scale *(26)*.

Efficacy and safety of GS were tested in several randomized, controlled, clinical trials of patients with OA, predominantly the knee or spine *(27)*. In OA of the knee, GS 400 mg intramuscularly twice a week for 6 wk was compared to placebo in a 155 patient study. There was a significant decrease in the Lequesne algofunctional index observed in the CS group when compared to placebo. This was both at the end of the treatment and 2 wk after drug discontinuation. A responder was considered someone with at least a three points reduction in the Lequesne index. GS was superior to placebo for evaluable patients (55% GS vs 33% placebo) or by intention-to-treat analysis (51% GS vs 30% placebo).

In 252 patients with Kellgren-Lawrence stage I to III OA of the knee, those treated with 1500 mg/d GS for 4 wk had a significantly greater reduction in the Lequesne index than those receiving a placebo *(28)*. The response rates (same criteria as in ref. *10*) approximated the improvement observed with the intramuscular formulation: i.e., 55% GC vs 38% placebo for evaluable patients and 52% GS vs 37% placebo patients in an intention-to-treat analysis.

In a 3-yr, 319 patient, randomized, placebo-controled trial comparing GS 1500 mg/d to placebo, there was significant improvement in those on GS when compared to the placebo group for the Lequesne algo-functional index *(29)*.

Interestingly, in an 8-wk double-blind, placebo-controlled study with an 8-wk posttreatment observation, GS hydrochloride was not as effective as GS sulfate *(30)*. GS hydrochloride was beneficial with respect to knee examination and on a daily diary pain questionnaire. In contrast with GS sulfate, GS hydrochloride was not effective in the primary endpoint (WOMAC questionnaire). More study is needed to determine if there is a clinical difference between these compounds, as GS hydrochloride is commonly available in countries where GS is a neutraceutical (e.g., the United States and United Kingdom).

GS 1500 mg/d was compared to placebo in 160 out-patients with spinal OA: 68 cervical, 57 lumbar, 37 cervical and lumbar *(31)*. There was a significant improvement in pain and function by VAS at both spinal sites. The improvement with GS persisted for up to 4 wk after drug discontinuation.

GS 1500 mg/d was compared to ibuprofen 1200 mg/d in a 4-wk study of 200 hospitalized patients with OA of the knee *(32)*. At 1 wk, ibuprofen was superior to GS in reduction of pain (GS 28% vs ibuprofen 48%). However, the agents provided equal improvement in pain at 4 wk (GS 48%; ibuprofen 52%). There were fewer adverse reactions in the GS group (GS 6% vs ibuprofen 35%), particularly gastrointestinal (GI) adverse reactions. Discontinuations also favored the GS group (GS 1% vs ibuprofen 7%). A similar study on 68 Chinese patients numerically favored GS vs ibuprofen for symptoms of OA with better tolerance of GS (adverse events GS 6% vs ibuprofen 16%), but without any discontinuations *(33)*.

GS 1500 mg/d, piroxicam 20 mg/d, both GS and piroxicam, and placebo were compared in a 19 patient, 12-wk study with an 8-wk follow-up without treatment *(34)*. Both GS groups had a reduction of Lequesne algofunctional index of 4.8 points, compared to piroxicam alone 2.9 points ($p < 0.001$) and placebo 0.7 points ($p < 0.001$). Adverse events favored the GS and placebo groups (GS 15%; placebo 24%; piroxicam 41%; GS and piroxicam 35%). The improvement in GS group persisted during the 8-wk follow-up period, whereas the improvement with piroxicam did not.

The potential of GS as a structure-modifying agent was studied in 212 patients with OA of the knee (American College of Rheumatology criteria) in a double-blind 3-yr program comparing GS 1500 mg/d to placebo *(35)*. The primary efficacy variable was change in medial tibio-femoral compartment joint-space width by weight bearing, anteroposterior radiographs obtained at baseline, 1 yr, and 3 yr. The width was measured by digital-image analysis using a validated computerized algorithm for the signal joint. The WOMAC was measured at 4-mo intervals. Although the overall data revealed no joint-space narrowing in the glucosamine sulfate group, there was an average joint-space narrowing of 0.08–0.10 mm narrowing each year in the placebo group.

In the placebo group, there was a slight worsening of symptoms by the end of the treatment period.

The safety profile of GS was evaluated in a systematic review of 12 randomized, controlled trials *(36)*. The conclusion was that safety was excellent. There were only 7 of 2486 patients withdrawn from clinical trials for GS-related adverse events. There were only 48 patients reporting any GS-related adverse events. Safety was further evaluated in an open study carried out by 252 Portugese physicians of 1208 patients on GS 500 mg three times daily for a mean of 50 d (range 13–99 d) *(37)*. Adverse reactions were reported in 12%, were mostly mild in severity and mostly gastroenterologic (e.g., epigastric pain, heart-burn, and diarrhea). All complaints remissed upon discontinuation of GS. There has been some concern about the role of glucosamine in glucose metabolism and the potential of increased insulin resistance *(38)*. Detailed review of existing scientific literature on GS find no evidence of glucose intolerance for both short- and long-term use of GS *(39)*.

OTHER AGENTS

Diacerein

The mechanism of action of diacerein differs from those of NSAIDs or corticosteroids. Studies in vitro and with animal models of OA suggest that diacerein as well as its active metabolite, rhein (1,8-dihydroxy-3-carboxyanthraquinone) inhibit the synthesis of cytokines (such as IL-1, IL-6, TNF, LIF) and metalloproteinases (such as collagenase and stromelysin). They also inhibit phagocytosis and migration of neutrophils and macrophages. All these effects are relevant to the anti-inflammatory effect on cartilage. In addition, diacerein also possesses moderate antipyretic and analgesic properties. Neither diacerein nor rhein inhibit prostaglandin biosynthesis *(40)* and diacerein has no inhibitory effects on the phospholipase, cyclooxygenase, or lipooxygenase pathways. The aforementioned actions support the clinical evidence of the beneficial effects of diacerein on the symptoms of OA *(41–47)*. After oral administration, diacerein is de-acetylated into rhein, which is the active metabolite, before entering the circulation. Oral bioavailability of diacerein is estimated at 35 and 56%.

In animal models of OA diacerein shows potential structure-modifying effects *(40–43)*. No reference molecules with pharmacological and clinical profiles comparable to those of diacerein are known at present.

Clinical experience *(48–52)* has confirmed diacerein as an agent for symptomatic treatment of OA. The delayed onset of action of diacerein *(40)* suggests that the molecule belongs to a class of Symptomatic Slow-Acting Drugs for the treatment of OA (SYSADOA) *(1)*. In comparative trials, the efficacy of diacerein was similar to that of NSAIDs, but with a slower onset of action. The use of diacerein seems to minimize (or even avoid) the major GI peptic ulcer concerns of NSAIDs.

In several studies, the efficacy of diacerein in patients with OA of the hip or the knee was determined by using a VAS for pain on movement, algofunctional index (Lequesne index), WOMAC index, global assessments by the patient and the investigator, and consumption of escape medications.

A multicenter randomized, placebo-controlled, dose-finding trial in 484 patients with OA of the hip was conducted in Canada and Israel. Patients received placebo or diacerein (50, 100, or 150 mg) in a divided dose daily for 4 mo *(48)*. The diacerein

100 mg/d group had marked decrease in pain (VAS for pain on movement) and improved function (WOMAC index), as compared to placebo. The onset of reduction in pain was generally not until the fourth week of treatment. Withdrawals for lack of efficacy were more common in the placebo group (18%) and diacerein 50 mg/d group (17%). Withdrawals were more frequent from adverse events (mostly changes in bowel habits or abdominal pain) in the diacerein 150 mg/d group (19%). The most common adverse event was related to transient changes in bowel habits in the diacerein groups (30%) over the placebo group (14%).

There were 288 patients with OA of the hip treated in an 8-wk randomized, double-blind, 2 × 2 factorial design trial comparing placebo, diacerein 100 mg/d, tenoxicam 20 mg, and diacerein 100 mg/d plus tenoxicam 20 mg/d (49). The VAS of pain and Lequesne index were improved in all treatment groups over placebo without significant differences between groups. Moderate, transient changes in bowel habits were the most frequent adverse events observed in the diacerein group (37%) as compared with the placebo (4%).

Diacerein was compared to naproxen in a study of 95 patients with OA of hip or knee, with a 2-mo placebo follow-up (50). The two agents were equal in reduction of pain (spontaneous, night, passive motion, active motion, tenderness). Epigastric distress was present in six patient on naproxen and diarrhea was present in six patients on diacerein. The onset of pain relief with diacerein was slower than naproxen, but the pain relief persisted in the placebo period, whereas it did not with naproxen.

The consumption of NSAIDs was assessed in a placebo-controlled, parallel-group study (51). In an 8-mo study, during the first phase, patients (n = 183) with OA of hip or knee received: (1) diacerein 100 mg/d with diclofenac 100 mg/d or (2) placebo with diclofenac 100 mg/d. At 2 mo, and during the second phase, the diclofenac was discontinued and the groups received: (1) diacerein or (2) placebo. Escape diclofenac was permitted. The third and final phase was 2 mo without treatment for either group. The VAS and Lequesne index response was similar in the first phase. In the second phase, when diclofenac was discontinued, the improvement persisted in the diacerein group. There was less consumption of escape NSAIDs in the diacerein group. The improvement also persisted in the third phase when the diacerein was discontinued for 2 mo. This study suggests that an NSAID may be of value in helping reduce pain for the first 4 wk of diacerein until the beneficial effects of the diacerein can be realized. It also supports the concomitant use of NSAIDs with diacerein, but any potential additive effect was not measured.

The influence of diacerein on quality of life and pharmaco-economics was assessed in an open, randomized, parallel-group, 207 patient, 6-mo clinical trial, comparing diacerein plus the standard treatment of OA to the standard treatment alone (52). Diacerein with standard treatment was superior to standard treatment alone in components of the Arthritis Impact Measurement Scale (AIMS2) and Nottingham Health Profile (NHP).

In all trials, the majority of the reported adverse events related to mild abdominal pain and a change in bowel habits involving mostly soft stools, loose stools, and diarrhea. These occurred in 20–40% of the patients on diacerein, vs 3% on placebo. In general, the changes in bowel habits occurred during the first 2 wk of treatment, were of mild-moderate intensity (loose stools, 2–3/d), and were well-tolerated. For the most part, patients regarded the event as a discomfort that did not influence their activities of daily living and often remitted, even with continued treatment with diacerein.

Initial reports on a 3-yr clinical trial involving 507 patients with OA of the hip suggests that diacerein may retard the progression of OA *(53)*.

Pentosan

Pentosan polysulfate is a hemicellulose isolated from the wood of the beech tree *(Fagus sylvatica) (54)*. It consists of repeating units of *(1–4)* linked β-D-xylanopyranoses in which α-D-4-methylglucopyranosyluronic acid residues are linked via oxygen to the 2-position of every tenth xylanopyranose unit. The high-charge density and rod-like conformation of pentosan polysulfate allows it to compete effectively with endogenous-sulfated glycosaminoglycans for protein and cellular-binding sites. Pentosan is prepared as a sodium salt for parenteral use or as a calcium salt that can be administered parenterally or orally. Pentosan had been shown to support chondrocyte anabolic activities and attenuate catabolic events responsible for loss of componenets of the cartilage extracellular matrix in OA joints. Some of these actions are through direct enzyme inhibition. They also enter chondrocytes and bind to promoter proteins and alter gene expression of MMPs. In rat models of arthritis, pentosan reduced joint swelling and inflammatory-mediator levels in pouch fluids. Synoviocyte biosynthesis of high molecular-weight hyaluronan was normalized when incubated with pentosan. In animal models of OA, pentosan improved blood flow to the subchondral bone. For dogs, the ideal dose of pentosan appeared to be 3 mg/kg weekly for 4 wk, based on a study of 40 dogs with OA of the stifle *(55)*. The beneficial effects of pentosan on articular cartilage seemed to be potentiated by the addition of insulin-like growth factor-1 (IGF-1) in a canine model of OA *(56)*.

Edelman et al. *(57)* studied 114 patients with OA in a double-blind, placebo-controlled trial of sodium pentosan 3 mg/kg intramuscularly once weekly for 4 wk and followed for a total of 6 mo. Pentosan was superior to placebo in 5 of the 7 measured parameters. Thirty-two percent of the placebo patients completed the trial in contrast to 61% of the pentosan group. There were no adverse effects reported in the trial.

Verbruggen et al. performed an open study of calcium pentosan 2 mg/kg intramuscularly once weekly for 5 wk in a 16-wk study in 23 patients with mild to moderate OA of the hand, hip, or knee *(58)*. Peak pentosan blood levels were achieved in 4 h post-injection with significant decrease by 8 h and no detectable blood levels by 24 h. When compared to baseline, there were significant reductions in global pain by 2 wk that persisted through the follow-up. Digital and knee pain was improved by 8 wk. Hip pain did not improve.

Verbruggen also studied calcium pentosan 20 mg/kg orally twice weekly for 6 wk in a double-blind, placebo-controlled, 50-patient study *(59)*. After a 6-wk hiatus, the agent was repeated for 6 wk, followed by 6 wk without drug (i.e., 24-wk study). There was a significant improvement after the second course of pentosan in global pain, morning stiffness, pain at night, hand function, and pain on palpation without a change in grip strength and analgesic use. Those on placebo did not achieve a 20% improvement, most improvement was early in the study. Those on pentosan all showed at least a 20% improvement relative to baseline at the end of the study.

Four weekly intraarticular injections of sodium pentosan 50 mg was studied in 31 patients with OA of the knee in a double-blind, controlled (Ringer's solution), 26-wk study *(60)*. The pentosan group had a greater change from baseline that the control group with demonstrated differences in stiffness, pain on walking, and pain for the previous

2 or 30 d. There was no change in synovial fluid metalloproteinase-3 or tissue inhibitor of metalloproteinase (TIMP). The pentosan group had a reduction in osteocalcin blood levels. This was a preliminary report on an 86-patient study.

Unsaponifiable Oils

An extract that is derived from one-third avocado and two-third soybean oils have shown some value in OA. They have been shown to stimulate the extracellular matrix synthesis by increasing collagen in cell cultures *(61)*, reducing IL-1 induced collagenolytic activity *(62)*, altering the cross-linking of collagen fibers in tissues *(63)*, and facilitating wound healing *(64)*. The avocado and soya unsaponifiables have also been shown to inhibit the stimulating action of IL-1β on stromelysin, IL-6, IL-8, and PGE2 production and IL-1β stimulated collagenase synthesis by human articular chondrocytes *(65)*. They also enhance TGF-β expression in cultured articular chondrocytes, increasing the production of PAI-1, promoting TGF-β induced matrix-repair mechanisms in articular cartilage *(66)*.

Following a pilot study suggesting efficacy *(67)*, Blotman et al. studied 164 patients with OA of the hip or knee in a prospective, 3-mo, randomized, double-blind, placebo-controlled trial *(68)*. The primary efficacy variable was the ability of the patients to not restart NSAIDs and the delay in restarting NSAIDs. There were 43% of those on avocado/soybean nonsaponifiables restarting NSAIDs vs 70% or those on placebo ($p < 0.001$). The time to restart NSAIDs was longer in the avocado/soybean non-saponifiable than the placebo group. Even though the overall rating was better for the avocado/soybean nonsaponifiables, the pain scores were similar between the two groups. There were no significant adverse events.

Maheu et al. studied 146 patients with knee or hip OA in a prospective, randomized, double-blind, placebo-controlled 8-mo study *(69)*. Following a 15-d washout, patients were treated with the avocado-soybean unsaponifiable or placebo for 6 mo with a 2-mo follow-up. The Lequesne algofunctional index decreased from a mean of 9.7 to 6.8 in the avocado-soybean unsaponifiable group vs 9.4 to 8.9 for the placebo, favoring the avocado-soybean unsaponifiable ($p < 0.001$). The reduction of knee pain by VAS was similarly significant. Fewer patients in the avocado-soybean group required NSAIDs than those on placebo. Hip OA seemed to respond more readily. Adverse events were infrequent and did not appear drug-related as they were no more frequent than in the placebo group.

REFERENCES

1. Lequesne, M., K. Brandt, N. Bellamy, R. Moskowitz, C.J. Menkes, J.P. Pelletier, and R.D. Altman. 1994. Guidelines for testing slow acting drugs in osteoarthritis. *J. Rheumatol.* 21 (Suppl. 41):65–73.

2. Points to consider on clinical investigation of medicinal products used in the treatment of osteoarthritis (CPMP/EWP/734/97, 07/I 993).

3. Food and Drug Administration. 1999. Guidance for industry: Clinical development programs for drugs, devices, and biological products intended for the treatment of osteoarthritis. FDA document 07/1999.

4. Dougados, M., J.P. Devogelaer, N'l. Annefeldt, B. Avouac, U. Bouvenot, C. Cooper, et al. 1996. (GREES). Recommendations for the registration of drugs used in the treatment of osteoarthritis. *Ann. Rheumatic Dis.* 55:552–557.

5. Hardingham, T.E. 1998. Chondroitin sulfate and joint disease. *Osteoarthritis Cartilage* 6 (Suppl. A):3–5.

6. Hardingham, T.B. and A.J. Fosang. 1992. Proteoglycans many forms, many functions. *FASEB J.* 6:861–870.

7. Hardingham, T.B. and M.T. Bayliss. 1991. Proteoglycans of articular cartilage: changes in ageing and in joint disease. *Semin. Arthritris Rheum.* 20 (Suppl. 1):12–33.

8. Bassleer, C.T., S.P.A. Comban, S. Bougaret, and M. Malaise. 1998. Effects of chondroitin sulfate and interleukin-Iβ on human articular chondrocytes cultivated in clusters. *Osteoarthritis Cartilage* 6:196–204.

9. Revelière, D., F. Mentz, H. Nterle-Beral, and X. Chevalier. 1999. Protective effect of chondroitin 4&6 sulfate on apoptosis of rabbit articular chondrocytes preliminary results. *In* New Approaches in OA: Chondroitin Sulfate (CS 4&6) Not Just a Symptomatic Treatment. U. Mautone, F. Tajana, S. Rovati, U. Vacher, editors. Litera Rheumatologica 24, Eular Publ, Zurich. 15–20.

10. Uebelhart, 0., I.N. Eugene, A. Thonar, Z. Jinwen, and J.M. Williams. 1998. Protective effect of exogenous chondroitin 4,6-sulfate in the acute degradation of articular cartilage in the rabbit. *Osteoarthritis Cartilage* 6 (Suppl. A):6–13.

11. Bourgeois, P., C. Chales, J. Dehais, B. Delcambrc, J.L. Kuntz, and S. Rozenberg. 1998. Efficacy and tolerability of chondroitin sulfate 1200 mg/day vs chondroitin sulfate 3×400mg vs placebo. *Osteoarthritis Cartilage* 6 (Suppl. A):25–30, 1285–1391.

12. Morreale, P., R. Manopulo, M. Galati, L. Boccanera, G. Saponati, and L. Bocchi. 1996. Comparison of the antiinflammatory efficacy of chondroitin sulfate and diclofenac sodium in patients with knee osteoarthritis. *J. Rheumatol.* 23:1385–1391.

13. Pavelka, K., R. Manopulo, and L. Bucsi. 1999. Double-blind, dose-effect study of oral Chondroitin 4&6 Sulfate 1200 mg, 800 mg, 200 mg and placebo in the treatment of knee osteoarthritis. In New Approaches in OA: Chondroitin Sulfate (CS 4&6) Not Just a Symptomatic Treatment. G. Mautone, E. Tajana, S. Rovati, and U. Vacher, editors. Litera Rheumatologica 24, Eular Publ, Zurich. 15–20.

14. Bucsi, L. and U. Poor. 1998. Efficacy and tolerability of oral chondroitin sulfate as a symptomatic slow-acting drug for osteoarthritis (SYSADOA) in the treatment of knee osteoarthritis. *Osteoarthritis Cartilage* 6 (Suppl. A):31–36.

15. Malaise, M., R. Mareolongo, 0. Uebelhart, and E. Vignon. 1999. Efficacy and tolerability of 800 mg oral Chondroitin 4&6 Sulfate in the treatment of knee osteoarthritis: a randomised, double-blind, multicentre study versus placebo. *In* New Approaches in OA: Chondroitin Sulfate (CS 4&6) Not Just a Symptomatic Treatment. U. Mautone, E. Tajana, S. Rovati, D. Vacher, editors. Litera Rheumatotogica 24, Eular Publ, Zurich. 15–20.

16. Setnikar, I., R. Cereda, M.A. Pacine, and L. Revel. 1991. Antireactive properties of glucosamine sulfate. *Arzneim-Forsch/Drug Res.* 41:157–161.

17. Verbruggen, G., S. Goemaere, and E.M. Veys. 1998. Chondroitin sulfate: S/DMOAD (structure modifying anti-osteoarthitis drug) in the treatment of finger joint OA. *Osteoarthritis Cartilage* 6 (Suppl. A):37–38.

18. Jimenez, S.A. and C.R. Dodge. 1997. The effects of glucosamine sulfate (CS04) on human chondrocyte gene expression. *Osteoarthritis Cartilage* 5 (Suppl. A):72.

19. Dodge, O.R., I.F. Hawkins, and S.A. Jimenez. 1999. Modulation of aggrecan MMP1 and MMP3 productions by glucosamine sulfate in cultured human osteoarthritis articular chondrocytes. *Arthritis Rheum.* 42 (Suppl.):253.

20. Basleer, C., L. Rovati, and P. Franchimont. 1998. Stimulation of proteoglycan production by glucosamine sulfate in chondrocytes isolated from human osteoarthritis articular cartilage in vitro. *Osteoarthritis Cartilage* 6:427–434.

21. Sandy, J.D., D. Gamett, V. Thompson, and C. Verscharen. 1998. Chondrocyte-mediated catabolism of aggrecan:aggreeanase-dependent cleavage induced by interleukin-1 or retinoic acid can be inhibited by glucosamine. *Biochem* 355:59–66.

22. Shikhman, A., N. Alaaeddine, and M.K. Lotz La Jolla. 1991. N-acetylglucosamine prevents IL-1 mediated activation of chondrocytes. *Arthritis Rheum.* 42 (Suppl.):381.

23. Abelda, S.M. and C.A. Buck. 1990. Integrins and other cell adhesion molecules. *FASEB J.* 4:2868–2880.

24. Piperno, M., P. Reboul, L. Hellio, M.P. Graverand, M.J. Peschard, M. Annefeld, et al. 1998. Maturation related compressive properties of rabbit knee articular cartilage and volume fraction of subchondral tissue. *Osteoarthritis Cartilage* 6:393–399.

25. Setnikar, I., R. Palumbo, S. Canali, and G. Zanolo. 1993. Pharmacokinetics of glucosamine in Man. *Arzneimittel/Forschung Drug Res.* 43:1109–1113.

26. Conrozier, I., P. Mathieu, M. Piperno, S. Richard, M. Annefeld, M. Richard, and E. Vignon. 1998. Glucosamine sulfate significantly reduced cartilage destruction in a rabbit model of osteoarthritis. *Arthritis Rheum.* 41(Suppl.):S147.

27. Reichelt, A., K.K. Forster, M. Fischer, L.C. Rovati, and I. Setnikar. 1994. Efficacy and safety of intramuscular glucosamine sulfate in osteoarthritis of the knee. *Arzneimittel/Forschung Drug Res.* 44:75–80.

28. Noack, W., M. Fischer, K.K. Former, I.C. Rovati, and I. Setnikar. 1994. Glucosamine sulfate in osteoarthritis of the knee. *Osteoarthritis Cartilage* 2:51–59.

29. Rovati, L.C. 1997. Clinical development of glucosamine sulfate as selective drug in osteoarthritis. *Rheumatol. Eur.* 26 (Suppl. 2):70.

30. Houpt, J.B., R. McMillan, C. Wein, and S.D. Paget-Dellio. 1999. Effect of glucosamine hydrochloride in the treatment of pain of osteoarthritis of the knee. *J. Rheumatol.* 26:11.

31. Rovati, L.C. 1993. Clinical efficacy of glucosamine sulfate in osteoarthritis of the spine. *Rev. Esp. Reumatol.* 20 (Suppl. 1):325.

32. Fassbender, H.M., G.L. Bach, W. Haase, L.C. Rovati, and I. Setnikar. 1994. Glucosamine sulfate compared to ibuprofen in osteoarthritis of the knee. *Osteoarthritis Cartilage* 2:61–69.

33. Qiu, O.X., S.N. Gao, U. Giacovelli, L. Rovati, and I. Setnikar. 1998. Efficacy and safety of glucosamine sulfate versus ibuprofen in patients with knee osteoarthritis. *Arzneimittel/Forschung Drug Res.* 48:469–474.

34. Rovati, L.C. 1997. The clinical profile of glucosamine sulfate as a selective symptom modifying drug in osteoarthritis: current data and perspectives. *Osteoarthritis Cartilage* 5 (Suppl. A):72.

35. Reginster, J.Y., R. Deroisy, I. Paul, R.L. Lee, Y. I-Ienrotin, U. Giacovelli, et al. 1999. Glucosamine sulfate significantly reduces progression of knee osteoarthritis over 3 years: a large, randomised, placebo-controlled, double-blind, prospective trial. *Arthritis Rheum.* 42 (Suppl.):S400.

36. Towheed, T.E. and T.P. Anastassiades. 1999. Glucosamine therapy for osteoarthritis. *J. Rheumatol.* 26:11–18.

37. Tapadinhas, M.J., I.C. Rivera, and A.A. Bignamini. 1982. Oral glucosamine sulphate in the management of arthrosis: report on a multi-centre open investigation in Portugal. *Pharmacotherapeutica* 3:157–168.

38. Adams. M.E. 1999. Hype about glucosarnine. *Lancet* 354:353–354.

39. Rovati, L.C., M. Annefeld, G. Giacovelli, K. Schrnid, I. Setnikar, A. Cumming, et al. 1999. Glucosamine in osteoarthritis. *Lancet* 4:1640.

40. Bendele, A.M., R.A. Bendele, J.F. Hulman, and B.P. Swann. 1996. Effets bénéfiques d'un traitement par la diacerhéine chez des cobayes atteints d'arthrose. *Rev. du Praticien* (Suppl. 6):35–39.

41. Mazières, B. 1997. Diacerhein in a post-contusive model of osteoarthritis. Structural results with "prophylactic" and "curative" regimens. *Osteoarthritis Cartilage* 5 (Suppl. A):73.

42. Brandt, K., G. Smith, S.Y. Kang, S. Myers, and M. Albrecht. 1997. Effects of diacerein in an accelerated canine model of osteoarthritis. *Osteoarthritis Cartilage* 5:438–449.

43. Smith, G., S. Myers, K.D. Brandt, E.A. Mickler, and M. Albrecht. 1999. Diacerein treatment reduces the severity of osteoarthritis in the canine cruciate-deficiency model of osteoarthritis. *Arthritis Rheum.* 42:545–554.

44. Martel-Pelletier, J., F. Mineau, F.C. Jolicoeur, J.M. Cloutier, and J.P. Pelletier. 1998. In vitro effects of diacerein and rhein on interleukin 1 and tumor necrosis factor-alpha systems in human osteoarthritic synovium and chondrocytes. *J. Rheumatol.* 25:753–762.

45. Pelletier, J.P. and J. Martel-Pelletier. 1997. Suppressive effects of Diacerein and Rhein on the synthesis of metalloproteases, interleukin-1B and leukemic inhibitory factor in human osteoarthritic synovial membrane. *Osteoarthritis Cartilage* 5 (Suppl. A):73.

46. Boitin, M., F. Redini, G. Loyau, and J.P. Pujol. 1993. Matrix deposition and collagenase release in cultures of rabbit articular chondrocytes (RAC) exposed to diacetylrhein (DAR). *Osteoarthritis Cartilage* 1:39–40.

47. Moore, A.R., K.J. Greenslade, C.A.S. Alam, and D.A. Willoughby. 1998. Effects of diacerhein on granuloma-induced cartilage breakdown in the mouse. *Osteoarthritis Cartilage* 6:19–23.

48. Pelletier, J.P., M. Yaron, and P. Cohen. 1999. Treatment of osteoarthritis of the knee with diacerein: a double-blind, placebo controlled trial. *Arthritis Rheum.* 42 (Suppl. 9):S295.

49. Nguyen, M., M. Dougados, L. Berdah, and B. Amor. 1994. Diacerein in the treatment of osteoarthritis of the hip. *Arthritis Rheum.* 37:529–536.

50. Marcolongo, R., A. Fioravanti, S. Adami, E. Tozzi, et al. 1988. Efficacy and tolerability of diacerein in the treatment of osteoarthritis. *Curr. Ther. Res.* 43:135–146.

51. Lequesne, M., L. Berdah, and I. Gerentes. 1998. Efficacité et tolerance de la diacerhéine dans le traitement de la gonarthrose et de la coxarthrose [Efficacy and tolerance of diacerein in the treatment of gonarthrosis and coxarthrosis]. *Rev. Prat.* 48 (Suppl. 17):S31–35.

52. Fagnani, F., G. Bouvenot, J.P. Valat, T. Bardin, et al. 1998. Medico-economic analysis of diacerein with or without standard therapy in the treatment of osteoarthritis. *Pharmacoeconomics* 13 (1, part 2): 135–146.

53. Dougados, M., M. Nguyen, L. Berdah, M. Lequesne, B. Mazieres, and E. Vignon. 1999. Evaluation of the structural (radiological) effect of diacerein in osteoarthritis of the hip: a 3 year placebo controlled study. *Osteoarthritis Cartilage* 7 (Suppl. A):S31.

54. Ghosh, P. 1999. The pathobiology of osteoarthritis and the rationale for the use of pentosan polysulfate for its treatment. *Semin. Arthritis Rheum.* 28:211–267.

55. Read, R.A., D. Cullis-Hill, and M.P. Jones. 1996. Systemic use of pentosan polysulphate in the treatment of osteoarthritis. *J. Small Anim. Pract.* 37:108–114.

56. Rogachefsky, R.A., D.D. Dean, D.S. Howell, and R.D. Altman. 1993. Treatment of canine osteoarthritis with insulin-like growth factor-1 (IGF-1) and pentosan polysulphate. *Osteoarthritis Cartilage* 1:105–114.

57. Edelman, J., L. March, and P. Ghosh. 1994. A double-blind placebo-controlled clinical study of a pleotropic osteoarthritis drug (pentosan polysulphate, Cartrophen) in 105 patients with osteoarthritis (OA) of the knee and hip joints. *Osteoarthritis Cartilage* 2:23.

58. Verbruggen, G., E.M. Veys, P. Ghosh, and D. Cullis-Hill. 1994. Pentosan polysulfate treatment in osteoarthritis, serological parameters which could correlate with clinical response. *Osteoarthritis Cartilage* 3:60.

59. Verbruggen, G., P. Ghosh, D. Cullis-Hill, and E. Veys. 1998. Xylan polysulphate has SMOAD activities in patients with inflammatory finger joint OA. *Osteoarthritis Cartilage* 6 (Suppl. A):6.

60. Rasaratnam, I., P. Ryan, L. Bowman, M. Smith, and P. Ghosh. 1996. A double-blind placebo-controlled study of intra-articular pentosan polysulphate (Cartrophen) in patients with gonarthritis: laboratory and clinical findings. *Osteoarthritis Cartilage* 4 (3):vi–vii.

61. Mauviel, A., M. Daireaux, D.J. Hartmann, P. Galera, G. Lohau, and J.-P. Pujol. 1989. Effets des insaponifiables d'avocat/soja (PIAS) sur la production de collagene par des cultures de synviocytes, chondrocytes articulaires it fibroblastes dermiques. *Rev. Rheum.* 56:207–211.

62. Mauviel, A., G. Loyau, and J.-P. Pujol. 1991. Effet des insaponifiables d'avacat/soja (piascledine) sur l'activite collagenolytique de cultures de synoviocytes rhumatoides humains et de chondrocytes articulaires de lapin trates par l'interleukine-1. *Rev. Rheum.* 58:241–245.

63. Werman, M.J., S. Mokady, M. E. Nimni, and I. Neeman. 1991. The effect of various avocado oils on skin collagen metabolism. *Connect Tissue Res.* 26:1–10.

64. Thiers, H., G. Zwingelstein, J. Fayole, and G. Moulin. 1961. Emploi therapeutique des insaponifiables d'huiles vegetales. *Therapie* 16:235–244.

65. Henroitin, Y., A. Labasse, S.X. Zheng, D. De Groote, J.-M. Jaspar, B. Guillou, et al. 1996. Effects of three avocado/soybean unsaponifiable mixtures on human articular chondrocytes metabolism. *Arthritis Rheum.* 29 (Suppl. 9):S226.

66. Boumediene, K., N. Felisaz, P. Bogdanowic, P. Galera, G.B. Guillou, and J-P. Pujol. 1999. Avocado/soya unsaponifiables enhance the expression of transforming growth factor beta 1 and beta 2 in cultured articular chondrocytes. *Arthritis Rheum.* 42:148–156.

67. Maheu, E. 1992. Les insaponifiables d'avocat-soja dans le traitement de la gonarthrose et de la coxarthrose. *Synoviale* 9:31–38.

68. Blotman, F., E. Maheu, A. Wulwik, H. Caspard, and A. Lopez. 1997. Efficacy and safety of avocado/soybean unsaponifiables in the treatment of symptomatic osteoarthritis of the knee and hip. A prospective, multicenter, three-month, randomized, double-blind, placebo-controlled trial. *Rev. Rheum. Engl. Ed.* 64:825–834.

69. Maheu, E., B. Mazieres, J.P. Valat, G. Loyau, X. Le Lo, and P. Bourgeois, et al. 1998. Symptomatic efficacy of avocado/soybean unsaponifiables in the treatment of osteoarthritis of the knee and hip: a prospective, randomized, double-blind, placebo-controlled, multicenter clinical trial with a six-month treatment period and two-month followup demonstrating a persistent effect. *Arthritis Rheum.* 41:81–91.

13 Intra-Articular Therapy in Osteoarthritis

Boulos Haraoui and Jean-Pierre Raynauld

CONTENTS

INTRODUCTION

Osteoarthritis (OA) is a degenerative disease involving mainly the hips, knees, spine, and the interphalangeal joints. Its clinical presentation is usually monoarticular or oligoarticular with fluctuations in intensity and localization over time. It is therefore logical to consider local therapeutic modalities in order to avoid untoward systemic effects. Several compounds have been used intra-articularly in open-label and in double-blind, randomized clinical trials.

CORTICOSTEROIDS

Intra-articular (IA) corticosteroid (CS) injections have been used for more than four decades for the symptomatic treatment of OA. A recent survey of rheumatologists in the United States suggested that more than 95% use this therapy sometimes and more than 50% frequently (1). Intra-articular CS is also recommended in the American College of Rheumatology (ACR) guidelines for the medical management of knee OA (2).

Different steroid formulations have been used over the years, with similar general efficacy: triamcinolone hexacetonide (THA), methylprednisolone, and prednisolone acetate were administered in single or multiple repetitive injection regimens (3–11). In one trial, THA had a long-standing effect superior to betamethasone (7); this observation, however, was not shared by other investigators who demonstrated a short-lived beneficial effect not lasting beyond 1 wk (5,9,12). Despite several observed flaws in the design of these trials, valuable information has been gathered, especially regarding the short-term safety of this approach. Moreover, the aspiration of the effusion, when present, seems to bring additional short term clinical benefit to THA injections (6). Despite their wide

From: *Modern Therapeutics in Rheumatic Diseases*
Edited by: G. C. Tsokos, et al. © Humana Press, Inc., Totowa, NJ

use in clinical practice, no predictors of response could be identified in two recent randomized, double-blind trials *(6,12)*.

The perceived efficacy and lack of major toxicity have made IA CS injections one of the mainstays of the management of OA, in particular knee OA.

HYALURONIC ACID

Hyaluronic acid (HA) (hyaluronan), a polysaccharide consisting of a long chain of disaccharides (β-D-glucuronyl-β-D-N-acethylglucosamine), is a natural component of cartilage and plays an essential role in the articular milieu. It is considered not only a joint lubricant, but also a physiological factor in the trophic status of cartilage. Balazs proposed HA as an effective agent in the treatment of patients with arthritic diseases *(13)*. Its clinical use was considered after determining that HA was reduced in concentration and in chain length in the synovial fluid of arthritis patients. Preliminary human clinical studies of sodium hyaluronate in human arthritic joints were performed by Peyron and Balazs in the early 1970s *(14)*. Several studies with various preparations of hyaluronan from different sources and molecular weights have since been conducted.

The efficacy of viscosupplementation—the replacement of pathological synovial fluid with a hyaluronan-based elastoviscous solution—depends on the physical properties of the solution used and its residence time in the joint. Preparations of hyaluronic acid or sodium hyaluronate with molecular weights between 500–700 kD, 600–1200 kD, and 4000–5000 kD have been used in clinical studies.

Intra-articular injections of hyaluronan or sodium hyaluronate with a molecular weight between 500,000 and 750,000 Daltons have been studied using corticosteroid injections *(15–18)* or nonsteroidal anti-inflammatory drugs (NSAIDs) *(19)* as control treatment, and by conducting placebo-controlled clinical trials *(20–25)*. A prospective study including 43 patients with knee OA showed good tolerance to HA treatment, without adverse side effects. This therapy was effective if OA was less than moderate in grade; it was not effective in cases with considerable effusion or in those with gross architectural changes *(25)*. A single-blind, parallel trial used two dosage regimens of HA (40 mg and 20 mg) to assess its efficacy *(20)*. The active treatments were shown to be equally highly effective in reducing pain; both were significantly superior to placebo, and beneficial effects lasted for more than a month, demonstrating the long-term action of the drug. Several double-blind, placebo-controlled trials suggest that intra-articular injection of sodium hyaluronate (Hyalectin) may improve the clinical condition and have a long-term beneficial effect in knee OA patients *(21–23)*. However, a double-blind, placebo-controlled study involving 91 patients with radiologically confirmed knee OA concluded that intra-articular administration of 750 kD hyaluronan offered no significant benefit over placebo during a 5-wk treatment period, but incurred a significantly higher morbidity *(24)*. The principal side effects were a transient increase in pain and swelling in the affected knee observed in 47% of the treatment group compared with 22% of the placebo group. Graf et al. conducted a single-blind, randomized clinical trial to compare both the efficacy and safety of HA with that of mucopolysaccharide polysulfuric acid ester (MPA) in OA patients *(26)*. Both HA and MPA demonstrated efficacy, with hyaluronic acid superior in the parameters investigated.

Furthermore, in a study that evaluated the effect of joint lavage with lactated Ringer's solution in 23 patients, the secondary goal was to determine if any additional benefit could be obtained by injecting the knee with HA following washout treatment *(27)*. Improvement was noted at 1- and 2-yr follow-ups, however, there were no statistically significant differences in outcome for the hyaluronan and placebo groups.

Others have used methylprednisolone acetate as the drug of comparison. The results showed that on a short-term basis, both HA and 6-methylprednisolone acetate were efficacious in controlling OA symptoms. In the long-term assessment, the results obtained at the end of treatment in the HA group persisted, and in some cases even improved *(16,18)*. It was concluded that sodium hyaluronate would appear to offer an alternative to steroids in intra-articular treatment of OA *(17)*. Grecomoro et al. evaluated the therapeutic synergism between HA and dexamethasone in intra-articular treatment by conducting an open randomized study *(15)*. Dexamethasone notably potentiated the clinical effectiveness of hyaluronic acid, even if used only during the first weekly infiltration of a 5-wk treatment regimen.

A 1-yr double-blind control study involving 52 patients compared the effect of intra-articular injections of hyaluronan (600–1200 kD) and placebo, both administrated weekly for 5 wk *(28)*. Though both groups improved from baseline, there was no statistically significant difference in any of the relevant variables at any time-point. Another large, randomized, double-blind, placebo-controlled trial also found no significant difference at 20 wk between the two groups when compared to their baseline evaluation. However, once stratified according to age and disease severity, HA proved more efficacious than placebo for patients over 60 yr of age who had the most severe knee OA *(29)*. On the other hand, in a recent randomized clinical trial of 495 patients with osteoarthritis of the knee, Altman et al. demonstrated that five weekly intra-articular injections of hyaluronan (500–730 kD, Hyalgan®) are at least as effective as continuous treatment with naproxen for 26 wk, with fewer adverse reactions *(30)*.

A review by Maheu looked at five different clinical trials, comparing different regimens of Hyalgan vs corticosteroid injections in the osteoarthritic knee, with follow-ups from 2–12 mo *(31)*. One study showed initial superiority of Hyalgan over steroid injections and in three studies, equal efficacy over time. The fifth study used a combination of Hyalgan and steroid injections initially. The steroid injections seemed to increase the long-term efficacy of the hyaluronan suggesting that the combination of these two local treatments would be promising.

The long-term, structure-modifying properties of HA (Hyalgan) were investigated through a double-blind, randomized, placebo-controlled trial using a standardized arthroscopic score after 1 yr of follow-up. HA proved superior to placebo in two out of three parameters used to quantify the severity of OA lesions *(32)*.

The efficacy of a weekly therapeutic regimen of either two or three injections of hylan G-F20 (a polymerized higher molecular-weight compound) was further demonstrated by Scale, Wobig and Dickson in three different randomized double-blind saline or arthrocentesis-controlled clinical trials that included a 3–6-mo follow-up *(33–35)*. Compared to the control groups, the two-injection or three-injection hylan treatment groups each showed statistically significantly greater improvement in pain outcome measurements, as well as overall evaluation of treatment at the 12-wk point. At 6-mo follow-up, results in the hylan treatment groups were superior to those in the control group. Adams et al. evaluated the safety and effectiveness of three weekly intra-articular injections of hylan G-F20 (Synvisc) in knee OA patients, and compared this treatment to continuous oral NSAID therapy in both the presence and absence of hylan G-F20 viscosupplementation *(19)*. The results support the hypothesis that treatment of knee OA pain with hylan is at least as effective as treatment with NSAIDs. Hylan G-F20 is a safe and effective treatment for knee OA, and can be used either as a replacement for or an adjunct to NSAID therapy. Dickson also reported that hylan injections were superior to diclofenac (100 mg daily) on knee pain and function at 3-mo follow-up *(35)*.

Intra-articular injection with hyaluronan or hylan is a relatively safe approach, however, some adverse events have been reported. One patient developed an haemarthrosis after sodium hyaluronate injection *(21)*. Other observed events were local reactions such as effusion, feeling of warmth, tingling, and pain following HA injections *(26)*. A transient adverse event of muscle pain was also mentioned *(33)*.

In conclusion, in the majority of studies, a clinical benefit of treatment was reported compared to the injected control group. Compared to treatment with local corticosteroids, the benefit of hyaluronan appeared somewhat less dramatic but longer-lasting.

OTHER INTRA-ARTICULAR THERAPIES FOR KNEE OA

Other substances such as orgotein, yttrium-90, silicone, somatostatin, and tenoxicam have been investigated as potentially therapeutic in the treatment of arthritic joints.

Orgotein is the pharmaceutical form of the bovine enzyme Cu-Zn superoxide dismutase (SOD). The anti-inflammatory properties of orgotein were discovered in 1965. Intra-articular injection of orgotein presents a potentially therapeutic alternative in the treatment of OA *(36)*. This study showed that four weekly injections of 4 mg orgotein were superior to four weekly injections of saline, and orgotein was safe and well-tolerated. Furthermore, three orgotein dose/regimens were compared with a placebo in terms of efficacy, safety, and duration of effect in 139 patients with knee OA. Orgotein was effective in reducing symptoms for up to 3 mo after treatment; 16 mg given twice was the most effective and best-tolerated regimen *(37)*.

A randomized, double-blind study comparing orgotein injections with intra-articular methylprednisolone acetate injections found that orgotein could be used safely and effectively without serious adverse reactions *(38)*. The efficacy of orgotein was compared to that of betamethasone over a 1-yr period in 419 patients with knee OA *(39)*. Though betamethasone acted more quickly, orgotein at low doses (4 or 8 mg) was comparable to the corticosteroid from wk four, and up to a year of follow-up.

The main adverse reactions to orgotein were pain, swelling, stiffness, prickling, or burning sensations, or a feeling of heaviness at the injection site *(38,39)*. Skin rashes and/or pruritus, and pain/swelling were also mentioned *(37)*.

An observational prospective study evaluating the effects of both radiation synovectomy and triamcinolone acetonide was conducted in 40 patients with knee OA over a 1-yr period *(40)*. A marked improvement in pain and evaluation scores occurred at three months, but had disappeared by 6 mo posttreatment. The safety and efficacy of dysprosium-165 hydroxide macroaggregate (165Dy) was compared to yttrium-90 silicate for radiation synovectomy of the knee in a multicenter, double-blind clinical trial, with no significant difference in clinical response between the two treatment groups. No clinically significant side effects were observed *(41)*.

Wright et al. conducted a pilot study in five patients, with a control of 25 outpatients, to evaluate intra-articular silicone as an artificial lubricant for OA joints *(42)*. Sequential analyses showed a significant benefit from saline compared to silicone at 1-wk follow-up, and no significant difference at 1 mo.

A randomized, placebo-controlled study with 20 patients was carried out to assess saline lavage of knee OA vs intra-articular saline injection without lavage *(43)*. Though both groups showed improvement, knee washout conferred no further benefit. However, in a recent randomized, single-blind study, tidal-knee irrigation with saline in 77 patients with knee OA showed a greater reduction in pain that did conservative medical management *(44)*.

In a 24-wk placebo-controlled study in 98 patients, Ravaud et al. compared joint lavage to a single corticosteroid injection and the combination of both interventions *(45)*. Intra-articular CS had a beneficial effect on pain as early as the first week, but which was lost by wk 12. On the other hand, joint lavage had a delayed onset of action (wk 4) but lasted up to the final 24-wk evaluation. Neither treatment had any long-term beneficial effect as assessed by Lequesne's index. No additional benefit was observed in the combination group.

Since pain is the main symptom in knee OA, IA analgesic agents were tested in two studies. In a single-blind trial, 20 patients were randomized to receive either IA bupivicaine or placebo *(46)*; the local anaesthetic agent had a short-lived significant effect (less than 24 h). In a crossover placebo-controlled design, IA morphine (100 mg) was shown to be superior to placebo and had a long-lasting effect, up to 9 d, which was the last evaluation period for this study *(47)*.

Several other compounds have been tested in single trials *(48–50)*. Glucosamine was shown to be safe and provided a greater benefit than placebo; a single tenoxicam IA injection was also superior to placebo with no local side effects. Somatostatin led to pain reduction and increased joint mobility with no reported adverse reactions. Finally, sodium pentosan polysulfate (NaPP) isolated from beechwood hemicellulose has anti-catabolic effects in OA by direct enzyme inhibition and gene-expression alteration of metalloproteinases. Four weekly injections of NaPP were administered intra-articularly in 15 patients with knee OA and showed better improvement of pain and mobility, as well as synovial-fluid viscosity at 2 mo vs a control group of 16 patients injected with saline *(51)*. However, data on long-term efficacy and safety is not available.

Despite the lack of strong, convincing, and reproducible evidence that any of these IA therapies significantly alters the short-term outcome and even less so the progression of OA, corticosteroids, and hyaluronic acid are widely used in patients who have failed other therapeutic modalities for lack of efficacy or toxicity. The virtual absence of serious side effects, coupled with the perceived benefits, make these approaches attractive. It remains to be proven if any agent has the potential for structural modification or to lengthen time to surgery.

ACKNOWLEDGMENTS

The authors thank Mariana Maier-Moldovan for her assistance in the research for this chapter.

REFERENCES

1. Hochberg, M.C., D.L. Perlmutter, J.I. Hudson, and R.D. Altman. 1996. Preferences in the management of osteoarthritis of the hip and knee: results of a survey of community-based rheumatologists in the United States. *Arthritis Care Res.* 9:170–176.

2. Hochberg, M.C., R.D. Altman, K.D. Brandt, B.M. Clark, P.A. Dieppe, M.R. Griffin, et al. 1995. Guidelines for the medical management of osteoarthritis. Part II. Osteoarthritis of the knee. American College of Rheumatology. *Arthritis Rheum.* 38:1541–1546.

3. Balch, H.W., J.M. Gibson, A.F. El-Ghobarey, L.S. Bain, and M.P. Lynch. 1977. Repeated corticosteroid injections into knee joints. *Rheumatol. Rehabil.* 16:137–140.

4. Dieppe, P.A., B. Sathapatayavongs, H.E. Jones, P.A. Bacon, and E.F. Ring. 1980. Intra-articular steroids in osteoarthritis. *Rheumatol. Rehabil.* 19:212–217.

5. Friedman, D.M. and M.E. Moore. 1980. The efficacy of intraarticular steroids in osteoarthritis: a double-blind study. *J. Rheumatol.* 7:850–856.

6. Gaffney, K., J. Ledingham, and J.D. Perry. 1995. Intra-articular triamcinolone hexacetonide in knee osteoarthritis: factors influencing the clinical response. *Ann. Rheum. Dis.* 54:379–381.

7. Valtonen, E.J. 1981. Clinical comparison of triamcinolonehexacetonide and betamethasone in the treatment of osteoarthrosis of the knee-joint. *Scand. J. Rheumatol.* (Suppl.) 41:1–7.

8. Sambrook, P.N., G.D. Champion, C.D. Browne, D, Cairns, M.L. Cohen, R.O. Day, et al. 1989. Corticosteroid injection for osteoarthritis of the knee: peripatellar compared to intra-articular route. *Clin. Exp. Rheumatol.* 7:609–613.

9. Cederlof, S. and G. Jonson. 1966. Intraarticular prednisolone injection for osteoarthritis of the knee. A double blind test with placebo. *Acta Chir. Scand.* 132:532–537.

10. Wada, J., T. Koshino, T. Morii, and K. Sugimoto. 1993. Natural course of osteoarthritis of the knee treated with or without intraarticular corticosteroid injections. *Bull. Hosp. Jt. Dis.* 53:45–48.

11. Towheed, T.E. and M.C. Hochberg. 1997. A systematic review of randomized controlled trials of pharmacological therapy in osteoarthritis of the knee, with an emphasis on trial methodology. *Semin. Arthritis Rheum.* 26:755–770.

12. Jones, A. and M. Doherty. 1996. Intra-articular corticosteroids are effective in osteoarthritis but there are no clinical predictors of response. *Ann. Rheum. Dis.* 55:829–832.

13. Balazs, E.A. and J.L. Denlinger. 1993. Viscosupplementation: a new concept in the treatment of osteoarthritis. *J. Rheum.* 39(Suppl.):3–9.

14. Peyron, J.G. and E.A. Balazs. 1974. Preliminary clinical assessment of Na-hyaluronate injection into human arthritis joints. *Pathol. Biol.* 22:731–736.

15. Grecomoro, G., F. Piccione, and G. Letizia. 1992. Therapeutic synergism between hyaluronic acid and dexamethasone in the intra-articular treatment of osteoarthritis of the knee: a preliminary open study. *Curr. Med. Res. Opin.* 13:49–55.

16. Leardini, G., L. Mattara, M. Franceschini, and A. Perbellini. 1991. Intra-articular treatment of knee osteoarthritis. A comparative study between hyaluronic acid and 6-methyl prednisolone acetate. *Clin. Exp. Rheumatol.* 9:375–381.

17. Leardini, G., M. Franceschini, L. Mattara, R. Bruno, and A. Perbellini. 1987. Intra-articular sodium hyaluronate in gonarthrosis. A controlled study comparing methylprednisolone acetate. *Clin. Trials J.* 24:341–350.

18. Pietrogrande, V., P.L. Melanotte, B. D'Agnolo, M. Ulivi, G.A. Benigni, L. Turchetto, et al. 1991. Hyaluronic acid versus methylprednisolone intra-articularly injected for the treatment of osteoarthritis of the knee. *Curr. Therap. Res.* 50:691–701.

19. Adams, M.E., M.H. Atkinson, A.J. Lussier, J.I. Schulz, K.A. Siminovitch, J.P. Wade, and M. Zummer. 1995. The role of viscosupplementation with Hylan G-F 20 (Synvisc) in the treatment of osteoarthritis of the knee: a Canadian multicenter trial comparing hylan G-F 20 alone, hylan G-F 20 with non-steroidal anti-inflammatory drugs (NSAIDs) and NSAIDs alone. *Osteoarthritis Cartilage* 3:213–225.

20. Bragantini, A. and M. Cassini 1987. Controlled single-blind trial of intra-articulary injected hyaluronic acid in osteoarthritis of the knee. *Clin. Trials J.* 24:333–340.

21. Dixon, A.S., R.K. Jacoby, H. Berry, and E.B. Hamilton. 1988. Clinical trial of intra-articular injection of sodium hyaluronate in patients with osteoarthritis of the knee. *Curr. Med. Res. Opin.* 11:205–213.

22. Dougados, M., M. Nguyen, V. Listrat, and B. Amor. 1993. High molecular weight sodium hyaluronate (hyalectin) in osteoarthritis of the knee: a 1 year placebo-controlled trial. *Osteoarthritis Cartilage* 1:97–103.

23. Grecomoro, G., U. Martorana, and C. Di Marco. 1987. Intra-articular treatment with sodium hyaluronate in gonarthrosis: a controlled clinical trial versus placebo. *Pharmatherapeutica* 5:137–141.

24. Henderson, E.B., E.C. Smith, F. Pegley, and D.R. Blake. 1994. Intra-articular injections of 750 kD hyaluronan in the treatment of osteoarthritis: a randomised single centre double-blind placebo- controlled trial of 91 patients demonstrating lack of efficacy. *Ann. Rheum. Dis.* 53:529–534.

25. Namiki, O., H. Toyoshima, and N. Morisaki. 1982. Therapeutic effect of intra-articular injection of high molecular weight hyaluronic acid on osteoarthritis of the knee. *Int. J. Clin. Pharm. Ther. Toxicol.* 20:501–507.

26. Graf, J., E. Neusel, E. Schneider, and F.U. Niethard. 1993. Intra-articular treatment with hyaluronic acid in osteoarthritis of the knee joint: a controlled clinical trial versus mucopolysaccharide polysulfuric acid ester. *Clin. Exp. Rheumatol.* 11:367–372.

27. Edelson, R., R.T. Burks, and R.D. Bloebaum. 1995. Short-term effects of knee washout for osteoarthritis. *Am. J. Sports Med.* 23:345–349.

28. Dahlberg, L., L.S. Lohmander, and L. Ryd. 1994. Intraarticular injections of hyaluronan in patients with cartilage abnormalities and knee pain: a one-year double-blind, placebo-controlled study. *Arthritis Rheum.* 37:521–528.

29. Lohmander, L.S., N. Dalen, G. Englund, M. Hamalainen, E.M. Jensen, K. Karlsson, et al. 1996. Intra-articular hyaluronan injections in the treatment of osteoarthritis of the knee: a randomised, double blind, placebo controlled multicentre trial. Hyaluronan Multicentre Trial Group. *Ann. Rheum. Dis.* 55:424–431.

30. Altman, R.D. and R. Moskowitz 1998. Intraarticular sodium hyaluronate (Hyalgan) in the treatment of patients with osteoarthritis of the knee: a randomized clinical trial. Hyalgan Study Group. *J. Rheumatol.* 25:2203–2212.

31. Maheu, E. 1995. Hyaluronan in knee osteoarthritis. A review of the clinical trials with Hyalgan®. *Eur. J. Rheumatol. Inflamm.* 15:17–24.

32. Listrat, V., X. Ayral, F. Patarnello, J.P. Bonvarlet, J. Simonnet, B. Amor, and M. Dougados. 1997. Arthroscopic evaluation of potential structure modifying activity of hyaluronan (Hyalgan) in osteoarthritis of the knee. *Osteoarthritis Cartilage* 5:153–160.

33. Scale, D., M. Wobig, and W. Wolpert. 1994. Viscosupplementation of osteoarthritic knees with hylan: a treatment schedule study. *Curr. Therap. Res.* 55:220–232.

34. Wobig, M., A. Dickhut, R. Maier, and G. Vetter. 1998. Viscosupplementation with hylan G-F 20: a 26-week controlled trial of efficacy and safety in the osteoarthritic knee. *Clin. Ther.* 20:410–423.

35. Dickson, J., G. Hosie, and Primary Care Rheumatism Society OA Knee Study Group. 1998. Double blind, double control comparison of viscosupplementation with hylan G-F20 (Synvisc®) against diclofenac and control in knee osteoarthritis. *Arthritis Rheum.* 41 (Suppl. 9):S197 (Abstract).

36. Huskisson, E.C. and J. Scott. 1981. Orgotein in osteoarthritis of the knee joint. *Eur. J. Rheumatol. Inflamm.* 4:212–218.

37. McIlwain, H., J.C. Silverfield, D.E. Cheatum, J. Poiley, J. Taborn, T. Ignaczak, and C.V. Multz. 1989. Intra-articular orgotein in osteoarthritis of the knee: a placebo-controlled efficacy, safety, and dosage comparison. *Am. J. Med.* 87:295–300.

38. Gammer, W. and L.G. Broback. 1984. Clinical comparison of orgotein and methylprednisolone acetate in the treatment of osteoarthrosis of the knee joint. *Scand. J. Rheumatol.* 13:108–112.

39. Mazieres, B., A.M. Masquelier, and M.H. Capron. 1991. A French controlled multicenter study of intraarticular orgotein versus intraarticular corticosteroids in the treatment of knee osteoarthritis: a one-year followup. *J. Rheumatol.* Suppl. 27:134–137.

40. Will, R., B. Laing, J. Edelman, F. Lovegrove, and I. Surveyor. 1992. Comparison of two yttrium-90 regimens in inflammatory and osteoarthropathies. *Ann. Rheum. Dis.* 51:262–265.

41. Edmonds, J., R. Smart, R. Laurent, P. Butler, P. Brooks, R. Hoschl, et al. 1994. A comparative study of the safety and efficacy of dysprosium-165 hydroxide macro-aggregate and yttrium-90 silicate colloid in radiation synovectomy--a multicentre double blind clinical trial. Australian Dysprosium Trial Group. *Br. J. Rheumatol.* 33:947–953.

42. Wright, V., D.I. Haslock, D. Dowson, P.C. Seller, and B. Reeves. 1971. Evaluation of silicone as an artificial lubricant in osteoarthrotic joints. *BMJ* 2:370–373.

43. Dawes, P.T., C. Kirlew, and I. Haslock. 1987. Saline washout for knee osteoarthritis: results of a controlled study. *Clin. Rheumatol.* 6:61–63.

44. Ike, R.W., W.J. Arnold, E.W. Rothschild, and H.L. Shaw. 1992. Tidal irrigation versus conservative medical management in patients with osteoarthritis of the knee: a prospective randomized study. Tidal Irrigation Cooperating Group. *J. Rheumatol.* 19:772–779.

45. Ravaud, P., L. Moulinier, B. Giraudeau, X. Ayral, C. Guerin, E. Noel, et al. 1999. Effects of joint lavage and steroid injection in patients with osteoarthritis of the knee: results of a multicenter, randomized, controlled trial. *Arthritis Rheum.* 42:475–482.

46. Creamer, P., M. Hunt, and P. Dieppe. 1996. Pain mechanisms in osteoarthritis of the knee: effect of intraarticular anesthetic. *J. Rheumatol.* 23:1031–1036.

47. Likar, R., M. Schafer, F. Paulak, R. Sittl, W. Pipam, H. Schalk, et al. 1997. Intraarticular morphine analgesia in chronic pain patients with osteoarthritis. *Anesth. Analg.* 84:1313–1317.

48. Vajaradul, Y. 1981. Double-blind clinical evaluation of intra-articular glucosamine in outpatients with gonarthrosis. *Clin. Ther.* 3:336–343.

49. Papathanassiou, N.P. 1994. Intra-articular use of tenoxicam in degenerative osteoarthritis of the knee joint. *J. Int. Med. Res.* 22:332–337.

50. Silveri, F., P. Morosini, D. Brecciaroli, and C. Cervini. 1994. Intra-articular injection of somatostatin in knee osteoarthritis: clinical results and IGF-1 serum levels. *Int. J. Pharmacol. Res.* 14:79–85.

51. Rasaratnam, I., P. Ryan, L. Bowman, M. Smith, and P. Ghosh. 1996. A double-blind placebo-controlled study of intra-articular pentosan polysulfate (cartrophen) in patients with gonarthrosis: laboratory and clinical findings. 8th APLAR Congress of Rheumatology. *Osteoarthritis Cartilage* 4:vi–vii (Abstract).

14 Promoting Articular Cartilage Repair

Joseph A. Buckwalter and James A. Martin

CONTENTS

INTRODUCTION
ARTICULAR-CARTILAGE LESIONS
PENETRATION OF SUBCHONDRAL BONE
DECREASED ARTICULAR SURFACE-CONTACT STRESS
SOFT-TISSUE GRAFTS
CELL TRANSPLANTATION
GROWTH FACTORS
ARTIFICIAL MATRICES
CONCLUSIONS
REFERENCES

INTRODUCTION

For more than 250 years, physicians and scientists have been seeking ways to repair or regenerate synovial-joint articular surfaces following articular-cartilage loss or degeneration *(1–3)*. (Repair refers to restoring a damaged articular surface with new tissue that resembles but does not duplicate the structure, composition, and function of articular cartilage; regeneration refers to forming new tissue indistinguishable from normal articular cartilage *[4–6]*.) They made little progress for the majority of these 250 years, but in the last three decades clinical and basic scientific investigations have shown that implantation of artificial matrices, growth factors, perichondrium, periosteum and transplanted chondrocytes, and mesenchymal stem cells can stimulate formation of cartilaginous tissue in synovial-joint osteochondral defects *(6–10)*. Other work has demonstrated that joint loading and motion can influence articular cartilage and joint healing *(11–13)*, and that mechanical-loading influences the repair process in all of the tissues that form parts of synovial joints *(5,14,15)*. In addition, review of several operative procedures used to treat osteoarthrosis (OA), including osteotomies, penetration of subchondral bone, and joint distraction and motion, has shown that these procedures can stimulate formation of new articular surfaces *(9)*. The apparent potential of these multiple methods for stimulating formation of cartilaginous-articular surfaces has created great interest on the part of patients, physicians, and scientists, however the wide variety of methods and approaches to assessing their results have made it

From: *Modern Therapeutics in Rheumatic Diseases*
Edited by: G. C. Tsokos, et al. © Humana Press, Inc., Totowa, NJ

difficult to evaluate their success in restoring joint function and to define their most appropriate current clinical applications.

ARTICULAR-CARTILAGE LESIONS

Better understanding of articular-cartilage lesions and degeneration has also contributed to the recent interest in cartilage repair and regeneration (1,9,16–18). Advances in synovial-joint imaging and arthroscopic techniques have increased understanding of the frequency and types of chondral defects and made it possible to diagnose and evaluate these lesions with greater accuracy (19). Age-related superficial cartilage fibrillation and focal lesions of the articular surface must be distinguished from cartilage degeneration occurring as part of the clinical syndrome of OA (2,18,20). Superficial articular-cartilage fibrillation occurs in many joints with increasing age and does not appear to cause symptoms or adversely affect joint function. Isolated articular-cartilage and osteochondral defects appear to result from trauma that often leaves the majority of the articular surface intact (17,19). They commonly occur in adolescents and young adults who wish to maintain a high level of activity and in some of these individuals cause joint pain, effusions, and mechanical dysfunction. Although the natural history of isolated chondral and osteochondral defects has not been well-defined (10,21,22). However, clinical experience shows that, in skeletally mature individuals, when these lesions are left untreated they fail to heal, and that defects that involve a significant portion of the articular surface may progress to symptomatic joint degeneration. For this reason treatment of selected isolated chondral and osteochondral defects may help delay or prevent the development of OA. Because treatment by debridement alone produces variable results (9,19), investigators have sought better methods of treating these focal defects.

PENETRATION OF SUBCHONDRAL BONE

Penetration of subchondral bone was the first method developed to stimulate formation of a new articular surface and is still the most commonly used (2,9,23). In regions with full thickness loss or advanced degeneration of articular cartilage, penetration of the exposed subchondral bone disrupts subchondral blood vessels leading to formation of a fibrin clot over the bone surface (2,5,9). If the surface is protected from excessive loading, undifferentiated mesenchymal cells migrate into the clot, proliferate, and differentiate into cells with the morphologic features of chondrocytes (24). In some instances they form a fibrocartilagenous articular surface (Fig. 1), but in others they fail to restore an articular surface (25,26).

Surgeons first debrided degenerated articular cartilage and drilled into the subchondral bone through arthrotomies and found that many patients reported a decrease in symptoms following recovery from the procedure (27–30). One group advocated treating patellar articular-surface degeneration by excising damaged cartilage along with underlying subchondral bone, a procedure they referred to as "spongialization." They found good or excellent results in a high percentage of their patients (31). Surgeons have developed a variety of other methods of penetrating subchondral bone to stimulate formation of a new cartilaginous surface including arthroscopic abrasion of the articular surface and making multiple small-diameter defects or fractures with an awl or similar instrument (9,19,23,25,26,32).

Prospective randomized controlled trials of arthroscopic abrasion treatment of osteoarthritic joints have not been reported, but several authors have reviewed series of patients and found that these procedures can decrease the symptoms owing to isolated articular-cartilage defects and OA of the knee *(19,25,26,32–35)*. One group of investigators reported less successful results in their series of 44 patients (49 knees): they found early treatment failures in 19 knees (39%), and 23 knees (47%) had failed at final follow-up examination *(36)*. In this same series, excellent results decreased from 20 knees (41%) at the time of maximum improvement to 12 knees (24%) at the time of final follow-up.

Examination of joint surfaces following arthroscopic abrasion has shown that in some individuals, it results in formation of fibrocartilagenous articular surface that varies in composition from dense fibrous tissue with little or no type II collagen to hyaline cartilage-like tissue with predominantly type II collagen *(25,26)*. Johnson also found that in many patients with radiographic evidence of cartilage joint-space narrowing, or no radiographically demonstrable joint space, the joint space increased following abrasion *(25,26)*. Although an increase in radiographic joint space following subchondral abrasion presumably indicates formation of a new articular surface, the development of this new surface does not necessarily result in symptomatic improvement. Bert and Maschka *(37,38)* found that 30 (51%) of 59 patients treated with abrasion arthroplasty had evidence of increased radiographic joint space 2 yr after treatment, but 18 (31%) of these individuals either had no symptomatic improvement or more severe symptoms.

Some of the variability in the clinical results of attempts to restore an articular surface by penetrating subchondral bone may result from differences in the extent and quality of the repair tissue. However, no studies have documented a relationship between the extent and type of repair tissue and symptomatic or functional results, suggesting that formation of a new articular surface following penetration of subchondral bone does not necessarily relieve pain *(9)*. The lack of predictable clinical benefit from formation of cartilage repair tissue may result from variability among patients in severity of the degenerative changes, joint alignment, patterns of joint use, age, perception of pain, pre-operative expectations, or other factors. It may also result from the inability of the newly formed tissue to replicate the properties of articular cartilage *(2,16)*. Examination of the tissue that forms over the articular surface following penetration of subchondral bone shows that it lacks the structure, composition, mechanical properties, and in most instances the durability of articular cartilage (Fig. 1) *(1,5,9,16,39)*. For these reasons, even though it covers the subchondral bone, it may fail to distribute loads across the articular surface in a way that avoids pain with joint loading and further degeneration of the joint.

Currently, it is not clear which method of penetrating subchondral bone produces the best new articular surface, and differences in patient selection and technique among surgeons using the same method may be responsible for variations in results making it difficult to compare techniques. However, comparison of bone abrasion with subchondral drilling for treatment of an experimental chondral defect in rabbits showed that although neither treatment predictably restored the articular surface, drilling appeared to produce better long-term results than abrasion *(40)*. This observation fits well with previous experimental work showing that chondral repair tissue that grows up through multiple drill holes that pass from the articular surface into vascularized bone will spread over exposed subchondral bone between holes and form a fibrocartilagenous articular

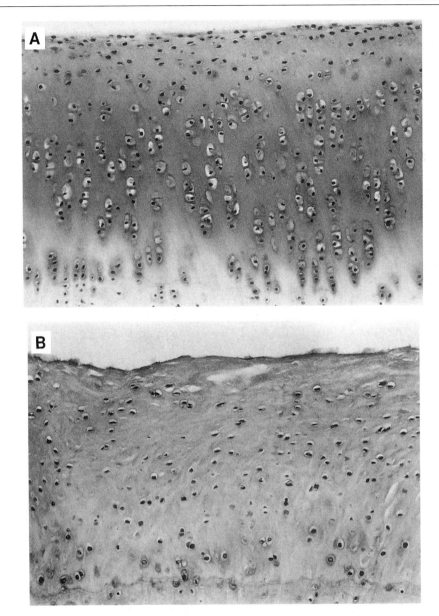

Fig. 1. Light micrographs of normal rabbit articular cartilage and repair cartilage. Reproduced from ref. *16* with permission. (**A**) Normal rabbit articular cartilage. The extracellular matrix appears homogenous. (**B**) Well-formed repair cartilage in a 6-mo-old osteochondral defect. The matrix appears fibrillar and has multiple clefts. Most of the cells are smaller than the normal chondrocytes in (A).

surface *(39)*. It also suggests that small diameter holes that leave the bone intact between defects lead to formation of more stable repair tissue than abraded bone surfaces *(40)*.

   One recent report suggests that the age of the patient may influence the results of attempts to stimulate articular cartilage repair by penetrating subchondral bone. Kumai and colleagues described the results of arthroscopic drilling of osteochondral

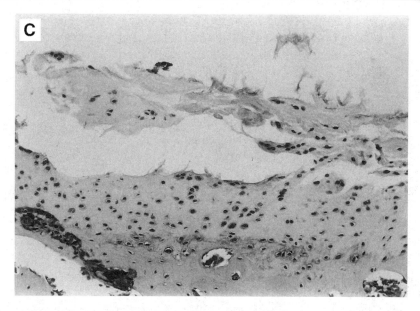

Fig. 1. (continued) **(C)** Fibrillation and fragmentation of articular-cartilage repair tissue 1 yr after experimental osteochondral injury.

lesions of the talus in 18 ankles (17 patients) *(41)*. They found that all patients had decreased pain at between 2 and 9.5 yr after treatment. Twelve of the thirteen ankles in patients less than 30 yr old had a good result, but only one of five ankles in patients over 50 yr old had a good result. This data supports the concept that with increasing age the probability of a good result of an attempt to repair or regenerate articular cartilage decreases *(2,42)*.

Despite the evidence that penetration of subchondral bone stimulates formation of fibrocartilagenous repair tissue, the clinical value of this approach remains uncertain. In contrast with reports of symptomatic improvement in patients with cartilage degeneration treated with penetration of subchondral bone *(25,26,33–35)*, one investigator has concluded that although joint debridement can improve symptoms in many patients, abrasion or drilling of subchondral bone does not benefit patients with OA of the knee, and may increase symptoms *(38)*. In addition, the short periods of follow-up; lack of well-defined evaluations of outcomes; lack of randomized, controlled trials; and the possibility for a significant placebo effect *(43)* or an improvement in symptoms owing to joint irrigation alone *(44–47)* make it difficult to define the indications for penetration of subchondral bone to stimulate formation of a new articular surface.

DECREASED ARTICULAR SURFACE-CONTACT STRESS

Several sets of observations suggest that decreased articular-surface contact stress combined with joint movement may stimulate restoration of an articular surface in osteoarthrotic joints. Before the development of artificial joints, surgeons found that resection of an osteoarthritic joint surface followed by decreased loading and joint motion resulted in the formation of fibrocartilagenous tissue over the bony surfaces *(9,16,48)*. When the surgeon resected the degenerated articular surfaces along with some underlying bone, the space between the bone surfaces filled with a fibrin clot, and then granulation tissue. Decreased loading and motion of resected joint facilitated formation of opposing fibrocartilagenous surfaces, immobilization and compression could lead to bony or fibrous ankylosis. Reports of the effects of releasing the muscles that act across degenerated hip joints in an attempt to decrease joint loading suggest that this procedure improved symptoms and increased the radiographic cartilage space in some patients (49–51); and, as noted in the discussion of osteotomies, examination of osteoarthrotic joints following osteotomies shows, in some instances, formation of a new articular surface.

Recently these observations concerning the effects of decreasing joint-contact pressures combined with motion have been supported by clinical studies of the effects of joint distraction and motion using external fixators. Aldegheri and colleagues used joint distraction that allowed joint motion to treat 80 patients with a variety of hip disorders (52). Twenty-four patients who either had inflammatory joint disease or were older than 45 yr had poor results, and only four patients over 45 yr of age had good results; however, 42 of 59 patients younger than 45 yr with OA, hip dysplasia, avascular necrosis, and chondrolysis had good results. These results suggest that, at least in people less than 45 yr of age, decreased contact pressure and motion of damaged hip-joint surfaces can decrease symptoms. A retrospective study by van Valburg and colleagues showed that joint distraction and motion treatment for patients with post-traumatic ankle osteoarthrosis produced favorable results (53). They treated advanced post-traumatic osteoarthrosis of the ankle with joint distraction in 11 patients (53). After application of an Ilizarov device, the authors distracted the joints 0.5 mm/d for 5 d and then maintained the distraction of the articular surfaces throughout the course of treatment. Patients were allowed to walk a few days after the operation, active joint motion was started between 6 and 12 wk after surgery. After 12–22 wk, the distraction device was removed. At an average of 20 mo after treatment, none of the patients had proceeded with an arthrodesis: all 11 patients had less pain, and 5 were pain-free; 6 had more motion; and, 3 of 6 that had radiographic studies had increased joint space. Subsequently, the same group of investigators treated 17 patients with advanced ankle OA with joint distraction for 3 mo. Thirteen of these patients had decreased pain and improved function more than 2 yr after treatment, four patients did not improve. Although these reports have important limitations (54), the symptomatic improvement and delay, if not avoidance, of arthrodesis in most patients indicates that distraction or other methods of decreasing joint-contact forces combined with motion deserve further evaluation.

SOFT-TISSUE GRAFTS

The potential benefits of soft-tissue grafts include introduction of a new cell population along with an organic matrix, a decrease in the probability of anklyosis before a new articular surface can form, and some protection of the graft or host cells from excessive loading. Treatment of osteoarthrotic joints by soft-tissue grafts involves debriding the joint and interposing soft-tissue grafts consisting of fascia, joint capsule, muscle, tendon, periosteum, or perichondrium between debrided or resected articular surfaces (9,55–60). The success of soft-tissue arthroplasty depends not only on the severity of the joint abnormalities and the type of graft, but on postoperative motion to facilitate generation of a new articular surface (11,55,56).

Animal experiments and clinical experience show that perichondrial and periosteal grafts placed in articular cartilage defects can produce new cartilage *(9,11)*. O'Driscoll has described the use of periosteal grafts for the treatment of isolated chondral and osteochondral defects, and in preliminary evaluation of a small series of patients he has found good or excellent results in more than three-quarters of the patients *(8,11,55,56)*. Other investigators have reported encouraging results with perichondrial grafts *(61,62)*. One study suggests that increasing patient age adversely affects the results of soft-tissue grafts. Seradge et al. studied the results of rib perichondrial arthroplasties in 16 metacarpophalangeal joints and 20 proximal interphalangeal joints at a minimum of 3 yr following the procedure *(63)*. Despite the small number of patients and joints, the results suggested that increasing age adversely affected the results for both metacarpalphalangeal and interphalangeal joints. Among the patients who had had an arthroplasty of the metacarpalphalageal joint, all three who were less than 20 yr old, three of four who were between 20 and 30, and only three of six who were more than 30 had a good result. Of the patients who had an arthroplasty of the interphalangeal joint, four of five who were less than 20, four of six who were between 20 and 30 and only one of three who was more than 30 yr old had a good result. None of the patients older than 40 yr had a good result with either type of arthroplasty. The authors concluded that perichondrial arthroplasty could be used for treatment of post-traumatic osteoarthrosis of the metacarpophalangeal joint and proximal interphalangeal joints of the hand in young patients.

The clinical observation that perichondrial grafts produced the best results in younger patients *(63)* agrees with the concept that age may adversely affect the ability of undifferentiated cells or chondrocytes to form an articular surface or that with age the population of cells that can form an articular-surface declines *(42)* and the evidence that with increasing age chondrocyte synthetic activity and response to anabolic growth factors decline *(64)*. The age-related differences in the ability of cells to form a new articular surface may also help explain some of the variability in the results of other procedures including osteotomies or procedures that penetrate subchondral bone; that is, younger people may have greater potential to produce a more effective articular surface when all other factors are equal *(64,65)*.

CELL TRANSPLANTATION

The limited ability of host cells to restore articular surfaces *(1,16)* has led investigators to seek methods of transplanting cells that can form cartilage into chondral and osteochondral defects *(66)*. Experimental work has shown that both chondrocytes and undifferentiated mesenchymal cells placed in articular cartilage defects survive and produce a new cartilage matrix *(9)*. Wakitani and associates estimated that hyaline cartilage developed in 75% of 40 rabbit osteochondral defects treated with allograft articular chondrocytes embedded in collagen gels while only fibrocartilage developed 24 control defects *(67)*. Other investigators have reported similar results with chondrocyte transplantation *(68–72)*. Brittberg and colleagues compared the results of treating chondral defects in rabbit patellar articular surfaces with periosteal grafts alone, carbon-fiber scaffolds and periosteum, autologous chondrocytes and periosteum and autologous chondrocytes, carbon-fiber scaffolds and periosteum *(73,74)*. They reported that the addition of autologous chondrocytes improved the histologic quality and amount of repair tissue. Other studies have shown that mesenchymal cells aspirated from bone can produce cartilagenous tissue in goats *(75)* and that cultured mesenchymal stem cells can repair large osteochondral defects in rabbits *(76,77)*.

In addition to these animal experiments, a group of investigators has reported using autologous chondrocyte transplants for treatment of localized cartilage defects in patients *(78,79)*. The investigators harvested chondrocytes from the patients, cultured the cells for 14–21 d, and then injected them into the area of the defect and covered them with a flap of periosteum. At two or more years following chondrocyte transplantation, 14 of 16 patients with condylar defects and 2 of 7 patients with patellar defects had good or excellent clinical results. Biopsies of the defect sites showed hyaline like cartilage in 11 of 15 femoral and one of seven patellar defects. More recently this group of investigators has reported the results in a larger groups of patients *(8,79)*. They found that 92% (23 of 25) patients with an average age of 32.2 yr had improved function at 2 yr or more after treatment for isolated articular-surface defects of femoral condyle. These results suggest that chondrocyte transplantation combined with a periosteal graft can promote restoration of an articular surface in humans, but more work is needed to assess the function and durability of the new tissue and determine if it improves joint function and delays or prevents joint degeneration, and if this approach will be beneficial in osteoarthritic joints *(66)*. Futhermore, as with other methods of promoting articular cartilage repair, with increasing age the potential for repairing articular cartilage may decline *(64,65)*.

GROWTH FACTORS

Growth factors influence a variety of cell activities including proliferation, migration, matrix synthesis and differentiation. Many of these factors, including the fibroblast growth factors (FGFs), insulin-like growth factors (IGFs) and transforming growth factor β (TGF-β), have been shown to affect chondrocyte metabolism and chondrogenesis *(5,9,80)*. Bone matrix contains a variety of these molecules including TGF-β, IGFs, bone morphogenic proteins, platelet-derived growth factors, and others *(5,81)*. In addition, mesenchymal cells, endothelial cells, and platelets produce many of these factors. Thus, osteochondral injuries and exposure of bone owing to loss of articular cartilage may release these agents that affect the formation of cartilage-repair tissue, and they probably have an important role in the formation of new articular surfaces after currently used operative procedures including resection arthroplasty, penetration of subchondral bone, soft-tissue grafts, and possibly osteotomies.

Local treatment of chondral or osteochondral defects with growth factors has the potential to stimulate restoration of an articular-surface superior to that formed after penetration of subchondral bone alone, especially in joints with normal alignment and range of motion and with limited regions of cartilage damage. A recent experimental study of the treatment of partial-thickness cartilage defects with enzymatic digestion of proteoglycans that inhibit adhesion of cells to articular cartilage followed by implantation of a fibrin matrix and timed release of TGF-β showed that this growth factor can stimulate cartilage repair *(82,83)*. The cells that filled the chondral defects migrated into the defects from the synovium and formed a fibrous matrix. Another study showed that treatment of experimental osteochondral defects in rabbit knees with a collagen sponge containing recombinant human bone morphogenetic protein improved the composition and appearance of the chondral repair tissue at 1 yr following treatment *(80)*. Despite the promise of this approach, the wide variety of growth factors, their multiple effects, the interactions among them, the possibility that the responsiveness of cells to growth factors may decline with age *(42,84,85)* and the limited understanding of their effects in osteoarthritic joints make it difficult to develop a simple strategy for using these agents to treat patients with osteoarthrosis. However, development of growth factor-based treatments for isolated chondral and osteochondral defects and early cartilage degenerative changes in younger people appears promising.

ARTIFICIAL MATRICES

Treatment of chondral defects with growth factors or cell transplants requires a method of delivering and in most instances at least temporarily stabilizing the growth factors or cells in the defect. For these reasons, the success of these approaches often depends on an artificial matrix. In addition, artificial matrices may allow, and in some instances stimulate ingrowth of host cells, matrix formation, and binding of new cells and matrix to host tissue *(86)*. Investigators have found that implants formed from a variety of biologic and nonbiologic materials including treated cartilage and bone matrices, collagens, collagens and hyaluronan, fibrin, carbon fiber, hydroxlyapatite, porous polylactic acid, polytetrafluoroethylene, polyester, and other synthetic polymers facilitate restoration of an articular surface *(2,9)*. Lack of studies that directly compare different types of artificial matrices makes it difficult to evaluate their relative merits, including the possibility that some implanted materials may cause synovitis *(87)*, but the available reports show that at least some types of artificial matrices can contribute to restoration of an articular surface. For example, in animal experiments, polyglycolic acid, collagen gels, and fibrin have proven to be effective ways of implanting cells and fibrin has been used to implant and allow timed release of a growth factor *(83,88–90)*. Treatment of osteochondral defects in rats and rabbits with carbon-fiber pads resulted in restoration of a smooth articular surface consisting of firm fibrous tissue that filled the pads *(91)*. Use of the same approach to treat osteochondral defects of the knee in humans produced a satisfactory result in 36 (77%) of 47 patients evaluated clinically and arthroscopically 3 yr after surgery *(91)*. Brittberg and colleagues also studied the use of carbon-fiber pads for treatment of articular-surface defects *(92)*. They found good or excellent results in 30 (83%) of 36 patients at an average of 4 yr after treatment.

CONCLUSIONS

A variety of methods have the potential to stimulate formation of a new articular surface including penetration of subchondral bone, osteotomies, joint distraction, soft-tissue grafts, cell transplantation, growth factors, and artificial matrices. The available evidence indicates that the results vary considerably among individuals, the potential for articular-cartilage repair declines with age and the tissue that forms following these treatments does not duplicate the composition, structure, and mechanical properties of normal articular cartilage. However, regeneration of normal articular may not be necessary for a procedure to be beneficial; in at least some instances stimulating formation of articular-cartilage repair tissue may decrease symptoms and improve joint function. Reports of the clinical results of procedures intended to restore a damaged or degenerated articular surface describe clinical improvement for a majority of the patients. Unfortunately these studies have serious limitations. The ages of patients treated and the types of articular-surface defects treated vary considerably. Some series included patients with advanced degenerative disease, whereas others only included patients with localized chondral defects in otherwise normal joints. None of them were controlled prospective studies and the lengths of follow-up and measures of outcome vary, thus it is difficult to compare the efficacy of these approaches to articular cartilage restoration. Nonetheless, review of the results of these procedures provides considerable insight into the potential for restoration of articular surfaces. Thus far none of these methods have been shown to predictably restore a durable articular surface in an osteoarthrotic joint, and it is unlikely that any one of them will be uniformly successful in the restoration of osteoarthrotic articular surfaces. Instead, the available clinical and experimental evidence indicates that future methods of restoring articular surfaces will begin with a detailed analysis of the structural and functional abnormalities of the involved joint, and the patient's expectations for future joint use. Based on this analysis, the surgeon will develop a treatment plan that potentially combines correction of mechanical abnormalities (including malalignment, instability, and intra-articular causes of mechanical dysfunction), debridement that may nor may not include limited penetration of subchondral bone, and applications of growth factors or implants that may consist of a synthetic matrix that incorporates cells or growth factors or transplants followed by a post-operative course of controlled loading and motion.

REFERENCES

1. Buckwalter, J.A., L.A. Rosenberg, and E.B. Hunziker. 1990. Articular cartilage: Composition, structure, response to injury, and methods of facilitation repair. *In* Articular Cartilage and Knee Joint Function: Basic Science and Arthroscopy. J.W. Ewing, editor. Raven Press, New York. 19–56.

2. Buckwalter, J.A. and H.J. Mankin. 1997. Articular cartilage II. Degeneration and osteoarthrosis, repair, regeneration and transplantation. *J. Bone Joint Surg.* 79A:612–632.

3. Buckwalter, J.A. 1997. Were the Hunter brothers wrong? Can surgical treatments repair articular cartilage. *Iowa Ortho. J.* 17:1–13.

4. Woo, S.L.-Y. and J.A. Buckwalter. 1988. Preface. *In* Injury and Repair of the Musculoskeletal Soft Tissues. S.L.-Y. Woo, and J.A. Buckwalter, editors. American Academy of Orthopaedic Surgeons, Park Ridge, IL.

5. Buckwalter, J.A., T.A. Einhorn, M.E. Bolander, and R.L. Cruess. 1996. Healing of musculoskeletal tissues. *In* Fractures. C.A. Rockwood, and D. Green, editors. Lippincott. Philadelphia. 261–304.

6. Buckwalter, J.A., V.C. Mow, and A. Ratliff. 1994. Restoration of injured or degenerated articular surfaces. *J. Am. Acad. Ortho. Surg.* 2:192–201.

7. Buckwalter, J.A. 1996. Regenerating articular cartilage: why the sudden interest? *Orthopaedics Today* 16:4–5.

8. Buckwalter, J.A. 1996. Cartilage researchers tell progress: Technologies hold promise, but caution urged. *Am. Acad. Ortho. Surg. Bull.* 44(2):24–26.

9. Buckwalter, J.A. and S. Lohmander. 1994. Operative treatment of osteoarthrosis: current practice and future development. *J. Bone Joint Surg.* 76A:1405–1418.

10. Messner, K. and J. Gillquist. 1996. Cartilage repair: a critical review. *Acta Orthop. Scand.* 67:523–529.

11. Salter, R.B. 1993. Continuous Passive Motion CPM: A Biological Concept for the Healing and Regeneration of Articular Cartilage, Ligaments and Tendons, from Original Research to Clinical Applications. Williams and Wilkins, Baltimore. 419.

12. Salter, R.B., D.B. Simmons, B.W. Malcolm, E.J. Rumble, D. MacMichael, and N.D. Clements. 1980. The biological effect of continuous passive motion on the healing of full-thickness defects in articular cartilage: an experimental investigation in the rabbit. *J. Bone Joint Surg.* 62A:1232–1251.

13. Moran, M.E., H.K. Kim, and R.B. Salter. 1992. Biological resurfacing of full-thickness defects in patellar articular cartilage of the rabbit. Investigation of autogenous periosteal grafts subjected to continuous passive motion. *J. Bone Joint Surg.* 74A:659–667.

14. Buckwalter, J.A. 1995. Activity vs. rest in the treatment of bone, soft tissue and joint injuries. *Iowa Orthop. J.* 15:29–42.

15. Buckwalter, J.A. 1995. Should bone, soft-tissue and joint injuries be treated with rest or activity? *J. Orthop. Res.* 13:155–156.

16. Buckwalter, J.A. and V.C. Mow. 1992. Cartilage Repair in Osteoarthritis. *In* Osteoarthritis: Diagnosis and Management 2nd ed. R.W. Moskowitz, D.S. Howell, V.M. Goldberg, and H.J. Mankin, editors. W.B. Saunders, Philadephia. 71–107.

17. Buckwalter, J.A. 1992. Mechanical Injuries of Articular Cartilage. *In* Biology and Biomechanics of the Traumatized Synovial Joint. G. Finerman, editor. American Academy of Orthopaedic Surgeons, Park Ridge, IL. 83–96.

18. Buckwalter, J.A. and J.A. Martin. 1995. Degenerative joint disease. *In* Clinical Symposia, vol. 47. Ciba Geigy, Summit, NJ. 2–32.

19. Levy, A.S., J. Lohnes, S. Sculley, M. LeCroy, and W. Garrett. 1996. Chondral delamination of the knee in soccer players. *Am. J. Sports Med.* 24:634–639.

20. Mankin, H.J. and J.A. Buckwalter. 1996. Restoring the osteoarthritic joint. *J. Bone Joint Surg.* 78A:1–2.

21. Messner, K. and W. Maletius. 1966. The long-term prognosis for severe damage to weight-bearing cartilage in the knee. A 14-year clinical and radiographic follow-up in 28 young athletes. *Acta Orthop. Scand.* 67:165–168.

22. Maletius, W. and K. Messner. 1996. The effect of partial menisectomy on the long-term prognosis of knees with localized severe chondral damage. A twelve- to fifteen-year follow-up. *Am. J. Sports Med.* 24:258–262.

23. Johnson, L.L. 1996. Arthroscopic arbrasion arthroplasty. *In* Operative Arthroscopy. J.B. McGinty, editor. Lippincott-Raven, Philadelphia. 427–446.

24. Shapiro, F., S. Koide, and M.J. Glimcher. 1993. Cell origin and differentiation in the repair of full-thickness defects of articular cartilage. *J. Bone Joint Surg.* 75A:532–553.

25. Johnson, L.L. 1986. Arthroscopic abrasion arthroplasty. Historical and pathologic perspective: present status. *Arthroscopy.* 2:54–59.

26. Johnson, L.L. 1990. The sclerotic lesion: Pathology and the clinical response to arthroscopic abrasion arthroplasty. Chap 22. *In* Articular Cartilage and Knee Joint Function. Basic Science and Arthroscopy. J.W. Ewing, editor. Raven Press, New York. 319–333.

27. Bentley, G. 1978. The surgical treatment of chondromalacia patellae. *J. Bone Joint Surg.* 60B:74–81.

28. Haggart, G.E. 1940. The surgical treatment of degenerative arthritis of the knee joint. *J. Bone Joint Surg.* 22:717–729.

29. Insall, J. 1974. The Pridie debridement operation for osteoarthritis of the knee. *Clin. Orthop.* 101: 61–67.

30. Magnuson, P.B. 1941. Joint debridement: surgical treatment of degenerative arthritis. *Surg. Gynecol. Obstet.* 73:1–9.

31. Ficat, R.P., C. Ficat, P.K. Gedeon, and J.B. Toussaint. 1979. Spongialization: a new treatment for diseased patellae. *Clin. Orthop.* 144:74–83.

32. Steadman, J.R., W.G. Rodkey, S.B. Singleton, and K.K. Briggs. 1997. Microfracture technique for full-thickness chondral defects: technique and clinical results. *Operative Tech. Orthopaed.* 7:294–299.

33. Friedman, M.J., D.O. Berasi, J.M. Fox, W.D. Pizzo, S.J. Snyder, and R.D. Ferkel. 1984. Preliminary results with abrasion arthroplasty in the osteoarthritic knee. *Clin. Orthop.* 182:200–205.

34. Ewing, J.W. 1990. Arthroscopic treatment of degenerative meniscal lesions and early degenerative arthritis of the knee. Chap. 9. *In* Articular Cartilage and Knee Joint Function. Basic Science and Arthroscopy. J.W. Ewing, editor. Raven Press, New York. 137–145.

35. Sprague, N.F. 1981. Arthroscopic debridement for degenerative knee joint disease. *Clin. Orthop.* 160:118–123.

36. Baumgaertner, M.R., W.D. Cannon, J.M. Vittori, E.S. Schmidt, and R.C. Maurer. 1990. Arthroscopic debridement of the arthritic knee. *Clin. Orth. Rel. Res.* 253:197–202.

37. Bert, J.M. and K. Maschka. 1989. The arthroscopic treatment of unicompartmental gonarthoisis. *J. Arthroscopy* 5:25.

38. Bert, J.M. 1993. Role of abrasion arthroplasty and debridement in the management of osteoarthritis of the knee. *Rheum. Dis. Clin. North Am.* 19:725–739.

39. Mitchell, N. and N. Shepard. 1976. The resurfacing of adult rabbit articular cartilage by multiple perforations through the subchondral bone. *J. Bone Joint Surg.* 58A:230–233.

40. Fenkel, S.R., D.S. Menche, B. Blair, N.F. Watnik, B.C. Toolan, and M.I. Pitman. 1994. A comparison of abrasion burr arthroplasty and subchondral drilling in the treatment of full-thickness cartilage lesions in the rabbit. *Trans. Ortho. Res. Soc.* 19:483.

41. Kumai, T., Y. Takakura, I. Higashiyama, and S. Tamai. 1999. Arthroscopic drilling for the treatment of osteochondral lesions of the talus. *J. Bone Joint Surg.* 81A:1229–1235.

42. Buckwalter, J.A., S.L.-Y. Woo, V.M. Goldberg, E.C. Hadley, F. Booth, T.R. Oegema, and D.R. Eyre. 1993. Soft tissue aging and musculoskeletal function. *J. Bone Joint Surg.* 75A:1533–1548.

43. Moseley, J.B., N.P. Wray, D. Kuykendall, K. Willis, and G.C. Landon. 1996. Arthroscopic treatment of osteoarthritis of the knee: a prospective, randomized, placebo-controlled trail: results of a pilot study. *Am. J. Sports Med.* 24:28–34.

44. Gibson, J.N.A., M.D. White, V.M. Chapman, and R.K. Strachan. 1992. Arthroscopic lavage and debridement for osteoarthritis of the knee. *J. Bone Joint Surg.* 74B:534–537.

45. Livesley, P.J., M. Doherty, M. Needoff, and A. Moulton. 1991. Arthroscopic lavage of osteoarthritic knees. *J. Bone Joint Surg.* 73B:922–926.

46. Chang, R.W., J. Falconer, S.D. Stulberg, W.J. Arnold, L.M. Manheim, and A.R. Dyer. 1993. A randomized, controlled trial of arthroscopic surgery versus closed-needle joint lavage for patients with osteoarthritis of the knee. *Arthritis Rheum.* 36:289–296.

47. Edelson, R., R.T. Burks, and R.D. Bloebaum. 1995. Short-term effects of knee washout for osteoarthritis. *Am. J. Sports Med.* 23:345–349.

48. Hass, J. 1944. Functional arthroplasty. *J. Bone Joint Surg.* 26:297–306.

49. Mensor, M.C. and M. Scheck. 1968. Review of six years experience with the hanging hip operation. *J. Bone Joint Surg.* 50A:1250–1254.

50. Radin, E.L., P. Maquet, and H. Park. 1975. Rationale and indications for the "hanging hip" procedure. A clinical and experimental study. *Clin. Orthop.* 112:221–230.

51. Scheck, M. 1970. Roentgenographic changes of the hip joint following extra-articular operations for dgenerative arthritis. *J. Bone Joint Surg.* 52A:99–104.

52. Aldegheri, R., G. Trivella, and M. Saleh. 1994. Articulated distraction of the hip. *Clin. Orthop. Rel. Res.* 301:94–101.

53. van-Valburg, A.A., P.M.v. Roermund, J. Lammens, J.v. Melkebeek, A.J. Verbout, F.P.J.G. Lafeber, and J.W.J. Bijlsma. 1995. Can Ilizarov joint distraction delay the need for an arthrodesis of the ankle? A preliminary report. *J. Bone Joint Surg.* 77A:720–725.

54. Buckwalter, J.A. 1996. Joint distraction for osteoarthritis. *Lancet* 347:279–280.

55. O'Driscoll, S.W., F.W. Keeley, and R.B. Salter. 1988. Durability of regenerated articular cartilage produced by free autogenous periosteal grafts in major full-thickness defects in joint surfaces under the influence of continuous passive motion. *J. Bone Joint Surg.* 70A:595–606.

56. O'Driscoll, S.W. and R.B. Salter. 1986. The repair of major osteochondral defects in joint surfaces by neochondrogenesis with autogenous osteoperiosteal grafts stimulated by continuous passive motion: An experimental investigation in the rabbit. *Clin. Orthop.* 208:131.

57. Ostgaard, S.E. and A. Weilby. 1993. Resection arthroplasty of the proximal interphalangeal joint. *J. Hand Surg.* 18B:613–615.

58. Hoikka, V.E., H.J. Jaroma, and V.A. Ritsila. 1990. Reconstruction of the patellar articulation with periosteal grafts. Four year follow-up of 13 cases. *Acta Ortho. Scand.* 61:36–39.

59. Jensen, L.J. and K.L. Bach. 1992. Periosteal transplantation in the treatment of osteochondritis dissecans. *Scan. J. Med. Sci. Sports.* 2:32–36.

60. Niedermann, B., S. Boe, J. Lauritzen, and J.M. Rubak. 1985. Glued periosteal grafts in the knee. *Acta Ortho. Scand.* 56:457–460.

61. Homminga, G.N., S.K. Bulstra, P.M. Bouwmeester, and A.J.V.D. Linden. 1990. Perichondrial grafting for cartilage lesions of the knee. *J. Bone Joint Surg.* 72 B:1003–1007.

62. Engkvist, O. and S.H. Johansson. 1980. Perichondrial arthroplasty: a clinical study in twenty-six patients. *Scand. J. Plast. Reconstr. Surg.* 14:71–87.

63. Seradge, H., J.A. Kutz, H.E. Kleinert, G.D. Lister, T.W. Wolff, and E. Atasoy. 1984. Perichondrial resurfacing arthroplasty in the hand. *J. Hand Surg.* 9A:880–886.

64. Martin, J.A., S.M. Ellerbroek, and J.A. Buckwalter. 1997. The age-related decline in chondrocyte response to insulin-like growth factor-I: the role of growth factor binding proteins. *J. Ortho. Res.* 15: 491–498.

65. Martin, J.A. and J.A. Buckwalter. 1996. Articular cartilage aging and degeneration. *Sports Med. Arthritis Rev.* 4:263–275.

66. Lohmander, L.S. 1998. Cell-based cartilage repair: do we need it, can we do it, is it good, can we prove it? *Curr. Opin. Orthoped.* 9:38–42.

67. Wakitani, S., T. Kimura, A. Hirooka, T. Ochi, M. Yoneda, N. Natsuo, et al. 1989. Repair of rabbit articular surfaces with allograft chondrocytes embedded in collagen gel. *J. Bone Joint Surg.* 71B:74–80.

68. Itay, S., A. Abramovici, and Z. Nevo. 1987. Use of cultured embryonal chick epiphyseal chondrocytes as grafts for defects in chick articular cartilage. *Clin. Orthop.* 220:284–303.

69. Itay, S., A. Abramovici, Z. Ysipovitch, and Z. Nevo. 1988. Correction of defects in articular cartilage by implants of cultures of embryonic chondrocytes. *Trans. Orthop. Res. Soc.* 13:112.

70. Noguchi, T., M. Oka, M. Fujino, M. Neo, and T. Yamamuro. 1994. Repair of osteochondral defects with grafts of cultured chondrocytes. Comparison of allografts and isografts. *Clin. Ortho. Rel. Res.* 302:251–258.

71. Robinson, D., N. Halperin, and Z. Nevo. 1990. Regenerating hyaline cartilage in articular defects of old chickens using implants of embryonal chick chondrocytes embedded in a new natural delivery substance. *Calcif. Tissue Int.* 46:246–253.

72. Shortkroff, S., L. Barone, H.P. Hsu, C. Wrenn, T. Gagne, T. Chi, et al. 1996. Healing of chondral and osteochondral defects in a canine model: the role of cultured chondrocytes in regeneration of articular cartilage. *Biomaterials* 17:147–154.

73. Brittberg, M., A. Nilsson, A. Lindahl, C. Ohlsson, and L. Peterson. 1996. Rabbit articular cartilage defects treated with autologous cultured chondrocytes. *Clin. Ortho. Rel. Res.* 326:270–283.

74. Brittberg, M. 1996. Cartilage Repair. Goteborg University, Sweden.

75. Butnariu-Ephrat, M., D. Robinson, D.G. Mendes, N. Halperin, and Z. Nevo. 1996. Resurfacing of goat articular cartilage by chondrocytes derived from bone marrow. *Clin. Ortho. Rel. Res.* 330: 234–243.

76. Wakitani, S., T. Goto, S.J. Pineda, R.G. Young, J.M. Mansour, A.I. Caplan, and V.M. Goldberg. 1994. Mesenchymal cell-based repair of large, full-thickness defects of articular cartilage. *J. Bone Joint Surg.* 76A:579–592.

77. Wakitani, S., T. Goto, J.M. Mansour, V.M. Goldberg, and A.I. Caplan. 1994. Mesenchymal stem cell-based repair of a large articular cartilage and bone defect. *Trans. Ortho. Res. Soc.* 19:481.

78. Brittberg, M., A. Lindahl, A. Nilsson, C. Ohlsson, O. Isaksson, and L. Peterson. 1994. Treatment of deep cartilage defects in the knee with autologous chondrocyte transplantation. *New Engl. J. Med.* 331:889–895.

79. Peterson, L., T. Minas, M. Brittberg, A. Nilsson, E. Sjogren-Jansson, and A. Lindahl. 2000. Two- to 9-year outcome after autologous chondrocyte transplantation of the knee. *Clin. Ortho. Rel. Res.* 374:212–234.

80. Sellers, R.S., R. Zhang, S.S. Glasson, H.D. Kim, D. Peluso, D.A. D'Augusta, K. Beckwith, and E.A. Morris. 2000. Repair of articular cartilage defects on year after treatment with recombinant human bone morphogenetic protein-2 (rhBMP-2). *J. Bone Joint Surg.* 82A:151–160.

81. Buckwalter, J.A., M.M. Glimcher, R.R. Cooper, and R. Recker. 1995. Bone biology II. formation, form, modeling and remodeling. *J. Bone Joint Surg.* 77A:1276–1289.

82. Hunziker, E.B. and L.C. Rosenberg. 1996. Repair of partial-thickness defects in articular cartilage: cell recruitment from the synovial membrane. *J. Bone Joint Surg.* 78A:721–733.

83. Hunziker, E.B. and R. Rosenberg. 1994. Induction of repair partial thickness articular cartilage lesions by timed release of TGF-Beta. *Trans. Ortho. Res. Soc.* 19:236.

84. Martin, J.A. and J.A. Buckwalter. 1996. Fibronectin and cell shape affect age related decline in chondrocyte synthetic response to IGF-I. *Trans. Ortho. Res. Soc.* 21:306.

85. Pfeilschifter, J., I. Diel, K. Brunotte, A. Naumann, and R. Ziegler. 1993. Mitogenic responsiveness of human bone cells in vitro to hormones and growth factors decreases with age. *J. Bone Miner Res.* 8:707–717.

86. Paletta, G.A., S.P. Arnoczky, and R.G. Warren. 1992. The repair of osteochondral defects using an exogenous fibrin clot. An experimental study in dogs. *Am. J. Sports Med.* 20:725–731.

87. Messner, K. and J. Gillquist. 1993. Synthetic implants for the repair of osteochondral defects of the medial femoral condyle: a biomechanical and histological evaluation in the rabbit knee. *Biomaterials* 14:513–521.

88. Freed, L.E., D.A. Grande, Z. Lingbin, J. Emmanual, J.C. Marquis, and R. Langer. 1994. Joint resurfacing using allograft chondrocytes and synthetic biodegradable polymer scaffolds. *J. Biomed. Materials Res.* 28:891–899.

89. Sams, A.E. and A.J. Nixon. 1995. Chondrocyte-laden collagen scaffolds for resurfacing extensive articular cartilage defects. *Osteoarthritis Cartilage* 3:47–59.

90. Hendrickson, D.A., A.J. Nixon, D.A. Grande, R.J. Todhunter, R.M. Minor, H. Erb, and G. Lust. 1994. Chondrocyte-fibrin matrix transplants for resurfacing extensive articular cartilage defects. *J. Ortho. Res.* 12:485–497.

91. Muckle, D.S. and R.J. Minns. 1990. Biological response to woven carbon fiber pads in the knee: A clinical and experimental study. *J. Bone Joint Surg.* 72B:60–62.

92. Brittberg, M., E. Faxen, and L. Peterson. 1994. Carbon fiber scaffolds in the treatment of early knee osteoarthritis. *Clin. Ortho. Rel. Res.* 307:155–164.

15

Using Molecular Markers to Monitor Osteoarthritis

Ivan G. Otterness and Mary J. Saltarelli

CONTENTS

INTRODUCTION

The diagnosis of osteoarthritis (OA) is currently based on clinical presentation and radiographic signs. However, because radiographic diagnosis is based on decreased joint space, it detects disease only after considerable cartilage damage has occurred. Yet, there is only a modest correlation between the extent of structural damage in the osteoarthritic joint and the pain and functional impairment that causes the patient to seek treatment. Still, there remains a fundamental belief that if further joint damage could be prevented, disease progression would be stopped, and if joint damage could be reversed, functionality would be restored. All of this means that a method of measuring disease activity in OA is critically important for rationalizing treatment of OA. A knowledge of disease activity is required for determining the need of treatment, the mode of treatment and the effectiveness of treatment. Ideally, this is a role for a molecular marker.*

Several recent reviews have discussed potential molecular markers for OA *(1–6)*. The marker measurement need not be particularly precise in its correlation with disease

---

*The terms bio-, biochemical, and molecular have been used as adjectives to describe the markers used to monitor OA. Although in the broad sense, all processes are biological, our measurements are not biological measurements, but are molecular measurements. These endpoints may be biochemical in nature (enzymatically driven, for example) or they may occur because of physical processes—tissue failure or inappropriate loading. We favor the term molecular marker because the marker is being used to monitor molecular events taking place without specifying the process.

From: *Modern Therapeutics in Rheumatic Diseases*
Edited by: G. C. Tsokos, et al. © Humana Press, Inc., Totowa, NJ

activity. The important criteria is that the marker be elevated when the patient is in need of therapy and that effective therapy reduces the marker to a near normal level. Moreover, rebound of the disease should be associated with rebound of the marker.

It is necessary to clarify what is meant by disease activity. To do so, we must add a complementary term: disease status. Disease status defines the patient's current state, in effect the accumulation of disease changes. For OA, disease status means the cartilage, subchondral bone, ligament, meniscal, and soft-tissue status. To this is added an assessment of the joint in terms of function and pain. Disease activity is by contrast a measure of the rate of pathological change.* It has an element of prognostic importance: it suggests what future joint status might be if there is no intervention *(5)*. Thus high disease activity suggests a rapid deterioration, low disease activity suggests slow progression, and stable disease suggest little or no progression.

There is a great ambiguity in definition of both disease status and disease activity. Different choices made in forming a global measure of disease status or activity will emphasize different aspects of the disease and will give different perspectives. Each clinical measure is a disease status indicator and the interpretation of disease status is different depending on whether status is assessed by walking ability, X-ray, magnetic resonance imaging (MRI), or visual analog scale (VAS). The relationship between clinical measures and how best they should be weighted in a global measure of disease status is a subject of considerable debate. Disease progression is commonly measured by change in disease status over a fixed time period, for example, X-rays over a 1- or 2-yr period, MRI or arthroscopy over 6–12 mo, or VAS measurements over 6–12 mo. Thus, the construction of a best measure of disease progression is a matter of considerable debate. Nonetheless, we live in a practical world, and practical determinations of joint status and disease progression are routinely made. Disease activity is simply the rate of disease progression. Ideally, the disease activity, i.e., the daily or hourly rates of disease progression, could be multiplied by the appropriate time interval and the disease progression determined. Here we use the terms disease status and disease activity primarily to denote two distinct classes of information about a patients disease recognizing both the practical use of the concepts and the alternative choices available in their practical application. In general, the use of molecular markers is limited to the estimation of disease activity; molecular markers measure neither disease status nor disease progression.

Currently, there are no validated measures of disease activity for OA. Disease progression is used instead. X-ray measurements of disease progression are considered the gold standard. As X-rays have limited sensitivity, 1–2 yr between radiographs are required to define progression in the majority of patients. MRI may provide a more

---

*Disease activity may be viewed as closely related to disease progression. It is the rate of disease progression. We measure disease progression in OA as the difference between two measurements separated by an extended time period, e.g., 6 or 12 or more months. By disease activity we mean the rate of disease progression as if it were measured at a single moment in time. Thus conceptually, the average disease activity for each day would be summed over the number of days to compute disease progression for an interval. Moreover, within a day, there can be a circadian rhythm of disease activity.

timely structural measure of disease progression, but these techniques are at the present time highly experimental. Thus, it is critical that a good molecular marker of disease activity be found to guide application of therapy prior to severe, irreversible disease and to facilitate discovery and validation of therapy.

Classification of Molecular Markers for OA

To facilitate an understanding of the use of molecular markers, we have categorized them into groups in which markers play similar roles.

CARTILAGE MARKERS

OA is considered a disease of cartilage failure. The cartilage components that include the collagens (types II, VI, IX, and XI), aggrecan (link protein, core protein, keratan sulfate, chondroitin sulfate [CS]) and the cartilage-associated molecules (matrilin, cartilage oligomeric protein [COMP], fibulin, etc.) are responsible for the physical properties of cartilage. Monitoring the breakdown of cartilage components and measuring their remnants in body fluids gives the best chance of assessing disease activity in OA. When the breakdown product measured is from one of the cartilage components primarily responsible for its physical properties, there is a chance that the appearance of breakdown products will correlate with disease activity.

DISEASE PROCESS MARKERS

These are not cartilage components, but mediators or indicators of processes that can lead to further deterioration of joint status. Thus changes in the skeletal components—bone, ligament, tendon, synovial lining—can each contribute to the severity of OA, but they are not a direct indication of OA. Likewise, an elevation of stromelysin or collagenase in synovial fluid suggests their possible participation in cartilage breakdown, but the elevation does not prove they are involved. Elevated levels of cytokines or decreased growth factors or increased levels of shed receptors could all be taken as a sign of increased disease activity. However, none of these markers are specific for OA; they can be elevated in many other diseases. Nonetheless, their elevation in the presence of a diagnosis of OA is suggestive of increased disease activity.

GENETIC MARKERS

These markers define genetic haplotypes that could predispose to or determine the occurrence of OA because of changed cartilage properties. One example is the well-characterized type II collagen Arg519Cys mutant, in which 100% of carriers have early onset OA *(7,8)*. At this time, there are no proven genetic markers for common OA, although some candidate genes have been identified *(9–12)*. These markers could be prognostically useful.

EPIDEMIOLOGICAL MARKERS

Obesity has a well-documented detrimental effect on the joint *(13)*, and thus hormonal imbalances that are associated with obesity such as elevated insulin *(14,15)*, are associated with OA. Higher levels of estrogens *(16)* and vitamin D *(17)* have been shown to be associated with less OA progression. Such markers can provide important information related to the occurrence of OA, but are not primary indicators of disease activity.

IRRELEVANT MARKERS

Most markers are simply irrelevant to the course of OA. Some of the markers thought important today may end up in this category when our knowledge improves, and some of our current irrelevant markers may likewise later be found useful. The important point is that the classification of markers is based on our best current knowledge.

Technical Criteria for Good Molecular Markers of OA

There are several technical requirements for a sound marker assay that should be met before it can be usefully applied to clinical samples. The assay should be reproducible and the error between independent measurements low. The standard curve should be valid in an appropriate medium, i.e., synovial fluid, serum, or urine. The specimens should dilute properly (the same values should be obtained independent of dilution) over the useful measurement range. Nonlinear dilution or the presence of inhibitors severely compromises the utility of any assay. The assay needs sufficient sensitivity to make measurements in both the normal and OA patients. The analyte should be stable during long-term storage. If not, samples must be run immediately and this drastically limits the utility of the assay. There should be a good recovery of spiked samples, i.e., spiking should add an appropriate amount to existing sample. The standard curve should be linked to some recognizable standard so that values can be readily interpreted. Finally, the analyte should be isolated and structural proof obtained of what is being measured. This last point may not always be possible because of the low level of analyte or because of the complexity of the analyte.

Clinical Criteria for Good Molecular Markers of OA

Ideally, a molecular marker should be extracellular, specific to the site of disease activity and relevant to the disease. Although the measurement of an intracellular marker can be useful for some diseases, lactic dehydrogenase (LDH), for example, in myocardial infarct, typical intracellular proteins are often not cell-specific, and like LDH, they are most likely to measure cell death. Specificity for the disease site means the ability to specify the source of the marker. An elevation of decorin in blood may not be able to be related back to the joint, because of its common occurrence elsewhere in the body.

Diurnal variation in marker levels should be examined and if evident, taken into account. Finally, the analyte should be detectable without the need for concentration, and levels of this analyte should be stable in the absence of disease modifying therapy. It is also extremely important that a marker differentiates the OA population from the nonarthritic controls. If it can't readily distinguish OA patients from controls, then there is nothing to measure in cross-sectional studies.*

*The marker might still have used if it is elevated during a specific disease stage and so could be used to define that disease stage.

Discernable marker differences in marker levels between controls and OA patients gives the window of opportunity for making meaningful measurements. Each population has a mean (m) and a standard deviation (SD). With the 24 markers we have so far examined in detail *(18,19)* and unpublished, the distribution of marker values failed to conform to a normal probability distribution. The nonstandard distribution of these markers can be corrected by using transformed variables, i.e., logarithm of the value rather than the value itself.

$$Y = \log(X) = \Sigma \log(X_i)/N \qquad (1)$$

And where

$$\sigma^2 = \Sigma (\log(X_i) - \log(X))^2 /(N - 1) \qquad (2)$$

Equally important, there is a standard statistical formula for defining the number of patients that would be required to reject a null hypothesis (i.e., hypothesis of no difference) and thus state with a given degree of assurance that the control and that the OA populations are different. The formula can be approximated as:

$$N = C \cdot I^2 \cdot (\sigma/\Delta)^2 \qquad (3)$$

where σ (the standard deviation of the OA population), $C = 12.5$, and $\Delta = \mu_1 - \mu_2$ (the differences between the mean values of the control and the OA populations). The formula can be used to determine the number of patients that would have to be treated with drug to detect a return of marker back to control levels ($I = 1$, $p = 0.05$). This is by far the most optimistic scenario because it assumes that the treatment will restore the marker back to control level. If instead, the treatment gave only half ($I = 2$), a third ($I = 3$), or a fourth ($I = 4$) improvement in the marker, the required number of patients for statistical significance would increase tremendously leading to a serious deterioration in the utility of the marker.

That brings us to a further problem—the specification of the error between measurements (σ). The important value is the error between marker values determined from independent clinical measurements, i.e., between patient visits in stable patients. We have found that error measured as the coefficient of variation (σ/average) between 4–5 patient visits to be around 25% for the better markers and higher for the poorer ones in stable patients. This is much higher than the error between independent replicates 3–6% run on different days, which is again higher than the error between replicates of the sample in the same assay (0.5–2%). Lohmander et al. *(20)* have also estimated the "between visit error" for a large number of markers sampled at eight times over a year. Synovial-fluid markers displayed higher levels of within patient variability (18–71%) than did serum or urine markers.

Validation of Molecular Markers

Validation of molecular markers requires proven clinical performance as determined by correlation with X-ray imaging, MRI, or other measures of clinical outcome. Thus if the marker has prognostic power, an elevated value should predict a deterioration of the patients outcome. At an elementary level, a simple correlation with outcome does not guarantee that the marker is truly prognostic. When there is deterioration in clinical status, there can be many correlated variables that also deteriorate. Some are obligatorily linked to disease activity and others have only secondary linkage. Thus C-reactive protein (CRP) is elevated during OA, but reduction in CRP alone is of little prognostic importance. CRP might be elevated because of unrelated inflammatory conditions and a reduction of CRP could be unrelated to any improvement OA. Conversely, type II collagen provides the tensile strength of cartilage. Inhibition of its breakdown could have significant prognostic importance for OA. Thus simple correlation with outcome in epidemiological studies is insufficient to validate a marker. There must be accompanying experimental evidence to show linkage to the disease process.

An even more useful validation criteria is the demonstration that a change in a molecular marker towards normal is associated with disease improvement. Such a demonstration would likely require the application of therapy that would preserve the cartilage as determined by some outcome measure such as MRI imaging. Unfortunately, effective therapy is still lacking in OA and thus so is the most efficient means of validating markers. However, a cartilage marker of OA may also have utility in rheumatoid arthritis (RA), in which case, the marker could be responsive to the initiation of disease-modifying anti-rheumatic drugs (DMARD) therapy (MTX, Enbrel, Remicade, Arava). In appropriate situations, marker validation in RA could be meaningful for OA and help validate the clinical utility of an OA marker.

Importance of Site for Sampling the Molecular Marker

It makes a substantial difference which body fluid is sampled to measure the molecular marker. Synovial fluid is closest to the site of generation of markers from articular cartilage and its concentration and molecular form is thus most likely to reflect events in the cartilage. As the marker diffuses from the cartilage into the synovial fluid, it is unlikely to undergo extensive metabolism. Marker concentration in synovial fluid depends not only on the rate of its release from the cartilage, but on its rate of clearance.

If the marker is of low molecular weight (<15–20 kD), it will be rapidly cleared through the capillaries ($t_{1/2} < 1/2$ h) and enter the blood stream. If it is of higher molecular weight, it will be cleared more slowly by the lymphatics with a clearance rate of 2 h or longer depending on the synovial volume. Hyaluronan is an exception. It has a high reflectance from the synovial lymphatics and a much slower than expected clearance.

Once the marker enters the circulation, it will be diluted many-fold (a mL cleared from synovial fluid will be diluted into a >10 L blood volume). Moreover, it will be mixed with marker coming from other body compartments. The elevation of marker attributable to articular cartilage may be diminished or even completely hidden by the amounts of the marker coming from other body compartments. Once a molecular marker enters the blood stream, it passes through the liver and the kidney. Both are sites of metabolism for many markers. For some, metabolism will destroy the marker; for others, it will blur the direct relationship between tissue damage and marker level. Thus if one samples blood or urine, there is always the potential that what is measured will no longer be a direct measure of the OA process because of metabolism or dilution in fragments from other body compartments.

All these qualifications suggest that sampling the synovial fluid would be the best way to monitor disease. Unfortunately, it is not a routine clinical procedure. Furthermore, as disease status improves, synovial fluid becomes increasingly difficult to obtain. Thus it behooves the investigator to understand the metabolism of the molecular marker and the contributions from other body compartments to know whether marker changes are a valid measure of joint disease in OA.

Immunological Assays for Measurement of Molecular Markers

Most molecular markers are measured by antibody assay in which each antibody recognizes a specific molecular epitope. Conceptually, there are four distinct types of epitopes recognized by antibodies and we briefly describe them.

CONFORMATIONAL EPITOPES

Most proteins in their native structure are constrained by folding into a specific conformation. Thus, collagen imbedded into the triple helix has a very defined rigid conformation and epitopes on triple-helical collagen are recognized by antibodies. Because collagen is normally in the helical conformation in mature tissues, these anti-helical antibodies recognize the native structure. Conversely, antibodies against helical epitopes usually fail to recognize the same amino acids when they are in a simple polypeptide chain and not constrained to the rigid helical conformation.

SEQUENTIAL EPITOPES

Antibodies against short amino acid sequences rarely react with the native conformation. Such antibodies recognize epitopes in newly synthesized proteins, in proteins cleaved by proteases and in denatured proteins. Such epitopes have been termed "denatured epitopes," "linear epitopes," or "sequential epitopes." We favor the latter, e.g., sequential epitopes, because they are defined by a sequence of amino acids generally too short to fold into a defined conformation.

CLEAVAGE NEO (NEW) EPITOPES

These antibodies are directed to new sequences that arise when a protein has been cut by a protease to give new N-terminal and C-terminal sequences. With aggrecan, neo-epitope specificity has been achieved by focusing on the aggrecanase cleavage site -NITEGE and ARGSVIL-. Defining an antibody as a neoepitope antibody means fulfilling additional specificity criteria: The antibody must be selective for the cleavage sequence and fail to recognize the extended epitope (epitope + Xn) or contracted epitope (epitope − Xn) where Xn is from 1 to *n* amino acids of the native sequence. Thus for the aggrecan epitope ..NITEGE, the antibody must not recognize the extended epitope …NITEGEA or …NITEGEAR, etc., or the truncated epitopes …NITEG or …NITE.

MODIFIED EPITOPES

Sometimes amino acids are chemically modified in ways that make them recognizable. The Gla containing peptides from bone, the pentosidine crosslinks of collagen, the collagen glu-gal-hydroxylysine fragments in urine and the pyridinoline crosslinks are examples. The type I collagen pyridinoline crosslinks have found great utility for monitoring bone loss in osteoporosis. Thus far, the most useful modified epitopes for OA have been assays for the pyridinoline crosslinks of fibrillar collagen. Because pyridinoline crosslinks are found in all three fibrillar collagens, there must be sufficient amino acid sequence attached to the crosslink for a detection antibody to clearly distinguish type II from type I and type III crosslinks.

EPITOPE YIELD

Ideally, one mole of a molecule will yield a maximum of one mole of a unique epitope. The yield of an epitope may be less than that maximum for two reasons. First, generation of the epitope is incomplete, or second, the epitope once generated is further fragmented and destroyed by hepatic or renal metabolism. Thus, usually whatever is measured is a minimal estimate of epitope generation. Some epitopes do not conform to that statement. Some epitopes are repeated multiply on the same molecule (chondroitin sulfate, and keratan sulfate on aggrecan and gal-hydroxylysine on type II collagen).

Further, some epitopes (generally in the class of C- or N-terminal neoepitopes) may be generated only by cleavage at a unique proteolytic site. Thus, the collagenase C-terminal neoepitope arises after collagenase cleavage (21,22), the bone type I crosslink fragment NTX after cleavage by cathepsin K (23). Such neoepitopes provide evidence for the pathway of generation of the fragment, and measure the amount of molecules fragmented by that enzyme. They are not a measure of total molecular fragmentation when other pathways are involved.

A SURVEY OF MOLECULAR MARKERS APPLIED TO OA

Type II Collagen (Col2) Assays

Type II collagen is the major structural cartilage component and the major determinant of its physical properties. It provides cartilage's tensile strength and, by providing structure to the cartilage, allows the aggrecan to respond to compressive forces as if it were under confined compression. Measurement of its degradation should be expected to provide a useful measure of disease activity because it is related to the loss of cartilage's physical properties.

COL2 SEQUENTIAL EPITOPE ASSAYS

When col2 is denatured, it loses its helical conformation. Antibodies can be made to the nonhelical peptides that react only with sequential epitopes. Such assays can be used to demonstrate the presence of nonhelical col2 and thus suggest its physical properties have been compromised.

COL2 3/4 m Assay of Dodge et al. (24) and Hollander et al. (25). Dodge et al. (24), and Hollander et al. (25) have provided an assay of nonhelical col2 that they describe as denatured collagen. The assay is useful for examining cartilage pieces from autopsy or at joint replacement. Dodge et al. (26) demonstrated the presence of nonhelical col2 in RA cartilage using immunogold staining. Using the COL2 3/4m monoclonal inhibition enzyme-linked immunosorbent assay (ELISA), Hollander et al. (25) have shown that the collagen in OA cartilage is more denatured than that of control cartilage. The data can be interpreted to suggest there may be an upper limit on the amount of denaturation in cartilage: If too much denaturation occurs, the nonhelical regions are processed by other proteases and removed from the cartilage. Thus, this assay substantially underestimates the amount of fragmentation that has occurred over time because it only measures the remaining sequential epitope.

E1E5:L25 Assay of Barrach et al. Barrach et al. *(27,28)* developed two monoclonal antibodies (MAbs), E1E5 and L25, against CNBr peptides of type II collagen for use in a capture ELISA with a lower limit of sensitivity of about 100 pM of col2 fragment (standardized in terms of CNBr generated col2 fragments). In the Hulth-Telhag rabbit model of OA *(29)*, levels of col2 fragments in synovial fluids rose from negligible to 9, 26, and 55 nM at 3, 5, and 8 wk after surgery.

The levels of collagen peptides found in normal rabbit plasma decreased with age presumably reflecting the fall in growth-plate activity with age. In 1 kg rabbits, 19 nM of fragment was found. That fell to 1.36 nM in 2.9–3.5 kg and to 220 pM in 4 kg rabbits. They used 3.5–5.0 kg rabbits for the Hulth-Telhag model and found plasma levels of 600, 900, and 800 pM at 3, 5, and 8 wk post-surgery. Barrach et al. *(30)* also measured col2 fragments in human synovial fluid.

The E1E5:L25 assay has the ability to measure col2 fragments in SF and blood in severe disease. Its utility under those circumstances seems clear, but it has only rarely been used for routine OA samples. It needs more extensive evaluation so that its utility can be properly defined.

TYPE II COLLAGEN CROSSLINK ASSAYS

Eyre et al. *(31)* and Osteometer *(32)* have developed similar assays for type II collagen crosslinks. The type I collagen crosslinks have found great utility for monitoring bone loss in osteoporosis *(33)* and it is hoped this success can be repeated with type II in OA. In nature, there is about 0.5–0.8 moles of crosslink/mole of chain. With fragmentation of col2, the crosslinks are released. They are nearly completely metabolized and appear in urine as the isolated crosslink or as the crosslink with a few attached amino acids. In the absence of the attached amino acids, the bone collagen crosslinks are indistinguishable from those of cartilage. However, with attached amino acids, the col2 crosslinks are uniquely detected. Here the antibody specificity becomes exceedingly critical for the interpretation. If it is a cleavage-site neoepitope antibody, it may detect only cross linking generated by that particular protease; if it recognizes a sequential epitope, it may be recognized independent of proteolytic origin.

Col2 CTx Assay of Eyre and Colleagues Using the 2B4 Antibody to Measure col2 Crosslinks (CTx). Atley et al. *(34)* compared col2 CTx the in urine between controls and OA patients. Control levels were 30 ± 10.4 ng/mg creatinine (Cr). Those values rose to 42.2 ± 15.2 in patients with OA. In patients with only knee OA levels were 36.6 ± 8.8 and with generalized OA (knee plus 5–10 digits) were 51.9 ± 20.7 ng/mg Cr. To obtain a 50% reduction toward control (*p* = 0.05), it would take 135 patients with knee OA only, but only 35 patients with generalized OA. The fine specificity of the antibody has not been published.

Lohmander et al. *(35)* have examined release of col2 CTx in synovial fluid in patients with traumatic joint injury. Crosslink levels rise promptly from less than 2 ng/mL to 17 ng/mL after injury and fall to a still elevated value of around 8–10 ng/mL where they remain for over 2 yr.

These data from the 2B4 assay suggests it will be very easily to identify elevated crosslink level in synovial fluid and that it will, in addition, be useful for monitoring more severe forms of OA.

Col2 CTx (CTC-II) Crosslink Assay of Osteometer. Garnero et al. *(32)* measured urinary crosslink levels in controls, and patients with both destructive and nondestructive

RA. This appears to be a cleavage neoepitope assay, but the protease of origin is not yet identified. Values for CTC-II were 6.9 ± 2.2 for controls vs 9.2 ± 5.4 and 16.5 ± 10 nmol/mmol creatinine for nondestructive and destructive RA, respectively. CTC-II levels do not correlate with CRP levels in either OA or RA patients. In spite of the localized bone loss in destructive RA, col1 CTx was decreased where as CTC-II was significantly elevated in destructive RA. To validate that CTC-II and TI CTx were in fact measuring different crosslinks, they also studied two additional populations of people: CT-II was 6.2 ± 0.9 in pre- vs 7.5 ± 2.8 in post-menopausal women, essentially unchanged, whereas col1 CTx increased over 100%. In Paget's disease, col1 CTx increased 4X whereas CTC-II failed to significantly increase. In OA patients, they examined 67 OA patients and 67 healthy controls *(36)*. They found urinary CTC-II increased by 25%. Most interesting, of the markers they examined (COMP, col1 CTx, YKL-40, HA, CRP), only CTC-II correlated with cartilage loss as assessed by joint space area (r = −0.40, $p > 0.0002$).

Col2: Collagenase Neoepitope Assays

When collagenase cleaves col2 producing a 1/4 and 3/4 piece, a new C-terminal and a new N-terminal sequence are formed. The new N-terminal can be degraded further by enzymes such as collagenase 3 *(37,38)* and tryptic enzymes. The new C-terminal sequence appears stable to further cleavage and can be detected in cartilage and in collagen fragments released from cartilage. Billinghurst et al. *(21)* and Otterness et al. *(22)* have described C-terminal collagenase-generated neoepitope antibodies that can be used for assays of collagenase cleavage of col2 in cartilage (Stoop et al. *[39]*, Hueber et al. *[40]*, and Otterness et al. *[22]*).

COL2 3/4C Assay (Billinghurst et al. [21]). A rabbit polyclonal antibody (PAb) against the new cleavage product C-terminal sequence -GPOGPQG (3/4C short) was used to establish a competitive inhibition ELISA. Standard curves show detectable inhibition by peptide 3/4C at about 600 nM with maximum inhibition at about 100 μ*M*. Using the methodology of Hollander et al. *(25)* and Billinghurst et al. *(21)* extracted the 3/4C epitope from cartilage with chymotrypsin and determined its concentration in cartilage. The amounts of 3/4C in cartilage were higher in OA cartilage (9×10^{-3} mole 3/4C epitope/mole of collagen col2 α1 chain) vs 4×10^{-3} mole/mole in nonarthritic human cartilage. Interestingly, the amounts of 3/4C epitope were about 30% of the 3/4m epitope in cartilage. This assay remains to be developed for body fluids.

TIINE Assay (Otterness et al. [22,41]). Two MAbs were developed in order to generate a sandwich assay for the collagenase neoepitope. 9A4 is a collagenase cleavage-site neoepitope antibody directed against the sequence –GPPGPQG *(22)*. The capture antibody 5109 is directed against a highly charged sequence EPGDDGP *(41,42)*. The capture ELISA format detects peptide–GEPGDDGPSGAEGPPGPQG. A liquid-phase assay has been developed that gives equivalent standard curves for the proline and hydroxyproline containing sequences *(43)*.

The TIINE assay detects very significant neoepitope concentration differences in urine between OA patients and controls *(44)*. Young controls averaged 500 pM, OA patients averaged 1900 pM and age-matched controls for the OA patients averaged 1100 pM. Treatment of RA patients with methotrexate lowers TIINE levels *(43)*. Power calculations using log transformed values show that to detect a 50% lowering of TIINE levels toward age-matched controls would require 26 patients whereas lowering half-way to control levels would requires only 12 patients. Drug effects are detectable in individual patients. The TIINE method appears to have characteristics that will make it a useful clinical assay.

COLLAGEN BIOSYNTHESIS ASSAYS

The chondrocyte synthesizes the procollagen chains that form triple-helical collagen, secretes it, and then clips off the N- and C-terminal propeptides. Studies have shown that the rate of C-propeptide release is proportional to the rate of synthesis of new collagen molecules in tissue culture *(45)*. Assays have been developed for the propeptide of type II collagen by Hinek *(46,47)* and Shinmei *(48)*. Increased levels of C-propeptide have been found in synovial fluid of OA and joint-injury patients *(49)*. Increased release of C-propeptide fragments from cartilage of OA patients has also been shown *(50)*. However, the C-propeptide is decreased in serum from OA patients *(19,50)* indicating that the serum level does not reflect events in the cartilage, but rather must reflect a systemic metabolic process.

TYPE IX COLLAGEN IN SYNOVIAL FLUID

An early report suggests that type IX collagen fragments may be released into synovial fluid *(51)*. Except for a much lower concentration in cartilage, type IX collagen also has much the same selective cartilage distribution as type II collagen. Thus this might offer another avenue for attaining specificity for OA changes.

Aggrecan Assays

Aggrecan is made up of a large number of sulfated polysaccharides (keratan sulfate [KS] and chondroitin sulfate [CS]) on a protein core linked to high molecular-weight hyaluronan. This huge, highly charge complex when confined by type II collagen gives cartilage its resiliency under compression.

The release of charged sulfated polysaccharides into synovial fluid as been routinely detected in biochemical assays using the dye dimethylmethylene blue. However, to get more mechanistic information, MAbs have been used to examine the metabolic fate of aggrecan and its fragments.

CS ASSAYS

CS is the predominate charged sulfated polysaccharide in aggrecan, but it exists in other body compartments. Using the 3B3 MAb of Ratcliffe et al. *(52)* showed elevation CS after ACLT in the dog. 3B3 was also used by Hazell et al. *(53)* to show that CS is elevated in OA synovial fluid following knee injury. Glant et al. *(54)* isolated a monoclonal antibody 846 which is essentially absent in adult cartilage but appears in OA *(55)*. The 846 epitope is increased in synovial fluid following ACL rupture (0.61 U/mL), meniscal injury (0.53 U/mL) and in primary OA (0.68 U/mL) compared to controls (0.28 U/mL) *(56)*. However, the ranges were quite broad. The change in serum levels is small and unlikely to be useful except in large OA patient populations *(18,57)*.

KERATAN SULFATE ASSAYS (5D4 AND AN9P1)

Early measurements in synovial fluid of OA patients showed elevation of keratan sulfate (KS) using the 5D4 monoclonal antibody of Caterson *(58–60)*, but Hazell et al. *(53)* found a significant decrease with 5D4 in traumatic joint injury. KS is also elevated in experimental canine OA *(61)*. In a large cross-sectional study, Champion et al. *(60)* found mean levels of 393 ± 124 ng/mL in OA patients. Most studies with 5D4 show a modest increase in levels, but not all *(62)*. By contrast, Poole using the KS MAb AN9P1, has found the KS epitope to be elevated in synovial fluid and decreased in OA blood *(19,57)*. Because of the small differences between OA patients and controls when measurements are made in blood and because of the discrepancy between changes in blood and synovial fluid, the KS assays are not useful for routine monitoring of the sera of OA patients.

AGGRECAN CORE PROTEIN

Heinegard first developed PAbs against the core protein of aggrecan for use in monitoring release of aggrecan fragments into synovial fluid in a canine model of OA *(63)*. Saxne et al. *(64)* were able to show the lowering of aggrecan fragments in human synovial fluid after glucocorticoid treatment. The elevation of aggrecan fragments after joint injury was shown by Lohmander et al. *(65)* using PAbs to study joint fluids. Controls (athletes) had synovial-fluid levels around 36 µg/mL; which rose more than 10-fold in the week following joint injury and then fell with time, but remained above normal indefinitely. However, the average elevation was only doubled in established knee OA and showed a coefficient of variation of approx one *(66)*. The I-F21 monoclonal *(67)* detects a core fragment and interestingly, its level is correlated with the 5D4 detection of keratan sulfate in synovial fluid. It detects increased aggrecan fragments in both knee injury and primary OA, but again only in the synovial fluid *(56)*.

AGGRECAN NEOEPITOPE ASSAYS

Fragments of aggrecan core can be analyzed using neoepitope antibodies that recognize cleavage sites of specific proteinases. Aggrecanase cleaves aggrecan leaving the fragments ...$NITEGE_{373}$ and $A_{374}RGSVIL$... matrix metalloproteinases (MMPs) cleave leaving the fragments ...$VDIPEN_{341}$ and $F_{342}FGVG$... Hughes et al. *(68)* produced the aggrecanase neoepitope antibody BC3 to ARGSVILT and the MMP neoepitope antibody BC4 to VDIPEN. Fosang developed antibody AF-28 to FFGVG. The VDIPEN and NITEGE C-terminal neoepitope antibodies have been primarily useful for staining residual aggrecan core left in cartilage and both fragments are detected in OA cartilage *(69)*. The N-terminal neoepitope antibodies have been primarily used for monitoring products released in synovial fluid or tissue culture. Fosang et al. *(70)* examined synovial fluid using AF-28 and found MMP-generated fragments that were small, but lacked the NITEGE site. The neoepitope antibodies have the potential to clarify aggrecan catabolic mechanisms and facilitate disease monitoring if they can be adapted to routine fluid-phase measurements.

Cartilage Component Markers

CARTILAGE OLIGOMERIC PROTEIN

COMP, a component of the articular cartilage extracellular matrix, is a >500 kD, homo-pentameric member of the thrombospodin family of extracellular calcium-binding proteins. It is found in high concentrations in articular cartilage (approx 0.1% wet weight), but it is also present in other tissues such as tendons. As this protein is made by activated synovial cells, elevated COMP may reflect synovitis. In a study of patients with clinical OA, those with progressive disease during the 5-yr follow-up had serum COMP levels that increased on the average of 6.4 µg/mL compared to only a 0.7 µg/mL increase in nonprogressive patients *(71)*. In a 3-yr study of individuals with chronic knee pain suggestive of early OA, those with evidence of radiographic progression at the studies end had significantly increased COMP levels over time. In a large study, Clark et al. *(72)*, using MAb 17-C10, found COMP levels significantly elevated in OA compared to control and in older (>65 yr) compared to younger individuals. Their study is of considerable interest in that they used log-transformed values to insure validity of the statistical tests and in addition showed data from other laboratories facilitating a comparison of COMP assay performance in other laboratories. In human synovial fluid, increased COMP is found after knee injury and in early OA *(73)*. Peterson et al. *(74)* reported examination of the serum of individuals without OA that progressed to OA had higher COMP levels than individuals who did not progress.

YKL-40 (Human Cartilage glycoprotein-39; HC gp-39)

YKL-40 is a major secretory protein of chondrocytes, synovial cells, macrophages, and neutrophils. It has been reported to be elevated in OA synovial fluid *(75,76)*, but the meaning of that elevation is unclear. Chondrocytes show elevated staining *(77)*, but because YKL-40 is a major constituent of neutrophil granules and is released when the granules are released, it may simply be a marker of inflammation.

Other Cartilage Components

There are a variety of other potential cartilage markers that could be examined in OA. A partial list would include decorin, biglycan, superficial zone protein (lubricin), matrilin, fibulin, fibromodulin, and so on. Some of these molecules have been tested for changes in cartilage during OA *(78)*, but as yet cartilage-specific assays have not been developed. The use of gene chips should lead to additional candidates. Because many of the potential markers are found outside of cartilage as well, e.g., decorin, biglycan, and so on, it is likely for some that a usable assay can be prepared only for synovial fluid.

Bone Markers

Bone markers that arise from the body's large bone mass are likely to provide little data of direct relevance to OA. It must be kept in mind that there is a huge menopausal effect on the levels of bone metabolites. This does not mean that measures of bone metabolism are without value. Metabolically active bone determined by scintigraphy is associated with OA progression *(79)*. Moreover, markers of bone metabolism may have a role in stratifying OA patients particularly when measured in synovial fluid where they might reflect bony changes in that joint.

Osteocalcin

Women with radiographically confirmed OA have higher bone mineral density (BMD) than do those without knee OA. This is reflected in lower bone turnover in these individuals as measured by serum osteocalcin, a marker of bone formation. Average serum osteocalcin levels were lower in incident cases of hand OA ($>60\%$, $p = 0.02$) or knee OA (20%, nonsignificant P) *(80)*. In a population of women over the age of 60 with clinically diagnosed OA awaiting total hip replacement, no difference in osteocalcin levels over controls were noted *(81)*.

TYPE I COLLAGEN METABOLITES

These are best characterized as markers of bone resorption. Either urinary pyridino-lines (hydroxylysylpyridinoline (Pyr) or deoxypyridinoline (D-Pyr) or telopeptides that contain these crosslinks are used routinely to assess changes in bone turnover. Type I crosslinks have been suggested to provide a measurement of disease activity *(82–84)*, but Graverand et al. *(85)* suggest that such changes are only seen in late disease.

BONE SIALOPROTEIN (BSP)

BSP appears to be released from the more superficial layers of bone and has been measured in a number of OA clinical trials. Lohmander et al. *(86)* showed it to be elevated in synovial fluid after joint injury. Petersson et al. found it elevated in synovial fluid of patients with joint pain *(74)* and in patients with bone-scan abnormalities *(87)*.

Disease Process Markers

METALLOPROTEINASE MARKERS

Molecules such as stromelysin, collagenase, the gelatinases, members of the adamalysin thrombospondin (ADAMTS) family, and so on, could contribute to the progression of OA. Thus, stromelysin rises 15–45-fold over control levels in OA synovial fluid *(66)* and in the synovial fluid from patients with join injury *(65,88)*. In joint injury, it remains elevated 2–4× for years after injury. In the normal and the athlete groups, ratios of stromelysin/tissue inhibitor of metalloproteinase (TIMP) were 0.5, suggesting an excess of TIMP, whereas the ratios reversed in the OA and knee groups (1.6–2.0) suggesting the potential for uninhibited enzyme. Because the stromelysin is in the proform, it is difficult to interpret this data. A determination of the amounts of active enzyme could help *(89)*. Also the source of the enzyme could be meniscus, cartilage, or synovial lining as all have increased message levels. The levels in blood are not elevated.

Collagenase by contrast, seems to be upregulated in blood *(90)* as well as synovial fluid in OA, but its levels are very low, making it a nonroutine maker. It, too, is in the proform.

CYTOKINE MARKERS

IL-1, TNF, and IL-6. Immunohistochemical analysis of synovial and cartilage biopsy following knee arthroscopy revealed IL-1β and TNF-α positive chondrocytes from almost all patients *(91)*. However, these markers were expressed at low levels or not at all in synovial membranes. In a study by Manicourt et al. *(92)*, synovial fluid TNF-α levels from OA patients were detectable at low levels in 20/31 subjects analyzed with undetectable levels in the remaining 11 subjects. In this same study, IL-6 levels positively correlated with TNF-α levels. Serum IL-6 and sTNF-RII levels were distinguishable in specimens from OA and control subjects *(18)*.

Chemokines. An apparently novel OA-specific increase in the chemokine MP-1β has been reported *(93)*. This could be of interest, but no further work has appeared.

INFLAMMATION MARKERS

CRP. Lowering of serum C-reactive protein (CRP) is one the ACR criteria for improvement in RA. However, as OA is less inflammatory in nature, CRP levels (~5 vs > 50 µg/mL in RA) may not be as useful an indicator. Sharif et al. *(94)* reported elevated CRP levels predicted knee radiographic progression 8 yr later. However, specimens obtain 5 yr prior to progression were not predictive raising questions about the meaning. In another long-term study (4 yr), Spector et al. *(95)* demonstrated a predictive value of small elevations in CRP levels in progressor vs nonprogressor women with mild to moderate knee OA. However, Garnero et al. *(36)* found that CRP (as well as serum type II collagen N-propeptide [PIIINP]) was correlated with the WOMAC, but not correlated with cartilage loss.

Hyaluronan. Synovial fluid hyaluronan is present at around 2–3 mg/mL. It rises in concentration during inflammation. It is produced by the synovial lining cells in sufficient amounts that it is unlikely there is any significant contribution to the elevation arising from degradation of aggrecan. HA has been reported elevated in OA and plasma HA levels were found to correlate with an objective functional capacity score and with an articular index based on the total amount of cartilage in the involved joints *(96)*. HA is also elevated in experimental models of OA *(97)*. A comparison has been made of various assays for monitoring HA levels *(98)*.

Glc-Gal-PYD. This glycosylated crosslink fragment has been recently reported as a marker of synovial inflammation and is measured in the urine *(98a)*. It, like PIIIPN, is elevated in OA *(36)*, but far more modestly than in RA *(98a)*.

GROWTH FACTORS

TGF-β. It has been reported increased in OA *(18)*, but the meaning remains to be determined.

IGF1. The data of Fraenkel et al. *(99)* suggest that serum IGF1 levels are not related to OA. Because of the variety IGF binding factors, it may well be that the binding factors have larger role in regulating the amount of available IGF1.

INTERPRETATION OF RESULTS FROM DISEASE MARKERS

Type II collagen seems to have some important characteristics that lend it to use as a measure of cartilage breakdown. It seems to be synthesized in early life and the extent of remodeling seems to be small. Its half-life in cartilage has been estimated to be over a 100 yr in man *(99a)*. While there is clear evidence for new synthesis of type II collagen in OA, the bulk of the fragments seem to come from breakdown of pre-existing collagen. If this assumption is validated, then type II collagen fragmentation could be an actual disease marker with fragment elevation related to actual loss of physical properties of cartilage, and the amount of cartilage compromise actually related to the total amount of fragment lost.

How rigidly should the interpretation of clinical functional loss being directly proportional to the collagen fragment be held? There would seem to be some clues from other markers. The oldest disease marker is fever. It is elevated in infectious disease. Whether or not the physician considers that there is some rough correlation between bacterial load and fever elevation is immaterial; fever signifies the need of therapy. Moreover, in spite of confounding effects of aspirin and other NSAID, which lower fever without affecting bacterial load, fever remains an effective and widely used measure of disease activity. Such practical considerations ought to guide marker interpretation in OA as well. High levels of marker should reflect high progression and the need for therapy; low levels, low progression, and the need of therapy more debatable.

Frequently, when examining clinical-marker data, one obtains a statistically significant association with disease status. It should be understood that this is a secondary correlation. It arises because it is likely that patients with a high marker level have had a high marker level for sometime and that those with a low marker level have not. Thus it is likely that those with high marker levels have more active disease for a longer time and have therefore experienced more joint damage over time.

If new synthesis is a major contributor to the level of collagen fragments in the urine, then the type II collagen fragment assays shift from being a disease marker to being a disease-process marker and the lowering of fragments in the urine may or may not indicate an improvement in outcome. Even so, there could be an exception to that category shift. If the bulk of fragments from new synthesis are generated by enzymes (cathepsins) different from those used in the pathological process (collagenases), then the use of neoepitope antibodies could potentially differentiate between the two pathways and make it possible to retain the disease-marker status.

Conversely, the data on aggrecan indicate there is a high level of normal turnover with a $t_{1/2}$ of around 3 yr *(100)*. In this case, aggrecan fragments become disease-process markers. There is no direct linkage between pathology and fragment concentrations. However, if again there is the involvement of an enzyme, for example one of the ADAMTS enzymes, that is pathological in the disease process, then it might be possible to tighten the disease linkage and improve the prognostic importance of the markers by use of antibodies that would specifically recognize breakdown fragments generated by that enzyme. This is work that is still to be done.

For markers based on other cartilage molecules, we simply have insufficient data. There is an indication that levels of COMP might be useful for predicting progression *(101)*, but the synovial-lining cells can synthesize COMP so the direct relationship to cartilage is obscured. At this stage of knowledge, it must be viewed as a disease-process marker rather than a disease marker.

For the disease-process markers, we can only say that we believe that their lowering toward normal would be beneficial. Some of the disease-process markers in synovial fluid can be associated closely with OA and are unlikely to be nonspecific indications of other disease, e.g., stromelysin, collagenase, aggrecanase, COMP. However, we don't know how to interpret their elevation in OA. If a drug were to lower this elevation, would it be an indication that the drug works? It would be suggestive, but one must wait for marker validation by application of an effective drug. Where the linkage to the disease is less clear, such as with CRP, IL-1, or TNF receptor elevation, then it becomes necessary to exclude contributions from secondary conditions that elevate these markers in a variety of diseases. Still, the same question must be asked. If the elevation is in fact owing to OA, would a lowering of the marker improve the prognosis? Again, we don't know the answers. For now, this leaves these markers as most useful for hypothesis testing and for mechanistic studies.

Finally, there is the question of how to use the data from markers. We have examined a variety of markers in a side by side comparison. Our results suggest that many of the markers give similar, if not comparable information *(19)*. If they do provide redundant data, then there is little point in running several markers that give essentially the same information. The question then arises, what marker(s) should be used to best estimate disease activity in OA in order to guide treatment and therapy. The data we have reviewed give no clear answers. Too few side by side comparisons of markers have been carried out. We suggest power analysis provides a powerful tool to winnow the field of markers, but that too has rarely been done. We think that of the cartilage markers, the collagen-fragment assays have the most promise, but that remains to be proven.

THE STATUS OF MOLECULAR MARKERS IN OA

The outlook for the use of markers for monitoring OA is perhaps better than it has ever been. There is clear utility of markers for clinical trials where populations of patients can be used. There are a few markers that could potentially be useful for monitoring of individual patients, but they have only been closely examined in population studies. Currently the primary use of markers is to give mechanistic information and to support (not prove) clinical utility of a drug. A substantial amount of work remains to be done before any marker is deemed useful for the determination of clinical efficacy and can be used to monitor therapy in an individual patient.

REFERENCES

1. Garnero, P., J.-C. Rousseau, and P.D. Delmas. 2000. Molecular basis and clinical use of biochemical markers of bone, cartilage, and synovium in joint diseases. *Arthritis Rheum.* 43:953–968.

2. Greenwald, R.A. 1996. Review: Monitoring collagen degradation in patients with arthritis: the search for suitable surrogates. *Arthritis Rheum.* 39:1455–1465.

3. Heinegård, D. and T. Saxne. 1991. Molecular markers of processes in cartilage in joint disease. *Br. J. Rheumatol.* 30 (Suppl.):21–4.

4. Lohmander, L.S. 1997. What is the current status of biochemical markers in the diagnosis, prognosis and monitoring of osteoarthritis? *Baillieres Clin. Rheum.* 11:711–726.

5. Lohmander, L.S. and D.T. Felson. 1997. Defining the role of molecular markers to monitor disease, intervention, and cartilage breakdown in osteoarthritis. *J. Rheumatol.* 24:782–785.

6. Poole, A.R. 1994. Immunochemical markers of joint inflammation, skeletal damage and repair: Where are we now? *Ann. Rheum. Dis.* 53:3–5.

7. Ala-Kokk, L., C.T. Baldwin, R.W. Moskowitz, and D.J. Prockop. 1990. Single base mutation in the type II procollagen gene (COL2A1) as a cause of primary osteoarthritis associated with a mild chondrodysplasia. *Proc. Natl. Acad. Sci. USA* 87:6565–6568.

8. Pun, Y.L., R.W. Moskowitz, S. Lie, W.R. Sundstrom, S.R. Block, C. McEwen, et al. 1994. Clinical correlations of osteoarthritis associated with a single-base mutation (arginine519 to cysteine) in type II procollagen gene: a newly defined pathogenesis. *Arthritis Rheum.* 37:264–269.

9. Horton, W.E., Jr., M. Lethbridge-Cejku, M.C. Hochberg, R. Balakir, P. Precht, C.C. Plato, et al. 1998. An association between an aggrecan polymorphic allele and bilateral hand osteoarthritis in elderly white men: data from the Baltimore Longitudinal Study of Aging (BLSA). *Osteoarth. Cart.* 6:245–251.

10. Meulenbelt, I., C. Bijkerk, S.C. de Wildt, H.S. Miedema, H.A. Valkenburg, F.C. Breedveld, et al. 1997. Investigation of the association of the CRTM and CRTL1 genes with radiographically evident osteoarthritis in subjects from the Rotterdam study. *Arthritis Rheum.* 40:1760–1765.

11. Meulenbelt, I., C. Bijkerk, H.S. Miedema, F.C. Breedveld, A. Hofman, H.A. Valkenburg, et al. 1998. A genetic association study of the IGF-1 gene and radiological osteoarthritis in a population-based cohort study (the Rotterdam Study). *Ann. Rheum. Dis.* 57:371–374.

12. Meulenbelt, I., C. Bijkerk, S.C. de Wildt, H.S. Miedema, F.C. Breedveld, H.A. Pols, et al. 1999. Haplotype analysis of three polymorphisms of the COL2A1 gene and associations with generalised radiological osteoarthritis. *Ann. Human Genet.* 63:393–400.

13. Oliveria, S.A., D.T. Felson, P.A. Cirillo, J.I. Reed, and A.M. Walker. 1999. Body weight, body mass index, and incident symptomatic osteoarthritis of the hand, hip, and knee. *Epidemiology* 10:161–166.

14. Silveri, F., D. Brecciaroli, F. Argentati, and C. Cervini. 1994. Serum levels of insulin in overweight patients with osteoarthritis of the knee [see comments]. *J. Rheumatol.* 21:1899–1902.

15. Denko, C.W., B. Boja, and R.W. Moskowitz. 1994. Growth promoting peptides in osteoarthritis and diffuse idiopathic skeletal hyperostosis: insulin, insulin-like growth factor-I, growth hormone. *J. Rheumatol.* 21:1725–1730.

16. Zhang, Y., T.E. McAlindon, M.T. Hannan, C.E. Chaisson, R. Klein, P.W. Wilson, et al. 1998. Estrogen replacement therapy and worsening of radiographic knee osteoarthritis: the Framingham Study. *Arthritis Rheum.* 41:1867–1873.

17. Lane, N.E., L.R. Gore, S.R. Cummings, M.C. Hochberg, J.C. Scott, E.N. Williams, et al. 1999. Serum vitamin D levels and incident changes of radiographic hip osteoarthritis: a longitudinal study. Study of Osteoporotic Fractures Research Group. *Arthritis Rheum.* 42:854–860.

18. Otterness, I.G., R.O. Zimmerer, A.C. Swindell, A.R. Poole, D. Heinegård, T. Saxne, et al. 1995. An examination of some molecular markers in blood and urine for discriminating patients with osteoarthritis of the knee from normal individuals. *Acta Orthop. Scand.* 66 (Suppl. 266):148–150.

19. Otterness, I.G., A.C. Swindell, R.O. Zimmerer, A.R. Poole, M. Ionescu, and E. Weiner. 2000. Analysis of 14 molecular markers for monitoring osteoarthritis. Segregation of the markers into clusters and distinguishing osteoarthritis at baseline. *Osteoarth. Cart.* 8:180–185.

20. Lohmander, L.S., L. Dahlberg, D. Eyre, M. Lark, E.J. Thonar, and L. Ryd. 1998. Longitudinal and cross-sectional variability in markers of joint metabolism in patients with knee pain and articular cartilage abnormalities. *Osteoarth. Cart.* 6:351–361.

21. Billinghurst, R.C., L. Dahlberg, M. Ionescu, A. Reiner, R. Bourne, C. Rorabeck, et al. 1997. Enhanced cleavage of type II collagen by collagenases in osteoarthritic articular cartilage. *J. Clin. Inv.* 99:1534–1545.

22. Otterness, I.G., J.T. Downs, C. Lane, M.L. Bliven, H. Stukenbrok, D.N. Scampoli, et al. 1999. Detection of collagenase-induced damage of collagen by 9A4, a monoclonal C-terminal neoeptiope antibody. *Matrix Biol.* 18:331–341.

23. Atley, L.M. J.S. Mort, M. Lalumiere, and D.R. Eyre. 2000. Proteolysis of human bone collagen by cathepsin K: characterization of the cleavage sites generating by cross-linked N-telopeptide neoepitope. *Bone* 26:241–247.

24. Dodge, G.R., I. Pidoux, and A.R. Poole. 1991. The degradation of type II collagen in rheumatoid arthritis: an immunoelectron microscopic study. *Matrix* 11:330–338.

25. Hollander, A.P., T.F. Heathfield, C. Webber, Y. Iwata, R. Bourne, C. Rorabeck, et al. 1994. Increased damage to type II collagen in osteoarthritic articular cartilage detected by a new immunoassay. *J. Clin. Inv.* 93:1722–1732.

26. Dodge, G.R. and A.R. Poole. 1989. Immunohistochemical detection and immunochemical analysis of type II articular cartilages and in explants of bovine articular cartilage cultured with interleukin 1. *J. Clin. Invest.* 83:647–661.

27. Srinivas, G.R., H.J. Barrach, and C.O. Chichester. 1993. Quantitative immunoassays for type II collagen and its cyanogen bromide peptides. *J. Immunol. Method* 159:53–62.

28. Srinivas, G.R., C.O. Chichester, H.J. Barrach, V. Pillai, and A.L. Matoney. 1994. Production of type II collagen specific monoclonal antibodies. *Immunol. Inv.* 23:85–98.

29. Felice, B.R., C.O. Chichester, and H.J. Barrach. 1999. Type II collagen peptide release from rabbit articular cartilage. *Ann. NY Acad. Sci.* 878:590–593.

30. Barrach, H.-J., C.O. Chichester, D.A. Sargetn, M.J. Saracen, S. Griggs, M. Hulstyn, et al. 1996. Quantification of collagen type II peptides in synovial fluid by an inhibition ELISA. *Transact. Orthop. Res. Soc.* 21:218.

31. Eyre, D.R., P. Shao, K. Vosberg-Smith, M. Weis, K. Shaffer, and P. Yoshihara. 1996. Cross-linked telopeptides from collagens type I, II and III in human urine. *Am. Soc. Bone Min. Res.* S1, Ps413.

32. Garnero, P., E. Gineyts, S. Christgau, and P.D. Delmas. 1999. Urinary type II collagen C-telepeptide breakdown products as markers of cartilage degradation in rheumatoid arthritis. *Arthritis Rheum.* 42:S128.

33. Calvo, M.S., D.R. Eyre, and C.M. Gundberg. 1996. Molecular basis and clinical application of biological markers of bone turnover. *Endocr. Rev.* 17:333–368.

34. Atley, L.M., L. Shyarma, J.D. Clemens, K. Shaffer, T.A. Pietka, H.A. Riggins, et al. 2000. The collagen II CTx degradation marker is generated by collagenase 3 and in urine reflects disease burden in knee OA patients. *Proc. Orthop. Res. Assoc.* 46th Annual Meeting:0168.

35. Lohmander, L.S., L.M. Atley, T.A. Pietka, and D.R. Eyre. 2000. The release of cross-linked peptides from type II collagen into joint fluid and serum is increased in osteoarthritis and after joint injury. *Proc. Orthop. Res. Assoc.* 46th Annual Meeting:0236.

36. Garnero, P., M. Piperno, S. Christgau, P.D. Delmas, and E. Vignon. 2001. Cross-sectional evaluation of biochemical markers of bone, cartilage, and synovial tissue metabolism in patients with knee osteoarthritis: relations with disease activity and joint damage. *Ann. Rheum. Dis.* 60:619–626.

36a. Garnero, P., M. Piperno, E. Gineyts, S. Christgau, P.D. Delmas, and E. Vignon. 2001. Cross-sectional evaluation of biochemical markers of bone, cartilage, and synovial tissue metabolism in patients with knee osteoarthritis: relations with disease activity and joint damage. *Ann. Rheum. Dis.* 60: 619–626.

37. Mitchell, P.G., H.A. Magna, L.M. Reeves, L.L. Lopresti-Morrow, S.A. Yocum, P.J. Rosner, et al. 1996. Cloning, expression, and type II collagenolytic activity of matrix metalloproteinase-13 from human osteoarthritic cartilage. *J. Clin. Inv.* 97:761–768.

38. Vankemmelbeke, M., P.M. Dekeyser, A.P. Hollander, D.J. Buttle, and J. Demeester. 1998. Characterization of helical cleavages in type II collagen generated by matrixins. *Biochem. J.* 330: 633–640.

39. Stoop, R., P.M. Van Der Kraan, P. Buma, A.P. Hollander, R.C. Billlinghurst, A.R. Poole, et al. 1999. Type II collagen degradation in spontaneous osteoarthritis in C57bl/6 and Balb/c mice. *Arthritis Rheum.* 42:2381–2389.

40. Huebner, J.L., I.G. Otterness, E.M. Freund, B. Caterson, and V.B. Kraus. 1998. Collagenase 1 and collagenase 3 expression in a guinea pig model of osteoarthritis [see comments]. *Arthritis Rheum.* 41:877–890.

41. Downs, J.T., C.L. Lane, N.B. Nestor, T.J. McLellan, M.A. Kelly, G.A. Karam, et al. 2001. Analysis of collagen cleavage of type II collagen using a neoepitope ELISA. *J. Immunol. Meth.* 247:25–34.

42. Andrews, G.C., R.T. Suleske, M.A. Kelly, B.C. Guarino, M.H. Rosner, T.J. McLellan, et al. 2000. Mapping critical amino acids in a linear epitope: A comparison of ELISA methods using a solid state peptide library with a fluorescent polarization solution phase binding assay. Submitted.

43. Saltarelli, M.J., K. Johnson, E. Pickering, I.G. Otterness, M.D. Vazquez-Abad, and T.G. Woodworth. 1999. Measurement of uninary type II collagen neoepitope levels in rheumatoid arthritis patients to assess joint status. *Arthritis Rheum.* 42 (Suppl. 9):S249.

44. Woodworth, T.G., I.G. Otterness, K. Johnson, E. Pickering, and M.J. Saltarelli. 1999. Urinary type II collagen neoepitope in osteoarthritis patients is associated with disease severity. *Arthritis Rheum.* 42 (Suppl. 9):S258.

45. Nelson, F., A. Reiner, M. Ionescu, E. Brooks, E. Bogoch, and A.R. Poole. 1994. The content of the C-propeptide of type II collagen in articular cartilage is an index of synthesis of this molecule which is increased in osteoarthritis. *Transact. Orthop. Res. Soc.* 19:216.

46. Hinek, A., A. Reiner, and A.R. Poole. 1987. The calcification of cartilage matrix in chondrocyte culture: studies of the C-propeptide of type II collagen (chondrocalcin). *J. Cell Biol.* 104: 1435–1441.

47. Hinek, A. and A.R. Poole. 1988. The influence of vitamin D metabolites on the calcification of cartilage matrix and the C-propeptide of type II collagen (chondrocalcin). *J. Bone Mineral Res.* 3:421–429.

48. Shinmei, M., K. Ito, S. Matsuyama, Y. Yoshihara, and K. Matsusawa. 1993. Joint fluid carboxy-terminal type II procollagen peptide as a marker of cartilage collagen biosynthesis. *Osteoarth. Cart.* 1:121–128.

49. Lohmander, L.S., Y. Yoshira, H. Roos, T. Kobayashi, H. Yamada, and M. Shinmei. 1966. Changes in joint cartilage aggrecan metabolism after knee injury and in osteoarthritis. *Arthritis Rheum.* 42:534–544.

50. Nelson, F., L. Dahlberg, S. Laverty, A. Reiner, I. Pidous, M. Ionescu, et al. 1998. Evidence for altered synthesis of type II collagen in patients with osteoarthritis. *J. Clin. Inv.* 102:2115–2125.

51. Wotton, S.F., P.A. Dieppe, and V.C. Duance. 1999. Type IX collagen immunoreactive peptides in synovial fluids from arthritis patients. *Rheumatology* (Oxford) 38:338–345.

52. Ratcliffe, A., W. Shurety, and B. Caterson. 1993. The quantitation of native chondroitin sulfate epitope in synovial fluid lavages and articular cartilage from canine experimental osteoarthritis and disuse atrophy. *Arthritis Rheum.* 36:543–551.

53. Hazell, P.K., C. Dent, J.A. Fairclough, M.T. Bayliss, and T.E. Hardingham. 1995. Changes in glycosaminoglycan epitope levels in knee joint fluid following injury. *Arthritis Rheum.* 38:953–959.

54. Glant, T.T., K. Mikecz, P.J. Roughley, E. Buzaz, and A.R. Poole. 1986. Age-related changes in protein-related epitopes of human articular cartilage proteoglycans. *Biochem. J.* 236:71–75.

55. Rizkalla, G., A. Reiner, E. Bogoch, and A. Poole. 1992. Studies of the articular cartilage proteoglycan aggrecan in health and osteoarthritis. Evidence for molecular heterogeneity and extensive molecular changes in disease. *J. Clin. Inv.* 90:2268–2277.

56. Lohmander, L.S., M. Ionescu, H. Jugessur, and A.R. Poole. 1999. Changes in joint cartilage aggrecan after knee injury and in osteoarthritis. *Arthritis Rheum.* 42:534–544.

57. Poole, A.R., M. Ionescu, A. Swan, and P. Dieppe. 1994. Changes in cartilage metabolism in arthritis are reflected by altered serum and synovial fluid levels of glycosaminoglycan epitopes on fragments of the cartilage proteoglycan aggrecan: implications for pathogenesis. *J. Clin. Invest.* 94:25–33.

58. Sweet, M.B.E., A. Coelho, C.M. Schnitzler, T.J. Schnitzer, M.E. Lenz, I. Jaki, et al. 1988. Serum keratan sulfate levels in osteoarthritis patients. *Arthritis Rheum.* 31:648–652.

59. Thonar, E.J.-M.A. and T. Glant 1992. Serum keratan sulfate-A marker of predisposition to polyarticular osteoarthritis. *Clin. Biochem.* 25:175–180.

60. Champion, G.V., F. McCrai, T.J. Schnitzer, M.E. Lenz, P.A. Dieppe, and E.J.-M.A. Thonar. 1991. Levels of keratan sulfate in the serum and synovial fluid of patients with osteoarthritis of the knee. *Arthritis Rheum.* 34:1254–1259.

61. Manicourt, D.H., M.-E. Leny, and E.J.-M.A. Thonar. 1991. Levels of serum keratan sulfate rise rapidly and remain elevated following anterior cruciate ligament transection in the dog. *J. Rheumatol.* 18:1872–1876.

62. Thonar, E.J.-M.A., M. Shinmei, and L.S. Lohmander. 1993. Body fluid markers of cartilage changes in osteoarthritis. *Rheum. Dis. Clin. North Am.* 19:635–657.

63. Heinegärd, D., S. Inerot, J. Wieslander, and G. Lindblad. 1985. A method for the quantification of cartilage proteoglycan structures liberated to the synovial fluid during developing degenerative joint disease. *Scand. J. Clin. Lab. Inv.* 45:421–427.

64. Saxne, T., D. Heinegard, and F.A. Wollheim. 1986. Therapeutic effects on cartilage metabolism in arthritis as measured by release of proteoglycan structures into the synovial fluid. *Ann. Rheum. Dis.* 45:491–497.

65. Lohmander, L.S., L.A. Hoerrner, L. Dahlberg, H. Roos, S. Björnsson, and M.W. Lark. 1993. Stromelysin, tissue inhibitor of metalloproteinases and proteoglycan fragments in human knee joint fluid after injury. *J. Rheumatol.* 20:1362–1368.

66. Lohmander, L.S., L.A. Hoerrner, and M.W. Lark. 1993. Metalloproteinases, tissue inhibitor, and proteoglycan fragments in knee synovial fluid in human osteoarthritis. *Arthritis Rheum.* 36:181–189.

67. Møller, H.J., F.S. Larsen, T. Ingemann-Hansen, and J.H. Poulsen. 1994. ELISA for the core protein of the cartilage large aggregating proteoglycan, aggrecan: comparison with the concentrations of immunogenic keratan sulfate in synovial fluid, serum and urine. *Clin. Chim. Acta* 225:43–55.

68. Hughes, C.E., B. Caterson, A.J. Fosang, P.J. Roughley, and J.S. Mort. 1995. Monoclonal antibodies that specifically recognize neoepitope sequences gererated by "aggrecanase" and matrix metalloproteinase cleavage of aggrecan: Application to catabolism *in situ* and *in vitro*. *Biochem. J.* 305:799–804.

69. Lark, M.W., E.K. Bayne, J. Flanagan, C.R. Harper, L.A. Hoerrner, N.I. Hutchinson, et al. 1997. Aggrecan degradation in human cartilage. Evidence for both matrix metalloproteinase and aggrecanase activity in normal, osteoarthritic, and rheumatoid joints. *J. Clin. Inv.* 100:93–106.

70. Fosang, A.J., K. Last, P. Gardiner, D.C. Jackson, L. Brown. 1995. Development of a cleavage-site-specific monoclonal antibody for detecting metalloproteinase-derived aggrecan fragments: detection of fragments in human synovial fluids. *Biochem. J.* 310:2337–2343.

71. Sharif, M., T. Saxne, L. Shepstone, J.R. Kirwan, C.J. Elson, D. Heinegard, et al. 1995. Relationship between serum cartilage oligomeric matrix protein levels and disease progression in osteoarthritis of the knee joint. *Br. J. Rheumatol.* 34:306–310.

72. Clark, A.G., J.M. Jordan, V. Vilim, J.B. Renner, A.D. Dragomir, G. Luta, et al. 1999. Serum cartilage oligomeric matrix protein reflects osteoarthritis presence and severity: the Johnston County Osteoarthritis Project. *Arthritis Rheum.* 42:2356–2364.

73. Lohmander, L.S., T. Saxne, and D.K. Heinegard. 1994. Release of cartilage oligomeric matrix protein (COMP) into joint fluid after knee injury and in osteoarthritis. *Ann. Rheum. Dis.* 53:8–13.
74. Petersson, I.F., T. Boegard, B. Svensson, D. Heinegard, and T. Saxne. 1998. Changes in cartilage and bone metabolism identified by serum markers in early osteoarthritis of the knee joint. *Br. J. Rheumatol.* 37:46–50.
75. Johansen, J.S., H.S. Jensen, and P.A. Price. 1993. A new biochemical marker for joint injury. Analysis of YKL-40 in serum and synovial fluid. *Br. J. Rheumatol.* 32:949–955.
76. Harvey, S., M. Weisman, J. O'Dell, T. Scott, M. Krusemeier, J. Visor, et al. 1998. Chondrex: new marker of joint disease. *Clin. Chem.* 44:509–516.
77. Volck, B., K. Ostergaard, J.S. Johansen, C. Garbarsch, and P.A. Price. 1999. The distribution of YKL-40 in osteoarthritic and normal human articular cartilage. *Scand. J. Rheumatol.* 28:171–179.
78. Cs-Szabo, G., L.I. Melching, P.J. Roughley, and T.T. Glant. 1997. Changes in messenger RNA and protein levels of proteoglycans and link protein in human osteoarthritic cartilage samples. *Arthritis Rheum.* 40:1037–1045.
79. Dieppe, P., J. Cushgnaghan, P. Young, and J. Dirwan. 1993. Prediction of the progression of joint space narrowing in osteoarthritis of the knee by bone scintigraphy. *Ann. Rheum. Dis.* 52:557–563.
80. Sowers, M., L. Lachance, D. Jamadar, M.C. Hochberg, B. Hollis, M. Crutchfield, et al. 1999. The associations of bone mineral density and bone turnover markers with osteoarthritis of the hand and knee in pre- and perimenopausal women [see comments]. *Arthritis Rheum.* 42:483–489.
81. Stewart, A., A. Block, S.P. Robins, and D.M. Reid. 1999. Bone density and bone turnover in patients with osteoarthritis and osteoporosis. *J. Rheumatol.* 26:622–626.
82. Thompson, P.W., T.D. Spector, I.T. James, E. Henderson, and D.J. Hart. 1992. Urinary collagen crosslinks reflect the radiographic severity of knee osteoarthritis. *Br. J. Rheumatol.* 31:759–761.
83. Sinigaglia, L., M. Varenna, L. Binelli, F. Bartucci, M. Arrigoni, R. Ferrara, et al. 1995. Urinary and synovial pyridinium crosslink concentrations in patients with rheumatoid arthritis and osteoarthritis. *Ann. Rheum. Dis.* 54:144–147.
84. MacDonald, A.G., P. McHenry, S.P. Robins, and D.M. Reid. 1994. Relationship of urinary pyridinium crosslinks to disease extent and activity in osteoarthritis [see comments]. *Br. J. Rheumatol.* 33:16–19.
85. Graverand, M.P., A.M. Tron, M. Ichou, M.C. Dallard, M. Richard, D. Uebelhart, et al. 1996. Assessment of urinary hydroxypyridinium cross-links measurement in osteoarthritis. *Br. J. Rheumatol.* 35:1091–1095.
86. Lohmander, L.S., T. Saxne, and D. Heinegard. 1996. Increased concentrations of bone sialoprotein in joint fluid after knee injury. *Ann. Rheum. Dis.* 55:622–626.
87. Petersson, I.F., T. Boegård, J. Dahlström, B. Svensson, D. Heinegård, and T. Saxne. 1998. Bone scan and serum markers of bone and cartilage in patients with knee pain and osteoarthritis. *Osteoarthritis Cart.* 6:33–39.
88. Lohmander, L.S., H. Roos, L. Dahlberg, L.A. Hoerrner, and M.W. Lark. 1994. Temporal patterns of stromelysin-1, tissue inhibitor, and proteoglycan fragments in human knee joint fluid after injury to the cruciate ligament or meniscus. *J. Orthop. Res.* 12:21–28.
89. Beekman, B., J.W. Drijfhout, W. Bloemhoff, H.K. Ronday, P.P. Tak, and J.M. te Koppele. 1996. Convenient fluorometric assay for matrix metalloproteinase activity and its application in biological media. *FEBS Lett.* 390:221–225.
90. Keyszer, G., I. Lavviri, R. Nagel, C. Keusser, M. Keysser, E. Gromnica-Ihle, et al. 1999. Circulating levels of matrix metalloproteinases MMP-3 and MMP-1, tissue inhibitor of metalloproteinases 1 (TIMP-1) and MMP-1/TIMP-1 comploex in rheumatic disease. Correlation with clinical activity of rheumatoid arthritis. *J. Rheumatol.* 26:251–258.
91. Melchiorri, C., R. Meliconi, L. Frizziero, T. Silvestri, L. Pulsatelli, I. Mazzetti, et al. 1998. Enhanced and coordinated in vivo expression of inflammatory cytokines and nitric oxide synthase by chondrocytes from patients with osteoarthritis. *Arthritis Rheum.* 41:2165–2174.
92. Manicourt, D.H., P. Vache, A. Egeren, J.-P. Devogelaer, M.E. Lenz, and E.J.-M.A. Thonar. 2000. Synovial fluid levels of tumor necrosis factor a and oncostatin M correlate with levels of markers of the degradation of crosslinked collagen and cartilage aggrecan inrheumatoid arthritis but not in osteoarthritis. *Arthritis Rheum.* 43:281–288.
93. Koch, A.E., S.L. Kunkel, M.R. Shah, R. Fu, D.D. Mazarakis, G.K.Haines, et al. 1995. Macrophage inflammatory protein-1 beta: a C-C chemokine in osteoarthritis. *Clin. Immunol. Immunopath.* 77:307–314.

94. Sharif, M., L. Shepstone, C.J. Elson, P.A. Dieppe, and J.R. Kirwan. 2000. Increased serum C reactive protein may reflect events that precede radiographic progression in osteoarthritis of the knee. *Ann. Rheum. Dis.* 59:71–74.

95. Spector, T.D., D.J. Hart, D. Nandra, D.V. Doyle, N. Mackillop, J.R. Gallimore, et al. 1997. Low-level increases in serum C-reactive protein are present in early osteoarthritis of the knee and predict progressive disease. *Arthritis Rheum.* 40:723–727.

96. Goldberg, R.L., J.P. Huff, M.E. Lenz, P. Glickman, R. Katz, and E.J. Thonar. 1991. Elevated plasma levels of hyaluronate in patients with osteoarthritis and rheumatoid arthritis. *Arthritis Rheum.* 34:799–807.

97. Manicourt, D.H., O. Cornu, M.E. Lenz, A. Druetz-van Egeren, and E.J. Thonar. 1995. Rapid and sustained rise in the serum level of hyaluronan after anterior cruciate ligament transection in the dog knee joint. *J. Rheumatol.* 22:262–269.

98. Lindqvist, U., K. Chichibu, B. Delpech, R.L. Goldberg, W. Knudson, A.R. Poole, et al. 1992. Seven different assays of hyaluronan compared for clinical utility. *Clin. Chem.* 38:127–132.

98a. Gineyts, E., P. Garnero, and P.D. Delmas. 2001. Urinary excretion of glucosyl-galactosyl puridinoline: a specific biochemical marker of synovium degradation. *Rheumatology* 40:5–23.

99. Fraenkel, L., Y. Zhang, S.B. Trippel, T.E. McAlindon, M.P. LaValley, A. Assif, et al. 1998. Longitudinal analysis of the relationship between serum insulin-like growth factor-I and radiographic knee osteoarthritis. *Osteoarthritis Cart.* 6:362–367.

99a. Verzijl, N., J. DeGroot, S.R. Thorpe, R.A. Bank, J.N. Shaw, T.J. Lyons, et al. 2000. Effect of collagen turnover on the accumulation of advanced glycation end products. *J. Biol. Chem.* 275:39,027–39,031.

100. Maroudas, A., M.T. Bayliss, N. Uchitel-Kaushansky, R. Schneiderman, and E. Gilav. 1998. Aggrecan turnover in human articular cartilage: use of aspartic acid racemization as a marker of molecular age. *Arch. Biochem. Biophys.* 350:61–71.

101. Sharif, M., C.J. Elson, P.A. Dieppe, and J.R. Kirwan. 1997. Elevated serum C-reactive protein levels in osteoarthritis. *Br. J. Rheumatol.* 36:140–141.

16

New Therapeutic Targets for Osteoarthritis

The Rewards of Research

Jean-Pierre Pelletier,
Johanne Martel-Pelletier,
and Pamela Manning

CONTENTS

INTRODUCTION

As the most common form of joint disease, osteoarthritis (OA) represents a major cause of morbidity and disability, particularly in the second half of life, as well as a significant burden on health-care resources. Although important advances in understanding the pathophysiologic processes of OA have been made, today's treatment of the disease still focuses mainly on improving its symptoms *(1)*. As the relationship between the etiology and pathology of OA have become more clearly defined, new concepts and molecular targets for the treatment of this arthritic condition have emerged and have permitted the development of new therapeutic agents. These agents are likely to provide significant progress toward modifying the progression of the structural changes of this disease. The pharmacological agents of this class are named disease-modifying anti-osteoarthritis drugs, or DMOAD, introducing the concept that some drugs may slow the rate of cartilage degeneration, and/or enhance the rate of cartilage repair. The discovery of new agents that have the potential to reduce or stop the progression of the structural

From: *Modern Therapeutics in Rheumatic Diseases*
Edited by: G. C. Tsokos, et al. © Humana Press, Inc., Totowa, NJ

changes observed in this disease in humans is most promising and likely to change the therapeutic approach in the near future.

Many different DMOAD agents are presently into preclinical and/or clinical development for the therapy of OA. These can be mainly classified within the following categories.

INHIBITORS OF METALLOPROTEASES

In OA cartilage there is now clear evidence that the earliest histopathological lesions, which are a depletion of proteoglycans and a breakdown of the collagen network, result from increased synthesis and/or activity of proteolytic enzymes. Current knowledge indicates a major involvement of the matrix metalloprotease (MMP) family in this disease process *(2)*. As MMP appear intimately involved in the degradation of cartilage matrix as well as in the structural changes occurring during the course of the disease, it is therefore no surprise that considerable attention has been devoted to developing strategies to reduce their levels and/or activity *in situ* in arthritic joints.

MMPs are enzymes implicated in the natural turnover of the extracellular macro-molecules *(3)*. They are produced by cells of the articular joint tissues, including chondrocytes, fibroblasts, osteoclasts, osteoblasts, and inflammatory cells. Collectively, they can degrade all the major macromolecules of the extracellular matrix: collagens, aggrecans, laminin, fibronectin, and other glycoproteins. These enzymes are synthesized as proenzymes, and must be activated by proteolytic cleavage *(3)*. Generally they are present as soluble forms, but some are membrane-bound. The activation of the latent secreted enzyme results from the proteolytic cleavage of the propeptide domain from the N-terminus of the enzyme.

MMP genes are generally expressed in cartilage and synovial-membrane cells in low levels, and their gene transcription induced by factors such as proinflammatory cytokines (interleukin-1β [IL-1β], tumor necrosis factor-α [TNF-α]) and some growth factors (epidermal growth factor [EGF], platelet-derived growth factor [PDGF], basic fibroblast growth factor [bFGF], transforming growth factor-β [TGF-β]) *(2)*. Their gene transcription can be suppressed by various factors, and those of physiological interest in articular tissues are the vitamin A analogs (retinoids) and glucocorticoids. Although each of these agents has its own pathway for inhibiting MMP gene transcription, the presence of an activator protein-1 (AP-1) site in their gene promoter appears to be a key element in the inhibitory effect *(4,5)*. Both factors first bind their respective hormone receptors and the ligand/receptor complexes translocate to the nucleus. One proposed pathway of repression is by the interaction of the ligand/receptor complexes with the Jun or Fos proteins, thus interfering with the transcriptional activation of AP-1. Another pathway found for the action of retinoids involves the downregulation of c-Fos protein expression.

The secreted pro-MMP are activated by a number of physiological activators. In turn, a number of agents that bind the active site of the enzyme can inhibit their catalytic activity. Among these are natural MMP inhibitors, such as tissue inhibitor of metalloproteases (TIMP) and α_2-macroglobulin *(6)*. The α_2-macroglobulin acts as a nonspecific inhibitor of proteases by trapping the enzyme and blocking its access to the substrate. Because of its high molecular weight, this inhibitor is unlikely to penetrate the cartilage and its relevance to tissue degradation appears doubtful. Its role appears to be restricted to the fluid or inflammatory exudates.

The balance between the level of activated MMP and the available TIMP determines the net enzyme activity, and is a key determinant of extracellular-matrix turnover. Increasing the local synthesis of TIMP would be an effective way to prevent connective-tissue turnover and OA progression (7). However, this natural inhibitor has narrow application as a therapeutic agent, mainly because of its limitation regarding the administration of proteins. Nonetheless, therapy with TIMP using recombinant protein and gene therapy has been shown to be effective in antimetastatic treatment (8).

The three dimensional structure of TIMP/stromelysin-1 complex has recently been demonstrated (9), and revealed that TIMP slots into the active MMP domain by the TIMP N-terminal part and binds in a substrate manner. Based on current knowledge of the TIMP/MMP complex structure, researchers have begun to look at engineering the TIMP molecule to be selective to a specific MMP; this can be achieved by specific point mutation of TIMP at the MMP contact site (10). Based on these findings, there might therefore be a regain of interest in the use of TIMP as treatment in the field of OA.

A large variety of synthetic approaches for the control of the level of MMP synthesis/activity have been the focus of very intensive research over the last decade. Developing protease inhibitors that are therapeutically active is very challenging. In addition to ensuring that the molecule has the required potency, it must also be bioavailable, orally active, specific for the targeted enzyme family, and have no significant toxicity. Encouragingly, many of these conditions have been met with the development of inhibitors of another protease family, the zinc-dependent, metalloexopeptidase, angiotensin-converting enzyme (ACE). These compounds form a model for the design of MMP inhibitors. This approach consists of choosing a zinc-chelating ligand and attaching it to a peptide that mimics the cleavage site of the MMP target substrates (11).

Although the prospects for the prevention of cartilage macromolecule breakdown using synthetic MMP inhibitors look promising, opinions differ as to the best MMP to target. One option points to stopping the degradation of the collagen network, as it has been shown that its loss leads to irreversible damage, and that proteoglycans and other proteins can be readily lost from cartilage but rapidly replaced. Collagenase and stromelysin have a premier role in the degradation process in OA (2). However, as to which of the MMP should be the main candidate for inhibition, at this time collagenase-3 seems to be a very attractive candidate, first because it is the most potent peptidolytic enzyme of the three collagenases, and second, because this enzyme is present in only a few normal human tissue cells, therefore, its inhibition should not be harmful to the function of normal tissues (12). Its main role is hypothesized to be related to the remodeling process of cartilage in the early stages of OA, in addition to degradation. Others suggest that the inhibitors should have a broad spectrum, the advantage being to inhibit yet undiscovered MMP that may be involved in the disease process.

The first rational approach to the design of synthetic inhibitors was made toward collagenase. Different chelating moieties were tested, and these included thiols, carboxyl-alkyls, phosphonic acids, phophonamides, and hydroxamate groups (13). The hydroxamate-based compounds are potent inhibitors of MMP. They are believed to work by interacting with the active site of the MMP molecule and binding with the zinc molecule, thus inactivating the enzyme. Thiols and carboxyl-alkyls have a similar mode of action. Some of these compounds are currently under investigation.

Antibiotics such as tetracycline and its semisynthetic forms (doxycycline and minocycline) have very significant inhibitory properties that impact MMP activity *(14)*. Their action is mediated by chelating the zinc present in the active site of MMP. Tetracycline is a poor inhibitor of MMP, whereas semisynthetic homologs are more potent, making them more attractive. A clinical trial is presently underway to explore the therapeutic efficacy of doxycycline in knee OA patients.

Based on the results of clinical trials, it would be interesting to see whether the blockage of MMP alone is sufficient to halt the progressive and chronic destruction of connective tissue seen in the arthritides. If the release of connective tissue fragments is responsible for increasing synovial-joint inflammation, leading to a chronic cycle of damage with further destruction of connective tissue, then perhaps these inhibitors could be effective on their own. However, it is also possible that it may be necessary to combine protease inhibitors, either in sequence or with other agents that block specific steps in the disease process, before the chronic cycle of joint destruction found in these diseases can be broken.

ANTI-PROINFLAMMATORY CYTOKINES

Proinflammatory cytokines are additional factors that favor the enhancement of the catabolic process in OA. They appear to be first produced by the synovial membrane and diffused into the cartilage through the synovial fluid, where they activate the chondrocytes to also produce proinflammatory cytokines through auto- and paracrine mechanisms *(2)*. In OA synovium, it is the synovial-lining cells that play a major role as producers of inflammatory effectors. Yet it is claimed, and has been substantiated by studies in animal models, that IL-1β plays a pivotal role in cartilage destruction and be considered the main cytokine responsible for processing of enzyme systems, whereas TNF-α seems to be responsible for the induction of the inflammatory process *(15–17)*. These cytokines are able to stimulate their own production, to increase the synthesis of enzymes and more specifically the MMP, to inhibit the synthesis of the major physiological inhibitors of these enzymes, and also to inhibit the synthesis of matrix constituents such as collagen and aggrecans, thus making these two cytokines prime targets for therapeutic approaches.

Anti-Inflammatory Cytokines

An interesting and normal approach to the control of cytokine production is the use of cytokines with anti-inflammatory properties. At least three such cytokines, IL-4, IL-10, and IL-13, have been identified as being able to effectively reduce the production of some proinflammatory cytokines *(18–20)*. In vitro in OA synovium explants, recombinant human (rh) IL-4 suppressed the synthesis of both IL-1β and TNF-α in the same manner as low-dose dexamethasone *(21)*. In OA synovial fibroblasts, IL-4, IL-10, and IL-13 inhibit the TNF-α-induced PGE$_2$ *(22)*. In rheumatoid arthritis (RA) tissues, IL-10 has also been shown to inhibit the synthesis of the above proinflammatory cytokines *(19)*. IL-13 significantly inhibits lipopolysaccharide (LPS)-induced TNF-α production by mononuclear cells from peripheral blood *(23)*. In OA synovial membranes treated with

LPS, IL-13 inhibited the synthesis of IL-1β, TNF-α, and stromelysin, while increasing the IL-1 receptor antagonist (IL1-Ra) production *(24)*. All these data suggest that these anti-inflammatory cytokines could potentially be useful for the treatment of OA. Clinical trials using one of these anti-inflammatory cytokines, namely IL-10, is now underway to test its effects in RA patients.

Inhibiting IL-1β and TNF-α Maturation

A better understanding of the regulation of mechanisms responsible for the increased synthesis of these proinflammatory cytokines in the OA tissues has led to the development of new and promising therapeutic strategies. IL-1β and TNF-α are synthesized as inactive precursors, and have to be activated by an enzyme before being released extracellularly in their active forms. For IL-1β one protease belonging to the cysteine-dependent protease family and named IL-1β converting enzyme (ICE or caspase-1) has been identified and can specifically generate the mature form of IL-1β *(25)*. It was recently demonstrated that ICE can be detected in both human synovial membrane and in cartilage, with a marked and significant increase of its expression and synthesis in OA tissues *(26)*.

The proteolytic cleavage of the membrane-bound pro-TNF-α appears to occur, at least in part, via the TNF-α converting enzyme (TACE), an enzyme belonging to a subfamily of adamalysin *(27)*. An upregulation of the TACE expression has also recently been shown in OA human articular cartilage *(28,29)*.

Based on these findings, it becomes obvious that inhibition of these cytokines' activity by inhibiting the convertase enzymes is an attractive therapeutic target. It was recently shown in vitro using OA cartilage and synovium explants that a specific ICE inhibitor can completely abrogate the formation of active IL-1β *(26)*. Likewise, a recent in vivo study has demonstrated that ICE inhibitor effectively reduces the progression of murine type II-collagen-induced arthritis (CIA) *(30)*.

Inhibition of IL-1β and TNF-α Activity

Cell signaling by proinflammatory cytokines such as IL-1β and TNF-α occurs through binding to specific membrane receptors. For each cytokine, two types of receptors have been identified, type I and type II IL-1R, and TNF-R55 and TNF-R75. Type I IL-1R and TNF-R55 are responsible for the signal transduction in articular tissue cells *(31–34)*. Modulating IL-1 and TNF-α activity is likely to be a promising strategy to reduce the progression of structural changes in OA. Therapeutic strategies of antagonizing IL-1β and TNF-α with either receptor blockade or molecular quenching appear to be of value in other arthritic diseases or in OA animal models.

The IL-1 system is regulated by a natural antagonist of the receptor, which has been named IL-1Ra *(35)*. This molecule interferes specifically with the binding of the ligand to its receptor by competing for the same binding site. This inhibitor does not bind to IL-1, and therefore is not a binding protein, but rather a competitive inhibitor of IL-1/IL-1 receptor. In OA synovium, a relative deficit in the production of IL-1Ra vis-à-vis IL-1 has been demonstrated *(36)*. In vitro addition of IL-1Ra demonstrated its ability to reduce IL-1-induced cartilage degradation. In vivo, intra-articular injections of IL-1Ra were also found to retard the progression of experimental OA *(15)*. These findings have elicited much attention concerning the use of this gene in OA therapy. Studies done with two experimental animal models of OA and using two different methodologies of gene transfection (viral and nonviral) have proved successful in inducing in vivo gene expression and reducing the progression of structural changes *(37,38)*.

The second line of inhibition for proinflammatory cytokines is the binding of the cytokine to free receptors. Such molecules are named soluble receptors and are shed receptors: types I and II IL-1 soluble receptors (IL-1sR) and TNF-sR55 and TNF-sR75 *(39,40)*. The shed receptors may function as a receptor antagonist because the ligand-binding region is preserved, thus being capable of competing with the membrane-associated receptors of the target cells. It is suggested that type II IL-1R serve as the main precursor for shed soluble receptors. Interestingly, the binding affinity of IL-1sR to IL-1 and IL-1Ra differs. Type II IL-1sR binds IL-1β more readily than IL-1Ra; in contrast, type I IL-1sR binds IL-1Ra with high affinity *(41)*. Hence, the simultaneous addition of both IL-1Ra and type II IL-1sR appears extremely beneficial, while the individual inhibitory effects of both IL-1Ra and type I IL-1sR are abrogated when present concurrently.

In vivo, both forms of TNF-sR, TNF-sR55, and TNF-sR75, are present. In arthritic tissues and in OA synovial fibroblasts, increased amounts of TNF-sR75 were found *(33)*. It is suggested that TNF-sR functions as an inhibitor of cytokine activity by rendering the cells less sensitive to the activity of the ligands or by scavenging free ligands. The administration of TNF-sR has been shown to be a very effective treatment in RA patients *(42)*.

Another option would be the use of specific antibodies against IL-1 or TNF-α to neutralize their activity. Although this technique has been successfully tested for IL-1 in a CIA murine model of inflammatory arthritis *(43)*, no data is yet available for OA. Anti-TNF-α treatment in the murine CIA has also been shown to significantly improve the disease *(44)*. Clinical trials using an anti-TNF-α chimeric monoclonal antibody (MAb) in RA patients have shown that this approach is also a very promising one *(45,46)*.

Specific Inhibition of Proinflammatory
Cytokine-Induced Signal Transduction Pathways

Several post-receptor signaling pathways have been implicated in the synthesis of cytokines. Better understanding of the pathway specifically involved in IL-1β and TNF-α intracellular signaling cascades, particularly in OA cells, will provide additional molecular targets for pharmacological intervention. Two of these pathways, which involve the p38 MAP kinase and the nuclear factor-κB (NF-κB), appear to be major ones involved in mediating the synthesis of inflammatory cytokines, although their exact role in OA remains to be determined.

The p38 MAP kinase, a member of the MAP kinase family of serine-threonine protein kinases, was first identified as a protein kinase activated in mouse macrophages in response to LPS *(47)*. Subsequently, the human ortholog of p38 was identified. The inhibition of p38 MAP kinase and subsequently the synthesis of a number of important proinflammatory proteins has been identified as the primary mechanism by which inhibitors to p38 exert anti-inflammatory activity. The p38 pathway is commonly associated with the early stages of host response to injury and infection, and its potential role in various pathologic conditions has made it a target for therapeutic intervention. The p38 MAP kinase signaling pathway is activated by a variety of stressful stimuli, including heat, ultraviolet (UV) light, LPS, inflammatory cytokines, and high osmolarity

(47). When activated, p38 phosphorylates a number of downstream substrates, which include kinases (MAPKAPK-2 and K-3, MST, MSK, PRAK) and transcription factors (CHOP, MEF2, CREB, and ATF-2), which are responsible for subsequently regulating the synthesis of several proinflammatory cytokines.

The pyridinyl imidazole compounds that inhibit p38 MAP kinase and block proinflammatory cytokine production have been named cytokine suppressive anti-inflammatory drugs, or CSAIDs. These compounds inhibit proinflammatory cytokine synthesis at the translational rather than the transcriptional level *(48)*. In general, the CSAIDs inhibit the two splice forms of p38 (CSBP1 and CSBP2) as well as another isoform of this kinase, p38β, but not other closely related isoforms p38γ and p38δ *(49)*. Of particular relevance to the inhibition of p38 MAP kinase is that several cell types from articular tissues, including chondrocytes, express this protein. Some CSAIDs which have shown their ability to inhibit the synthesis of a number of proinflammatory cytokines in vitro translate into pharmacological activity in vivo, as some have proved their therapeutic activity in a number of animal models in the absence of generalized immunosuppression *(50–52)*. In addition to the inhibition of cytokines such as IL-1β and TNF-α, some CSAIDs were also shown to inhibit the production of nitric oxide (NO) from IL-1β or IL-17 stimulated cartilage explants and chondrocytes *(53,54)* or downregulated the spontaneous release of NO from human OA cartilage *(55)*. However, one must be cautious as there are instances where CSAID inhibition of certain metabolic pathways is not consistent across cells, stimuli, or species.

Development of drugs targeted against NF-κB activity/activation is also considered as a potential novel therapy for arthritis. NF-κB is a heterodimeric DNA binding protein that appears to be a major element in the regulation of proinflammatory cytokine production, by activating a coordinated transactivation of their genes. NF-κB consists of at least five members (p50, p52, p65, Rel B, c-Rel) which form complexes. NF-κB activation by the cytokines IL-1β and TNF-α has been found in many cells including OA chondrocytes and synovial fibroblasts. Moreover, it is quite likely that cyclooxygenase (COX)-2 and IL-1β are but two of several genes modulated, at least in part, by TNF-α-induced NF-κB activation. A recent report showed that specifically blocking the activation of this factor suppresses the severity of joint destruction in the rat CIA model *(56)*. Indeed, this study showed that transfection into joint synovial cells of synthetic decoy oligodeoxynucleotides containing the NF-κB *cis* element that binds NF-κB induced a marked reduction in the proinflammatory cytokine IL-1β and TNF-α at the gene level in joint synovium, as well as suppressing the degradation of bone and cartilage of the arthritic joint.

ANTI-NITRIC OXIDE (NO) AGENT

In addition, the inorganic free radical NO has been suggested as a factor that promotes cartilage catabolism in OA. NO is synthesized from L-arginine by the action of an enzyme, NO synthase (NOS). At present, the major isoforms of NO include the constitutive type (cNO) and an inducible type (iNO). It is the latter that is expressed after cell activation by cytokines or inflammatory factors. The constitutive NO production was shown to be necessary for the regulation of numerous physiological processes including blood pressure, platelet adhesiveness, gastrointestinal (GI) motility, and neurotransmission.

Compared to normal cartilage, OA cartilage produces a larger amount of NO, both under spontaneous and proinflammatory cytokine-stimulated conditions resulting in enhanced expression and protein synthesis of the inducible NO synthase (iNOS) *(57,58)*. A high level of nitrite/nitrate has also been found in the synovial fluid and serum of arthritic patients *(59)*. NO produced in response to cytokine stimulation exerts a number of catabolic effects that promote the degradation of articular cartilage. Indeed, NO has been shown to reduce proteoglycan synthesis, enhance MMP activity, and decrease synthesis of IL-1Ra, which are likely factors contributing to cartilage damage in OA *(57,60,61)*. This factor has also been reported to inhibit chondrocyte proliferation and induce apoptosis. The increased production of NO may be an additional factor contributing to the excess production of PGE_2 by OA tissues. In vitro inhibition of iNOS showed that it relieves the inhibition of matrix synthesis that otherwise occurs in response to IL-1. NO was also shown to inhibit the production of TGF-β by chondrocytes treated with IL-1, as well as to decrease matrix production in response to IGF-1. In OA cartilage, the involvement of NO in chondrocyte IGF-1 nonresponse was also confirmed from data obtained using iNOS$^{-/-}$ mice *(62)*.

Hence, the discovery and characterization of the functions of the iNOS isoenzyme has provided the impetus for novel therapeutic approaches toward developing a potential new class of drugs. The challenge was to have a selective inhibitor targeting only the inducible form of NOS in order not to downregulate the constitutive isoform. Even though iNOS inhibitors lag behind in their clinical development, there have been recent investigations into the in vivo potential of a selective iNOS inhibitor in a surgically induced OA animal model *(63,64)*. These studies examined the in vivo effect of a specific and selective iNOS inhibitor, the L-N^6-imminoethyl-L-lysine (L-NIL), under prophylactic conditions on the progression of experimentally induced OA. Selective inhibition of iNOS was demonstrated to reduce the progression of early lesions in an experimental OA model, and the inhibition of NO production was associated with a reduction in MMP activity in the cartilage. Moreover, it was shown that L-NIL decreased *in situ* the level of chondrocyte apoptosis and, more particularly, reduced the level of caspase-3. This data provides additional support for the hypothesis that the excess production of NO is related to cell apoptosis. Treatment with the selective iNOS inhibitor was also associated with a reduction in the level of proinflammatory mediators IL-1β and PGE_2 and nitrite/nitrate in the OA synovial fluid, as well as in a marked reduction of the volume of joint effusion. Collectively, these data suggest that selective iNOS inhibitors may not only be effective agents for treatment of the signs and symptoms of OA, but may also possess disease-modifying activity.

ANTI-APOPTOTIC THERAPY

Recent findings suggest that chondrocyte apoptosis may play a role in the pathogenesis of OA. Chondrocytes show several morphologic changes in OA cartilage. Cell cloning is a well-known phenomenon characterizing OA changes. Moreover, there is often an increase in the number of intracytoplasmic organelles that reflect the hypersynthetic state of these cells. There is also an increase in the number of cells exhibiting signs of degeneration or even death, a phenomenon that has been shown to be related to both cell necrosis and apoptosis, also called programmed cell death. This is a complex process related to the activation of several intercellular-signaling pathways *(65–68)*, including the caspase cascade. Caspases are a family of proteases that have been demonstrated to play a prominent role in inducing DNA damage *(69)*. On the other hand, a number of factors have been shown to exert a "protective effect" against apoptosis *(68,69)*. Such factors include proteins from the Bcl-2 family, which can prevent the efflux of cytochrome c from mitochondria and, secondarily, activation of the caspase cascade *(70,71)*. It has also been shown to prevent apoptosis through a caspase activation-independent mechanism that is not yet fully understood *(71)*. Excess production of NO has been linked with cartilage chondrocyte apoptosis both in vitro and in vivo *(64,72,73)*. Results of studies using cell lines indicate that NO might induce apoptosis via mitochondria damage and, more precisely, by cytochrome c release leading to activation of the caspase enzymes *(74)*. As mentioned earlier, in chondrocytes the NO effect on apoptosis appears related to a decreased level of caspase-3 activity *(64)*. The loss of chondrocytes reduces the ability of cartilage to repair itself and may in fact accelerate the progression of lesions, particularly in the early stages of OA, when the repair process predominates. In articular cartilage, chondrocyte apoptosis is associated with a reduction in the amount of the pericellular matrix and accumulation of apoptotic bodies in chondrocyte lacunae and in the interterritorial space. These apoptotic bodies may share functional properties with matrix vesicles and contain enzymatic activities that are involved in the deposition of calcium, thus promoting the calcification of pathologic cartilage observed in OA *(75)*. Moreover, the very weak capacity for chondrocytes to replicate makes cell loss in cartilage a very significant problem, particularly in conditions such as OA where the need for chondrocytes to produce an increased amount of macromolecules is dramatically increased.

Our increased knowledge about the mechanisms regulating chondrocyte apoptosis now makes it possible to plan strategy for therapeutic approaches that could be targeted for future OA treatment.

TARGETING SUBCHONDRAL BONE AS A STRATEGY FOR OA THERAPY

In an ideal world, drug therapy for OA should target the early pathogenic events of the disease process. It is currently suggested that subchondral bone remodeling may be more intimately related to the progression and/or onset of OA rather than merely a consequence of this disease. Recent work indicates that very early in the OA process, biological and morphological disturbances occur at the subchondral bone, and may have a role in modulating articular cartilage metabolism. However, the "myth" of harder subchondral bone explaining the sclerosis in this tissue must be put aside as emerging data indicate a generalized undermineralization of this tissue, as in osteoporosis *(76,77)*. This situation of subchondral bone appears to result from abnormal osteoblast metabolism. Because there is evidence that subchondral bone is involved early in OA *(78,79)*, attempts to interfere with bone metabolism are of special interest.

A potential pharmacological approach may target the reduction of abnormal subchondral bone-metabolism activities, particularly in early disease. As this tissue is now believed to be undermineralized, two lines of intervention may be taken: prevent the removal of mineralized matrix, and/or increase mineralization. The mechanisms controlling the mineralization process are currently not well-known, yet abnormal collagen production is a recognized factor that could be targeted in this process.

It is obviously easier to target the removal of mineralized matrix. However current antiresorptive drugs, which could inhibit the formation of cancellous subchondral bone, would not be effective on the formation of marginal osteophytes that occur through enchondral ossification.

It is also important to note that osteoblasts obtained from OA patients do not behave similarly in in vitro culture, and two populations of patients can be discriminated based on cytokine and prostaglandin production *(80)*. Hence, medication aimed at curbing IL-1β or IL-6 signaling, or reducing TGF-β and PGE$_2$ production, could be effective in about half the patients with OA. In that respect, using nonsteroidal anti-inflammatory drugs (NSAIDs) would be beneficial for those patients that produce high endogenous levels of PGE$_2$. On the other hand, corticosteroids may prove effective in subchondral bone. Indeed, a retrospective observational study evaluating radiographic changes over 4–15 yr following repeated intra-articular injections *(81)*, as well as a study with an animal model of OA *(82)* showed that corticosteroids may be adequate to retard cartilage degeneration along with osteophyte formation. Indeed, corticosteroids are known to retard bone formation via the inhibition of cell growth and collagen deposition, and abnormal collagen production that is undermineralized is observed in OA bone tissue.

GENE THERAPY

A major stumbling block in the use of biological molecules as therapeutic agents is the limitation in the methods that can be used to deliver these agents and its applicability to the clinical scenario. Degradation of the protein after oral administration poses a problem and, if injected systematically, the large amount required and the need for frequent injections are often deterrents. This last route of administration can induce adverse effects including an immunological reaction with the appearance of a neutralizing antibody. The necessity of maintaining a sustained level of the agents systemically or logically over time is the major concern with this type of therapy.

Over the last few years, much attention has been focused on the use of gene-transfer techniques as a method of delivery. Many techniques have been developed using various genes, and a great deal of work is currently devoted to these techniques to facilitate the transfer of genes into joint cells and tissues both in vitro and in vivo. The advantages of gene transfer for the treatment of OA are multiple and include the identification of a very specific target, a consistently high local concentration in the joint of the therapeutic protein, and the maintenance of sustained delivery over time. Moreover, there is also hope that this type of therapy could reduce the incidence of side effects.

Treatment can be effected in various ways: by ex vivo modification, with the gene being reintroduced into the body after modification, or by in vivo modification. Regardless of the approach being adopted, the treatment will probably involve one of the following strategies: gene replacement, in which the substitution of a nonactive or defective gene by a new or additional functional copy of the gene will be used to restore the production of a required protein, or, the insertion into the cell of a gene to enable the production of a protein not normally expressed or expressed in low amounts by the cell: a convertase gene that activates a pro-factor (example, some growth factors) or *IL-1Ra* gene. A third approach could be the use of a control gene (example, a gene that will be turned on by a specific stimulus) in which protein production will control production of another gene to increase or alter the expression of a given gene.

Two main systems, viral and nonviral, are currently used for gene transfer to cells *(83)*. At this time, the viral system is favored for some proteins because it generally allows for a very effective transfer to a large percentage of cells, while maintaining a sustained high level of protein expression that can be extended over significant periods of time. For the nonviral system, the simplest are plasmids encoding the gene of interest and named naked DNA. Usually their expression is low and transient. However, their efficacy can be improved by combining them with carriers, such as liposomes.

The potential tissue targets for gene therapy in OA are synovial membrane, cartilage, and bone. However, based on previous work in RA and OA in animal models, the lining cells of the synovium remain the easier target for gene delivery. Moreover, it is well-established that secreted transgene products are able to diffuse from the synovium into cartilage and modulate chondrocyte metabolism. Ex vivo transfer of marker genes to the articular cartilage has been demonstrated in animals with the use of retroviral and adenoviral vectors *(37,83)*. In vivo gene delivery to chondrocytes has been proven to be technically difficult, owing in part to the extracellular matrix thickness, except in advanced OA. Nevertheless, successful in vivo liposome-mediated delivery to chondrocytes in the superficial and mid-zones of the articular cartilage of rat knees by a combination of a virus and liposomes or of rabbit knees by a plasmid-liposome vector liposomes has been reported *(84)*.

Although the treatment of OA using gene therapy is very promising, this technique is still in the very early stages of development, and much work remains to be done, particularly on the in vivo development of this technology for humans. Moreover, although some gene transfers such as IL-1Ra, IL-10, IL-13 have been studied using OA or inflammatory animal models and have shown interesting data, the selection or combination of the gene(s) that would offer the best protection against OA remains to be determined.

As mentioned earlier, the relevance of subchondral bone to OA pathophysiology has become much appreciated in recent years. The increased level of synthesis of cytokines, proteases and growth factors such as TGF-β that have been identified in OA subchondral bone tissue as well as in cartilage and synovial membrane have the potential for adverse effects in each of these joint tissues. Therefore, the modulation of their synthesis by gene therapy could prove an interesting target.

CONCLUSION

Despite an extensive armamentarium of treatment options available, OA remains incurable. An improved approach in the development of remittive treatment is imperative. The current understanding of the factors involved in this disease has evolved greatly in recent years. A clearer understanding of the pathophysiology of OA has permitted a better comprehension of the modulating factors as well as the major regulators, which may have potential therapeutic value in treatment to specifically and effectively retard the progression of this disease. The future holds great promise for the development of new and successful approaches to the treatment of this disease.

Appropriate goals for the development of new therapies to treat OA should include better-tolerated and more effective drugs to treat the symptoms of OA, and treatment to slow, arrest, prevent, or repair the inevitable pathologic changes associated with OA, i.e., structure-modifying agents. Recent evidence points to a significant role for anti-inflammatory, cytokine-related drugs. They may represent a promising approach although clinical studies in humans are awaited. Further data on the therapeutic effects of selective MMP and iNOS inhibitors on the progression of lesions in OA is emerging.

Basic and clinical studies have shown that there is some continuity between both bone and cartilage changes as OA progresses, suggesting cross-talk between these tissues. If bone response to injury and the associations with bone proteins could be elucidated, it may be possible to identify factors associated with OA progression. Moreover, studies have also shown that synovial-membrane inflammation results in the "full-blown" clinical situation. However, the exact sequence of pathological events in OA remains unclear; the temporal relationship between bone damage, chronic inflammation of synovial tissue and cartilage erosion is still very much unknown.

Findings from basic science research are progressing at an exponential rate. Discovery of new mediators and pathways that may be relevant to OA are continually being discovered. Investigation of these parameters and the beneficial effects of new drugs and agents may be provided by in vitro testing assessing the processes involved in OA and its treatment. However, in vitro studies might not always be relevant to the in vivo situation. A number of animal models have been developed and can provide some useful in vivo information about OA processes and new experimental treatments. However, regardless of the methodology used for eliciting a process that is similar to human OA, all such studies must be equivalent to studies in humans in terms of predetermined outcome measures.

Drug delivery is a major weakness of existing anti-arthritic therapies. Local delivery of anti-arthritic factors or the in vivo induction of their expression using gene transfer may provide a novel approach for the treatment of OA. Evidence of efficacy of gene therapy in OA remains, for the moment, at the experimental level.

It is clear that considerable progress has been made towards greater understanding of the underlying mechanisms involved in OA. The outlook for finding a cure for OA is more promising than ever. However, as OA progression is alluded to as being the advancement of a series of pathological features resulting from aberrant biochemistry in the joint, a question that remains to be answered is what causes the joint to progress from dormancy to an active disease, and whether there is any way in which this can be accurately evaluated. Based on the discovery of major pathophysiological pathways leading to the structural changes observed in OA, one is confident that it will be possible, through new ways, to treat this disease.

REFERENCES

1. Felson, D.T. and Y. Zhang, 1998. An update on the epidemiology of knee and hip osteoarthritis with a view to prevention. *Arthritis Rheum.* 41:1343–1355.

2. Pelletier, J.P., J. Martel-Pelletier, and D.S. Howell. 2000. Etiopathogenesis of osteoarthritis. In Arthritis and Allied Conditions. A Textbook of Rheumatology, 14th edition. W.J. Koopman, editor. Williams & Wilkins, Baltimore. 2195–2245.

3. Birkedal-Hansen, H., W.G. Moore, M.K. Bodden, L.J. Windsor, B. Birkedal-Hansen, A. DeCarlo, and J.A. Engler. 1993. Matrix metalloproteinases: a review. *Crit. Rev. Oral Biol. Med.* 4:197–250.

4. Vincenti, M.P., L.A. White, D.J. Schroen, U. Benbow, and C.E. Brinckerhoff. 1996. Regulating expression of the gene for matrix metalloproteinase-1 (collagenase): mechanisms that control enzyme activity, transcription, and mRNA stability. *Crit. Rev. Eukaryot. Gene Expr.* 6:391–411.

5. Benbow, U. and C.E. Brinckerhoff. 1997. The AP-1 site and MMP gene regulation: what is all the fuss about? *Matrix Biol.* 15:519–526.

6. Gomez, D.E., D.F. Alonso, H. Yoshiji, and U.P. Thorgeirsson. 1997. Tissue inhibitors of metalloproteinases: structure, regulation and biological functions. *Eur. J. Cell Biol.* 74:111–122.

7. Cawston, T.E. 1996. Metalloproteinase inhibitors and the prevention of connective tissue breakdown. *Pharmacol. Ther.* 70:163–182.

8. Wojtowicz-Praga, S.M., R.B. Dickson, and M.J. Hawkins. 1997. Matrix metalloproteinase inhibitors. *Invest. New Drugs* 15:61–75.

9. Gomis-Ruth, F.X., K. Maskos, M. Betz, A. Bergner, R. Huber, K. Suzuki, N. Yoshida, H. Nagase, K. Brew, G.P. Bourenkov, et al. 1997. Mechanism of inhibition of the human matrix metalloproteinase stromelysin-1 by TIMP-1. *Nature* 389:77–81.

10. Huang, W., Q. Meng, K. Suzuki, H. Nagase, and K. Brew. 1997. Mutational study of the amino-terminal domain of human tissue inhibitor of metalloproteinases 1 (TIMP-1) locates an inhibitory region for matrix metalloproteinases. *J. Biol. Chem.* 272:22,086–22,091.

11. Beckett, R. and M. Whittaker. 1998. Matrix metalloproteinase inhibitors. *Exp. Opin. Ther. Patents* 8:259–282.

12. Martel-Pelletier, J. and J.P. Pelletier. 1996. Wanted: the collagenase responsible for the destruction of the collagen network in human cartilage! *Br. J. Rheumatol.* 35:818–820.

13. Vincenti, M.P., I.M. Clark, and C.E. Brinckerhoff. 1994. Using inhibitors of metalloproteinases to treat arthritis. Easier said than done? *Arthritis Rheum.* 37:1115–1126.

14. Yu, L.P. Jr., G.N. Smith, Jr., K.D. Brandt, S.L. Myers, B.L. O'Connor, and D.A. Brandt. 1992. Reduction of the severity of canine osteoarthritis by prophylactic treatment with oral doxycycline. *Arthritis Rheum.* 35:1150–1159.

15. Caron, J.P., J.C. Fernandes, J. Martel-Pelletier, G. Tardif, F. Mineau, C. Geng, and J.P. Pelletier. 1996. Chondroprotective effect of intraarticular injections of interleukin-1 receptor antagonist in experimental osteoarthritis: suppression of collagenase-1 expression. *Arthritis Rheum.* 39:1535–1544.

16. Van de Loo, F.A.J., L.A. Joosten, P.L. van Lent, O.J. Arntz, and W.B. van den Berg. 1995. Role of interleukin-1, tumor necrosis factor alpha, and interleukin-6 in cartilage proteoglycan metabolism and destruction. Effect of *in situ* blocking in murine antigen- and zymosan-induced arthritis. *Arthritis Rheum.* 38:164–172.

17. Plows, D., L. Probert, S. Georgopoulos, L. Alexopoulou, and G. Kollias. 1995. The role of tumour necrosis factor (TNF) in arthritis: studies in transgenic mice. *Rheumatol. Eur.* (Suppl. 2):51–54.

18. Hart, P.H., G.F. Vitti, D.R. Burgess, G.A. Whitty, D.S. Piccoli, and J.A. Hamilton. 1989. Potential antiinflammatory effects of interleukin 4: suppression of human monocyte tumor necrosis factor alpha, interleukin 1, and prostaglandin E_2. *Proc. Natl. Acad. Sci. USA* 86:3803–3807.

19. Jenkins, J.K., M. Malyak, and W.P. Arend. 1994. The effects of interleukin-10 on interleukin-1 receptor antagonist and interleukin-1β production in human monocytes and neutrophils. *Lymphokine Cytokine Res.* 13:47–54.

20. de Waal Malefyt, R., C.G. Figdor, R. Huijbens, S. Mohan-Peterson, B. Bennett, J.A. Culpepper, et al. 1993. Effects of IL-13 on phenotype, cytokine production, and cytotoxic function of human monocytes. Comparison with IL-4 and modulation by IFN-gamma or IL-10. *J. Immunol.* 151:6370–6381.

21. Bendrups, A., A. Hilton, A. Meager, and J.A. Hamilton. 1993. Reduction of tumor necrosis factor alpha and interleukin-1 beta levels in human synovial tissue by interleukin-4 and glucocorticoid. *Rheumatol. Int.* 12:217–220.

22. Alaaeddine, N., J.A. Di Battista, J.P. Pelletier, K. Kiansa, J.M. Cloutier, and J. Martel-Pelletier. 1999. Inhibition of tumor necrosis factor alpha-induced prostaglandin E_2 production by the antiinflammatory cytokines interleukin-4, interleukin-10, and interleukin-13 in osteoarthritic synovial fibroblasts: distinct targeting in the signaling pathways. *Arthritis Rheum.* 42:710–718.

23. Hart, P.H., M.J. Ahern, M.D. Smith, and J.J. Finlay-Jones. 1995. Regulatory effects of IL-13 on synovial fluid macrophages and blood monocytes from patients with inflammatory arthritis. *Clin. Exp. Immunol.* 99:331–337.

24. Jovanovic, D., J.P. Pelletier, N. Alaaeddine, F. Mineau, C. Geng, P. Ranger, and J. Martel-Pelletier. 1998. Effect of IL-13 on cytokines, cytokine receptors and inhibitors on human osteoarthritic synovium and synovial fibroblasts. *Osteoarthritis Cart.* 6:40–49.

25. Black, R.A., S.R. Kronheim, M. Cantrell, M.C. Deeley, C.J. March, K.S. Prickett, et al. 1988. Generation of biologically active interleukin-1 beta by proteolytic cleavage of the inactive precursor. *J. Biol. Chem.* 263:9437–9442.

26. Saha, N., F. Moldovan, G. Tardif, J.P. Pelletier, J.M. Cloutier, and J. Martel-Pelletier. 1999. Interleukin-1β-converting enzyme/caspase-1 in human osteoarthritic tissues: localization and role in the maturation of IL-1β and IL-18. *Arthritis Rheum.* 42:1577–1587.

27. Gearing, A.J., P. Beckett, M. Christodoulou, M. Churchill, J. Clements, A.H. Davidson, et al. 1994. Processing of tumour necrosis factor-alpha precursor by metalloproteinases. *Nature* 370:555–557.

28. Patel, I.R., M.G. Attur, R.N. Patel, S.A. Stuchin, R.A. Abagyan, S.B. Abramson, and A.R. Amin. 1998. TNF-alpha convertase enzyme from human arthritis-affected cartilage: isolation of cDNA by differential display, expression of the active enzyme, and regulation of TNF-alpha. *J. Immunol.* 160:4570–4579.

29. Amin, A.R. 1999. Regulation of tumor necrosis factor-alpha and tumor necrosis factor converting enzyme in human osteoarthritis. *Osteoarthritis Cart.* 7:392–394.

30. Ku, G., T. Faust, L.L. Lauffer, D.J. Livingston, and M.W. Harding. 1996. Interleukin-1β converting enzyme inhibition blocks progression of the type II collagen-induced arthritis in mice. *Cytokine* 8:377–386.

31. Martel-Pelletier, J., R. McCollum, J.A. Di Battista, M.P. Faure, J.A. Chin, S. Fournier, et al. 1992. The interleukin-1 receptor in normal and osteoarthritic human articular chondrocytes. Identification as the type I receptor and analysis of binding kinetics and biologic function. *Arthritis Rheum.* 35:530–540.

32. Sadouk, M., J.P. Pelletier, G. Tardif, K. Kiansa, J.M. Cloutier, and J. Martel-Pelletier. 1995. Human synovial fibroblasts coexpress interleukin-1 receptor type I and type II mRNA: The increased level of the interleukin-1 receptor in osteoarthritic cells is related to an increased level of the type I receptor. *Lab. Invest.* 73:347–355.

33. Alaaeddine, N., J.A. Di Battista, J.P. Pelletier, J.M. Cloutier, K. Kiansa, M. Dupuis, and J. Martel-Pelletier. 1997. Osteoarthritic synovial fibroblasts possess an increased level of tumor necrosis factor-receptor 55 (TNF-R55) that mediates biological activation by TNF-alpha. *J. Rheumatol.* 24:1985–1994.

34. Westacott, C.I., R.M. Atkins, P.A. Dieppe, and C.J. Elson. 1994. Tumour necrosis factor-alpha receptor expression on chondrocytes isolated from human articular cartilage. *J. Rheumatol.* 21:1710–1715.

35. Arend, W.P. 1993. Interleukin-1 receptor antagonist. *Adv. Immunol.* 54:167–227.

36. Pelletier, J.P., R. McCollum, J.M. Cloutier, and J. Martel-Pelletier. 1995. Synthesis of metalloproteases and interleukin 6 (IL-6) in human osteoarthritic synovial membrane is an IL-1 mediated process. *J. Rheumatol.* 22:109–114.

37. Pelletier, J.P., J.P. Caron, C.H. Evans, P.D. Robbins, H.I. Georgescu, D. Jovanovic, et al. 1997. *In vivo* suppression of early experimental osteoarthritis by IL-Ra using gene therapy. *Arthritis Rheum.* 40:1012–1019.

38. Fernandes, J.C., G. Tardif, J. Martel-Pelletier, V. Lascau-Coman, M. Dupuis, F. Moldovan, et al. 1999. *In vivo* transfer of interleukin-1 receptor antagonist gene in osteoarthritic rabbit knee joints: prevention of osteoarthritis progression. *Am. J. Pathol.* 154:1159–1169.

39. Giri, J.G., R.C. Newton, and R. Horuk. 1990. Identification of soluble interleukin-1 binding protein in cell-free supernatants. Evidence for soluble interleukin-1 receptor. *J. Biol. Chem.* 265: 17,416–17,419.

40. Lantz, M., U. Gullberg, E. Nilsson, and Olsson. I. 1990. Characterization *in vitro* of a human tumor necrosis factor-binding protein. A soluble form of a tumor necrosis factor receptor. *J. Clin. Invest.* 86:1396–1342.

41. Svenson, M., M.B. Hansen, P. Heegaard, K. Abell, and K. Bendtzen. 1993. Specific binding of interleukin-1 (IL-1)-β and IL-1 receptor antagonist (IL-1ra) to human serum. High-affinity binding of IL-1ra to soluble IL-1 receptor type I. *Cytokine* 5:427–435.

42. Franklin, C.M. 1999. Clinical experience with soluble TNF p75 receptor in rheumatoid arthritis. *Semin. Arthritis Rheum.* 29:172–181.

43. Joosten, L.A.B., M.M. Helsen, F.A. van de Loo, and W.B. van den Berg. 1996. Anticytokine treatment of established type II collagen-induced arthritis in DBA/1 mice. A comparative study using anti-TNF alpha, anti- IL-1 alpha/beta, and IL-1Ra. *Arthritis Rheum.* 39:797–809.

44. Williams, R.O., J. Ghrayeb, M. Feldmann, and R.N. Maini. 1995. Successful therapy of collagen-induced arthritis with TNF receptor-IgG fusion protein and combination with anti-CD4. *Immunology* 84:433–439.

45. Elliott, M.J., R.N. Maini, M. Feldmann, J.R. Kalden, C. Antoni, J.S. Smolen, et al. 1994. Randomised double-blind comparison of chimeric monoclonal antibody to tumour necrosis factor alpha (cA2) versus placebo in rheumatoid arthritis. *Lancet* 344:1105–1110.

46. Maini, R., St. E.W. Clair, F. Breedveld, D. Furst, J. Kalden, M. Weisman, et al. 1999. Infliximab (chimeric anti-tumour necrosis factor alpha monoclonal antibody) versus placebo in rheumatoid arthritis patients receiving concomitant methotrexate: a randomised phase III trial. ATTRACT Study Group. *Lancet* 354:1932–1939.

47. Han, J., J.D. Lee, L. Bibbs, and R.J. Ulevitch. 1994. A MAP kinase targeted by endotoxin and hyperosmolarity in mammalian cells. *Science* 265:808–811.

48. Young, P., P. McDonnell, D. Dunnington, A. Hand, J. Laydon, and J. Lee,. 1993. Pyridinyl imidazoles inhibit IL-1 and TNF production at the protein level. *Agents Actions* 39 Spec No:C67–69.

49. Cuenda, A., J. Rouse, Y.N. Doza, R. Meier, P. Cohen, T.F. Gallagher, et al. 1995. SB 203580 is a specific inhibitor of a MAP kinase homologue which is stimulated by cellular stresses and interleukin-1. *FEBS Lett.* 364:229–233.

50. Lee, J.C., A.M. Badger, D.E. Griswold, D. Dunnington, A. Truneh, B. Votta, et al. 1993. Bicyclic imidazoles as a novel class of cytokine biosynthesis inhibitors. *Ann. NY Acad. Sci.* 696:149–170.

51. Reddy, M.P., E.F. Webb, D. Cassatt, D. Maley, J.C. Lee, D.E. Griswold, and A. Truneh. 1994. Pyridinyl imidazoles inhibit the inflammatory phase of delayed type hypersensitivity reactions without affecting T-dependent immune responses. *Int. J. Immunopharmacol.* 16:795–804.

52. Badger, A.M., D.E. Griswold, R. Kapadia, S. Blake, B.A. Swift, S.J. Hoffman, et al. 2000. Disease-modifying activity of SB 242235, a selective inhibitor of p38 mitogen-activated protein kinase, in rat adjuvant-induced arthritis. *Arthritis Rheum.* 43:175–183.

53. Badger, A.M., M.N. Cook, M.W. Lark, T.M. Newman-Tarr, B.A. Swift, A.H. Nelson, et al. 1998. SB 203580 inhibits p38 mitogen-activated protein kinase, nitric oxide production, and inducible nitric oxide synthase in bovine cartilage-derived chondrocytes. *J. Immunol.* 161:467–473.

54. Martel-Pelletier, J., F. Mineau, D. Jovanovic, J.A. Di Battista, and J.P. Pelletier. 1999. Mitogen-activated protein kinase and nuclear factor-κB together regulate interleukin-17-induced nitric oxide production in human osteoarthritic chondrocytes: possible role of transactivating factor mitogen-activated protein kinase-activated protein kinase (MAPKAPK). *Arthritis Rheum.* 42:2399–2409.

55. Attur, M.G., I.R. Patel, R.N. Patel, S.B. Abramson, and A.R. Amin. 1998. Autocrine production of IL-1 beta by human osteoarthritis-affected cartilage and differential regulation of endogenous nitric oxide, IL-6, prostaglandin E2, and IL-8. *Proc. Assoc. Am. Physicians* 110:65–72.

56. Tomita, T., E. Takeuchi, N. Tomita, R. Morishita, M. Kaneko, K. Yamamoto, et al. 1999. Suppressed severity of collagen-induced arthritis by *in vivo* transfection of nuclear factor kappaB decoy oligodeoxynucleotides as a gene therapy. *Arthritis Rheum.* 42:2532–2542.

57. Pelletier, J.P., F. Mineau, P. Ranger, G. Tardif, and J. Martel-Pelletier. 1996. The increased synthesis of inducible nitric oxide inhibits IL-1Ra synthesis by human articular chondrocytes: possible role in osteoarthritic cartilage degradation. *Osteoarthritis Cart.* 4:77–84.

58. Amin, A.R., P.E. Di Cesare, P. Vyas, M.G. Attur, E. Tzeng, T.R. Billiar, et al. 1995. The expression and regulation of nitric oxide synthase in human osteoarthritis-affected chondrocytes: evidence for an inducible "neuronal-like" nitric oxide synthase. *J. Exp. Med.* 182:2097–2102.

59. Farrell, A.J., D.R. Blake, R.M. Palmer, and S. Moncada. 1992. Increased concentrations of nitrite in synovial fluid and serum samples suggest increased nitric oxide synthesis in rheumatic diseases. *Ann. Rheum. Dis.* 51:1219–1222.

60. Järvinen, T.A.H., T. Moilanen, T.L.N. Järvinen, and E. Moilanen. 1995. Nitric oxide mediates interleukin-1 induced inhibition of glycosaminoglycan synthesis in rat articular cartilage. *Mediators Inflamm.* 4:107–111.

61. Murrell, G.A.C., D. Jang, and R.J. Williams. 1995. Nitric oxide activates metalloprotease enzymes in articular cartilage. *Biochem. Biophys. Res. Commun.* 206:15–21.

62. Van de Loo, F.A.J., O.J. Arntz, van F.H. Enckevort, P.L. van Lent, and W.B. van den Berg. 1998. Reduced cartilage proteoglycan loss during zymosan-induced gonarthritis in NOS2-deficient mice and in anti-interleukin-1-treated wild-type mice with unabated joint inflammation. *Arthritis Rheum.* 41:634–646.

63. Pelletier, J.P., V. Lascau-Coman, D. Jovanovic, J.C. Fernandes, P. Manning, M.G. Currie, and J. Martel-Pelletier. 1999. Selective inhibition of inducible nitric oxide synthase in experimental osteoarthritis is associated with reduction in tissue levels of catabolic factors. *J. Rheumatol.* 26:2002–2014.

64. Pelletier, J.P., D.V. Jovanovic, V. Lascau-Coman, J.C. Fernandes, P.T. Manning, J.R. Connor, et al. 2000. Selective inhibition of inducible nitric oxide synthase reduces the progression of experimental osteoarthritis *in vivo*: Possible link with the reduction in chondrocyte apoptosis and caspase-3 level. *Arthritis Rheum.* 43:1290–1299.

65. Blanco, F.J., R. Guitian, E. Vazquez-Martul, F.J. de Toro, and F. Galdo. 1998. Osteoarthritis chondrocytes die by apoptosis. A possible pathway for osteoarthritis pathology. *Arthritis Rheum.* 41:284–289.

66. Horton, W.E. Jr., L. Feng, and C. Adams. 1998. Chondrocyte apoptosis in development, aging and disease. *Matrix Biol.* 17:107–115.

67. Vaishnaw, A.K., J.D. McNally, and K.B. Elkon. 1997. Apoptosis in the rheumatic diseases (review). *Arthritis Rheum.* 40:1917–1927.

68. Nagata, S. 1997. Apoptosis by death factor. *Cell* 88:355–365.

69. Thornberry, N. and Y.A. Lazebnik. 1998. Caspases: enemies within. *Science* 281:1312–1316.

70. Swanton, E., P. Savory, S. Cosulich, P. Clarke, and P. Woodman. 1999. Bcl-2 regulates a caspase-3/caspase-2 apoptotic cascade in cytosolic extracts. *Oncogene* 18:1781–1787.

71. Okuno, S., S. Shimizu, T. Ito, M. Nomura, E. Hamada, Y. Tsujimoto, and H. Matsuda. 1998. Bcl-2 prevents caspase-independent cell death. *J. Biol. Chem.* 273:34,272–34,277.

72. Hashimoto, S., K. Takahashi, D. Amiel, R.D. Coutts, and M. Lotz. 1998. Chondrocyte apoptosis and nitric oxide production during experimentally induced osteoarthritis. *Arthritis Rheum.* 41:1266–1274.

73. Blanco, F.J., R.L. Ochs, H. Schwarz, and M. Lotz. 1995. Chondrocyte apoptosis induced by nitric oxide. *Am. J. Pathol.* 146:75–85.

74. Ushmorov, A., F. Ratter, V. Lehmann, W. Droge, V. Schirrmacher, and V. Umansky. 1999. Nitric-oxide-induced apoptosis in human leukemic lines requires mitochondrial lipid degradation and cytochrome C release. *Blood* 93:2342–2352.

75. Hashimoto, S., R.L. Ochs, F. Rosen, J. Quach, G. McCabe, J. Solan, et al. 1998. Chondrocyte-derived apoptotic bodies and calcification of articular cartilage. *Proc. Natl. Acad. Sci. USA* 95:3094–3099.

76. Grynpas, M.D., B. Alpert, I. Katz, I. Lieberman, and K.P.H. Pritzker. 1991. Subchondral bone in osteoarthritis. *Calcif. Tissue Int.* 49:20–26.

77. Li, B. and R.M. Aspden. 1997. Composition and mechanical properties of cancellous bone from the femoral head of patients with osteoporosis or osteoarthritis. *J. Bone Miner. Res.* 12:614–651.

78. Hilal, G., J. Martel-Pelletier, J.P. Pelletier, P. Ranger, and D. Lajeunesse. 1998. Osteoblast-like cells from human subchondral osteoarthritic bone demonstrate an altered phenotype *in vitro*: Possible role in subchondral bone sclerosis. *Arthritis Rheum.* 41:891–899.

79. Hilal, G., J. Martel-Pelletier, J.P. Pelletier, N. Duval, and D. Lajeunesse. 1999. Abnormal regulation of urokinase plasminogen activator by insulin-like growth factor-1 in human osteoarthritic subchondral osteoblasts. *Arthritis Rheum.* 42:2112–2122.

80. Benderdour, M., G. Hilal, D. Lajeunesse, J.P. Pelletier, N. Duval, and J. Martel-Pelletier. 1999. Osteoarthritic osteoblasts show variable levels of cytokines production despite similar phenotypic expression. *Arthritis Rheum.* 42:S251 (Abstract).

81. Balch, H.W., J.M. Gibson, A.F. El-Ghobarey, L.S. Bain, and M.P. Lynch. 1977. Repeated corticosteroid injections into knee joints. *Rheumatol. Rehabil.* 16:137–140.

82. Pelletier, J.P., F. Mineau, J.P. Raynauld, J.F. Woessner Jr., Z. Gunja-Smith, and J. Martel-Pelletier. 1994. Intraarticular injections with methylprednisolone acetate reduce osteoarthritic lesions in parallel with chondrocyte stromelysin synthesis in experimental osteoarthritis. *Arthritis Rheum.* 37:414–423.

83. Evans, C.H. and P.D. Robbins. 1994. Gene therapy for arthritis. *In* Gene Therapeutics: Methods and Applications of Direct Gene Transfer. J.A. Wolff, editor. Birkhauser, Boston. 320–343.

84. Tomita, T., H. Hashimoto, N. Tomita, R. Morishita, S.B. Lee, K. Hayashida, et al. 1997. *In vivo* direct gene transfer into articular cartilage by intraarticular injection mediated by HVJ (sendai virus) and liposomes. *Arthritis Rheum.* 40:901–906.

17

Recent Developments in the Therapy of Osteoarthritis

Jean-Pierre Pelletier
and Johanne Martel-Pelletier

CONTENTS

INTRODUCTION

INTRODUCTION

The last decade has been the scene of several interesting advances in the treatment of osteoarthritis (OA). Improved understanding regarding the pathophysiology of OA has contributed to the development of new strategies for treatments aimed at specifically and effectively retarding or stopping the progression of this disease.

The drugs in development for the treatment of OA can be classified as being either symptomatic or structure (disease)-modifying. Greater comprehension of the mechanisms responsible for joint damage and repair has led to the development of several new classes of molecules that inhibit one or more OA catabolic processes, whereas some of the drugs now used are being evaluated for their potential to alter the degenerative process.

Although nonsteroidal antiinflammatory drugs (NSAIDs) are effective for acute and chronic pain, their use in the treatment of OA is not completely resolved. Some of the hesitation regarding the use of NSAIDs for the treatment of OA is related mainly to their side effects. A significant level of gastrointestinal (GI) complications have been well-documented and are related in part to the local inhibition of prostaglandin synthesis. NSAIDs appear to share some degree of similarity, in that they inhibit prostaglandin synthesis, which are produced by cyclooxygenase (COX). At least two isoforms of this enzyme have been identified: COX-1, which plays a constitutive role, and COX-2, which plays a critical role in the inflammatory disease process. The recent discovery of these isoforms has allowed the synthesis of a new generation of drugs that specifically block COX-2 but spare COX-1. These anti-inflammatory drugs have proven to be much safer compared to the classic NSAIDs, which inhibit both COX-1 and COX-2. The new specific COX-2 inhibitors have so far fared as well as the old ones in terms of efficacy in OA. It is hoped that these new NSAIDs will have a better risk-to-benefit ratio than classic NSAIDs, given their lower morbidity toward the GI tract. It is obvious that a large

From: *Modern Therapeutics in Rheumatic Diseases*
Edited by: G. C. Tsokos, et al. © Humana Press, Inc., Totowa, NJ

number of patients suffering from OA cannot function with anti-inflammatory therapy. Rather than avoiding NSAIDs or resorting to combination prophylactic therapies, the COX-2 specific inhibitors may solve the problem that has plagued the easy handling of this therapy, especially in older, high-risk patients.

The agents used for the treatment of OA can also be arbitrarily classified into at least two categories based on their time of onset of action: fast-acting, such as NSAIDs and corticosteroids, and slow-acting, having a few weeks delay of action. There are a number of such agents that, through clinical trials, have been shown effective at relieving the symptoms of the disease. Several of those agents are now in use for the symptomatic treatment of knee and hip OA and include diacerein, glucosamine sulphate, chondroitin sulphate (CS), and the avocado/soybean unsaponifiables. Their potential mode of action has been the subject of a number of in vitro and in vivo studies. These agents present several interesting properties including an extremely low incidence of side effects, a carryover effect of several weeks, with some having an additive effect with NSAIDs. These agents could provide an alternative for the symptomatic treatment of OA alone or in combination with an NSAID.

Among the local agents used for the symptomatic treatment of OA at the present time, the most popular are those given by intra-articular injection. Corticosteroids and hyaluronic acid (HA) are probably the most frequently used although their effectiveness, particularly over the long term, is still the subject of debate. A number of studies have been done and have demonstrated their usefulness and safety. Compared to HA, corticosteroids have a more rapid onset of action but their effect is much shorter. Their potential effect on disease progression is still hypothetical and is the subject of clinical evaluation.

The possibility of successfully inducing cartilage repair as a treatment for OA has been the dream of many scientists and physicians. It is a well-known fact that the repair capacity of cartilage is very limited, even more so during OA. There have been many approaches proposed including cell and tissue grafts and the use of synthetic matrices and biological agents, including growth factors. Interesting experimental results have been obtained. Although application in humans remain very limited at this time, the potential for the future is tremendous.

The development of noninvasive methods for observing the progression of OA has and would provide a very significant advance in this field of research. The development of new methods to measure biological markers to accurately and specifically estimate the degradative and/or the anabolic process in OA joints has been the subject of a large number of studies. These markers should ideally allow quantification of the metabolism of cartilage and other joint tissues such as the synovium and the subchondral bone to prognosticate and measure the response to treatment. Studies have already allowed identification of some molecules that may have some value as markers of disease progression. The usefulness of such markers is obvious and it is hoped that ongoing research will introduce more definite developments in this field. The primary use of molecular markers today is to facilitate the understanding of the disease process. Markers are used in epidemiological and genetic studies to clarify the OA processes and are used in clinical trials to strengthen efficacy arguments. Nonetheless, a goal for the clinical management of OA is to identify molecular markers that can be used for diagnosis and the monitoring of therapy. New tests measuring cartilage breakdown and other OA-related disease parameters are promising. A number of these tests, their interpretation and relevance to OA will be reviewed. Importantly, test validation should demonstrate good clinical performance as determined by correlation with imaging and other measures of patient outcome. Unfortunately, clinical validation is currently lacking. However, with current progress in clinical testing, there is a good chance that some of these molecular markers will move from the academic into clinical practice.

The main objectives in the management of OA are to reduce symptoms, minimize functional disability, and limit progression of the structural changes. The first two objectives have so far had much more success than the last. We have a much better understanding of the role of proteases in cartilage degradation, the implication of synovial inflammation and cytokines in disease progression and also the possible interaction between the subchondral bone and cartilage. These findings have made possible more precise identification of target pathways that may have potential therapeutic value and can be modified to effectively retard the progression of the disease. A number of such new agents are now the subject of pre-clinical and clinical trials.

With the aging of the population, OA has become a medical, social, and economic burden, which is progressively becoming heavier. Owing to very intensive research, there has recently been a significant improvement in the number of new diagnostic and therapeutic tools available to more precisely evaluate the disease progression and also provide better treatment for patients. All of these developments in the field of OA makes us realize the importance of medical research to therapeutic progress.

III   SYSTEMIC AUTOIMMUNE DISEASES

18 Treatment of Systemic Lupus Erythematosus

Peter H. Schur and Gary M. Kammer

Contents

INTRODUCTION

Systemic lupus erythematosus (SLE) is a chronic multi-system, autoimmune disorder of unknown etiology that is occasionally life threatening. Persons with SLE suffer from a wide array of symptoms and have a variable prognosis, depending upon the severity and type of organ involvement. Owing to its uncertain course, effective treatment requires ongoing patient-doctor communication to correctly interpret symptoms and signs of disease activity and ancillary tests, to limit or treat relapses, and to minimize side effects related to drug therapy *(1,2)*.

In this chapter, we will review current management and discuss issues related to the treatment of subjects with SLE. When applicable, we will also briefly summarize clinical trials of new therapies for SLE.

DETERMINATION OF ACTIVITY AND SEVERITY OF SLE

An effective therapeutic regimen first requires the accurate determination of both disease activity and severity *(3–6)*. Disease activity refers to the degree of inflammation, whereas severity denotes impairment of organ structure and/or function. The degree of organ dysfunction has been referred to as the "damage index" *(7)*.

A number of research/academic protocols (SLEDAI, SLAM, BILAG, etc.) have been designed in an attempt to accurately monitor disease activity *(3–5,8)*. These

From: *Modern Therapeutics in Rheumatic Diseases*
Edited by: G. C. Tsokos, et al. © Humana Press, Inc., Totowa, NJ

protocols synthesize information from the history, physical examination, and laboratory data. Although these protocols may have general applicability once they are further refined and simplified, they are currently being used to monitor responses to therapy in clinical trials.

For many patients monitoring their CBC (complete blood count), urinalysis, anti-dsDNA Abs, and complement levels may be useful. Erythrocyte sedimentation rate (ESR) and C-reactive protein (CRP) are rarely useful in assessing activity.

GENERAL TREATMENT CONSIDERATIONS

Although organ involvement requires specific drug therapy, a number of general issues are applicable to every patient with SLE.

Diet and Nutrition

Limited data exist concerning the effect of dietary modification on SLE disease activity. One study reported that frequent intake of meat was associated with more active and progressive disease *(9)*. In contrast, dietary fish oil may be efficacious. One double-blind, randomized study found that 14 of 17 patients who ingested 20 g/d of eicosapentaenoic acid achieved either a useful or ideal status; in contrast, 13 of 17 receiving placebo were worse or had not changed *(10)*. These findings await confirmation; at present, we do not recommend fish-oil supplements in the treatment of SLE. A conservative approach is to recommend a balanced diet consisting of carbohydrates, proteins, and fats. However, the diet should be modified based upon disease activity and the response to therapy. Patients with active inflammatory disease and fever may require an increase in caloric intake.

Corticosteroids enhance appetite, resulting in potentially significant weight gain. Hunger can be somewhat lessened by the ingestion of water, antacids, and/or H_2 blockers. If, however, weight gain is significant, patients should receive instruction on low-calorie diets.

Significant hyperlipidemia may be induced by the nephrotic syndrome or the administration of corticosteroids *(11)*. Increasing the dose of prednisone by 10 mg/d is associated with a 7.5 mg/dL (0.2 mmol/L) elevation in serum cholesterol *(12)*. It is currently recommended that hyperlipidemia be actively managed by a low-fat diet *(13)* and a lipid-lowering agent (usually a statin) if cholesterol levels remain high despite a change in diet.

Vitamins are rarely needed when patients eat a balanced diet. However, persons who cannot eat an adequate diet or who are dieting to lose weight should take a daily multivitamin. Persons with lupus who are advised to avoid the sun should also take a diet adequate in Vitamin D.

Use of long-term steroids and postmenopausal women should also ingest 400–800 U of Vitamin D plus 1000 mg of calcium/d to help prevent development of osteoporosis.

Exercise

Inactivity produced by illness causes a rapid loss of muscle mass and stamina. Fatigue may therefore ensue once the illness subsides. This can usually be treated with graded exercise *(14)*. In selected refractory cases, relief of fatigue can be obtained with prednisone *(15)*, antimalarials, or dehydroepiandrosterone (DHEA) *(16)*.

Immunizations

It was previously thought that immunizations might exacerbate SLE. However, influenza vaccine has now been shown to be safe and effective *(17)*; pneumococcal vaccine is also safe, but resultant antibody (Ab) titers are lower in subjects with SLE than in controls *(18)*. In contrast, it is inadvisable to immunize potentially immunosuppressed patients with live vaccines. The efficacy and safety of hepatitis B vaccination has not been determined *(19)*.

AVOIDANCE OF MEDICATIONS

Anecdotal data suggest that sulfonamides and penicillin (but not the synthetic penicillins) may cause exacerbations of SLE and should therefore be avoided *(20)*. In contrast, medications that cause drug-induced lupus, such as procainamide and hydralazine, do not cause exacerbations of idiopathic SLE. This observation is a presumed reflection of the pathogenetic differences between the two disorders.

PREGNANCY AND CONTRACEPTION

Pregnancy should be avoided during active disease (especially with significant organ impairment) owing to the high risk of miscarriage. Women with SLE should be counseled not to become pregnant until the disease has been quiescent for at least 6 mo.

Oral contraceptives containing high-dose estrogens can cause exacerbations of SLE. However, this complication rarely occurs with the current use of low-dose estrogen- or progesterone-containing compounds. Lupus subjects with a history of migraine headaches, Raynaud's syndrome, thrombophlebitis, or antiphospholipid Abs probably should not be treated with oral contraceptives. We also recommend avoidance of intrauterine devices owing to the increased risk of infection.

Pregnant women with active lupus are generally managed with corticosteroids. Other drugs used during pregnancy include nonsteroid anti-inflammatory drugs (NSAIDs) and hydroxychloroquine (probably safe). Cyclophosphamide and methotrexate are contraindicated; however, azathioprine can be cautiously used.

MEDICATIONS

A number of medications are commonly used in the treatment of SLE, including nonsteroidal anti-inflammatory drugs (NSAIDs), antimalarials (primarily hydroxychloroquine), corticosteroids, and immunosuppressive agents (primarily cyclophosphamide and azathioprine). What follows is a general overview of which drugs are preferred in selected clinical settings.

NSAIDs are generally effective for musculoskeletal complaints and mild serositis.

Antimalarials are most useful for skin manifestations (e.g., rashes) and for musculoskeletal disorders that do not adequately respond to NSAIDs alone.

Systemic corticosteroids used alone or in combination with immunosuppressive (e.g., cyclophosphamide, azathioprine, methotrexate) agents are reserved for subjects

Table 1
Mucocutaneous Manifestations of SLE

- Photosensitivity
- Acute, erythematosus, edematous rash
    Butterfly rash
- Discoid lupus
- Neonatal lupus
- Subacute cutaneous lupus
    Annular or polycyclic
    Psoriaform
- Lupus profundus/panniculitis
- Alopecia
- Bullous lesions
- Mucous membranes
- Vascular lesions
    Periungal erythema
    Livedo reticularis
    Telangiectasia
    Raynaud's phenomenon
- Urticarial or purpuric vasculitis
- Atrophic blanche
- Chilblain lupus

From UpToDate® © 2001.

with significant organ involvement, particularly renal and central nervous system (also termed neuropsychiatric SLE [NPSLE]) disease. Treatment with prednisone as soon as a significant rise in anti-dsDNA Abs levels occurred prevented relapses in most cases in a study of 156 subjects *(21)*. Notwithstanding, we recommend that such individuals, with rising or high titers of anti-dsDNA Abs in the absence of clinical evidence of active disease, be closely monitored.

A number of other therapeutic approaches have been used or are under investigation in SLE. These include intravenous immune globulin (IVIG), DHEA, thalidomide, bromocriptine, zileuton, cyclosporine, anti-CD40 MAb, LJP 394, anti-C5 complement MAb, anti-IL-10 MAb, mycophenolate mofetil, and stem cell transplantation *(16,22–26)*.

TREATMENT OF SPECIFIC ORGAN INVOLVEMENT

Cutaneous Manifestations of SLE

The skin and mucous membranes are symptomatically involved at some point in over 80% of subjects with SLE *(27)*. Such lesions include the classical butterfly rash, atrophic hyperkeratotic discoid lesions, bullae, cicatrizing and noncicatrizing alopecia, and arteriolar and/or venular vasculitis (Table 1). In the chronic, progressive form of discoid lupus, the rash can be disfiguring and require aggressive therapy to prevent scarring and hypopigmentation and/or hyperpigmentation. Many of the cutaneous lesions are worsened by exposure to ultraviolet (UV) light.

The goal of treatment in the different forms of cutaneous lupus is to prevent long-term skin sequelae, such as telangiectasia, hyperpigmentation or hypopigmentation, alopecia, and scarring. Preventive measures will prevent skin lesions in most patients. The following measures are currently recommended:

Avoid high sun exposure, and if feasible, medications that are associated with photosensitivity (Table 2) *(28)*.

Sunscreens of at least SPF15 should be used; higher SPFs are available if required. A current list of commercially available sunscreens can be found in the May, 1998 volume of Consumer Reports.

A lupus rash should initially be treated with topical corticosteroids. Hydrocortisone will often suffice, but more potent steroids (particularly the fluorinated preparations) are available for thicker lesions. There are several points that deserve emphasis:

Fluorinated steroids may be used for facial lesions, but should be used very cautiously and probably for no more than 2 wk.

Ointments are more effective than creams.

Lotions should be used on scalp lesions.

Chronic use of topical steroids may lead to skin atrophy, thinning, telangiectasia, hypertrichosis, striae, and depigmentation.

Subjects with persistent rashes should be treated with an antimalarial agent, such as hydroxychloroquine or quinacrine. One of these drugs should be used only when the diagnosis is secure with the following precautions:

Antimalarial agents may be associated with flares of psoriasis.

Antimalarial drugs should not be given to the rare individual with G6PD deficiency.

Antimalarial agents may potentially cause serious ocular changes, including macular degeneration; as a result, all subjects should have ophthalmologic examinations at 6-mo intervals *(29)*.

Currently, the most commonly prescribed antimalarial agent for SLE is hydroxychloroquine. The recommended dosage is <6.5 mg/kg/d. Overall improvement of erythema, infiltration, scaling, and hyperkeratosis occurs in 50% of subjects *(30)*. Chloroquine (250–500 mg/d) is somewhat more potent, but has a higher risk of eye damage *(31)*. Quinacrine (100 mg/d) is even more effective and has a much lower risk of eye damage *(32)*; however, the skin of many individuals turns somewhat yellow and bone marrow depression is a rare complication. Subacute cutaneous lupus erythematosus (SCLE) and lupus panniculitis respond best to antimalarial drugs, but higher doses may be needed. Combination therapy with chloroquine or hydroxychloroquine and quinacrine was found to be effective among most patients with chronic cutaneous lupus and/or SCLE resistant to antimalarial monotherapy *(33)*. Improvement with antimalarials may not be seen until 6–12 wk of use.

Systemic steroids or immunosuppressive agents are rarely needed to clear skin lesions, except for bullous lesions. Systemic drugs that have been used when local therapy fails include oral steroids, dapsone, azathioprine, thalidomide, gold, retinoids, methotrexate, cyclophosphamide, chlorambucil, IVIG, diphenylhydantoin, anti-CD4 Abs, and clofazimine *(30,32,34–37)*.

Alopecia in active SLE usually responds well to treatment of the disease, especially with antimalarials (*see* above), whereas hair loss owing to steroids recovers as the steroid dose is lowered. In comparison, the hair loss is usually permanent when associated with scarring owing to discoid lesions of the scalp *(38)*. Topical minoxidil may be beneficial in a limited number of persons *(38)*.

Table 2
Some Agents That May Cause Photosensitivity Reactions

Anticancer drugs
Dacarbazine
Fluorouracil
Flutamine
Methotrexate
Vinblastine

Antidepressants
Amitriptyline
Amoxapine
Clomipramine
Desipramine
Doxepin
Imipramine
Maprotiline
Nortriptyline
Phenelzine
Protriptyline
Trazodone
Trimipramine

Antimicrobials
Ciprofloxacin
Clofazimine
Dapsone
*Demeclocycline
*Doxycycline
Enoxacin
Flucytosine
Griseofulvin
*Lomefloxacin
Minocycline
*Nalidixic acid
Norfloxacin
Ofloxacin
Oxytetracycline
Pyrazinamide
Sulfonamides
Tetracycline
Trimethopterin

Antiparasitic drugs
Chloroquine
Quinine

Antipsychotic drugs
*Chlorpromazine
Fluphenazine
Haloperidol
Perphenazine
*Prochlorperazine
Thioridazine
Thiothixene
Trifluoperazine
Triflupromazine

Diuretics
Acetazolamide
Amiloride
Bendroflumethiazide
Benzthiazide
*Chlorthiazide
*Furosemide
*Hydrochlorothiazide
Hydroflumethiazide
Methyclothiazide
Metolazone
Polythiazide
Trimterene
Trichlormethiazide

Hypoglycemics
Acetohexamide
Chlorpropamide
Glipizide
Glyburide
Tolazamide
*Tolbutamide

NSAIDs
Difluisal
Ibuprofen
Indomethacin
Ketoprofen
Nabumetone
Naproxen
Phenylbutazone
*Piroxicam
Sulindac

Sunscreens
*Aminobenzoic acids
Avobenzone
*Benzophenonones
Cinnamates
Homosalate
Menthyl anthranilate
*PABA esters

Antihistamine
Cyproheptadine
Diphenhydramine

Antihypertensives
Captopril
Diltiazem
Methyldopa
Minoxidil
Nifedipine

Others
Alpazolam
Amantadine
*Amiodarone
Benzocaine
Benzyl peroxide
*Bergamol oil, oils of citron,
  lavender, lime, sandalwood,
  cedar
Carbamazepine
Chlordiazepoxide
Clofibrate
Desoximetasone
Disopyramide
Etretinate
Fluoroscein
Gold salts
Hexachlorophene
Isotretinoin
*6-methylcoumRIN
*Musk ambrette
Oral contraceptives
*Promethazine
Quinidine sulfate
Tretinoin
Trimeprazine

*Reactions which occur more frequently.
From UpToDate® © 2001.

Mucous membrane lesions respond well to topical steroids and systemic antimalarial drugs. The response to topical steroids (usually Orabase with either hydrocortisone or triamcinolone) takes a few days to weeks, whereas the response to hydroxychloroquine takes weeks to months.

Raynaud's phenomenon can often be prevented by educating individuals about trigger factors, such as avoidance of smoking, caffeine, vasopressors, vasoconstrictors, and, for cold-induced Raynaud's, wearing warm clothing. More severe or resistant disease can be treated with vasodilators, such as nifedipine, nicardipine, and/or prazosin, and topical nitroglycerine. Intravascular treatment with prostacyclin may be effective *(39)*.

Treatment of urticarial or purpuric vasculitis with indomethacin or hydroxychloroquine yields complete or partial remissions in some subjects with mild lesions; prednisone at doses of 25–60 mg/d is recommended for more severe disease *(40)*.

Musculoskeletal Manifestations of SLE

Involvement of the musculoskeletal system is extremely common in persons with SLE. This disorder can involve joint spaces (e.g., arthralgia and arthritis), osteonecrosis, and myopathy. Osteoporosis is also a common manifestation that is usually due to corticosteroid therapy.

Multiple drugs are available to treat arthralgias and the pain syndromes of SLE. NSAIDs and/or acetaminophen are the staples typically used initially. If these are ineffective, acetaminophen/propoxyphene HCl, tramadol HCl, and/or amitriptyline may be added and/or substituted.

If arthritis, i.e., inflammation (swelling, redness, and warmth), is the most prominent feature, we recommend NSAIDs rather than full-dose aspirin (which requires too many pills). Typical doses are ibuprofen (800 mg QID pc), naproxen (500 mg BID pc), and nabumetone (1 g/d or BID pc). In those at risk for NSAID-induced gastrointestinal (GI) toxicity, a selective COX-2 inhibitor may be more appropriate; three are currently available.

Antimalarial drugs (e.g., hydroxychloroquine 200–400 mg/d) are very effective for the amelioration of joint symptoms and prevention of clinical relapse *(41–43)*. Hydroxychloroquine is typically given to persons with articular manifestations, rashes, and fatigue, often in combination with a NSAID.

Dehydroepiandrosterone (DHEA, 200 mg/d) has shown promising results in preliminary studies, and may be of benefit in mild to moderate SLE *(44)*. However, further clinical trials will be required to establish the efficacy of DHEA.

Corticosteroids are needed infrequently, and should be avoided for the treatment of pain not associated with inflammation. In subjects who have already been treated with steroids with a positive response, we recommend a NSAID and hydroxychloroquine and gradually tapering the steroid.

For resistant inflammatory arthritis, methotrexate 7.5–15 mg/wk has been shown to be useful *(45,46)*. In a prospective, double-blind trial, 41 individuals were randomized to methotrexate plus prednisone or prednisone alone *(46)*. Compared to those given prednisone, methotrexate plus prednisone was more effective in controlling articular activity, while permitting a lower prednisone dosage.

Low-dose tricyclic antidepressants (e.g., amitriptyline 5–75 mg QHS) are often useful in combination with other therapy when pain is only partially responsive or completely unresponsive to the above measures.

OSTEONECROSIS

The management of osteonecrosis is problematic. The best initial approach is prevention by avoiding high-dose chronic steroid therapy. Once the condition develops, however, it may only be recognized after bony collapse has occurred, and joint replacement may be necessary.

The treatment of early osteonecrosis, demonstrable by magnetic resonance imaging (MRI) but not conventional X-ray, remains controversial. Some studies have reported good results (e.g., prevention of femoral head collapse) by core decompression of the femoral-head in such persons *(47)* whereas others have not achieved this benefit *(48)*.

OSTEOPOROSIS

Certain general principles should be followed in all patients, particularly those receiving prolonged steroid therapy, to minimize bone loss. These include:

1. Modification of lifestyle factors: elimination of cigarette smoking, limitation of alcohol consumption, and maintenance of an exercise regimen.
2. Administration of 1 g of elemental calcium and 400–800 IU of vitamin D/d.
3. Limitation of steroid therapy to the lowest possible dose and duration.
4. Measurement of bone mineral density (BMD) of the spine and hip.

Baseline values of BMD more than one SD below the mean (e.g. osteopenia) may be at increased risk for the development of osteoporosis. The test may be repeated yearly for as long as the patient is receiving steroids. More aggressive therapy (e.g., bisphosphonates) should be undertaken if bone loss exceeds 5%/yr or with fractures in osteopenic sites. In the postmenopausal woman, hormonal replacement with estrogen is also effective, but must be balanced against the risk for breast malignancy.

MUSCLE DISEASE

Lupus myositis responds to treatment with steroids (using a regimen similar to that in polymyositis), whereas steroid-induced myopathy responds to a reduction in or withdrawal of steroid therapy. Antimalarial myopathy responds to stopping the drug, but it may take months for the myopathy to improve, partly owing to the long half-life of hydroxychloroquine (months).

Hematologic Manifestations of SLE

Abnormalities of the formed elements of the blood, and of the clotting, fibrinolytic, and related systems, are very common in SLE. The major clinical manifestations are anemia, leukopenia, thrombocytopenia, and the antiphospholipid Ab syndrome (APLS).

ANEMIA

The anemia of chronic inflammation in SLE usually responds to high dose corticosteroids (1 mg/kg/d of prednisone or its equivalent in divided dose). Immunosuppressive agents also may be efficacious, although there is a risk of further bone marrow suppression.

Red cell aplasia has rarely been observed. This form of anemia generally responds to steroids, although cyclophosphamide and cyclosporine have also been used. Even rarer are isolated case reports of aplastic anemia that is presumably mediated by autoabs against bone marrow precursors; immunosuppressive therapy also may be effective in this setting (49,50).

The anemia owing to chronic renal disease generally responds to erythropoietin.

Hemolytic anemia responds to steroids (1 mg/kg/d of prednisone or its equivalent in divided doses) in approx 75% of patients (51). Once the hematocrit begins to rise and the reticulocyte count falls, steroids can be rapidly tapered. If there is no response, one can consider pulse steroids (51), azathioprine (up to 2 mg/kg/d) (52), cyclophosphamide (up to 2 mg/kg) (53), or splenectomy. Success rates for splenectomy as high as 60% have been reported (54), although others have found no benefit (55).

Persons with thrombotic microangiopathic hemolytic anemia should probably be treated with plasma exchange as in other cases of thrombotic thrombocytopenic purpura or the hemolytic-uremic syndrome. In a review of 28 SLE subjects, those treated with plasma infusions or plasmapheresis, corticosteroids alone, or no therapy had mortality rates of 25, 50, and 100%, respectively (56).

LEUKOPENIA

Leukopenia in SLE rarely needs treatment, with the exception of persons having recurrent pyogenic infections. One problem is the toxicity of the usual therapies. Prednisone (10–60 mg/d) and immunosuppressive agents (azathioprine or cyclophosphamide) can raise the white blood cell count, but can also result in an increased risk of infections and worsening of leukopenia via bone marrow suppression, respectively (57).

Newer potential therapies for leukopenia may also result in significant adverse results. One study of nine SLE subjects with neutropenia and refractory infections found that treatment with recombinant granulocyte colony-stimulating factor (GC-SF) increased the polymorphonuclear cell count, but caused a disease flare in three patients.

THROMBOCYTOPENIA

Platelet counts of less than 50,000/µL rarely cause more than a prolonged bleeding time, whereas counts of less than 20,000/µL can be associated with (and account for) petechiae, purpura, ecchymoses, epistaxis, gingival, and other clinical bleeding. Treatment of thrombocytopenia is recommended for counts <50,000/µL associated with bleeding phenomena and for all subjects with counts of <20,000/µL.

The treatment of ITP in SLE is the same as that in subjects without lupus. The mainstay of treatment is prednisone 1 mg/kg/d in divided doses (58,59). Most patients respond within 1–8 wk (60). If there is no significant increase in the platelet count within 1–3 wk or side effects are intolerable, the following options may be considered. The order in which they are used depends in part on the severity of the thrombocytopenia and the presence or absence of other manifestations of SLE.

Azathioprine (0.5–2 mg/kg/d) (60).

Cyclophosphamide, given as daily oral or IV pulse therapy. Pulse cyclophosphamide is preferred when there is severe active lupus nephritis. In one report of six such individuals, all had normal platelet counts within 2–18 wk, after the onset of pulse cyclophosphamide (61).

IVIG is very effective and may be preferred to azathioprine or cyclophosphamide when a rapid rise in platelet count is necessary (as in the patient who is actively bleeding or requires emergent surgery) (62).

Splenectomy. Surgery should be preceded by immunization with pneumococcal vaccine. Although splenectomy can raise the platelet count *(54,63)*, it does not cure the disease, because relapse is common and occurs 1–54 mo after surgery *(64)*. Splenectomy in ITP was originally thought to predispose to the development of SLE; however, this hypothesis was refuted in subsequent studies.

Danazol (400–800 mg/d) *(65,66)*. In one analysis, all subjects who were refractory to other therapies responded to danazol (200 mg QID) within 6 wk; this benefit occurred without a change in platelet-bound IgG Abs *(65)*. The dose could be tapered without relapse in five of the six persons.

Vincristine *(67)*.

Lymphadenopathy and Splenomegaly

Even though lymphadenopathy and splenomegaly are common in SLE, their presence should make one consider the possibility of a lymphoproliferative malignancy. One study found an increased risk of cancer in subjects with SLE; the relative risk at 11 yr was 2.6 for all tumors and 44 for non-Hodgkin's lymphoma *(68)*. However, an overall increase in risk of malignancy was not confirmed in two later reports *(69,70)*. The largest, 724 subjects followed prospectively for an average of 10 yr, did find a fourfold increase in risk of non-Hodgkin's lymphoma compared to the general population *(70)*. Thus, a lymph-node biopsy may be warranted when the degree of lymphadenopathy is out of proportion to the activity of the lupus.

Cardiac Manifestations of SLE

Cardiac disease is common among individuals with SLE; valvular, pericardial, myocardial, and coronary-artery involvement are the commonest cardiovascular manifestations.

Valvular disease requires no specific therapy, unless hemodynamically significant. Serial echocardiograms are a convenient way of monitoring the process. In addition, one can consider antibiotic prophylaxis when SLE subjects with valvular disease undergo procedures associated with a risk of developing bacteremia (such as dental care) *(71)*.

Verrucous endocarditis may produce systemic emboli, and infective endocarditis can complicate preexisting vegetations on damaged valves *(72,73)*. Affected persons should be tested for antiphospholipid Abs, which are often associated. Treatment for infection is as for any SBE; without infection, treatment is usually with IV heparin.

Pericardial Disease

Pericardial involvement is the second most common echocardiographic lesion in SLE, and is the most frequent cause of symptomatic cardiac disease *(74)*.

In the majority of affected persons, the course of lupus pericardial disease is benign. Symptomatic pericarditis often responds to a NSAID, especially indomethacin *(72)*. When there is intolerance or lack of response to a NSAID, prednisone (0.5–1 mg/kg/d in divided doses) can be substituted. The most serious consequence is the development of purulent pericarditis in the immunosuppressed, debilitated patient *(75)*. Large effusions, tamponade, and constrictive pericarditis are rare in SLE *(76)*.

Myocarditis

Myocarditis is an uncommon manifestation of SLE with a prevalence of 8–25% in different studies *(72)*. It may be asymptomatic, but should be suspected in persons with tachycardia, EKG abnormalities (such as ST- and T-wave abnormalities), cardiomegaly, and signs of congestive failure. There may be diffuse abnormalities demonstrated by echocardiogram.

Myocarditis should be treated with prednisone (1 mg/kg/d in divided doses) in addition to contemporary therapy for congestive heart failure, if present. Cyclophosphamide or azathioprine have been used when necessary with good, albeit slower responses *(77,78)*. Cardiomyopathy with fibrosis is usually resistant to steroids and/or immunosuppressive drugs.

Coronary Artery Disease

Coronary-artery disease (CAD) has been recognized in 2–16% of individuals with SLE *(79,80)*, and can lead to acute myocardial infarction in young women *(80,81)*. In some cases, however, thrombi rather than coronary disease is responsible for the ischemia *(82)*. Coronary-artery vasculitis is rare.

People with lupus should be advised to stop smoking, exercise, consider the use of hormone-replacement therapy, and follow measures designed to improve lipid profiles. Hydroxychloroquine should be used in preference to prednisone whenever possible and aspirin should be prescribed for its antiplatelet properties. The utility of newer agents, such as clopidogrel (Plavix) and cilostazol (Pletal), remain to be established.

Hypertension is an important risk factor in SLE *(83)*. We recommend aggressive therapy, aiming for a diastolic pressure below 85 mm Hg, especially in younger persons. The choice of antihypertensive agent depends in part on coexisting disorders. One consideration is nifedipine in subjects with Raynaud's phenomenon and an angiotensin-converting enzyme (ACE) inhibitor in persons with renal disease. Steroids may contribute to hypertension and diabetes, so the steroid dosage should be reduced, if possible.

Symptomatic coronary artery disease should be evaluated and managed as one would in the absence of lupus.

Pulmonary Manifestations of SLE

SLE is commonly associated with involvement of the lung, its vasculature, the pleura, and/or the diaphragm *(84)*. Pleurisy, coughing, and/or dyspnea are often the first clues to either lung involvement or SLE itself *(85)*. Pulmonary abnormalities do not appear to correlate with the extent of immune dysfunction *(86)*.

Musculoskeletal Chest Wall Pain

In general experience, the most common cause of chest pain in SLE is from muscles, other supporting tissues, and/or the costochondral joints (costochondritis or Tietze's syndrome)*(87)*. The chest pain is characterized by painful deep breaths, is aggravated by motion or change of position (especially during sleep), and is elicited by palpation of the painful areas. The person can be reassured that this specific pain does not represent lung and/or heart involvement.

Chest-wall pain generally responds to local heat, NSAIDs, topical analgesics, and acetaminophen. Local trigger-point injections may be helpful in refractory cases; steroids are rarely necessary.

PLEURITIS

Inflammation of the pleura may cause chest pain in the absence of a friction rub or radiographic pleural effusion. In this setting, it is often difficult to determine whether or not the chest pain represents pleuritis. However, the presence of a rub, often very transient, and/or a pleural effusion facilitates the diagnosis. The effusion is usually small or moderate, although large effusions have been noted. They tend to be evanescent and recurrent, and are often bilateral.

Pleural disease in SLE often responds to therapy with NSAIDs. If there is no response within a few days, moderate- to high-dose steroids will generally be effective. Immunosuppressive agents are rarely indicated.

ACUTE PNEUMONITIS

Acute lupus pneumonitis is an uncommon (1–12%) manifestation of SLE (88). It is characterized by fever, cough (sometimes with hemoptysis), pleurisy, dyspnea, pulmonary infiltrates on X-ray, hypoxia, basilar rales, pleural effusion, serum anti-dsDNA Abs, and no apparent infection (that is, a pathogen cannot be cultured or isolated). Chest X-ray often reveals diffuse acinar infiltrates, especially in the lower lung fields. Pleural effusion is relatively common, occurring in about one-half of cases. The prognosis is poor in this disorder. Lupus pneumonitis developing in the postpartum period has a particularly poor outcome.

Acute lupus pneumonitis needs prompt intervention if the outcome is to be improved. Broad-spectrum antibiotic coverage should be given pending culture results. The mainstay of therapy is systemic prednisone (1–1.5 mg/kg/d in divided doses). If no response is seen within 72 h, the administration of intravenous pulse steroids (which act quickly) and slower acting immunosuppressive drugs should be considered (87,88).

Survivors often have persistent pulmonary function abnormalities, including severe restrictive ventilatory defects.

CHRONIC PNEUMONITIS

Chronic (fibrotic) lupus pneumonitis has been noted in up to 9% of patients with SLE in some series (89,90). Patients with longstanding SLE (87), and possibly those with anti-Ro Abs, are more likely to develop chronic pneumonitis (91). An episode of acute lupus pneumonitis frequently precedes the development of this disorder.

In treating chronic pneumonitis, it is important to determine if the primary process is inflammation or scarring, a distinction that can often be made by high-resolution CT (HRCT) scan, 67 gallium scintigraphy, and BAL (92). Treatment is begun with oral prednisone in a dose of 1 mg/kg/d if inflammation is predominant. Patients treated with steroids tend to improve slowly or to stabilize with time. Immunosuppressive agents should be considered if no response is seen within a few weeks.

PULMONARY HYPERTENSION

Severe, symptomatic pulmonary hypertension is thought to be a rare complication of SLE (87), being more frequently associated with scleroderma or overlap syndromes.

However, a recent study found that mild to moderate pulmonary hypertension developed in 12 of 28 subjects followed for 5 yr *(93)*.

The management of patients with secondary pulmonary hypertension and SLE is similar to that in primary pulmonary hypertension *(94)*. Therapies that have been used include the administration of oxygen, anticoagulants, and vasodilators (calcium-channel blockers). Recently, efficacy of continuous IV infusions of prostacyclin has been reported in primary systemic sclerosis *(95)*, although a practical note of caution was raised *(96)*. However, current evidence suggests that pulmonary hypertension associated with SLE is generally resistant to treatment and is associated with a poor prognosis.

SHRINKING LUNG SYNDROME

The shrinking or vanishing lung syndrome has been noted in some patients with SLE. This syndrome is characterized by dyspnea, persistent episodes of pleuritic chest pain, a progressive decrease in lung volume, and no evidence of interstitial fibrosis or significant pleural disease on chest CT *(97)*. Corticosteroid therapy can improve both symptoms and pulmonary function, although its efficacy is often debated *(98)*.

PULMONARY HEMORRHAGE

Pulmonary hemorrhage, not necessarily with hemoptysis, is a rare complication in SLE *(99)*. Previous treatment regimens (primarily high-dose corticosteroids) were associated with a very high mortality. A combination of corticosteroids, cyclophosphamide, mechanical ventilation, and/or antibiotics appears to reduce mortality.

Pregnancy in Women with SLE

SLE occurs frequently in women of childbearing age. Although patients with SLE are as fertile as women in the general population, their pregnancies may be complicated. The prognosis for both mother and child is best when the disorder has been quiescent for at least 6 mo prior to the pregnancy, and the patient's underlying renal function is adequate. Thus, contraception and family planning are important so that pregnancy and delivery can occur in a scheduled manner; in addition, these should be followed by an obstetrician knowledgeable in high-risk pregnancies *(100)*.

There are two issues related to therapy of women with lupus who become pregnant: (1) monitoring of disease activity in both asymptomatic and symptomatic patients, and (2) treatment of active disease. Mothers should be assessed for disease activity at least once each trimester, and more often if active. The schedule for monitoring includes:

1. Physical examination, including blood pressure.
2. Renal function, urinalysis, plasma creatinine concentration, and 24-h urine collection for protein.
3. Complete blood count, anti-dsDNA titer, and C4/C3 complement levels.
4. Pelvic ultrasonography to monitor fetal growth.
5. Anti-Ro/SSA, anti-La/SSB, and antiphospholipid Abs (at onset of pregnancy).

Treatment of SLE during pregnancy is associated with some unique problems. Consideration must be given to the following issues:

Medications used to treat SLE may cross the placenta and cause fetal disorders. Thus, the risks and benefits of treatment during pregnancy must be repeatedly weighed against the risk of lupus activity on the mother and fetus *(101,102)*.

Nephritis in pregnancy requires special consideration because of its potential morbidity and possible confusion with preeclampsia.

Treatment of the mother with antiphospholipid Abs is important because of the risk of both fetal demise and low birth weight.

Drugs that are typically used to treat persons with SLE may be divided into three categories: (1) those that should be avoided in pregnancy; (2) those that are probably safe to use; and, (3) those that are safe.

Certainly, drugs that can potentially cause birth defects should be avoided, such as cyclophosphamide and methotrexate. However, azathioprine may be used cautiously. Antimalarials theoretically may cause problems to the fetus, although none have been documented *(103)*. Thus, hydroxychloroquine is probably safe to use. NSAIDs are safe, but should be discontinued in the last few weeks of pregnancy (to facilitate closure of the ductus arteriosus). Likewise, prednisone is "safe" in that no fetal defects develop other than rare temporary neonatal adrenal suppression. Steroid side effects in the mother may be reduced by recommending a low-salt diet (to prevent weight increase and hypertension), an exercise program (to prevent bone loss and depression), and calcium supplementation (to prevent osteoporosis).

Serological markers (complement, anti-dsDNA Abs) should be monitored closely. Increasing abnormality of these markers is not necessarily a rationale for a change in therapy, but is an indication that closer observation is necessary for possible exacerbation of lupus. If treatment of a flare is deemed necessary, high-dose prednisone is the therapy of choice.

Persons with a significant flare of lupus nephritis should be treated with high-dose prednisone and an antihypertensive agent(s) (e.g., hydralazine, methyldopa, and calcium-channel blockers, but not diuretics, angiotensin converting enzyme inhibitors, or some beta blockers). In addition, the fetus should be delivered as soon as possible *(102,104)*. Signs of a renal flare include renewed activity of the urine sediment and an increase in the plasma creatinine concentration. In comparison, an isolated elevation in protein excretion is a common, probably hemodynamically mediated finding in all glomerulopathies during pregnancy and should not necessarily be considered a finding of increased lupus activity.

There is little if any experience with pulse methylprednisolone in pregnancy, and its effects on the fetus are unknown. Azathioprine can be used with relative safety as long as the white blood cell count is normal.

Thrombocytopenia during lupus pregnancies may have multiple causes, including antiplatelet Abs, toxemia, and antiphospholipid Abs *(101,102)*. Treatment includes high-dose prednisone and intravenous immune globulin *(102)*.

As previously mentioned, individuals with antiphospholipid Abs may be at high risk for recurrent fetal loss, especially after 10 wk. Therefore, patients with these Abs without a history of such fetal loss are usually treated with aspirin 81 mg/d. Those women with a previous history of a fetal loss after 10 wk should be managed with subcutaneous heparin (10,000–12,000 U BID, especially for wk 12 through 32) plus low-dose aspirin (81 mg/d) *(105,106)*. A frequent complication of this regimen is heparin-induced osteoporosis. Recovery of bone density occurs postpartum after the heparin is discontinued; it is unclear, however, if the recovery is complete.

If heparin and aspirin therapy do not prevent fetal loss, intravenous gamma globulin should be tried during the next pregnancy (0.4 g/kg/d for five consecutive days of each month) *(107,108)*. If IVIG fails, prednisone (20–40 mg/d) and low-dose aspirin can be tried in the next pregnancy *(105,109)*. However, use of steroids during pregnancy may be associated with increased morbidity *(110–112)*. Importantly, pregnant women with the antiphospholipid antibody syndrome (APLS) should be monitored carefully by sonography early in pregnancy, and at about 20 wk for fetal heart rate. Women with a history of intravascular clotting events unassociated with APLS should probably be anticoagulated for a few months postpartum *(102)*. By contrast, current evidence suggests that women who have documented hypercoagulability associated with the APLS should probably be on warfarin for life.

Menstrual Function, Menopause, and Oral Contraceptives

Menstrual irregularities are common in women with SLE. Their treatment is dependent on finding an underlying cause, and is basically similar to that in women without SLE. Factors to be considered include (1) thrombocytopenia, (2) antiphospholipid Abs, and (3) the use of corticosteroids and/or NSAIDs.

Temporary or even permanent amenorrhea has been noted in 17–24% of women with SLE. Two major mechanisms have been identified: (1) SLE disease activity, leading to autoimmune ovarian injury and (2) the administration of immunosuppressive agents (especially cyclophosphamide) *(113,114)*. A gynecologist should evaluate amenorrhea. If owing to active SLE, its treatment often restores normal menses. By contrast, amenorrhea secondary to treatment is rarely reversible. It is more likely to happen in women over age 25. Thus, in the woman over 25 (and especially over 30) who is still considering having children, using an immunosuppressive agent other than cyclophosphamide may be preferable.

Menopause is often associated with a diminution in the symptoms and signs and signs of SLE. However, it brings on several new concerns. Both normal women and those with SLE who are postmenopausal have a greater risk of CAD. Corticosteroid therapy increases this risk *(115)*. In addition, both normal women and those with SLE who are postmenopausal have a greater risk of osteoporosis. Corticosteroid therapy increases this risk.

Hormone-replacement therapy with estrogen and a progestin can decrease the risk of both CAD and osteoporosis, improve mood and a sense of well-being, and enhance libido. However, these benefits must be weighed against the potential risk of exacerbation of SLE *(116)*. Via mechanisms that may be mediated via estrogen receptors *(117,118)*, estrogen increases the susceptibility to SLE, which probably explains the marked female preponderance in this disorder. However, the risk of estrogen-replacement therapy appears to be small. Two reports compared women on hormone replacement to untreated women *(119,120)*. There was no difference in lupus activity between the two groups.

Similar concerns about exacerbation of SLE have been raised with the use of oral contraceptives. In the past, the use of estrogen-containing oral contraceptives was associated with an increased risk of activation of lupus *(121)*. However, most currently available oral contraceptives are primarily comprised of progesterone and/or low-dose estrogens; these preparations are not generally associated with adverse affects in women with SLE *(122)*.

Thus, current oral contraceptives are probably safe in most women with SLE, but should probably be avoided in women already at an increased risk of clotting. This includes subjects with antiphospholipid Abs, the nephrotic syndrome, and/or a history of thrombophlebitis *(123,124)*. Persons with active nephritis also may be at increased risk of renal exacerbation *(123)*. In these individuals, barrier methods are the contraceptive method of choice, because intrauterine devices can be complicated by hemorrhage or infection.

A separate issue is whether oral contraceptives promote the development of SLE as may occur with estrogen-replacement therapy. A prospective analysis found that the relative risk (RR) of developing SLE was not significantly different in past users and never users of oral contraceptives when ACR criteria alone were used for the diagnosis of lupus *(125)*. However, a small but significant increase in RR (1.9) was noted when more stringent criteria were used for the diagnosis *(125)*. It was concluded that concerns about the development of SLE should not be a limiting factor in the use of oral contraceptives.

Treatment of Lupus Nephritis

FOCAL PROLIFERATIVE GN

In focal proliferative glomerulonephritis (GN), fewer than 50% of glomeruli are affected on light microscopy *(126)*. The prognosis and optimal therapy in focal proliferative disease is less clear *(127)*. Death directly attributable to renal disease or progression to advanced renal failure within 5 yr appears to occur in less than 5% of patients with relatively mild focal involvement (fewer than 25% of glomeruli affected, primarily with segmental areas of proliferation) *(126)*. Specific immunosuppressive therapy may not be indicated in this setting, although many persons are treated with corticosteroids for extrarenal symptoms. The net effect is that the plasma creatinine concentration is relatively stable for at least 5 yr *(126)*.

In contrast, more widespread or severe focal disease (40–50% of glomeruli affected with areas of necrosis or crescent formation, significant subendothelial immune deposits, nephrotic range proteinuria, and/or hypertension) has a worse long-term outcome that is probably similar to that of diffuse proliferative lupus GN *(127)*. The incidence of renal death or advanced renal failure at 5 yr in the latter disorder is as high as 15–25% *(126,127)*. Thus, these patients should probably treated in a manner similar to those with diffuse proliferative GN *(see* below).

MEMBRANOUS GN

Like focal proliferative GN, the renal prognosis is variable with membranous lupus GN *(128)*. The natural history of this disorder is uncertain, because most reported subjects have been treated with corticosteroids (often for extrarenal disease). Partial or complete remissions in proteinuria can occur, and the plasma creatinine concentration often remains normal or near normal for 5 or more yr.

Worsening renal function or severe nephrotic syndrome and its associated complications (marked edema, hyperlipidemia, and possible thromboembolic disease) are indications for employing the regimens described below. These subjects often respond well to immunosuppressive therapy with the 10-yr kidney-survival rate approaching 93% *(128)*. However, worsening renal function can occur *(128,129)*. Clinical features associated with a poor outcome included black race, hypertension, elevated plasma creatinine concentration at presentation, and heavy proteinuria; no initial histologic feature was clearly predictive, although progression was more likely in those who also had proliferative lesions *(130)*.

Optimal therapy of membranous lupus is uncertain. Asymptomatic patients are often not treated, those with moderate disease may be treated with prednisone, and those with a rising plasma creatinine concentration or marked nephrotic syndrome are often treated with the same regimen as diffuse proliferative GN. An NIH study randomized 22 patients with membranous nephropathy but no proliferative disease to 1 yr of prednisone alone, pulse cyclophosphamide (as described below), or cyclosporine (5 mg/kg/d) *(130)*. Although each therapy appeared to be effective, cyclophosphamide was perhaps most beneficial. There was a trend favoring intravenous cyclophosphamide; however, more patients must be evaluated to fully define the role of such therapy in this condition.

Diffuse Focal Proliferative GN

Aggressive therapy is primarily indicated in persons at high risk for progressive renal failure: those with diffuse or severe focal proliferative GN and those with severe or progressive membranous GN. It had been proposed that subjects with diffuse proliferative GN and a moderate degree of irreversible chronic changes (such as glomerular scarring, interstitial fibrosis, and tubular atrophy) are at particular risk and may derive the greatest benefit from cytotoxic agents such as cyclophosphamide *(131)*. However, other studies have not confirmed the predictive value of the severity of either chronic or acute (cellular proliferation, necrosis, or crescent formation) histologic changes; both the activity and chronicity indices are often similar in subjects who progress to renal failure and in those who maintain stable renal function *(127,132)*. The limited utility of these indices is in part owing to the subjective nature of their determination, leading to variable and irreproducible results *(132)*.

Thus, the presence of diffuse proliferative GN alone seems to be a sufficient indication for aggressive therapy *(127,132)*. Despite optimal therapy, however, some patients will progress to renal insufficiency *(see* below). Clinical risk factors for progression include a plasma creatinine concentration above 2.4 mg/dL (212 µmol/L) at the time of renal biopsy, anemia with a hematocrit below 26%, and black race *(see* Importance of Race section) *(133)*. The severity of tubulointerstitial disease and crescent formation also correlate with long-term prognosis in lupus nephritis, as they do in other chronic progressive glomerular diseases *(133)*.

Although some individuals with diffuse proliferative lupus GN respond to corticosteroids alone, most studies suggest that renal survival is significantly enhanced by the addition of a cytotoxic agent, such as cyclophosphamide *(134,135)*. A meta-analysis of multiple controlled trials found that the addition of cyclophosphamide or azathioprine lowered the incidence of progression to end-stage renal disease by 40% when compared to therapy with corticosteroids alone *(136)*. High-risk individuals may derive even greater benefit; the probability of avoiding renal failure at 10–12 yr in high-risk patients was 90% with cyclophosphamide, 60% with azathioprine (this was not significantly different from cyclophosphamide), and only 20% with prednisone *(131)*. Although patients may do better with azathioprine than prednisone alone during the first 10 yr of follow-up *(131)*, there is no significant difference in the incidence of renal failure in the longer term and the results are clearly inferior to those in patients initially treated with cyclophosphamide *(137)*.

These trials also suggested that, rather than being given orally on a daily basis (2–2.5 mg/kg/d), cyclophosphamide may be less toxic when given as monthly intravenous boluses *(131)*: beginning with 0.75 g/m^2 of body-surface area and, assuming the white blood cell count remains above 3000/mm^3, increasing to a maximum of 1 g/m^2 given in a saline solution over 30–60 min. Even obese patients have generally been treated according to body surface area; a lower initial dose of 0.5 g/m^2 minimizes the risk of overdosing in this setting. An oral pulse cyclophosphamide regimen may also be effective, but this regimen is still experimental.

Effective immunosuppressive therapy is associated with a diminution in the inflammatory manifestations of lupus, resulting in control of extrarenal symptoms and a tendency to normalization of the plasma complement level and the anti-dsDNA Ab titer *(138)*. Within the kidney, cessation of inflammation reduces the activity of the urine sediment (fewer red and white cells and casts) and decreases or at least stabilizes the plasma creatinine concentration *(135)*. However, a stable plasma creatinine concentration over a period of time does not necessarily imply inactive disease, because progressive glomerulosclerosis can occur in the absence of inflammation.

Monitoring Disease Activity

Monitoring proteinuria is another important marker of the response to therapy. Successful therapy should lead to an often-marked reduction to protein excretion. However, there may be some degree of irreversible proteinuria, because healing of the inflammatory process can lead to permanent glomerular scarring. On the other hand, increasing protein excretion usually reflects continued active disease.

Selection of Therapy

The likelihood of a successful outcome is greater if therapy is initiated relatively early in the course of the disease. Delaying therapy is often associated with increased glomerular injury and fibrosis and, therefore, a lesser response to immunosuppressive drugs *(139)*.

The optimal duration of pulse cyclophosphamide therapy (which is usually accompanied by low-dose prednisone) is not known. However, results of a National Institutes of Health (NIH) clinical trial revealed the following:

The incidence of a doubling of the plasma creatinine concentration at 3 yr was much higher in the methylprednisolone group than in the cyclophosphamide groups: 48% vs 25%.

The likelihood of relapse was significantly higher in the short-course as opposed to the long-course cyclophosphamide regimen *(135)*.

One potential criticism of this study is that the pulse methylprednisolone course was too short. A follow-up report from the NIH compared 1 yr of monthly pulse methylprednisolone to monthly pulse cyclophosphamide (for 6 mo and then quarterly) to combination therapy *(140)*. Renal remission occurred in 17 of 20 patients treated with combination therapy, 13 of 21 treated with cyclophosphamide alone, and only 7 of 24 treated with methylprednisolone alone (*p* = 0.03). Combination therapy was associated with a higher incidence of adverse events than either form of monotherapy. Avascular necrosis occurred almost as frequently as with methylprednisolone alone and infections and amenorrhea were most frequent in this group.

Although these observations suggest that prolonged maintenance cyclophosphamide is associated with the best outcome, the Lupus Nephritis Collaborative Study attempted to control disease activity with a much shorter and therefore less toxic course of therapy *(141)*. Patients in this trial were treated with 60–80 mg of prednisone/d for 4 wk, followed by tapering to 20–25 mg every other day over a period of 32 wk. Oral cyclophosphamide (1–2 mg/d) was given for only 8 wk. Exacerbations were treated with increasing doses of prednisone. Almost 40% of 55 patients with an initial plasma creatinine concentration above 1.2 mg/dL (106 µmol/L) had at least a 3 mg/dL (254 µmol/L) elevation in the plasma creatinine concentration at 3–4 yr; these persons might well have benefited from the more aggressive pulse cyclophosphamide regimen described earlier. In comparison, the great majority of persons with an initial plasma creatinine concentration of 1.2 mg/dL (106 µmol/L) were either in remission (55%) or had stable disease; only 16% (5 of 31) had a rise in the plasma creatinine concentration at 3–4 yr.

In summary, once an individual has attained a complete remission, the optimal choice of immunosuppressive agent and the duration of treatment are unclear. Those with initially mild disease may be maintained on oral azathioprine (*see* next section). By comparison, investigators at the NIH continue quarterly cyclophosphamide in persons with initially severe disease until the patient has been in complete remission for one year *(142)*. However, a paucity of data exists suggesting that such therapy is superior to maintenance therapy with oral azathioprine.

Despite its efficacy, concerns about toxicity often limit the use of cytotoxic agents. There are three major complications that can occur: infection (particularly with neutropenia), malignancy, and infertility. The risk of the last two side effects is dose-dependent, increasing with prolonged therapy. A possibly safer alternative than cyclophosphamide for maintenance therapy in lupus nephritis is oral azathioprine (2 mg/kg/d), which has a much lower risk of late neoplasia and no risk of ovarian dysfunction. Azathioprine can also be used as initial therapy in persons who refuse (because of the potential complications) or cannot tolerate cyclophosphamide *(131)*.

RELAPSING DISEASE

Relapse is primarily defined as renewed clinical activity, as manifested in the kidney by either an active urine sediment, increasing proteinuria, and/or a rise in the plasma creatinine concentration. The new finding of red cell and/or white cell casts is a particularly strong predictor of relapse. In one report, these findings were noted before or at the onset of 35 of 43 relapses; the sensitivity was even greater (24 of 25) when seen in individuals excreting more than 1 g of protein/d *(143)*. It remains unknown whether early therapy would be beneficial when new cellular casts are seen in persons who had been in remission.

The role of serologic abnormalities in predicting relapse is less clear. An elevation/rise in the titer of anti-dsDNA Abs and, to a lesser degree, a fall in circulating complement levels are associated with a high likelihood (over 75%) of subsequent clinical relapse, which typically occurs within the ensuing 8–10 wk *(144)*.

It is unclear, however, how to translate these findings into the clinical setting. Many relapses do not involve the kidney, and most physicians do not routinely monitor anti-dsDNA Ab and complement titers at monthly intervals as was performed in the above study *(144)*. Furthermore, although plasma C3 and C4 levels tend to vary inversely with disease activity, there may be a prolonged reduction in C4 levels long after clinical remission has been induced *(145)*. It has been suggested that a fall in complement levels is a more valuable predictor of subsequent relapse than is the absolute plasma level *(145)*.

A recent study monitored the course of 106 patients with clinically quiescent but serologically active lupus *(146)*. Over a 1-yr period, 60 remained in clinical remission. There were no predictive factors that identified subjects who subsequently relapsed. We currently recommend that an increase in anti-dsDNA Ab levels or new hypocomplementemia should be monitored carefully, but should not be treated solely for changes in serologic activity.

In subjects with an acute flare, the initial regimen may be altered when disease is (1) severe, (2) complicated by acute renal failure, and (3) associated with very high levels of circulating immune complexes and high anti-dsDNA Ab levels. In this setting, IV pulse methylprednisolone (500–1000 mg given over 30 min for 3 d) is administered to induce a rapid immunosuppressive effect; conventional doses of oral prednisone may be ineffective in these patients and a response to IV cyclophosphamide is not seen for 10–14 d *(147)*. Although pulse steroids appear to be effective as adjunctive therapy for acute, severe lupus nephritis, this modality is not as effective when given as monotherapy when compared to cyclophosphamide plus conventional dose prednisone *(135,140)*.

How pulse corticosteroids downregulate the inflammatory response remains speculative. In the kidney, acute lupus glomerular inflammation is mediated in part by the release of cytokines (such as interferon-gamma) from activated T cells and by the upregulation of class II MHC molecules on the surface of the glomerular endothelial cells. Recent studies suggest that a principal immunosuppressive effect of corticosteroids is to inhibit the synthesis of almost all known cytokines. Steroids appear to act by inducing the synthesis of IkBα, a protein that traps and thereby inactivates the transcription factor, nuclear factor kappa B (NF-κB) *(148,149)*. As a transcription factor, NF-κB translocates to the nucleus where it initiates transcriptional activation of particular cytokine genes, including the proinflammatory cytokine, tumor necrosis factor (TNF). Pulse corticosteroids may more effectively impair cytokine generation *(150)*.

Importantly, persons with hypertension should be vigorously treated with antihypertensives. ACE inhibitors appear to delay the onset of renal failure as well as diminish proteinuria.

Prognosis

Therapy with cyclophosphamide and steroids leads, in most subjects, to improvement in the clinical and serologic signs of SLE, decreased activity of the urine sediment, and a reduction in or stabilization of the plasma creatinine concentration *(131,134,135,140,151)*.

Importance of Race

Recent reports have found that, among individuals with diffuse proliferative lupus GN, blacks are much more likely than whites to have aggressive, cyclophosphamide-resistant disease *(152,153)*. The renal survival rate was 95% at 5 yr in whites, whereas it progressively declined from 79% at 1 yr to 58% at 5 yr in blacks. This difference was independent of other risk factors such as age, hypertension, and activity or chronicity indices *(153)*. From these studies, it is unclear whether the adverse outcome in black patients is due to socioeconomic or biologic-genetic factors or both.

NEWER THERAPIES

Cyclosporine. There is only a limited reported experience with cyclosporine in the treatment of different types of lupus nephritis. An uncontrolled prospective study of 17 patients with type IV diffuse proliferative lupus GN evaluated the efficacy of prednisolone plus cyclosporine at an initial dose of 5 mg/kg/d, which was lowered to 2.5 mg/kg/d after 6 mo *(154)*. Benefits of this regimen included stabilization of the plasma creatinine concentration, a significant reduction in proteinuria (except for three patients who had relapsing nephrotic syndrome), and corticosteroid-sparing.

A second study analyzed treatment of nephrotic syndrome and membranous GN with cyclosporine, usually in combination with low-dose prednisone, for 3–4 yr *(155)*. All patients had decreased lupus activity and a substantial reduction in proteinuria; six went into complete remission. Three patients had a lupus flare during therapy that responded to standard treatment. Repeat renal biopsy in five patients showed decreased active disease but more advanced interstitial fibrosis, presumably owing to scarring of previous inflammatory injury.

At present, cyclosporine is a reasonable consideration in subjects with refractory disease or those who cannot tolerate more conventional therapies. Cost is always an important issue with this agent. Studies in adult renal transplant recipients suggest that the concurrent administration of the antifungal agent ketoconazole markedly diminishes the cyclosporine dose by slowing hepatic metabolism and reduces the total cost (cyclosporine plus ketoconazole vs cyclosporine alone) by over 70%. A similar but less pronounced effect can be attained with the calcium-channel blockers diltiazem and verapamil. The applicability of these findings to the treatment of lupus nephritis remains to be determined.

Mycophenolate Mofetil (MMF). The effectiveness of MMF as immunosuppressive therapy in renal transplant patients has prompted its evaluation in the treatment of primary renal disorders, including lupus nephritis *(156,157)*. After 1 yr of treatment of resistant lupus GN, combined MMF (dose range of 0.5–2 g/d) and prednisone resulted in significant decreases in proteinuria (–2.53 change in the urine protein/creatinine ratio) and in the serum creatinine concentration (–0.3 mg/dL [27 µmol/L]). MMF was discontinued in only one subject because of recurrent pancreatitis.

Preliminary evidence suggests that MMF may also have a role in maintenance therapy following remission after induction therapy using cyclophosphamide. In one study of proliferative lupus GN, subjects were randomized to 1–3 yr of one of the following therapies: mycophenolate (500–3000 mg/d), azathioprine (0.5–4 mg/kg/d), or IV cyclophosphamide (given once every 3 mo) *(158)*. The three regimens were similarly effective based on changes in the serum creatinine concentration and proteinuria.

Plasmapheresis. Plasmapheresis appears to be of no added benefit to immunosuppressive therapy in most persons *(159)*. A randomized controlled trial of 86 individuals with severe lupus nephritis showed that treatment with plasmapheresis, prednisone, and short-term oral cyclophosphamide led to a more rapid decline in circulating autoAb levels (such as anti-dsDNA Abs) but no difference in outcome when compared to treatment with prednisone and cyclophosphamide alone *(160)*. The percentage of subjects progressing to renal failure (25 vs 17%) and going into clinical remission (30 vs 28%) was the same in both groups.

These findings, however, do not mean that selected subjects might not benefit from plasmapheresis. It has also been suggested that the regimen used was not optimized to prevent rebound autoab production, thereby minimizing its possible efficacy. An uncontrolled study of severe lupus (and active but not severe lupus GN) refractory to conventional immunosuppressive therapy utilized an aggressive regimen consisting of plasmapheresis synchronized with pulse IV cyclophosphamide followed by oral cyclophosphamide and prednisone *(161)*. All subjects responded and eight remained off therapy for 5–6 yr. The main side effects were five episodes of herpes zoster and irreversible amenorrhea. However, a second analysis found a high number of significant adverse effects, including serious infection and death, in association with plasmapheresis and pulse cyclophosphamide therapy *(162)*. Thus, there is no proven role for plasmapheresis in subjects with lupus GN given the limited evidence of efficacy and possible increased toxicity when given with cyclophosphamide.

IVIG. The administration of IVIG can diminish immunologic activity in certain autoimmune diseases, perhaps by interacting with Fc receptors on effector cells or by the presence of anti-idiotypic Abs directed against idiotypes on the patient's own autoAbs. A small uncontrolled study found that IVIG led to histologic, immunologic, and clinical improvement *(163)*. However, other observations in lupus GN suggest that disease activity may be increased, perhaps owing to enhanced immune-complex formation mediated by the infused IgG. Thus, the efficacy of this regimen must be evaluated in controlled studies.

Cladribine. Cladribine (2-deoxyadenosine, 2-CdA), an agent with an excellent safety profile, which is currently utilized in the management of B-cell neoplasms, is being evaluated for the treatment of autoimmune diseases, including lupus GN. A pilot study evaluating the efficacy of cladribine in proliferative lupus GN revealed reductions in proteinuria and urinary evidence of glomerular inflammation with continuous infusions of 0.05 mg/kg/d *(164)*. This encouraging preliminary result warrants further study.

Cytokine-Directed Therapies. Recent data suggest that multiple cytokines have significant roles in the pathogenesis and manifestations of SLE. Treatment aimed at manipulating these cytokines may therefore prove fruitful. As examples:

Because elevated levels of interleukin-10 (IL-10) have been observed in many subjects with SLE, one study of a murine model of lupus GN evaluated the effectiveness of AS101, an immunomodulator shown to significantly decrease IL-10 levels in mice and humans *(165)*. The administration of AS101 for 6 mo to NZB/NZW F1 mice markedly diminished the incidence of proteinuria (30 vs 100% for untreated mice).

The recruitment of monocytes into the glomerulus in SLE is due in part to the production of chemoattractant molecules, particularly monocyte chemoattractant protein-1 (MCP-1) *(166)*. In a murine model of lupus GN, the administration of bindarit, an agent that completely prevents the upregulation of MCP-1, significantly limited glomerular inflammation and improved survival *(167)*.

Gastrointestinal Manifestations of SLE

Gastrointestinal (GI) manifestations occur in approx 25–40% of patients with SLE *(168)*. Many of these symptoms are nonspecific, and often reflect either lupus of the GI tract or the effects of medications.

Dysphagia

The esophagus is involved in 1.5–25% of persons with SLE *(168,169)*. Dysphagia is the most frequent complaint and is usually due to esophageal hypomotility.

Abdominal Pain

Abdominal pain, accompanied by nausea and vomiting, occurs in up to 30% of patients with SLE *(168,170)*. The differential diagnosis does not differ significantly from that in subjects without SLE. However, special consideration should be given to disorders that may be associated with lupus, including peritonitis, peptic ulcer disease, mesenteric vasculitis with intestinal infarction, pancreatitis, and inflammatory bowel disease. The specific cause of abdominal pain is usually established through the use of computed tomography (CT) scan, endoscopy, barium studies, ultrasound, angiography, and paracentesis. The role of *Helicobacter pylori* infection in peptic ulcers in individuals with lupus is not well-defined. However, Helicobacter infection should be excluded.

Prophylactic therapy also may be beneficial in certain settings, such as dyspepsia, a history of peptic ulcer disease, or combined therapy with an NSAID and high-dose corticosteroids. Such persons can be given prophylactic therapy with either misoprostol or H2 blockers.

Mesenteric Vasculitis and Infarction

Lower abdominal pain secondary to mesenteric vasculitis is generally an insidious symptom that may be intermittent for months prior to the development of an acute abdomen with nausea, vomiting, diarrhea, GI bleeding, and fever *(168,170)*. Risk factors for the development of mesenteric vasculitis include peripheral vasculitis and central nervous system (CNS) lupus *(170)*. An acute presentation may also be associated with mesenteric thrombosis and infarction, often in association with antiphospholipid Abs *(171)*.

In addition to broad-spectrum antibiotics, some authors have advocated treatment with 1–2 mg prednisone/kg/d *(168)*. The following regimen in mesenteric vasculitis without perforation is currently recommended *(172)*:

One to three courses of IV pulse steroids (1000–1500 mg methylprednisolone over 2 h/d) PLUS a bolus of pulse cyclophosphamide (1000 mg IV) are administrated immediately to suppress the inflammatory response. After 7–10 d, if feasible, a second bolus of IV cyclophosphamide (750 mg/m^2 body-surface area) should be administered.

Surgery to remove ischemic bowel is performed if the patient with acute disease has evidence of perforation or fails to respond promptly to medical therapy *(168)*.

Pancreatitis

Pancreatitis occurs in as many as 2–8% in persons with active SLE *(168,173)*. Pancreatitis generally responds to usual medical treatment. In persons who do not respond, systemic prednisone (1 mg/kg/d in divided doses) may be given, particularly if there is clear evidence for active SLE elsewhere. Steroids can be continued without any apparent delay in resolution of pancreatitis *(174)*.

Protein-Losing Enteropathy

Protein-losing enteropathy is an uncommon complication of SLE. The entity typically occurs in young women, and is characterized by the onset of profound edema and hypoalbuminemia. It may represent the first manifestation of SLE. Diarrhea is present in

50% of subjects. The disorder typically responds well to treatment with corticosteroids, although immunosuppressive drugs have also been used *(175)*.

Neuropsychiatric Manifestations of SLE (NPSLE)

Neurologic and psychiatric symptoms occur in 10–80% of persons either prior to or during the course of SLE *(176,177)*. The American College of Rheumatology (ACR) has formulated case definitions, reporting standards, and diagnostic testing recommendations for the 19 neuropsychiatric SLE syndromes *(178)*.

The most common neurologic manifestations of SLE are stroke, seizures, headaches, and peripheral neuropathies. Treatment varies with the manifestation.

Stroke Syndromes

Cerebrovascular accidents (CVAs) have been reported in up to 15% of persons with SLE *(179)*. Chronic warfarin therapy is indicated in most patients with stroke syndromes owing to antiphospholipid Abs once they are stable and if there is no evidence of hemorrhage. The INR is generally maintained between 3 and 4 *(180)*. The administration of corticosteroids and perhaps cyclophosphamide (*see* below) may be warranted if there is an associated lupus flare (including vasculitis). By contrast, steroids are not used in subjects with a stroke and antiphospholipid Abs, but no evidence of active SLE.

Seizures

Seizures develop in approx 15–20% of individuals with SLE *(179)*. Both generalized and partial seizures can occur. The latter may be complex (temporal lobe epilepsy) or simple (focal epilepsy). Seizures may be the first manifestation of lupus or develop during the course of the illness.

Seizures can be treated with a variety of medications:

Generalized seizures are usually managed with phenytoin and barbiturates.

Partial complex seizures and psychosis related to seizures are best treated with carbamazepine, klonopin, valproic acid, and gabapentin.

If new onset seizures are thought to reflect an acute inflammatory event or if a concomitant flare exists, a short course of steroids (prednisone, 1 mg/kg in divided doses) may be given in an attempt to prevent the development of a permanent epileptic focus.

Headaches

Tension and migraine headaches are frequent complaints in SLE. These headaches may result from numerous etiologies.

The treatment of headaches in SLE does not differ from that in persons without this disease, unless there are other manifestations of CNS lupus. Most patients respond to nonsteroidal anti-inflammatory drugs and/or acetaminophen. Corticosteroids and narcotics are rarely warranted, although they may be beneficial in persons with severe migraine. Tricyclic antidepressants (e.g., amitriptyline at 5–100 mg/d) are often helpful for frequently recurring headaches.

Peripheral Neuropathy

Approximately 10–15% of subjects with SLE develop a peripheral neuropathy that is probably due to vasculopathy of small arteries supplying the affected nerves

(181). Autonomic neuropathy also occurs, resulting in multiple GI, bladder, cardiac, pupillary, and sweating disorders *(182)*. Neuropathies generally respond to therapy with corticosteroids in relatively high doses (30–60 mg/d). A complete response, however, may take weeks to months.

CHOREA AND OTHER MOVEMENT DISORDERS

The frequency of movement disorders is <5% in SLE. Symptoms may include chorea, ataxia, choreoathetosis, dystonia, and hemiballismus; there are usually other associated signs of active organic brain involvement. Movement abnormalities are thought to reflect lesions in the cerebellum and/or basal ganglia. Some association with antiphospholipid Abs has been made, raising the question of whether these persons should be treated with anticoagulants *(183)*. In our experience, however, this is a self-limited and reversible disorder, and therefore may not require therapy.

EYE INVOLVEMENT

Ocular involvement in SLE includes a lupus rash of the eyelids, conjunctivitis (usually infectious), and keratoconjunctivitis (usually mild). The most characteristic finding is the presence of cotton wool exudates (i.e., cytoid bodies) that are usually near the disc, and reflect microangiopathy of the retinal capillaries and localized microinfarction of the superficial nerve fiber layers of the retina. Microaneurysms may also be demonstrated by fluorescein dye angiography.

Altered visual acuity may occasionally result from a vasculitis of the retinal vessels. Ophthalmoscopy or angiography can detect retinal vasculitis, but the latter procedure is the superior technique.

A number of therapeutic agents have been used to treat retinal vasculitis. In one retrospective study, various combinations of corticosteroids, hydroxychloroquine, and cytotoxic agents were found to be effective *(184)*. The long-term use of cytotoxic agents was associated with a corticosteroid-sparing effect.

TRANSVERSE MYELITIS

Transverse myelitis may present with the sudden onset of lower extremity weakness and/or sensory loss, plus loss of rectal and urinary bladder sphincter control. The onset usually coincides with other signs of active SLE. Transverse myelitis must be treated very aggressively and quickly if there is to be significant recovery. Treatment has been successful when combined therapy of prednisone 1.5 mg/kg, plasmapheresis, and cyclophosphamide has been used *(185,186)*. The mortality rate is high, and for those who survive, full recovery is rare. One report found that use of IV pulse methylprednisolone and pulse cyclophosphamide resulted in recovery of walking and partial or complete sphincter control *(186)*.

USE OF MORE AGGRESSIVE THERAPY IN NEUROPSYCHIATRIC SLE

The preceding discussion has primarily emphasized the use of specific therapy for different forms of neurologic manifestations of SLE. This may or may not include the use of corticosteroids. To date, the role of more aggressive therapy, especially with cyclophosphamide, has only been evaluated in a limited number of studies *(186)*.

Two studies assessed the outcome of severe neuropsychiatric lupus unresponsive to previous therapy with corticosteroids and/or oral cytotoxic drugs *(187,188)*. Substantial improvement was seen in 61–95%. Although promising, additional, prospective analyses should be undertaken.

RECOMMENDATIONS

The role of cyclophosphamide and/or plasmapheresis in the management of NPSLE is not well-defined. We consider these modalities in people with the following characteristics:

- Acute or recent onset of neurologic symptoms, such as seizures or organic brain syndromes, in the absence of another cause.
- Evidence of active inflammation in the brain, such as increased cells and protein in the cerebrospinal fluid, brain swelling on MRI or CT scan, and vascular injury on MR angiography.
- Failure to respond to a one to two week course of high dose oral corticosteroids (e.g., prednisone in a dose of 1–2 mg/kg/d) or to pulse methylprednisolone (1000 mg/d for 3 d).

PSYCHIATRIC DISTURBANCES OWING TO NPSLE

Psychiatric manifestations occur frequently in subjects with NPSLE. These clinical features are characterized by some investigators as either diffuse (e.g., organic brain syndrome, coma, depression, and psychosis) or complex (e.g., organic brain syndrome with stroke or seizure, and psychiatric presentation with stroke or seizure) *(189)*. Disturbances of mental function are the most common symptom.

A psychiatric disturbance owing to NPSLE is a diagnosis of exclusion; all other possible causes of the observed symptoms must, therefore, be considered, including infection, electrolyte abnormalities, renal failure, drug effects, mass lesions, arterial emboli, and primary psychiatric disorders (such as bipolar disorder or severe stress disorder resulting from a chronic and life-threatening disease) *(190)*. One clue to the diagnosis is that most acute psychiatric episodes occur during the first 2 yr after the onset of SLE *(191)*.

Primary Psychiatric Disturbances. Psychosis, cognitive defects, and dementia are the primary psychiatric disturbances in CNS lupus.

Psychosis owing to (active) organic involvement by SLE usually responds to steroids. Treatment should be initiated as soon as possible to prevent permanent damage. Prednisone (1–2 mg/kg/d) given for a few weeks in divided doses is usually sufficient. If no improvement is seen within two to three weeks, a trial of cytotoxic therapy (e.g., pulse cyclophosphamide) is warranted *(192)*. While waiting for steroids or immunosuppressive drugs to take effect, psychologic manifestations are best treated with antipsychotic drugs (such as haloperidol), as well as with active support by health caretakers and family.

Cognitive Defects. Cognitive dysfunction is an organic mental syndrome characterized by any combination of the following symptoms: difficulty in short- or long-term memory; impaired judgment and abstract thinking; aphasia; apraxia; agnosia; and personality changes *(193)*.

Treatment of cognitive defects is based on the presumed etiology of the cognitive abnormalities. If owing to medications, such as steroids, consider reducing the dose or stopping therapy. If associated with antiphospholipid Abs, begin anticoagulation. If associated with anti-neuronal Abs, a short course of steroids (0.5 mg/kg for a few weeks) may be beneficial *(194)*. Cognitive retraining may be effective if symptoms persist.

Dementia. Dementia is characterized by severe cognitive dysfunction, resulting in impaired memory, abstract thinking, and a decreased ability to perform simple manual tasks. There may also be difficulty making decisions or controlling impulses. In NPSLE, this syndrome can reflect multiple small ischemic strokes associated with antiphospholipid Abs *(195)*.

The exact therapeutic regimen is unclear. Although symptoms occasionally abate without treatment, the following general recommendations can be made:

Consideration should be given to discontinuing or lowering the dose of medications that may aggravate symptoms, including NSAIDs, antimalarial drugs, anti-anxiety drugs, and corticosteroids *(196)*.

Coexisting depression should be treated by conventional means.

Low-dose prednisone (0.5 mg/kg/d) may be efficacious *(194)*. We recommend a trial using this regimen if the aforementioned modalities are ineffective.

Support by family and health professionals, plus reminder prompts, will usually help patients deal with this problem.

Secondary Psychiatric Manifestations. Although depression, anxiety, and manic behavior may occasionally reflect organic involvement, these symptoms are more typically functional. The distinction between organic and functional disease is based on a psychiatric interview and psychological testing. Further testing may be appropriate, including CT scan, MRI, SPECT scans, evoked potentials, electroencephalograms, and/or cerebrospinal fluid analysis *(197)*. Treatment usually includes counselling, anxiolytic and/or anti-depressant therapy. In particular, consultation with and concurrent therapy by a psychiatrist is recommended.

SLE IN THE ELDERLY

Historically, SLE has been regarded as a disease of women in the childbearing years. Although this characterization is epidemiologically accurate, we now appreciate that SLE can occur during childhood as well as in older people *(198,199)*. Defined as disease onset over the age of 55, the female: male ratio is still a striking 7:1. Also notable is the long duration between onset of symptoms/signs of SLE and diagnosis, ranging from 18–48 mo. Of particular interest is the shift of racial predominance away from African-American to Caucasian in the United States in older SLE subjects.

Although the clinical features of late-onset SLE are similar to those observed in younger-onset disease, the frequency of certain manifestations vary considerably. In older-onset SLE, there is an increased prevalence of interstitial pulmonary disease, serositis, myositis, Sjögren's syndrome and thrombocytopenia. Like younger-onset SLE, however, arthralgia/arthritis (60.2%) and rashes (46.8%) remain the most frequent symptoms.

In general, disease activity tends to be milder in late-onset SLE *(198,199)*. Therefore, selection of treatment agents that are better-tolerated and tend to cause fewer adverse effects in this age group can be given higher priority. Arthritis and serositis can often be effectively treated by use of nonacetylated aspirin or lower dosages of NSAIDs. A history of congestive heart failure, peptic ulcer disease, renal or hepatic insufficiency, or warfarin therapy is a relative contraindication to the use of NSAIDs. The antimalarial agents, hydroxychloroquine and quinacrine, are very effective for treatment of both rashes and arthritis. As long as these agents are monitored appropriately, there is no contraindication to their use in older subjects. By contrast, lupus pneumonitis, thrombocytopenia, and hemolytic anemia require corticosteroid therapy. Corticosteroid dosages similar to that prescribed in younger adults may be necessary. As expected, there is a higher incidence of debilitating steroid complications in this population, particularly osteoporosis, cataracts, and skin atrophy. Under some conditions, the dosage of steroids can be lowered more quickly in order to obviate side effects. And other anti-inflammatory or immunosuppressive agents, such as dapsone or azathioprine, can be prescribed concomitantly in order to reduce steroid dosage. Notwithstanding, when this population is managed with steroids, a pretreatment BMD scan should be obtained and aggressive preventive treatment for steroid-induced osteoporosis must be initiated.

SUMMARY

The prognosis of SLE is unpredictable owing to the widely divergent disease patterns. The disease can run a varied clinical course, ranging from a relatively benign illness to a rapidly progressive disease with fulminant organ failure and death. Most persons with SLE have a relapsing and remitting course, which may necessitate use of high-dose steroids and/or immunosuppressive agents during the treatment of severe flares.

The survival rate in SLE has dramatically increased over the last several decades from approx 40% at 5 yr in the 1950s to approx 90% at 10 yr at the present time *(200)*. The improvement in survival is probably owing to multiple factors. These include: (1) increased disease recognition with more sensitive diagnostic tests *(201)*; (2) earlier diagnosis or treatment; (3) the inclusion of milder cases; and (4) increasingly judicious therapy and prompt treatment of complications *(202)*.

Serious infection is most often owing to immunosuppressive therapy. Individuals at particular risk are those treated with both corticosteroids and cyclophosphamide, especially if the white blood cell count is <3000/dL and/or high-dose steroids are given *(203)*.

Premature CAD is being increasingly recognized as a cause of late mortality; this has been primarily attributed to accelerated atherosclerosis associated with corticosteroid use *(204)*.

The causes of death in SLE include active lupus (29–34%), infection (22–29%), cardiovascular disease (including thromboses, 16–27%), and cancer (6%)*(202,205,206)*. Deaths, which resulted directly from SLE and infection, were common among younger patients; the risk of death directly owing to SLE was highest in the first 3 yr after diagnosis.

Poor prognosis for survival in SLE include *(207,208)*:

- Renal disease (especially diffuse proliferative GN).
- Hypertension.
- Male sex.
- Young age.
- Older age at presentation.
- Black race, which may primarily reflect low socioeconomic status *(205)*.

- Poor socioeconomic status.
- Presence of antiphospholipid Abs.
- High overall disease activity.

Despite the reduction in long-term mortality, patients with SLE are still at risk for significant morbidity owing both to active disease and the untoward effects of drugs such as corticosteroids and cytotoxic agents. Steroid-induced avascular necrosis of the hips and knees, osteoporosis, fatigue, and cognitive dysfunction have become particularly important problems as persons live longer with their illness. To enhance control of disease activity, prolong remissions, and obviate adverse effects, new therapies must be developed. With the imminent completion of the Human Genome Project and the identification of lupus disease-susceptibility genes, gene therapy may be possible within the decade. Discovery of new classes of pharmacologic agents that can modify the expression of multiple genes that predispose to and promote disease activity is the most practical current approach to new innovative therapy.

REFERENCES

1. Boumpas, D.T., H.A. Austin, III, B.J. Fessler, et al. 1995. Systemic lupus erythematosus. Emerging concepts, Part 1: Renal, neuropsychiatric, cardiovascular, pulmonary, and hematologic disease. *Ann. Intern. Med.* 122:940–950.
2. Boumpas, D.T., B.J. Fessler, H.A Austin, III, et al. 1995. Systemic lupus erythematosus. Emerging concepts, Part 2: Dermatologic and joint disease, the antiphospholipid antibody syndrome, pregnancy and hormonal therapy, morbidity and mortality and pathogenesis. *Ann. Intern. Med.* 123:42–53.
3. Vitali, C., W. Bencivelli, D.A. Isenberg, et al. 1992. Disease activity in systemic lupus erythematosus: report of the consensus study group of the European workshop for rheumatology research. I. A descriptive analysis of 704 European lupus patients. European consensus study group for disease activity in SLE. *Clin. Exp. Rheumatol.* 10:527–539.
4. Vitali, G., W. Bencivelli, D.A. Isenberg, et al. 1992. Disease activity in systemic lupus erythematosus: Report of the consensus study group of the European workshop for rheumatology research. II. Identification of the variables indicative of Disease activity and their use in the development of an activity score. The European consensus study group for disease activity in SLE. *Clin. Exp. Rheumatol.* 10:541–547.
5. Bencivelli, W., C. Vitali, D.A. Isenberg, et al. 1992. Disease activity in systemic lupus erythematosus: Report of the consensus study group of the European workshop for rheumatology research. III. Development of a computerized clinical chart and its application to the comparison of different indices of disease activity. The European consensus study group for disease activity in SLE. *Clin. Exp. Rheumatol.* 10:549–554.
6. Gladman, D.D. 1995. Prognosis and treatment of systemic lupus erythematosus. *Curr. Opin. Rheumatol.* 7:402–408.
7. Gladman, D., E. Ginzler, C. Goldsmith, et al. 1996. The development and initial validation of The Systemic Lupus International Collaborating Clinics/American College of Rheumatology Damage Index for SLE. *Arthritis Rheum.* 39:363–369.
8. Liang, M.H., S.A. Socher, M.G. Larsen, and P.H. Schur. 1989. Reliability and validity of 6 systems for the clinical assessment of disease activity in SLE. *Arthritis Rheum.* 32:1107–1118.
9. Minami, Y., T. Sasaki, S. Komatsu, et al. 1993. Female SLE in Miyagi Prefecture, Japan: a case-control study of dietary and reproductive factors. *Tohoku J. Exp. Med.* 169:245–252.
10. Walton, A.J., M.L. Snaith, M. Locniskar, et al. 1991. Dietary fish oil and the severity of symptoms in patients with SLE. *Ann. Rheum. Dis.* 50:463–466.
11. Ettinger, W.H., A.P. Goldberg, D. Applebaum-Bowden, and W.R. Hazzard. 1987. Dyslipoproteinemia in SLE. Effect of corticosteroids. *Am. J. Med.* 83:503–508.
12. Petri, M., C. Lakatta, L. Magder, and D. Goldman. 1994. Effect of prednisone and hydroxychloroquine on coronary artery disease risk factors in SLE: a longitudinal data analysis. *Am. J. Med* 96:254–259.

13. Hearth-Holmes, M., B.A. Baethge, L. Broadwell, and R.E. Wolf. 1995. Dietary treatment of hyperlipidemia in patients with SLE. *J. Rheumatol.* 22:450–454.

14. Robb-Nicholson, L.C., L. Daltroy, H. Eaton, et al. 1989. Effects of aerobic conditioning in lupus fatigue: a pilot study. *Br. J. Rheumatol.* 28:500–505.

15. Rothfield, N. 1981. Clinical features of systemic lupus erythematosus, in Textbook of Rheumatology. W.N. Kelley, E.D. Harris, S. Ruddy, C.B. Sledge, (editors). W.B. Saunders, Philadelphia.

16. van Vollenhoven, R.F., E.G. Engleman, and J.L. McGuire. 1995. Dehydroepiandrosterone in SLE: Results of a double-blind placebo-controlled, randomized clinical trial. *Arthritis Rheum.* 38:1826–1831.

17. Brodmann, R., R. Gilfillan, D. Glass, and P.H. Schur. 1978. Influenzal vaccine response in SLE. *Ann. Intern. Med.* 88:735–740.

18. Battafarano, D.F., N.J. Battafarano, L. Larsen, et al. 1998. Antigen-specific antibody responses in lupus patients following immunization. *Arthritis Rheum.* 41:1828–1834.

19. Ioannou, Y. and D.A. Isenberg. 1999. Immunization of patients with sytemic lupus erythematosus: the current state of play. *Lupus* 8:497–501.

20. Petri, M. and J. Allbritton. 1992. Antibiotic allergy in SLE: a case control study. *J. Rheumatol.* 19: 265–269.

21. Bootsma, H., P. Spronk, R. Derksen, et al. 1995. Prevention of relapses in SLE. *Lancet* 345: 1595–1599.

22. Schroeder, J.O., R.A. Zeuner, H.H. Euler, and H. Loffler. 1996. High dose intravenous immuno-globulins in SLE: Clinical and serologic results of a pilot study. *J. Rheumatol.* 23:71–75.

23. McMurray, R.W., D. Weidensaul, S.H. Allen, and S.E. Walker. 1995. Efficacy of Bromocriptine in an open label therapeutic trial for SLE. *J. Rheumatol.* 22:2084–2091.

24. Hackshaw, K.V., Y. Shi, S.R. Brandwein, et al. 1995. A pilot study of zileuton, a novel selective 5-lipoxygenase inhibitor in patients with SLE. *J. Rheumatol.* 22:462–468.

25. Strand, V. 1999. Biologic agents and innovative interventional approaches in the management of systemic lupus erythematosus. *Curr. Opin. Rheumatol.* 11:330–340.

26. Caccavo, D., B. Lagana, A.P. Mitterhofer, et al. 1997. Long-term treatment of systemic lupus erythematosus with cyclosporin A. *Arthritis Rheum.* 40:27–35.

27. McCauliffe, D.P. and R.D. Sontheimer. 1996. Cutaneous Lupus Erythematosus, in The Clinical Management of Systemic Lupus Erythematosus, 2nd ed. P.H. Schur, editor. Lippincott, Philadelphia. pp. 67–82.

28. 1995. Drugs that cause photosensitivity. *Med. Lett.* 37:35–36.

29. Jones, S.K. 1999. Ocular toxicity and hydroxychloroquine: guideline for screening. *Br. J. Dermatol.* 140:3–7.

30. Ruzicka, T., C. Sommerburg, G. Goerz, et al. 1992. Treatment of cutaneous lupus erythematosus with acitretin and hydroxychloroquine. *Br. J. Dermatol.* 127:513–518.

31. Sjolin-Forsberg, G., B. Berne, T.A. Eggelte, and A. Karlsson-Parra. 1995. In situ localization of chloroquine and immunohistological studies in UVB-irradiated skin of photosensitive patients. *Acta Derm. Venereol.* 75:228–231.

32. Wallace, D.J. 1994. Antimalarial agents and lupus. *Rheum. Dis. Clin. North Am.* 20:243–263.

33. Feldman, R., D. Salomon, and J. Saurat. 1994. The association of the two antimalarials chloroquine and quinacrine for treatment-resistant chronic and subacute cutaneous lupus erythematosus. *Dermatology* 189:425–427.

34. Laman, S.D. and T.T. Provost. 1994. Cutaneous manifestations of lupus erythematosus. *Rheum. Dis. Clin. North Am.* 20:195–212.

35. Stevens, R.J., C. Andujar, C.J. Edwards, et al. 1997. Thalidomide in the treatment of the cutaneous manifestations of lupus erythematosus: experience in sixteen consecutive patients. *Br. J. Rheumatol.* 36: 353–359.

36. Bottomley, W.W. and M. Goodfield. 1995. Methotrexate for the treatment of severe mucocutaneous lupus erythematosus. *Br. J. Dermatol.* 133:311–314.

37. Duna, G.F. and J.M. Cash. 1995. Treatment of refractory cutaneous lupus erythematosus. *Rheum. Dis. Clin. North Am.* 21:99–115.

38. Price, V.H. 1999. Treatment of hair loss. *N. Engl. J. Med.* 341:964–973.

39. Clifford, P.C., M.F. Martin, E.J. Sheddon, et al. 1980. Treatment of vasospastic disease with prostaglandin E1. *BMJ* 281:1031–1034.

40. Senecal, J.L., S. Chartier, and N. Rothfield. 1995. Hypergammaglobulinemic purpura in systemic autoimmune rheumatic diseases: Predictive value of anti-Ro (SSA) and anti-La (SSB) antibodies and treatment with indomethacin and hydroxychloroquine. *J. Rheumatol.* 22:868–875.

41. The Canadian Hydroxychloroquine Study Group. 1991. A randomized study of the effect of withdrawing hydroxychloroquine sulfate in systemic lupus erythematosus. *N. Engl. J. Med.* 324:150–154.

42. Williams, H.B., M.J. Egger, J.Z. Singer, et al. 1994. Comparison of hydroxychloroquine and placebo in the treatment of the arthropathy of mild systemic lupus erythematosus. *J. Rheumatol.* 21:1457–1462.

43. Tsakonas, E., L. Joseph, J.M. Esdaile, et al. 1998. A long-term study of hydroxychloroquine withdrawal on exacerbations in systemic lupus erythematosus. The Canadian Hydroxychloroquine Study Group. *Lupus* 7:80–85.

44. van Vollenhoven, R.F., L.M. Morabito, E.G. Engleman, and J.L. McGuire. 1998. Treatment of systemic lupus erythematosus with dehydroepiandrosterone: 50 patients treated up to 12 months. *J. Rheumatol.* 25:285–289.

45. Rahman, P., S. Humphrey-Murto, D.D. Gladman, and M.B. Urowitz. 1998. Efficacy and tolerability of methotrexate in antimalarial resistant lupus arthritis. *J. Rheumatol.* 25:243–246.

46. Carneiro, J.R.M. and E.I. Sato. 1999. Double blind, randomized, placebo controlled clinical trial of methotrexate in systemic lupus erythematosus. *J. Rheumatol.* 26:1275–1279.

47. Zizic, T.M. 1991. Osteonecrosis. *Curr. Opin. Rheumatol.* 3:481–489.

48. Kalla, A.A., I.D. Learmonth, and P. Klemp. 1986. Early treatment of avascular necrosis in systemic lupus erythematosus. *Ann. Rheum. Dis.* 45:649–652.

49. Brooks, B.J. Jr., H.E. Broxmeyer, C.F. Bryan, and S.H. Leech. 1984. Serum inhibitor in systemic lupus erythematosus associated with aplastic anemia. *Arch. Intern. Med.* 144:1474–1477.

50. Winkler, A., R.W. Jackson, D.S. Kay, et al. 1988. High dose intravenous cyclophosphamide treatment of systemic lupus erythematosus associated aplastic anemia. *Arthritis Rheum.* 31:693–694.

51. Jacob, H.S. 1985. Pulse steroids in hematologic disease. *Hosp. Pract. (Off. Ed.)* 20(8):87–94.

52. Corley, C.C., Jr., H.E. Lessner, W.E. Larsen. 1966. Azathioprine therapy of "autoimmune" diseases. *Am. J. Med.* 41:404–412.

53. Murphy, S. and A.F. LoBuglio. 1976. Drug therapy of autoimmune hemolytic anemia. *Semin. Hematol.* 13:323–334.

54. Coon, W.W. 1988. Splenectomy for cytopenias associated with SLE. *Am. J. Surg.* 155:391–394.

55. Rivero, S.J., M. Alger, and D. Alarcon-Segovia. 1979. Splenectomy for hemocytopenia in systemic lupus erythematosus: A controlled reappraisal. *Arch. Intern. Med.* 39:773–776.

56. Nesher, G., V.E. Hanna, T.L. Moore, et al. 1994. Thrombotic microangiopathic hemolytic anemia in systemic lupus erythematosus. *Semin. Arthritis Rheum.* 24:165–172.

57. Boumpas, D.T., G.P. Chrousos, R.L. Wilder, et al. 1993. Glucocorticoid therapy for immune-mediated diseases: Basic and clinical correlates. *Ann. Intern. Med.* 119:1198–1208.

58. George, J.N., S.H. Woolf, G.E. Raskob, et al. 1996. Idiopathic thrombocytopenic purpura: a practice guideline developed by explicit methods for the American Society of Hematology. *Blood* 88:3–40.

59. Blanchette, V., J. Freedman, and B. Garvey. 1998. Management of chronic immune thrombocytopenic purpura in children and adults. *Semin. Hematol.* 35(Suppl. 1):36–51.

60. Goegel, K.M., W.D. Gassel, and F.D. Goebel. 1973. Evaluation of azathioprine in autoimmune thrombocytopenia and lupus erythematosus. *Scand. J. Haematol.* 10:28–34.

61. Boumpas, D.T., S. Barez, J.H. Klippel, and J.E. Balow. 1990. Intermittent cyclophosphamide for the treatment of autoimmune thrombocytopenia in systemic lupus erythematosus. *Ann. Intern. Med.* 112:674–677.

62. Maier, W.P., D.S. Gordon, R.F. Howard, et al. 1990. Intravenous immunoglobulin therapy in systemic lupus erythematosus-associated thrombocytopenia. *Arthritis Rheum.* 33:1233–1239.

63. Karpatkin, S. 1985. Autoimmune thrombocytopenic purpura. *Semin. Hematol.* 22:260–288.

64. Hall, S., J.L. McCormick, Jr., P.R. Greipp, et al. 1985. Splenectomy does not cure the thrombocytopenia of systemic lupus erythematosus. *Ann. Intern. Med.* 102:325–328.

65. West, S.G. and S.C. Johnson. 1988. Danazol for the treatment of refractory autoimmune thrombocytopenia in systemic lupus erythematosus. *Ann. Intern. Med.* 108:703–706.

66. Cervera, H., L.J. Jara, S. Pizarro, et al. 1995. Danazol for SLE with refractory autoimmune thrombocytopenia or Evan's syndrome. *J. Rheumatol.* 22:1867–1871.

67. Ahn, Y.S., W.J. Harrington, R.C. Seelman, and C.S. Eytel. 1974. Vincristine therapy of idiopathic and secondary thrombocytopenias. *N. Engl. J. Med.* 291:376–380.

68. Pettersson, T., E. Pukkala, L. Teppo, and C. Friman. 1992. Increased risk of cancer in patients with SLE. *Ann. Rheum. Dis.* 51:437–439.

69. Sweeney, D.M., S. Manzi, J. Janosky, et al. 1995. Risk of malignancy in women with SLE. *J. Rheumatol.* 22:1478–1482.

70. Abu-Shakra, M., D.D. Gladman, and M.B. Urowitz. 1996. Malignancy in SLE. *Arthritis Rheum.* 39:1050–1054.

71. Zysset, M.K., M.T. Montgomery, S.W. Redding, and L.J. Dell'Italia. 1987. Systemic lupus erythematosus: a consideration for antimicrobial prophylaxis. *Oral Surg. Oral Med. Oral Pathol.* 64:30–34.

72. Mandell, B.F. 1987. Cardiovascular involvement in systemic lupus erythematosus. *Semin. Arthritis Rheum.* 17:126–141.

73. Roldan, C.A., B.K. Shively, and M.H. Crawford. 1996. An echocardiographic study of valvular heart disease associated with systemic lupus erythematosus. *N. Engl. J. Med.* 335:1424–1430.

74. Moder, K.G., T.D. Miller, and H.D. Tazellar. 1999. Cardiac involvement in systemic lupus erythematosus. *Mayo Clin. Proc.* 74:275–284.

75. Klacsmann, P.G., B.H. Bulkley, and G.M. Hutchins. 1977. The changed spectrum of purulent pericarditis: An 86 year autopsy experience in 200 patients. *Am. J. Med.* 63:666–673.

76. Kahl, L.E. 1992. The spectrum of pericardial tamponade in systemic lupus erythematosus. *Arthritis Rheum.* 35:1343–1349.

77. Borenstein, D.G., W.B. Fye, F.C. Arnett, and M.B. Stevens. 1978. The myocarditis of systemic lupus erythematosus. *Ann. Intern. Med.* 89:619–624.

78. Fairfax, M.J., T.G. Osborn, G.A. Williams, et al. 1988. Endomyocardial biopsy in patients with systemic lupus erythematosus. *J. Rheumatol.* 15:593–596.

79. Rosner, S., E.M. Ginzler, H.S. Diamond, et al. 1982. A multicenter study of outcome in systemic lupus erythematosus. *Arthritis Rheum.* 25:612–617.

80. Manzi, S., E.N. Meilahn, J.E. Rairie, et al. 1997. Age-specific incidence rates of myocardial infarction and angina in women with systemic lupus erythematosus: comparison with the Framingham study. *Am. J. Epidemiol.* 145:408–415.

81. Petri, M., S. Perez-Gutthann, D. Spence, and M.C. Hochberg. 1992. Risk factors for coronary artery disease in patients with systemic lupus erythematosus. *Am. J. Med.* 93:513–519.

82. Kutom, A.H. and H.R. Gibbs. 1991. Myocardial infarction due to intracoronary thrombi without significant coronary artery disease in systemic lupus erythematosus. *Chest* 100:571–572.

83. Petri, M., C. Lakatta, L. Magder, and D. Goldman. 1994. Effect of prednisone and hydroxychloroquine on coronary risk factors in SLE: a longitudinal data analysis. *Am. J. Med.* 96:254–259.

84. Orens, J.B., F.J. Martinez, and J.P. Lynch, III. 1994. Pleuropulmonary manifestations of systemic lupus erythematosus. *Rheum. Dis. Clin. North Am.* 20:159–193.

85. Hellman, D.B., C.M. Kirsch, Q. Whiting-O'Keefe, et al. 1995. Dyspnea in ambulatory patients with SLE: prevalence, severity, and correlation with incremental exercise testing. *J. Rheumatol.* 22:455–461.

86. Silberstein, S.L., P. Barland, A.I. Grayzel, et al. 1980. Pulmonary dysfunction in systemic lupus erythematosus: prevalence classification and correlation with other organ involvement. *J. Rheumatol.* 7:187–195.

87. Cheema, G.S., and E.P., Jr. Quismorio. 2000. Interstitial lung disease in systemic lupus erythematosus. *Curr. Opin. Med.* 6:424–429.

88. Matthay, R.A., M.I. Schwarz, T.L. Petty, et al. 1975. Pulmonary manifestations of systemic lupus erythematosus: review of twelve cases of acute lupus pneumonitis. *Medicine* 54:397–409.

89. Weinrib, L., O.P. Sharma, and F.P. Quismorio, Jr. 1990. A long-term study of interstitial lung disease in systemic lupus erythematosus. *Semin. Arthritis Rheum.* 20:48–56.

90. Wiedemann, H.P. and R.A. Matthay. 1992. Pulmonary manifestations of systemic lupus erythematosus. *J. Thorac. Imag.* 7:1–18.

91. Hedgpeth, M.T. and D.W. Boulware. 1988. Interstitial pneumonitis in antinuclear antibody-negative SLE: a new clinical manifestation and possible association with anti-Ro (SS-A) antibodies. *Arthritis Rheum.* 31:545–548.

92. Witt, C., T. Dorner, F. Hiepe, A.C. Borges, et al. 1996. Diagnosis of alveolitis in interstitial lung manifestation in connective tissue diseases: importance of late inspiratory crackles, 67 gallium scan and bronchoalveolar lavage. *Lupus* 5:606–612.

93. Winslow, T.M., M.A. Ossipov, G.P. Fazio, et al. 1995. Five-year follow-up study of the prevalence and progression of pulmonary hypertension in systemic lupus erythematosus. *Am. Heart J.* 129:510–515.

94. Palevsky, H.I. and A.P. Fishman. 1991. The management of primary pulmonary hypertension. *JAMA* 265:1014–1020.

95. Badesch, D.B., V.F. Tapson, M.D. McGoon, et al. 2000. Continuous intravenous epoprostenol for pulmonary hypertension due to the scleroderma spectrum of disease. A randomized, controlled trial. *Ann. Int. Med.* 132:425–434.

96. Fishman, A.P. 2000. Epoprostenol (prostacyclin) and pulmonary hypertension. *Ann. Int. Med.* 132:500–502.

97. Laroche, C.M., D.A. Mulvey, P.N. Hawkins, et al. 1989. Diaphragm strength in the shrinking lung syndrome of SLE. *Q. J. Med.* 71:429–439.

98. Walz-Leblanc, B.A., M.B. Urowitz, D.D. Gladman, and P.J. Hanly. 1992. The "shrinking lungs syndrome" in systemic lupus erythematosus? improvement with corticosteroid therapy. *J. Rheumatol.* 19:1970–1972.

99. Eagen, J.W., V.A. Memoli, J.L. Roberts, et al. 1978. Pulmonary hemorrhage in SLE. *Medicine* 57:545–560.

100. Mintz, G., J. Niz, G. Gutierrez, et al. 1986. Prospective study of pregnancy in systemic lupus erythematosus. Results of a multidisciplinary approach. *J. Rheumatol.* 13:732–739.

101. Lockshin, M.D., P.C. Harpel, M.L. Druzin, et al. 1985. Lupus pregnancy. II. Unusual pattern of hypocomplementemia and thrombocytopenia in the pregnant patient. *Arthritis Rheum.* 28:58–66.

102. Boumpas, D.T., B.J. Fessler, H.A. Austin, III, et al. 1995. Systemic lupus erythematosus: Emerging concepts Part 2: Dermatologic and joint disease, the antiphospholipid antibody syndrome, pregnancy and hormonal therapy, morbidity and mortality, and pathogenesis. *Ann. Intern. Med.* 123:42–53.

103. Buchanan, N.M., E. Toubi, M.A. Khamashta, et al. 1996. Hydroxychloroquine and lupus pregnancy: review of a series of 36 cases. *Ann. Rheum. Dis.* 55:486–488.

104. Bobrie, G., F. Liote, P. Houillier, et al. 1987. Pregnancy in lupus nephritis and related disorders. *Am. J. Kidney Dis.* 9:339–343.

105. Cowchock, F.S., E.A. Reece, D. Balaban, et al. 1992. Repeated fetal losses associated with antiphospholipid antibodies: a collaborative randomized trial comparing prednisone with low-dose heparin treatment. *Am. J. Obstet. Gynecol.* 166:1318–1323.

106. Branch, D.W., R.M. Silver, J.L. Blackwell, et al. 1992. Outcome of treated pregnancies in women with antiphospholipid syndrome: an update of the Utah experience. *Obstet. Gynecol.* 80:614–620.

107. Scott, J.R., W.D. Branch, N.K Kochenour,. and K. Ward. 1988. Intravenous immunoglobulin treatment of pregnant patients with recurrent pregnancy loss caused by antiphospholipid antibodies and Rh immunization. *Am. J. Obstet. Gynecol.* 159:1055–1056.

108. Spinatto, J.A., A.L. Clark, S.S. Pierangeli, E.N. Harris. 1995. Intravenous immunoglobulin therapy for the antiphospholipid syndrome in pregnancy. *Am. J. Obstet. Gynecol.* 172:690–694.

109. Buchanan, N.M., M.A. Khamashta, K.E. Morton, et al. 1992. A study of 100 high risk lupus pregnancies. *Am. J. Reprod. Immunol.* 28:192–194.

110. Lockshin, M.D., M.L. Druzin, and T. Qamar. 1989. Prednisone does not prevent recurrent fetal death in women with antiphospholipid antibody. *Am. J. Obstet. Gynecol.* 160:439–443.

111. Silveira, L.H., C.L. Hubble, L.J. Jara, et al. 1992. Prevention of anticardiolipin antibody-related pregnancy losses with prednisone and aspirin. *Am. J. Med.* 93:403–411.

112. Silver, R.K., S.N. MacGregor, J.S. Shol, et al. 1993. Comparative trial of prednisone plus aspirin versus aspirin alone in the treatment of anticardiolipin antibody-positive obstetric patients. *Am. J. Obstet. Gynecol.* 169:1411–1417.

113. LaBarbera, A.R., M.M. Miller, C. Ober, and R.W. Rebar. 1988. Autoimmune etiology in premature ovarian failure. *Am. J. Reprod. Immunol.* 16:115–122.

114. Boumpas, D.T., H.A. Austin, 3d, E.M. Vaughn, et al. 1993. Risk for sustained amenorrhea in patients with systemic lupus erythematosus receiving intermittent pulse cyclophosphamide therapy. *Ann. Intern. Med.* 119:366–369.

115. Petri, M., D. Spence, L.R. Bone, and M. Hochberg. 1992. Coronary artery disease risk factors in the Johns Hopkins lupus cohort: prevalence, recognition by patients, and preventive practices. *Medicine* 71:291–302.

116. Kreidstein, S., M.B. Urowitz, D.D. Gladman, and J. Gough. 1997. Hormone replacement therapy in systemic lupus erythematosus. *J. Rheumatol.* 24:2149–2152.

117. Rider, V., R.T. Foster, M. Evans, R. Suenaga, and N.I. Abdou. 1998. Gender differences in autoimmune diseases: estrogen increases calcineurin expression in systemic lupus erythematosus. *Clin. Immunol. Immunopathol.* 89:171–180.

118. Rider, V., S.R. Jones, M. Evans, and N.I. Abdou. 2000. Molecular mechanisms involved in the estrogen-dependent regulation of calcineurin in systemic lupus erythematosus T cells. *Clin. Immunol.* 95:124–134.

119. Arden N.K., M.E. Lloyd, T.D. Spector, and G.R. Hughes. 1994. Safety of hormone replacement therapy (HRT) in systemic lupus erythematosus. *Lupus* 3:11–13.

120. Kreidstein, S., M.B. Urowitz, D.D. Gladman, and J. Gough. 1997. Hormone replacement therapy in systemic lupus erythematosus. *J. Rheumatol.* 24:2149–2152.

121. Jungers, P., M. Dougados, C. Pelissier, et al. 1982. Influence of oral contraceptive therapy on the activity of systemic lupus erythematosus. *Arthritis Rheum.* 25:618–623.

122. Petri, M. and C. Robinson. 1997. Oral contraceptives and systemic lupus erythematosus. *Arthritis Rheum.* 40:797–803.

123. Julkunen, H.A. 1991. Oral contraceptives in systemic lupus erythematosus: side-effects and influence on the activity of SLE. *Scand. J. Rheumatol.* 20:427–433.

124. Julkunen, H.A., R. Kaaja, and C. Friman. 1993. Contraceptive practice in women with systemic lupus erythematosus. *Br. J. Rheumatol.* 32:227–230.

125. Sanchez-Guerrero, J., E.W. Karlson, M.H. Liang, et al. 1997. Past use of oral contraceptives and the risk of developing systemic lupus erythematosus. *Arthritis Rheum.* 40:804–808.

126. Schwartz, M.M., K.S. Kawala, H. Corwin, and E.J. Lewis. 1987. The prognosis of segmental glomerulonephritis in systemic lupus erythematosus. *Kidney Int.* 32:274–279.

127. Appel, G.B., D.J. Cohen, C.L. Pirani, et al. 1987. Long-term follow-up of lupus nephritis: a study based on the WHO classification. *Am. J. Med.* 83:877–885.

128. Pasquali, S., G. Banfi, A. Zucchelli, et al. 1993. Lupus membranous nephropathy: long-term outcome. *Clin. Nephrol.* 39:175–182.

129. Sloan, R.P., M.M. Schwartz, S.M. Korbet, et al. 1996. Long-term outcome in systemic lupus erythematosus membranous glomerulonephritis. *J. Am. Soc. Nephrol.* 7:299–305.

130. Austin, H.A., E.M. Vaughan, D.T. Boumpas, et al. 1996. Lupus membranous nephropathy: Controlled trial of prednisone, pulse cyclophosphamide, and cyclosporine A (abstract). *J. Am. Soc. Nephrol.* 7:1328.

131. Steinberg, A.D. 1986. The treatment of lupus nephritis. *Kidney Int.* 30:769–787.

132. Schwartz, M.M., S.P. Lan, J. Bernstein, et al. 1992. The role of pathology indices in the management of severe lupus glomerulonephritis. *Kidney Int.* 42:743–748.

133. Austin, H.A., 3d, D.T. Boumpas, E.M. Vaughan, and J.E. Balow. 1994. Predicting renal outcomes in severe lupus nephritis: Contributions of clinical and histologic data. *Kidney Int.* 45:544–550.

134. Austin, H.A., 3d, J.H. Klippel, J.E. Balow, et al. 1986. Therapy of lupus nephritis. Controlled trial of prednisone and cytotoxic drugs. *N. Engl. J. Med.* 314:614–619.

135. Boumpas, D.T., H.A. Austin, 3d, E.M. Vaughn, et al. 1992. Controlled trial of pulse methyl-prednisolone versus two regimens of pulse cyclophosphamide in severe lupus nephritis. *Lancet* 340:741–745.

136. Bansal, V.K. and J.A. Beto. 1997. Treatment of lupus nephritis: a meta-analysis of clinical trials. *Am. J. Kidney Dis.* 29:193–199.

137. Steinberg, A.D. and S.C. Steinberg. 1991. Long-term preservation of renal function in patients with lupus nephritis receiving treatment that includes cyclophosphamide versus those treated with prednisone only. *Arthritis Rheum.* 34:945–950.

138. McCune, W.J., J. Golbus, W. Zeldes, et al. 1988. Clinical and immunologic effects of monthly administration of intravenous cyclophosphamide in severe systemic lupus erythematosus. *N. Engl. J. Med.* 318:1423–1431.

139. Esdaile, J.M., L. Joseph, J. Mackenzie, et al. 1994. The benefit of early treatment with immunosuppressive agents in lupus nephritis. *J. Rheumatol.* 21:2046–2051.

140. Gourley, M.F., H.A. Austin, III, D. Scott, et al. 1996. Methylprednisolone and cyclophosphamide, alone or in combination, in patients with lupus nephritis. A randomized, controlled trial. *Ann. Intern. Med.* 125:549–557.

141. Levey, A.S., S.P. Lan, H.L. Corwin, et al. 1992. Progression and remission of renal disease in the Lupus Nephritis Collaborative Study. Results of treatment with prednisone and short-term oral cyclophosphamide. *Ann. Intern. Med.* 116:114–123.

142. Austin, H.A. and J.E. Balow. 1999. Natural history and treatment of lupus nephritis. *Semin. Nephrol.* 19:2–11.

143. Hebert, L.A., J.J.Dillon, D.F. Middendorf, et al. 1995. Relationship between appearance of urinary red blood cell/white blood cell casts and onset of renal relapse in systemic lupus erythematosus. *Am. J. Kidney Dis.* 26:432–438.

144. ter Borg, E.J., G. Horst, E.J. Hummel, et al. 1990. Predictive values of rise in anti-double stranded DNA antibody levels for disease exacerbation in systemic lupus erythematosus: a long term prospective study. *Arthritis Rheum.* 33:634–643.

145. West, C.D. 1991. Relative value of serum C3 and C4 levels in predicting relapse in systemic lupus erythematosus (editorial). *Am. J. Kidney Dis.* 18:686–688.

146. Leblanc, B.A., D.D. Gladman, and M.B. Urowitz. 1994. Serologically active clinically quiescent systemic lupus erythematosus: predictors of clinical flares. *J. Rheumatol.* 21:2239–2241.

147. Kimberly, R.P., M.D. Lockshin, R.L. Sherman, et al. 1981. High-dose intravenous methylpred-nisolone pulse therapy in systemic lupus erythematosus. *Am. J. Med.* 70:817–824.

148. Scheinman, R.I., P.C. Cogswell, A.K. Lofquist, and A.S. Baldwin, Jr. 1995. Role of transcriptional activation of IkBa in mediation of immunosuppression by glucocorticoids. *Science* 270:283–286.

149. Auphan, N., J.A. DiDonato, C. Rosette, et al. 1995. Immunosuppression by glucocorticoids: inhibition of NF-κB activation through induction of I kappa B synthesis. *Science* 270:286–290.

150. Yokoyama, H., T. Takabatake, M. Takaeda, et al. 1992. Up-regulated MHC-class II expression and gamma-IFN and soluble IL-2R in lupus nephritis. *Kidney Int.* 42:755–763.

151. Valeri, A., J. Radhakrishnan, D. Estes, et al. 1994. Intravenous pulse cyclophosphamide treatment of severe lupus nephritis: a prospective five-year study. *Clin. Nephrol.* 42:71–78.

152. Austin, H.A., 3d, D.T. Boumpas, E.M. Vaughan, and J.E. Balow. 1994. Predicting renal outcomes in severe lupus nephritis: contributions of clinical and histologic data. *Kidney Int.* 45:544–550.

153. Dooley, M.A., S. Hogan, C. Jennette, and R. Falk. 1997. Cyclophosphamide therapy for lupus nephritis: poor renal survival in black Americans. *Kidney Int.* 51:1188–1195.

154. Tam, L.S., E.K. Li, C.B. Leung, et al. 1998. Long-term treatment of lupus nephritis with cyclosporin A. *QJM* 91:573–580.

155. Radhakrishnan, J., C.L. Kunis, V. D'Agati, and G.B. Appel. 1994. Cyclosporine treatment of lupus membranous nephropathy. *Clin. Nephrol.* 42:147–154.

156. Nachman, P.H., M.A. Dooley, S.L. Hogan, et al. 1997. Mycophenolate mofetil therapy in patients with cyclophosphamide-(CyP) resistant or relapsing diffuse proliferative lupus nephritis (SLE-DPGN) (abstract). *J. Am. Soc. Nephrol.* 8:94A.

157. Glicklich, D. and A. Acharya. 1998. Mycophenolate mofetil therapy for lupus nephritis refractory to intravenous cyclophosphamide. *Am. J. Kidney Dis.* 32:318–322.

158. Contreras, G., D. Roth, M. Berho, et al. 1999. Immunosuppressive therapy for proliferative lupus nephritis: Preliminary report of a prospective, randomized clinical trial with mycophenolate mofetil (MMF). *J. Am. Soc. Nephrol.* 10:99A (Abstract).

159. Berden, J.H. 1997. Lupus nephritis. *Kidney Int.* 52:538–558.

160. Lewis, E.J., L.G. Hunsicker, S.P. Lan, et al. 1992. A controlled trial of plasmapheresis therapy during severe lupus nephritis. *N. Engl. J. Med.* 326:1373–1379.

161. Euler, H.H., J.O. Schroeder, P. Harten, et al. 1994. Treatment-free remission in severe systemic lupus erythematosus following synchronization of plasmapheresis with subsequent pulse cyclophosphamide. *Arthritis Rheum.* 37:1784–1794.

162. Arainger, M., J.S. Smolen, and W.B. Graninger. 1998. Severe infections in plasmapheresis-treated systemic lupus erythematosus. *Arthritis Rheum.* 41:414–420.

163. Lin, C.Y., H.C. Hsu, and H. Chiang. 1989. Improvement of histological and immunological changes in steroid and immunosuppressive drug-resistant lupus nephritis by high dose IgG. *Nephron* 53:303–310.

164. Davis, J.C., Jr., H. Austin, III, D. Boumpas, et al. 1998. A pilot study of 2-chloro-2'-deoxyadenosine in the treatment of systemic lupus erythematosus-associated glomerulonephritis. *Arthritis Rheum.* 41:335–343.

165. Kalechman, Y., U. Gafter, J.P. Da, M. Albeck, D. Alarcon-Segovia, and B. Sredni. 1997. Delay in the onset of systemic lupus erythematosus following treatment with the immunomodulator AS101: association with IL-10 inhibition and increase in TNF-α levels. *J. Immunol.* 159:2658–2667.

166. Wada, T., H. Yokoyama, S.B. Su, et al. 1996. Monitoring urinary levels of monocyte chemotactic and activating factor reflects disease activity of lupus nephritis. *Kidney Int.* 49:761–767.

167. Zoja, C., D. Corna, G. Benedetti, et al. 1998. Bindarit retards renal disease and prolongs survival in murine lupus autoimmune disease. *Kidney Int.* 53:726–734.

168. Hoffman, B.I. and W.A. Katz. 1980. The gastrointestinal manifestations of systemic lupus erythematosus: A review of the literature. *Semin. Arthritis Rheum.* 9:237–247.

169. Gutierrez, F., J.E. Valenziuela, G.R. Ehresmann, et al. 1982. Esophageal dysfunction in patients with mixed connective tissue diseases and systemic lupus erythematosus. *Dig. Dis. Sci.* 27:592–597.

170. Zizic, T.M., J.N. Classen, and M.B. Stevens. 1982. Acute abdominal complications of systemic lupus erythematosus and polyarteritis nodosa. *Am. J. Med.* 73:525–531.

171. Sanchez-Guerrero, J., E. Reyes, and D. Alarcon-Segovia. 1992. Primary anti-phospholipid antibody syndrome as a cause of intestinal infarction. *J. Rheumatol.* 19:623–625.

172. Petri, M. 1996.Gastrointestinal manifestations, in The Clinical Management of Systemic Lupus Erythematosus, 2nd ed., P.H. Schur, editor. Lippincott, Philadelphia, pp. 127–140.

173. Reynolds, J.C., R.D. Inman, R.P. Kimberly, et al. 1982. Acute pancreatitis in systemic lupus erythematosus: Report of twenty cases and a review of the literature. *Medicine* 61:25–32.

174. Saab, S., M.P. Corr, and M.H. Weisman. 1998. Corticosteroids and systemic lupus erythematosus. *J. Rheumatol.* 25:801–806.

175. Perednia, D.A. and N.A. Curosh. 1990. Lupus-associated protein-losing enteropathy. *Arch. Intern. Med.* 150:1806–1810.

176. Wong, K.L., E.K. Woo, Y.L. Yu, and R.W. Wong. 1991. Neurologic manifestations of systemic lupus erythematosus: A prospective study. *QJM* 81:857–870.

177. Hanly, J.G. and M.H. Liang. 1997. Cognitive disorders in systemic lupus erythematosus. Epidemiologic and clinical issues. *Ann. NY Acad. Sci.* 823:60–68.

178. ACR Ad Hoc Committee on Neuropsychiatric Lupus Nomenclature. 1999. The American College of Rheumatology nomenclature and case definitions for neuropsychiatric syndromes. *Arthritis Rheum.* 42:599–608.

179. Moore, P.M. 1997. Neuropsychiatric systemic lupus erythematosus: stress, stroke, and seizures. *Ann. NY Acad. Sci.* 823:1–17.

180. Moore, P.M. and T.R. Cupps. 1983. Neurological complications of vasculitis. *Ann. Neurol.* 14:155–167.

181. Huynh, C., S.L. Ho, K.Y. Fong, R.T. Cheung, C.C. Mok, and C.S. Lau. 1999. Peripheral neuropathy in systemic lupus erythematosus. *J. Clin. Neurophysiol.* 16:164–168.

182. Straub, R.H., M. Zeuner, G. Lock, et al. 1996. Autonomic and sensorimotor neuropathy in patients with SLE and systemic sclerosis. *J. Rheumatol.* 23:87–92.

183. Cervera, R., R.A. Asherson, J. Font, et al. 1997. Chorea in the antiphospholipid syndrome. Clinical, radiologic, and immunologic characteristics of 50 patients from our clinics and the recent literature. *Medicine* 76:203–212.

184. Neumann, R. and C.S. Fostert. 1995. Corticosteroid-sparing strategies in the treatment of retinal vasculitis in SLE. *Retina* 15:201–212.

185. Boumpas, D.T., N.J. Patronas, M.C. Dalakas, et al. 1990. Acute transverse myelitis in systemic lupus erythematosus: magnetic resonance imaging and review of the literature. *J. Rheumatol.* 17:89–92.

186. Barile, L. and C. Lavalle. 1992. Transverse myelitis in systemic lupus erythematosus ? The effect of IV pulse methylprednisolone and cyclophosphamide. *J. Rheumatol.* 19:370–372.

187. Neuwelt, C.M., S. Lakcs, B.R. Kaye, et al. 1995. Role of intravenous cyclophosphamide in the treatment of severe neuropsychiatric systemic lupus erythematosus. *Am. J. Med.* 98:32–41.

188. Ramos, P.C., M.J. Mendez, P.R. Ames, et al. 1996. Pulse cyclophosphamide in the treatment of neuropsychiatric SLE. *Clin. Exp. Rheumatol.* 14:295–299.

189. West, S.G., W. Emlen, M.H. Wener, and B.L. Kotzin. 1995. Neuropsychiatric lupus erythematosus: a 10-year prospective study on the value of diagnostic tests. *Am. J. Med.* 99:153–163.

190. Miguel, E.C., R.M.R. Pereira, C.A. Pereira, et al. 1994. Psychiatric manifestations of SLE: clinical features, symptoms, and signs of central nervous system activity in 43 patients. *Medicine* 73:224–232.

191. Ward, M.M. and S. Studenski. 1991. The time course of acute psychiatric episodes in systemic lupus erythematosus. *J. Rheumatol.* 18:535–539.

192. Boumpas, D.T., H. Yamada, N.J. Patronas, et al. 1991. Pulse cyclophosphamide for severe neuropsychiatric lupus. *QJM* 81:975–984.

193. Rogers, M.P. 1996. Psychiatric aspects, in The Clinical Management of Systemic Lupus Erythematosus, 2nd ed., P.H. Schur, editor. Lippincott, Philadelphia, pp. 155–173.

194. Denburg, S.D., R.M. Carbotte, and J.A. Denburg. 1994. Corticosteroids and neuropsychological functioning in patients with systemic lupus erythematosus. *Arthritis Rheum.* 37:1311–1320.

195. Asherson, R.A., D. Mercey, G. Philips, et al. 1987. Recurrent stroke and multi-infarct dementia in systemic lupus erythematosus: association with antiphospholipid antibodies. *Ann. Rheum. Dis.* 46:605–611.

196. Hoppman, R.A., J.G. Peden, and S.K. Ober. 1991. Central nervous system side effects of nonsteroidal anti-inflammatory drugs. Aseptic meningitis, psychosis, and cognitive dysfunction. *Arch. Intern. Med.* 151:1309–1313.

197. Carbotte, R.M., S.D. Denburg, and J.A. Denburg. 1986. Prevalence of cognitive impairment in systemic lupus erythematosus. *J. Nerv. Ment. Dis.* 174:357–364.

198. Mishra, N. and G.M. Kammer. 1998. Clinical expression of autoimmune diseases in older adults. *Clin. Geriatric Med.* 14:515–542.

199. Kammer, G.M. and N. Mishra. 2000. Systemic lupus erythematosus in the elderly. *Rheum. Dis. Clin. North Am.* 26:475–492.

200. Urowitz, M.B., D.D. Gladman, M. AbuShakra, and V.T. Farewell. 1997. Mortality studies in systemic lupus erythematosus. Results from a single center. 3. Improved survival over 24 years. *J. Rheumatol.* 24:1061–1065.

201. Seleznick, M.J. and J.F. Fries. 1991. Variables associated with decreased survival in systemic lupus erythematosus. *Semin. Arthritis Rheum.* 21:73–80.

202. Ward, M.M., E. Pyun, and S. Studenski. 1996. Mortality risks associated with specific clinical manifestations of SLE. *Arch. Intern. Med.* 157:1337–1344.

203. Pryor, B.D., S.G. Bologna, and L.E. Kahl. 1996. Risk factors for serious infection during treatment with cyclophosphamide and high-dose corticosteroids for systemic lupus erythematosus. *Arthritis Rheum.* 39:1475–1482.

204. Sturfelt, G., J. Eskilsson, O. Nived, et al. 1992. Cardiovascular disease in systemic lupus erythematosus. A study of 75 patients from a defined population. *Medicine* 71:216–223.

205. Ward, M.M., E. Pyun, and S. Studenski. 1995. Causes of death in SLE. Long-term followup of an inception cohort. *Arthritis Rheum.* 38:1492–1499.

206. Cerbera, R., M.A. Khamashta, J. Font, et al. 1999. Morbidity and mortality in systemic lupus erythematosus during a 5-year period. *Medicine* 78:167–175.

207. Cohen, M.G. and E.K. Li. 1992. Mortality in systemic lupus erythematosus: active disease is the most important factor. *Aust. NZ J. Med.* 22:5–8.

208. Miller, M.H., M.D. Urowitz, D.D. Gladman, and D.W. Killinger. 1983. Systemic lupus erythematosus in males. *Medicine* 62:327–334.

19

Treatment of the Antiphospholipid Syndrome

Joan T. Merrill

CONTENTS

WHOM TO TREAT AND WHEN?
USE OF CURRENTLY AVAILABLE CLINICAL PREDICTORS OF OUTCOME
ANTICOAGULATION: THE FIRST LINE OF DEFENSE
REFERENCES

WHOM TO TREAT AND WHEN?

The antiphospholipid syndrome is a blood-clotting disorder characterized by a range of autoantibodies, which bind to phospholipids and coagulation proteins *(1–3)*. This disease, which can lead to life-threatening thrombotic events, is strongly associated with systemic lupus, but may also occur in the absence of other known illness, or associated with infections or neoplasms *(4–19)*.

Benign, nonthrombotic antiphospholipid antibodies may be common in some infectious states *(20,21)*. Similar nonthrombotic antiphospholipid antibodies have been described circulating as masked, natural autoantibodies, in healthy individuals *(22)*. It is possible, therefore, that the antiphospholipid syndrome may not represent an aberrant repertoire of antibodies, totally unique to autoimmune patients, but more subtle gradations in the specificity of natural antibodies that arise in chronic inflammatory states. In this disease model, persistent antibody spreading, coupled to the background of impaired tolerance found in autoimmune disorders, might lead to increasing avidity of antibodies targeted at critical coagulation structures *(22,23)*.

Because of the heterogeneity of autoantibodies found in patients with this syndrome, the detection of antiphospholipid antibodies by currently available tests does not predict the likelihood of thrombosis or when such an event may occur *(24–26)*. Nevertheless, a direct pathogenic role for the antibodies is supported by the observation that high titer and IgG isotype confer an increased risk of thrombosis *(27)*. Additionally, isolated patient antibodies can interfere with various elements of the coagulation cascade *(28–48)*. Antibodies that bind specifically to β_2-glycoprotein 1 or prothrombin, as well as antibodies that display the confusing in vitro phenomena known as the lupus anticoagulant effect, appear to correlate better with morbidity in the antiphospholipid syndrome than the general range of antiphospholipid antibodies do *(49–53)*. It is

From: *Modern Therapeutics in Rheumatic Diseases*
Edited by: G. C. Tsokos, et al. © Humana Press, Inc., Totowa, NJ

hypothesized (but not yet proven) that pathologic, epitope-specific antibodies may eventually be identified that selectively interfere with important coagulation structures on these proteins. This could make a profound difference in the diagnosis and treatment of the antiphospholipid syndrome.

Meanwhile, given mounting evidence that many of the more pathologic antiphospholipid antibodies might be directed against specific epitopes on β_2-glycoprotein I and/or prothrombin, and that pure antiphospholipid antibodies, which are frequently associated with infections, may not confer the same thrombotic risk, can the battery of tests now available to detect antiphospholipid antibodies be narrowed down? More importantly, are there any currently available assays that can at least improve the prediction of pathogenicity and allow treatments to be initiated for some patients prior to a life-threatening thrombotic event?

The answer is no. The sensitivity, specificity, and consistency of currently available diagnostic tests remain inadequate for this purpose. Even if they were, epidemiologic study of this syndrome is woefully lacking. Definitive prospective studies to define antibody-associated risk markers remain to be performed. It must particularly be stressed that, despite subsets of phospholipid-binding antibodies, such as those associated with syphilis and HIV infections, that do not appear to confer thrombotic risk *(20,21,54)*, it has not been demonstrated that all pure antiphospholipid antibodies are nonpathogenic. Furthermore, no epidemiologic study of appropriate design or power to address this problem has yet been undertaken.

In fact, despite cross-sectional evidence suggesting that the subset of antiphospholipid antibodies that are associated with some infections are not prothrombotic, the phospholipids themselves are not irrelevant to currently accepted theories of pathogenicity. Dynamic changes in phospholipid environments that occur in inflammation or in cellular apoptosis provide critical modulation of the combined, interactive protein-lipid structures upon which anticoagulant functions and/or antibody binding depend *(55–60)*. Some evidence suggests that antibodies that bind to either β_2-glycoprotein I or prothrombin are low-affinity antibodies *(61,62)*. Such antibodies may require their targets to be either densely packed or conformationally modulated in order to achieve optimal binding and detection *(61)*. This depends on the presence of negatively charged phospholipids, but can be mimicked in commercial assays using specially prepared γ-irradiated polystyrene plates, which function very much like plastic phospholipids *(62)*.

In vivo, coagulation-regulating proteins are in close association with phospholipids and arrays of these proteins may be tightly complexed along a phospholipid surface during hemostatic events. By targeting either phospholipid or proximate cofactor proteins, antibodies may interfere with the roles of both in coagulation. It would follow that changes in the different phospholipid-membrane environments, created by various disease states or various degrees of immune activation, might have profound effects on the pathogenicity of antiphospholipid antibodies, which might circulate harmlessly in the bloodstream at other times. This illustrates the complexity of the search for specific pathologic antiphospholipid antibodies, and why current diagnostic tests cannot differentiate in advance those patients at risk for thrombosis from those who are not.

Because of this, a clinician is left in doubt as to when and for whom anticoagulant therapy is useful. Given such widespread uncertainty combined with the potential complications of anticoagulant medications, patients are generally not treated until after some significant morbidity has occurred. Then, because of an apparent high rate of reoccurrence *(30)* most patients remain on aggressive anticoagulant therapy indefinitely.

A better understanding of pathologic antiphospholipid antibodies and the epitopes they bind may someday lead to safer and more specific therapies for this disorder. However, given the limited therapeutic options at this time, and the limited scope of predictive testing, therapeutic issues primarily revolve around when and for whom to initiate global anticoagulant treatment and how aggressive the treatment should be. Critical to these decisions is the ability to utilize the available tests wisely.

USE OF CURRENTLY AVAILABLE CLINICAL PREDICTORS OF OUTCOME

Available Antiphospholipid Antibody Assays: What to Order and How to Interpret It

Despite laudable international efforts to introduce conformity into both enzyme-linked immunosorbent assay (ELISA) and lupus anticoagulant tests, current assays are not well-standardized *(63,64)*. Nevertheless these inconsistent measures are the only means of distinguishing patients with this syndrome, and current understanding of the epidemiologic features of the disorder rests upon them.

The association of thrombotic risk with high titer IgG anticardiolipin or antiphospholipid antibodies, especially if combined with a positive assay for lupus anticoagulant, has been confirmed in several different studies *(27,65–68)*. In one 4-yr follow-up of 321 women with antiphospholipid antibodies, patients with IgM or lower-level IgG anticardiolipin antibodies were not at risk for antiphospholipid-related disorders *(67)*. However, 12 of 129 patients who had either IgM or low IgG at the start of this study developed higher levels of IgG or lupus anticoagulants during the 4-yr period. Of these, half experienced at least one thrombotic complication *(67)*. This indicates that lupus patients or other patients at risk should be retested for antiphospholipid antibodies over time if negative or borderline, particularly if they develop new or recurrent clinical symptoms suggestive of the antiphospholipid syndrome.

This brings up the question of whether it makes sense to test each patient by multiple techniques to increase the sensitivity of these assays, as has been suggested repeatedly in the literature *(62,69–73)*. In one study of 1513 sera from 399 patients *(71)*, 60% of the samples containing antiphospholipid antibodies reacted to phospholipids other than cardiolipin, the most commonly used phospholipid in commercial assays. Considering only the more (probably) pathologic IgG subtypes, reactivity to phosphatidylserine was more prevalent than reactivity to cardiolipin. Reactivity to phosphatidylethoanolamine was also relatively common *(71)*. In another report of 141 sera tested using both anionic and zwitterionic phospholipids 79 phospholipid-reactive sera were found. Of these 11 reacted with noncardiolipin phospholipid, of which seven patients had a history of ether recurrent fetal loss or thrombotic events *(70)*. This confirms the need to use more than just the anticardiolipin assay in obtaining a diagnosis for patients for whom there is strong suspicion. In one intriguing study, IgG from women with clinical features suggestive of the antiphospholipid syndrome but negative at one point in time in both antiphospholipid antibodies and lupus anticoagulant assays, were tested in a murine passive-immunization model, causing significantly more fetal loss in the mice than control IgG *(72)*. Either low-titer anticardiolipin or antiphosphatidylserine antibodies were subsequently found in some, but not all of these women.

It seems likely that the laboratory analysis of antiphospholipid antibodies will continue to evolve over the coming years. Bilayer phospholipids of varying composition may be used increasingly to provide a more physiologic substrate in the detection of these antibodies in combination with various lipid-binding proteins *(74)*. Given the multiple protein antigens now associated with the antiphospholipid syndrome, assays to detect antibodies specific for prothrombin or other lipid-binding proteins using negatively charged plates may also become available in the near future, although their ultimate usefulness in juxtaposition to current (and less expensive) assays remains to be determined.

Positivity in a specific anti-β_2-glycoprotein I immunoassay has been more closely associated with the clinical manifestations of the antiphospholipid syndrome than positivity in conventional anticardiolipin ELISA *(54,75)*. Unlike the anticardiolipin assay, there appears to be less chance of false-positive results for syphilis patients using the assay specific for β_2-glycoprotein I *(36,54,76)*. This assay has recently become commercially available. Some commercial antiphospholipid assays incorporate mixed phospholipids and β_2-glycoprotein into one ELISA. Because it is now thought that different phospholipid environments may differentially affect detection of anti-β_2-glycoprotein antibodies, it is not clear that the net effect of this mixture would increase the range or sensitivity of this assay.

In patients for whom there is reasonable suspicion for the antiphospholipid syndrome, it seems logical to use up to three different assays from the more easily available common testing methods first, such as an anticardiolipin and/or antiphosphatidylserine test plus lupus anticoagulant assays (here, too, sensitivity may be increased employing different LA tests, including both the Kaolin Clotting Time assay (KCT) and dilute Russel Viper Venom Time assay (dRVVT), and/or an lupus anticagulants (LA) test employing hexagonal-phase phospholipids). Where available, an anti-β_2-glycoprotein immunoassay should be employed, which, by eliminating many of the nonthrombotic, phospholipid-specific antibodies associated with infections, may be at least marginally more selective for the autoimmune syndrome. To analyze further the sera of patients for whom there is a high suspicion of this syndrome but the aforementioned tests are negative, it might be worth obtaining a more comprehensive testing battery, particularly if a laboratory can be found capable of testing for antibodies to β_2-glycoprotein and/or prothrombin against different phospholipid backgrounds.

In summary, the lack of standardization in the tests currently available to clinicians, coupled with evidence that patient results may change over time using these assays, indicates that patients in whom there is a high suspicion for the antiphospholipid syndrome but who test negative in a preliminary assay for antiphospholipid antibodies, should be tested using more than one technique. They should also be retested over time if still negative, particularly if they develop new or recurrent clinical symptoms suggestive of active antiphospholipid syndrome. It seems obvious, however, that to avoid excessive false-positive diagnoses, the use of more than one assay in the detection of the antiphospholipid syndrome should only be used for patients at apparent high clinical risk, and in the absence of other explanations for thrombosis. Multiple assays may not only increase the sensitivity of detection. In certain situations, positive results on multiple assays might be prognostic. For example, three assays positive for antiphospholipid antibodies at conception has been associated with a major risk for obstetric complications *(73)*. Once a patient tests positive in any standardized assay for antiphospholipid antibodies and has had a major thrombotic complication, the standard of care is permanent anticoagulation and there is no need for further testing. When detectable antiphospholipid antibodies disappear, it is not known whether risk for thrombosis lessens. This too is a subject pressing for study.

Other Considerations to Help Establish Thrombotic Risk

Immunologic tests such as the assays discussed earlier do not establish thrombotic risk for patients until some morbidity, usually a life-threatening thrombotic event, has occurred. There are a few additional tests that might indicate the likelihood of thrombotic risk prior to clinically obvious disease, but it has not as yet been determined in prospective studies whether these should be used either routinely in lupus patients with high-titer antiphospholipid antibodies or to initiate anticoagulation earlier than might occur under the current standard of care. In certain clinical situations, these tests might also be helpful in establishing a diagnosis when the testing and/or history suggests the antiphospholipid syndrome but evidence remains equivocal.

PREGNANCY LOSS

Spontaneous abortion in the antiphospholipid syndrome is strongly associated with fetal loss, as opposed to earlier first-trimester loss, but first-trimester loss is also well-described in this syndrome. In one study of patients with recurrent pregnancy loss *(77)*, the specificity of fetal death for patients with antiphospholipid antibodies was 76%. Conversely, the specificity of two or more early first-trimester abortions for the ability to select patients with antiphospholipid antibodies was 6%. Nevertheless, in the same study, although more than 80% of women with antiphospholipid antibodies had at least one fetal death by history, only 50% of overall antiphospholipid antibody-related abortion involved fetal death. This leaves some doubt about what to do in a second pregnancy when a lupus patient with high-titer IgG anticardiolipin antibodies suffers a first-trimester pregnancy loss. It is not considered warranted to initiate heparin in a subsequent pregnancy on the basis of this insufficient evidence *(78)*. However, this is often a highly charged issue for patients, who request to know if anything more can be done diagnostically.

One strategy, if the initial loss is late enough and tissue available, is to have the placenta examined. Given the fact that villous infarction is rare in first-trimester abortion, finding this clear-cut clue in the placenta from a patient with antiphospholipid antibodies might alter the strategy for the next pregnancy *(79)*. One study also indicates that IgG anticardiolipin antibodies can be eluted from placentae of patients with the antiphospholipid syndrome but not from controls *(80)*. Not surprisingly, β_2-glycoprotein I is also found bound to both normal and control placentae, located in the syncytiotrophoblast *(80)*.

There is evidence that placental pathology in the antiphospholipid syndrome is repeated in subsequent pregnancies *(81)*. Therefore, when antiphospholipid-positive lupus patients with past early first-trimester loss reach term or near-term in a subsequent pregnancy, placental pathology should not be overlooked owing to the happy outcome, especially with low birth-weight infants. Similarly, when a subsequent pregnancy reaches the second trimester in a patient for whom there is some but not definitive suspicion of the antiphospholipid syndrome, fetal size should be closely monitored. One study also suggests that abnormal resistance of uterine arteries at 18–24 wk gestation (measured by velocimetry) may predict pregnancies at increased risk for obstetric complications *(73)*.

CEREBROVASCULAR MONITORING

Optimally, patients with high-titer IgG antiphospholipid antibodies and established transient ischemic attacks should be anticoagulated before serious cerebrovascular accidents occurred. However, in practice, TIAs may or may not be clearcut from a patients description, if they are described at all. A thorough history is obviously of primary importance, but even so, there is a large grey zone between the description of fearful, but equivocal symptoms, and making a commitment to lifelong, or at least indefinitely long anticoagulation. Computed tomography (CT) or magnetic resonance imaging (MRI) neuroimaging findings in patients with possible TIAs may also be difficult to interpret. Results range from cerebral atrophy to focal infarcts, which appear to be fairly common and are of uncertain significance *(82)*. On the other hand angiography of these patients may demonstrate more dramatic abnormalities, including clearcut stenosis and subclinical occlusions *(82)*. There is one report suggesting that single photon-emission computerized tomography (SPECT) may be useful in demonstrating decreased cerebral blood flow in patients with the antiphospholipid syndrome *(83)*, and in an addtional report SPECT revealed hypoperfusion lesions in 16 of 22 patients with primary antiphospholipid syndrome, mild neuropsychiatric manifestations, and normal brain MRI findings *(84)*. Again, the usefulness of this interesting approach in predictive testing remains to be evaluated. Lockshin's group has found strong evidence for a cardioembolic etiology in antiphospholipid-related stroke *(85)*, so the importance of obtaining an echocardiogram for patients with known or suspected TIA cannot be over stressed. In an additional study either anticardiolipin antibody or lupus anticoagulant were found in 35 of 41 patients with Sneddon's syndrome (defined as cerebrovascular disease and livedo reticularis). Thirty-four percent of these patients had evidence of ischemic heart disease and 13/32 of these patients were found to have mitral valve thickening, again suggesting a link between the heart and the brain. Although arterial occlusion accounts for most reports of cerebrovascular accidents in the antiphospholipid syndrome, hemorrhagic venous infarction (in the context of dural sinus thrombosis) has also been described *(86)*, stressing the importance of confirming a pure thrombotic event prior to initiating anticoagulation, even in patients with this syndrome.

MONITORING THE KIDNEY

There is evidence to suggest that the kidney may be a more frequent target organ in the antiphospholipid syndrome than may have been previously appreciated *(87)*. Clinical manifestations may easily be confused with lupus nephritis, including proteinuria, hypertension, and/or acute renal failure. The pathology is clearly thrombotic, however, indicating the importance of renal biopsy in patients with systemic lupus erythromatosis (SLE) and apparent renal disease, because the first line of therapy for thrombotic kidney disease is probably anticoagulation rather than immune suppression. Furthermore, under conditions of stress, there may be enhanced risk for kidney vasculature. Patients with antiphospholipid antibodies appear to be at high risk of post-transplant renal thrombosis and anticoagulation therapy appears to prevent this *(88)*.

DRUG-INDUCED ANTIPHOSPHOLIPID ANTIBODIES

Antiphospholipid antibodies have now been found in association with medications known to induce lupus-like syndromes *(89,90)* Our laboratory found a high incidence of antiphospholipid antibodies in patients taking procainamide, whether or not there was clinically evident drug-related lupus *(89)*. These antibodies have characteristics similar to autoimmune antiphospholipid antibodies, as opposed to the infectious type *(89,90)*, including specificity for β_2-glycoprotein I *(90)*. It remains to be determined whether these antibodies increase risk for thrombosis in a population that may already be at high risk for heart and vascular disease.

THE EPIDEMIOLOGY OF RECURRENCE: IS RISK PREDICTABLE?

It was recently widely accepted that recurrent thrombosis in the antiphospholipid syndrome has a tendency to mimic the original thrombotic event, with arterial thrombosis following arterial occlusion and venous following venous *(91)*. However, the study cited involved only 20 patients, and none were followed during subsequent pregnancies. Several studies performed in an attempt to predict risk factors for pregnancy, confirm the intuitive impression that there are multifactorial outcomes in this multifactorial disease, citing, along with the known risks of high IgG antiphospholipid antibodies and history of previous miscarriage, the additional factors of thrombocytopenia and/or other previous thrombotic events as predictors of adverse pregnancy outcome *(92–94)*.

The antiphospholipid syndrome was identified as a poor prognostic factor for survival in one cohort of 667 patients, and a stepwise cox multivariate analysis suggested that this was primarily attributable to either thrombocytopenia or arterial occlusions *(95)*. A different group of 360 patients with lupus anticoagulants with or without antiphospholipid antibodies were followed in a 4-yr prospective study. Thirty-four developed thrombotic complications, suggesting an overall incidence of 2.5%/patient yr. Two independent risk factors identified were history of previous thrombosis or presence of an IgG anticardiolipin antibody with a binding strength of greater than 40 international units (IU) *(93)*. Of some concern, 4 patients in the original group of 360 developed non-Hodgkins lymphoma.

In one study with a historic cohort design, obstetric and medical histories were taken from 130 women with lupus anticoagulant and/or IgG anticardiolipin antibodies at a mean of 3.7 yr after the initial positive assay. In the interim period, 63 (48%) had developed at least one new disorder consistent with the antiphospholipid syndrome or risk thereof, including CVAs, amaurosis fugax, TIAs, SLE, and thrombocytopenia. There were 34 thrombotic events in all, eight of which were pregnancy related *(96)*. Eight of the 34 thrombotic events were also reported while patients were on anticoagulant therapy *(96)*.

ANTICOAGULATION: THE FIRST LINE OF DEFENSE

It is now generally accepted that patients with the antiphospholipid syndrome are at higher risk for recurrent thrombosis than other patients with thrombotic disease *(97)*, and require long-term and possibly lifelong treatment *(98)*. Because the pathologic vasculopathy of the antiphospholipid syndrome is predominantly thrombotic, anticoagulation remains the treatment of choice *(99)*. Current possible options include antiplatelet therapy and anticoagulation with warfarin, heparin, or low molecular-weight heparins *(100)*. The best available evidence suggests that long-term therapy with oral anticoagulation does prevent recurrent thrombosis, but prospective studies are still lacking *(101)*. Given the retrospective nature of most of the literature and the potential morbidity of high-dose warfarin therapy, there is still no widespread consensus of treatment strategies *(102)*.

Warfarin for Non-Gravid Patients

The most widely accepted recommendation for treatment of thrombosis and ongoing prophylaxis against recurrent thrombosis is higher dose warfarin anticoagulation, aiming to keep an international normalized ratio (INR) greater than 3.0 with or without aspirin *(103,104)*. However the appropriateness of INR for warfarin monitoring has been questioned in the presence of lupus anticoagulant activity *(97)*. Furthermore there may be assay-dependency of INR values in LA patients on oral anticoagulation. For these patients, accurate INR values may be obtained using combined thromboplastin reagents that permit testing at high plasma dilution *(105)*. In one small study, it was observed that patients with deep venous thrombosis had higher incidence of complications during anticoagulant therapy than those with cerebrovascular symptoms *(106)*. Prospective studies on a scale that enables appropriate subgroup analysis have not been done.

Other risks arise when the patients medical condition becomes more complicated. For example, there may be significant problems with recurrent thromboses when warfarin is withdrawn for surgery, despite attempts to cover patients with heparin *(106)*. Thrombocytopenia is a complication of the antiphospholipid syndrome itself, occurring in 20–40% of patients *(107)*. The actual drop in platelet count is usually mild and it has been suggested that this should not modify the policy for treatment of thrombosis *(107)*. However, platelet-function abnormalities have been described even with normal platelet counts, associated with a detectably prolonged bleeding time *(108)*. It therefore seems advisable, where thrombocytopenia exists, to at least obtain a bleeding time prior to making the ultimate decision regarding an anticoagulant regimen.

Where specific treatment is required for thrombocytopenia in the antiphospholipid syndrome, it is usually handled similarly to idiopathic thrombocytopenic purpura (ITP) *(107)*. There is one anecdotal description of thrombocytopenia in a patient with SLE and antiphospholipid syndrome that actually responded to warfarin after only a partial response to immunosuppressive therapy *(109)*. However, it would be premature to draw any general conclusions from this report.

Comparative Anticoagulation Treatments: Lack of Data

Other than the short-term use of heparin during the initial thrombotic incidence, there is little published data to allow a systematic evaluation of treatment alternatives in nonpregnant patients with the antiphospholipid syndrome. It is now apparent that for the acute treatment of established venous thrombosis in general, not associated with this syndrome, low molecular-weight heparin is at least as safe and effective as unfractionated heparin *(110,111)*, and might be considered preferable by virtue of the potential for substantial cost savings and fewer side effects *(110–117)*. One case series suggests that long-term dalteparin may be safe and effective *(118)* in the antiphospholipid syndrome, although there is no direct comparison to alternative treatments.

One anecdotal report observed response to fibrinolytic treatment of an extensive common femoral/iliac thrombosis after failure to improve during high-dose heparin therapy *(119)*. In another report, acute myocardial infarction was successfully treated with tissue plasminogen activator in a patient with the antiphospholipid syndrome *(120)*. Other than these sporadic reports, it is quite clear that testing of new anticoagulant drugs is lacking in this syndrome, as is any formal testing of the hypothesis that anticoagulation strategy might be selected for the different types of thrombosis observed.

A particular deficit in our knowledge is the lack of epidemiologic rationale for the use of aspirin. It is common to suggest low-dose aspirin therapy for patients with antiphospholipid syndrome who do not meet criteria for the syndrome. Clinical experience suggests that aspirin alone may not be sufficient after many years of follow-up in preventing a first episode of thrombosis. However, this has not been formally tested, or considered with regards to arterial vs venous disease. The usefulness of low doses of aspirin as an addition to other forms of anticoagulation is now well-demonstrated in the prevention of obstetric complications *(121)* in which pathology of uteroplacental arteries may play some role. Aspirin may also be useful in stroke-recurrence prevention in patients with antiphospholipid antibodies *(121)*, although this remains to be established in prospective studies.

Special Case of Pregnancy

The standard of care in pregnancy is better delineated than treatment of other complications of the antiphospholipid syndrome *(122)*, and the benefits of treating patients known to be at risk are generally accepted *(122,123)*. However, even with anticoagulant or immunosuppressive therapies, there appears to be high incidence of pregnancy complications in affected women, including intrauterine growth retardation, preeclampsia, fetal distress, and premature birth *(73,94,123)*. Optimal treatment in pregnancy involves the use of aspirin plus heparin, which is usually adjusted to a higher dose than the 5000 IU bid used in nonpregnant thrombotic prophylaxis. This can be monitored by use of a nadir aPTT or a factor Xa inhibition assay at 2 h post-injection *(114,122)*. Both heparin and pregnancy may contribute to decreased bone density *(110,114,124–126)*, although the extent of long-term clinical significance remains unclear. Other heparin side effects include thrombocytopenia, eosinophilia, skin reactions, alopecia, transaminasemia, hyperkalemia, and hypoaldosteronism *(110–114,117,126,127)*. Warfarin, unlike heparin, crosses the placenta. It is a known teratogen when used in early pregnancy and can also be associated with bleeding problems in the fetus, particularly at the time of delivery. Thus, warfarin has a limited use in the antenatal period *(126)*. However, in some countries, where options are limited, it is still used successfully later in pregnancy, and can be considered in patients with heparin-induced thrombocytopenia. Prednisone is no longer favored in pregnancy owing to increased potential for morbidity *(114)*, but its use is still considered when other options are ruled out or insufficient, given a good efficacy record.

Initial reports of the use of low molecular-weight heparin in antiphospholipid pregnancy suggests that it is both safe and effective *(94,110,115,122,128)*. Low molecular-weight heparin may have significant advantages over unfractionated heparin, including better bioavailability, longer half-life, and a more predictable anticoagulant response that eliminates the need for frequent laboratory monitoring *(111)*. The common side effects of unfractionated heparin, including bleeding, thrombocytopenia, and osteoporosis, may be less common with low molecular-weight heparin *(110–117)*, although one meta-analysis did not support the hypothesis that there are actually fewer bleeding complications *(116)*.

As mentioned previously, aspirin is an established conjunctive treatment for antiphospholipid pregnancy *(114,121)*. An additional theoretical rationale for the use of aspirin is provided by evidence that prostaglandin metabolites have been implicated in the pregnancy disorder *(42,129,130)*. Low-dose aspirin inhibits cyclooxygenase (COX) and shifts metabolism of arachidonic acid towards leukotrienes, which in turn stimulate interleukin-3 (IL-3) production. IL-3, an important cytokine in support of placental growth and development, has been found to be low in SLE patients in general and in pregnant patients with the antiphospholipid syndrome *(130)*.

Immune Modulation: Steroids, Cytotoxic Therapy, Plasmapheresis, IVIG

In lupus patients, vasculitis may coexist with the antiphospholipid syndrome and contribute to a generalized prethrombotic state *(99)*. Also, underlying endothelial damage may contribute to a favorable environment for aPL to induce thrombotic complications *(100)*. Although autoimmunity and inflammation may be important to the pathogenesis of the syndrome, immunosuppressive therapy in and of itself is not the initial standard of care *(100)*, and is generally reserved for refractory situations.

Whether or not immunosuppressive therapy has any role in lowering or eliminating thrombotic risk remains unknown, but immunosuppression has been used empirically by many physicians, either alone or in conjunction with anticoagulant measures, particularly when aggressive anticoagulation has failed. Sporadic reports indicate the possibility that plasmapheresis or plasma exchange might also be a more or less successful treatment *(131,132)* but these interventions are usually reserved for catastrophic cases.

Another argument for immunosuppressive therapy is based on evidence that autoantibodies may arise from imbalance or excess of immune factors. This is supported by the observation that the induction of antiphospholipid antibodies can accompany immune-enhancing therapy. In one study of 30 patients under treatment for disseminated melanoma, antiphospholipid antibodies were detected in 0/10 who received no therapy, 0/18 who received IL-2 alone, 2/4 who received α interferon (IFN-α) alone, and 3/8 who were treated with a combination of IL-2 and IFN-α. Of the five patients who developed antiphospholipid antibodies in this study, all five had prolonged PTT, and four developed deep-vein thrombosis *(133)*.

The pregnancy literature further supports the possibility that immunosuppression is an effective treatment for the thrombotic complications of the antiphospholipid syndrome. Equivalent live birth rates have been seen in patients receiving combinations of aspirin with either heparin or prednisone, but prednisone is associated with increased maternal and obstetric risks, and is therefore considered a second line of treatment in pregnancy *(122)*. It is not known whether antithrombotic treatment is superior to immune modulation in prevention of recurrent neurologic complications *(134)*, although there is some suggestion that combined anticoagulation and immunosuppression may prevent further cerebral ischemic events *(135)*.

Further support for the concept of treatment strategies that interfere with the antibodies themselves has been provided by initial therapeutic successes using intravenous immune globulin (IVIG). IVIG, which is thought to contain anti-idiotypic antibodies that bind to patient antiphospholipid antibodies, was first shown to ameliorate an antiphospholipid syndrome-like state in a mouse model *(136)*. It has subsequently been found to be well-tolerated in pregnancy, although definitive comparitive studies have not been performed *(137–142)*. In one larger pilot study, 38 women with three or more consecutive first-trimester abortions and antiphospholipid antibodies received 300 mg/kg q 3 wk from the time pregnancy was confirmed to the 16th or 17th wk. Pregnancy proceeded beyond the first trimester in 89.4% and healthy infants were born in 81.4% *(141)*.

Untested Treatments

Novel, but as yet unproven, strategic therapies for the antiphospholipid syndrome have recently been explored using murine models. These include IL-3 *(143)*, a thromboxane receptor antagonist *(144)*, anti-idiotype or anti-CD4 antibodies *(66)*, bone marrow transplantation *(145)* ciprofloxacin, and bromocryptine *(146)*. Because association with phospholipids seems to enhance the interaction between β_2-glycoprotein I and autoantibodies, one recently suggested strategy (as yet untested) for development of therapeutic agents is based on the use of small cyclic, organic oligoanions such as inositol derivatives, which might act as ligands for lysine residues at the phospholipid-binding site of β_2-glycoprotein I *(147)*. It remains unclear what the coagulation effects of this sort of therapy would be, if any.

An additional new concept in immune-modulating therapeutics, which may have wide applicability to autoimmune disease is the use of toleragens, tetravalent conjugates of antigenic material linked to a common platform. LJP 394, a toleragen aimed at antibodies to dsDNA, was created by La Jolla Pharmaceuticals by attaching four oligonucleotides to a triethylene glycol-based platform *(148)*. This was shown to reduce anti-dsDNA specific plaque-forming cells in an immunized mouse model *(148)*, possibly by crosslinking B-cell surface immunoglobulins. LJP 394 was subsequently found to inactivate anti-dsDNA-specific B cells in vivo in both murine-immunized and spontaneous disease models of nephritis, enhancing survival and lessening renal pathology in BXSB mice *(149)*. Clinical trials are currently underway to study the potential of this therapy in human lupus nephritis.

An appropriate definition of the epitopes of pathologic antiphospholipid antibodies might create a similar opportunity for toleragen therapy in the near future. Presumably, such an agent would have the potential to recognize and remove coagulation-enhancing antibodies from the circulation, along with the B cells that give rise to them. In toleragen development, one problem is that the construct developed needs to lack T-cell epitopes, so that it does not trigger its own immune response *(149)*. Another problem that would need to be addressed is that there is some risk that an antiphospholipid toleragen might resemble an important coagulation functional site, and, by competition, interfere with intravascular hemostasis in a dose-responsive manner.

Summary

Treatment of the antiphospholipid syndrome is currently hampered by lack of clear prognostic indicators and the potentially serious side effects of either global anticoagulation or global immune suppression. As immune-modulating therapeutics become more sophisticated and as the pathophysiology of this syndrome becomes better-clarified, it can be hoped that safer and more specific medications will be developed to replace the current standard of care, which in most cases involves lifelong warfarin therapy.

REFERENCES

1. Hughes, G.R., E.N. Harris, and A.E. Gharavi. 1986. The anticardiolipin syndrome. *J. Rheum.* 13:486–489.

2. Alarcon-Segovia, D., M.H. Cardiel, and E. Reyes. 1989. Antiphospholipid arterial vasculopathy. *J. Rheum.* 16:762–767.

3. Boey, M.L., C.B. Colaco, and A.E. Gharavi. 1983. Thrombosis in systemic lupus erythematosus: striking association with the presence of circulating lupus anticoagulant. *Brit. Med. J.* 287: 1021–1023.

4. Sorice, M., V. Pittoni, T. Griggi, A. Losardo, O. Leri, Magno M.S., et al. 2000. Specificity of anti-phospholipid antibodies in infectious mononucleosis: a role for anti-cofactor protein antibodies. *Clin. Exp. Immunol.* 120:301–306.

5. Loizou, S., J.K. Cazabon, M.J. Walport, D. Tait, and A.K. So. 1997. Similarities of specificity and cofactor dependence in serum antiphospholipid antibodies from patients with human parvovirus B19 infection and from those with systemic lupus erythematosus. *Arthritis Rheum.* 40:103–108.

6. Keung, Y.K., E. Cobos, G,E. Meyerrose, and G.H. Roberson. 1996. Progressive thrombosis after treatment of diffuse large cell non-Hodgkin's lymphoma and concomitant lupus anticoagulant. *Leuk. Lymphoma* 20:341–345.

7. Mengarelli, A., C. Minotti, G. Palumbo, P. Arcieri, G. Gentile, A.P. Iori, et al. 2000. High levels of antiphospholipid antibodies are associated with cytomegalovirus infection in unrelated bone marrow and cord blood allogeneic stem cell transplantation. *Br. J. Haematol.* 108:126–131.

8. Uthman, I., Z.Tabbarah, and A.E. Gharavi. 1999. Hughes syndrome associated with cytomegalovirus infection. *Lupus* 8:775–777.

9. Viallard, J.F., G. Marit, J. Reiffers, A. Broustet, and M. Parrens. 2000. Antiphospholipid syndrome during chronic myelomonocytic leukemia [letter] *Am. J. Hematol.* 63:60.

10. Ghirarduzzi, A., M. Silingardi, M. D'Inca, and A. Tincani. 1999. The antiphospholipid syndrome during chronic lymphatic leukemia. An association with anti-factor VIII antibodies. *Ann. Ital. Med. Int.* 14:46–50.

11. Naschitz, J.E., I. Rosner, M. Rozenbaum, E. Zuckerman, and D. Yeshurun. 1999. Rheumatic syndromes: clues to occult neoplasia. *Semin. Arthritis. Rheum.* 29:43–55.

12. Samadian, S. and L. Estcourt. 1999. Recurrent thrombo-embolic episodes: the association of cholangiocarcinoma with antiphospholipid syndrome. *Postgrad. Med. J.* 75:45–46.

13. Hayem, G., N. Kassis, P. Nicaise, P. Bouvet, A. Andremont, C. Labarre, et al. 1999. Systemic lupus erythematosus-associated catastrophic antiphospholipid syndrome occurring after typhoid fever: a possible role of Salmonella lipopolysaccharide in the occurrence of diffuse vasculopathy-coagulopathy.*Arth. Rheum.* 42:1056–1061.

14. Kupferwasser, L.I., G. Hafner, S. Mohr-Kahaly, R. Erbel, J. Meyer, and H. Darius. 1999. The presence of infection-related antiphospholipid antibodies in infective endocarditis determines a major risk factor for embolic events. *J. Am. Coll. Cardiol.* 33:1365–1371.

15. Gharavi, A.E. and S.S. Pierangeli. 1998. Origin of antiphospholipid antibodies: induction of aPL by viral peptides. *Lupus* 7(Suppl. 2):S52–4.

16. Quintanilla, S., S. Ferrer, and M. Bravo. 1998. Myxoma and antiphospholipid antibody syndrome *Rev. Med. Chil.* 126:670–676.

17. Tucker, S.C., I.H. Coulson, W. Salman, J.R. Kendra, and C.E. Johnson. 1998. Mesothelioma-associated antiphospholipid antibody syndrome presenting with cutaneous infarction and neuropathy *Br. J. Dermatol.*138:1092–1094.

18. Peyton, B.D., B.S. Cutler, and F.M. Stewart. 1998. Spontaneous tibial artery thrombosis associated with varicella pneumonia and free protein S deficiency. *J. Vasc. Surg.* 27:563–567.

19. D. Rodriguez Gonzalez, R. Hernandez Camarena, R. Velarde Ibarra, and D. Urzua Orozco. 1998. Antiphospholipid antibody syndrome, molar pregnancy and cerebral infarct. A case report. *Ginecol. Obstet. Mex.* 66:18–20.

20. de Larranaga, G.F., R.R. Forastiero, L.O. Carreras, and B.S. Alonso. 1999. Different types of antiphospholipid antibodies in AIDS: a comparison with syphilis and the antiphospholipid syndrome. *Thromb. Res.* 96:19–25.

21. Petrovas, C., P.G. Vlachoyiannopoulos, T. Kordossis, and H.M. Moutsopoulos. 1999. Antiphospholipid antibodies in HIV infection and SLE with or without anti-phospholipid syndrome:comparisons of phospholipid specificity, avidity and reactivity with beta2-GPI. *J. Autoimmun.*13:347–355.

22. Cabiedes, J., A.R. Cabral, and D. Alarcon-Segovia. 1998. Hidden anti-phospholipid antibodies in normal human sera circulate as immune complexes whose antigen can be removed by heat, acid, hypermolar buffers or phospholipase treatments. *Eur. J. Immunol.* 28:2108–2114.

23. Celli, C.M., A.E. Gharavi, and H. Chaimovich. 1999. Opposite beta2-glycoprotein I requirement for the binding of infectious and autoimmune antiphospholipid antibodies to cardiolipin liposomes is associated with antibody avidity. *Biochim. Biophys. Acta.* 1416:225–238.

24. Buchanen, R.C., J.R. Wardlow, and A. Riglar. 1989. Antiphospholipid antibodies in the connective tissue diseases: their relation to the antiphospholipid syndrome and forme fruste disease. *J. Rheum.* 16: 757–761.

25. Harris, E.N. 1989. Anticardiolipin antibodies and autoimmune diseases. *Curr. Opin. Rheum.* 1:215–220.

26. Hendra, T.J., E. Baguley, and E.N. Harris. 1989. Anticardiolipin antibody levels in diabetic subjects with and without coronary artery disease. *Postgrad. Med. J.* 65:140–143.

27. Harris, E.N. 1992. Serologic detection of antiphospholipid antibodies. *Stroke* 23:SI3.

28. Bevers, E.M., M. Galli, and T. Barbui. 1991. Lupus anticoagulant IgG's [LA] are not directed to phospholipids only but to a complex of lipid-bound human prothrombin. *Thromb. Haem.* 66:629–632.

29. Oosting, J.D., R.H. Derksen, I.W. Bobbink, T.M. Hackeng, B,N. Bouma, and P.G. de Groot. 1993. Antiphospholipid antibodies directed against a combination of phospholipids with prothrombin, protein C or protein S: an explanation for their pathogenic mechanism? *Blood* 81:2618–2625.

30. Oosting, J.D., R.H.W.M. Derksen, and T.I. Entjes. 1992. Lupus anticoagulant activity is frequently dependent on the presence of β_2-glycoprotein-1. *Thromb. Haem.* 67:499–502.

31. Triplett, D.A. 1992. Antiphospholipid antibodies:proposed mechanisms of action. *Am. J. Reprod. Immunol.* 28:211–215.

32. Malia, R.G., S. Kitchen, M. Graves, and F.E. Preston. 1990. Inhibition of activated protein C and its cofactor protein S by antiphospholipid antibodies. *Br. J. Haem.* 76:101–107.

33. Killeen, A.A., K.C. Meyer, J.M. Vogt, and J.R. Edson. 1987. Kallikrein inhibition and C1-esterase inhibitor levels in patients with the lupus inhibitor. *Am. J. Clin. Pathol.* 88:223–228.

34. Keeling, D.M., S.J. Campbell, and I.J. Mackie. 1991. The fibrinolytic response to venous occlusion and the natural anticoagulants in patients with antiphospholipid antibodies both with and without systemic lupus erythematosus. *Br. J. Haem.* 77:354–357.

35. Triplett, D.A. 1993. Antiphospholipid antibodies and thrombosis. A consequence, coincidence or cause? *Arch. Path. Lab. Med.* 117:78–88.

36. Roubey, R.A.S., C.W. Pratt, J.P. Buyon, and J.B. Winfield. 1992. Lupus anticoagulant activity of autoimmune antiphospholipid antibodies is dependent on beta 2-glycoprotein 1. *J. Clin. Invest.* 90: 1100–1104.

37. Shibata, S., P,C, Harpel, A. Gharavi, J. Rand, and H. Fillit. 1994. Autoantibodies to heparin from patients with antiphospholipid antibody syndrome inhibit formation of antithrombin III-thrombin complexes. *Blood* 83:2389–2391.

38. Fillit, H., S. Shibata, T. Sasaki, H. Spiera, L.D. Kerr, and M. Blake. 1993. Autoantibodies to the protein core of vascular basement membrane heparan sulfate proteoglycan in systemic lupus erythematosus. *Autoimmunity* 14:243–249.

39. Aron, A.L., A.E. Gharavi, and Y. Shoenfelfd. 1995. Mechanisms of action of antiphospholipid antibodies in the antiphospholipid syndrome. *Int. Arch. Allergy Immunol.* 106:8–12.

40. Martini, F., A. Farsi, A.M. Gori, M. Boddi, S. Fedi, M,P. Domeneghetti, et al. 1996. Antiphospholipid antibodies [aPL] increase the potential monocyte procoagulant activity in patients with systemic lupus erythematosus. *Lupus* 5:206–211.

41. Reverter, J.C., D. Tassies, J. Font, J. Monteagudo, G. Escolar, M. Ingelmo, and A. Ordinas. 1996. Hypercoagulable state in patients with antiphospholipid syndrome is related to high induced tissue factor expression on monocytes and to low free protein S. *Arterioscler. Thromb. Vasc. Biol.* 16:1319–1326.

42. Wisbey, H.L. and A.C. Klestov. 1996. Thrombocytopenia corrected by warfarin in antiphospholipid syndrome. *J. Rheum.* 23:769–771.

43. Barquinero, J., J. Ordi-Ros, A. Selva, P. Perez-Peman, M. Vilardell, and Khamashta. M. 1994. Antibodies against platelet-activating factor in patients with antiphospholipid antibodies. *Lupus* 3:55–58.

44. Machin, S.J. 1996. Platelets and antiphospholipid antibodies. *Lupus* 5:386–387.

45. Meroni, P.L., N.D. Papa, B. Beltrami, A. Tincani, G. Balestrieri, and S.A. Krilis. 1996. Modulation of endothelial cell function by antiphospholipid antibodies. *Lupus* 5: 448–450.

46. Mizutani, H., Y. Kurata, S. Kosugi, M. Shiraga, H. Kashiwagi, Y.Tomiyama, et al. 1995. Monoclonal anticardiolipin autoantibodies established from the [New Zealand white x BXSB]F1 mouse model of antiphospholipid syndrome cross-react with oxidized low-density lipoprotein. *Arthritis Rheum.* 38:1382–1388.

47. Sorice, M., P. Arcieri, T. Griggi, A. Circella, R. Misasi, L. Lenti, et al. 1996. Inhibition of protein S by autoantibodies in patients with acquired protein S deficiency. *Thromb. Haem.* 75:555–559.

48. Merrill, J.T., E. Rivkin, C. Shen, and R.G. Lahita. 1995. Selection of a gene for apolipoprotein A1 using autoantibodies from a patient with SLE. *Arthritis Rheum.* 38:1655–1659.

49. Arvieux, J., B. Roussel, D. Ponard, and M.G. Colomb. 1994. IgG2 subclass restriction of anti-beta 2 glycoprotein 1 antibodies in autoimmune patients. *Clin. Exp. Immunol.* 95: 310–315.

50. Pengo, V., A. Biasiolo, T. Brocco, S. Tonetto, and A. Ruffatti. 1996. Autoantibodies to phospholipid-binding plasma proteins in patients with thrombosis and phospholipid-reactive antibodies. *Thromb. Haem.* 75:721–724.

51. Pierangeli, S.S., E.N. Harris, S.A. Davis, and G. DeLorenzo. 1992. Beta 2-glycoprotein 1 enhances cardiolipin binding activity but is not the antigen for antiphospholipid antibodies. *Br. J. Haem.* 82:565–570.

52. Viard, J.P., Z. Amoura, and J.F. Bach. 1991. Anti-beta 2 glycoprotein I antibodies in systemic lupus erythematosus: a marker of thrombosis associated with a circulating anticoagulant. *Comptes Rend L'Acad. Sci.* 313:607–612.

53. Puurunen, M., O. Vaarala, H. Julkunen, K. Aho, and T. Palosuo. 1996. Antibodies to phospholipid-binding plasma proteins and occurrence of thrombosis in patients with systemic lupus erythematosus. *Clin. Immunol. Immunopathol.* 80:16–22.

54. Forastiero, R.R., M.E. Martinuzzo, L.C. Kordich, and L.O. Carreras. 1996. Reactivity to beta 2 glycoprotein I clearly differentiates anticardiolipin antibodies from antiphospholipid syndrome and syphilis. *Thromb. Haem.* 75:717–720.

55. Pierangeli, S,S,, G.H. Goldsmith, D.W. Branch, and E.N. Harris. 1997. Antiphospholipid antibody: functional specificity for inhibition of prothrombin activation by the prothrombinase complex. *Br. J. Haem.* 97:768–774.

56. Gharavi, A.E., L.R. Sammaritano, J.L. Bovastro, Jr., and W.A. Wilson. 1995. Specificities and characteristics of beta 2 glycoprotein 1-induced antiphospholipid antibodies. *J. Lab. Clin. Med.* 125:775–778.

57. Shibata, S., P. Harpel, C. Bona, and H. Fillit. 1993. Monoclonal antibodies to heparan sulfate inhibit the formation of thrombin-antithrombin III compexes. *Clin. Immunol. Immunopathol.* 67:264–272.

58. Qamar, T., A.E. Gharavi, R.A. Levy, and M.D. Lockshin. 1990. Lysophosphatidyl-ethanolamine is the antigen to which apparent antibody to phosphatidylethanolamine binds. *J. Clin. Immunol.* 10:200–203.

59. Casciola-Rosen, L., A. Rosen, M. Petri, and M. Schlissel. 1996. Surface blebs on apoptotic cells are sites of enhanced procoagulant activity: implications for coagulation events and antigenic spread in systemic lupus erythematosus. *Proc. Natl. Acad. Sci. USA* 93:1624–1629.

60. Price, B.E., J. Rauch, M.A. Shia, M.T. Walsh, W. Lieberthal, H.M. Gilligan, et al. 1996. Antiphospholipid antibodies bind to apoptotic, but not viable, thymocytes in a beta 2-glycoprotein I-dependent manner. *J. Immunol.* 157:2201–2208.

61. Roubey, R.A.S., R.A. Eisenberg, M.F. Harper, and J.B. Winfield. 1995. Anticardiolipin autoantibodies recognize beta 2-glycoprotein 1 in the absence of phospholipid. Importance of Ag density and bivalent binding. *J. Immunol.* 154:954–960.

62. Galli, M., G. Beretta, M. Daldossi, E.M. Bevers, and T. Barbui. 1997. Different anticoagulant and immuological properties of anti-prothrombin antibodies in patients with antiphospholipid antibodies. *Thromb. Haemost.* 77:486–491.

63. Lockshin, M.D. 1991. Antiphospholipid antibody and antiphospholipid antibody syndrome. *Curr. Opin. Rheumatol.* 3:797–802.

64. Capel, P., J. Arnout, P. Cauchie, B. Chatelain, A. Criel, J.L. David, et al. 1997. Comparative study of antiphospholipid antibody detection in eleven Belgian laboratories. *Acta. Clin. Belg.* 52:84–91.

65. Gattorno, M., A. Buoncompagni, A.C. Molinari, G.C. Barbano, G. Morreale, F. Stalla, et al. 1995. Antiphospholipid antibodies in paediatric systemic lupus erythematosus, juvenile chronic arthritis and overlap syndromes: SLE patients with both lupus anticoagulant and high-titre anticardiolipin antibodies are at risk for clinical manifestations related to the antiphospholipid syndrome. *Br. J. Rheum.* 34:873–881.

66. Levine, S.R., R.L. Brey, K.L. Sawaya, L. Salowich-Palm, J. Kokkinos, B.Kostrzema, et al. 1995. Recurrent stroke and thrombo-occlusive events in the antiphospholipid syndrome. *Ann. Neurol.* 38:119–124.

67. Silver, R.M., T.F. Porter, I. van Leeuween, G. Jeng, J.R. Scott, and D.W. Branch, 1996. Anticardiolipin antibodies:clinical consequences of "low titers." *Obstet. Gynecol.* 87:494–500.

68. Ghirardello, A., A. Doria, A. Ruffatti, A.M. Rigoli, P. Vesco, A. Calligaro, and P.F. Gambari. 1994. Antiphospholipid antibodies [aPL] in systemic lupus erythematosus. Are they specific tools for the diagnosis of aPL syndrome? *Ann. Rheum. Dis.* 53:140–142.

69. Vivancos, J., A. Lopez-Soto, J. Font, J. Balasch, R. Cervera, J.C. Reverter, et al. 1994. Primary antiphospholipid syndrome:clinical and biological study of 36 cases. *Med. Clin.* 102:561–565.

70. Laroche, P., M. Berard, A.M. Rouquette, C. Desgruelle, and M.C. Boffa. 1996. Advantage of using both anionic and zwitterionic phospholipid antigens for the detection of antiphospholipid antibodies. *Am. J. Clin. Pathol.* 106:549–554.

71. Gilman-Sachs, A., J. Lubinski, A.E. Beer, S. Brend, and K.D. Beaman. 1991. Patterns of anti-phospholipid specificities. *J. Clin. Lab. Immunol.* 35:83–88.

72. Silver, R.M., S.S. Pierangeli, S.S. Edwin, F. Umar, E.N. Harris, J.R. Scott, and D.W. Branch. 1997. Pathogenic antibodies in women with obstetric features of antiphospholipid syndrome who have negative test results for lupus anticoagulant and anticardiolipin antibodies. *Am. J. Obstet. Gynecol.* 176:628–633.

73. Caruso, A., S. De Carolis, S. Ferrazzani, G. Valesini, L. Caforio, and S.Mancuso. 1993. Pregnancy outcome in relation to uterine artery flow velocity waveforms and clinical characteristics in women with antiphospholipid syndrome. *Obstet. Gynecol.* 82:970–977.

74. Eschwege, V., I. Laude, F. Toti, J.L. Pasquali, and J.M. Freyssinet. 1996. Detection of bilayer phospholipid-binding antibodies using flow cytometry. *Clin. Exp. Immunol.* 103:171–175.

75. Amengual, O., T. Atsumi, M.A. Khamashta, T. Koike, and G.R. Hughes. 1996. Specificity of ELISA for antibody to beta 2-glycoprotein I in patients with antiphospholipid syndrome. *Br. J. Rheum.* 35:1239–1243.

76. Roubey, R.A.S. 1996. Antigenic specificities of antiphospholipid antibodies: implications for clinical laboratory testing and diagnosis of the antiphospholipid syndrome. *Lupus* 5:425–430.

77. Oshiro, B.T., R.M. Silver, J.R. Scott, H. Yu, and D.W. Branch. 1996. Antiphospholipid antibodies and fetal death. *Obstet. Gynecol.* 87:489–493.

78. Cowchock, S. and E.A. Reece. 1997. Do low-risk women with antiphospholipid antibodies need to be treated? Organizing Group of the Antiphospholipid Antibody Treatment Trial. *Am. J. Obstet. Gynecol.* 176:1099–1100.

79. Nayer, R. and J.M. Lage. 1996. Placental changes in a first trimester missed abortion in maternal systemic lupus erythematosus with antiphospholipid syndrome; a case report and review of the literature. *Human Pathol.* 27:201–206.

80. Chamley, L.W., N.S. Pattison, and E.J. McKay. 1993. Elution of anticardiolipin antibodies and their cofactor beta 2-glycoprotein 1 from the placentae of patients with a poor obstetric history. *J. Reproduct. Immunol.* 25:2–7.

81. Salafia, C.M. and A.M. Parke. 1997. Placental pathology in systemic lupus erythematosus and phospholipid antibody syndrome. *Rheum. Dis. Clin. North Am.* 23:85–97.

82. Weingarten, K., C. Filippi, D. Barbut, and R.D. Zimmerman. 1997. The neuroimaging features of the cardiolipin antibody syndrome. *Clin. Imaging* 21:6–12.

83. Kato, T., A. Morita, and Y. Matsumoto. 1997. Hypoperfusion of brain single photon emission computerized tomography in patients wih antiphospholipid antibodies. *J. Dermatol. Sci.* 14:20–28.

84. Kao, C.H., J.L. Lan, J.F. Hsieh, Y.J. Ho, S.P. ChangLai, J.K. Lee, and H.J. Ding. 1999. Evaluation of regional cerebral blood flow with 99mTc-HMPAO in primary antiphospholipid antibody syndrome. *J. Nucleic Med.* 40:1446–1450.

85. Barbut, D., J.S. Borer, D. Wallerson, O. Ameisen, and M. Lockshin. 1991. Anticardiolipin antibody and stroke:possibe relation of valvular heart disease and embolic events. *Cardiology* 79:99–109.

86. Provenzale, J.M. and H.A. Loganbill. 1994. Dural sinus thrombosis and venous infarction associated with antiphospholipid antibodies:MR findings. *J. Comput. Assist. Tomogr.* 18:719–723.

87. Piette, J.C., Cacoub, P. and B. Wechsler. 1994. Renal manifestations of the antiphospholipid syndrome. *Semin. Arth. Rheum.* 23:357–366.

88. Vaidya, S., R. Sellers, P. Kimball, T. Shanahan, J. Gitomer, K. Gugliuzza, and J.C. Fish. 2000. Frequency, potential risk and therapeutic intervention in end-stage renal disease patients with antiphospholipid antibody syndrome: a multicenter study. *Transplantation* 69:1348–1352.

89. Merrill, J.T., C. Shen, R.G. Lahita, and A-B. Mongee. 1997. High prevalence of antiphospholipid antibodies in patients taking procainamide. *J. Rheum.* 24:1083–1088.

90. Gharavi, A.E., L.R. Sammaritano, J. Wen, N. Miyawaki, J.H. Morse, M.H. Zarrabi, and M.D. Lockshin. 1994. Characteristics of human immunodeficiency virus and chlorpromazine induced antiphospholipid antibodies:effect of beta 2 glycoprotein I on binding to phospholipid. *J. Rheum.* 21:94–99.

91. Vlachoyiannopoulos, P.G., E. Tsiakou, G. Chalevelakis, S.A. Raptis, and H.M. Moutsopuolos. 1994. Antiphospholipid syndrome: clinical and therapeutic aspects. *Lupus* 3:91–96.

92. Finazzi, G. 1997. The Italian Registry of antiphospholipid antibodies. *Haematologica* 82: 101–105.

93. Finazzi, G., V. Brancaccio, M. Moia, N. Ciaverella, M.G. Mazzucconi, P.C. Schinco, et al. 1996. Natural history and risk factors for thrombosis in 360 patients with antiphospholipid antibodies:a four year prospective study from the Italian Registry. *Am. J. Med.* 100:530–536.

94. Lima, F., M.A. Khamashta, N.M. Buchanan, S. Kerslake, B.J. Hunt, and G.R. Hughes. 1996. A study of sixty pregnancies in the antiphospholipid syndrome. *Clin. Exp. Rheum.* 14:131–136.

95. Drenkard, C., A.R. Villa, D. Alarcon-Segovia, and M.E. Perez-Vazquez. 1994. Influence of the antiphospholipid syndrome in the survival of patients with systemic lupus erythematosus. *J. Rheum.* 21:1067–1072.

96. Silver, R.M., M.L. Draper, J.R. Scott, J.L. Lyon, J. Reading, and D.W. Branch. 1994. Clinical consequences of antiphospholipid antibodies: an historic cohort study. *Obstet. Gynecol.* 83:372–377.

97. Della Valle, P., L. Crippa, O. Safa, L. Tomassini, E. Pattarini, S. Vigano-D'Angelo, et al. 1996. Potential failure of the International Normalized Ratio [INR] System in the monitoring of oral anticoagulation in patients with lupus anticoagulants. *Ann. Med. Intern.* 147:10–14.

98. Kamashta, M.A. 1996. Management of thrombosis in the antiphospholipid syndrome. *Lupus* 5:463–466.

99. Lie, J.T. 1996. Vasculopathy of the antiphospholipid syndrome revisited: thrombosis is the culprit and vasculitis the consort. *Lupus* 5:368–371.

100. Myones, B.L. and D. McCurdy. 2000. The antiphospholipid syndrome: immunologic and clinical aspects. Clinical spectrum and treatment. *J. Rheumatol.* (Suppl. 58):20–28.

101. Derkson, R.H. 1996. Clinical manifestations and management of the antiphospholipid syndrome. *Lupus* 5:167–169.

102. McCrae, K.R. 1996. Antiphospholipid antibody associated thrombosis:a concensus for treatment? *Lupus* 5:560–570.

103. Rivier, G., M.T. Herranz, M.A. Khamashta, and G.R. Hughes. 1994. Thrombosis and antiphospholipid syndrome:a preliminary assessment of three antithrombotic treatments. *Lupus* 3:85–90.

104. Piette, J.C. and B. Wechsler. 1997. Antiphospholipid syndrome. A better codified treatment. *Presse Med.* 26:108–109.

105. Della Valle, P., L. Crippa, A.M. Garlando, E. Pattarini, O. Safa, S.Vigano D'Angelo, and A. D'Angelo. 1999. Interference of lupus anticoagulants in prothrombin time assays: implications for selection of adequate methods to optimize the management of thrombosis in the antiphospholipid-antibody syndrome *Haematologica* 84:1065–1074.

106. Asherson, R.A., E. Baguley, C. Pal, and G.R. Hughes. 1991. Antiphospholipid syndrome: five year follow up. *Ann. Rheum. Dis.* 50:805–810.

107. Galli, M., G. Finazzi, and T. Barbui. 1996. Thrombocytopenia in the antiphospholipid syndrome: pathophysiology, clinical relevance and treatment. *Ann. Med. Interne.* 147: 24–27.

108. Orlando, E., S. Cortelazzo, M. Marchetti, R. Sanfratello, and T. Barbui. 1992. Prolonged bleeding time in patients with lupus anticoagulant. *Thromb. Haemost.* 68:495–499.

109. Wiener, H.M., N. Vardinon, and I. Yust. 1991. Platelet antibody binding and spontaneous aggregation in 21 lupus anticoagulant patients. *Vox Sang* 61:111–121.

110. Pineo, G.F. and R.D. Hull. 1998. Heparin and low-molecular-weight heparin in the treatment of venous thromboembolism. *Baillieres Clin. Haematol.* 11:621–637.

111. Hauer, K.E. 1998. Low-molecular-weight heparin in the treatment of deep venous thrombosis. *West. J. Med.* 169:240–244.

112. Bar, J., B. Cohen-Sacher, M. Hod, D. Blickstein, J. Lahav, and P. Merlob. 2000. Low-molecular-weight heparin for thrombophilia in pregnant women. *Int. J. Gynaecol. Obstet.* 69:209–213.

113. Bick, R.L. and E.P. Frenkel. 1999. Clinical aspects of heparin-induced thrombocytopenia and thrombosis and other side effects of heparin therapy. *Clin. Appl. Thromb. Hemost.* (Suppl. 1):S7–S15.

114. Wechsler, B., Du L.T. Huong, and J.C. Piette. 1999. Is there a role for antithrombotic therapy in the prevention of pregnancy loss? *Haemostasis* (Suppl. S1):112–120.

115. Bates, S.M. 1999. Optimal management of pregnant women with acute venous thromboembolism. *Haemostasis* (Suppl. S1):107–111.

116. Martineau, P. and N. Tawil. 1998. Low-molecular-weight heparins in the treatment of deep-vein thrombosis. *Ann. Pharmacother.* 32:588–598.

117. Nelson-Piercy, C. 1997. Hazards of heparin: allergy, heparin-induced thrombocytopenia and osteoporosis. *Baillieres Clin. Obstet. Gynaecol.* 11:489–509.

118. Bick, R.L. and J. Rice. 1999. Long-term outpatient dalteparin (fragmin) therapy for arterial and venous thrombosis: efficacy and safety—a preliminary report. *Clin. Appl. Thromb. Hemost.* 5(Suppl. 1): S67–S71.

119. Camps Garcia, M.T., M. Guil, J. Sanchez-Lora, M.I. Grana, J. Martinez, and E. de Ramon. 1996. Fibrinolytic treatment in primary antiphospholipid syndrome. *Lupus* 5:627–629.

120. Ho, Y.L., M.F. Chen, C.C. Wu, W.J. Chen, and Y,T. Lee. 1996. Successful treatment of acute myocardial infarction by thrombolytic therapy in a patient with primary antiphospholipid syndrome. *Cardiology* 87:354–357.

121. Hachulla, E., A.M. Piette, P.Y. Hatron, and O. Bletry. 2000. Aspirin and antiphospholipid syndrome. *Rev. Med. Interne.* Mar. 21 (Suppl. 1):83s–88s.

122. Cowchock, S. 1996. Prevention of fetal death in the antiphospholipid syndrome: *Lupus* 5:467–472.

123. Welsch, S. and D.W. Branch. 1997. Antiphospholipid syndrome in pregnancy. Obstetric concerns and treatment. *Rheum. Dis. Clin. North Am.* 23:71–84.

124. Backos, M., R. Rai, E. Thomas, M. Murphy, C. Dore, and L. Regan. 1999. Bone density changes in pregnant women treated with heparin: a prospective, longitudinal study. *Human Reprod.*14: 2876–2880.

125. Shefras, J. and R.G. Farquharson. 1996. Bone density studies in pregnant women receiving heparin. *Eur. J. Obstet. Gynecol. Reprod. Biol.* 65:171–174.

126. Greer, I.A. 1998. The special case of venous thromboembolism in pregnancy. *Haemostasis* 28(Suppl. 3):22–34.

127. Cancio, L.C. and D.J. Cohen. 1998. Heparin-induced thrombocytopenia and thrombosis. *J. Am. Coll. Surg.* 186:76–91.

128. Sanson, B.J., A.W. Lensing, M.H. Prins, J.S. Ginsberg, Z.S.Barkagan, E. Lavenne-Pardonge, et al. 1999. Safety of low-molecular-weight heparin in pregnancy: a systematic review. *Thromb. Haemost.* 81:668–672.

129. Fishman, P., E. Faach-Vaknin, B. Sredni, P.L. Meroni, C. Rudniki, and Y. Shoenfeld. 1995. Aspirin modulates interleukin-3 production:additional explanation for the preventative effects of aspirin in antiphospholipid antibody syndrome. *J. Rheum.* 22:1086–1090.

130. Fishman, P., E. Falach-Vaknin, B. Sredni, P.L. Meroni, A. Tincani, D. Dicker, and Y. Shoenfeld. 1996. Aspirin-interleukin-3 interrelationships in patients with anti-phospholipid syndrome. *Am. J. Reprod. Immunol.* 35:80–84.

131. Waterer, G.W., B. Latham, J.A. Waring, and E. Gabbay. 1999. Pulmonary capillaritis associated with the antiphospholipid antibody syndrome and rapid response to plasmapheresis. *Respirology* 4:405–408

132. Flamholz, R., T. Tran, G.I. Grad, A.M. Mauer, O.I. Olopade, M.H. Ellman, et al. 1999. Therapeutic plasma exchange for the acute management of the catastrophic antiphospholipid syndrome: beta(2)-glycoprotein I antibodies as a marker of response to therapy. *J. Clin. Apheresis* 14:171–176.

133. Becker, J.C., B. Winkler, S. Klingert, and E.B. Brocker. 1994. Antiphospholipid syndrome associated with immunotherapy for patients with melanoma. *Cancer* 73:1621–1624.

134. Brey, R.L. and S.R. Levine. 1996. Treatment of neurologic complications of antiphospholipid antibody syndrome. *Lupus* 5:473–476.

135. Braune, S., R. Siekmann, P. Vaith, and C.H. Lucking. 1993. Primary antiphosphlipid antibody syndrome and cerbral ischemia: report on acute intervention in two cases and literature review with emphasis on therapeutic options. *Rheum. Int.* 13:169–174.

136. Bakimer, R., B. Guilburd, N. Zurgil, and Y. Shoenfeld. 1993. The effect of intravenous gamma globulin on the induction of experimental antiphospholipid syndrome. *Clin. Immunol. Immunopath.* 69:97–102.

137. Clark, A.L. 1999. Clinical uses of intravenous immunoglobulin in pregnancy. *Clin. Obstet. Gynecol.* 42:368–380.

138. Clark, A.L., D.W. Branch, R.M. Silver, E.N. Harris, S. Pierangeli, and J.A. Spinnato. 1999. Pregnancy complicated by the antiphospholipid syndrome: outcomes with intravenous immunoglobulin therapy. *Obstet. Gynecol.* 93:437–441.

139. Spinnato, J.A., A.L. Clark, S.S. Pierangeli, and E.N. Harris. 1995. Intravenous immunoglobulin therapy for the antiphospholipid syndrome in pregnancy. *Am. J. Obstet. Gynecol.* 172:690–694.

140. Arnout, J., B. Spitz, C. Wittevrongel, M. Vanrusselt, A. Van Assche, and J. Vermylen. 1994. High dose intravenous immunoglobulin treatment of a pregnant patient with an antiphospholipid syndrome: immunologic changes associated with a successful outcome. *Thromb. Haem.* 71:741–747.

141. Marzusch, K., J. Dietl. R. Klein, D. Hornung, A. Neuer, and P.A. Berg. 1996. Recurrent first trimester spontaneous abortion associated with antiphospholipid antibodies: a pilot study of treatment with intravenous immunoglobulin. *Acta. Obstet. Gynecol. Scand.* 75:922–926.

142. Branch, D.W., A.M. Peaceman, M. Druzin, R.K. Silver, Y. El-Sayed, R.M. Silver, et al. 2000. A multicenter, placebo-controlled pilot study of intravenous immune globulin treatment of antiphospholipid syndrome during pregnancy. *Am. J. Obstet. Gynecol.* 182:122–127.

143. Espinoza, L.R. 1996. Antiphospholipid antibody syndrome:treatment. *Lupus* 5:456–457.

144. Shoenfeld, Y. and M. Blank. 1994. Effect of long-acting thromboxane receptor antagonist on experimental antiphospholipid syndrome. *Lupus* 3:397–400.

145. Adachi, Y., M. Inaba, Y. Amoh, H. Yoshifusa, Y. Nakamura, H. Suzuka, et al. 1995. Effect of bone marrow transplantation on antiphospholipid antibody syndrome in murine lupus mice. *Immunobiology* 192:218–230.

146. Krause, I., M. Blank, and Y. Shoenfeld. 1996. Immunomodulation of experimental APS:lessons from murine models [rev.] *Lupus* 5:458–462.

147. Kohles, J.D., M. Petersheim, and V.A. DeBari. 1999. Inhibition of beta 2glycoprotein I binding to anionic phospholipids: a strategy for the development of antiphospholipid syndrome-specific drugs. *Drug Des. Discov.* 16:227–236.

148. Jones, D.S., P.A. Barstead, M.J. Feild, J.P. Hachmann, M.S. Hayag, K.W. Hill, et al. 1995. Immunospecific reduction of antioligonucleotide antibody-forming cells with a tetrakis-oligonucleotide conjugate [LJP 394], a therapeutic candidate for the treatment of lupus nephritis. *J. Med. Chem.* 38:2138–2144.

149. Coutts, S.M., M.L. Plunkett, G.M. Iverson, P.A. Barstad, and C.M. Berner. 1996. Pharmacological intervention in antibody mediated disease. *Lupus* 5:158–159.

20

Treatment of Systemic Lupus Erythematosus by Blocking T-Cell Costimulation

David I. Daikh and David Wofsy

CONTENTS

INTRODUCTION
T-CELL COSTIMULATION VIA CD28
T-CELL COSTIMULATION VIA CD40-LIGAND
SIMULTANEOUS BLOCKADE OF T-CELL COSTIMULATION VIA CD28
  AND CD40L
COMBINATION THERAPY WITH CTLA4IG PLUS PULSE
  CYCLOPHOSPHAMIDE
BLOCKADE OF T-CELL COSTIMULATION IN HUMANS
SUMMARY
ACKNOWLEDGMENTS
REFERENCES

INTRODUCTION

The era of biologic therapies for chronic inflammatory and autoimmune rheumatic diseases has begun. Biologic agents have already had a dramatic impact on the treatment of rheumatoid arthritis (RA), where inhibitors of tumor necrosis factor α (TNF-α) are now widely used. In addition, numerous other biologically based therapies are in the late stages of development for RA.

The success of new therapies for RA has paved the way for the introduction of biologic therapies for other rheumatic diseases, such as systemic lupus erythematosus (SLE). At present, the therapeutic strategies that seem most promising in SLE are based on the two-signal model for T-cell activation (Fig. 1). According to this model, the nature of the T-cell response to antigen (Ag) is determined by how the T cell integrates two kinds of signals (1,2). The first signal is antigen-specific. It is generated when T-cell receptors (TCR) recognize antigenic fragments on the surface of antigen-presenting cells (APC), such as macrophages. This signal is critical for T-cell responses, but it does not by itself determine whether the T cell will be activated to mount an immune response, as it should if the Ag originates from an infectious agent, or whether the T cell will be

From: *Modern Therapeutics in Rheumatic Diseases*
Edited by: G. C. Tsokos, et al. © Humana Press, Inc., Totowa, NJ

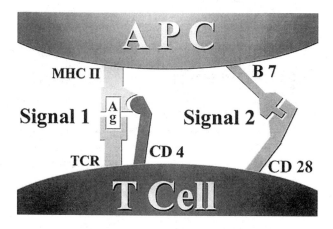

Fig. 1. The T-cell response to antigen is determined by two signals. The first signal is generated when the T-cell receptor (TCR) recognizes an antigenic peptide (Ag) in the context of major histocompatibility complex (MHC) molecules on antigen-presenting cells (APC). The second signal is generated by other receptor-ligand pairs on the surface of T cells and APC. One pair that can provide the second signal consists of CD28 on T cells and members of the B7 family of molecules on APC.

rendered hyporesponsive (or anergic), as it should if the antigen originates from self. Rather, T cells make this distinction based on other receptor-ligand interactions at the T cell/APC interface. These interactions constitute the second signal, which is also called costimulation. In general, the simultaneous occurrence of both signals (stimulation plus costimulation) activates T cells to mount an immune response. In contrast, the occurrence of the first signal in the absence of the second signal may cause antigen-specific hyporesponsiveness. This principle forms the foundation for new therapeutic strategies for SLE that are designed to render autoreactive T cells unresponsive by blocking T-cell costimulation.

T-CELL COSTIMULATION VIA CD28

Several T-cell surface molecules can transmit signals that promote T-cell costimulation. Among them, a molecule designated CD28 plays a particularly important role. CD28 is a 44-kDa homodimeric glycoprotein that is constitutively expressed on the majority of T cells *(3)*. Signaling via CD28 is crucial not only for the activation of normal T-cell responses, but apparently also for the activation of autoreactive T cells *(3,4)*.

The ligands for CD28 are designated B7-1 and B7-2 *(3)*. These ligands are expressed in low density, if at all, on resting APC. However, upon interaction with Ag, APC upregulate the expression of the B7 molecules, which then can mediate T-cell costimulation by binding to CD28. Thus, in people with autoimmune diseases, blockade of B7-CD28 interactions might preferentially inhibit autoreactive T cells without adversely affecting resting T cells.

The development of new therapies designed to block signaling via CD28 have taken advantage of the homology between CD28 and another T-cell surface molecule, designated CTLA4 (Fig. 2). Unlike CD28, CTLA4 appears to be a negative regulator of T-cell function *(5,6)*. Moreover, it binds to B7-1 and B7-2 with considerably higher avidity than does CD28 *(7)*. Therefore, a fusion protein consisting of the extracellular

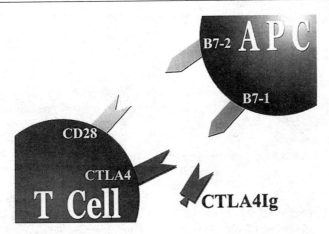

Fig. 2. One new therapeutic strategy is based on the homology between CD28 and CTLA4. CTLA4 binds tightly to the B7 ligands for CD28. Therefore, a fusion protein composed of the extracellular domain of CTLA4 linked to the constant region of an immunoglobulin molecule (CTLA4Ig) can bind to B7-1 and B7-2 and, by so doing, prevent them from costimulating T cells via CD28.

domain of CTLA-4 bound to an immunoglobulin Cγ1 chain (CTLA4Ig) blocks the interaction between the B7 molecules and CD28 and thereby inhibits T-cell activation *(8,9)*. This fusion protein has been used successfully in vivo to prolong acceptance of allografts and xenografts, to inhibit B-cell differentiation into immunoglobulin-secreting cells, to suppress antibody responses to T-dependent antigens, and even to induce long-term unresponsiveness to autoantigens *(10,11)*.

Based on the profound immunologic effects of CTLA4Ig in numerous experimental systems, we treated lupus-prone NZB/NZW F_1 (B/W) mice with CTLA4Ig for 4 mo beginning at the onset of disease *(12)*. Treatment prevented autoantibody production, retarded lupus nephritis, and significantly prolonged life (Fig. 3). Subsequently, we showed that, even when treatment was delayed until severe disease had been established, CTLA4Ig had substantial beneficial effects *(12)*. However, the benefits of treatment with CTLA4Ig were not permanent. When treatment with CTLA4Ig was discontinued, murine lupus remained quiescent for several months but then relapsed *(13)*. Thus, although CTLA4Ig is effective against murine lupus, it is not curative. Autoreactive T-cell responses are blunted for a while, but then they recur.

T-CELL COSTIMULATION VIA CD40-LIGAND

Just as B7-1 and B7-2 are upregulated on activated but not on resting APC, other molecules are expressed on activated but not on resting T cells. One such molecule, designated CD154 or gp39, plays an important role in T-cell costimulation and in B-cell differentiation. CD154 is more commonly called CD40-ligand (CD40L), because it binds to CD40 on all B cells *(14)*. The interaction between CD40 and CD40L contributes to T-cell costimulation in part by facilitating antigen-induced upregulation of B7-1 and B7-2 *(14)*. In addition, the CD40-CD40L interaction provides a critical stimulus for B-cell proliferation, immunoglobulin production, and ultimately isotype switching *(14)*. Like the B7-CD28 costimulation pathway, the CD40-CD40L pathway also plays a role in cytokine regulation *(15,16)*.

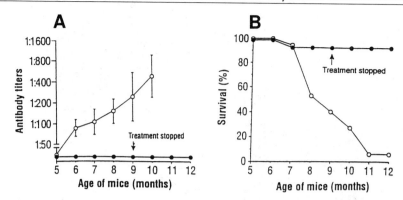

Fig. 3. Female B/W mice were treated with CTLA4Ig (●) or a control MAb (○) from age 5 mo to age 9 mo (50 μg ip three times/wk). **(A)** Geometric mean titer of antibodies to double-stranded DNA. **(B)** Percent survival. Adapted with permission from ref. *12*. Copyright 1994, American Association for the Advancement of Science.

Recent studies indicate that, like agents that selectively block B7-CD28 interactions, agents that selectively block CD40-CD40L interactions can suppress autoimmunity in murine models for several autoimmune diseases *(17–19)*. For example, Monoclonal Antibody (MAb) to CD40L can prevent collagen-induced arthritis (CIA) in mice *(18)*. To determine whether selective inhibition of CD40-CD40L interactions could also inhibit murine lupus, Mohan et al. *(19)* treated lupus-prone SWR/NZB (SNF₁) mice with three injections of MAb to CD40L at age 3 mo, prior to the onset of autoimmune disease. Although treatment was brief, anti-CD40L delayed the development of lupus by several months without any further immunosuppressive therapy. However, the beneficial effect was not permanent, and the mice eventually went on to develop lupus nephritis. Early et al. *(20)* subsequently showed that chronic administration of anti-CD40L could retard murine lupus in B/W mice but, in this study, some of the mice eventually developed lupus nephritis despite ongoing therapy, at least in part because they developed an immune response to the hamster anti-CD40L MAb.

SIMULTANEOUS BLOCKADE OF T-CELL COSTIMULATION VIA CD28 AND CD40L

Treatment of SNF₁ mice with anti-CD40L suppresses lupus nephritis without eliminating pathogenic T-cell clones, apparently by preventing autoantibody production by B cells *(19)*. This observation is consistent with findings in an experimentally induced model for autoimmune oophoritis, in which MAb to CD40L prevented autoantibody production and autoimmune disease without preventing proliferation of autoantigen-specific T cells *(17)*. CTLA4Ig also prevented autoimmune disease in this model without reducing Ag-specific T cells. However, when anti-CD40L and CTLA4Ig were administered together, there was a marked synergistic effect that blocked clonal expansion of effector T cells *(17)*.

To determine whether antiCD40L and CTLA4Ig might produce similar synergistic benefit in murine lupus, we treated 5-mo-old B/W females for 2 wk only with either CTLA4Ig alone, anti-CD40L alone, or both CTLA4Ig and anti-CD40L *(13)*. The beneficial effects of the short course of CTLA4Ig alone or anti-CD40L alone were

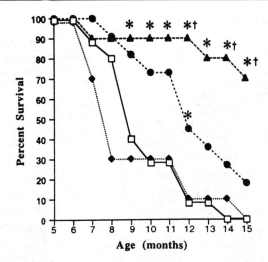

Fig. 4. Female B/W mice were treated for 2 wk at age 5 mo with either CTLA4Ig alone (◆), MAb to CD40L alone (●), a combination of both CTLA4Ig and MAb to CD40L (▲), or control Ig (◻). Asterisks (*) denote points at which there is a statistically significant difference from control mice ($p < 0.05$). Daggers (=) denote points at which there is a statistically significant difference from mice that received MAb to CD40L alone ($p < 0.05$). Reprinted with permission from ref. *13*. Copyright 1997, The American Association of Immunologists.

relatively brief. However, when CTLA4Ig and anti-CD40L were combined, there was sustained suppression of murine lupus that lasted for many months without the need for chronic, generalized immune suppression (Fig. 4). Specifically, 10 mo after cessation of therapy, 70% of the mice that received CTLA4Ig plus anti-CD40L were still alive, compared to only 18% survival among mice that received anti-CD40L, and 0% survival among mice that received CTLA4Ig. These findings provide support for the hope that brief blockade of T-cell costimulation, if sufficiently thorough, may provide long-lasting benefit in SLE.

COMBINATION THERAPY WITH CTLA4IG
PLUS PULSE CYCLOPHOSPHAMIDE

The combination of anti-CD40L and CTLA4Ig is not the only combination that has shown promise in murine models for SLE. Recent studies have shown that CTLA4Ig and pulse cyclophosphamide (CTX) also act synergistically in the treatment of lupus nephritis in mice *(21,22)*. In these studies, 6-mo-old B/W females with advanced renal disease received either pulse CTX, CTLA4Ig, both pulse CTX and CTLA4Ig, or saline. After 12 wk of treatment, none of the saline-treated mice survived, compared to 36% survival among mice treated with either CTX or CTLA4Ig alone *(21)*. In contrast, 93% of mice treated with both agents were alive. Although mice treated with either CTX or CTLA4Ig alone had prolonged survival relative to saline-treated control mice, there was no reduction in their severe proteinuria. However, there was a striking reduction in proteinuria in mice treated with both agents together. Careful examination of renal pathology in a separate cohort of mice confirmed that treatment with both agents reduced renal injury from baseline, whereas treatment with either agent alone merely slowed the rate of progression *(22)*. The demonstration that renal damage can be reversed in murine lupus is unprecedented, but it remains to be determined whether the addition of CTLA4Ig to pulse CTX in humans with lupus nephritis will have similarly profound effects.

BLOCKADE OF T-CELL COSTIMULATION IN HUMANS

Anti-CD40L Trials in Humans

Based on the encouraging results in murine models, several groups have begun to explore the possibility of treating autoimmune diseases in humans by blocking T-cell costimulation. In the past two years, two companies have sponsored trials of anti-CD40L in people with SLE, using different MAb directed against different epitopes on CD40L. The first phase I trial of a MAb to CD40L in patients with active SLE demonstrated that treatment was well-tolerated, without any significant short-term toxicity *(23)*. This single-dose, dose-escalating trial was not designed to assess efficacy. Subsequently, there have been two phase II trials of anti-CD40L in SLE, both of which have raised concerns about this approach. One trial examined several doses of anti-CD40L administered over a 4-mo period to a total of 88 subjects with diverse manifestations of SLE *(24)*. Treatment was again well-tolerated, as it had been in the phase I trial, but the primary clinical goal (reduction in the systemic lupus erythematosus disease activity index (SLEDAI) score) was not achieved. The other trial was suspended before completion owing to the occurrence of unexplained thrombotic complications. The mechanism responsible for the thrombotic complications has not yet been determined, nor is it clear whether this problem will be limited to the particular MAb used in this study or whether it will apply generally to all anti-CD40 MAb independent of the target epitope.

CTLA4Ig Trials in Humans

Unlike anti-CD40L, CTLA4Ig has not yet been studied in humans with SLE. However, it is currently the subject of clinical investigation in two other autoimmune diseases of humans: psoriasis and RA. In a phase I trial of patients with psoriasis, CTLA4Ig was not only well-tolerated, but it also appeared to be clinically effective *(25)*. Although this was not a blinded or controlled trial, the dose-escalating design was used successfully to demonstrate that CTLA4Ig can suppress immune function in humans. This study also strongly suggested that CTLA4Ig can reduce disease severity in patients with psoriasis. Based on the encouraging results in this T-cell-mediated autoimmune disease, controlled phase II trials have been initiated in people with RA. The results of these studies are expected soon, and they will undoubtedly play a major role in determining whether studies of CTLA4Ig are initiated in people with SLE.

SUMMARY

Recent studies in murine models for SLE have raised the hope that blockade of T-cell costimulation may provide an effective new form of therapy for people with SLE. Based on these animal studies, trials have been initiated in humans to assess the safety and efficacy of new treatments that block T-cell costimulation via CD28 and/or CD40L. Early results have demonstrated promise, but they have also raised important concerns.

Further studies will be needed before we know whether the promising findings in murine models can be safely translated into effective treatments for people.

ACKNOWLEDGMENTS

This work was supported by grants from the Department of Veterans Affairs and the National Institutes for Health, and by the Rosalind Russell Medical Research Center for Arthritis at UCSF.

REFERENCES

1. Marrack, P. and J.W. Kappler. 1993. How the immune system recognizes the body. *Sci. Am.* 269:80–89.

2. Harding, F.A., J.G. McArthur, J.A. Gross, D.H. Raulet, and J.P. Allison. 1992. CD28-mediated signaling co-stimulates murine T cells and prevents induction of anergy in T cell clones. *Nature* 356:607–610.

3. Bluestone, J.A. 1995. New perspectives of CD28-B7-mediated T cell costimulation. *Immunity* 2:555–559.

4. Oliveira-dos-Santos, A.J., A. Ho, Y. Tada, J.J. Lafaille, S. Tonegawa, T.W. Mak, and J.M. Penninger. 1999. CD28 costimulation is crucial for the development of spontaneous autoimmune encephalomyelitis. *J. Immunol.* 162:4490–4495.

5. Krummel, M.F. and J.P. Allison. 1995. CD28 and CTLA-4 have opposing effects on the response of T cells to stimulation. *J. Exp. Med.* 182:459–465.

6. Waterhouse, P.J., M. Penninger, E. Timms, A. Wakeham, A. Shahinian, K.P. Lee, et al. 1995. Lymphoproliferative disorders with early lethality in mice deficient in CTLA-4. *Science* 270:985–988.

7. Lenschow, D.J., S.C. Ho, H. Sattar, L. Rhee, G. Gray, N. Nabavi, et al. 1995. Differential effects of anti-B7-1 and anti-B7-2 monoclonal antibody treatment on the development of diabetes in the nonobese diabetic mouse. *J. Exp. Med.* 181:1145–1155.

8. Linsley, P.S., P.M. Wallace, J. Johnson, M.G. Gibson, J.L. Greene, J.A. Ledbetter, et al. 1992. Immunosuppression in vivo by a soluble form of the CTLA-4 T cell activation molecule. *Science* 257:792–795.

9. Tan, P., C. Anasetti, J.A. Hansen, J. Melrose, M. Brunvand, J. Bradshaw, et al. 1993. Induction of alloantigen-specific hyporesponsiveness in human T lymphocytes by blocking interaction of CD28 with its natural ligand B7/BB1. *J. Exp. Med.* 177:165–173.

10. Lenschow, D.J., Y. Zeng, J.R. Thistlethwaite, A. Montag, W. Brady, M.G. Gibson, et al. 1992. Long-term survival of xenogeneic pancreatic islet grafts induced by CTLA4Ig. *Science* 257:789–792.

11. Milich, D.R., P.S. Linsley, J.L. Hughes, and J.E. Jones. 1994. Soluble CTLA-4 can suppress autoantibody production and elicit long term unresponsiveness in a novel transgenic model. *J. Immunol.* 153:429–435.

12. Finck, B.K., P.S. Linsley, and D. Wofsy. 1994. Treatment of murine lupus with CTLA4Ig. *Science* 265:1225–1227.

13. Daikh, D.I., B.K. Finck, P.S. Linsley, D. Hollenbaugh, and D. Wofsy. 1997. Long-term inhibition of murine lupus by brief simultaneous blockade of the B7/CD28 and CD40/gp39 costimulation pathways. *J. Immunol.* 159:3104–3108.

14. Durie, F.H., T.M. Foy, S.R. Masters, J.D. Laman, and R.J. Noelle. 1994. The role of CD40 in the regulation of humoral and cell-mediated immunity. *Immunol. Today* 15:406–411.

15. Struber, E., W. Strober, and M. Neurath. 1996. Blocking the CD40L-CD40 interaction in vivo specifically prevents the priming of T helper cells through the inhibition of interleukin 12 secretion. *J. Exp. Med.* 183:693–698.

16. Campbell, K.A., P.J. Ovendale, M.K. Kennedy, W.C. Fanslow, S.G. Reed, and C.R. Maliszewski. 1996. CD40 ligand is required for protective cell-mediated immunity to Leishmania major. *Immunity* 4:283–289.

17. Griggs, N.D., S.S. Agersborg, R.J. Noelle, J.A. Ledbetter, P.S. Linsley, and K.S.K. Tung. 1996. The relative contribution of the CD28 and gp39 costimulatory pathways in the clonal expression and pathogenic acquisition of self reactive T cells. *J. Exp. Med.* 183:801–810.

18. Durie, F.H., R.A. Fava, T.M. Foy, A. Aruffo, J.A. Ledbetter, and R.J. Noelle. 1993. Prevention of collagen-induced arthritis with an antibody to gp39, the ligand for CD40. *Science* 261:1328–1330.

19. Mohan, C., Y. Shi, J.D. Laman, and S.K. Datta. 1995. Interaction between CD40 and its ligand gp39 in the development of murine lupus nephritis. *J. Immunol.* 154:1470–1480.

20. Early, G.S., W. Zhao, and C.M. Burns. 1996. Anti-CD40 ligand antibody treatment prevents the development of lupus-like nephritis in a subset of New Zealand Black x New Zealand White mice. *J. Immunol.* 157:3159–3164.

21. Daikh, D.I. and D. Wofsy. 2001. Reversal of murine lupus nephritis with CTLA4Ig and cyclophosphamide. *J. Immunol.* 166:2913–2916.

22. Cunnane, G., B. Yen, G. Cassifer, S. Brindis, D. Wofsy, and D.I. Daikh. 1999. Effects of combined CTLA4Ig and cyclophosphamide on renal pathology in advanced murine lupus. *Arthritis Rheum.* 42:S359 (Abstract).

23. Davis, J.C., M.C. Totoritis, J. Rosenberg, T.A. Sklenar, and D. Wofsy. 2001. A phase I clinical trial of a monoclonal antibody against CD40-ligand (IDEC-131) in patients with systemic lupus erythematosus. *J. Rheum.* 28:95–101.

24. Kalunian, K.C., J. Davis, J.T. Merill, M. Petri, J. Buyon, E. Ginzler, et al. 2000. Treatment of systemic lupus erythematosus by inhibition of T cell costimulation. *Arthritis Rheum.* (Abstract) 43:S271.

25. Abrams, J.R., M.G. Lebwohl, C.A. Guzzo, B.V. Jegasothy, M.T. Goldfarb, B.S. Goffe, et al. 1999. CTLA4Ig-mediated blockade of T cell costimulation in patients with psoriasis vulgaris. *J. Clin. Invest.* 103:1243–1252.

21

Current Management of Systemic Sclerosis

*Clarence W. Legerton III
and Richard M. Silver*

CONTENTS

INTRODUCTION
RAYNAUD PHENOMENON
RENAL INVOLVEMENT
PULMONARY INVOLVEMENT
GI MANIFESTATIONS
CONCLUSION
REFERENCES

INTRODUCTION

Systemic sclerosis (SSc) is a multi-system disease characterized by increased synthesis and deposition of extracellular matrix that results in fibrosis of the skin (scleroderma) and visceral organs. Although often used interchangeably, the terms "scleroderma" and "systemic sclerosis" are not synonymous. Scleroderma, literally meaning "hard skin," can occur in discrete areas without visceral or systemic involvement and in such cases is classified as "localized" scleroderma (morphea, linear, en coup de sabre, guttate). Nearly always, the digits are spared, i.e., there is no sclerodactyly, and Raynaud phenomenon (RP) is absent. In contrast, scleroderma may occur in concert with visceral organ involvement, in which case it is called "systemic sclerosis."

In SSc, skin involvement usually begins acrally with sclerodactyly and progresses proximally. Systemic sclerosis is classified into two types, which are principally distinguished by the extent of skin involvement. In one form, skin disease is usually "limited" to the distal extremities and face and is called "limited" cutaneous systemic sclerosis (lcSSc), previously known as the CREST syndrome (calcinosis, Raynaud phenomenon, esophageal dysmotility, sclerodactyly, telangiectasis). In contrast, more widespread skin involvement (proximal to the elbows or knees and inferior to the clavicles) is classified as "diffuse" cutaneous systemic sclerosis (dcSSc) and is characterized by more extensive visceral involvement and a higher mortality rate. Because

From: *Modern Therapeutics in Rheumatic Diseases*
Edited by: G. C. Tsokos, et al. © Humana Press, Inc., Totowa, NJ

localized scleroderma (e.g., morphea) is immunologically and clinically distinct, this chapter will address systemic sclerosis only.

Owing in part to the fact that the pathogenesis of SSc is complex and incompletely understood, no therapies exist that modify the underlying disease process. Fibrosis is most certainly a late manifestation that results from the response of the mesenchymal cell to aberrations of the immune and vascular systems, possibly with a contribution from environmental triggers. No current therapies are both safe and effective at degrading mature collagen without damage to surrounding tissues. Therefore, any antifibrotic therapy would need to be instituted early in the course of disease to be effective.

Much of the unwarranted pessimism that surrounds treatment of the patient with SSc results, it seems, from the failure of therapies to halt the dermal fibrosis, the most outwardly visible feature. However, great strides have been made in the management of organ-specific visceral involvement in this disease; witness the dramatic reduction in scleroderma renal crisis after the introduction of drugs that inhibit angiotensin converting enzyme.

The extensive list of failed therapies might serve to heighten one's pessimism regarding our ability to treat this disease (Table 1). Instead, the physician should appreciate the difficulties of gauging improvement in SSc, especially the improvement of fibrotic manifestations such as the skin. In addition to the difficulty of reversing established fibrosis, distinguishing therapeutic effects from the natural history of scleroderma can be difficult. Skin disease often progresses rapidly early in the disease course, particularly in dcSSc, only to stabilize and then gradually atrophy and soften over time. Such improvement may lead to the appearance of success for any particular intervention, when the change is actually owing to the thinning of the skin that may occur naturally. In addition, the clinical course varies widely between individual patients and measurements of outcome are difficult. Thus, the results of uncontrolled trials should be viewed with extreme caution. The literature on SSc is replete with reports of successful therapies in uncontrolled trials, only to see these same therapies fail when studied more rigorously. The recent experience with D-penicillamine (DPA) serves as but one example.

DPA has long been utilized to treat SSc because of its ability to inhibit crosslinking of collagen, as well as its possible immunomodulating effects. Uncontrolled studies of DPA appeared promising, resulting in a decrease in skin scores and even an improvement in survival and a decreased incidence of scleroderma renal crisis (1,2). However, a large, randomized, controlled, blinded trial comparing therapeutic doses of DPA (750–1000 mg/d) to low-dose DPA (125 mg every other day) failed to meet the primary endpoint, a difference in skin involvement between the two groups as measured by the modified Rodnan Skin Score (3). Similarly, secondary endpoints including mortality and renal crisis were not different. Another anti-fibrotic therapy, interferon-α (IFN-α) was recently reported not to improve outcome when studied in a randomized, double-blind, placebo-controlled trial in 35 patients with early dcSSc (4). Some experts believe that DPA remains effective and, based on the trial results, they employ low doses, as opposed to the prior practice of escalating to higher doses. Caution must prevail, as discussed earlier, until controlled trials prove the efficacy of these or other therapies.

Thus, treatment of skin involvement in this disease remains experimental and symptomatic. The authors stress the use of emollients and aggressive physical and occupational therapy in an attempt to reduce or prevent flexion contractures, which

Table 1
Promising Treatments of Skin Disease That Have Failed
in Controlled Clinical Trials

Treatment	Proposed Action
Plasmapheresis	Immunosuppression
Photopheresis	Immunosuppression
Aminobenzoate potassium	Antifibrotic
Anti-thymocyte globulin	Immunosuppression
Factor XIII	Antifibrotic
Colchicine	Anti-inflammatory
Chlorambucil	Immunosuppression
Dimethyl sulfoxide	Antifibrotic
Dipyridamole	Antiplatelet
Ketotifen	Mast-cell inhibition
Ketansarin	Antiplatelet
Methotrexate	Immunosuppression
Interferon α	Anti-inflammatory
D-Penicillamine	Immunosuppressive and antifibrotic

Adapted with permission from ref. *38.*

result in loss of function, especially in the hands. Reassurance to the patient that the skin disease often softens with time provides hope and reinforces the fact that although the skin disease itself can result in disfigurement and dysfunction, it is not a direct cause of mortality.

A number of therapies for skin fibrosis have been reported to be effective, or are currently under study. Methotrexate was reported effective in a small controlled trial, but only 5 patients had dcSSc and the blinded phase of the trial continued only for 6 mo *(5)*. Minocycline received much publicity in the lay press based on a small uncontrolled study in which only 6 patients completed the study *(6)*. Hematopoietic stem cell transplantation (HSCT) is another experimental therapy undergoing clinical testing. Generally felt to be safer than classical bone marrow transplantation, HSCT allows rescue of marrow function after immunoablative chemotherapy with or without radiotherapy and is being attempted in different autoimmune diseases. Depending on the center, differences exist in patient selection, conditioning regimens, and techniques of stem cell mobilization. At present, only anecdotal reports are available *(7)* and the aforementioned differences make comparison across centers difficult. However, it is hoped that databases of treated patients will provide some conclusions on which therapeutic decisions may be based *(8)*.

Currently underway are two trials of note. Relaxin is a hormone that seems to have several physiologic roles related to uterine growth and parturition. Relaxin loosens pelvic ligaments and stimulates uterine growth *(9)*. Recombinant human relaxin decreases collagen synthesis by cultured scleroderma fibroblasts *(10)*. A recently published randomized, double-blind, pilot study compared placebo to two different doses of relaxin (25 μg/kg/d or 100 μg/kg/d) given as a continuous subcutaneous infusion over 24 wk in 64 patients with dcSSc with a disease duration of 5 yr or less *(11)*. Results were encouraging, with the patients receiving the 25 μg/kg dose demonstrating a significant reduction in skin score compared to those receiving placebo. However, patients treated with the higher dose of relaxin did not differ from the placebo patients. A larger, phase III trial was halted when relaxin failed to reach the primary endpoint, i.e., reduction in skin score. Evidence suggests a role for an autoimmune response to type I collagen in patients with systemic sclerosis. *(12–14)* In another trial recently funded, the hypothesis that tolerance to type I collagen by oral feeding of type I collagen will result in clinical improvement is to be tested in patients with dcSSc.

RAYNAUD PHENOMENON

RP is the most frequent initial symptom and occurs in virtually all patients with systemic sclerosis. Its near universal presence reflects the primary role for an altered vascular response in this disease. In response to cooling, but sometimes after stress or other factors, the digits change color with a clear line of demarcation between the affected part of the digit and the palm. Characteristically, the digits turn pale, reflecting ischemia secondary to arterial vasospasm. Alternatively, cyanosis may be present. Again, the clearly demarcated distinction in color between the digit and the palm helps to distinguish to RP from acrocyanosis. RP may be unassociated with any underlying disease, so-called primary RP. A minority of patients may have an associated disease and are classified as having secondary RP. A number of features may assist the clinician in distinguishing primary RP from RP secondary to SSc. These features may include clinical manifestations of SSc itself (sclerodactyly or tendon friction rubs), positive serological tests (anti-nuclear antibodies, anti-centromere antibodies, anti-topoisomerase antibodies), the presence of organ involvement (bibasilar fibrosis, esophageal disease), or abnormalities of the nailfold capillary bed (dilated or drop-out). Overt digital ischemia manifested as ulceration, pitting, or gangrene is associated with secondary causes of RP and is not seen in primary RP.

RP may range in severity from mild to severe. Mild cases often cause little morbidity and may not require any specific pharmacological therapy. Severe RP may result in gangrene and auto-amputation of digits. Behavioral and environmental modifications should be prescribed for all patients to prevent the vasoconstrictive response to body cooling. Behavioral measures should be directed at the prevention of cooling of the body's core temperature so as preclude the resultant peripheral vasoconstriction. Additionally, gloves should be worn in cool indoor places such as grocery stores or movie theaters. Although symptoms are generally more severe in the winter, dramatic shifts in temperature from outdoor summer heat to a cool indoor environment may precipitate severe attacks even in warm weather. Obviously, the home and workplace need to be maintained at warm temperatures. Secondly, pharmacologic agents that may exacerbate vasoconstriction should be discontinued, such as beta-blockers or ergot alkaloids. Nicotine is a potent vasoconstrictor and will contribute to severe complications of RP including gangrene of the digits. When this occurs, the authors' experience suggests that other therapies will prove ineffective as long as the patient continues the use of nicotine.

Pharmacologic therapy most commonly utilizes calcium-channel blockers which have been studied in RP. A recent controlled study of 313 patients with primary RP compared sustained-release nifedipine to temperature biofeedback and demonstrated a

66% reduction in verified attacks of RP in the nifedipine treated group *(15)*. Patients treated with temperature biofeedback fared no better than their control group. Like many protocols, this study examined patients with primary RP, i.e., those patients without evidence for an underlying connective tissue disease, and supporting evidence for efficacy in secondary RP is less convincing.

Additional pharmacologic therapy may be required if tissue loss such as fingertip ulceration or gangrene occurs. Anti-platelet therapy has not been well-studied, although there is evidence of platelet activation in SSc *(16)*. The newer glycoprotein IIb/IIIa inhibitors may be instituted but have not been studied for this manifestation of SSc. Vasodilation with drugs such as alpha-adrenergic blockers may be tried. Often, nitroglycerin paste is applied topically to the base of the most severely affected digits, but there is no reason to believe that its systemic vasodilating effect would be less if applied elsewhere. Narcotic analgesics alleviate the severe pain of ischemia and have the added benefit of vasodilation as well, but such therapy must be used with caution because it may exacerbate intestinal hypomotility. Lastly, the use of the prostacyclin analog iloprost has generally been favorable when given intravenously, but results have not been consistently positive *(17,18)*.

Another approach involves disruption of the vasoconstricting input of the sympathetic nervous system. Options include digital sympathectomy, in which the sympathetic nerves specifically to the affected digits are interrupted. Stellate ganglion block is less invasive and may be effective in reducing acute pain, although theoretical concern exists over inducing a "steel phenomenon" and shunting blood away from the most severely affected digits. A similar result can be performed via a cervical epidural catheter through which a narcotic analgesic and a low-dose of local anesthetic are infused, usually for three continuous days. Benefits of surgical cervical sympathectomy are felt to be transient and this procedure is no longer recommended. None of these measures has been studied prospectively in a controlled manner, in part owing to the inherent difficulties of measuring responses.

Local treatment of any open wound should occur, as well as utilization of antibiotics for infection. We generally attempt to avoid surgical resection, in the hope that less tissue will ultimately be lost; however, intractable pain, extensive gangrene, or infection may be treated best by removing the diseased tissue.

RENAL INVOLVEMENT

Advances in the prevention and management of scleroderma renal crisis (SRC) exemplify the tremendous progress that has occurred and is occurring in the treatment of SSc, despite our lack of success at treating the outwardly visible skin disease. Formerly the principal cause of death in patients with scleroderma, renal failure is now much less common since the advent of therapy with angiotensin-converting enzyme (ACE) inhibitors.

Pathologically, SRC develops as a result of intimal proliferation and thickening in the renal vasculature. The resultant decrease in cortical blood flow induces a state of increased renin release, malignant hypertension, and renal insufficiency. Vasculopathy manifests as schistocytes on peripheral blood smear, sometimes with thrombocytopenia. Any of these clinical features (increasing blood pressure, worsening renal function, hemolysis, or declining platelet count) should prompt immediate intervention as discussed below. Other manifestations of this syndrome may include headaches, proteinuria, or active urine sediment.

Early sustained therapy with ACE inhibitors may prevent renal failure and allow recovery of renal function. SRC occurs almost exclusively in the diffuse variant of systemic sclerosis, and patients with dcSSc should comply with rigorous home monitoring of blood pressure (at least several times weekly). Any elevation from baseline, even if the pressure remains within the "normal" range, should prompt immediate institution of ACE inhibitor therapy. Owing to the catastrophic nature of SRC and its high mortality, any patient with manifestations of SRC should be hospitalized and treated immediately with short-acting ACE inhibitors, with rapid upward titration of the dose to regain control of blood pressure. Owing to the tremendous hyperreninemic state, ACE inhibitors must be continued despite worsening renal failure, a practice counter to the more common perception in which ACE inhibitors contribute to renal failure, e.g., in patients with bilateral renal-artery stenosis. Once blood pressure is controlled, therapy can be switched to ACE inhibitors with a longer half-life.

Several factors may indicate a risk of SRC. Patients early in the course of diffuse disease with rapidly advancing skin disease are most at risk of developing SRC and this population should have regular monitoring of blood pressure and early institution of ACE inhibitors. Secondly, any insult to renal perfusion such as hypotension may precipitate SRC. Among pharmaceutical agents, the use of glucocorticoids, in particular, has been associated with the development of SRC. Glucocorticoids have little proven therapeutic efficacy in SSc, and the use of glucocorticoids in patients at risk for SRC should be minimized. Musculoskeletal complications such as myositis or arthritis in patients with dcSSc should be treated early with second-line agents (e.g., methotrexate) in order to minimize the use of glucocorticoids. Rarely, SRC may occur without significant increase in blood pressure, so called "normotensive" SRC. In our experience and that of others *(19)*, this rare disease subset has a particularly poor prognosis.

Dialysis, either hematological or peritoneal, may be utilized in patients with SSc, just as for patients with other causes of renal failure. Gradual recovery of renal function after SRC is well-described and, therefore, ACE inhibition therapy should be continued even in the face of end-stage renal disease. Renal transplantation should be considered if renal failure persists beyond 1 yr. Recurrence of SRC in a transplanted kidney has been reported in one case only *(20)*.

PULMONARY INVOLVEMENT

Reflecting the success of preventing and treating renal crisis, pulmonary disease now ranks as the leading cause of mortality in SSc. Two distinct types of scleroderma pulmonary disease predominate. In keeping with the systemic fibrosis occurring in scleroderma is the development of interstitial pulmonary fibrosis, primarily occurring in patients with the diffuse variant of the disease. Fibrosis is felt to develop as a result of inflammation present in the alveoli, called alveolitis. The presence of increased numbers of activated alveolar macrophages, neutrophils, and eosinophils in bronchoalveolar lavage (BAL) fluid is a marker of alveolitis, which is associated with greater pulmonary dysfunction and a higher propensity for decline in pulmonary function than in SSc patients whose BAL fluid is of normal cellularity *(21)*. Additionally, high-resolution computed tomography (HRCT) scans of the lungs may demonstrate ground glass attenuation, which correlates with alveolitis.

Pulmonary fibrosis may present with symptoms of dyspnea on exertion, a nonproductive cough, or with physical exam findings of bibasilar rales. However, because a significant degree of pulmonary reserve exists, symptoms may not occur until late in the disease course. Thus, screening for pulmonary involvement by means of baseline chest radiograph (CXR) and pulmonary function testing (PFT) for spirometry, lung volumes, and diffusion capacity of carbon monoxide should be performed on all newly diagnosed patients. The authors recommend repeat annual CXR and PFT testing in patients with newly diagnosed or rapidly progressive disease. Either symptoms or abnormalities on testing (radiographs or PFTs) should prompt further evaluation with BAL or HRCT. Although BAL is more invasive and requires expertise at cellular analysis, it is generally felt to be more sensitive and predictive of alveolitis than HRCT. Smoking increases the number of alveolar macrophages and neutrophils recovered in BAL fluid and renders this test of little benefit in patients who smoke; either smoking or lack of expertise in the analysis of BAL fluid would favor performance of HRCT instead.

No therapy has been shown by prospective controlled trial to be effective in altering the course of interstitial fibrosis in scleroderma, but immunosuppressive therapy is often employed in patients with evidence of alveolitis on either BAL or HRCT in an attempt to suppress inflammation and thereby retard fibrosis. Uncontrolled studies suggest the efficacy of cyclophosphamide treatment in improving forced vital capacity (FVC) *(22–24)* and in regression of interstitial lesions as documented by HRCT scan. A multi-center, prospective placebo-controlled trial of daily oral cyclophosphamide has been initiated. High-dose glucocorticoid therapy is to be avoided owing to concern over adverse effects, e.g., the induction of SRC. Usually, cyclophosphamide is prescribed orally in the range of 1–2 mg/kg/d to a slight lowering of the white blood cell count (approx 3000 cells/mm^3) and is continued for up to 2 yr if symptoms, pulmonary function, and radiographic changes stabilize or improve. Other supportive and preventive measures also should be instituted as indicated, such as supplemental oxygen therapy and vaccination against pneumococcus and influenza. Lung transplantation is an effective option for those patients without severe esophageal or renal disease.

Pulmonary hypertension (PHT) is the other major form of pulmonary disease seen in SSc. Isolated pulmonary hypertension almost exclusively occurs in limited systemic sclerosis. However, it may occur secondary to pulmonary fibrosis in either the diffuse (more common) or limited (less common) variants. Ten percent of patients with lcSSc (CREST) syndrome develop isolated PHT, usually many years after the onset of RP. Symptoms may include dyspnea, chest pain, or syncope. Reduced diffusion capacity for carbon monoxide (DLCO) should alert the clinician to the presence of this condition, and either unexplained symptoms or a reduced DLCO should prompt further study by echocardiography with Doppler estimation of pulmonary-artery pressure.

Patients with lcSSc and pulmonary hypertension have a significantly reduced survival rate of 40% over 2 yr, compared with a survival rate of 88% of patients with lcSSc in the absence of PHT*(25)*. Therapy has been largely unsuccessful in the management of this condition. The main goal of treatment has been to attempt vasodilation of the pulmonary vascular bed, thus reducing pulmonary pressures and increasing cardiac output, all while maintaining peripheral vascular tone and pressure. Therapy with nifedipine and other calcium-channel blockers results in a reduction in pulmonary artery resistance, but the fact that some patients will have an adverse effect (decreased cardiac output or decline in systemic blood pressure) requires that this therapy be instituted with appropriate monitoring. A meta-analysis *(26)* demonstrated a decline in pulmonary-artery pressure in response to nifedipine therapy that was statistically significant when given over a period of at least several weeks. However, the studies were not blinded, nor randomized, and attrition rates were high. Other studies reflect that only a minority of patients respond to vasodilators but, at least in the case of nifedipine, survival might be improved among those patients who do experience a hemodynamic response *(27)*.

The availability of the potent vasodilator, prostacyclin, has generated much enthusiasm regarding the treatment of pulmonary hypertension. In addition to its vasodilating properties, prostacyclin also functions as an inhibitor of platelet aggregation and smooth-muscle proliferation. Prostacyclin (epoprostenol, Flolan®) has a short half-life of 3–5 min and, therefore, must be given via continuous intravenous infusion. Its potency is exemplified by the dramatic improvements in pulmonary hemodynamics, even among patients with primary pulmonary hypertension who failed trials of adenosine *(28)*.

Moreover, it is now recognized that the effects of prostacyclin extend beyond its ability to vasodilate the pulmonary vasculature. Even patients who fail to respond to vasodilators with an acute decline in pulmonary vascular resistance may improve in symptoms and in other hemodynamic measures following prostacyclin infusion. The reason for this is unclear but is hypothesized to involve vascular remodeling. Trials in primary pulmonary hypertension suggest an improvement in symptoms such as exercise tolerance, measures of quality of life, and survival *(29)*.

Although most of these studies have been performed in primary pulmonary hypertension, most experts have extrapolated the results to pulmonary hypertension associated with connective tissue diseases owing to the similarity of the clinical and histopathologic pictures. Fortunately, studies that include patients with collagen vascular disease are now being published. Most notable among these is a randomized controlled trial comparing epoprostenol plus conventional therapy to conventional therapy alone in 111 patients with scleroderma-spectrum disease *(30)*. The primary outcome variable in this study was exercise capacity as determined by distance walked in 6 min. The epoprostenol plus conventional therapy group improved steadily and continuously throughout the 12 wk of the study, whereas the patients receiving conventional therapy alone suffered a steady decline in exercise capacity (Fig. 1). Secondary measures, which also improved significantly, included hemodynamic data and pulmonary symptoms. In contrast with previous studies in primary pulmonary hypertension *(29)*, the study involving patients with scleroderma-spectrum disease failed to demonstrate a difference in survival between the two groups, although the study was not powered to detect his difference and was only 12 wk in duration *(30)*.

Adverse effects of epoprostenol include jaw pain, nausea, and gastrointestinal (GI) upset, headache, and rash. Additionally, complications of the continuous infusion can include infection, sepsis, pneumothorax, and mechanical-pump failure. To circumvent these problems, as well as to provide selective pulmonary effects, other trials have utilized inhaled iloprost, a more stable prostacyclin analog. One small uncontrolled trial of 19 patients with pulmonary hypertension treated with inhaled iloprost, including

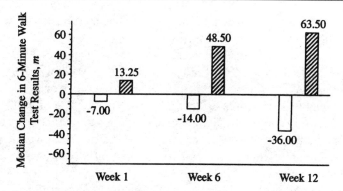

Fig. 1. Median change from baseline in results of the 6-min walk test at wk 1, 6, and 12. Nonparametric analysis of covariance with adjustment for 6-min walk values and use of vasodilators at baseline showed that the median distance walked in 6 min increased in patients who received epoprostenol (striped bars) compared with patients who received conventional therapy (white bars) at wk 6 ($p = 0.003$) and 12 ($p < 0.001$). Reprinted with permission from ref. *30*.

three with collagen vascular disease, demonstrated improved exercise tolerance and hemodynamic data over 3 mo *(31)*.

GI MANIFESTATIONS

The GI tract is involved in nearly all patients with SSc, the esophagus being the most commonly affected segment. Most patients are clinically symptomatic, and the vast majority can be shown to have abnormalities of esophageal function. A moderate amount of evidence supports the hypothesis that the early manifestations of scleroderma GI involvement are due to autonomic dysfunction. From the standpoint of motility, peristalsis is uncoordinated and, because the smooth muscle remains normal, patients are more likely to respond to therapy during this stage. Motility is further impaired as smooth muscle becomes atrophic and is replaced by fibrous tissue; obviously treatment is much more difficult at this stage.

Esophageal symptoms present as gastroesophageal reflux disease (GERD) or substernal dysphagia. Several factors contribute to GERD and are targets for therapy. Although many otherwise healthy people have reflux, the motility disorder in patients with scleroderma results in an inability to clear the refluxed acid from the esophagus. Thus, acid remains in contact with the esophageal mucosa for prolonged periods, as compared with reflux in patients without SSc. In addition, loss of tone of the lower esophageal sphincter and delayed gastric emptying also contribute to this common symptom complex.

Therapy for GERD includes physical anti-reflux measures such as consumption of small frequent meals, avoidance of recumbency after eating, and elevation of the head of the bed. Acid-lowering drugs such as histamine-2 blockers are prescribed in nearly all patients initially. If symptoms persist, proton-pump inhibitors are significantly more effective *(32)*. Promotility agents such as metoclopramide appear to have little effect on esophageal motility directly, but ameliorate reflux symptoms by increasing the tone of the lower esophageal sphincter and by increasing gastric motility and emptying *(33)*.

The use of cisapride has been restricted lately, but it is an alternative in the refractory patient without contraindications to its use.

Often overlooked is the contribution of drugs with adverse effects on GI motility, such as calcium-channel blockers. Endoscopy or other studies are indicated in the patient with persistent or progressive symptoms or so-called "alarm symptoms" such as weight loss. Esophageal strictures are common and respond to dilation. Symptoms of GERD may improve in the presence of a stricture, only to worsen after the stricture is dilated. Candidiasis may occur in patients on longstanding therapy which raises gastric pH. The development of Barrett's esophagus, a potentially premalignant condition, requires regular screening.

Gastric involvement resulting in delayed gastric emptying is common in patients with SSc and is often not recognized. Capillary dilation (telangiectasis) can occur throughout the GI tract, and may cause overt or occult blood loss. In the stomach, gastric antral vascular ectasia (GAVE), also called "watermelon stomach," is a characteristic finding that is most commonly treated by endoscopic ablation.

Bowel dysmotility may result in intestinal symptoms of bloating, distension, and abdominal pain. Abnormal peristalsis results in an inability to clear gut flora, resulting in bacterial overgrowth and the aforementioned symptoms. Malabsorption may develop, resulting in symptoms of diarrhea and weight loss. We often treat empirically for bacterial overgrowth with a course of oral antibiotics such as tetracycline. In the case of symptom recurrence or a failure to respond, a rotating course of antibiotics such as metronidazole, ampicillin, or trimethoprin-sulfamethoxazole may be given, one antibiotic for 1 wk each month in a rotating fashion. Bacterial overgrowth can be detected formally by hydrogen breath testing or culture of duodenal aspirates, the latter of which may allow a more targeted choice of antibiotics based on results of sensitivity testing, but this is rarely required.

Pseudo-obstruction of the small bowel or colon (megacolon) presents very difficult management situations for the rheumatologist and surgeon. Intraluminal decompression, antibiotics, and supportive measures such as bowel rest and oxygen are the recommended therapies. Surgery should be undertaken only as a last resort as it often fails to disclose a mechanical obstruction and will result in a prolonged postoperative ileus. One must be aware of the complication of pneumatosis cystoides intestinalis, in which air infiltrates the bowel wall, which is also treated conservatively. Octreotide has been used in both idiopathic and scleroderma-associated pseudo-obstruction *(34–37)*. Wide-mouthed diverticula are characteristic to SSc and are usually asymptomatic, though they may be foci for bacterial overgrowth or perforation. Of course, true obstruction or perforation necessitates appropriate surgical intervention.

As is the case for gastric involvement, disease of the rectum is often unappreciated, both by physicians who fail to ask and patients who are embarrassed to comment. The most common complication is anal sphincter incompetence, which is difficult to manage either medically or surgically.

Importantly, nutritional support may be required in the patient with malabsorption or progressive unexplained weight loss. A guideline of therapy is that it is often better to feed in a way that avoids the affected segment than to attempt a difficult surgical repair. Commonly, refractory upper-GI involvement will necessitate the use of a jejunal feeding tube to bypass the dysfunctional esophagus and poorly emptying stomach. A

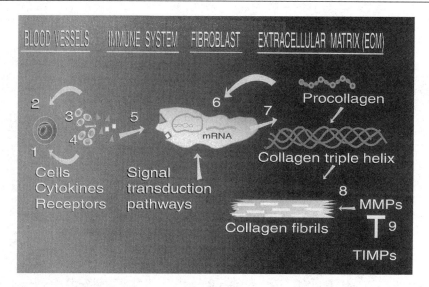

Fig. 2. Pathophysiologic events of SSc where future therapeutic modalities might act: (1) inhibition of adhesion molecules; (2) anti-platelet agents; (3) mast cell inhibitors; (4) anti-cytokines; (5) inhibitors of growth factors or growth factor receptor blockers; (6) inhibitors of signal transduction; (7) inhibitors of procollagen secretion; (8) collagenase and other metalloproteases (MMPs); (9) neutralization of TIMPs, tissue inhibitors of metalloproteinases.

number of patients have done well for long periods with total parenteral nutrition, often provided as nighttime feedings.

CONCLUSION

Much progress has been made in recent years in the control of visceral involvement of systemic sclerosis. Although skin disease remains difficult to treat, new therapies are currently under active investigation. Other therapies have dramatically reduced morbidity and mortality for complications such as renal crisis. Novel therapies such as prostacyclin, relaxin, cytokine inhibitors, and other biological agents are being studied and hold great promise for the future. As the pathophysiology of SSc is better understood (Fig. 2), rational therapies will be developed to halt the activation of dermal and visceral fibroblasts, thus blocking the process of fibrosis, which ultimately will improve morbidity and mortality. We have great reason to be optimistic that improved therapies for our patients are on the horizon.

REFERENCES

1. Steen, V.D., T.A. Medsger, Jr., and G.P. Rodnan. 1982. D-Penicillamine therapy in progressive systemic sclerosis (scleroderma): a retrospective analysis. *Ann. Intern Med.* 97(5):652–659.

2. Jimenez, S.A. and S.H. Sigal. 1991. A 15-year prospective study of treatment of rapidly progressive systemic sclerosis with D-penicillamine. *J. Rheumatol.* 18(10):1496–1503.

3. Clements, P.J., D.E. Furst, W.K. Wong, M. Mayes, B. White, F. Wigley, et al. 1999. High-dose versus low-dose D-Penicillamine in early diffuse systemic sclerosois: analysis of a two-year, double-blind, randomized, controlled clinical trial. *Arthritis Rheum.* 42(6):1194–1203.

4. Black, C.M., A.J. Silman, A.I. Herrick, C.P. Denton, H. Wilson, J. Newman, et al. 1999. Interferon-alpha does not improve outcome at one year in patients with diffuse cutaneous scleroderma: results of a randomized, double-blind, placebo-controlled trial. *Arthritis Rheum.* 42(2):299–305.

5. van den Hoogen, F.H., A.M. Boerbooms, A.J. Swaak, J.J. Rasker, H.J. van Lier, and L.B. van de Putte. 1996. Comparison of methotrexate with placebo in the treatment of systemic sclerosis: a 24 week randomized double-blind trial, followed by a 24 week observational trial. *Br. J. Rheumatol.* 35(4): 364–372.

6. Lee, C.H., A. Morales, and D.E. Trentham. 1998. Minocycline in early diffuse scleroderma. *Lancet* 352:1755–1756.

7. Tyndall, A., C. Black, J. Finke, J. Winkler, R. Merthesmann, H.H. Peter, and A. Gratwohl. 1997. Treatment of systemic sclerois with autologous haemopoietic stem cell transplantation. *Lancet* 349(9047):254.

8. Tyndall, A. 1999. Haematological stem cell transplantation in the treatment of severe autoimmune diseases: first experiences from an international project. *Rheumatology* 38:774–776.

9. Sherwood, O.D. 1988. Relaxin, in The Physiology of Reproduction. E. Knobil and J.D. Neill, editors. Raven Press New York. 585–673.

10. Unemori, E.N., E.A. Bauer, and E.P. Amento. 1992. Relaxin alone and in conjunction with interferon-gamma decreases collagen synthesis by cultured human scleroderma fibroblasts. *J. Invest. Dermatol.* 99(3):337–342.

11. Seibold, J.R., J.H. Korn, R. Simms, P.J. Clements, L.W. Moreland, M.D. Mayes, et al. 2000. Recombinant human relaxin in the treatment of scleroderma; a randomized, double-blind, placebo-controlled trial. *Ann Intern Med.* 132:871–879.

12. Stuart, J.M., A.E. Postlethwaite, and A.H. Kang. 1976. Evidence for cell-mediated immunity to collagen in progressive systemic sclerosis. *J. Lab. Clin. Med.* 88:601–607.

13. Hawrylko, E., A. Spertus, C.A. Mele, N. Oster, and M. Frieri. 1991. Increased interleukin-2 production in response to human type I collagen stimulation in patients with systemic sclerosis. *Arthritis Rheum.* 34:580–587.

14. Gurram, M., S. Pahwa, and M. Frieri. 1994. Augmented interleukin-6 secretion in collagen-stimulated peripheral blood mononuclear cells from patients with systemic sclerosis. *Ann. Allergy* 73(6):493–496.

15. Raynaud's Treatment Study Investigators. 2000. Comparison of sustained-release nifedipine and temperature biofeedback for treatment of primary Raynaud's phenomenon. *Arch. Intern. Med.* 160:1101–1108.

16. Kahaleh, M.B., I. Osborn, and E.C. Leroy. 1982. Elevated levels of circulating platelet aggregates and beta-thromboglobulin in scleroderma. *Ann. Intern. Med.* 96(5):610–613.

17. Wigley, F.M., R.A Wise,. J.R. Seibold, D.A. McCloskey, G. Kujala, T.A. Medsger, Jr., et al. 1994. Intravenous iloprost infusion in patients with Raynaud phenomenon secondary to systemic sclerosis. A multicenter, placebo-controlled, double-blind study. *Ann. Intern. Med.* 120(3):199–206.

18. Wigley, F.M., J.H. Korn, M.E. Csuka, T.A. Medsger, Jr., N.F. Rothfield, M. Ellman, et al. 1998. Oral iloprost treatment in patients with Raynaud's phenomenon secondary to systemic sclerosis: a multicenter, placebo-controlled, double-blind study. *Arthritis Rheum.* 41(4):670–677.

19. Helfrich, D.J., B. Banner, V.D. Steen, and T.A. Medsger, Jr. 1989. Normotensive renal failure in systemic sclerosis. *Arthritis Rheum.* 32:1128–1134.

20. Wood, P.B., R.C. McCoy, J.C. Gunneles, and H.F. Seiguler. 1976. Apparent reoccurrence of progressive systemic sclerosis in a renal allograft. *JAMA* 236:1032–1034.

21. Silver, R.M., K.S. Miller, M.B. Kinsella, and E.A. Smith. 1990. Evaluation and management of scleroderma lung disease using bronchoalveolar lavage. *Am. J. Med.* 88:470–475.

22. Silver, R.M., J.H. Warrick, M.B. Kinsella, L.S. Staudt, M.H. Baumann, and C. Strange. 1993. Cyclophosphamide and low dose prednisone therapy in patients with systemic sclerosis (scleroderma) with interstitial lung disease. *J. Rheumatol.* 20:838–844.

23. Akesson, A., A. Scheja, A. Lundin, and F.A. Wollheim. 1994. Improved pulmonary function in systemic sclerosis after treatment with cyclophosphamide. *Arthritis Rheum.* 38(1):147.

24. White, B., W.C. Moore, F.M. Wigley, H.Q. Xizo, and R.A. Wise. 2000. Cyclophosphamide is associated with pulmonary function and survival benefit in patients with scleroderma and alveolitis. *Ann. Intern. Med.* 132:947–954.

25. Stupi, A.M., V.D. Steen, G.R. Owens, E.L. Barnes, G.P. Rodnan, and T.A. Medsger, Jr. 1986. Pulmonary hypertension in the CREST syndrome variant of systemic sclerosis. *Arthritis Rheum.* 29(4):515–524.

26. Malik A.S. S. Warshafsky, and S. Lehrman. 1997. Meta-analysis of the long term effect of nifedipine for pulmonary hypertension. *Arch. Intern. Med.* 157:621–625.

27. Rich, S., E. Kaufman, and P.S. Levy. 1992. The effect of high doses of calcium-channel blockers on survival in primary pulmonary hypertension. *NEJM* 327:76–81.

28. McLaughlin, V.V., D.E. Genthner, M.M. Panella, and S. Rich. 1998. Reduction in pulmonary vascular resistance with long-term epoprostenol (prostacyclin) therapy in primary pulmonary hypertension. *NEJM* 338(5):273–277.

29. Barst, R.J., L.J. Rubin, W.A. Long, M.D. McGoon, S. Rich, D.B. Badesch, et al. 1996. A comparison of continuous intravenous epoprostenol (prostacyclin) with conventional therapy for primary pulmonary hypertension. *NEJM* 334:296–301.

30. Badesch, D.B., V.F. Tapson, M.D. McGoon, B.H. Brundage, L.J. Rubin, F.M. Wigley, et al. 2000. Continuous intravenous epoprostenol for pulmonary hypertension due to the scleroderma spectrum of disease. *Ann. Intern. Med.* 132(6):425–434.

31. Olschewski H., A. Ghofrani, T. Schmehl, J. Winkler, H. Wilkens, M.M. Hoper, et al. 2000. Inhaled iloprost to treat severe pulmonary hypertension. *Ann. Intern. Med.* 132(6):435–448.

32. Hendel, L., E. Hage, J. Hendel, and P. Stentoft. 1992. Omeprazole in the long-term treatment of severe gastro-oesophageal reflux disease in patients with systemic sclerosis. *Aliment. Pharmacol.* 6(5):565–577.

33. Johnson, D.A., W.E. Drane, J. Curran, S.B. Benjamin, S.J. Chobanian, K. Karvelis, and E.L. Cattau, Jr. 1987. Metoclopramide response in patients with progressive systemic sclerosis. Effect on esophageal and gastric motility abnormalities. *Arch. Intern. Med.* 147(9):1597–1601.

34. Verne, G.N., E.Y. Eaker, E. Hardy, and C.A. Sninsky. 1995. Effect of octreotide and erythromycin on idiopathic and scleroderma-associated intestinal pseudoobstruction. *Dig. Dis. Sci.* 40(9):1892–1901.

35. Kobayashi, T., M. Kobayashi, M. Naka, K. Nakajima, A. Momose, and M. Toi. 1993. Response to octreotide of intestinal pseudoobstruction and pneumatosis cystoides intestinalis associated with progressive systemic sclerosis. *Intern. Med.* 32(7):607–609.

36. Soudah, H.C., W.L. Hasler, and C. Owyang. 1991. Effect of octreotide on intestinal motility and bacterial overgrowth in scleroderma. *NEJM* 325(21):1461–1467.

37. Perlemuter, G., P. Cacoub, S. Chaussade, B. Wechsler, D. Couturier, and J.C. Piette. 1999. Octreotide treatment of chronic intestinal pseudoobstruction secondary to connective tissue diseases. *Arthritis Rheum.* 42(7):1545–1549.

38. Smith, E.A. and R.M. Silver. 2000. Can we improve outcome in systemic sclerosis? *J. Clin. Outcomes Management* 7(2):43–47.

22 Sjögren's Syndrome

Robert W. Hoffman and Eric L. Greidinger

CONTENTS

INTRODUCTION

The disease entity now widely recognized by the name Sjogren's syndrome (SS) was first fully characterized by Henrik Sjögren, who in 1933 described 13 women with xerostomia, keratoconjunctivitis, and rheumatoid arthritis (RA) *(1)*. Although SS is now widely recognized, the differences between classification criteria for the disease that was proposed by investigators from the United States, Europe, and Japan have yet to be resolved *(2–6)*. The disease is characterized by signs and symptoms attributable to infiltration and destruction of lacrimal and salivary glands by inflammatory cells, resulting in ocular and oral dryness. Systemic symptoms including fatigue are now also recognized to be significant features of SS. Extraglandular features of SS that may occur include: arthralgia, arthritis, Raynaud's phenomenon, myalgia, pulmonary disease, gastrointestinal (GI) disease, leukopenia, anemia, lymphadenopathy, neuropathy, vasculitis, renal tubular acidosis, and lymphoma *(7,8)*. SS can occur as a primary disease entity or be secondary to another disease, most commonly a rheumatic disease. SS appears to be a common disease having prevalence similar to that of RA. Prevalence rates of 0.05–3.00% have been published using different criteria for disease classification among different study populations *(9–12)*. Features indistinguishable from classically defined primary SS have been recently reported associated with viral infections with hepatitis C virus (HCV) *(13,14)*, the human immunodeficiency virus (HIV) *(15)*, and the human T-cell lymphotrophic virus (HTLV) *(16)*. Currently, however, neither these

From: *Modern Therapeutics in Rheumatic Diseases*
Edited by: G. C. Tsokos, et al. © Humana Press, Inc., Totowa, NJ

viruses or other known viruses are implicated as the cause of SS in the majority of patients classified as primary SS.

PATHOGENIC MECHANISMS THAT RATIONALIZE THE USE OF NEW TREATMENTS

There are at least five processes that may contribute to the pathogenesis of SS: glandular inflammation and immune destruction of tissues, hormonal abnormalities, autonomic dysfunction, viral infection, and abnormalities of programmed cell death (apopotosis).

Based on a large body of histopathologic studies in human disease and animal models, immune destruction of salivary and lacrimal glands is thought to be central to the pathogenesis of SS *(8)*. There is infiltration of these glands with CD4 positive T cells and there is oligoclonal expansion of T cells possessing select T-cell receptor (TCR) β-chain variable region genotypes *(17)*. There is also evidence of clonal proliferation of B cells, which appears to be antigen-driven *(18)*, and costimulatory molecules such as B7 are upregulated on salivary-gland epitaliel cells *(19)*. Controlled clinical trials of immune modulation using immunosuppressive or immunomodulatory drugs have been based on the premise of stopping glandular inflammation and destruction.

Some features of SS suggest that sex hormones and pituitary hormones could be important factors in disease pathogenesis. SS is increased in prevalence among women (with approximately a 9:1 female to male ratio), it has an increased frequency of onset after menopause and there are abnormalities in the serum levels of estrogens, androgens, and their metabolites in SS *(20)*. Also, the lactotrophic hormone prolactin has been shown to be abnormally elevated in some patients with SS *(21)*. Studies of hormonal replacement or hormonal suppression are based on the concept that hormones have a contributory role in the pathogenesis of SS. Estrogen and prolactin can have direct effects on the immune system, so their impact on SS could be mediated through the autoimmune mechanisms described earlier.

Another area of investigation in SS concerns functional abnormalities of glandular secretion, including effects of the autonomic nervous system on secretion. Normal salivary and lacrimal output has been shown to be maintained in animals and in humans until the gland is over 90% destroyed. However, this degree of destruction is not present in most patients with symptomatic SS. Inflammatory destruction of salivary and lacrimal glands may therefore not fully account for the symptoms of SS. Evidence has been presented of functional denervation of salivary glands in addition to varying degree of glandular destruction *(22)*. Such autonomic dysfunction could in part explain why the glands do not function normally, despite only moderate tissue destruction. Functional abnormalities of the sympathetic and parasympathetic nervous system could contribute to gland dysfunction and could also contribute to fatigue and other systemic symptoms *(23,24)*. One possible mechanism of autonomic nerve dysfunction is through antibody-mediated disruption of muscarinic receptors. Recently, investigators have reported that M3 muscarinic acetylcholine receptor-reactive antibodies can be detected in SS and suggest this may be their mechanism of action *(25,26)*. Studies on the role of the autonomic dysfunction in the pathogenesis of SS provide a conceptual basis for clinical trials of agents directed at restoring normal autonomic function in SS.

There has been long-standing interest in the hypothesis that SS has a viral etiology. In fact, studies have demonstrated that patients infected with HCV, HIV, and HTLV can have features of SS *(13–16)*. In addition, a viral infection triggering event resulting in unregulated or perpetuated immune recognition of self or altered-self antigen has been proposed as another related mechanism of disease *(27)*. Apoptosis or abnormalities of apoptosis could also be directly involved in the pathogenesis of SS; for example, by generating altered self-antigen or by failing to downregulate an antiviral immune response *(see* below) *(28,29)*. These concepts in part form the rationale for the empiric use of agents with antiviral activity in treating SS.

Finally, the process of programmed cell death called apoptosis has become the focus of much current research on the pathogenesis of autoimmunity *(30)*. For example, Fleck et al. have reported that murine cytomegalovirus (CMV) can induce a SS-like disease in C57Bl/-*lpr/lpr* mice *(28)*. Using congenic mice possessing the defective apoptosis-related gene Fas *(lpr)* on the C57 background, they found that a defect in Fas-mediated apoptosis (which is necessary for downregulation of the immune response) can result in a chronic inflammatory destruction of the salivary glands that resembles SS.

ANIMAL DATA

There are a large number of spontaneous and induced animal models of SS that have been reported *(31)*. Jonsson and Skarstein have recently published an excellent review of this topic *(32)*. Animal data have provided important new insights into such applications as the use of hormonal manipulation and immunosuppressive agents to treat SS. Topical androgen-therapy treatment in a rabbit model has suggested that these compounds may be beneficial to treat SS *(33)*. Administration of androgenic compounds to murine models of SS has also shown beneficial effects on salivary- and lacrimal-gland inflammation *(34,35)*. Topical administration of cyclosporin A to the eye in murine models of SS has been shown to reduce inflammation in the lacrimal and submandibular glands *(36,37)*. Recently, the use of CLT4Ig has been reported to be highly effective in treating the New Zealand black/New Zealand white (NZB/NZW) model of SS *(38)*. Preliminary gene-therapy studies have demonstrated that recombinant adenovirus vectors can be used for gene delivery into animal models of SS *(39)*. Future studies propose to use this approach to deliver and locally express cDNA encoding functionally important genes that might restore salivary secretion in SS models, such as aquaporin 1.

REVIEW OF CLINICAL TRIALS

Although many questions remain in the overall management of SS, results from recently published clinical trials have provided direction for an evidenced-based approach to therapy in SS. The present summary is the result of a comprehensive MEDLINE search for all articles relating to SS and therapy as of July 2001, with a focus on recent studies. The evidence-based record presented here for the management of SS consists of controlled trials, open-label trials and highly selected case reports.

A randomized, placebo-controlled, fixed-dose, multicenter trial of pilocarpine tablets for the treatment of dry-mouth and dry-eye symptoms in SS has demonstrated that 5 mg of pilocarpine taken four times a day results in subjective and objective improvement of SS *(40)*. Subjective features of patient and physician global assessment of dry eyes and dry mouth were improved, as were objective measures of salivary-flow rates in this study involving 373 patients. Open-label trials have demonstrated that parentally administered interferon-α (IFN-α) resulted in improvement in salivary production *(41)*. Furthermore, a single-blinded, placebo-controlled, fixed dose trial of low-dose oral IFN-α involving 60 patients demonstrated significant increase in salivary-flow rates, decreased salivary-gland lymphocytic infiltration, as well as improvement of subjective symptoms of SS *(42)*. The lozenge formulation of oral IFN-α is currently available only through clinical trials. An open-label trial of methotrexate taken orally at a dose of 0.2 mg/kg body weight weekly, involving 18 patients with primary SS, reported improvement of subjective symptoms, such as dry eyes and mouth, but did not result in improvement of any of the objective parameters measured *(43)*.

An open-label trial of the antiviral agent zidovudine (AZT) performed on seven patients was reported to result in improvement in patient global assessment and physician global assessment, the subjective symptoms of, dry eyes, dry mouth, fatigue, and the objective measures of Schirmer's test, tear break-up time (TBUT), and Rose Bengal score *(44)*. Topical treatment of the parotid gland using corticosteroid irrigation has been reported to increase salivary-gland flow rates in a study that included 24 patients with primary SS and seven patients with secondary SS *(45)*. For connective-tissue disease patients (including one with primary SS) with interstitial lung disease, treatment with intravenous-pulse cyclophosphamide combined with prednisone has been reported to beneficial in a study of six patients *(46)*. A case report has also described successful treatment of steroid-resistant interstitial lung disease in primary SS using low-dose cyclosporin *(47)*. A case report has also claimed successful treatment of the peripheral neuropathy associated with primary SS using high-dose, intravenous immunoglobulin *(48)* in several patients. A double-blinded, placebo-controlled trial of azathioprine *(49)* and a 2-yr, double-blind, crossover trial of hydroxychloroquine failed to demonstrate clinical benefit in SS *(50)*.

CURRENT RECOMMENDATION

Treatment of SS should be individualized on a case-by-case basis, concentrating on stopping debilitating and life-threatening disease expression whenever possible. Most patients have mild disease that requires minimal intervention. For this group, the use of with potentially toxic therapy is not justified. A challenge for the clinician is to identify the minority of patients who may develop life-threatening manifestations that require aggressive treatment. This section is a summary drawn from insights learned from the Animal Data section, the Review of Clinical Trials section, extrapolations from other conditions, personal communications, and the longitudinal experience of practitioners who have followed cohorts of SS patients.

Oral Cavity and Nose

The goal of preventative oral care is to stop both tooth decay and the development of periodontal disease. Preventative care consists of good oral hygiene; regular professional dental preventative care, including fluoride application; supplemental oral fluoride;

and a diet low in sugar content. Symptomatic palliative care consists of oral hydration, nighttime humidification of the air and salivary stimulants, including: sugar-free gum, sugarless hard candies, systemic secreatogogues (e.g., pilocarpine), or low-voltage electrical stimulation (i.e., Salitron™ device). Detection and therapy of oral microbial pathogens, especially *Candida* species, is believed to be important is slowing or stopping tooth decay and periodontal disease. The identification and use of a disease-modifying drug that reduces many or all of the clinical features of SS is of course ultimately desired.

Eye

The systemic secretogogue pilocarpine has been demonstrated beneficial in controlled trials to relieve ocular symptoms. Clinical experience suggests that topical tear-conservation methods, such as tear-duct occlusion, and the use of topical tear substitutes may provide symptomatic relief in some patients. Similarly, topical application of mucolytic agents, steroids, cyclosporin A, or androgens are felt to be of benefit in select patients.

Joints and Muscle

Arthralgia and arthritis may respond to nonsteroidal, anti-inflammatory drugs (NSAID). The newer cyclooxygenase-2 (COX-2) specific NSAID appear to have potential advantage of a lower risk of serious gastrointestinal complications *(51,52)*. Disease-modifying, anti-rheumatic drugs (DMARDs), including hydroxychloroquine and methotrexate, may be effective for arthritis. Patients with primary and secondary fibromyalgia have been demonstrated to respond to the antidepressant imipramine, as well as cyclobenzaprine, aerobic exercise, and biofeedback in controlled trials. In SS imipramine may be intolerable owing to its drying effects, however. Although the newer serotonin-release inhibitors have less drying effect and are effective in treating depression, they have been variably reported to have efficacy for fibromyalgia in controlled trials *(53,54)*.

Skin

Itching: Aggressive use of skin moisturizers is often helpful. Itching can be manifestation of autoimmune liver disease, which can be associated with SS.

Reproductive

Pregnancy: Patients possessing anti-Ro/SS-A antibodies are now known to be at increased risk for fetal loss, complete congenital heart block in the fetus, and neonatal lupus syndrome in the newborn. This topic has recently been reviewed *(55)* and information on National Instiues of Health (NIH)-sponsored registries and clinical trials for this and other rheumatic diseases can be found at: www. nih.gov/niams. Vaginal dryness and dyspareunia can be treated with water-soluble gels, such as KY™ gel.

Lungs

Fibrosing alveolitis: Document in suspicious cases with high-resolution computed tomography (HRCT). At centers with expertise in bronchoalveolar lavage (BAL), this may provide useful information to guide diagnosis and treatment. In advanced or progressive cases consider aggressive immunosuppression with high-dose corticosteroids plus cyclophosphamide or cyclosporin A.

Infection prophylaxis: Patients should receive influenza and pneumococcal vaccines. It is uncertain if currently available hemophilus vaccines benefit adults with rheumatic diseases.

Nervous System

Depression is common and has been proven to be increased in some rheumatic diseases, such as RA. Depression, when sought for and diagnosed, is highly treatable. Serious central nervous system (CNS) involvement can uncommonly occur in SS and may require aggressive therapy with moderate-high dose corticosteroid and immunosuppressive agents, such as cyclophosphamide *(56)*.

Systemic

Fatigue/fever: Fatigue is a common symptom among SS patients. It remains a challenging feature of disease to treat in many patients. Evidence of depression and fibromyalgia should be sought and treated, as these may contribute to the symptoms of fatigue. Exercise deconditioning may contribute to fatigue and a program of supervised regular exercise can provide health benefits to all patients including those with fatigue. Fever and fatigue may respond to NSAID or hydroxychloroquine. Careful evaluation for unrecognized pulmonary disease, thyroid disease, or cardiac disease should also be performed in such patients.

Vasculitis: Evidence for infection with HCV should be sought and treated if detected and liver disease of appropriate stage is documented by biopsy. Infection with HIV should also be considered. Small-vessel vasculitis may not require therapy. Various unproven treatments have been proposed including corticosteroids, immunosuppressive, antimalarial and pulse immunoglobulin.

Cryoglobulinemia: Evidence for infection with HCV should be sought. Treatment with IFN-α can be effective. Association of HCV and SS is currently controversial with associations described in Italy and France but not in a number of other countries. Plasmapheresis or plasma exchange may be beneficial in severe cases of cryoglobulinemia.

Psychosocial: Patient support organizations can help patients cope with their illness, and organizations such as the Sjögren's Syndrome Foundation and the Arthritis Foundation can be found in many larger cities or accessed through their publications and web sites (www.sjogrens.com, www.arthritisfoundation.org).

SIDE EFFECTS AND PRECAUTIONS

Many of the drugs used to treat SS are the same as those used to treat the other rheumatic diseases. All of the hazards these drugs present in other contexts should be anticipated in SS. There are concerns that estrogen-containing compounds, and perhaps other hormones, should not be used in patients with the lupus anticoagulant or anti-phospholipid antibodies.

Pilocarpine is contraindicated in patients with uncontrolled asthma, unstable cardiovascular disease, closed-angle glaucoma, uveitis, gastric or duodenal ulcers, and during pregnancy.

CONCLUSIONS

The synopsis of the state-of-the-art SS treatment is drawn from insights learned from basis studies of animal models, clinical trials data, personal communications, and the longitudinal experience of practitioners who have followed cohorts of SS patients. Most patients will have mild disease that requires a balanced approach in therapy, concentrating potentially toxic therapies on mitigating debilitating and life-threatening disease expression. Fortunately, a minority of patients may develop life-threatening manifestations that require aggressive treatment. The establishment of widely accepted classification would assist investigators in future clinical trials in SS. Ultimately, additional clinical trials specifically targeting the management of SS are needed to bring the management of this very common disorder into the era of evidenced-based medicine.

ACKNOWLEDGMENTS

This work was supported by the Medical Research Service, Department of Veterans Affairs and NIH Grant AR43308.

REFERENCES

1. Sjögren, H. 1933. Zur kenntnis der keratoconjunctivitis sicca. *Acta Opthalmol.* 11:1–151.

2. Fox, R.I., C. Robinson J. Curd, P. Michelson, R. Bone, and F.V. Howell. 1986. Suggested criteria for classification of Sjögren's syndrome. *Scand. J. Rheumatol.* 61:28–30.

3. Manthorpe, R., P. Oxholm, J.U. Prause, and M. Schiodt. 1986. The Copenhagen criteria for Sjögren's syndrome. *Scand. J. Rheumatol.* 61:19–21.

4. Yamada, K., S. Hayasaka, and T. Setogawa. 1990. Test results in patients with Sjögren's syndrome defined by the Japanese criteria. *Acta. Ophthalmol.* (Copenh.) 68:80–86.

5. Vitali, C., S. Bombardieri, H. Moutsopoulos, G. Balestrieri, W. Bencivelli, R.M. Bernstein, et al. 1993. Preliminary criteria for the classification of Sjögren's syndrome: results of a prospective concerted action supported by the European Community. *Arthritis Rheum.* 36:340–347.

6. Vitali, C., S. Bombardieri, H.M. Moutsopoulos, J. Coll, R. Gerli, P.Y. Hatron, et al. 1996. Assessment of the European classification criteria for Sjögren's syndrome in a series of clinically defined cases: results of a prospective multicentre study. *Ann. Rheum. Dis.* 55:116–121.

7. Bloch, K.J., W.W. Buchanan M.J. Wohl, and J.J. Bunim. 1965. Sjögren's syndrome: a clinical, pathological and serological study of sixty-two cases. *Medicine* 44:187–231.

8. Sharp, G.C. and R.W. Hoffman. 1999. Mixed connective tissue disease, overlap syndromes and Sjögren's syndrome. *In* Systemic Lupus Erythematosus, 3rd ed. R.G. Lahita, editor. Academic Press, New York, pp. 551–573.

9. Jacobsson, L.T.H., T.E. Axell, B.U. Hansen, V.J. Henricsson, A. Larsson, K. Lieberkind, et al. 1989. Dry eyes or mouth. An epidemiological study in Swedish adults, with special reference to primary Sjögren's syndrome. *J. Autoimmun.* 2:521–527.

10. Bjerrum, K. 1997. Keratoconjunctivitis sicca and primary Sjögren's syndrome in a Danish population aged 30–60 years. *Acta. Ophthalmol. Scand.* 75:281–286.

11. Dafni, U.G., G. Tzioufas, P. Staikos, F.N. Skopouli, and H.M. Moutsopoulos. 1997. Prevalence of Sjögren's syndrome in a closed rural community. *Ann. Rheum. Dis.* 56:521–525.

12. Hochberg, M.C., J. Tielsch, B. Munoz, K. Bandeen-Roche, S.K. West, and O.D. Schein. 1998. Prevalence of symptoms of dry mouth and their relationship to saliva production in community dwelling elderly: the SEE project. *J. Rheumatol.* 25:486–491.

13. Haddad, J., P. Deny, C. Munz-Gotheil, J.C. Ambrosini, J.C. Trinchet, D. Pateron, et al. 1992. Lymphocytic sialadenitis of Sjögren's syndrome associated with chronic hepatitis C virus liver disease. *Lancet* 339:321–323.

14. Garcia-Carrasco M., M. Ramos R. Cervera J. Font, J. Vidal, F.J. Munoz, et al. 1997. Hepatitis C virus infection in primary Sjögren's syndrome: prevalence and clinical significance in a series of 90 patients. *Ann. Rheum. Dis.* 56:173–175.

15. Itescu, S. and R. Winchester. 1992. Diffuse infiltrative lymphocytosis syndrome: a disorder occurring in human immunodeficiency virus-1 infection that may present as a sicca syndrome. *Rheum. Dis. Clin. North. Am.* 18:683–697.

16. Terada, K., S. Katamine, K. Eguchi, R. Moriuchi, M. Kita, H. Shimada, et al. 1994. Prevalence of serum and salivary antibodies to HTLV-1 in Sjögren's syndrome. *Lancet.* 344:1116–1119.

17. Sumida, T., F. Yonaha, T. Maeda, E. Tanabe, T. Koike, H. Tomioka, and S. Yoshida. 1992. T-cell receptor repertoire of infiltrating T-cells in lips of Sjögren's syndrome patients. *J. Clin. Invest.* 89:681–685.

18. Stott, D.I., F. Hiepe, M. Hummel, G. Steinhauser, and C. Berek. 1998. Antigen-driven clonal proliferation of B cells within the target tissue of an autoimmune disease: the salivary glands of patients with Sjögren's syndrome. *J. Clin. Invest.* 102:938–946.

19. Manoussakis, M.N., I.D. Dimitriou, E.K. Kapsogeorgou, G. Xanthou, S. Paikos, M. Polihronis, and H.M. Moutsopoulos. 1999. Expression of B7 costimulatory molecules by salivary gland epithelial cells in patients with Sjögren's syndrome. *Arthritis Rheum.* 42:229–239.

20. Lahita, R.G. 1996. The connective tissue disease and the overall influence of gender. *Int. J. Fertil. Menopausal. Stud.* 41:156–165.

21. Haga, H.J. and T. Rygh. 1999. The prevelance of hyperprolactinemia in patients with primary Sjögren's syndrome. *J. Rheumatol.* 26:1291–1295.

22. Mandl, T., L. Jacobsson, B. Lilja, G. Sundkvist, and R. Manthorpe. 1997. Disturbances of autonomic nervous function in primary Sjögren's syndrome. *Scand. J. Rheumatol.* 26:401–406.

23. Bonafede, R.P., D.C. Downey, and R.M. Bennett. 1995. An association of fibromyalgia with primary Sjögren's syndrome: a prospective study of 72 patients. *J. Rheumatol.* 22:133–136.

24. Yunus, M.B., F.X. Hussey, and J.C. Aldag. 1993. Antinuclear antibodies and connective tissue disease features in fibromyalgia syndrome: a controlled study. *J. Rheumatol.* 20:1557–1560.

25. Bacman, S., C. Perez Leiros, L. Sterin-Borda, O. Hubscher, R. Arana, and E. Borda. 1998. Autoantibodies against lacrimal gland M3 muscarinic acetylcholine receptors in patients with primary Sjögren's syndrome. *Invest. Opthalmol. Vis. Sci.* 39:151–156.

26. Robinson, C.P., J. Brayer, S. Yamachika, T.R. Esch, A.B. Peck, C.A. Stewart, et al. 1998. Transfer of human serum IgG to NOD.Igμ^{null} mice reveals a role for autoantibodies in the loss of secretory function of exocrine tissues in Sjögren's syndrome. *Proc. Natl. Acad. Sci. USA* 95:7538–7543.

27. Scofield, R.H., W.D. Dickey, K.W. Jackson, J.A. James, and J.B. Harley. 1991 A common autoepitope near the carboxyl terminus of the 60-kD Ro ribonucleoprotein: sequence similarity with a viral protein. *J. Clin. Immunol.* 11:378–388.

28. Fleck, M., E.R. Kern, T. Zhou, B. Lang, and J.D. Mountz. 1998. Murine cytomegalovirus induces a Sjögren's syndrome-like disease in C57Bl/6-*lpr/lpr* mice. *Arthritis Rheum.* 41:2175–2184.

29. Kong, L., N. Ogawa, T. Nakabayashi, G.T. Liu, E. D'Souza, H.S. McGuff, et al. 1997. *Fas* and *Fas* ligand expression in the salivary glands of patients with primary Sjögren's syndrome. *Arthritis Rheum.* 40:87–97.

30. Rosen, A. and L. Casciola-Rosen. 1999. Clustering and proteolytic cleavage of autoantigens in surface blebs of apoptotic cells. *In* Lupus: Molecular and Cellular Pathogenesis. G.M. Kammer and G.C. Tsokos, editors. Humana Press, Totowa, NJ. 65–78.

31. Hoffman, R.W. and S.E. Walker. 1987. Animal models in Sjögren's syndrome. *In* Sjögren's Syndrome: Clinical and Immunologic Aspects. N. Talal and H.J. Moutopoulos, editors. Springer-Verlag, New York. 266–290.

32. Jonsson, R. and K. Skarstein. 2001. Experimental models of Sjögren's syndrome, in The Molecular Pathology of Autoimmune Diseases, in press.

33. Sullivan, D.A., L.A. Wickham, E.M. Rocha, K.L. Krenzer, B.D. Sullivan, R. Steagall, et al. 1999. Androgens and dry eye in Sjögren's syndrome. *Ann. NY Acad. Sci.* 22:312–324.

34. Sullivan, D.A. and J.A. Edwards. 1997. Androgen stimulation of lacrimal gland function in mouse models of Sjögren's syndrome. *J. Steroid Biochem. Mol. Biol.* 60:237–245.

35. Toda, I., L.A. Wickham, and D.A. Sullivan. 1998. Gender and androgen treatment influence the expression of proto-oncogenes and apoptotic factors in lacrimal and salivary tissues of MRL/lpr mice. *Clin. Immunol. Immunopathol.* 86:59–71.

36. Jabs, D.A., B. Lee, C.L. Burek, A.M. Saboori, and R.A. Predergast. 1996. Cyclosporine therapy suppresses ocular and lacrimal gland disease in MRL/Mp-lpr/lpr mice. *Invest. Ophthalmol. Vis. Sci.* 37: 377–383.

37. Tsubota, K., I. Saito, N. Ishimaru, and Y. Hayashi. 1998. Use of topical cyclosporin A in a primary Sjögren's syndrome mouse model. *Invest. Ophthalmol. Vis. Sci.* 39:1551–1559.

38. Sugai, S. 1999. Suppression of the Sjögren's syndrome-like disease in NZB/W F1 mice by blockade of the CD40L/CD40 interaction. VII International Symposium on Sjögren's Syndrome, Venice. December 2, 1999 (Abstract).

39. Kefalides, P.T. 1999. Saliva research leads to new diagnostic tools and therapeutic options. *Ann. Int. Med.* 131:992–993.

40. Vivino, F.B., I. Al-Hashimi, Z. Khan, F.G. LeVeque, P.L. Salisbury, T.K. Tran-Johnson, et al. 1999. Pilocarpine tablets for the treatment of dry mouth and dry eye symptoms in patients with Sjögren's syndrome. *Arch. Intern. Med.* 159:174–181.

41. Shiozawa, S., Y. Tanaka, and K. Shiozawa. 1998. Single-blinded controlled trial of low-dose oral IFN-α for the treatment of xerostomia in patients with Sjögren's syndrome. *J. Interferon Cytokine Res.* 18:255–262.

42. Ship, J.A., P.C. Fox, J.E. Michalek, M.J. Cummins, and A.B. Richards. IFN Protocol Study Group. 1999. Treatment of primary Sjögren's syndrome with low-dose national human interferon-α administered by the oral mucosal route: a phase II clinical trial. *J. Interferon Cytokine Res.* 19:943–951.

43. Skopouli, F.N., P. Jagiello, N. Tsifetaki, and H.M. Moutsopoulos. 1996. Methotrexate in primary Sjögren's syndrome. *Clin. Exp. Rheumatol.* 14:555–558.

44. Steinfeld, S.D., P. Demols, J.-P. Van Vooren, E. Cogan, and T. Appelboom. 1999. Zidovudine in primary Sjögren's syndrome. *Rheumatology* (Oxford) 38:814–817.

45. Izumi, M., K. Eguchi, H. Nakamura, Y. Takagi, Y. Kawabe, and T. Nakamura. 1998. Corticosteroid irrigation of parotid gland for treatment of xerostomia in patients with Sjögren's syndrome. *Ann. Rheum. Dis.* 57:464–469.

46. Schnabel, A., M. Reuter, and W.L. Gross. 1998. Intravenous pulse cyclophosphamide in the treatment of interstitial lung disease due to collagen vascular diseases. *Arthritis Rheum.* 41:1215–1220.

47. Ogasawara, H., M. Sekiya, A. Murashima, T. Hishikawa, Y. Tokano, I. Sekigawa, et al. 1998. Very low-dose cyclosporin treatment of steroid-resistant interstitial pneumonitis associated with Sjögren's syndrome. *Clin. Rheumatol.* 17:160–162.

48. Pascual, J., C. Cid, and J. Berciano. 1998. High-dose IV immunoglobulin for peripheral neuropathy associated with Sjögren's syndrome. *Neurology* 51:650–651.

49. Price, E.J., S.P. Rigby, U. Clancy, and P.J.W. Venables. 1998. A double blind placebo controlled trial of azathioprine in the treatment of primary Sjögren's syndrome. *J. Rheum.* 25:896–899.

50. Kruize, A.A., R.J. Hené, C.G.M. Kallenberg, O.P. van Bijsterveld, A. van der Heide, L. Kater, and J.W.J. Bijlsma. 1993. Hydroxychloroquine treatment for primary Sjögren's syndrome: a two year double blind crossover trial. *Ann. Rheum. Dis.* 52:360–364.

51. Simon, L.S., A.L. Weaver, D.Y. Graham, A.J. Kivitz, P.E. Lipsky, R.C. Hubbard, et al. 1999. Anti-inflammatory and upper gastrointestinal effects of celecoxib in rheumatoid arthritis: a randomized controlled trial. *JAMA* 282:1921–1928.

52. Laine, L., S. Harper, T. Simon, R. Bath, J. Johanson, H. Schwartz, et al. 1999. A randomized trial comparing the effect of rofecoxib, a cyclooxygenase 2-specific inhibitor, with that of ibuprofen on the gastroduodenal mucosa of patients with osteoarthritis. *Gastroenterology* 117:1002–1005.

53. Goldenberg, D., M. Mayskiy, C. Mossey, R. Ruthazer, and C. Schmid. 1996. A randomized, double-blind crossover trial of fluoxetine and amitriptyline in the treatment of fibromyalgia. *Arthritis Rheum.* 39:1852–1859.

54. Norregaard, J., H. Volkmann, and B. Danneskiold-Samsoe. 1995. A randomized controlled trial of citalopram in the treatment of fibromyalgia. *Pain* 61:445–449.

55. Buyon, J.P. 1998. Neonatal lupus and autoantibodies reactive with SSA/Ro-SSB/La. *Scand. J. Rheumatol.* (Suppl.) 107:23–30.

56. Niemela, R.K. and M. Hakala. 1999. Primary Sjögren's syndrome with severe central nervous system disease. *Semin. Arthritis Rheum.* 29:4–13 (Review).

23   Mixed Connective Tissue Disease

Robert W. Hoffman and Eric L. Greidinger

CONTENTS

INTRODUCTION
PATHOGENIC MECHANISMS THAT RATIONALIZE THE USE OF NEW
    TREATMENTS
ANIMAL DATA
CLINICAL TRIALS
CURRENT RECOMMENDATIONS
SIDE EFFECTS AND PRECAUTIONS
CONCLUSIONS
ACKNOWLEDGMENTS
REFERENCES

INTRODUCTION

In the early 1970s, Sharp and colleagues described a series of patients in whom features of Systemic lupus erythematosis (SLE), scleroderma, and inflammatory myositis were found in association with autoantibodies to the U1-ribonucleoprotein (RNP) antigen *(1)*. This syndrome complex was called mixed connective tissue disease (MCTD). Although several classification criteria for MCTD have been published, there remains no universally accepted definition of the condition *(2–5)*. The existence of MCTD as a clinically, immunogenetically, and serologically distinct entity remains a subject of controversy. An excellent review of MCTD and the controversy surrounding its classification has recently been published *(6)*. In support of the concept of MCTD, recent published data demonstrate the distinctive serologic associations of anti-U1-70kD-specific, anti-U1-RNA-specific, and anti-heteronuclear ribonucleoprotein (hnRNP) A2/RA33-specific antibodies with MCTD *(7–9)*. Furthermore, the association of anti-RNP and/or MCTD with the genetic marker HLA-DR4 has been reported from studies done in a number of different countries *(6,7,10,11)*. Finally, it would appear that the concept of MCTD is useful to the clinician regardless of the controversy over nomenclature, because MCTD identifies a group of patients in whom increased surveillance for specific end-organ manifestations may improve patient care *(12)*.

The most common systems affected in MCTD that lead to significant mortality or morbidity are the lungs, the joints, the peripheral vasculature, and the gastrointestinal

From: *Modern Therapeutics in Rheumatic Diseases*
Edited by: G. C. Tsokos, et al. © Humana Press, Inc., Totowa, NJ

(GI) tract *(12)*. Skin disease and mild myositis are also common in MCTD patients, whereas central nervous system (CNS) or renal disease is uncommon *(12)*. Regrettably, few methodologically strong studies have investigated treatment interventions for these or other target organs in MCTD. Advances in the management of MCTD have developed anecdotally from treatments used in SLE, scleroderma, polymyositis, rheumatoid arthritis (RA), and related disorders. Insights into the immune pathophysiology expressed in MCTD patients does suggest investigational treatments for the underlying auto-immune process that may be helpful in the future.

PATHOGENIC MECHANISMS THAT RATIONALIZE THE USE OF NEW TREATMENTS

Several lines of evidence implicate autoimmunity in the pathogenesis of MCTD. MCTD shares clinical manifestations with other autoimmune conditions *(8)*. Also, MCTD patients and family members of MCTD patients may have an increased incidence of other autoimmune diseases *(13)*. Most importantly, antibodies to RNP are an essential element of MCTD *(8)*. Moreover, the anti-RNP immune response in MCTD shows features of being antigen driven: anti-RNP antibodies undergo isotype switching, B-cell and T-cell responses develop to the same antigens, and the immune response spreads over time to additional epitopes on the same antigen *(14,15)* as well as to other physically associated RNP antigens *(16,17)*. Anti-RNP responses often first develop against the U1-70kD RNP antigen *(12,18)*. U1-70kD has been shown to be uniquely susceptible to post-translational modifications by apoptotic cell death, by metal-catalyzed oxidation, and by granzyme B-induced cleavage *(19,20)*. Antigen modification by apoptotic cell death has been associated with self-immunity in lupus *(21)*, antigen modification by metal-catalyzed oxidation has been associated with self-immunity in scleroderma *(20)*, and antigen modification by granzyme B-induced cleavage has been may be linked to self-immunity in inflammatory myositis *(22)*. The ability to bridge multiple modalities of self-immunity may explain why subjects with anti-U1-70kD immunity show features of lupus, scleroderma, and myositis. The clinical expression of disease in patients with U1-70kD antibodies follows with the form(s) of modified U1-70kD to which they mount an autoimmune response. A higher proportion of patients who strongly recognize the apoptotic form of U1-70kD have lupus-like skin disease, whereas a higher proportion of patients who strongly recognize the oxidatively modified form of U1-70kD have scleroderma-like Raynaud's phenomenon *(23)*. A molecular link through RNP autoimmunity has been similarly drawn between MCTD and RA via the hnRNP-A2/RA33 molecule, an antigen recognized at different epitopes by MCTD and RA sera *(6)*. Thus, a feature of autoimmunity in MCTD may be overlap with the autoimmune responses seen in other rheumatic conditions, manifesting in the unique immunogenetic context observed for MCTD *(7,24,25)*. Emerging approaches to the control of the autoimmune process have one of three goals: reducing the amount of immunologically active antigen that is produced, modulating the proimmune context in which antigen is encountered, and limiting the damage produced by inflammatory pathways.

Treatments to reduce the amount of immunologically active antigen are in an early phase of development, because the antigens that drive the immune response in MCTD are still incompletely understood. There are at least two ways of reducing the amount of immunologically active antigen: decreasing production of antigen or increasing clearance. One (anecdotally) effective therapy for photosensitive skin disease in MCTD already acts to decrease antigen production: sun avoidance and sunscreen use reduces the production of apoptotic antigens from keratinocytes. Preliminary studies are investigating pharmacologic inhibitors of the production of modified forms of RNP antigens (unpublished data). Recent observations that early complement components facilitate the clearance of apoptotic material (26), and that impaired clearance of apoptotic material is seen in autoimmune disease patients (27) has led to study of whether supplementation of antigen-clearance pathways may also have a role in MCTD therapy.

A dramatic increase in the number of immunomodulators being studied for rheumatic-disease therapy has followed the recent boom in understanding of immune pathophysiology. Some of the approaches that may hold promise in MCTD include anergizing antigen exposure, T-cell second-signal blockade, and alteration of the balance of proinflammatory vs anti-inflammatory cytokines. Clinical trials of agents with these actions are at a more advanced stage in other rheumatic diseases than in MCTD, and are discussed elsewhere in this book.

Approaches to limiting inflammatory damage in MCTD are also expanding as inflammatory pathways become further elucidated. Inhibitors of proinflammatory cytokines such as tumor necrosis factor (TNF) and interleukin-1 (IL-1) are available for clinical study. Inhibitors of complement-mediated inflammation are also becoming available. Cyclooxygenase COX-2 inhibitors may be only the first step toward the development of more specific and effective inhibitors of eicosanoid-associated inflammatory responses (28,29).

Emerging treatments specific for MCTD may place particular emphasis on the control of pulmonary hypertension. Pulmonary hypertension is a frequent finding in MCTD patients, and is an important cause of disability and death (12). The vasculopathy of MCTD that has been linked to pulmonary hypertension is characterized by intimal thickening and medial muscular hypertrophy of the arteries and arterioles without a cellular inflammatory infiltrate (12,30–32). Thus, the vascular lesion in MCTD is often reminiscent of the lesion described in primary pulmonary hypertension. Although an autoimmune basis for this lesion may exist in MCTD, treatments that have relevance in primary pulmonary hypertension may merit special attention in the management of MCTD.

ANIMAL DATA

There is currently no animal model that fully encompasses the clinical manifestations of MCTD. Models in which RNP immunity develops that have been used to study other autoimmune conditions may have relevance to MCTD, however. Animal models with RNP immunity including MRL/lpr mice, NZB/W mice, Palmerston North mice, pristane-treated BALB/C mice, xeno-RNP immunized mice, and RNP-peptide immunized rabbits are characterized by a high prevalence of glomerulonephritis (33,34), unlike human MCTD. A number of treatment interventions have been reported in these models to attenuate nephritis and to improve survival. The relevance of these treatment trials to human MCTD absent renal disease is uncertain. Graft-vs-host disease (GVHD) has been proposed as a model of some features of scleroderma, and anti-RNP immunity has been reported in graft-vs-host models *(34)*, but the Raynaud's phenomenon-like peripheral vasculopathy typical of MCTD has not been observed in these models. The hepatic and cutaneous lesions of GVHD also differ from those commonly reported in MCTD, so the relevance to MCTD of treatments that may benefit these manifestations of GVHD are also uncertain. On the other hand, various animal models do demonstrate features consistent with MCTD. In some, inflammatory pulmonary disease, erosive arthritis, and/or myositis are observed *(35)*. Improvements in extra-renal manifestations of autoimmunity have been reported with protocols, such as cytotoxic drug therapy *(36)* and antibody-mediated T-cell depletion *(37)*. Combined blockade of the B7.1 and B7.2 molecules that provide T-cell costimulatory signals in MRL/lpr mice led to decreased levels of RNP antibodies *(38)*.

CLINICAL TRIALS

To our knowledge, no randomized, controlled clinical trials of therapeutics in the management of MCTD have been published. This reflects personal communications, plus the results of comprehensive MEDLINE searches for all articles relating to MCTD, mixed connective-tissue disease, or the topic "RNP and autoimmunity" as of July 2001. The evidence-based record for the management of MCTD consists of case reports, extrapolations from other conditions, and the longitudinal experience of practitioners who have followed cohorts of MCTD patients. Specific barriers to performing systematic trials in MCTD have hindered progress compared to other rheumatic diseases. First, longitudinal follow-up of MCTD cohorts has only recently pointed out the hazards of MCTD and the inadequacies of traditional corticosteroid-based management schemes *(12)*. Second, multicenter collaborative efforts at patient recruitment for MCTD studies have been infrequent. Finally, validated clinical indices of disease activity and damage have not yet emerged in MCTD as they have in lupus and SS *(39,40)*. Previous studies investigating the relationship of autoantibodies to activity have relied on SLE-activity indices, which may underreport MCTD manifestations including pulmonary and gastrointestinal (GI) involvement. Case reports of treatment specifically for MCTD have generally reported organ-specific responses to therapy, rather than improvements in global disease scores.

Two general approaches to disease management are discussed in the bulk of case reports of MCTD treatment: immunosuppression and treatment of vasculopathy. Because publication bias in favor of successful outcomes is expected, it is uncertain how to interpret positive outcomes in these reports. The natural history of MCTD includes a waxing and waning component in some patients, and some in some individuals MCTD may enter apparent remission irrespective of therapy *(12)*.

The most frequent immunosuppressant drugs reported for treatment of MCTD are steroids and cytotoxic agents *(8–12)*. In a cohort studied at the University of Missouri, roughly two-thirds of patients who received these drugs were felt by their rheumatologists to have responded to corticosteroids and/or cytotoxic agents *(12)*. Failure of such regimens has been reported in MCTD, however *(41)*. Clinical manifestations of MCTD that overlap with lupus and inflammatory myositis have been reported to respond to similar treatment protocols *(8–12)*. Cytotoxic agents, typically cyclophosphamide, have been used in conjunction with higher doses of corticosteroids for major organ-threatening disease. Relatively mild manifestations including skin disease, serositis, nonerosive synovitis, and myositis have been reported to be responsive to nonsteroidal, anti-inflammatory drugs (NSAIDs), antimalarials, and/or steroids *(7–12)*. Some MCTD manifestations that are less typical for lupus or myositis have also been reported to improve with steroid and cytotoxic therapy. These include pulmonary hypertension, protein-losing enteropathy, and esophageal disease *(42–44)*. Methotrexate use, derived from the management of RA and inflammatory myositis, has been reported to be helpful for erosive arthritis and severe myositis in MCTD *(8–12)*. Published reports have not yet evaluated the potential utility of biologic response modifying agents such as anti-TNF therapies. Other potentially immunomodulatory treatments for MCTD have been reported. The lack of demonstrated efficacy for these treatments in other rheumatic diseases with which MCTD overlaps makes their role in MCTD therapy more questionable. Such therapies include plasmapheresis, intravenous gamma-globulin, photopheresis, and hyperbaric oxygen. The role of a vast range of other potential immunomodulators—ranging from nutritional supplements to immunoablation/hematopoietic stem cell transplantation—have not been examined in MCTD.

Treatment of vasculopathy in MCTD has concentrated on the use of vasodilators. Although vasculopathy leading to ischemia-reperfusion injury has been postulated as a mechanism inducing autoimmunity in scleroderma-spectrum diseases, the impact of vasoactive agents on the immune manifestations of MCTD have not been described. At least three distinct microvascular environments exist that show different patterns of response to vasodilators: the peripheral vasculature, the kidneys, and the lungs. Peripheral vasculopathy manifesting as Raynaud's phenomenon in MCTD responds to calcium-channel blockers and to prostaglandin-infusion therapy *(8–12,45)*. As in scleroderma, hypertensive renal crisis can occur in MCTD, and responds to therapy including angiotensin-converting enzyme (ACE) inhibitors *(46)*. Pulmonary hypertension in MCTD, like primary pulmonary hypertension, has responded in some cases to therapies including prostacyclin infusion, calcium-channel blockers, and ACE inhibitors *(47–50)*.

Published data exists for some additional therapies that are not presumed to be immunosuppressive or primarily vasoactive. Cisapride has been reported to be ineffective for lower esophageal dysfunction in MCTD *(51)*. Octreotide but not the promotility agents domperidone or cisapride have been beneficial for chronic intestinal pseudo-obstruction in two patients with MCTD *(52)*. Improved healing of digital ulcers owing to Raynaud's phenomenon in MCTD has been described with the use of a sargramostim graulocyte-monocyte colony stimulating factor (GM-CSF) topical cream *(53)*.

CURRENT RECOMMENDATIONS

Treatment for MCTD should be individualized on a case-by-case basis, concentrating on mitigating organ-specific disease expression. Some patients may have mild disease that requires minimal intervention, whereas others may develop life-threatening manifestations that require aggressive care. History and physical examination are felt to be adequate screening tools for clinically significant manifestations of MCTD with two exceptions: pulmonary hypertension and erosive arthritis. By the time that pulmonary hypertension or erosive arthritis become clinically evident, the ideal window to initiate therapy has already passed. Thus, additional studies, such as radiographs to assess for early joint erosions and diagnostic testing to assess for early evidence of pulmonary hypertension should be considered. A fall in carbon monoxide-diffusing capacity has been associated with the onset of pulmonary hypertension and findings on two-dimensional echocardiography have also been associated with pulmonary hypertension and therefore serial testing with these may identify patients at an early stage of disease. In our experience, the use of these tests alone or in combination are neither sensitive nor specific. However, they remain the best methods currently available. Recently, it has been reported that the presence of anti-cardiolipin antibodies identifies a subset of patients at risk of developing pulmonary hypertension *(12)*.

Lung

PULMONARY HYPERTENSION

Document and follow mild cases with serial pulmonary function testing and echocardiography. In severe or progressive cases, consider referral to a pulmonary hypertension specialist for right heart catheterization and vasodilator trial. Consider immunosuppression for vasodilator-unresponsive cases.

FIBROSING ALVEOLITIS

In suspicious cases, document with high-resolution computed tomography (HRCT) and/or bronchoalveolar lavage. Consider aggressive immunosuppression, as in scleroderma fibrosing alveolitis.

INFECTION PROPHYLAXIS

Patients should receive influenza and pneumococcal vaccines. It is uncertain if currently available hemophilus vaccines benefit adults with rheumatic diseases. Consider the potential for esophageal dysfunction to cause aspiration pneumonia.

Joints

EROSIVE ARTHRITIS

Early aggressive disease-modifying therapy patterned after the management of RA is appropriate. Bracing and surgery may be helpful in select cases to maintain function.

SYNOVITIS

NSAIDs and hydroxychloroquine are first-line options. In refractory cases, treat as with erosive disease.

Skin

PHOTOSENSITIVITY/LUPUS SKIN DISEASE

Sun avoidance and smoking cessation can help to control lesions. Antimalarials are often effective. Corticosteroids topically or systemically are helpful for self-limited flares. Anecdotally, azathioprine seems particularly effective if immunosuppressive therapy is required.

RAYNAUD'S PHENOMENON

Maintaining total body warmth and extremity warmth are essential. Calcium-channel blockers are effective at reducing the frequency and severity of episodes. For more severe cases, options taken from scleroderma management, including prostaglandin infusion, may have a role.

FIBROSIS/THICKENING

Relaxin, a promising agent for control of fibrosis in scleroderma, may have a role in MCTD. Localized regions may respond to Psoralin Ultra Violet A (PUVA) therapy. Physical therapy can help to maintain and restore mobility.

ITCHING

Aggressive use of skin moisturizers is often helpful. In some cases, itching is a manifestation of ongoing inflammation in the skin.

SUBCUTANEOUS NODULES

MCTD patients can develop rheumatoid nodules or calcinosis lesions. Surgery is effective for management of bothersome lesions.

Gut

ESOPHAGEAL REFLUX

Proton-pump inhibitors are effective. In some patients, high doses of proton-pump inhibitors or chronic therapy may be necessary to control symptoms. Referral for upper endoscopy to screen for Barrett's esophagus may be appropriate. Dilatation can be helpful for dysphagia.

CONSTIPATION

This common difficulty often is not mentioned by patients unless they are specifically asked. Fiber, fluids, and exercise should be emphasized. More severe lower GI manifestations of MCTD including pseudo-obstruction and pneumatosis intestinalis may require hospitalization and bowel rest. Octreotide may also be useful.

SICCA SYNDROME

As in other rheumatic diseases, secondary Sjögren's Syndrome can occur with MCTD.

Muscle

MYOSITIS

Steroids and, if needed, methotrexate are the standard of care. Some patients will have mild myositis with mild chronic elevation in creatine phosphokinase but without progression to clinically significant weakness, and can have their treatment titrated down.

FIBROMYALGIA

As in other inflammatory rheumatic diseases, the incidence of noninflammatory musculoskeletal aches may be increased in MCTD. This dimension of a patient's complaints should be addressed with multimodal chronic-pain management, rather than increasing aggressiveness of anti-rheumatic therapy. Assessment for depression, which also has increased incidence in rheumatic diseases, is also appropriate.

Systemic

Fever/Fatigue/Serositis

Steroids or NSAIDs can control a disease flare. Before increasing long-term, anti-rheumatic therapy, the possibility of occult infection or neoplasm should be excluded.

Hematologic

The spectrum of autoimmune cytopenias that can present in lupus are managed as in SLE when they occasionally occur in MCTD. Leukopenia is frequent and often requires no therapy. Mild to moderate thrombocytopenia may respond to treatment with low-dose corticosteroids.

Nephritis/Vasculitis

Aggressive immunosuppression is the standard of care for these unusual MCTD manifestations. Hypertension and renal insufficiency should be treated with ACE inhibitor for possible scleroderma renal crisis until proven otherwise if tolerated.

Reproductive Issues

Altered Sexual Response and Erectile dysfunction

Common in scleroderma patients, the prevalence in MCTD may also be high. Sildenafil may be beneficial.

Pregnancy

The effect of pregnancy on MCTD activity has not been studied. Avoidance of drugs that may be toxic to the fetus, close clinical follow-up, and referral to high-risk obstetrician are appropriate. Neonatal lupus can occur with RNP antibodies in the absence of Ro or La, but has been reported to cause only self-limited skin disease, not cardiac disease.

SIDE EFFECTS AND PRECAUTIONS

The drugs used to treat MCTD are the same as those used to treat the other rheumatic diseases with which it overlaps. All of the hazards these drugs present in other contexts should be anticipated in MCTD.

The use of some therapeutic agents for other conditions may lead to exacerbations in the context of MCTD. Some nonsteroidals, notably ibuprofen, may pose an increased risk of inducing aseptic meningitis in MCTD. A variety of other agents have been reported to be possibly associated with SLE flares, and are thus suspect in MCTD. These include photosensitizing drugs, external beam radiation, sulfa-containing antibiotics, estrogens, alfalfa, and echinacea.

CONCLUSIONS

The state of the art in the management of MCTD is taken from approaches to treating the other rheumatic diseases with which MCTD overlaps. In addition to applying treatment approaches taken from lupus, scleroderma, RA, and inflammatory myositis, MCTD is managed most effectively by remembering the target organs that are most at risk in this disease spectrum to guide surveillance and treatment. Improvements in therapy for MCTD in particular may emerge in the future from antigen-specific immunomodulation, or from improved understanding and therapy for the unique aspects of MCTD-associated pulmonary hypertension. Clinical trials specifically targeting the management of MCTD are needed to bring the management of MCTD into the era of evidence-based medicine.

ACKNOWLEDGMENTS

This work was supported by the Medical Research Service, Department of Veterans Affairs, and NIH Grant AR43308.

REFERENCES

1. Sharp, G.C., W.S. Irvin, E.M. Tan, R.G. Gould, and H.R. Holman. 1972. Mixed connective tissue disease: an apparently distinct rheumatic disease syndrome associated with a specific antibody to an extractable nuclear antigen (ENA). *Am. J. Med.* 52:148–159.

2. Sharp, G.C. 1987. Diagnostic criteria for classification of MCTD, in *Mixed Connective Tissue Disease and Antinuclear Antibodies.* R. Kasukawa and G.C. Sharp, editors. Elsevier, Amsterdam. 23–32.

3. Alarcón-Segovia, D. and M. Villareal. 1987. Classification and diagnostic criteria for mixed connective tissue disease, in *Mixed Connective Tissue Disease and Antinuclear Antibodies.* R. Kasukawa and G.C. Sharp, editors. Elsevier, Amsterdam. 33–40.

4. Kasukawa, R., T. Tojo, and S. Miyawaki. 1987. Preliminary diagnostic criteria for classification of mixed connective tissue disease, in *Mixed Connective Tissue Disease and Antinuclear Antibodies.* R. Kasukawa and G.C. Sharp, editors. Elsevier, Amsterdam. 41–47.

5. Porter, J.F., L.C. Kingsland, III, D.A.B. Lindberg, I. Shah, J.M. Benge, S.E. Hazelwood, et al. 1988. The AI/RHEUM knowledge-based computer consultant system in rheumatology: performance in the diagnosis of 59 connective tissue disease patients from Japan. *Arthritis Rheum.* 31:219–226.

6. Smolen, J.S. and G. Steiner. 1998. Mixed connective tissue disease: to be or not to be? *Arthritis Rheum.* 41:768–777.

7. Sharp, G.C. and R.W. Hoffman. 1999. Mixed connective tissue disease, overlap syndromes and Sjögren's syndrome, in *Systemic Lupus Erythematosus,* 3rd ed. R.G. Lahita, editor. Academic Press, New York.

8. Hoffman, R.W. 2001. Mixed connective tissue disease, in *Textbook of Nephrology,* 4th ed. S.G. Massry and R.J. Glassock, editors, pp. 787–790.

9. Hoffman, R.W. and E.L. Greidinger. 2000. Mixed connective tissue disease. *Curr. Opin. Rheum.,* 12:386–390.

10. Sharp, G.C. and R.W. Hoffman. 1995. Mixed connective tissue disease, in *Connective Tissue Diseases.* J. Belch and R. Zurier, editors. Chapman and Hall, London, pp. 151–178.

11. Hoffman, R.W. and G.C. Sharp. 1995. Is Anti-U1-70kD Autoantibody-positive connective tissue disease genetically distinct? *J. Rheumatol.* 22:586–589.

12. Burdt, M.A., R.W. Hoffman, S.L. Deutscher, G.S. Wang, J.C. Johnson, and G.C. Sharp. 1999. Long-term outcome in mixed connective tissue disease: longitudinal clinical and serologic findings. *Arthritis Rheum.* 42:899–909.

13. Ramos-Niembro, F. and D. Alarcon-Segovia. 1978. Familial aspects of mixed connective tissue disease (MCTD). *J. Rheumatol.* 5:433–440.

14. Nyman, U., I. Lundberg, E. Hedfors, M. Wahern, and I. Pettersson. 1992. IgG and IgM anti-sn-RNP reactivity in sequentially obtained serum samples from patients with connective tissue diseases. *Ann. Rheum. Dis.* 51:1307–1312.

15. Holyst, M-M., D.L. Hill, S.O. Hoch, and R.W. Hoffman. 1997. Analysis of human T cell and B cell responses against U small nuclear ribonucleoprotein 70-kd, B, and D polypeptides among patients with systemic lupus erythematosus and mixed connective tissue disease. *Arthritis Rheum.* 40:1493–1503.

16. James, J.A., T. Gross, H. Scofield, and J.B. Harley. 1995. Immunoglobulin epitope spreading and autoimmune disease after peptide immunization: Sm B/B′-derived PPPGMRPP and PPPGIRGP induce spliceosome autoimmunity. *J. Exp. Med.* 181:453–461.

17. Fatenejad, S., M. Bennett, J. Moslehi, and J. Craft. 1998. Influence of antigen organization on the development of lupus autoantibodies. *Arthritis Rheum.* 41:603–612.

18. Greidinger, E.L. and R.W. Hoffman. 1999. The U1-70kDa protein is often the first snRNP to which humoral immunity develops in patients with U1-70kDa antibodies. *Arthritis Rheum.* 42:S110 (Abstract).

19. Casciola-Rosen, L., F. Andrade, D. Ulanet, W.B. Wong, and A. Rosen, 1999. Cleavage by granzyme B is strongly predictive of autoantigen status: implications for initiation of autoimmunity. *J. Exp. Med.* 190:815–826.

20. Casciola-Rosen, L., F. Wigley, and A. Rosen. 1997. Scleroderma autoantigens are uniquely fragmented by metal-catalyzed oxidation reactions: Implications for pathogenesis. *J. Exp. Med.* 185: 71–79.

21. Utz, P.J. and P. Anderson. 1998. Posttranslational protein modifications, apoptosis, and the bypass of tolerance to autoantigens. *Arthritis Rheum.* 41:1152–1160.

22. Casciola-Rosen, L., A. Pluta, P. Plotz, K. Nagaraju, A. Cox, S. Morris, and A. Rosen. 1998. HPMS1 is a novel, frequently targeted myositis autoantigen which is cleaved by granzyme B but not by caspases during apoptosis. *Arthritis Rheum.* 41:S127 (Abstract).

23. Greidinger, E.L., Casciola-Rosen, L. Morris, S.A. Hoffman, R.W. and A. Rosen. 2000. Auto-antibody recognition of distinctly modified forms of the U1-70kDa antigen are associated with different clinical disease manifestations. *Arthritis Rheum.* 43:881–888.

24. Hoffman, R.W., L.J. Rettenmaier, Y. Takeda, J.E. Hewett, I. Pettersson, U. Nyman, et al. 1990. Human autoantibodies against the 70-kd polypeptide of U1 small nuclear RNP are associated with HLA-DR4 among connective tissue disease patients. *Arthritis Rheum.* 33:666–673.

25. Kaneoka, H., K.C. Hsu, Y. Takeda, G.C. Sharp, and R.W. Hoffman. 1992. Molecular genetic analysis of HLA-DR and HLA-DQ genes among anti-U1-70kD autoantibody-positive connective tissue disease patients. *Arthritis Rheum.* 35:83–94.

26. Botto, M., C. Dell'Agnola, A.E. Bygrave, E.M. Thompson, H.T. Cook, F. Petry, et al. 1998. Homozygous C1q deficiency causes glomerulonephritis associated with multiple apoptotic bodies. *Nature Genet.* 19:56–59.

27. Herrmann, M., R.E. Voll, O.M. Zoller, M. Hagenhofer, B.B. Ponner, and J.R. Kalden. 1998. Impaired phagocytosis of apoptotic cell material by monocyte-derived macrophages from patients with systemic lupus erythematosus. *Arthritis Rheum.* 41:1241–1250.

28. Simon, L.S., A.L. Weaver, D.Y. Graham, A.J. Kivitz, P.E. Lipsky, R.C. Hubbard, et al. 1999. Anti-inflammatory and upper gastrointestinal effects of celecoxib in rheumatoid arthritis: a randomized controlled trial. *JAMA* 282:1921–1928.

29. Laine, L., S. Harper, T. Simon, R. Bath, J. Johanson, H. Schwartz, et al. 1999. A randomized trial comparing the effect of rofecoxib, a cyclooxygenase 2-specific inhibitor, with that of ibuprofen on the gastroduodenal mucosa of patients with osteoarthritis. *Gastroenterology* 117:1002–1005.

30. Hosoda, Y., Y. Suzuki, M. Takano, T. Tojo, and M. Homma. 1987. Mixed connective tissue disease with pulmonary hypertension: a clinical and pathological study. *J. Rheumatol.* 14:826–830.

31. Nishimaki, T., S. Aotsuka, H. Kondo, K. Yamamoto, Y. Takasaki, M. Sumiya, and R. Yokohari. 1999. Immunological analysis of pulmonary hypertension in connective tissue diseases. *J. Rheumatol.* 26: 2357–2362.

32. Okawa-Takatsuji, M., S. Aotsuka, M. Fujinami, S. Uwatoko, M. Kinoshita, and M. Sumiya. 1999. Up-regulation of intercellular adhesion molecule-1 (ICAM-1), endothelial leucocyte adhesion molecule-1 (ELAM-1) and class II MHC molecules on pulmonary artery endothelial cells by antibodies against U1-ribonucleoprotein. *Clin. Exp. Immunol.* 116:174–180.

33. Satoh, M., H.B. Richards, and W.H. Reeves. 1999. Pathogenesis of Autoantibody Production and Glomerulonephritis in Pristane-Treated Mice, in *Lupus: Molecular and Cellular Pathogenesis,* G.M. Kammer and G.C. Tsokos, editors. Humana Press, Totowa, NJ. 399–416.

34. Shustov, A., V. Rus, P. Nguyen, and C.S. Via. 1999. Murine Graft-vs-Host Disease, in *Lupus: Molecular and Cellular Pathogenesis*. G.M. Kammer and G.C. Tsokos, editors. Humana Press, Totowa, NJ. 140–151.

35. Kono, D.H. and A.N. Theofilopoulos. 1997. The genetics of murine systemic lupus erythematosus, in *Dubois' Systemic Lupus Erythematosus,* 5th ed. D.J. Wallace and B.H. Hahn, editors. Williams Wilkins, Baltimore. 119–132.

36. Russell, P.J., J.D. Hicks, and F.M. Burnet. 1966. Cyclophosphamide treatment of mouse systemic lupus erythematosus. *Lancet* 1:1280–1284.

37. Daikh, D.I. and D. Wofsy. 1999. Treatment of systemic lupus erythematosus by selective inhibition of T cell function, in *Lupus: Molecular and Cellular Pathogenesis*. G.M. Kammer and G.C. Tsokos, editors. Humana Press, Totowa, NJ. 642–655.

38. Liang, B., R.J. Gee, M.J. Kashgarian, A.H. Sharpe, and M.J. Mamula. 1999. B7 costimulation in the development of lupus: autoimmunity arises either in the absence of B7.1/B7.2 or in the presence of anti-B7.1/B7.2 blocking antibodies. *J. Immunol.* 163:2322–2329.

39. Sutcliffe, N., T. Stoll, S. Pyke, and D.A. Isenberg. 1998. Functional disability and end organ damage in patients with systemic lupus erythematosus (SLE), SLE and Sjögren's syndrome (SS), and primary SS. *J. Rheumatol.* 25:63–68.

40. Gladman, D.D., C.H. Goldsmith, M.B. Urowitz, P. Bacon, P. Fortin, E. Ginzler, et al. 2000. The systemic lupus international collaborating clinics/American College of Rheumatology (SLICC/ACR) Damage index for systemic lupus erythematosus international comparison. *J. Rheumatol.* 27:373–376.

41. Hendra, T.J. 1988. Failure of steroid and immunosuppressant therapy to halt progression of mixed connective tissue disease. *Br. J. Clin. Pract.* 42:256–257.

42. Dahl, M., A. Chalmers, J. Wade, D. Calverly, and B. Munt. 1992. Ten year survival of a patient with advancing pulmonary hypertension and mixed connective tissue disease treated with immunosuppressive therapy. *J. Rheumatol.* 19:1807–1809.

43. Furuya, T., T. Suzuki, N. Onoda, K. Tamura, K. Sato, H. Demura, and S. Kashiwazaki. 1992. Mixed connective tissue disease associated with protein losing enteropathy: successful treatment with intravenous cyclophosphamide therapy. *Intern. Med.* 31:1359–1362.

44. Pines, A., N. Kaplinsky, E. Goldhammer, and O. Bregman. 1982. Corticosteroid induced remission of oesophageal involvement in mixed connective tissue disease. *Postgrad. Med. J.* 58:297–298.

45. Cohen, L.E., I. Faske, and M.A. Greist. 1989. Prostaglandin infusion therapy for intermittent digital ischemia in a patient with mixed connective tissue disease. Case report and review of the literature. *Am. Acad. Dermatol.* 20:893–897.

46. Satoh, J., H. Imai, T. Yasuda, H. Wakui, A.B. Biura, and Y. Nakamoto. 1994. Sclerodermatous renal crisis in a patient with mixed connective tissue disease. *Am. J. Kidney Dis.* 24:215–218.

47. Badesch, D.B., V.F. Tapson, and M.D. McGoon. 2000. Continuous intravenous epoprostenol for pulmonary hypertension due to scleroderma spectrum disease: A randomized, controlled trial. *Ann. Int. Med.* 132:425–434.

48. Lahaye, I.E., P.E. Rogiers, J.M. Nagler, and R. Chappel. 1999. Vanishing pulmonary hypertension in mixed connective tissue disease. *Clin. Rheumatol.* 18:45–47.

49. Alpert, M.A., T.A. Pressly, V. Mukerji, C.R. Lambert, B. Mukerji, H. Panayiotou, and G.C. Sharp. 1991. Acute and long-term effects of nifedipine on pulmonary and systemic hemodynamics in patients with pulmonary hypertension associated with diffuse systemic sclerosis, the CREST syndrome and mixed connective tissue disease. *Am. J. Cardiol.* 68:1687–1691.

50. Alpert, M.A., T.A. Pressly, V. Mukerji, C.R. Lambert, and B. Mukerji. 1992. Short- and long-term hemodynamic effects of captopril in patients with pulmonary hypertension and selected connective tissue disease. *Chest* 102:1407–1412.

51. Limburg, A.J., A.J. Smit, and J.H. Kleibeuker. 1991. Effects of cisapride on the esophageal motor function of patients with progressive systemic sclerosis or mixed connective tissue disease. *Digestion* 49:156–160.

52. Perlemuter, G., P. Cacoub, S. Chaussade, B. Wechsler, D. Couturier, and J.C. Piette. 1999. Octreotide treatment of chronic intestinal pseudoobstruction secondary to connective tissue diseases. *Arthritis Rheum.* 42:1545–1549.

53. Gaches, F., A.S. Blanc, B. Couret, and E. Arlet-Suau. 1998. Digital necrosis and Sharp's syndrome: the success of topical application of granulocyte/macrophage-colony stimulating factor in promoting healing after amputation of three toes. *Br. J. Dermatol.* 138:550–551.

24 Vasculitis

Dimitrios Vassilopoulos and Leonard H. Calabrese

INTRODUCTION

Among the various rheumatic diseases, vasculitides are notably associated with multi-organ involvement leading frequently to severe organ dysfunction and death. Vasculitis is defined as inflammation of the vessel wall that causes narrowing/occlusion of the lumen or occasionally aneurysm formation, resulting in ischemia of the supplied tissue(s). The size, number, and location of the involved vessels are the main factors determining the degree of individual organ damage. Taking into account the propensity of certain vasculitides to affect vessels of various sizes in different organs, one can easily explain the often devastating effects that these inflammatory processes have on multiple organs and systems.

Although the term "vasculitis" collectively refers to the histologic appearance of vascular-wall inflammation, there are clearly distinct patterns of vascular-wall injury that are observed in the various vasculitides. These distinct features most likely reflect different immune-mediated mechanisms that are involved in the pathogenesis of each syndrome. On the other hand, there is considerable overlap in the histologic findings between certain vasculitides with clearly discrete clinical presentations, making the distinction between them a difficult task even for experienced clinicians. These

From: *Modern Therapeutics in Rheumatic Diseases*
Edited by: G. C. Tsokos, et al. © Humana Press, Inc., Totowa, NJ

problems are exemplified by the inability to establish a widely accepted scheme for the classification of vasculitides.

The treatment of vasculitides has been problematic for many reasons. Lack of diagnostic homogeneity, marked individual variation in disease severity, lack of uniformly acceptable diagnostic criteria, difficulty in agreeing on disease activity markers, small numbers of patients, and lack of large randomized trials have all contributed. Progress, however, has been evident in recent years as a result of advancement in many of these areas and beginning of multicenter randomized controlled clinical trials in the field.

Furthermore, recent advances in our understanding of the pathogenetic mechanisms of these complex processes have provided the rational for the design and application of new therapeutic schemes aimed at specific steps of the inflammatory cascade that lead to vessel wall inflammation. Theoretically, the development of such treatments could result in reduction of the serious and common side effects of the currently used immunosuppressive medications.

In this chapter, we will review the available data on the pathogenetic mechanisms that rationalize the use of the new treatments, summarize the available animal and human clinical data and provide recommendations regarding the treatment of vasculitides. For the shake of discussion a modified classification scheme based on the classification criteria of the American College of Rheumatology (ACR) (1990) *(1)* and the clinical definitions of the Chapel Hill Consensus Conference (1992) *(2)*, is utilized (*see* Table 1). Vasculitides associated with various diseases (*see* Table 1) are beyond the scope of this chapter and will not be discussed here.

GIANT-CELL VASCULITIS

Pathogenesis

Giant-cell (temporal) arteritis (GCA) involves predominantly large and medium-size vessels with a well-defined internal and external elastic lamina *(3)*. A specific predilection for the extracranial vessels of the head and the aorta and its branches in the upper extremities, in individuals older than 50 yr has been noted in numerous clinical studies, although convincing scientific data explaining this pattern of involvement are missing.

Histologically, inflammatory cells comprised exclusively from monocytes/macrophages and T lymphocytes infiltrate all layers of the arterial wall, resulting in characteristic granuloma formation in 50% of the cases, fragmentation of the internal and external elastic lamina, thinning of the arterial media, neoangiogenesis in the media and intima *(4)* as well as intimal hyperplasia *(3)*. In-depth work by Weyand and her group over the last decade has indicated the oligoclonal nature of the artery infiltrating T lymphocytes, suggesting an antigen-driven immune response *(5,6)*. According to this model, unknown (auto)-antigen(s) presented by macrophages to CD4 (+) T cells in the adventitial layer of the arteries is the critical initial event in the inflammatory process that leads to arterial-wall injury *(3)*. T cells activated through this pathway in the adventitia produce cytokines like interferon-γ (IFN-γ) and interleukin-2 (IL-2), whereas activated macrophages from the same area secrete interleukin-1β (IL-1β), interleukin-6 (IL-6), and transforming growth factor β (TGF-β) *(3,7)*. IFN-γ is considered crucial in the pathogenesis of the arterial-wall pathology because it has been implicated in the

Table 1
Classification of Vasculitides

Large-vessel vasculitis
  Giant-cell arteritis
  Takayasu's arteritis
Systemic necrotizing vasculitis
  Polyarteritis nodosa
  Churg-Strauss syndrome
  Wegener's granulomatosis
  Microscopic polyangiitis
Hypersensitivity vasculitis
  Cutaneous leucocytoclastic vasculitis
  Henoch-Schönlein purpura
  Cryoglobulinemic vasculitis
  Hypocomplementemic urticarial vasculitis
Kawasaki disease
Isolated central nervous system vasculitis
Vasculitis associated with various diseases
  Vasculitis associated with rheumatic/autoimmune diseases (e.g., SLE. RA,
  Behcet's syndrome, etc.)
  Vasculitis associated with malignancies
  Vasculitis associated with infections
  Radiation vasculitis
  Transplant vasculitis

formation of multinucleated giant cells, stenosis of the arterial lumen, and amplification of the localized inflammatory response *(3)*. Other locally released substances such as platelet-derived growth factor (PDGF), vascular endothelial growth factor (VEGF), matrix metalloproteinases (MMPs), reactive oxygen species, toxic aldehydes, and nitric oxide synthase-2 (NOS-2) have been also implicated as important mediators in the complex inflammatory cascade that results in the typical arterial-wall lesion *(3)*. Recently, tumor necrosis factor α (TNF-α), a cytokine with known proinflammatory activity, has been localized by immunohistochemical methods in the intima and media of inflamed arteries, suggesting a potential role in GCA *(8)*.

Animal Data

So far there have been no good animal models for GCA. In an attempt to circumvent this problem, Weyand and her colleagues established a xenotransplant model by engrafting inflamed temporal arteries from patients with GCA into severe combined immunodeficiency diseased (SCID) mice *(9)*. Using this novel approach, they were able to show persistent inflammation of the engrafted arteries in these immunodeficient mice. Moreover, they studied the effects of corticosteroid (CS) treatment on the inflammatory infiltrates and pattern of cytokine expression in the involved arteries. Long-term CS treatment did not significantly alter the inflammatory lesions of the temporal arteries, despite significant reduction in the levels of proinflammatory cytokines such as IFN-γ, IL-2, IL-6, and IL-1β. These effects were mediated through inhibition of the transcription factor NFκB, a known target of CS action. On the contrary, CS had no effect on the levels of TGF-β1, a cytokine derived mainly by tissue-infiltrating macrophages. The authors postulated that this probably explains the inability of CS to efficiently control arterial-wall inflammation (9).

Clinical Data

CS remain the mainstay of treatment of patients with GCA. Several studies have shown that treatment with prednisone or its equivalent with initial doses ranging between 40–60 mg/d and gradual tapering, is usually sufficient to control the systemic inflammatory response and prevent serious complications such as visual loss (10). Despite this favorable effect, 5–10% of patients do not adequately respond to the initial CS treatment, active inflammatory arterial lesions persist in certain patients with apparent clinical remission and more importantly long-term treatment (>2 yr) with CS is necessary for the majority of patients with GCA (11). Prolonged treatment with CS has been associated with increased morbidity and mortality in this group of patients.

These observations in combination with the recent findings regarding the pathogenesis of the disease, emphasize the need for medications that could suppress arterial-wall inflammation in a more specific fashion and function as steroid-sparing agents. So far there have not been any well-designed controlled trials evaluating the efficacy of other immunosuppressive agents alone or in combination with CS for the treatment of GCA. Small studies have suggested a favorable effect of methotrexate (MTX) (12,13) and azathioprine (AZA) (14). A multi-center trial comparing CS to CS and MTX is currently under way and its results are anticipated in the near future. Cyclosporine A (CsA), an agent with known suppressive effect on activated T cells, had no additional effects compared to CS alone in a small study (15).

Potential agents that could be proven useful in this group of patients include agents that inhibit TNF-α or IL-1 action and possibly neoangiogenesis.

TAKAYASU'S ARTERITIS

Pathogenesis

Takayasu's arteritis (TA) is a chronic inflammatory arteritis involving predominantly the aorta, aortic arch vessels, and pulmonary arteries (16). In contrast to GCA, it primarily affects younger patients (<40 yr) with a strong female predominance (16). Clinically, two phases of the disease have been observed including an early-systemic phase characterized by a systemic inflammatory response and a late-chronic occlusive phase with evidence of vascular occlusions.

A prominent granulomatous panarteritis with inflammatory infiltrates involving large arteries in a continuous or patchy fashion is observed histologically during the active stages of the disease (11,17). The infiltrating cells include variable numbers of giant cells, lymphocytes, and plasma cells. Following the active phase, fibrosis of the adventitial and intima layers of the arterial wall ensues.

Immunological studies looking into the pathogenesis of TA are limited. During the systemic inflammatory phase of the disease, certain markers of inflammation and angiogenesis are upregulated systemically, including IL-6 (18), Regulated upon Activation Normal T-cell Expressed and Secreted (RANTES) factor (18), vascular cell adhesion molecule-1 (VCAM-1) (19), VEGF (20), and thrombomodulin (21). These findings have not been reproduced by other investigators (22) and most likely reflect active arterial inflammation without providing specific information regarding the pathogenesis of the arterial lesions.

Recent studies have suggested a prominent role of T cells in the pathogenesis of this arteritis. Seko and colleagues, demonstrated increased numbers of cytotoxic (CTLs) and γδ T lymphocytes secreting perforin in the arterial wall of patients with TA *(23)*. The same group also found that these infiltrating T cells demonstrated a restricted usage of T-cell receptors (TCR), indicating a T-cell-mediated, antigen-driven immune response in the arterial wall *(24)*. Expansions of certain subsets of CD4 and CD8 T cells have been noted also in the circulation of patients with TA *(25)* as well as enhanced proliferative activity of peripheral blood mononuclear cells (PBMC) to aortic extracts *(26)*, further supporting the role of T-cell immunity in this process. Although a strong expression of the heat-shock protein-65 (HSP-65) has been observed in the media of the inflamed arteries *(27,28)*, the nature of the arterial antigen(s) to whom the T cells react have not been identified yet.

Anti-endothelial cell antibodies (AECA) frequently found in the serum of patients with TA *(27,28)* demonstrate specific reactivity against aortic and not microvascular endothelial cells in vitro *(29)*. Moreover, these antibodies had a direct stimulatory effect on aortic endothelial cells in vitro *(29)*, implying a direct role of AECA in the pathogenesis of TA. On the other hand, the frequent presence of AECA in a number of other connective-tissue diseases and the absence of significant endothelial injury in the involved large arteries, question their direct contribution to arterial-wall inflammation.

Animal Data

The evaluation of different treatment strategies in animals is hampered by the absence of a suitable animal model of large-vessel arteritis. Recently, a group of investigators were able to show severe aortic-wall inflammation in mice infected with different herpesviruses including cytomegalovirus (CMV) *(30)* and γ-herpesvirus 68 *(31)*. Histologically, arteritis in both animal models had the characteristics of a panarteritis with prominent mononuclear-cell inflammation in the adventitia and intima layers, with few inflammatory cells in the media. Manipulation of the expression of different cytokine genes had profound effects on the clinical expression of the vasculitic process. Specifically, the absence of IFN-γ or its receptor, was associated with more severe inflammation and increased mortality. Similarly, the absence of T and B cells was associated with limited vascular inflammation, emphasizing the importance of T cells in the development of the arteritic lesions.

In a different model, Nicklin et al. generated mice that were genetically deficient for the IL-1 receptor antagonist, a naturally circulating anti-inflammatory cytokine *(32)*. They observed a large-vessel arteritis involving the aorta and its major branches with development of characteristic stenotic and aneurysmal lesions. The vessel wall of the involved arteries showed transmural infiltration by macrophages, CD4+ T lymphocytes and neutrophils, especially around areas of turbulent flow. The observed lesions emphasize the potential crucial role of a predominantly macrophage-derived cytokine like IL-1 in the development of large-vessel vasculitis.

Obviously these findings are highly provocative and open new roads in the studying of pathogenesis and treatment of large-vessel vasculitides. However, the absence of granuloma formation, the clear association with a known chronic persistent viral infection, or the genetic deficiency of an anti-inflammatory cytokine in these animal models, question their relevance to large-vessel human vasculitides at the moment.

Clinical Data

Treatment of patients with TA includes medical treatment with immunosuppressive medications in combination with surgical treatment or interventional techniques such as angioplasty *(33,34)*. Large studies from North America and Japan, have indicated that treatment with CS at a dose of approx 1 mg/kg/d induces remission in about 60% of patients with active disease *(16)*. Despite this initial response rate, approx half of the patients are not adequately controlled or require high doses of CS for maintenance of remission.

For this sizeable group of patients, different immunosuppressive agents have been employed in an uncontrolled manner with variable success. In the National Institutes of Health (NIH) series, MTX, AZA, and cyclophosphamide (CYC) were used with limited success, i.e., only 30% of patients achieving remission *(16)*. In an open-label trial from the same center, CS in combination with weekly MTX at a mean dose of 17 mg, was utilized in a small group of patients. The combination was effective in half of the patients, but approx 20% of the patients progressed despite treatment *(35)*. Overall, these studies show that approx 20–25% of patients treated with CS alone or in combination with various immunosuppressive agents, never achieve a complete long-lasting remission.

Mycophenolate mofetil (MMF), a new immunosuppressive agent with specific action on activated T and B lymphocytes, has been recently used successfully in three patients with TA *(36)*. MMF is a compound that inhibits the proliferation of T and B lymphocytes through specific inhibition of the *de novo* pathway of purine biosynthesis. This pathway is considered critical for the proliferation of T and B lymphocytes *(37)*. Additionally, an inhibitory activity on monocytes/macrophages has been demonstrated in vitro and in animal models *(37,38)*. These properties of MMF make it an attractive candidate for the treatment of large-vessel vasculitides, which are characterized by infiltration of the vessel wall, by activated T cells, and by monocytes/macrophages. Controlled studies are obviously needed in order to elucidate its efficacy in these diseases.

POLYARTERITIS NODOSA

Pathogenesis

Definitions regarding polyarteritis nodosa (PAN) have been met with significant controversy. The Chapel Hill Consensus Conference defined PAN as a "necrotizing inflammation of medium-sized or small arteries without glomerulonephritis or vasculitis in arterioles, capillaries or venules" *(2)*. Using this definition, capillaries, venules, or arterioles are not affected and patients who demonstrate such involvement are considered as having microscopic polyangiitis (MPA).

Small- and medium-size arteries show a characteristic focal, segmental involvement with frequent coexistence of active inflammatory and healed lesions *(39)*. Active lesions show evidence of transmural infiltration by different inflammatory cells including granulocytes, macrophages, and T lymphocytes *(39)*. Fibrinoid necrosis is frequently present, especially in cases with prominent granulocyte infiltration. Thrombosis of the inflammed vessel often results, whereas formation of microaneurysms of the arterial wall represents one of the angiographic hallmarks of the disease.

PAN is considered a paradigm of an immune complex (IC)-mediated vasculitis. The initial description of PAN in association with hepatitis B virus (HBV) infection *(40)*, led to a number of studies examining the potential role of IC in this process. IC containing hepatitis B surface antigen (HBsAg) and antibodies against HBsAg (anti-HBs) are found in increased levels in the circulation and they are detected in vessel walls *(40,41)*. Immunofluorescent (IF) studies of active vascular lesions identified the presence of HBsAg, IgM, IgG, and complement (C3), whereas healed lesions did not demonstrate similar findings. Furthermore, levels of the complement components –3 and –4 (C3/C4) are frequently decreased in patients with PAN, further emphasizing the pathogenetic role of IC *(40,41)*.

Cases of PAN have been reported in patients with other viral infections such as human immunodeficiency virus (HIV) infection *(42)*, hepatitis C virus (HCV) infection *(43)*, and in patients with neoplasms like hairy-cell leukemia *(44)*, underscoring the variable nature of antigens that can induce the formation of pathogenic IC.

The prevailing theory of IC mediated vascular injury, suggests that IC deposition in the vessel wall induces localized activation of the complement cascade, through the classical or alternative pathway, leading to formation of the membrane attack complex (MAC) and release of chemotactic factors like C3a and C5a. These locally released substances induce further vessel damage and recruit inflammatory cells such as polymorphonuclear leucocytes (PMN) in these areas. IC can also bind directly to endothelial and inflammatory cells (monocytes/granulocytes) through their Fc receptors, leading to the release of proinflammatory cytokines such as IL-1α, IL-6, and TNF-α, which further amplify arterial-wall inflammation by increasing endothelial-cell permeability and recruiting more inflammatory cells at these sites.

Although these findings support a role of IC in PAN, do not explain the absence of an underlying triggering factor (i.e., infection, neoplasia, etc.) in the majority of patients with PAN *(45)* as well as the frequent presence of circulating IC, without development of PAN, in patients with HBV or HCV infection. Moreover, they don't account for the ability of IC with similar antigenic properties to induce different vasculitic syndromes as is the case with IC containing HBsAg/anti-HBs in HBV infection that can either induce PAN or small vessel (hypersensitivity) vasculitis *(46)*.

Cell-mediated immune mechanisms are also participating in the pathogenesis of PAN lesions, as evidenced by immunohistochemical studies showing equal amounts of infiltrating macrophages and CD4+ T lymphocytes with variable numbers of PMN in the vessel walls *(47)*. As expected, most of the infiltrating cells display an activated phenotype with high expression of IL-2 receptor (IL-2R) and MHC class II molecules. Neo-angiogenesis with formation of microvessels in advanced inflammatory lesions with upregulated expression of adhesion molecules has also been demonstrated in these lesions *(48)*.

Animal Data

The most widely used animal model of IC-mediated arteritis is that of acute serum sickness described initially by Germuth in 1953 *(49)*. According to this model, a single intravenous (iv) injection of an antigen-like bovine serum albumin (BSA) leads to the formation of IC after a period of 12–18 d, and subsequent deposition of these IC in medium-size arteries of different organs. Vascular lesions resemble those of PAN, with frequent fibrinoid necrosis of the media, fragmentation of the elastic lamina, and infiltration of the vessel wall by PMN. Immunohistochemical studies reveal transient deposits of antigen, Ig, and complement in the subintima of the vessel wall. IC deposition has been also demonstrated in other sites like the glomerular basement membrane (GBM), synovial membranes, and the endocardium with variable local inflammatory responses.

Similar findings of IC-mediated arteritis have been also observed during the course of various chronic viral infections from lymphocytic choriomeningitis virus *(50)* and Aleutian disease virus *(51)* and spontaneously in susceptible strains of MRL/lpr *(52)* and SL/Ni mice *(53)*. In all these animal models, a strong and sustained antibody response is mounted against certain viral or auto-antigens, leading to IC formation/deposition in the arterial wall with subsequent activation of complement and development of vasculitis. Although the location, type, and severity of the vascular lesions vary widely between these animals, hypergammaglobulinemia and decreased complement levels accompanied by IF showing characteristic Ig and complement deposition in the wall of medium-size arteries, are universal findings.

The specific characteristics of the antigens and antibodies that lead to the formation of pathogenic IC have been delineated under various experimental conditions. Different antigen and antibody properties have been identified as important including the size, concentration, charge, and vascular tropism of the antigen(s) as well as the class, size, charge, affinity/avidity, and specificity of the antibody *(54)*. Furthermore, the ratio of antigen-antibody in IC and the ability of the host to efficiently clear circulating IC appear critical in IC-mediated vascular injury *(54)*.

Therapeutic interventions have been also attempted in some of these models. Specifically, in mink infected by the Aleutian disease virus, administration of CYC led to decreased Ig levels and absence of the characteristic arterial lesions, despite the persistence of viremia *(55)*. Similar results have been obtained in MRL/lpr mice treated with different immunosuppressive agents including CS, CYC, CsA, FK-506 *(56)*, and recently MMF *(57)*. These immunosuppressive regimens ameliorate the vasculitic process mainly through suppression of the pathogenic (auto)-antibody production but also via inhibition of the influx of inflammatory cells in the vessel wall, regardless of the nature of the inciting antigenic stimulus.

Clinical Data

The prognosis of severe PAN in untreated patients is dismal with a 5-yr survival rate of 15% in older series *(58)*. The introduction of immunosuppressive regimens such as CS and CYC has significantly improved the outcome of these patients with 5-yr survival rates reaching 80 % in recent series *(59)*.

Although the percentage of PAN cases that are currently associated with certain viral infections (HBV, HIV, HCV) is small (<10%) *(45)*, a distinction should be made regarding the management of patients with "virus associated PAN" compared to patients with "nonvirus associated PAN."

Patients with PAN not associated to known viral infections are traditionally treated with CS either in the form of oral prednisone at a starting dose of 1 mg/kg/d or iv pulse methylprednisolone of short duration (1–3 d) followed by oral prednisone, with gradual tapering *(59)*. In patients that relapse after initial treatment (~20%) or present with severe target organ involvement (i.e., cardiac, gastrointestinal [GI], central nervous system [CNS], or renal), the addition of CYC seems necessary *(59,60)*. CYC has been administered orally or with monthly iv pulses with comparable results in patients with PAN *(61)*. Similarly to other forms of systemic vasculitis such as Wegener's granulomatosis (WG), the selection of the most appropriate route of its administration remains a controversial issue.

Using this combination approach, most patients achieve complete remission and withdraw from therapy after 12–18 mo. Relapses after initial remission are uncommon (~18%) with 10-yr survival rates reaching 80% *(62)*.

In the setting of virus-associated PAN, therapy should be aimed at both the underlying viral infection that leads to the development and persistence of the vasculitic process as well as towards the harmful host-immune response *(63)*. Use of immunosuppressive agents in patients with chronic viral infections are associated with increased levels of viremia (HBV and HCV infection), deterioration of underlying major-organ function (liver in chronic HBV infection), and development of life-threatening opportunistic infections (HIV infection). Assessing the severity of the vasculitic involvement and the status of the underlying viral infection appears critical in the therapeutic decision-making *(63)*.

In patients with HBV-associated PAN, combination therapies including antiviral agents such as interferon-α (IFN-α) or vidarabine and plasma exchanges (PE) with or without the addition of CS, led to a 10-yr survival rate of 83%, similar to that achieved in patients with nonvirus associated PAN *(45)*. The relapse rate was much lower in these patients (~6%) most likely reflecting the monophasic pattern of this vasculitic process *(45)*. Successful use of new antiviral agents like lamivudine *(64)* or famciclovir *(65)* in the treatment of HBV-associated PAN have been recently reported.

In the few cases of HIV-associated PAN that have been reported in the literature, different therapeutic agents have been tried in an uncontrolled manner including CS, PE, and antiretrovirals, with favorable results *(42,66,67)*. Given the rarity and complexity of HIV-associated vasculitis, thorough assessment of these patients by experienced physicians is the preferred approach.

CHURG-STRAUSS SYNDROME

Pathogenesis

Originally described by Churg and Strauss in 1951, Churg-Strauss Syndrome (CSS) is a necrotizing vasculitis involving small- and medium-size vessels (arteries and veins) accompanied by asthma and eosinophilia *(68,69)*. Typical histological findings include, except the vasculitic lesions, granulomas, and tissue infiltration by eosinophils, although the constellation of all three lesions is uncommon (15–25%) *(69)*. Compared to PAN, a wider range of vessels are involved ranging from small venules to medium-size muscular arteries displaying a characteristic eosinophilic infiltration *(39)*.

Clinically, patients with CSS present with a prodromal phase manifested by peripheral and/or tissue eosinophilia and development of allergic rhinitis and/or asthma. This phase can last for several years and is followed by the appearance of constitutional symptoms and the various organ manifestations of systemic vasculitis (vasculitic phase). Churg has described elegantly the stages of the vascular injury in patients with CSS *(70)*. Initially, there is prominent edema of the vascular wall followed by eosinophilic infiltration of the outer layers (adventitia/media) with subsequent development of fibrinoid necrosis and, in some cases, granulomas in the affected vessels *(70)*. In patients with progressive disease, the intima layer may become thickened and fibrotic giving the characteristic histologic appearance of "healing" arteritis *(70)*. Whether or not this sequence of pathologic changes occurs in every patient with CSS is unknown.

Until now there have not been any suitable animal models of CSS, so information regarding the pathogenesis of this syndrome is derived mainly from scarce human studies including small number of patients. The presence of peripheral and/or tissue eosinophilia in patients with CSS suggests a critical role for eosinophils in the pathogenesis of this systemic vasculitis.

Eosinophils are bone marrow-derived cells that participate in the complex system of mucosal immunity and also in the host immune response against parasites *(71)*. Their role in certain allergic diseases and immediate hypersensitivity reactions is also well established *(71)*. Eosinophils possess a number of surface receptors for various cytokines (e.g., IL-2, IL-4, IL-16), immunoglobulins (Ig), complement components (C1q, complement receptor –1 and –3), chemoattractants (C5a, eotaxin), and IFN-α. Their effector action is exerted through the release of a number of preformed mediators such as the eosinophilic cationic protein (ECP), the eosinophil-derived neurotoxin and so on, various cytokines (IL-1, IL-2, IL-3, IL-5), growth factors such as granulocyte-monocyte colony stimulating factor (GM-CSF), and chemokines (RANTES, MIP-1a, eotaxin).

Immunological studies in patients with CSS show clear evidence of eosinophil activation with increased serum levels of ECP *(72)* whereas analysis of bronchoalveolar lavage (BAL) fluid revealed elevated levels of ECP and myeloperoxidase (MPO) indicating concomitant neutrophil activation *(73)*. Clonal analysis of eosinophils from patients with CSS showed a polyclonal pattern of expansion in contrast to patients with the idiopathic hypereosinophilic syndrome (HES) *(74)*. In patients with HES, a critical role of T cells in the development of eosinophilia through secretion of soluble factors has been identified. These T-cell clones display a predominant Th-2 phenotype secreting IL-4 and IL-5. Similarly, Muschen et al. found an oligoclonal expansion of T cells in the periphery of patients with CSS *(75)*. Furthermore, in these patients increased levels of soluble Fas (CD95), which could lead to the rescue of eosinophils from Fas-induced apoptosis, were detected *(75)*.

Collectively, these limited findings suggest that oligoclonal T-cell expansion (predominantly Th2) in response to unidentified antigen(s), locally or systemically, may lead to an initial polyclonal eosinophilic activation and expansion followed by eosinophilic-tissue infiltration and vasculitis. A direct role of T lymphocytes in vascular injury is also suggested by the presence of activated T cells (CD4 and CD8) in the arterial wall of patients with CSS-associated nerve involvement *(76)*. Whether these T lymphocytes were the cells that initially led to the recruitment of eosinophils in the vessel wall or vice versa is currently unknown.

Anti-neutrophil cytoplasmic antibodies (ANCA) are frequently detected in patients with CSS (~40%) with a predominant perinuclear pattern (p-ANCA) *(77)*. A direct role though of these antibodies in the pathogenesis of this vasculitic syndrome has not been specified.

Clinical Data

The response of CSS to treatment with high-dose oral CS (prednisone 1 mg/kg/d) is dramatic *(68,69,78)*. Ninety to 100% of patients achieve clinical remission with significant decrease in the eosinophil count *(68,69,78)*. This effect is mediated through the pronounced CS-induced decrease in the absolute eosinophil count and inhibition of eosinophil-mediated injury and chemotaxis. Despite this initial response, relapses are not rare, occurring in 25–40% of patients, especially when cardiac or GI involvement is present *(68,78)*.

For patients that display resistance to CS or present with serious target-organ involvement, other immunosuppressive agents have been tried in small numbers of patients. These included traditional immunosuppressive agents like CYC, MTX, and AZA with variable success *(68,78)*. CsA inhibits in vitro production of T-cell-released soluble factors that cause eosinophilia. McDermott et al. have reported the case of a patient with severe CSS resistant to CS and iv pulses of CYC, who responded promptly to CsA *(79)*. Studies with larger number of patients are needed in order to support this initial observation.

Recently, Tatsis et al. reported that IFN-α in high doses had a favorable effect in patients with CSS *(80)*. IFN-α is a known agent with a wide spectrum of immunomodulatory and antiviral activities. IFN-α acting through its specific receptor on eosinophils, leads to a significant reduction in the release of inflammatory mediators from these cells *(81)*. Furthermore, treatment with IFN-α leads to a decrease in eosinophil count either through inhibition of eosinophil release from the bone marrow *(82)* or by induction of apoptosis *(83)*. An indirect mode of action, via inhibition of secretion of T-cell-derived cytokines such as IL-5 and GM-CSF *(84,85)*, may also contribute to this profound effect of IFN-α on eosinophils.

WEGENER'S GRANULOMATOSIS

Pathogenesis

WG is a multisystemic inflammatory disorder with a specific predilection for the upper/lower respiratory tract and kidneys *(86)*. Characteristic pathologic findings include tissue necrosis, vasculitis, and granulomatous inflammation. This classical triad of pathologic features is found more often in patients with lung involvement (90%) but uncommonly in upper respiratory-tract lesions (~15%) *(86,87)*.

Several authors propose that the earlier lesions in WG are small foci of collagen necrosis, especially in the lung *(88)*. In these necrotic areas, a prominent neutrophilic and histiocytic infiltration is typically seen, defined as a "microabscess" *(87)*. In some cases, around these areas of necrosis, histiocytes and T lymphocytes accumulate, giving the distinctive appearance of "palisading granulomas." This granulomatous inflammation surrounding necrotic areas, indicates the presence of a strong Th1 response with localized release of cytokines such as TNF-α and IFN-γ, that play a critical role in granuloma formation. However, it remains to be ascertained which are the factor(s) that initiate this localized and often generalized necro-inflammatory response. Environmental and infectious triggers may be directly or indirectly involved in this process but these have not yet been identified.

Vasculitis of small- and medium-size vessels (arteries and veins) is a common feature of tissue biopsies from patients with WG *(87,89)*. It can be present in three different forms, including:

1. Granulomatous vasculitis, involving small- and medium-size arteries and veins, characterized by the presence of histiocytes or giant cells in the vessel wall with or without associated necrosis. Typically, it is observed in areas with surrounding parenchymal granulomatous inflammation (lung).
2. Neutrophilic capillaritis, characterized by neutrophilic infiltration of capillaries, arterioles or venules, with or without associated fibrinoid necrosis. Inflammation of these small vessels in different organs is responsible for the clinical manifestations of necrotizing glomerulonephritis (kidneys), leucocytoclastic vasculitis (skin), or diffuse alveolar hemorrhage (lung) that are frequently encountered during the clinical course of WG.
3. Necrotizing vasculitis, involving small- and medium-size arteries and veins, in the absence of giant cells or surrounding granulomatous inflammation.

Some authors hypothesize that vasculitis represents a secondary event in the pathophysiological sequence of events in WG rather than the primary cause of the syndrome *(88)*. This hypothesis is mainly based on the variable frequency of typical vasculitic lesions in tissue specimens from patients with typical clinical manifestations of WG. Whether this is true or just reflects the limitations of tissue biopsy in regards to timing and sampling errors is unclear.

Existing theories regarding the pathogenesis of WG are primarily focusing on the pathogenetic role of ANCA and/or T-cell-mediated mechanisms. ANCA are antibodies directed against different cytoplasmic components of neutrophils and monocytes *(90)*. A strong association between ANCA and WG has been established in several studies. Specifically, serum from most patients with WG produces a characteristic cytoplasmic staining of ethanol-fixed neutrophils (c-ANCA) as detected by indirect immunofluorescence (IIF) *(90)*. The predominant target antigen of these c-ANCA is proteinase-3 (PR3), a serine cytoplasmic neutrophilic protease. In vitro studies have demonstrated that priming of resting neutrophils by cytokines like TNF-α or induction of apoptosis, leads to the translocation of PR3 to the cell surface, where it is accessible to specific anti-PR3 antibodies *(90)*. The mechanism(s) by which tolerance to a self-protein like PR3 is lost and generation of anti-PR3 antibodies occurs, is unknown.

Anti-PR3 binding to PR3 with co-engagement of Fc-receptors (IIa and IIIb) on the surface of neutrophils leads to neutrophil activation. Neutrophil activation is prominent in WG lesions, especially in the kidney *(91)*. These activated neutrophils may subsequently bind to primed endothelium, through their surface PR3 causing endothelial detachment and lysis. Anti-PR3 can also bind directly to PR3 expressed on primed endothelial cells leading to further endothelial injury and release of various cytokines (IL-1β) or chemoattractants (IL-8) *(90)*. Similar interaction of circulating ANCA with monocytes promotes the release of various proinflammatory and chemoattractant substances, leading to the recruitment of additional inflammatory cells at the sites of the initial vascular injury. Furthermore, epidemiological data have demonstrated that in two-thirds of patients with WG, there is a correlation between ANCA titers and disease activity *(90)*.

Although these in vitro findings and clinical observations strongly support a contributing role of ANCA in the pathogenesis of WG, do not prove a causal relationship. Apart from the controversy regarding the primary or secondary role of vasculitis in the pathogenesis of WG, immunofluorescent studies have failed to detect Ig or complement deposition in the vascular wall, whereas endothelial damage does not appear to be a prominent early histologic feature of WG. Moreover, a number of patients with limited biopsy-proven WG do not have circulating ANCA, whereas certain patients with quiescent disease display persistently elevated ANCA titers *(90)*. The absence of a suitable animal model of "ANCA-associated vasculitis" (*see* below) limits the delineation of the exact role of ANCA in the pathogenesis of WG *(92)*.

On the other hand, the critical role of cell-mediated immunity has emerged from a number of studies. The absence of detectable IC and the predominance of T cells and macrophages at inflammatory sites (especially granulomatous) *(93,94)* firmly supports this concept. Furthermore, isolated peripheral T cells react to purified PR3 *(95,96)*, whereas markers of T-cell activation like sIL2R *(97–99)* or circulating activated T cells (CD25 or HLA-DR+) are elevated in patients with WG *(100–102)*. In addition, two recent studies have shown a predominant IFN-γ secretion (Th1 response) in the peripheral blood *(103,104)* and local inflammatory lesions *(103)* from patients with WG.

Animal Models

Although a number of animal models have been generated, none of these reproduces the characteristic histologic and clinical features of WG *(92)*. The majority of these models are focusing on the pathogenetic role of ANCA under various experimental conditions including manipulation of the different components of the animal immune system. Nevertheless, these animal models represent valuable tools in the study of diseases like WG and MPA. Because most of these models are studying the effects of antibodies against myeloperoxidase (MPO), they will be discussed separately in the MPA section.

Regarding WG, the only animal model that has been developed so far is based on the theory of dysregulation of the idiotypic network that leads to the development of autoimmune diseases like systemic lupus erythematosus (SLE), scleroderma, and WG *(105)*. According to the work performed by Shoenfeld and his colleagues, immunization of BALB/c mice with purified human IgG anti-PR3 (antibody-1 or Ab-1) from patients with WG, led to the development of anti-human anti-PR3 (Ab-2) and later of anti-anti-human anti-PR3 (Ab-3) antibodies *(106)*. The mouse antibodies (Ab-3) presumably share the same characteristic binding for PR3 with the initial human Ab-1. Nevertheless, studies so far have not detected any reactivity of the mouse anti-PR3 against the murine homolog of PR3 *(107)*. In addition, the pathologic lesions that were observed in these animals, were either mild perivascular mononuclear infiltrates in the lungs and mild proteinuria or sterile microabscesses in the lung, without the characteristic granulomatous lesions or the pauci-immune necrotizing glomerulonephritis of human WG. Similarly, infusion of active PR3 in Brown-Norway rats caused no demonstrable binding to GBM or induction of proteinuria *(108)*. In the absence of a suitable animal model of WG, there have not been any experiments examining the effect of different therapeutic interventions.

Clinical Data

Untreated WG carries the worst prognosis among vasculitides, with a mean survival of 5 mo and a 2-yr survival rate of just 10% *(109)*. The addition of CS increased the mean survival time to only 12 mo. The pioneer work by Wolf and Fauci at NIH in the early 1970s established that addition of daily oral CYC to CS, significantly improves survival *(110)*. In a recent update of a large cohort of patients treated with this regimen at the same center by Hoffman et al., the mortality rate was 13% after a mean follow-up of 8 yr *(86)*.

According to the NIH protocol, CYC is started at a dose of 2 mg/kg/d and is continued for 1 yr after remission *(109)*. The dose can be gradually increased (by 25 mg/wk) for persistently active disease while avoiding leukopenia (white blood cell count ≤ 3000/mm^3). CS are used in combination, starting with 1 mg/kg/d of prednisone for 1 mo with gradual tapering. Using this approach a 90% initial remission rate was achieved but the number of relapses was almost 50% *(86)*.

In a recent randomized trial from France, steroids plus iv pulses of CYC were compared to CS plus oral CYC *(111)*. There were no statistically significant differences in terms of remission or 5-yr survival rates between the two groups. The group of patients that received iv pulses of CYC had fewer side effects but a higher number of relapses. Both groups of patients had a high rate of infectious complications, most likely related to the intensity of the CYC treatment. Similar results showing equal efficacy with decreased side effects of iv pulse vs oral CYC were reported in a smaller study by Haubitz et al. *(112)*. These two studies suggest that for patients with nonimmediately life-threatening disease or contraindications to oral CYC, pulse iv CYC could offer an alternative vital option.

In patients treated with the combination of CYC (oral or iv) and CS, most authors suggest the concomitant use of trimethoprim/sulfomethoxazole (T/S) as prophylaxis for *Pneumocystis carinii* pneumonia *(109)*. Whether or not the use of T/S offers an additional benefit in these patients by preventing disease relapses is unclear *(113)*.

Prolonged use of CYC in patients with WG has been associated with a number of serious side effects including infections and malignancies like carcinoma of the bladder *(86)*. In an effort to reduce these hazardous side effects a number of alternative regimens have been tried. MTX in combination with steroids has been used either as induction therapy for patients with nonlife-threatening WG or as maintenance therapy after induction with CS and CYC.

In two studies including patients with nonlife-threatening WG, the combination of CS and MTX induced remission in ~70% of patients but the relapse rate was high, ranging from 36–50% *(114,115)*. In contrast, the use of MTX as maintenance therapy for WG appears more promising. Langford et al. used MTX at doses ranging from 15–25 mg/wk in patients that have achieved complete remission after induction therapy with CS and CYC, with gradual tapering of CS *(116)*. After a median follow-up of 13 mo, only 16% of patients have experienced relapse with few side effects.

Experience with other agents like CsA, AZA and intravenous immunoglobulins (IVIG) remains limited and anecdotal *(117)*. Recently, MMF in combination with CS has been used as maintenance therapy in 9 patients with predominantly renal involvement with promising results *(118)*. Similarly, good results have been achieved in a preliminary study of 20 patients with generalized WG with leflunomide (20–40 mg/d), an immunosuppressive agent currently in use for patients with RA *(119)*.

Based on the potential role of TNF-α in WG pathogenesis through its effects on granuloma formation, neutrophil and/or endothelial-cell priming, and cell-mediated immune responses, therapeutic strategies aiming at antagonizing its actions are currently underway. Specifically, in an open-label trial, Etanercept, a recombinant fusion protein consisting of soluble TNF-α receptors and the Fc portion of human IgG1, was used in conjunction with standard-of-care regimens (120). Preliminary results revealed that the agent was well-tolerated and efficacious. The final results of this ongoing trial are eagerly anticipated in the near future.

Collectively, the results from these small studies emphasize the importance of "step down" regimens, including induction therapy with CS and CYC followed by a "less toxic" maintenance regimen (MTX, MMF, leflunomide, etc.) for the long-term treatment of patients with WG. A similar approach may be of value in other systemic vasculitides such as MPA, CSS, and PAN.

MICROSCOPIC POLYANGIITIS

Pathogenesis Definition

According to the Chapel Hill Consensus Conference, MPA is defined as a necrotizing vasculitis affecting capillaries, venules, and arterioles (small vessels) and occasionally small- or medium-size arteries, with few or no immune deposits (2). This mode of vascular involvement differentiates MPA from PAN, which by definition does not involve capillaries, venules, or arterioles (2). Furthermore, kidney and lung are characteristically involved in the form of necrotizing crescentic rapidly progressive glomerulonephritis and capillaritis, respectively.

Small vessels are involved in a focal segmental fashion with areas of necrosis and inflammation by a mixture of inflammatory cells (2,62). In contrast to WG and CSS, granulomas are absent (2,62). Similarly, aneurysm formation in medium-size arteries is rare, although aneurysms have been observed in small arteries of the kidneys (121). D'Agati et al., examining kidney biopsies from patients with MPA, proposed that the earlier pathological finding of vessel-wall injury was the presence of endothelial-cell edema and focal degeneration followed by subendothelial-fibrin deposition and infiltration by a variety of inflammatory cells including PMN and mononuclear cells (MNCs) (122). As mentioned earlier, several studies confirmed the relative absence of IC deposition in vessel walls (62,122,123).

Studies examining the pathogenesis of MPA in humans are limited. Pathogenetic theories that have been proposed are identical to those of WG, emphasizing the role of ANCA and cell-mediated processes. ANCA are detected in 50–75% of patients with MPA (77). Most of patient's sera display a characteristic perinuclear IIF pattern (p-ANCA) reacting specifically to MPO. In vitro purified IgG (p-ANCA) or anti-MPO antibodies induce endothelial activation (124), activation of primed neutrophils (125) with release of proinflammatory cytokines like IL-1β (126,127), and release of monocyte chemoattractant protein-1 (MCP-1) from monocytes (128).

Certain markers of cell-mediated immunity like serum levels of sIL-2R (97) and TNF-α (129), as well as transcripts of TNF-α and IL-1β in localized kidney lesions (129), are upregulated in patients with MPA. Likewise, Simpson et al. observed an increased expression of the TCR Vβ 2.1 gene in patients with MPA (130), whereas Griffith et al. showed T-cell reactivity to MPO *(131)*, indicating a major role of T-cell-mediated responses in MPA pathogenesis.

Animal Models

Several animal models have been developed based on the presence of anti-MPO antibodies and their clinical and histological features that resemble human MPA *(92)*. These models include necrotizing vasculitis developing in Brown Norway rats after exposure to mercuric chloride ($HgCl_2$), spontaneous necrotizing vasculitis in MRL/lpr and SCG/Ki mice and necrotizing vasculitis, crescentic glomerulonephritis, or lung disease developing in Brown-Norway rats after immunization with human MPO *(92)*. In the spontaneous and after exposure to $HgCl_2$ models, anti-MPO antibodies are generated among numerous antibodies reacting against dsDNA, ssDNA, smooth muscle, and GBM antigens *(92)*. Thus, it is unclear whether anti-MPO are the only antibodies involved in tissue injury in these models. Recently, Harper et al. showed that infusion of anti-MPO antibodies in MRL mice induced a neutrophilic vasculitis in 1/3 of the animals, only if preceded by neutrophil activation (by TNF-α priming) and endothelial injury *(132)*.

Similar results have been obtained in Brown Norway rats immunized with human MPO *(132)*. These animals develop, a few weeks later, anti-human MPO antibodies crossreacting with rat MPO. Anti-MPO antibodies alone are not pathogenic in the immunized animals; in order to provoke tissue injury, neutrophil and monocyte activation accompanied by endothelial activation locally or systemically, are obligatory *(92)*. Even under these optimal conditions, combined lung and kidney lesions resembling human MPA have not been observed in these animals.

Collectively, these data indicate a clear ability of anti-MPO antibodies to enhance and perpetuate tissue injury initially triggered by activated neutrophils in sites of endothelial injury, but do not prove a direct pathogenic role for these antibodies.

Therapeutic interventions were limited in these models. In rats exposed to $HgCl_2$ administration of CsA during the early phases delayed the rise in anti-MPO antibodies and had an ameliorating effect on the development of necrotizing vasculitis. On the contrary, when given later, vasculitic lesions were exacerbated despite the absence of anti-MPO antibodies *(133)*.

Clinical Data

Patients with MPA generally are treated similarly to patients with WG, although large controlled trials comparing different treatment immunosuppressive regimens have not been performed *(59)*. In older studies, patients with MPA were grouped together with patients with PAN or patients with crescentic glomerulonephritis who were ANCA (+), so clear conclusions can not be easily drawn.

Combination treatment with CS and CYC is clearly superior to treatment with CS alone as initial treatment for patients with MPA *(59,134)*. CS are used at similar doses with WG, except in cases with severe lung and/or kidney involvement where iv pulses of methylprednisolone are administered for a few days. iv pulses and oral CYC have been used with similar success in patients with MPA *(59,134)*. Addition of plasma exchanges may be indicated in patients presenting with fulminant pulmonary-renal syndrome, although adequate clinical data to support their use are lacking. IVIG has also been tried in patients with resistant disease with conflicting results *(59)*.

Relapses after initial remission are observed in 30–46% of patients with MPA *(59,134,135)*, emphasizing the need for maintenance immunosuppressive therapy in certain patients. Different agents including oral CYC *(134)*, AZA *(62)*, CsA *(136)*, and MMF *(118)*, have been used with variable success in small numbers of patients. As mentioned in the section regarding WG treatment, the use of new agents like leflunomide or anti-TNF-based therapies may be proven useful in these patients.

HYPERSENSITIVITY VASCULITIS

Definition-Pathogenesis

The term "hypersensitivity vasculitis" encompasses a heterogeneous group of vasculitides with characteristic predominant involvement of the small vessels of the skin (capillaries, venules, and occasionally arterioles). Skin may be the only site (termed "cutaneous leucocytoclastic vasculitis" according to the Chapel Hill Consensus Conference definition) *(2)* or one of multiple sites of vasculitic involvement (e.g., Henoch-Schönlein purpura-HSP or cryoglobulinemic vasculitis-CV). In 50–60% of the cases an initiating factor or associated disease can be identified *(137,138)*. Certain features of hypersensitivity vasculitis like the localized IC and/or complement deposition and the presence of leukocytoclasis, are distinctive and may help differentiate it from other forms of systemic vasculitides with occasional skin involvement such as WG, CSS, and MPA.

A variety of exogenous or endogenous antigens can elicit the generation and deposition of pathogenic IC, leading to the characteristic vasculitic skin lesions. Igs, DNA, and tumor antigens are common examples of endogenous antigens causing hypersensitivity vasculitis, whereas among the exogenous antigens, drugs, food products, and viral or bacterial proteins have been also identified as frequent causes *(137)*.

Histologically, a predominant neutrophilic vasculitis involving mainly the post-capillary venules is present in skin biopsies *(139)*. Biopsies of uninvolved skin sites from patients with hypersensitivity vasculitis show initially IC deposition in the vessel wall *(139–141)*. The factors that lead to this vascular precipitation of IC are diverse, including the different physicochemical properties of the inciting IC, localized permeability of the endothelium and regional blood-flow characteristics *(54,142)*. The majority of deposited Igs are of the IgM or IgG class, except in the case of HSP, where IgA is found. IC deposition is followed by activation of the complement cascade with release of chemotactic substances like C5a and generation of MAC *(139–141)*. MAC deposition has been demonstrated in endothelial cells of clinically uninvolved skin *(143)*, indicating that complement activation is an early event in the development of the vasculitic lesions. In vitro MAC has a deleterious effect on endothelium, causing endothelial-cell detachment *(144)*.

Sequential skin biopsies from affected individuals have demonstrated an influx of PMN, following IC and complement deposition, in the vessel wall *(139,145)*. Activated neutrophils release locally proteolytic enzymes and free-oxygen radicals, leading to vessel injury and fibrin deposition *(146)*. The specific signals that recruit PMN in the post-capillary venule walls are unknown, but the recently identified chemokines like

IL-8 and cytokines like IL-1 may be of paramount importance. Elevated serum levels of IL-8 in patients with hypersensitivity vasculitis support this hypothesis *(147)*.

Zax et al. in sequential biopsies from skin lesions from a patient with cutaneous vasculitis showed that after the neutrophilic-phase, MNCs appear in the vessel wall *(145)*. Their ability to clear apoptotic material such as apoptotic neutrophils and cellular debris, may assist in the gradual spontaneous clearance of the vasculitic lesions that is observed in the majority of patients with hypersensitivity vasculitis *(148)*. Persistence of the pathogenic IC as it commonly occurs in chronic viral infections like hepatitis B *(149)* or C *(150)*, may be responsible for persistent skin or other organ lesions.

Animal Models

The best-studied model of IC-mediated vascular injury resembling hypersensitivity vasculitis is that of Arthus reaction *(151)*. In this model, sensitized animals to a specific antigen-like BSA receive a localized skin injection of BSA, with local formation of BSA/anti-BSA IC. Immunohistochemical studies reveal early deposition of IC in the vessels walls, where they bind to Fc receptors present on various cells and also activate complement. Release of C5a and other factors lead to the increased vascular permeability and influx of PMN in the vascular wall as well as local accumulation of platelets that release additional vasoactive amines. Activated neutrophils bind and phagocytose IC with subsequent release of proteinases (proteases, collagenases, and elastases) and free-oxygen radicals. These locally liberated substances amplify the vascular injury, giving the characteristic appearance of small-vessel vasculitis.

Depletion experiments have clearly shown that the Arthus reaction requires the combined presence of antigen, precipitating antibody, neutrophils, intact complement system, and presence of Fc-receptors on cell surfaces *(152)*. The role of lymphocytes and macrophages is less clear regarding skin injury, but they may be involved in IC-mediated injury in other organs like kidneys, lung, joints, and so on. Inhibition of macrophage-released cytokines has given contrasting results. Inhibition of TNF-α had limited effect on skin vasculitis *(153–155)*, whereas antagonism of IL-1 had an ameliorating effect on dermal vascular injury *(153)*.

Manipulation of neutrophil, complement, and Fc-receptor function is associated with decreased Arthus reaction. Older studies have clearly shown that depletion of neutrophils leads to dimished neutrophil influx in the vascular wall *(156)*. Recently, Hazenbos et al. showed that mice deficient for the Fc receptor III (CD16) had a diminished Arthus reaction *(157)*. Similar but less striking results were obtained in mice deficient for the C5a receptor *(158)*.

Clinical Data

CUTANEOUS LEUCOCYTOCLASTIC ANGIITIS

A thorough clinical and laboratory evaluation is mandatory in patients with hyper-sensitivity vasculitis in order to identify precipitating factors or associated conditions and also to evaluate the extent of organ involvement *(60)*. Removal of the responsible factor (e.g., drug) or treatment of the associated condition (e.g., infection) may suffice as initial treatment for patients with disease confined exclusively to the skin *(60)*. The prognosis of cutaneous leucocytoclastic angiitis is overall very good with most patients requiring no additional treatment *(159)*. In some cases, symptomatic treatment with nonsteroidal anti-inflammatory drugs (NSAIDs) and anti-histamines may be indicated. Whether or not short courses of oral CS (≤1 mo) shortens the duration or prevents chronicity of the skin vasculitic lesions is unknown. Their use should be probably reserved for severe symptomatic skin lesions and given for a short period of time (≤1 mo). Anecdotally colchicine has been suggested as an efficacious agent, but a recent prospective randomized controlled trial failed to show any benefit *(160)*.

In patients with recurrent or chronic cutaneous vasculitis, immunosuppressive agents may be required. A number of agents have been tried in an uncontrolled manner including CS, CYC, MTX, NSAIDs, and AZA with variable success *(60)*. The selection of the most efficacious and less toxic agent seems appropriate.

Systemic involvement in cases of hypersensitivity vasculitis has been demonstrated mainly in patients with HSP and CV, so their management is discussed separately below.

Henoch-Schönlein Purpura

HSP predominantly affects children and carries a favorable prognosis, although relapses are observed in 30–40% of the cases *(161)*. The role of immunosuppressive agents in the treatment of HSP is a highly controversial issue. CS are extensively used in patients with severe GI or renal involvement, although their ability to shorten the duration of symptoms and prevent abdominal complications or severe renal involvement has not been established *(162,163)*.

For patients with severe renal involvement defined by the presence of >50% crescents in kidney biopsy, nephrotic syndrome, or renal insufficiency *(164)*, high-dose CS or combination immunosuppressive therapy is indicated. Controlled trials are lacking, but results from uncontrolled or retrospective studies suggest a favorable effect of these therapies. Niaudet et al. recently showed that iv pulses of methylprednisolone followed by oral CS for ~3 mo resulted in clinical response in 70% of HSP cases with severe nephritis, with only 10% of the patients progressing to end-stage renal disease *(165)*. Combination of CS with CYC has also given favorable results in two small studies *(166,167)*. A less aggressive approach by combining CS with AZA appears as a promising combination for these predominantly young patients with severe renal involvement *(168,169)*. Other modes of treatment include PEs *(170)* and IVIG administration *(171)*, but given the small number of patients enrolled, additional studies are needed for evaluation of their efficacy.

In conclusion, for patients with severe renal involvement iv methylprednisolone followed by oral CS combined with AZA or CYC is recommended. For resistant cases, PE or IVIG may be tried.

Cryoglobulinemic Vasculitis

CV is an immune-complex-mediated, small-vessel vasculitis caused by circulating cryoglobulins *(150)*. Cryoglobulins are classified according to their Ig composition as type I (monoclonal Ig), II (mixed, monoclonal, and polyclonal Ig), and III (mixed polyclonal Ig). Cryoglobulinemia is detected in different infections, neoplastic and connective-tissue disorders, whereas in certain cases the etiology is unknown (essential mixed cryoglobulinemia) *(150)*. Despite the frequent presence of serum cryoglobulins, CV is rather uncommon. Over the last decade, it has been shown that most cases of CV are owing to an underlying chronic HCV infection *(172)*.

In cases of CV related to a known condition, therapy is aimed at treating the underlying disorder (e.g. infection, neoplasia, etc.) *(60)*. A similar approach is followed in patients with an underlying HCV infection, who represent the majority of patients with CV. An initial assessment of the target-organ involvement by the vasculitic process is an essential first step in the treatment of these patients. For patients, with mild disease involving mainly skin or joints, a trial of antiviral therapy is indicated *(173)*. In most trials, so far, IFN-α in standard doses (3 million units three times a week for 6–12 mo) has been used with favorable results *(173)*. Typically, patients who clear the virus show good clinical response, although relapses are frequent after the end of therapy *(173)*. Recently, the combination of IFN-α with ribavirin (1000–1200 mg/d) has been found to be superior to IFN-α monotherapy for the treatment of HCV infection, so this combination should be the current treatment of choice. Nevertheless, clinical experience in patients with CV is limited *(174)*. In resistant cases, short courses of oral CS may be beneficial *(60,150)*.

For patients with severe organ dysfunction, i.e., renal, nerve, GI, and so on, a combination of antiviral and immunosuppressive agents is appropriate. CS in combination with oral CYC have been used successfully in these patients *(60)*. In cases with life-threatening or progressive disease, the addition of plasmapheresis offers an additional benefit *(60,150)*. Close monitoring of the renal and liver function is mandatory in these patients, while physicians should be aware of the potential of IFN-α treatment to worsen underlying vasculitic lesions *(175)*.

KAWASAKI DISEASE

Pathogenesis-Definition

Kawasaki disease (KD) is an acute vasculitic syndrome that affects primarily children under the age of 5, with involvement of small, medium, and large arteries *(176)*. A specific predilection for the coronary arteries is characteristic with formation of aneurysms. The pattern of involvement resembles PAN, while the absence of involvement of arterioles, capillaries, and venules differentiates KD from MPA.

Clinically, four phases of the disease have been described *(176,177)*. Phase 1 is characterized by the acute onset of fever; conjunctivitis; cervical lymphadenopathy; and edema of the hands, feet, and tongue (1–10 d). During that phase vasculitis of the small vessels is observed followed by vascular inflammation of medium- and large-size arteries. In phase 2, the inflammation in small vessels decreases but the characteristic aneurysms of medium-size vessels (i.e., coronary, iliac arteries) and thrombus formation occurs (10–25 d). In phase 3, further decrease of the inflammatory process ensues while fibrosis of the affected vessels develops (25–40 d). During phase 4, stenosis of involved blood vessels in areas of previous scar formation develops with prominent intimal thickening (40 d–4 yr).

During the acute phase of KD, a marked immune activation of lymphocytes (T and B cells), macrophages, and vascular endothelial cells is evident *(176,177)*. The infiltrating cells of the vessel walls are composed primarily of T lymphocytes (CD4 and CD8) and monocytes/macrophages, indicating a strong cellular immune response. Furthermore, circulating levels of cytokines like TNF-α, IL-1, IL-6, and IFN-γ, cytokine receptors like IL-2R *(177)*, chemokines like MCP-1 *(178)* and VEGF *(179)* are elevated, indicating a dominant endothelial and cell-mediated activation. Successful treatment of KD patients with IVIG leads to a decrease of the elevated pro-inflammatory cytokine levels and endothelial activation, further supporting their role in disease pathogenesis *(177,178)*. AECA emerge during the acute phase of KD with cytotoxic activity against endothelial cells, which can further contribute to the vascular injury *(177)*.

It is still unknown what triggers this profound cellular and endothelial-cell activation of young patients with KD. An infectious cause has long been suspected based on epidemiological observations of large-scale epidemics of KD in Japan, its self-limited course, the almost exclusive involvement of young children and the obvious therapeutic effect of IVIG *(177)*. The selected expansion of TCR-bV2 (+) T cells in the peripheral blood and/or involved tissues, led to the hypothesis that a number of toxins with superantigen activity may be the initial trigger for immune activation *(177)*. A number of candidate toxins released during staphylococcal and streptococcal infections have been identified providing strong evidence for their pathogenetic role *(177)*. On the other hand, the occasional association of KD with a number of other bacterial (*Propionobacterium acnes, Streptococcus sanguis*) or viral (Epstein-Barr virus [EBV], parvovirus, adenovirus, varicella-zoster virus) infections, implies that other agents may be involved *(176)*.

Animal Models

Lehman et al. have developed an animal model that closely resembles human KD *(180)*. In this model, mice are injected intraperitoneally with a single dose of *Lactobacillus casei* (*L. casei*) cell wall fragments. Three to four weeks later, all mice develop an asymmetric coronary vasculitis characterized by endothelial and smooth-muscle proliferation as well as by prominent MNC infiltration. Typical lumen narrowing or stenotic lesions are frequent findings *(180)*.

Recently, Brahn et al. reported that early treatment of mice, injected with *L. casei* cell-wall fragments, with an angiogenesis inhibitor (AGM-1470), resulted in 70% reduction of the coronary vasculitic lesions *(181)*. The preliminary results of this study are encouraging and indicate a role of agents that interfere with endothelial activation at least during the early acute phase of the disease.

Clinical Data

Current recommendations regarding the treatment of KD include the combination of aspirin (ASA) and IVIG *(177)*. ASA is given at a daily dose of 80–100 mg/kg (in 4 divided doses) during the acute phase of the disease, until the patient becomes afebrile. At that point, ASA dose is reduced to 3–5 mg/kg/d and is continued for 6–8 wk. In patients that develop coronary aneurysms, therapy is continued indefinitely *(177)*. IVIG is given as single infusion at a dose of 2 g/kg over 10–12 h. For patients with recurrent fever, retreatment with IVIG at the same dose has been proposed *(177)*.

Recently, the role of CS in the treatment of KD has been reevaluated *(182)*. In a small study of four patients, Wright et al. observed a favorable effect of iv pulse methylprednisolone (30 mg/kg/d × 1–3 d) in patients with IVIG-resistant disease *(183)*. Similarly, in a retrospective study, Shinohara et al. found that addition of prednisolone to ASA or ASA + IVIG, led to a statistical decrease in the development of coronary aneurysms *(184)*. An ongoing study of patients with acute KD comparing the standard regimen of IVIG + ASA to IVIV + ASA + iv pulse methylprednisolone, will help clarify the role of CS in the treatment of KD *(185)*.

The use of new agents aiming at the action of proinflammatory cytokines like TNF-α or IL-1 may also be useful in these patients. Similarly, based on the animal model of *L. casei*, inhibitors of neoangiogenesis offer another potential target of future therapies.

CONCLUSIONS

The treatment of vasculitides is still based on traditional regimens containing CS in combination with different immunosuppressive agents. Despite their crucial impact on patient survival and preservation of major organ function as is the case in patients with WG, their long-term use is associated with significant morbidity and mortality. New immunosuppressive agents targeting different elements of the harmful host-immune response are gradually entering clinical trials, as is the case with anti-TNF-based strategies. Better delineation of the pathogenetic steps that culminate in vascular-wall inflammation will certainly identify new targets of therapy. Agents that act as inhibitors of neutrophil or lymphocyte recruitment in the vessel wall, inhibitors of neoangiogenesis, suppressors of endothelial-cell activation, or modulators of complement activation, are promising therapeutic candidates.

Furthermore, the discovery of infectious agents that are responsible for a number of different vasculitic syndromes (e.g., HCV for cryoglobulinemic vasculitis) provide the rational for the design of specific treatments aiming at complete eradication of these causative agents. Additional research in this fascinating area may lead to the discovery of new microorganisms or identify old agents that are causally related to until now considered "idiopathic" vasculitic syndromes. The enormous advances in the molecular techniques that are used for the identification and discovery of infectious agents over the last decade, provide a powerful tool in this direction.

REFERENCES

1. Bloch, D.A., B.A. Michel, G.G. Hunder, D.J. McShane, W.P. Arend, L.H. Calabrese, et al. 1990. The American College of Rheumatology 1990 criteria for the classification of vasculitis. Patients and methods. *Arthritis Rheum.* 33:1068–1073.
2. Jennette, J.C., R.J. Falk, K. Andrassy, P.A. Bacon, J. Churg, W.L. Gross, et al. 1994. Nomenclature of systemic vasculitides. Proposal of an international consensus conference. *Arthritis Rheum.* 37:187–192.
3. Weyand, C.M. and J.J. Goronzy. 1999. Arterial wall injury in giant cell arteritis. *Arthritis Rheum.* 42: 844–853.
4. Kaiser, M., B. Younge, J. Bjornsson, J.J. Goronzy, and C.M. Weyand. 1999. Formation of new vasa vasorum in vasculitis. Production of angiogenic cytokines by multinucleated giant cells. *Am. J. Pathol.* 155:765–774.
5. Weyand, C.M., J. Schonberger, U. Oppitz, N.N. Hunder, K.C. Hicok, and J.J. Goronzy. 1994. Distinct vascular lesions in giant cell arteritis share identical T cell clonotypes. *J. Exp. Med.* 179:951–960.
6. Brack, A., A. Geisler, V.M. Martinez-Taboada, B.R. Younge, J.J. Goronzy, and C.M. Weyand. 1997. Giant cell vasculitis is a T cell-dependent disease. *Mol. Med.* 3:530–543.
7. Weyand, C.M., K.C. Hicok, G.G. Hunder, and J.J. Goronzy. 1994. Tissue cytokine patterns in patients with polymyalgia rheumatica and giant cell arteritis. *Ann. Intern. Med.* 121:484–491.
8. Field, M., A. Cook, and G. Gallagher. 1997. Immuno-localisation of tumour necrosis factor and its receptors in temporal arteritis. *Rheumatol. Int.* 17:113–118.
9. Brack, A., H.L. Rittner, B.R. Younge, C. Kaltschmidt, C.M. Weyand, and J.J. Goronzy. 1997. Glucocorticoid-mediated repression of cytokine gene transcription in human arteritis-SCID chimeras. *J. Clin. Invest.* 99:2842–2850.
10. Hazleman, B.L. 1998. Polymyalgia rheumatica and giant cell arteritis, in Rheumatology. J.H. Klippel and P.A. Dieppe, editors. Mosby, London. 7.21.1–7.21.8

11. Wilke, W.S. and G.S. Hoffman. 1995. Treatment of corticosteroid-resistant giant cell arteritis. *Rheum. Dis. Clin. North Am.* 21:59–71.

12. Langford, C.A., M.C. Sneller, and G.S. Hoffman. 1997. Methotrexate use in systemic vasculitis. *Rheum. Dis. Clin. North Am.* 23:841–853.

13. Hernandez-Garcia, C., C. Soriano, C. Morado, P. Ramos, B. Fernandez-Gutierrez, M. Herrero, et al. 1994. Methotrexate treatment in the management of giant cell arteritis. *Scand. J. Rheumatol.* 23: 295–298.

14. De Silva, M. and B.L. Hazleman. 1986. Azathioprine in giant cell arteritis/polymyalgia rheumatica: a double-blind study. *Ann. Rheum. Dis.* 45:136–138.

15. Schaufelberger, C., R. Andersson, and E. Nordborg. 1998. No additive effect of cyclosporin A compared with glucocorticoid treatment alone in giant cell arteritis: results of an open, controlled, randomized study [letter]. *Br. J. Rheumatol.* 37:464–465.

16. Kerr, G.S., C.W. Hallahan, J. Giordano, R.Y. Leavitt, A.S. Fauci, M. Rottem, and G.S. Hoffman. 1994. Takayasu arteritis. *Ann. Intern. Med.* 120:919–929.

17. Lie, J.T. 1990. Diagnostic histopathology of major systemic and pulmonary vasculitic syndromes. *Rheum. Dis. Clin. North Am.* 16:269–292.

18. Noris, M., E. Daina, S. Gamba, S. Bonazzola, and G. Remuzzi. 1999. Interleukin-6 and RANTES in Takayasu arteritis: a guide for therapeutic decisions? *Circulation* 100:55–60.

19. Noguchi, S., F. Numano, M.B. Gravanis, and J.N. Wilcox. 1998. Increased levels of soluble forms of adhesion molecules in Takayasu arteritis. *Int. J. Cardiol.* 66 (Suppl. 1):S23–S33

20. Harada, M., H. Yoshida, K. Mitsuyama, M. Sakamoto, H. Koga, K. Matsuo, et al. 1998. Aortitis syndrome (Takayasu's arteritis) with cataract and elevated serum level of vascular endothelial growth factor. *Scand. J. Rheumatol.* 27:78–79.

21. Boehme, M.W., W.H. Schmitt, P. Youinou, W.R. Stremmel, and W.L. Gross. 1996. Clinical relevance of elevated serum thrombomodulin and soluble E-selectin in patients with Wegener's granulomatosis and other systemic vasculitides. *Am. J. Med.* 101:387–394.

22. Hoffman, G.S. and A.E. Ahmed. 1998. Surrogate markers of disease activity in patients with Takayasu arteritis. A preliminary report from The International Network for the Study of the Systemic Vasculitides (INSSYS). *Int. J. Cardiol.* 66 (Suppl. 1):S191–S194

23. Seko, Y., S. Minota, A. Kawasaki, Y. Shinkai, K. Maeda, H. Yagita, et al. 1994. Perforin-secreting killer cell infiltration and expression of a 65-kD heat-shock protein in aortic tissue of patients with Takayasu's arteritis. *J. Clin. Invest.* 93:750–758.

24. Seko, Y., O. Sato, A. Takagi, Y. Tada, H. Matsuo, H. Yagita, et al. 1996. Restricted usage of T-cell receptor Valpha-Vbeta genes in infiltrating cells in aortic tissue of patients with Takayasu's arteritis. *Circulation* 93:1788–1790.

25. Nityanand, S., R. Giscombe, S. Srivastava, P. Hjelmstrom, C.B. Sanjeevi, N. Sinha, et al. 1997. A bias in the alphabeta T cell receptor variable region gene usage in Takayasu's arteritis. *Clin. Exp. Immunol.* 107:261–268.

26. Sagar, S., N.K. Ganguly, M. Koicha, and B.K. Sharma. 1992. Immunopathogenesis of Takayasu arteritis. *Heart Vessels* (Suppl. 7):85–90.

27. Dhingra, R., K.K. Talwar, P. Chopra, and R. Kumar. 1993. An enzyme linked immunosorbent assay for detection of anti-aorta antibodies in Takayasu arteritis patients. *Int. J. Cardiol.* 40:237–242.

28. Eichhorn, J., D. Sima, B. Thiele, C. Lindschau, A. Turowski, H. Schmidt, et al. 1996. Anti-endothelial cell antibodies in Takayasu arteritis. *Circulation* 94:2396–2401.

29. Blank, M., I. Krause, T. Goldkorn, A. Praprotnik, A. Livneh, P. Langevitz, et al. 1999. Monoclonal anti-endothelial cell antibodies from a patient with Takayasu arteritis activate endothelial cells from large vessels. *Arthritis Rheum.* 42:1421–1432.

30. Presti, R.M., J.L. Pollock, A.J. Dal Canto, A.K. O'Guin, and H.W. Virgin. 1998. Interferon gamma regulates acute and latent murine cytomegalovirus infection and chronic disease of the great vessels. *J. Exp. Med.* 188:577–588.

31. Weck, K.E., A.J. Dal Canto, J.D. Gould, A.K. O'Guin, K.A. Roth, J.E. Saffitz, et al. 1997. Murine gamma-herpesvirus 68 causes severe large-vessel arteritis in mice lacking interferon-gamma responsiveness: a new model for virus-induced vascular disease. *Nature Med.* 3:1346–1353.

32. Nicklin, M.J., D.E. Hughes, J.L. Barton, J.M. Ure, and G.W. Duff. 2000. Arterial inflammation in mice lacking the interleukin 1 receptor antagonist gene. *J. Exp. Med.* 191:303–312.

33. Kerr, G.S. 1995. Takayasu's arteritis. *Rheum. Dis. Clin. North Am.* 21:1041–1058.

34. Wilke, W.S. 1997. Large vessel vasculitis (giant cell arteritis, Takayasu arteritis). *Baillieres Clin. Rheumatol.* 11:285–313.

35. Hoffman, G.S., R.Y. Leavitt, G.S. Kerr, M. Rottem, M.C. Sneller, and A.S. Fauci. 1994. Treatment of glucocorticoid-resistant or relapsing Takayasu arteritis with methotrexate. *Arthritis Rheum.* 37:578–582.

36. Daina, E., A. Schieppati, and G. Remuzzi. 1999. Mycophenolate mofetil for the treatment of Takayasu arteritis: report of three cases. *Ann. Intern. Med.* 130:422–426.

37. Allison, A.C. and E.M. Eugui. 1993. The design and development of an immunosuppressive drug, mycophenolate mofetil. *Springer Semin. Immunopathol.* 14:353–380.

38. Durez, P., T. Appelboom, C. Pira, P. Stordeur, B. Vray, and M. Goldman. 1999. Antiinflammatory properties of mycophenolate mofetil in murine endotoxemia: inhibition of TNF-alpha and upregulation of IL-10 release. *Int. J. Immunopharmacol.* 21:581–587.

39. Lie, J.T. 1995. Histopathologic specificity of systemic vasculitis. *Rheum. Dis. Clin. North Am.* 21: 883–909.

40. Dienstag, J.L. 1981. Immunopathogenesis of the extrahepatic manifestations of hepatitis B virus infection.. *Springer Semin. Immunopathol.* 3:461–472.

41. Nowoslawski, A. 1979. Hepatitis B virus-induced immune complex disease. *Prog. Liver Dis.* 6:393–406.

42. Calabrese, L.H. 1991. Vasculitis and infection with the human immunodeficiency virus. *Rheum. Dis. Clin. North Am.* 17:131–147.

43. Carson, C.W., D.L. Conn, A.J. Czaja, T.L. Wright, and M.E. Brecher. 1993. Frequency and significance of antibodies to hepatitis C virus in polyarteritis nodosa. *J. Rheumatol.* 20:304–309.

44. Hasler, P., H. Kistler, and H. Gerber. 1995. Vasculitides in hairy cell leukemia. *Semin. Arthritis Rheum.* 25:134–142.

45. Guillevin, L., F. Lhote, P. Cohen, F. Sauvaget, B. Jarrousse, O. Lortholary, et al. 1995. Polyarteritis nodosa related to hepatitis B virus. A prospective study with long-term observation of 41 patients. *Medicine* (Baltimore) 74:238–253.

46. Gupta, R.C. and P.F. Kohler. 1984. Identification of HBsAg determinants in immune complexes from hepatitis B virus-associated vasculitis. *J. Immunol.* 132:1223–1228.

47. Cid, M.C., J.M. Grau, J. Casademont, E. Campo, B. Coll-Vinent, A. Lopez-Soto, et al. 1994. Immunohistochemical characterization of inflammatory cells and immunologic activation markers in muscle and nerve biopsy specimens from patients with systemic polyarteritis nodosa. *Arthritis Rheum.* 37: 1055–1061.

48. Coll-Vinent, B., M. Cebrian, M.C. Cid, C. Font, J. Esparza, M. Juan, et al. 1998. Dynamic pattern of endothelial cell adhesion molecule expression in muscle and perineural vessels from patients with classic polyarteritis nodosa. *Arthritis Rheum.* 41:435–444.

49. Germouth, F.G.J. 1953. Comparative histologic and immunologic study in rabbits of induced hypersensitivity of serum sickness type. *J. Exp. Med.* 97:257–269.

50. Kajima, M. and M. Pollard. 1969. Arterial lesions in gnotobiotic mice congenitally infected with LCM virus. *Nature* 224:188–190.

51. Porter, D.D., A.E. Larsen, and H.G. Porter. 1980. Aleutian disease of mink. *Adv. Immunol.* 29:261–286.

52. Moyer, C.F., J.D. Strandberg, and C.L. Reinisch. 1987. Systemic mononuclear-cell vasculitis in MRL/Mp-lpr/lpr mice. A histologic and immunocytochemical analysis. *Am. J. Pathol.* 127:229–242.

53. Miyazawa, M., M. Nose, M. Kawashima, and M. Kyogoku. 1987. Pathogenesis of arteritis of SL/Ni mice. Possible lytic effect of anti-gp70 antibodies on vascular smooth muscle cells. *J. Exp. Med.* 166:890–908.

54. Gauthier, V.J. and M. Mannik. 1992. Immune complexes in the pathogenesis of vasculitis, in Systemic vasculitis. The biological basis. C.E. LeRoy, editor. Marcel Dekker, Inc., New York. 401–420.

55. Cheema, A., J.B. Henson, and J.R. Gorham. 1972. Aleutian disease of mink. Prevention of lesions by immunosuppression. *Am. J. Pathol.* 66:543–556.

56. Hahn, B.H. 1997. Animal models of systemic lupus erythematosus, in Dubois' lupus erythematosus. D.J. Wallace and B.H. Hahn, editors. Williams & Wilkins, Baltimore. 339–380.

57. Jonsson, C.A., M. Erlandsson, L. Svensson, J. Molne, and H. Carlsten. 1999. Mycophenolate mofetil ameliorates perivascular T lymphocyte inflammation and reduces the double-negative T cell population in SLE-prone MRLlpr/lpr mice. *Cell. Immunol.* 197:136–144.

58. Frohnert, P. and S. Sheps. 1967. Long term follow-up study of polyarteritis nodosa. *Am. J. Med.* 48:8–14.

59. Guillevin, L. and F. Lhote. 1998. Treatment of polyarteritis nodosa and microscopic polyangiitis. *Arthritis Rheum.* 41:2100–2105.

60. Calabrese, L.H., G.S. Hoffman, and L. Guillevin. 1995. Therapy of resistant systemic necrotizing vasculitis. Polyarteritis, Churg-Strauss syndrome, Wegener's granulomatosis, and hypersensitivity vasculitis group disorders. *Rheum. Dis. Clin. North Am.* 21:41–57.

61. Gayraud, M., L. Guillevin, P. Cohen, F. Lhote, P. Cacoub, P. Deblois, et al. 1997. Treatment of good-prognosis polyarteritis nodosa and Churg-Strauss syndrome: comparison of steroids and oral or pulse cyclophosphamide in 25 patients. French Cooperative Study Group for Vasculitides. *Br. J. Rheumatol.* 36:1290–1297.

62. Lhote, F., P. Cohen, and L. Guillevin. 1998. Polyarteritis nodosa, microscopic polyangiitis and Churg-Strauss syndrome. *Lupus* 7:238–258.

63. Mandell, B.F. and L.H. Calabrese. 1998. Infections and systemic vasculitis. *Curr. Opin. Rheumatol.* 10:51–57.

64. Maclachlan, D., M. Battegay, A.L. Jacob, and A. Tyndall. 2000. Successful treatment of hepatitis B-associated polyarteritis nodosa with a combination of lamivudine and conventional immunosuppressive therapy: a case report [letter]. *Rheumatology* (Oxford) 39:106–108.

65. Kruger, M., K.H. Boker, H. Zeidler, and M.P. Manns. 1997. Treatment of hepatitis B-related polyarteritis nodosa with famciclovir and interferon alfa-2b. *J. Hepatol.* 26:935–939.

66. Font, C., O. Miro, E. Pedrol, F. Masanes, B. Coll-Vinent, J. Casademont, et al. 1996. Polyarteritis nodosa in human immunodeficiency virus infection: report of four cases and review of the literature. *Br. J. Rheumatol.* 35:796–799.

67. Gisselbrecht, M., P. Cohen, O. Lortholary, B. Jarrousse, M. Gayraud, I. Lecompte, et al. 1998. Human immunodeficiency virus-related vasculitis. Clinical presentation of and therapeutic approach to eight cases. *Ann. Med. Interne.* (Paris) 149:398–405.

68. Guillevin, L., P. Cohen, M. Gayraud, F. Lhote, B. Jarrousse, and P. Casassus. 1999. Churg-Strauss syndrome. Clinical study and long-term follow-up of 96 patients. *Medicine* (Baltimore) 78:26–37.

69. Lanham, J.G., K.B. Elkon, C.D. Pusey, and G.R. Hughes. 1984. Systemic vasculitis with asthma and eosinophilia: a clinical approach to the Churg-Strauss syndrome. *Medicine* (Baltimore) 63:65–81.

70. Lanham, J.G. and J. Churg. 1991. Churg-Strauss syndrome, in Systemic Vasculitides. A. Churg and J. Churg, editors. Igaku-Shoin, New York. 101–120.

71. Costa, J.J., P.F. Weller, and S.J. Galli. 1997. The cells of the allergic response: mast cells, basophils, and eosinophils. *JAMA* 278:1815–1822.

72. Schmitt, W.H., E. Csernok, S. Kobayashi, A. Klinkenborg, E. Reinhold-Keller, and W.L. Gross. 1998. Churg-Strauss syndrome: serum markers of lymphocyte activation and endothelial damage. *Arthritis Rheum.* 41:445–452.

73. Schnabel, A., E. Csernok, J. Braun, and W.L. Gross. 1999. Inflammatory cells and cellular activation in the lower respiratory tract in Churg-Strauss syndrome. *Thorax* 54:771–778.

74. Chang, H.W., K.H. Leong, D.R. Koh, and S.H. Lee. 1999. Clonality of isolated eosinophils in the hypereosinophilic syndrome. *Blood* 93:1651–1657.

75. Muschen, M., U. Warskulat, A. Perniok, J. Even, C. Moers, B. Kismet, et al. 1999. Involvement of soluble CD95 in Churg-Strauss syndrome. *Am. J. Pathol.* 155:915–925.

76. Hattori, N., M. Ichimura, M. Nagamatsu, M. Li, K. Yamamoto, K. Kumazawa, et al. 1999. Clinicopathological features of Churg-Strauss syndrome-associated neuropathy. *Brain* 122:427–439.

77. Vassilopoulos, D. and G.S. Hoffman. 1999. Clinical utility of testing for antineutrophil cytoplasmic antibodies. *Clin. Diagn. Lab. Immunol.* 6:645–651.

78. Abu-Shakra, M., H. Smythe, J. Lewtas, E. Badley, D. Weber, and E. Keystone. 1994. Outcome of polyarteritis nodosa and Churg-Strauss syndrome. An analysis of twenty-five patients. *Arthritis Rheum.* 37:1798–1803.

79. McDermott, E.M. and R.J. Powell. 1998. Cyclosporin in the treatment of Churg-Strauss syndrome [letter]. *Ann. Rheum. Dis.* 57:258–259.

80. Tatsis, E., A. Schnabel, and W.L. Gross. 1998. Interferon-alpha treatment of four patients with the Churg-Strauss syndrome. *Ann. Intern. Med.* 129:370–374.

81. Aldebert, D., B. Lamkhioued, C. Desaint, A.S. Gounni, M. Goldman, A. Capron, et al. 1996. Eosinophils express a functional receptor for interferon alpha: inhibitory role of interferon alpha on the release of mediators. *Blood* 87:2354–2360.

82. Ernstoff, M.S. and J.M. Kirkwood. 1984. Changes in the bone marrow of cancer patients treated with recombinant interferon alpha-2. *Am. J. Med.* 76:593–596.

83. Morita, M., B. Lamkhioued, G.A. Soussi, D. Aldebert, E. Delaporte, A. Capron, and M. Capron. 1996. Induction by interferons of human eosinophil apoptosis and regulation by interleukin-3, granulocyte/macrophage-colony stimulating factor and interleukin-5. *Eur. Cytokine. Netw.* 7:725–732.

84. Krishnaswamy, G., J.K. Smith, S. Srikanth, D.S. Chi, J.H. Kalbfleisch, and S.K. Huang. 1996. Lymphoblastoid interferon-alpha inhibits T cell proliferation and expression of eosinophil-activating cytokines. *J. Interferon Cytokine Res.* 16:819–827.

85. Nakajima, H., A. Nakao, Y. Watanabe, S. Yoshida, and I. Iwamoto. 1994. IFN-alpha inhibits antigen-induced eosinophil and CD4+ T cell recruitment into tissue. *J. Immunol.* 153:1264–1270.

86. Hoffman, G.S., G.S. Kerr, R.Y. Leavitt, C.W. Hallahan, R.S. Lebovics, W.D.R. Travis, and A.S. Fauci. 1992. Wegener granulomatosis: an analysis of 158 patients. *Ann. Intern. Med.* 116:488–498.

87. Travis, W.D., G.S. Hoffman, R.Y. Leavitt, H.I. Pass, and A.S. Fauci. 1991. Surgical pathology of the lung in Wegener's granulomatosis. Review of 87 open lung biopsies from 67 patients. *Am. J. Surg. Pathol.* 15:315–333.

88. Mark, E.J., O. Matsubara, N.S. Tan-Liu, and R. Fienberg. 1988. The pulmonary biopsy in the early diagnosis of Wegener's (pathergic) granulomatosis: a study based on 35 open lung biopsies. *Human Pathol.* 19:1065–1071.

89. Ledford, D.K. 1997. Immunologic aspects of vasculitis and cardiovascular disease. *JAMA* 278: 1962–1971.

90. Hoffman, G.S. and U. Specks. 1998. Antineutrophil cytoplasmic antibodies. *Arthritis Rheum.* 41: 1521–1537.

91. Brouwer, E., M.G. Huitema, A.H. Mulder, P. Heeringa, H. van Goor, J.W. Tervaert, et al. 1994. Neutrophil activation in vitro and in vivo in Wegener's granulomatosis. *Kidney Int.* 45:1120–1131.

92. Heeringa, P., E. Brouwer, T.J. Cohen, J.J. Weening, and C.G. Kallenberg. 1998. Animal models of anti-neutrophil cytoplasmic antibody associated vasculitis. *Kidney Int.* 53:253–263.

93. Cunningham, M.A., X.R. Huang, J.P. Dowling, P.G. Tipping, and S.R. Holdsworth. 1999. Prominence of cell-mediated immunity effectors in "pauci-immune" glomerulonephritis. *J. Am. Soc. Nephrol.* 10:499–506.

94. Gephardt, G.N., M. Ahmad, and R.R. Tubbs. 1983. Pulmonary vasculitis (Wegener's granulomatosis). Immunohistochemical study of T and B cell markers. *Am. J. Med.* 74:700–704.

95. Ballieux, B.E., S.H. van der Burg, E.C. Hagen, F.J. van der Woude, C.J. Melief, and M.R. Daha. 1995. Cell-mediated autoimmunity in patients with Wegener's granulomatosis (WG). *Clin. Exp. Immunol.* 100:186–193.

96. Brouwer, E., C.A. Stegeman, M.G. Huitema, P.C. Limburg, and C.G. Kallenberg. 1994. T cell reactivity to proteinase 3 and myeloperoxidase in patients with Wegener's granulomatosis (WG). *Clin. Exp. Immunol.* 98:448–453.

97. Arranz, O., J. Ara, R. Rodriguez, A. Saurina, E. Mirapeix, and A. Darnell. 2000. Serum levels of soluble interleukin-2 receptor in patients with ANCA-associated vasculitis. *J. Nephrol.* 13:59–64.

98. Schmitt, W.H., C. Heesen, E. Csernok, A. Rautmann, and W.L. Gross. 1992. Elevated serum levels of soluble interleukin-2 receptor in patients with Wegener's granulomatosis. Association with disease activity. *Arthritis Rheum.* 35:1088–1096.

99. Stegeman, C.A., J.W. Tervaert, M.G. Huitema, and C.G. Kallenberg. 1993. Serum markers of T-cell activation in relapses of Wegener's granulomatosis. *Adv. Exp. Med. Biol.* 336:389–392.

100. Popa, E.R., C.A. Stegeman, N.A. Bos, C.G. Kallenberg, and J.W. Tervaert. 1999. Differential B- and T-cell activation in Wegener's granulomatosis. *J. Allergy Clin. Immunol.* 103:885–894.

101. Schlesier, M., T. Kaspar, J. Gutfleisch, G. Wolff-Vorbeck, and H.H. Peter. 1995. Activated CD4+ and CD8+ T-cell subsets in Wegener's granulomatosis. *Rheumatol. Int.* 14:213–219.

102. Ikeda, M., Y. Watanabe, S. Kitahara, and T. Inouye. 1993. Distinctive increases in HLA-DR+ and CD8+57+ lymphocyte subsets in Wegener's granulomatosis. *Int. Arch. Allergy Immunol.* 102:205–208.

103. Csernok, E., A. Trabandt, A. Muller, G.C. Wang, F. Moosig, J. Paulsen, A. Schnabel, and W.L. Gross. 1999. Cytokine profiles in Wegener's granulomatosis: predominance of type 1 (Th1) in the granulomatous inflammation. *Arthritis Rheum.* 42:742–750.

104. Ludviksson, B.R., M.C. Sneller, K.S. Chua, C. Talar-Williams, C.A. Langford, R.O. Ehrhardt, et al. 1998. Active Wegener's granulomatosis is associated with HLA-DR+ CD4+ T cells exhibiting an unbalanced Th1-type T cell cytokine pattern: reversal with IL-10. *J. Immunol.* 160:3602–3609.

105. Shoenfeld, Y. 1994. Idiotypic induction of autoimmunity: a new aspect of the idiotypic network. *FASEB J.* 8:1296–1301.

106. Blank, M., Y. Tomer, M. Stein, J. Kopolovic, A. Wiik, P.L. Meroni, et al. 1995. Immunization with anti-neutrophil cytoplasmic antibody (ANCA) induces the production of mouse ANCA and perivascular lymphocyte infiltration. *Clin. Exp. Immunol.* 102:120–130.

107. Jenne, D.E., L. Frohlich, A.M. Hummel, and U. Specks. 1997. Cloning and functional expression of the murine homologue of proteinase 3: implications for the design of murine models of vasculitis. *FEBS Lett.* 408:187–190.

108. Heeringa, P., J. van den Born, E. Brouwer, K.M. Dolman, P.A. Klok, M.G. Huitema, et al. 1996. Elastase, but not proteinase 3 (PR3), induces proteinuria associated with loss of glomerular basement membrane heparan sulphate after in vivo renal perfusion in rats. *Clin. Exp. Immunol.* 105: 321–329.

109. Hoffman, G.S. 1997. Treatment of Wegener's granulomatosis: time to change the standard of care? *Arthritis Rheum.* 40:2099–2104.

110. Wolff, S.M., A.S. Fauci, R.G. Horn, and D.C. Dale. 1974. Wegener's granulomatosis. *Ann. Intern. Med.* 81:513–525.

111. Guillevin, L., J.F. Cordier, F. Lhote, P. Cohen, B. Jarrousse, I. Royer, et al. 1997. A prospective, multicenter, randomized trial comparing steroids and pulse cyclophosphamide versus steroids and oral cyclophosphamide in the treatment of generalized Wegener's granulomatosis. *Arthritis Rheum.* 40:2187–2198.

112. Haubitz, M., S. Schellong, U. Gobel, H.J. Schurek, D. Schaumann, K.M. Koch, and R. Brunkhorst. 1998. Intravenous pulse administration of cyclophosphamide versus daily oral treatment in patients with antineutrophil cytoplasmic antibody-associated vasculitis and renal involvement: a prospective, randomized study. *Arthritis Rheum.* 41:1835–1844.

113. Stegeman, C.A., T.J. Cohen, P.E. de Jong, and C.G. Kallenberg. 1996. Trimethoprim-sulfamethoxazole (co-trimoxazole) for the prevention of relapses of Wegener's granulomatosis. Dutch Co-Trimoxazole Wegener Study Group. *N. Engl. J. Med.* 335:16–20.

114. Sneller, M.C., G.S. Hoffman, C. Talar-Williams, G.S. Kerr, C.W. Hallahan, and A.S. Fauci. 1995. An analysis of forty-two Wegener's granulomatosis patients treated with methotrexate and prednisone. *Arthritis Rheum.* 38:608–613.

115. Stone, J.H., W. Tun, and D.B. Hellman. 1999. Treatment of non-life threatening Wegener's granulomatosis with methotrexate and daily prednisone as the initial therapy of choice. *J. Rheumatol.* 26:1134–1139.

116. Langford, C.A., C. Talar-Williams, K.S. Barron, and M.C. Sneller. 1999. A staged approach to the treatment of Wegener's granulomatosis: induction of remission with glucocorticoids and daily cyclophosphamide switching to methotrexate for remission maintenance. *Arthritis Rheum.* 42:2666–2673.

117. de Groot, K. and W.L. Gross. 1998. Wegener's granulomatosis: disease course, assessment of activity and extent and treatment. *Lupus* 7:285–291.

118. Nowack, R., U. Gobel, P. Klooker, O. Hergesell, K. Andrassy, and F.J. van der Woude. 1999. Mycophenolate mofetil for maintenance therapy of Wegener's granulomatosis and microscopic polyangiitis: a pilot study in 11 patients with renal involvement. *J. Am. Soc. Nephrol.* 10:1965–1971.

119. Metzler, C., I. Loew-Friedrich, E. Reinhold-Keller, C. Fink, and W.L. Gross. 1999. Maintenance of remission with leflunomide in Wegener's Granulomatosis. *Arthritis Rheum.* 42:S315(Abstract).

120. Stone, J.H., D.B. Hellman, M.L. Uhlfelder, N.M. Bedocs, S.I. Crook, J. Holbrook, and G.S. Hoffman. 1999. Etanercept in Wegener's Granulomatosis: Results of an open-label trial. *Arthritis Rheum.* 42:S315(Abstract).

121. Inoue, M., B. Akikusa, Y. Masuda, and Y. Kondo. 1998. Demonstration of microaneurysms at the interlobular arteries of the kidneys in microscopic polyangiitis: a three-dimensional study. *Human Pathol.* 29:223–227.

122. D'Agati, V., P. Chander, M. Nash, and R. Mancilla-Jimenez. 1986. Idiopathic microscopic polyarteritis nodosa: ultrastructural observations on the renal vascular and glomerular lesions. *Am. J. Kidney Dis.* 7:95–110.

123. Guillevin, L., B. Durand-Gasselin, R. Cevallos, M. Gayraud, F. Lhote, P. Callard, et al. 1999. Microscopic polyangiitis: clinical and laboratory findings in eighty-five patients. *Arthritis Rheum.* 42:421–430.

124. Muller, K.A., R.T. van Wijk, C.F. Franssen, G. Molema, C.G. Kallenberg, and J.W. Tervaert. 1999. In vitro up-regulation of E-selectin and induction of interleukin-6 in endothelial cells by autoantibodies in Wegener's granulomatosis and microscopic polyangiitis. *Clin. Exp. Rheumatol.* 17:433–440.

125. Falk, R.J., R.S. Terrell, L.A. Charles, and J.C. Jennette. 1990. Anti-neutrophil cytoplasmic autoantibodies induce neutrophils to degranulate and produce oxygen radicals in vitro. *Proc. Natl. Acad. Sci. USA* 87:4115–4119.

126. Reumaux, D., P.J. Vossebeld, D. Roos, and A.J. Verhoeven. 1995. Effect of tumor necrosis factor-induced integrin activation on Fc gamma receptor II-mediated signal transduction: relevance for activation of neutrophils by anti-proteinase 3 or anti-myeloperoxidase antibodies. *Blood* 86:3189–3195.

127. Brooks, C.J., W.J. King, D.J. Radford, D. Adu, M. McGrath, and C.O. Savage. 1996. IL-1 beta production by human polymorphonuclear leucocytes stimulated by anti-neutrophil cytoplasmic autoantibodies: relevance to systemic vasculitis. *Clin. Exp. Immunol.* 106:273–279.

128. Casselman, B.L., K.S. Kilgore, B.F. Miller, and J.S. Warren. 1995. Antibodies to neutrophil cytoplasmic antigens induce monocyte chemoattractant protein-1 secretion from human monocytes. *J. Lab. Clin. Med.* 126:495–502.

129. Noronha, I.L., C. Kruger, K. Andrassy, E. Ritz, and R. Waldherr. 1993. In situ production of TNF-alpha, IL-1 beta and IL-2R in ANCA-positive glomerulonephritis. *Kidney Int.* 43:682–692.

130. Simpson, I.J., M.A. Skinner, A. Geursen, J.S. Peake, W.G. Abbott, J.D. Fraser, et al. 1995. Peripheral blood T lymphocytes in systemic vasculitis: increased T cell receptor V beta 2 gene usage in microscopic polyarteritis. *Clin. Exp. Immunol.* 101:220–226.

131. Griffith, M.E., A. Coulthart, and C.D. Pusey. 1996. T cell responses to myeloperoxidase (MPO) and proteinase 3 (PR3) in patients with systemic vasculitis. *Clin. Exp. Immunol.* 103:253–258.

132. Harper, J.M., D.G. Healey, S. Thiru, C. Gordon, and A. Cook. 1999. Factors involved in the pathogenesis of neutrophilic vasculitis in MRL/Mp-lpr/lpr mice: a model for human microscopic angiitis. *Autoimmunity* 31:133–145.

133. Qasim, F.J., P.W. Mathieson, S. Thiru, and D.B. Oliveira. 1995. Cyclosporin A exacerbates mercuric chloride-induced vasculitis in the brown Norway rat. *Lab. Invest.* 72:183–190.

134. Nachman, P.H., S.L. Hogan, J.C. Jennette, and R.J. Falk. 1996. Treatment response and relapse in antineutrophil cytoplasmic autoantibody-associated microscopic polyangiitis and glomerulonephritis. *J. Am. Soc. Nephrol.* 7:33–39.

135. Westman, K.W., P.G. Bygren, H. Olsson, J. Ranstam, and J. Wieslander. 1998. Relapse rate, renal survival, and cancer morbidity in patients with Wegener's granulomatosis or microscopic polyangiitis with renal involvement. *J. Am. Soc. Nephrol.* 9:842–852.

136. Haubitz, M., K.M. Koch, and R. Brunkhorst. 1998. Cyclosporin for the prevention of disease reactivation in relapsing ANCA-associated vasculitis. *Nephrol. Dial Transplant.* 13:2074–2076.

137. Blanco, R., V.M. Martinez-Taboada, V. Rodriguez-Valverde, and M. Garcia-Fuentes. 1998. Cutaneous vasculitis in children and adults. Associated diseases and etiologic factors in 303 patients. *Medicine* (Baltimore) 77:403–418.

138. Gyselbrecht, L., F. De Keyser, K. Ongenae, J.M. Naeyaert, M. Praet, and E.M. Veys. 1996. Etiological factors and underlying conditions in patients with leucocytoclastic vasculitis. *Clin. Exp. Rheumatol.* 14:665–668.

139. Braverman, I.M. and A. Yen. 1975. Demonstration of immune complexes in spontaneous and histamine-induced lesions and in normal skin of patients with leukocytoclastic angitis. *J. Invest. Dermatol.* 64:105–112.

140. Gower, R.G., W.M.J. Sams, E.G. Thorne, P.F. Kohler, and H.N. Claman. 1977. Leukocytoclastic vasculitis: sequential appearance of immunoreactants and cellular changes in serial biopsies. *J. Invest. Dermatol.* 69:477–484.

141. Herrmann, W.A., R.H. Kauffmann, L.A. van Es, M.R. Daha, and C.J. Meijer. 1980. Allergic vasculitis. A histological and immunofluorescent study of lesional and non-lesional skin in relation to circulating immune complexes. *Arch. Dermatol. Res.* 269:179–187.

142. Gross, W.L. 1998. Immunopathogenesis of vasculitis, in Rheumatology. J.H. Klippel and P.A. Dieppe, editors. Mosby, London. 7.19.1–7.19.8

143. Boom, B.W., M. Mommaas, M.R. Daha, and B.J. Vermeer. 1989. Complement-mediated endothelial cell damage in immune complex vasculitis of the skin: ultrastructural localization of the membrane attack complex. *J. Invest. Dermatol.* 93:68S–72S.

144. Kawana, S. 1996. The membrane attack complex of complement alters the membrane integrity of cultured endothelial cells: a possible pathophysiology for immune complex vasculitis. *Acta Derm. Venereol.* 76:13–16.

145. Zax, R.H., S.J. Hodge, and J.P. Callen. 1990. Cutaneous leukocytoclastic vasculitis. Serial histopathologic evaluation demonstrates the dynamic nature of the infiltrate. *Arch. Dermatol.* 126:69–72.

146. Claudy, A. 1998. Pathogenesis of leukocytoclastic vasculitis. *Eur. J. Dermatol.* 8:75–79.

147. Grunwald, M.H., O. Shriker, S. Halevy, M. Alkan, and R. Levy. 1997. Impaired neutrophil functions in patients with leukocytoclastic vasculitis. *Int. J. Dermatol.* 36:509–513.

148. Shi, Y., M. Honma, and F. Koizumi. 1998. Cutaneous allergic vasculitis: clinicopathological characterization and identification of apoptosis. *Pathol. Int.* 48:705–716.

149. Bonkovsky, H.L., T.J. Liang, K. Hasegawa, and B. Banner. 1995. Chronic leukocytoclastic vasculitis complicating HBV infection. Possible role of mutant forms of HBV in pathogenesis and persistence of disease. *J. Clin. Gastroenterol.* 21:42–47.

150. Lamprecht, P., A. Gause, and W.L. Gross. 1999. Cryoglobulinemic vasculitis. *Arthritis Rheum.* 42: 2507–2516.

151. Theofilopoulos, A.N. 1993. Immune complexes in autoimmunity, in The molecular pathology of autoimmune diseases. C.A. Bona, K.A. Siminovitch, M. Zanetti, and A.N. Theofilopoulos, editors. Harwood Academic Publishers, Switzerland. 229–243.

152. Sylvestre, D.L. and J.V. Ravetch. 1994. Fc receptors initiate the Arthus reaction: redefining the inflammatory cascade. *Science* 265:1095–1098.

153. Mulligan, M.S. and P.A. Ward. 1992. Immune complex-induced lung and dermal vascular injury. Differing requirements for tumor necrosis factor-alpha and IL-1. *J. Immunol.* 149:331–339.

154. Norman, K.E., T.J. Williams, M. Feldmann, and A.G. Rossi. 1996. Effect of soluble P55 tumour-necrosis factor binding fusion protein on the local Shwartzman and Arthus reactions. *Br. J. Pharmacol.* 117:471–478.

155. Warren, J.S. 1991. Disparate roles for TNF in the pathogenesis of acute immune complex alveolitis and dermal vasculitis. *Clin. Immunol. Immunopathol.* 61:249–259.

156. Cochrane, C.G. and D. Koffler. 1973. Immune complex disease in experimental animals and man. *Adv. Immunol.* 16:185–264.

157. Hazenbos, W.L., J.E. Gessner, F.M. Hofhuis, H. Kuipers, D. Meyer, I.A. Heijnen, et al. 1996. Impaired IgG-dependent anaphylaxis and Arthus reaction in Fc gamma RIII (CD16) deficient mice. *Immunity* 5:181–188.

158. Hopken, U.E., B. Lu, N.P. Gerard, and C. Gerard. 1997. Impaired inflammatory responses in the reverse arthus reaction through genetic deletion of the C5a receptor. *J. Exp. Med.* 186:749–756.

159. Martinez-Taboada, V.M., R. Blanco, M. Garcia-Fuentes, and V. Rodriguez-Valverde. 1997. Clinical features and outcome of 95 patients with hypersensitivity vasculitis. *Am. J. Med.* 102: 186–191.

160. Sais, G., A. Vidaller, A. Jucgla, F. Gallardo, and J. Peyri. 1995. Colchicine in the treatment of cutaneous leukocytoclastic vasculitis. Results of a prospective, randomized controlled trial. *Arch. Dermatol.* 131:1399–1402.

161. Saulsbury, F.T. 1999. Henoch-Schonlein purpura in children. Report of 100 patients and review of the literature. *Medicine* (Baltimore) 78:395–409.

162. Mollica, F., V.S. Li, R. Garozzo, and G. Russo. 1992. Effectiveness of early prednisone treatment in preventing the development of nephropathy in anaphylactoid purpura. *Eur. J. Pediatr.* 151:140–144.

163. Saulsbury, F.T. 1993. Corticosteroid therapy does not prevent nephritis in Henoch-Schonlein purpura. *Pediatr. Nephrol.* 7:69–71.

164. Austin, H.A. and J.E. Balow. 1983. Henoch-Schonlein nephritis: prognostic features and the challenge of therapy. *Am. J. Kidney Dis.* 2:512–520.

165. Niaudet, P. and R. Habib. 1998. Methylprednisolone pulse therapy in the treatment of severe forms of Schonlein-Henoch purpura nephritis. *Pediatr. Nephrol.* 12:238–243.

166. Faedda, R., M. Pirisi, A. Satta, L. Bosincu, and E. Bartoli. 1996. Regression of Henoch-Schonlein disease with intensive immunosuppressive treatment. *Clin. Pharmacol. Ther.* 60:576–581.

167. Oner, A., K. Tinaztepe, and O. Erdogan. 1995. The effect of triple therapy on rapidly progressive type of Henoch-Schonlein nephritis. *Pediatr. Nephrol.* 9:6–10.

168. Bergstein, J., J. Leiser, and S.P. Andreoli. 1998. Response of crescentic Henoch-Schoenlein purpura nephritis to corticosteroid and azathioprine therapy. *Clin. Nephrol.* 49:9–14.

169. Foster, B.J., C. Bernard, K.N. Drummond, and A.K. Sharma. 2000. Effective therapy for severe Henoch-Schonlein purpura nephritis with prednisone and azathioprine: a clinical and histopathologic study. *J. Pediatr.* 136:370–375.

170. Hattori, M., K. Ito, T. Konomoto, H. Kawaguchi, T. Yoshioka, and M. Khono. 1999. Plasmapheresis as the sole therapy for rapidly progressive Henoch-Schonlein purpura nephritis in children. *Am. J. Kidney Dis.* 33:427–433.

171. Rostoker, G., D. Desvaux-Belghiti, Y. Pilatte, M. Petit-Phar, C. Philippon, L. Deforges, et al. 1994. High-dose immunoglobulin therapy for severe IgA nephropathy and Henoch-Schonlein purpura. *Ann. Intern. Med.* 120:476–484.

172. Agnello, V., R.T. Chung, and L.M. Kaplan. 1992. A role for hepatitis C virus infection in type II cryoglobulinemia. *N. Engl. J. Med.* 327:1490–1495.

173. Hadziyannis, S.J. and D. Vassilopoulos. 2000. Complex management issues: management of HCV in the atypical patient. *Baillieres Clin. Gastroenterol.* 14:277–291.

174. Donada, C., A. Crucitti, V. Donadon, L. Chemello, and A. Alberti. 1998. Interferon and ribavirin combination therapy in patients with chronic hepatitis C and mixed cryoglobulinemia [letter]. *Blood* 92:2983–2984.

175. Cid, M.C., J. Hernandez-Rodriguez, J. Robert, A. Rio, J. Casademont, B. Coll-Vinent, et al. 1999. Interferon-a may exacerbate cryoglobulinemia-related ischemic manifestations. An adverse effect potentially related to its anti-angiogenic activity. *Arthritis Rheum.* 42:1051–1055.

176. Kawasaki, T. 1998. Kawasaki disease. *In* Rheumatology. J.H. Klippel and P.A. Dieppe, editors. Mosby, London. 7.27.1–7.27.4

177. Leung, D.Y., P.M. Schlievert, and H.C. Meissner. 1998. The immunopathogenesis and management of Kawasaki syndrome. *Arthritis Rheum.* 41:1538–1547.

178. Terai, M., T. Jibiki, A. Harada, Y. Terashima, K. Yasukawa, S. Tateno, et al. 1999. Dramatic decrease of circulating levels of monocyte chemoattractant protein-1 in Kawasaki disease after gamma globulin treatment. *J. Leukoc. Biol.* 65:566–572.

179. Terai, M., K. Yasukawa, S. Narumoto, S. Tateno, S. Oana, and Y. Kohno. 1999. Vascular endothelial growth factor in acute Kawasaki disease. *Am. J. Cardiol.* 83:337–339.

180. Lehman, T.J., R. Warren, D. Gietl, V. Mahnovski, and M. Prescott. 1988. Variable expression of Lactobacillus casei cell wall-induced coronary arteritis: an animal model of Kawasaki's disease in selected inbred mouse strains. *Clin. Immunol. Immunopathol.* 48:108–118.

181. Brahn, E., T.J.A. Lehman, D.J. Peacock, C. Tang, and M.L. Banquerigo. 1999. Suppression of coronary vasculitis in a murine model of Kawasaki disease using an angiogenesis inhibitor. *Clin. Immunol.* 90:147–151.

182. Newburger, J.W. 1999. Treatment of Kawasaki disease: corticosteroids revisited. *J. Pediatr.* 135:411–413.

183. Wright, D.A., J.W. Newburger, A. Baker, and R.P. Sundel. 1996. Treatment of immune globulin-resistant Kawasaki disease with pulsed doses of corticosteroids. *J. Pediatr.* 128:146–149.

184. Shinohara, M., K. Sone, T. Tomomasa, and A. Morikawa. 1999. Corticosteroids in the treatment of the acute phase of Kawasaki disease. *J. Pediatr.* 135:465–469.

185. Sundel, R.P., A. Baker, D.R. Fulton, B.A. Eberhard, and J.W. Newburger. 1999. Corticosteroid therapy in Kawasaki disease: preliminary report of a pilot study of combined IVIG and pulse methylprednisolone as initial treatment. *Arthritis Rheum.* 42:S315(Abstract).

Treatment of Juvenile Rheumatoid Arthritis

Laura J. Mirkinson and Ildy M. Katona

CONTENTS

INTRODUCTION: PATHOGENESIS OF DISEASE AND GOALS OF THERAPY

Juvenile rheumatoid arthritis (JRA) is a term that encompasses a number of chronic inflammatory conditions of childhood that, in many ways, are distinct entities in and of themselves. Age, gender, ethnicity, genetic factors, and geographic regions may all influence disease expression. Recent nomenclature, such as juvenile chronic arthritis and juvenile inflammatory (or idiopathic) arthritis, reflect attempts to recognize the variety

From: *Modern Therapeutics in Rheumatic Diseases*
Edited by: G. C. Tsokos, et al. © Humana Press, Inc., Totowa, NJ

of diseases that now fall under this name. Traditionally, JRA subtypes were named based on the type of onset and/or the number of affected joints at the time of disease. Thus, the terms systemic onset, pauciarticular (oligoarticular), and polyarticular JRA became familiar in the lexicon of pediatric rheumatology. Recently, a new classification is being considered by the International League of Associations of Rheumatologists (ILAR) to more closely reflect clinically homogenous groups rather than onset type or clinical characteristics (1). The American College of Rheumatology (ACR) still holds as its classification criteria age of onset less than 16 yr; arthritis in one or more joints, duration of disease equal to or greater than 6 wk; oligoarticular, polyarticular, or systemic onset; and exclusion of other forms of juvenile arthritis. Of these subtypes, approx 10–20% present as systemic onset (prominent systemic symptoms such as fever and rash precede arthritis), about 40–60% as polyarthritis (>5 joints affects at time of onset), and about 40–50% as pauciarticular (<5 joints affected at time of onset). Of those who present with pauciarticular arthritis, there appear to be two predominant groups. The first group consists of girls less than 7 yr old, many of whom are antiniclear antibody (ANA) positive and have a higher risk of inflammatory uveitis. The second group, previously considered type-II pauciarticular onset, are male, often HLA-B27 positive, and go on to develop one of the diseases which belong to the spondlyloarthropathy group. Of note, patients with juvenile psoriatic arthritis and a positive ANA, have a clinical course that closely mimics pauci- or polyarticular JRA with arthritis (that can precede the development of a psoriatic rash) accompanied by uveitis.

It is important to note that systemic-onset JRA (SOJRA) is a diagnosis of exclusion, with a long differential diagnosis including viral syndromes, fever of unknown origin, and malignancy. Fever spikes in SOJRA typically return to normal at least once per day. There is a widely varied outcome for this subset of patients, who may recover fully, go on to have mild pauciarticular disease, or an especially aggressive systemic and polyarticular course. Of all the subtypes of JRA, systemic onset remains the most resistant to all forms of therapy and the most difficult therapeutic challenge. In its aggressive form, the extreme difficulty in controlling its extensive systemic and articular manifestations have prompted the use of most intensive and experimental therapies. This is also the form in which significant drug reactions are most commonly experienced.

Treatment of pediatric disease has long been hampered by the lack of drug trials of new medications in the pediatric population. The Food and Drug Administration (FDA) Modernization Act, "Pediatric Final Rule," published in 1994, initiated specific requirements to provide information in product labeling for dosages and therapies in pediatric patients. More recently, pediatric provisions of the FDA Modernization Act require sponsors to include pediatric studies of drugs that are likely to be of therapeutic benefit to children (2). Any drug utilized in the pediatric population has to be studied with regard to its safety profile, pharmacokinetics, and efficacy. Many of the drugs used in pediatric rheumatology have been studied by the Pediatric Rheumatology Collaborative Study Group.

In fact, patients rarely adhere to the definitions of the subtypes as closely as the terminology would suggest. Although some patients tend to follow a much more clearly defined course, such as those with systemic-onset and polyarticular rhematoid factor (RF)-positive JRA, the progression of disease, response to treatment, and overall prognosis of the vast majority of other patients is highly variable. Several subtypes can be identified as having a poorer outcome. These include adolescent girls who have an adult-like RA, with erosive, polyarticular disease with involvement of large and small joints, systemic onset patients with severe polyarticular disease, and oligoarticular patients who continue to add on involved joints over time. Overall, the pauciarticular-onset patients who are ANA-negative and who do not progress to polyarticular disease (about 30%) have the most favorable outcome. Any patient, regardless of type of onset of JRA, can progress to polyarticular disease resulting in a more guarded prognosis. Like adult RA, the goals of treatment are aimed at preservation of joints, overall mobility, and quality of life. In addition, unique to pediatric patients, the promotion of growth and development is of paramount importance.

A number of features of patients with malignancy overlap with rheumatic disease including fever, fatigue, weight loss, hepatomegaly, and arthritis (3). The presence of leukopenia, thrombocytopenia, or elevated lactase dehydrogenase should immediately suggest the need for bone marrow examination. The presence of significant nonarticular pain, especially back pain that is out of proportion with the physical findings, should also raise the suspicion of a diagnosis of malignancy. It is of importance to note that the articular pain of some patients with malignancy may respond favorably to anti-inflammatory therapy, thereby delaying the diagnosis.

EPIDEMIOLOGY AND GENETICS OF DISEASE

The occurrence of JRA has ethnic and geographic variations. Although reporting bias and patterns of referral can influence prevalence rates, there is a general consensus in the rheumatology community that there are true ethnic differences in diagnostic types of disease. In the United States, pauciarticular JRA is most common in young Caucasian females, whereas African-American children are more likely to present at an older age and have polyarticular disease. In addition, African-American children are more likely to be ANA-negative than Caucasian children (4).

The genetic predisposition to JRA is likely complex and multifactorial. Although JRA has been described in sibpairs (5), familial disease is quite rare. Several chromosomal syndromes have associations with JRA, including 22q11 deletion (6), 22q11.2 deletion, and Trisomy 21 and 18q- syndromes (7). Genetic differences may influence not only disease expression, but therapeutic responses as well. Of the different groups, pauciarticular disease appears most easily identifiable as an immunogenetically distinct entity and has been closely associated with a number of HLA antigens such as DR5, DR6, DR8, and DPw2.1 (8). As summarized by Glass and Giannini (9), DR1 and DR4 have been reported to be associated with polyarticular disease, and interestingly, DR1 is associated with pauciarticular patients who later extend to polyarticular disease. Combinations of major histocompatibility genes are also associated with different subgroups of JRA. In older males with pauciarticular disease, HLA-B27 is associated with later development of spondyloarthropathy. The proposal that JRA is a complex genetic trait is based on the idea that in diseases that show genetic predisposition, although not significant familial tendency, interactions of multiple genes are necessary for disease to occur (9).

POTENTIAL IMMUNOPATHOLOGICAL MECHANISMS OF DISEASE

Recent research has provided preliminary evidence regarding the relationships between immunogenetic factors and the pro- and anti-inflammatory effects of cytokines in JRA. Study of the immunopathogenesis of JRA has revealed a possible mixed T-helper 1 and TH2 cell response pattern in children with JRA. T cells produce a variety of factors that promote cell-mediated immunity and humoral antibody-mediated responses. TH1 cells stimulate the production of proinflammatory cytokines such as interleukin-2 (IL-2), interferon-γ (IFN-γ), tumor necrosis factor-α (TNF-α) and tumor necrosis factor-β (TNF-β). TH2 cells promote production of anti-inflammatory cytokines including IL-4, IL-10, and transforming growth factor-β (TGF-β). Raziuddin et al. *(10)* studied 10 children with active systemic-onset disease and found enhanced IL-4 and IL-10 production. In another study, Murray et al. *(11)* noted differences in synovial-fluid levels of IL-4 and IL-10 in patients of different subtypes and in patients with and without erosive disease. They also noted that, on the whole, type 1 cytokines, such as IL-2 and INF-γ were more uniformly associated with all forms of JRA than type 2 cytokines. Elevated IL-6 levels have been found to be associated with SOJRA and to correlate with disease activity *(12)*. A mixed pattern of production of TH1 and TH2 cells in JRA has implications for therapeutic strategies that seek to restore the persistent imbalances of proinflammatory and anti-inflammatory cytokines. How this loss of normal homeostasis is triggered, whether by an acute infectious event and/or by a genetic predisposition or other mechanism, is still unclear.

Recent research has also highlighted the differences between the subgroups of JRA by demonstrating differences in cellular activation for different types. For example, Gattorno et al. *(13)* found a relationship between IL-12 concentrations in JRA patients and activity of disease, positively correlating with disease activity, erythrocyte sedimentation rate (ESR), and C-reative protein (CRP). IL-8 and MCP-1 (monocyte chemoattractant protein-1) were found to be elevated in patients with active SOJRA *(14)*. IL-6 has also been implicated as having a role in disease activity in SOJRA, after being shown by Keul et al. to be present in higher concentrations in patients with systemic-onset disease and to correlate with the presence of fever in these patients *(15)*. Differences in cytokine profiles between systemic-onset and polyarticular JRA were also seen by Rooney et al. *(12)*, who found that IL-6 levels were higher in the systemic onset group and correlated with febrile phases of disease in five patients. Grom and colleagues detected TNF-α and TNF-β in synovial tissues of patients with JRA, and the presence of TNF-β was unique to JRA as compared to adult RA. In addition, they noted that expression of TNF-α was more intense in polyarticular JRA than persistent pauciarticular-course JRA *(16)*. Woo has observed significantly higher TNF-α levels in the synovial fluid of patients with polyarticular vs pauciarticular or spondlyloarthropathy disease *(17)*. Mangge et al. *(18)* has found elevated serum levels of sTNFR in patients with all subtypes of JRA, with the highest values demonstrated in patients with SOJRA. In 1995, Horneff et al *(19)* attempted to interrupt T-cell activation by treating two children with refractory SOJRA with monoclonal CD4 antibodies. They found that the anti-CD4 treatment resulted in decreases in the number of CD4 T cells in the peripheral blood and significant but transient improvements of clinical disease-activity markers. De Benedetti et al. *(14)*, also studying patients with systemic JRA had higher serum levels of IL-8 and MCP-1 as compared to controls or patients with polyarticular or pauciarticular disease.

CORRELATES OF DISEASE ACTIVITY

In general, unlike in RA, traditional markers of disease activity such as ESR and CRP have not measured well against clinical evidence of arthritis in JRA. Thus, there is a continuing search for objective and reliable markers of disease activity specific to JRA. Bakkaloglu et al. *(20)* observed alterations in lipoprotein patterns that correlated with disease activity. In their study, HDL, ApoA, and ApoA1/ApoB ratios inversely correlated with laboratory indices of inflammation such as ESR and CRP. This finding was most strongly noted in patients with polyarticular disease. A correlation between increased serum hyaluronic acid (HA) levels and severity of joint symptoms was seen in polyarticular and systemic JRA patients by Takei et al. *(21)*. This finding was not seen in patients with pauciarticular disease, presumably because these patients have a smaller synovitis mass and produce lower levels of HA in response to inflammatory cytokines such as IL-1 and TNF-α. This same group, in a separate study *(22)*, noted significantly higher levels of vascular endothelial growth factor (VEGF) in systemic and polyarticular JRA. In addition, they reported that serum VEGF levels correlated with disease activity, ESR, and serum HA levels in patients with polyarticular disease. Increased levels of serum IL-1Ra, noted in patients with systemic-onset disease, have been correlated with disease activity *(23)*. A relationship between serum concentrations of prolactin and antinuclear antibody seropositivity in prepubertal girls with JRA was seen by McMurray et al. *(24)*, but levels did not correlate with disease duration, subtype, severity, ANA titer, or uveitis.

Comparisons of clinical data with indices of clinical disease have identified potential synovial-fluid correlates of disease activity. In patients with systemic JRA, increased levels of synovial-fluid level of IL-6 and significant increases in synovial IL-1α in patients with pauciarticular JRA have been reported *(25)*. Differing synovial-fluid cytokine profiles in different forms of JRA were seen by Murray et al. *(11)* who found IL-4 more closely associated with pauciarticular vs polyarticular or systemic-onset disease. In addition, they noted that the combination of IL-4 and IL-10 was more commonly found in patients with nonerosive vs erosive disease. Reduced levels of testosterone and dehydroepiandrosterone sulphate (DHEA-S) has been noted in the synovial fluid (and serum) of pubertal JRA patients *(26)*. Falcini et al. *(27)* documented increased concentrations of nerve growth factor (NGF) in 80 children in the active and inactive phases of systemic, polyarticular, and pauciarticular disease, and found a correlation of increased levels with clinical and laboratory indices of clinical activity.

THERAPEUTIC CHOICES

Current approaches to therapy recognize that a number of broad categories of JRA exist and that, in a very general way, strategies for therapy can be guided by what group best fits the patients' clinical presentation and course. These categories include SOJRA with polyarticular joint disease, pauciarticular disease in younger patients (<9 yr), extended pauciarticular disease (pauciarticular at time of onset with subsequent progression to polyarticular disease), polyarticular rheumatoid factor-negative disease (a very diverse group), and polyarticular, RF-positive disease (primarily seen in teenage girls). Other identified subgroups such as arthritis associated with psoriasis and arthritis associated with enthesitis or a spondyloarthropathy will not be discussed here. With the exception of the children with mild pauciarticular disease who respond to nonsteroidal, anti-inflammatory drugs (NSAID) therapy and/or intra-articular steroids, other patients frequently require combination therapy that incorporates NSAID; second-line agents such as methotrexate and glucocorticoids; immunosuppressants such as cyclosporin; and possibly biologics such as etanercept, or newer experimental interventions such as hematopoeitic stem cell transplantation. Hydroxychloroquine and sulfasalazine are still used as part of combination therapy, but methotrexate now holds the position as the drug of choice of the second-line agents for patients with moderate to severe disease who fail NSAID therapy, and etanercept is prescribed increasingly. Second-line agents such as penicillamine and intramuscular gold no longer serve as therapy after NSAIDs.

NONSTEROIDAL ANTI-INFLAMMATORY DRUGS

NSAIDs inhibit prostaglandin synthesis, specifically by inhibiting the enzyme cyclooxygenase (COX). Two COX isoforms exist: COX-1 is thought to function in gastric mucosa, kidneys, and platelets, and COX-2 is thought to be produced in areas of inflammation. Selective inhibition of COX-2 preserves the normal gastric mucosal protection by prostaglandins while mediating anti-inflammatory actions (28).

NSAIDs remain first-line therapy for patients with all types of JRA. Aspirin is now infrequently used owing to its association with Reye's Syndrome. Of the classic NSAIDs, several have been approved for pediatric use (see Table 1). Of those that are not approved, an appropriate dose based on body weight is calculated from the adult recommendations. There is considerable clinical experience in the use of the other well-known NSAIDs such as naproxyn, tolmentin, ibuprofen, indocin, diclofenac, and sulindac. Occasionally, and especially in the adolescent age group, oxaprozin, nabumetone, and diclofenac are useful. As in any group of patients, compliance is lower with medications requiring frequent dosing schedules. This is particularly true for children of school age who must have separate medications dispensed to them by identified individuals at school. Naproxyn, in particular, is useful as it comes in liquid and tablet preparations and has a BID-dosing schedule that encourages compliance in younger school-aged children and adolescents. NSAIDs have been noted to cause an unusual rash that may appear initially as small vesicles or blisters and evolve into small linear scars, particularly on the face. Facial scarring is more common in light-skinned children with blue or green eyes and may not be apparent to the patient or parent (29). The appearance of scarring should prompt discontinuation of the medication, as it may not resolve over time. Originally described as a "pseudo-porphyria" type of rash, the etiology is still unclear. Various reports in the literature indicate naproxyn as the most common cause. Indomethacin appears to be very efficacious in older children and adolescents, but its significant central nervous system side effects can limit its use. A pediatric patient may respond better to one of the classic NSAIDs than another. NSAID-associated gastrointestinal (GI) toxicity in children appears to be less common than in adults, but it is our experience that it increases as children approach adolescent age. Vigilance in instructing parents and patients of the signs and symptoms of GI toxicity is critical and we recommend that our patients always take these medications with meals. In addition, we use many of the medications used for GI protection such as H2-blockers and proton-pump inhibitors for our patients.

COX-2 inhibitors, now used widely in the adult population, are being used for selected pediatric patients, but no clinical trials of their efficacy for treatment of JRA have been reported as yet. Their value, as with adults, is the limited gastric complications such as erosions, ulcerations, and bleeding that occur with COX-1 NSAIDs. They may not, however, be completely free of gastric toxicity, particularly in patients with a prior history of GI mucosal problems or *Helicobacter pylori* infection *(30)*. It is reasonable to consider their use for individual pediatric patients who clinically respond to a classic NSAIDs but are unable to tolerate their GI side effects, or for patients who have the more adult-like form of RF-positive polyarticular JRA.

SECOND-LINE AGENTS: METHOTREXATE, LEFLUNOMIDE, HYDROXYCHLOROQUINE, SULFASALAZINE, GOLD, AND PENICILLAMINE

Second-line agents typically have slower anti-inflammatory effects than NSAIDs, but over time they can delay the destructive nature of erosive articular disease. In the literature they have been classified as disease-modifying drugs (DMARDs), slow-acting antirheumatic drugs (SAARDs), or second-line agents. Their optimal therapeutic effects are often not seen for 3–6 mo, but if after that period of time, the patient has not responded at all, the drug should be discontinued and an alternate therapy instituted. If the response was partial, an additional drug should be added to the regimen. At this time, methotrexate (MTX) is the most widely used for children with any form of moderate or severe JRA. In randomized, placebo-controlled trials of the comparative efficacy of four therapeutic agents used to treat JRA—D-penicillamine, hydroxychloroquine, auranofin, and MTX—only MTX resulted in a significantly greater improvement than placebo *(31)*. In a rare individual patient, hydroxychloroquine is still used as a form of therapy. Patients with systemic-onset disease may be more predisposed to adverse drug reactions from SAARDs *(32)*, including macrophage-activation syndrome (MAS) *(33)*.

The efficacy of MTX as a disease-modifying, second-line drug in JRA has been established by several studies, and it is currently the most widely used second-line therapy for JRA. It is still not entirely clear what the action of MTX is as a DMARD. Cronstein et al. *(34)* have suggested that the anti-inflammatory mechanism of MTX is increased adenosine release at inflamed sites rather than its more well-known effect of binding to dihydrofolate reductase and depleting folic acid. It has also been proposed that MTX promotes apoptosis of activated peripheral T cells *(35)*.

Depletion of folate may be one factor responsible for MTX action, and in a randomized double-blind placebo crossover (DBPC) study of 18 patients with active JRA over a 12-wk period, standard folic-acid supplementation did not alter the clinical efficacy of weekly oral MTX *(36)*. Folic acid is used often as a supplement to MTX therapy with the presumption that it will decrease the toxicity of the drug without compromising its efficacy.

In an unexpected finding, Falcini et al. *(37)* reported a single case of accelerated nodulosis in a young girl with RF-, ANA-, systemic-onset JRA as a side effect of MTX therapy. Reports in the adult literature, as noted by Wallace *(38)*, suggest that rheumatoid nodules that develop during MTX therapy may stabilize or regress with or without discontinuation of MTX. The MTX that accelerated rheumatoid nodulosis is possibly

Table 1
Drugs Used in the Treatment of Juvenile Rheumatoid Arthritis

Drug	Dosage form	Dose and route of administration	Initial labs	Follow-up labs	Contraindications and precautions	Adverse drug reactions
Prednisone	1, 2.5, 5, 10, 20, 50 mg tabs 5 mg/5 mL solution	Variable Low dose: <0.5 mg/kg/d High dose: 2 mg/kg/d divided TID-QID	Varies	Varies	Systemic infection, CHF, HTN, diabetes, seizure disorder, osteoporosis, abnormal LFTs	Adrenal insufficiency steroid psychosis, immunosuppression, GI upset, peptic ulcer osteoporosis, pseudotumor cerebri, pancreatitis, anaphylaxis, edema, appetite changes, mood changes, insomnia, anxiety, headache, dizziness, HTN, acne, skin atrophy, cushingoid features, menstrual changes, electrolyte abnls.
Prednisolone	15 mg/5 mL syrup	Variable	Varies	Varies	"	"
Naproxen	200 mg (OTC) 250, 375, 500 mg tabs, 125/5cc suspension	10-20 mg/kg/d PO, div. BID, 1000 mg/d max. dose	AST ALT UA BUN Creat	AST ALT UA Q 3–4 mo	Viral syndrome, influenza, varicella, ASA sensitivity	Elevated AST/ALT, gastritis, ulcers, hematuria, elevated BUN, hypertension, rash, facial scarring
Ibuprofen	200 mg (OTC) 400, 600, 800 mg tabs, 100 mg/5cc suspension	30–40 mg/kg/d PO, div. QID 2400 mg/d max. dose	"	"	"	"
Tolmentin	200 mg tab 400 mg cap	20–30 mg/kg/d PO, div. TID, 1600 mg/d max. dose	"	"	"	"
Indomethacin	25 mg cap 75 mg SR cap 25/5cc suspension	1–3 mg/kg/d PO, div. TID (BID–SR) 150 mg/d max. dose	"	"	"	"
Sulindac	150, 200 mg tab	4–6 mg/kg/d PO, div. BID 400 mg/d max. dose	"	"	"	"
Celecoxib	100, 200 mg capsules	100–200 mg PO BID 400 mg/d max. dose	AST ALT BUN Creat	"	Sulfonamide allergy, NSAID allergy including ASA triad, edema	Renal toxicity, GI irritation, elevation AST, ALT, bone marrow toxicity
Refecoxib	12.5, 25 mg tablets, 12.5 mg/5cc and 25 mg/5cc suspension	12.5–25 mg PO Q day 25 mg/d max. dose	"	"	"	"

Table 1 *(continued)*

Drug	Dosage form	Dose and route of administration	Initial labs	Follow-up labs	Contraindications and precautions	Adverse drug reactions
Hydroxy-chloroquine	200 mg tab	5–7 mg/kg PO Q day 400 mg/d max. dose	Eye exam	Eye exam q 4 mo	Retinal or visual field changes, inability to be tested for color vision	Retinopathy including blurred vision, photophobia, visual field defects GI irritation, bone marrow suppression, dermatitis
Sulfasalazine	500 mg tab	40-60 mg/kg/d PO, div. TID-QID, 3 g/d max. dose Optimal dose should be achieved over 6–8 wk	G6PD test, CBC AST ALT BUN Creat	CBC q 4 wk × 2 mo, then q 3 mo	G6P deficiency sulfonamide allergy	GI irritation, rash, mucosal ulcers, LFT abnormalities, BM suppression, poor folate absorption, reversible oligospermia, CNS effects (HA, nausea, dizziness, depression, anorexia)
Methotrexate	2.5 mg tab 25 mg/1 mL suspension	0.3–1.0 mg/kg/wk PO or SC, 40 mg/wk max. dose	CBC AST ALT	CBC, AST, ALT q month	Alcohol use pregnancy, or at risk for pregnancy	Headache, nausea, dizziness, mood changes, rash, weight loss, oligospermia, interstitial pneumonitis, hepatic fibrosis, bone marrow suppression
Etanercept	25 mg in single use vial, reconstituted with diluent given SC	0.4 mg/kg (max. 25 mg per dose), given twice weekly given SC 72–96 h apart	Update immuni-zations prior to use CBC AST ALT	''	Serious infection or sepsis, do not give concurrently with live vaccines. Liver enzyme elevation, autoimmune syndromes, thrombotic events	Immunosuppression, infection, gastroenteritis, depression, personality disorder, cutaneous ulcer, esophagitis, gastritis, emesis, headache, nausea, abdominal pain, injection site reaction
Infliximab	100 mg in 20-mL vial	3 mg/kg (approx 200 mg) IV per infusion Given at 0, 2, and 6 wk, and q 4 wk thereafter	PPD	''	Positive PPD test	Infusion reactions, headache, rash, URI, anti-dsDNA antibodies with drug-induced lupus-like illness
Gold (water or oil soluble)	50 mg/mL	1 mg/kg/wk IM	CBC, UA	CBC, UA, with Q dose	Renal disease, leukopenia, thrombocytopenia	Dermatitis, stomatitis, proteinuria, hematuria, bone marrow depression

mediated by the engagement of adenosine receptors. A similar cellular mechanism is thought to be responsible for CNS toxicity such as headaches, lightheadedness, and cognitive dysfunction *(39)*.

Critical decisions in MTX use continue to focus on timing of initiation of therapy, length of therapy, timing of discontinuation of treatment, its use in combination with other drugs, and identifying the relationship between the onset type of JRA and response to therapy.

In a double-blind, placebo-controlled study in 1992, Giannini et al. *(40)* established MTX as a disease-modifying agent for use in JRA. In this study, children treated once weekly with MTX in oral doses of 10 mg/m^2 showed significantly reduced indexes of articular severity as compared to patients treated with placebo. These findings were strengthened by the work of Ravelli et al. *(41)* who evaluated 26 patients treated for 2 yr with an average of 9.5 mg/m^2/wk of MTX. Patients who were responders to the therapy not only showed clinical improvement but improved radiologic outcomes as well, as measured by the degree of deterioration of carpal length. Harel et al. *(42)* had previously concluded that MTX could be viewed as a disease-modifying drug by noting an improvement in carpal length (no progression of erosions or joint-space narrowing) in pediatric patients responsive to MTX after 2.5 yr of treatment.

In addition to improving clinical and laboratory indicators of inflammation (joint mobility, swelling, pain, and tenderness, morning stiffness, elevation of acute-phase reactants), MTX has been demonstrated to simultaneously improve direct measures of functional improvement, a major goal in the treatment of children *(43)*. MTX is now the most commonly used second-line agent for patients who have failed to respond to NSAID therapy. In patients with very aggressive polyarticular JRA, MTX is started early after the establishment of the diagnosis. In some patients, MTX is used in combination with other second-line therapies in cases where patients have failed to respond adequately to a single agent.

Overall, MTX has an excellent safety profile in the pediatric population. This is likely owing, in part, to the lower prevalence of risk factors such as diabetes, obesity, alcohol consumption, and preexisting liver disease. Early experience in treating pediatric patients did reveal, as expected from reports in the adult literature, that pediatric patients on MTX therapy had elevations in serum liver aminotransferases, which resolved after stopping the medication. As in adults, once weekly (vs every 2nd or 3rd d) doses decreases the length of exposure to high plasma levels, and reduces toxicity *(44)*. Although the complication of MTX-induced hypersensitivity pneumonitis is well-documented in the adult literature, it is exceptionally rare in the pediatric population. A report by Cron et al. in 1998 *(45)* described one patient with polyarticular JRA who developed pulmonary complications that resolved with corticosteroid therapy and discontinuation of MTX. In 1996, Kugathasan et al. *(46)* evaluated nine children by liver biopsy to address the concern about subclinical liver toxicity. After receiving MTX 10 mg/m^2/wk for at least 3 yr, biopsy findings showed no evidence of liver fibrosis, hepatocyte necrosis, or inflammation. Hashkes et al. *(47)* reviewed 33 biopsy specimens from 25 patients with JRA for MTX-induced liver toxicity. Although a significant association was noted between abnormalities in liver transaminases and fibrosis, only two patients showed mild fibrosis (Roenigk Classification IIIA), and no patient showed severe fibrosis (Grade IIIB or IV). Additionally, 27 specimens (82%) had normal histology or mild changes (Grade I) and 4 specimens (6%) demonstrated hepatocellular, inflammatory, fatty, or necrotic changes (Grade II). Because identifying risk factors for hepatotoxicity in pediatric patients are still elusive, serial aminotransferase determinations, considered acceptable indicators of hepatocellular damage, remain an integral part of care. However, concerns regarding potential long-term complications such as hepatotoxicity, risk of infection, pulmonary fibrosis, and malignancy owing to prolonged MTX therapy have led investigators to discontinue the treatment after patients had been well-controlled for variable periods of time. Although efforts to define the optimal time to discontinue therapy have thus far eluded investigators, a number of studies have revealed important considerations of therapy. In a retrospective review of 101 children, Gottleib et al. *(48)* demonstrated that a significant proportion (40–58%) of their patients in all onset groups, who had achieved apparent remission with MTX therapy, relapsed when MTX was discontinued. Follow-up data suggested that these same patients were unable to achieve remission at their previous MTX doses. Ravelli et al. *(49)* reviewed the outcome of children responsive to MTX therapy whose MTX was discontinued after remission was achieved. Their retrospective review revealed that discontinuation of MTX therapy was least successful in the subgroup of patients with extended pauciarticular JRA (oligoarticular JRA that has progressed to a polyarticular form). In summary, the aforementioned studies have helped to establish MTX as a disease-modifying agent, and shed light on the possibility of relapse after discontinuation of MTX therapy. In fact, the variability of the disease in individual patients makes it difficult to apply an interpretation of outcomes of therapy to a broader group of patients. As it stands, the optimal method, timing, and patient selection for discontinuation of MTX therapy is still uncertain.

MTX has the additional advantage of being beneficial in the treatment of resistant uveitis in children with JRA. Despite diligent surveillance with slit-lamp exam and early detection of the asymptomatic uveitis strongly associated with JRA, chronic inflammatory anterior uveitis is still a potentially severe complication of JRA in a few patients. MTX offers an addition and/or alternative to chronic systemic steroid use that has previously been the mainstay of treatment for uveitis. As Kotaniemi *(50)* has noted, a significant proportion of patients, up to 25%, respond poorly to topical corticosteroids, and may develop complications of cataracts, glaucoma, macular edema, and severe visual loss. Weiss et al. *(51)* found that six of seven patients with severe chronic uveitis (all pauciarticular onset) who failed both topical and subsequent systemic or periocular (injection) corticosteroid therapy responded to MTX (0.5–1.0 mg/kg/wk administered subcutaneously), showing significant reduction in the severity of uveitis. MTX has also been used as part of a combination therapy with oral corticosteroids and cyclosporin A to control uveitis that occurred in patients with long-standing arthritis *(50)*.

MTX dosing in pediatric patients is based, most conveniently, on a mg per kg weight calculation. MTX is most commonly administered in the 2.5 mg tablet form. However, in pediatric patients who require small doses, cannot swallow tablets, or cannot tolerate the tablets, the injectable form of MTX (25 mg/mL) may be taken by mouth (administered by a syringe). Taken orally, MTX is given once weekly at 0.3–1.0 mg/kg/dose. In prepubertal children, the typical starting dose is 0.4–0.5 mg/kg/wk with a maximum dose of 40 mg/wk. The optimal dose for an individual patient is usually reached within a few months from the start of therapy. MTX may be better absorbed if taken without food, particularly at the higher doses. In each individual, oral MTX may reach a saturation point, so that absorption is limited despite an increase in the dose. Peak serum levels are reached approx 1–2 h after ingestion and are highly variable. If a patient does not respond adequately to oral doses (especially above 0.6 mg/kg/wk), or cannot tolerate the GI effects (primarily nausea and emesis), a subcutaneous dose can be substituted. Absorption by the subcutaneous route differs from oral absorption of MTX at about 10 mg/m² *(52)*. In our experience, there are a few patients who develop such an exceptional aversion to MTX that they are unable to tolerate even the look or smell of the medication.

Leflunomide, a new second-line agent, inhibits *de novo* pyrimidine synthesis, thus inhibiting reversible cell-cycle arrest in cells particularly sensitive to this effect, such as activated lymphocytes involved with joint inflammation. In the adult population, it has been found to be well-tolerated *(53)* and an equally effective single agent as MTX and sulfasalazine for the signs and symptoms of RA, and phase III trials showed slowing of the radiologic parameters of disease progression *(54)*. Because leflunomide inhibits T-cell proliferation, which MTX does not, the combination of both drugs have been evaluated in a small open study. Although found to be well-tolerated by patients, it was associated with elevation of serum transaminase levels *(55)*. Its use as a single or combination drug in the pediatric population has not been studied in controlled trials, and it is not currently being recommended for this population. It may, in the future, be considered for treatment of individual patients with RF-positive, adult-like JRA who are not responding to other therapies.

Hydroxychloroquine, an antimalarial drug, has a good safety profile in the pediatric population. Its taste and availability as a 200-mg tablet, however, can limit its usefulness in smaller children, and it is not considered highly efficacious as a single agent. The pediatric dose is 5–7 mg/kg/d (maximum 400 mg/d). Among its side effects is a retinopathy that affects color vision, thus it should not be used in children who cannot cooperate with color-vision testing, which needs to be done routinely every 4–6 mo *(56)*. As noted earlier, it is no longer common practice to use this medication as single therapy, but it can be useful in certain individual patients or as part of a combination therapy with MTX and/or sulfasalazine.

Sulfasalazine has been widely used as a second-line agent for adult and pediatric arthritis since the 1970s. A combination sulfonamide and salicylate preparation, the mechanism of its effectiveness in treating JRA is not well-understood, but may be related to effects on folate transport, like MTX, or inactivation of prostaglandins. Its recommended dosage is 40–60 mg/kg/d. The drug is available as a 500-mg enteric-coated and nonenteric-coated tablet. The dose is gradually built up over 6–8 wk starting as one tablet/d or one tablet BID, with gradual increases every 2 wk up to the desired dose or maximum of 3 g/d. Side effects are predominantly GI and are less common with the enteric-coated preparation. Rashes occur in up to 5% of patients and a reversible oligospermia has been reported *(57)*. It is contraindicated in patients with sulfa allergy or G6PD deficiency. When used as combination therapy with MTX or azathioprine, folic-acid supplementation is recommended to reduce bone marrow suppression and GI side effects *(58)*. Recently, its use has been studied in 32 seronegative patients with JRA as a second-line medication along with NSAID therapy in an open prospective study *(59)*. Of the patients studied (21 with pauciarticular, 10 with polyarticular, and 1 with systemic-onset disease), a significant response, as measured by a disease activity index improvement of greater than 50%, was observed in 24 of 31 patients at the end of a 6-mo period. The small numbers of patients were inadequate to evaluate the relationship between efficacy and type of disease. It is our experience that patients with spondlyloarthropathy and/or moderate to severe polyarticular or oligoarticular JRA may respond well to sulfasalazine as a single drug when it is used in combination with MTX and/or hydroxychloroquine. Penicillamine is now a very rarely, if ever, used medication for JRA.

Gold compounds are available in water and oil-based preparations, and can be given intramuscularly. Prior to the recent practice of MTX use as second-line treatment, gold was considered an excellent choice as second-line treatment for the patient with polyarticular disease that failed NSAID or other SAARD therapy. As noted by Cassidy *(56)*, the average response rate to intramuscular gold is about 50%, but there are also adverse effects that can lead to discontinuation of therapy. An initial test dose of 2.5 or 5 mg is given as the first dose, followed by a weekly increasing dosage schedule up to 1 mg/kg/wk to a maximum of 50 mg/dose. Over time, and with improvement, the dosage schedule can be gradually expanded to an every 2–4 wk regimen. Surveillance requires a complete blood count (CBC) and urinalysis prior to each dose to monitor for hematologic and renal adverse effects. Microscopic hematuria, and more often, proteinuria, occurs not infrequently and is usually resolved by reducing the dose to the previous level. However, severe leukopenia, thrombocytopenia, eosinophilia, hematuria, proteinuria, or dermatitis may warrant discontinuation of therapy *(56)*. Intramuscular gold therapy was safe and well-tolerated by many children, however, the inconvenience of weekly laboratory investigation and supervised injection schedule made its use undesirable in children of our modern society.

CORTICOSTEROID THERAPY

Oral glucocorticoid therapy is frequently used as a potent anti-inflammatory medication in children with systemic manifestations, those with severe articular disease and patients with uveitis. It is often used to provide an initial burst of anti-inflammatory activity for patients with a new diagnosis or a flare of articular disease, and is tapered as quickly as disease activity and other therapy allows. Typical adverse side effects of high-dose or prolonged steroid use are of particular concern in the pediatric population as they include growth failure, aseptic necrosis of the hip, osteoporosis, cataracts, hyperlipidemia, atherosclerosis, hypertension, and diabetes. Initial doses may begin at 0.5–2.0 mg/kg/d of oral prednisone, with a typical maximum dosage of 40–60 mg/d. If the dose is administered once daily, AM administration has to be stressed to parents. Improved efficacy can be achieved by dividing the daily dose. For patients with relatively well-controlled disease an every-other-day regimen can be utilized before discontinuation of steroids. Similarly, low-dose steroids can be used for occasional flares in patients with otherwise well-controlled disease.

Intra-articular corticosteroid (IAS) therapy is used with increasing frequency in patients with monoarticular or pauciarticular disease who have not responded adequately to NSAIDs. Several recent studies support the safety of IAS in the pediatric population. In a study of 21 patients treated with intra-articular steroids, Huppertz et al. *(60)*

followed patients, primarily with chronic knee arthritis, by examining with magnetic resonance imaging (MRI) (enhanced with gadolinium diethylenetriaminetetraacetic acid, [Gd-DTPA]) prior to the therapy, after the therapy (mean 49 d) and again at approx 1–2 yr after treatment. In addition, standing height was measured before injection and about 1 yr later. Patients were treated with triamcinolone hexacetonide, approx 1 mg/kg, with a minimum dose of 20 mg and a maximum dose of 60 mg. Treatment resulted in suppression of synovial inflammation and reduction of pannus formation, often up to a year later. In some patients, concomitant therapy with NSAIDs or chloroquine was used, and no deviations in standardized height scores were seen. Similar findings were reported by Padeh and Passwell *(61)* who, in a study of 71 patients with juvenile arthritis, found IAS to be a highly successful form of therapy as evidenced by findings of rapid resolution of swelling and effusions, remissions of joint inflammation for greater than 6 mo, decreased pain, increased joint mobility, discontinuation of oral medications (this was limited by inflammation in other joints), and correction of joint contractures. None of the potential adverse reactions such as infection, thrombophlebitis, weakness, calcification, cartilage damage, joint destruction, avascular necrosis, or permanent subcutaneous lipolysis occurred in this group of patients. Although the majority of children with pauciarticular JRA have a good prognosis, excepting the complications of uveitis in this group, leg-length discrepancy (LLD) is one of the few long-term sequelae of this disease. It is not uncommon to see accelerated growth of an affected extremity, usually owing to knee arthritis, in children with JRA. Sherry et al. *(62)* found that IAS therapy resulted in less LLD in 30 Caucasian children with pauciarticular JRA. In general, common practice is to limit IAS injections to two per year, because of concerns of potential toxicity of IAS for articular cartilage, but this possibility must always be weighed against the potential for long-term destruction of cartilage in joints with persistent inflammation.

Intravenous (IV) pulse corticosteroid therapy is generally reserved for the treatment of systemic onset JRA, particularly for the nonarticular manifestations, such as myocarditis, or macrophage-activation syndrome that often respond poorly to NSAID and DMARD or oral-steroid therapy. In an open study, evaluating 18 children with systemic flare of disease, Adebajo and Hall *(63)* evaluated systemic features (fever, rash, hepatosplenomegaly, lymphadenopathy, serositis, and myocarditis) and articular findings (duration of morning stiffness, number of active joints, and functional status) before and after 1–3 doses of IV pulsed methylprednisolone (30 mg/kg, maximum dose 1 g). Using a standard of response defined as >50% improvement in measured variables at 1 mo posttreatment, they found a 72% rate of response (13 patients) and no adverse effects of therapy. Picco et al. *(64)* had previously studied the use of "Mini-pulses" of IV methylprednisolone (5 mg/kg/d for 3 d, then 2.5 mg/kg/d for 3 d followed by 1 mg/kg/d of oral prednisone thereafter) vs oral prednisone (1 mg/kg/d) in systemic onset JRA. Patients admitted to the study had significant symptoms of disease such as hepatosplenomegaly, pericarditis, myocarditis, pleurisy, long-standing fever, anemia, CNS manifestations, and severe articular disease. Both groups of patients showed marked decrease in disease activity, fever score, improvement in Hb concentration, as well as improvement of articular symptoms within 1 mo of treatment. Patients undergoing IV therapy had a more rapid resolution of fever and reduction in CRP (after

1 wk) and had significantly lower cumulative daily steroid requirements at the end of 6 mo. However, at the end of 12 mo, no differences in disease activity or cumulative daily dosage of steroids were noted between the two groups.

BIOLOGIC AGENTS: TUMOR NECROSIS FACTOR INHIBITORS AND INTRAVENOUS IMMUNOGLOBULIN THERAPY

TNF is one of the naturally synthesized protein mediators of the innate immune system. It is a principal player in normal immune function and in autoimmune disorders. Along with other cytokines, its contributes to the overall function of the cellular immune system. TNF is one of a number of cytokines that work in concert with receptors that influence cell proliferation and apoptosis, or programmed cell death. It is secreted by T lymphocytes, synovial cells, and mononuclear phagocytes (65,66). Of particular importance in arthritis, where the effects of cytokine abnormalities are prominent, TNF increases synoviocyte proliferation, influences migration of inflammatory cells, and directly effects the process of joint destruction. It is found in significantly higher levels in synovial fluid than plasma in patients with RA (67). Many different therapeutic modalities have been developed or are under development, which interfere with the TNF-α function. Recently approved by the FDA and the most widely used for the treatment of arthritis is Etanercept, which uses two identical chains of a recombinant soluble TNF receptor bound to the Fc receptor of immunoglobulin (sTNFR:Fc). Etanercept binds TNF thus inactivating it by preventing its ability to connect with cell-membrane receptors. The IgG component increases of the half-life of the molecule from minutes to days. It is dosed as 0.4/kg/dose (maximum 25 mg/dose), given subcutaneously twice weekly at home. In clinical trials etanercept was found to be an effective inhibitor of TNF activity. In addition, it proved to be safe and efficacious in decreasing disease activity, increasing functional ability, and improving quality of life in patients with RA (68). The most common side effects noted have been mild reactions at the site of injection. Patients can be at risk for severe infections owing to immunosuppression and it should not be given concurrently with live vaccines such as oral polio, varicella, and measles, mumps, and rubella (MMR). As with all new therapies, the full array of side effects is probably not known at the current time.

TNF receptor inhibitors, such as etanercept, are categorized as biologic response modifiers, and represent the recent focus on treatment aimed at inhibiting the specific biologic processes that effect cellular immune mechanisms (cytokine-mediated immunity). This is in contrast to previous efforts that focused primarily on understanding and mediating humoral immunity. Of interest, many of the drugs long used in rheumatic disease, such as glucocorticoids, gold compounds, MTX, cyclosporin-A, and D-penicillamine, heavily influence cytokine activity in general (69). Etanercept is now being approved for use in the pediatric population. In a two-part study starting with open-label TNRF:Fc treatment followed by randomized, blinded TNRF:Fc or placebo, Lovell et al. (70) found the drug to be well-tolerated with a good clinical response (74%) after 3 mo of treatment during the open-label phase. In the second, double-blind phase of the study, those patients who had responded to treatment were randomly assigned to receive etanercept or placebo for an additional 4 mo, or until a flare of previously controlled disease occurred. A significantly greater number of patients treated with placebo withdrew early from the study owing to disease flare (81 vs 28% treated with etanercept). In addition, the mean time to disease flare was significantly shorter in the placebo group (28 d) as compared with the etanercept treatment group (116 d) *(71)*. Patients participating in this study had severe polyarticular disease and responded well to therapy regardless of the onset type (systemic, pauciarticular, or polyarticular) of their arthritis. Several further studies of use of Etanercept in children are ongoing.

Infliximab, a chimeric IgG1 monoclonal antibody (MAb) TNF inhibitor initially indicated for the treatment of inflammatory bowel disease, is also approved for use in adult RA. It is given as an intravenous infusion at predetermined intervals. Currently, there are no reports of studies of its efficacy in the pediatric population.

Intravenous immunoglobulin (IVIG) therapy is costly, but considered a safe therapy used successfully in some patients with JRA, as well as several other pediatric diseases such as Kawasaki disease and idiopathic thrombocytopenic purpura. The mechanism of action of the high doses of immunoglobulin provided by IVIG is not well-understood in any individual setting, and is likely multifactorial.

The value of IVIG therapy has been studied in patients with refractory systemic-onset disease. Uziel et al. *(72)* used major outcome measures of fever, prednisone dose, and number of active joints to evaluate 27 patients at time of entry to study, and subsequently at 6 mo (*n* = 25), 12 mo (*n* = 24), 24 mo (*n* = 20), and >24 mo (*n* = 17). Two patients had worsening of systemic disease during IVIG therapy and dropped out of the study after <5 mo of treatment. Patients received 1–1.5 g/kg/d either 2 d monthly, or 1 d every 2 wk for the first 5 doses followed by once monthly for at least 6 mo. They found that the majority of patients had, by 1 yr after therapy, resolution of fever and significant decrease in steroid dose, suggesting a steroid-sparing effect. Fewer patients showed response in articular disease. Owing to lack of controls, the particular effects of the IVIG therapy were difficult to differentiate from the effects of other medications or the natural history of the disease, which does tend to improve over the long term, whatever the treatment. This same difficulty was experienced by Prieur, who has recommended caution in recommending therapy that, after a number of years, has still not been shown to have a long-term effect on the outcome of systemic JRA *(73)*.

The safety and efficacy of IVIG in 25 patients with refractory polyarticular JRA was tested in a multicenter, randomized, blinded-withdrawal study by Giannini et al. in 1996 *(74)*. Outcome measures were total number of joints with active arthritis, overall articular severity score, and global assessment of overall disease activity. Patients were permitted to continue stable doses of up to two NSAIDs, two slow-acting antirheumatic drugs and/or low dose prednisone at the time of therapy with IVIG. Nineteen of 25 patients responded favorably to the open phase of the study and proceeded to the double-blind phase. Of the 10 patients who went on to receive IVIG, 8 completed and 2 became eligible to "escape" to higher doses of IVIG. Of the 9 patients who received placebo, 4 completed, 4 "escaped" to IVIG, and 1 dropped out. Benefits produced by IVIG in the open phase of the study did not appear to be maintained in patients treated with placebo in the double-blind phase. Although the short-term safety of the therapy was promising, in that no patient developed clinically significant adverse reactions to therapy, long-term efficacy was not demonstrated.

IMMUNOSUPPRESSIVE DRUGS: AZATHIOPRINE, CYCLOPHOSPHAMIDE, CYCLOSPORIN, AND MYCOPHENOLATE MOFETIL

Immunosuppressive drugs are rarely used for the treatment of JRA, but are occasionally needed in selected patients with severe disease that is refractory to other therapy. Azathioprine is an immunosuppressive antimetabolite that primarily inhibits T-cell growth. Its effect on autoimmune diseases is not well-understood. In the adult population, it is indicated for patients with erosive RA refractory to other therapy and is recognized to spare glucocorticoid use. In the pediatric literature, the bulk of information regarding azathioprine precedes the recent surge in the use of MTX. In an uncontrolled, prospective study of 129 patients with JRA refractory to therapy starting in 1980, Savolainen et al. *(75)* found a strong glucocorticoid-sparing effect with the use of azathioprine, and speculated that its use had a positive influence on disease remissions. Side effects included GI symptoms, elevated liver enzymes, and potentially increased risk for severe infections and malignancies. At this time, it is unlikely that azathioprine would be used except for a patient with the most severe, refractory disease.

In a trial of IV pulse cyclophosphamide and methyprednisolone, Wallace and Sherry *(76)* reported the therapy to be useful in controlling severe uncontrolled disease in four patients with systemic JRA. Prior to treatment all patients had severe erosive disease, were corticosteroid-dependent, and had severe growth retardation. They had undergone maximum therapy including combinations of MTX, sulfasalazine, hydroxychloroquine, weekly IV pulse methylprednisolone, NSAIDs, gold, azathioprine and IVIG. All four patients demonstrated improvement by the third to fifth treatment. After 6–10 monthly treatments and an additional 6–10 every 3 wk treatments of IV pulsed cyclophosphamide (500–1000 mg/m^2) and methylprednisolone (30 mg/kg, max. 1 g), all patients showed clinical improvement, improved linear growth, and were eventually able to discontinue corticosteroids. Three patients were able to achieve apparent remission with the continuation of other medications including MTX, sulfasalazine, and hydroxychloroquine.

In an effort to treat refractory JRA, cyclosporin A has been used alone and in combination with MTX. The dose of Cyclosporin is 3–5 mg/kg/d orally. Side effects include renal toxicity, hypertrichosis and gingival hyperplasia. In a study by Reiff et al. *(77)*, Cyclosporin A, an inhibitor of T cell-derived cytokines and possible inhibitor of synovial T-cell proliferation, was used to treat 22 patients, 17 of whom had refractory systemic JRA. Ninety-one percent (11 of 17 patients) with SOJRA had resolution of fever, 70% (12 patients) had a significant decrease in number of swollen joints, and 50% (6 patients) a significant decrease or resolution of morning stiffness. Concomitant therapy of prednisone was reduced in 11 patients and discontinued in 5 patients. Concomitant methotrexate therapy was discontinued in 2 patients, and was well tolerated in combination with Cyclosporin A. Additional improvements in hematologic cell lines and ESR were seen in some patients.

Mycophenolate mofetil (CellCept) is the ester prodrug of mycophenolic acid. Taken orally, it is quickly absorbed and converted to mycophenolic acid. Mycophenolate mofetil was approved in 1995 for the prevention of acute renal allograft rejection, and is used in combination with cyclosporine and steroids. It selectively prevents the proliferation of rapidly dividing cells, particularly lymphocytes, by inhibiting guanosine nucleotide biosynthesis *(78)*. Mycophenolate mofetil is currently being used for the treatment of adult lupus nephritis refractory to other therapy *(79)* and adult RA *(80)*, but its use in JRA has not yet been studied.

ANTIMICROBIAL THERAPY: MINOCYCLINE

The ongoing debate regarding the efficacy of minocycline for the treatment of RA in the adult literature has raised questions for pediatric rheumatologists. Long used as a standard therapy for the treatment of acne, minocycline is a tetracycline drug that has antimicrobial, anti-inflammatory, and immunomodulatory effects. It is able to inhibit metalloproteinases *(81)* and collagenase activity *(82)* associated with joint-space narrowing and joint destruction. In addition to well-known mild side effects such as sun sensitivity and GI upset, it has been reported to cause drug-induced lupus in adolescents *(83)* and acute polyarthritis in adults *(84)*. There are neither controlled studies of pediatric patients comparing minocycline to other established therapies, nor studies defining its use in combination therapy. In the adult literature, where radiographic assessment of disease progression in RA is reported as an important outcome measure, there is insufficient data to evaluate minocycline *(85)*. In a double-blind, placebo-controlled study of 46 adults with early RA (<1 yr), O'Dell et al. *(86)* found minocycline to be superior to placebo. In this study, patients were treated with 100 mg minocycline BID or placebo for 3 mo, then 3 mo extension if they fulfilled criteria for 50% improvement in improving signs and symptoms of arthritis.

AUTOLOGOUS STEM CELL TRANSPLANTATION

A report of the first four children who underwent autologous hemopoietic stem cell transplantation (AHSCT) for severe JRA refractory to conventional and combination therapy showed interesting short-term results *(87)*. The patients included three children with systemic JRA and one with polyarticular JRA. The patients chosen had disease histories of 3.5–6.5 yr, severe systemic symptoms, erosive polyarticular disease, and growth failure, despite multiple medication trials with NSAIDS, DMARDs such as methotrexate and gold, immunosuppressive therapy with cyclosporin, and oral and pulsed IV corticosteroids. In preparation for AHSCT, patients were continued on NSAID therapy, but MTX and cyclosporin were discontinued. Prednisone was stopped 2 mo after AHSCT. Intense immunosuppression preceded AHSCT including antithymocyte globulin, high-dose cyclophosphamide, and low-dose total body irradiation. All patients had marked improvement in morning stiffness, joint swelling, and pain within 2 wk of stem-cell transplant. By 4 wk after AHSCT, hematologic abnormalities of ESR, CRP, and hemoglobin normalized. During the follow-up period of 6–18 mo, remarkable improvement in growth following AHSCT was reported for two patients: 10 cm/18 mo (previous growth 2 cm/36 mo) and 6 cm/11 mo (previous growth 1 cm/12 mo). Noted complications included transient thrombocytopenia treated with platelet transfusion for 28 d in one patient and uncomplicated Varicella infection 3 and 6 mo after treatment in two patients. Two patients had mild flares of disease (transient synovitis) treated only with NSAIDs. How much of the improvements can be attributed to the intense immunosuppression prior to the therapy will remain unclear until randomized trials are performed. Quartier et al., in a letter of response to the findings noted earlier, reported a patient with very severe SOJRA and erosive polyarticular arthritis who underwent AHSCT and died of complications of disseminated toxoplasmosis *(88)*.

APPROACHES TO THERAPY

The care of a child with JRA requires an understanding of the multiple personalities of this disease and the unique responses children with different types of JRA have to the variety of medications, both in terms of efficacy and toxicity. JRA is almost always a nonlethal disease, and can be self-limiting, but in a large number of cases it leads to severe disability from joint or eye disease if not managed appropriately. A generally aggressive approach to therapy that recognizes the significant risks to normal growth and development is appropriate in the pediatric population. Of paramount importance is the recognition that, in this group of patients, articular disease is often minimally symptomatic and eye disease (uveitis) is silent. The clinician who does not aggressively seek clinical evidence of disease may miss its most damaging manifestations and late consequences.

In general, a step-wise approach to therapy is influenced by the subtype of JRA and the severity of disease. For the purposes of determining therapy, the groups can be described in the following way: systemic-onset disease, oligoarticular disease in children less than 9 yr old, extended oligoarticular disease, polyarticular RF-negative disease, and polyarticular RF-positive disease. As noted earlier, any patient can progress to polyarticular disease. Unfortunately, the severity of the course of illness, the response to therapy, the potential for joint destruction and the remitting and relapsing nature of the chronic arthritis are very difficult to predict. In a recent survey of US and Canadian pediatric rheumatologists *(89)*, NSAIDs remained the mainstay of therapy, and MTX (DMARD) and sulfasalazine (SAARD) were the most commonly used second-line drugs. Gold was found to be used less frequently after 1991 when MTX supplanted its use.

With the exception of patients with mild pauciarticular disease, patients usually require combination therapy. With MTX now considered first choice of second-line therapy, combination therapy will inevitably consist of this drug and NSAIDs. In patients who respond only partially, a third agent might be added. Another option may be to discontinue MTX and start another agent. A new option is available now because etanercept has been approved for pediatric use. It is prudent practice in pediatrics that drugs with an established long-term safety record are tried first. There is considerable information in the adult literature supporting the use of combination therapy such as MTX and sulfasalazine and/or hydroxychloroquine, and MTX with azathioprine or cyclophosphamide. There are few or no pediatric studies evaluating the use of these combination therapies. However, combination therapy is frequently used by physicians caring for patients with JRA.

The initial therapy for patients with systemic-onset disease is NSAIDs singly, or in combination with corticosteroids. Based on the practice of some pediatric rheumatologists, hydroxychloroquine is a reasonable strategy early in therapy. Patients with SOJRA who have systemic and articular features generally do not respond very well to second-line agents. Additionally, patients with very active disease are at highest risk for developing drug reactions and macrophage-activation syndrome. MTX use has mixed results in SOJRA. Although it may be very beneficial for articular disease, it may not resolve the systemic manifestations. Sulfasalazine may have some beneficial effects in these patients. In patients with aggressive SOJRA, disease can be extremely difficult to control and combinations of NSAIDs, corticosteroids and second-line drugs, immunosuppressants, and biologics might be used. As noted earlier, it is in this group of patients that AHSCT has been attempted. There is growing experience with the use of etanercept in pediatric patients, and patients with systemic-onset disease are being studied. The severity of disease and long-term corticosteroid therapy can lead to severe growth retardation in patients with SOJRA. Administration of growth hormone has been tried in this population with limited success.

Patients with mild pauciarticular disease generally respond well to some type of NSAID therapy. This tends to be a large joint asymmetrical disease, generally sparing the small joints and hips. Oligoarticular disease of the knee is a common finding. In this group, initial episodes or periodic flares can be treated with intra-articular steroids. Intraarticular steroids should not be the initial approach because Lyme disease always needs to be ruled out. DMARDs such as MTX and gold and oral corticosteroids are not indicated for therapy. Most importantly, patients with mild pauciarticular disease, especially those who are ANA-positive, are still at risk for severe visual impairment, even blindness, from unrecognized uveitis. Regular surveillance for uveitis is a critical part of their medical therapy.

Pauciarticular disease can progress to extended pauciarticular JRA. This is quite a diverse group of patients, encompassing mild to extensive articular problems, and second-line, or commonly a combination therapy is usually indicated. These patients may progress to require a trial of etanercept or other immunosuppressive therapy. In this group, drug cessation is usually unsuccessful.

Polyarticular, RF-negative, JRA is also a very diverse group of patients. There may be features of this group that overlap with SOJRA including a long, insidious evolution of findings and systemic signs of disease such as occasional low-grade fevers, hepatosplenomegaly, and lymphadenopathy. In contrast to SOJRA, there is no characteristic rash. This is usually a large-joint, symmetrical arthritis, but small-joint disease can also occur. Therapy for these patients needs to be aggressive and follows the same rationale as those with extended pauciarticular disease. Etanercept has been found to be very effective in this group *(70,71)* and is tolerated alone or in combination with other medications including MTX *(90)*.

In the polyarticular, RF-positive group, teenage girls tend to predominate, and the arthritis takes an adult RA-like course with multiple-joint involvement and erosive articular changes. This form of JRA may show significant involvement of small joints such as the hands, feet, and cervical spine as well as large joints, including the hips. Although some of these patients are also ANA-positive, they do not have a predilection for the development of uveitis. As with other forms of polyarticular disease, therapy starts with the use of NSAIDs. It is unlikely that NSAIDs alone will control this disease, and many of these patients require combination therapy. Medications that have been found to be effective in adult RA such as the COX-2 inhibitors and leflunomide might be appropriate considerations in this group of patients with RA-like disease.

COMPLICATIONS OF JUVENILE RHEUMATOID ARTHRITIS: UVEITIS AND MACROPHAGE-ACTIVATION SYNDROME

The optimal therapy for the silent, chronic, anterior uveitis of JRA is prevention. Specific guidelines for ophthalmologic examination in children with JRA have been published by the sections on rheumatology and ophthalmology of the American Academy of Pediatrics *(91)*. In these recommendations, the risk criteria for the chronic asymptomatic iridocyclitis typical of JRA are based on JRA subtype at onset and age of onset. The recommended frequency of slitlamp exams, looking for the presence of inflammatory cells in the anterior chamber, is based on whether the patient is at high, medium, or low risk for uveitis. Patients who present at <7 yr of age and are ANA-positive are at high risk regardless of polyarticular or pauciarticular disease. These patients should have a slit-lamp exam every 3–4 mo. Patients who are ANA positive and present at >7 yr of age are at medium risk and require slit-lamp exam every 6 mo. Patients who are ANA-negative, with either polyarticular or pauciarticular arthritis, and regardless of age of onset are considered at medium risk and should be examined every 6 mo. Patients with systemic-onset disease, regardless of age of onset, are considered at low risk and require slit-lamp exam every 12 mo. Over time, risk for uveitis changes. For patients with age of onset <7 yr, they are at low risk 7 yr after the onset of arthritis and should have slit-lamp exams every 12 mo indefinitely. Similarly, patients who had onset of disease at >7 yr are considered at low risk 4 yr after onset of arthritis and should have slit-lamp exams every 12 mo indefinitely. All high-risk patients are considered at medium risk 4 yr after onset of arthritis. With the best possible care and follow-up, there are still patients who initially present with uveitis of differing degree. The treatment of these patients, as previously noted, includes topical, oral and periocular glucocorticoids and MTX.

Macrophage activation syndrome (MAS), is now recognized as a known, and potentially lethal, complication of childhood rheumatic diseases, particularly SOJRA. MAS is a clinical syndrome caused by production and activation of well-differentiated macrophages that actively phagocytize hematopoeitic elements *(92)*. Clinical presentation includes persistent and unremitting fever, mental-status changes, hepatosplenomegaly, elevation of liver enzymes, profound pancytopenia, low ESR, prolonged bleeding times, and hypofibrinogenemia. Problems induced by activation of macrophages include phagocytosis of cellular elements, and vasculitis with intravascular coagulation. Sporadic forms may be triggered by common intercurrent viral infections, such as Parvovirus B19 *(93)*. In JRA, a viral syndrome or specific drugs including gold, MTX, and NSAIDs may precipitate MAS. The diagnosis is made by bone marrow examination demonstrating hematophagocytic histiocytes, and traditional first-line therapy for MAS is high-dose corticosteroids *(94)*. Ravelli et al. *(95)* and Mouy et al. *(96)* have reported the successful use of cyclosporin as a therapeutic intervention for MAS in patients with SOJRA who failed standard high-dose intravenous corticosteroid therapy.

MEDICATION CONSIDERATIONS UNIQUE TO PEDIATRIC PATIENTS

As with all populations of patients, pediatric age groups pose unique problems with respect to medication compliance. In all stages of childhood, from toddlers to adolescents, developmental milestones, both motor and psychosocial, have a significant impact on successful medical management of chronic disease. For example, most children under the age of five are unable to swallow tablets. Similarly, busy schedules for school children and adolescents prompt weekend MTX dosing that better conforms to school and social activities. Of interest, most of our patients on MTX take their medication on one weekend night (Friday or Saturday). Medications that are available in liquid preparations, require infrequent dosing schedules, do not interfere with school performance or after school activities, and do not require frequent laboratory evaluation or administration by a health professional have the best chance of being used consistently and successfully.

Counseling for chronic drug use must include a specific schedule of laboratory and ophthalmologic surveillance and a discussion of known mechanism of action and long-term side effects of the medications. Parents may have questions and concerns regarding effects on growth and development and future fertility. Adolescents must be privately counseled regarding the specific hazards of concurrent drug use, either illicit or over-the-counter, sexual activity, contraceptive use, and risks associated with pregnancy. Pediatric patients on chronic medications must be followed not only for the progression and activity of their disease, but for the overall status of their growth, development, school performance, and psychosocial well-being.

REFERENCES

1. Petty, R.E. 1998. Classification of childhood arthritis: a work in progress. *Baillieres Clin. Rheumatol.* 12(2):181–190.

2. Robie-Suh, K. 1999. 'New Advisory Panel, Associate Director Tackle Host of Issues.' "News Along the Pike," March 31, 1999. (www.fda.gov/cder/pediatric 4/20/99).

3. Cabral, D.A. and L.B. Tucker. 1999. Malignancies in children who initially present with rheumatic complaints. *J. Pediatr.* 134(1):53–57.

4. Schwartz, M.M., P. Simpson, K.L. Kerr, and J.N. Jarvis. 1997. Juvenile Rheumatoid Arthritis in African Americans. *J. Rheumatol.* 24(9):1826–1829.

5. Moroldo, M.B., B.L. Tague, E.S. Shear, D.N. Glass, and E.H. Giannini. 1997. Juvenile Rheumatoid Arthritis in affected sibpairs. *Arthritis Rheum.* 40(11):1962–1966.

6. Verloes, A., C. Curry, M. Jamar, C. Herens, P. O'Lague, J. Marks, et al. 1998. Juvenile rheumatoid arthritis and del(22q11)syndrome: a non-random association. *J. Med. Genet.* 35:943–947.

7. Sullivan, K.E., D.M. McDonald-McGinn, D.A. Driscoll, C.M. Zmijewski, A.S. Ellabban, L. Reed, et al. 1997. Juvenile Rheumatoid Arthritis-like polyarthritis in chromosome 22q11.2 deletion syndrome (DiGeorge Anomalad/Velocardiofacial Syndrome/Conotruncal Anomaly Face Syndrome). *Arthritis Rheum.* 40(3):430–436.

8. Nepom, B. 1991. The immunogenetics of juvenile rheumatoid arthritis. *Rheum. Dis. Clin. North Am.* 17(4):825–842.

9. Glass, D.N. and E.H. Giannini. 1999. Juvenile Rheumatoid Arthritis as a complex genetic trait. *Arthritis Rheum.* 42(11):2261–2268.

10. Raziuddin, S., S. Bahabri, A. Al-Dalaan, A.K. Siraj, and S. Al-Sedairy. 1998. A Mixed Th1/Th2 Cell cytokine response predominates in systemic onset Juvenile Rheumatoid Arthritis: immunoregulatory IL-10 function. *Clin. Immunol. Immunopathol.* 86(2):192–198.

11. Murray, K.J., A.A. Grom, S.D. Thompson, D. Lieuwen, M.H. Passo, and D.N. Glass. 1998. Contrasting cytokine profines in the synovium of different forms of Juvenile Rheumatoid Arthritis and Juvenile Spondyloarthropathy: prominence of interleukin 4 in restricted disease. *J. Rheumatol.* 25:1388–1398.

12. Rooney, M., J. David, J. Symons, F. Di Giovine, H. Varsani, and P. Woo. 1995. Inflammatory cytokine responses in Juvenile Chronic Arthritis. *Br. J. Rheumatol.* 34(5):454–460.

13. Gattorno, M., P. Picco, S. Vignola, F. Stalla, A. Buoncompagni, and V. Pistoia. 1998. Serum interleukin 12 concentration in juvenile chronic arthritis. *Ann. Rheum. Dis.* 57(7):425–458.

14. DeBenedetti F, P. Pignatti, S. Bernasconi, V. Gerloni, K. Matsushima, R. Caporali, et al. 1999. Interleukin 8 and monocyte chemoattractant protein-1 in patients with Juvenile Rheumatoid Arthritis. Relation to onset types, disease activity, and synovial fluid leukocytes. *J. Rheum.* 26:425–431.

15. Keul , R., P.C. Heinrich, G. Muller-newen, K. Muller, and P. Woo. 1998. A possible role for soluble IL-6 receptor in the pathogenesis of systemic onset juvenile chronic arthritis. *Cytokine* 10(9):729–734 .

16. Grom, A.A., K.J. Murray, L. Luyrink, H.L. Emery, M.H. Passo, D.N. Glass, et al. 1996. Patterns of expression of tumor necrosis factor α, tumor necrosis factor β, and their receptors in synovia of patients with Juvenile Rheumatoid arthritis and Juvenile Spondyloarthropathy. *Arthritis Rheum.* 39(10):1703–1710.

17. Woo, P. 1997. The cytokine network in Juvenile Chronic Arthritis. *Ann. Med.* 29:145–147.

18. Mangge, H., H. Kenzian, Sl. Gallistl, G. Neuwirth, P. Liebmann, W. Kaulfersch, et al. 1995. Serum cytokines in Juvenile Rheumatoid Arthritis. *Arthritis Rheum.* 38(2):211–220.

19. Hornett, G., U. Dirksen, H. Schulze-Koops, R. Emmrich, and V. Wahn. 1995. Treatment of refractory juvenile chronic arthritis by monoclonal CD4 antibodies: a pilot study in two children. *Ann. Rheum. Dis.* 54:846–849.

20. Bakkaloglu, A., B. Kirel, S. Ozen, U. Saatci, R. Topaloglu, and N. Besbas. 1996. Plasma lipis and lipoproteins in Juvenile Chronic Arthritis. *Clin. Rheum.* 15(4):341–345.

21. Takei, S., H. Imanaka, N. Maeno, M. Shigemori, M. Kiminori, M. Hokonohara, and K. Miyata. 1996. Serum levels of hyanoronic acid indicate the severity of joint symptoms in patients with systemic and polyarticular Juvenile Rheumatoid Arthritis. *J. Rheumatol.* 23(11):1956–1962.

22. Maeno, N., S. Take, H. Imanaka, I. Takasaki, I. Kitajima, I. Maruyama, et al. 1999. Increased circulating vascular endothelial growth factor is correlated with disease activity in polyarticular Juvenile Rheumatoid Arthritis. *J. Rheumatol.* 26(10):2244–2248.

23. De Benedetti, F., P. Pignatti, M. Massa, P. Sartirana, A. Ravelli, and A. Martini. 1995. Circulating levels of interleukin 1B(beta) and of interleukin 1 receptor anatgonist in systemic juvenile chronic arthritis. *Clin. Exp. Rheum.* 13:779–784.

24. McMurray, R.W., S.H. Allen, P.H. Pepmueller, D. Keisler, and J.T. Cassidy. 1995. Elevated serum prolactin levels in children with Juvenile Rheumatoid Arthritis and antinuclear antibody seropositivity. *J. Rheumatol.* 22(8):1577–1580.

25. De Benedetti, F., P. Pignatti, V. Gerloni, M. Mass, P. Sartirana, R. Caporali, et al. 1997. Differences in synovial fluid cytokine levels between Juvenile and Adult Rheumatoid Arthritis. *J. Rheumatol.* 24(7):1403–1409.

26. Khalkhali-Ellis, A., T.L. Moore, and M.J.C. Hendrix. 1998. Reduced levels of testosterone and dehydroepiandrosterone sulphate in the serum and synovial fluid of juvenile rheumatoid arthritis patients correlates with disease severity. *Clin. Exp. Rheumatol.* 16:753–756.

27. Falcini, F., M.M. Cerinic, A. Lombardi, S. Generini, A. Pignone, P. Tirassa, et al. 1996. Increased circulating nerve growth factor is directly correlated with disease activity in juvenile chronic arthritis. *Ann. Rheum. Dis.* 55(10):745–748.

28. Silas, S. and D.O. Clegg. 1999. Selective COX-2 inhibition. *Bull. Rheum. Dis.* 48(2):1–4.

29. Wallace, C.A., D. Farrow, and D.D. Sherry. 1994. Increased risk of facial scars in children taking nonsteroidal antiinflammatory drugs. *J. Pediatr.* 125(5 part1):819–822.

30. Mandell, B.F. 1999. Cox 2-selective NSAIDS: Biology, promises, and concerns. *Clev. Clin. J. Med.* 66(5):285–292.

31. Giannini, E.H., J.T. Cassidy, E.J. Brewer, A. Shaikov, A. Maximov, and N. Kuzmina. 1993. Comparative efficacy and safety of advanced drug therapy in children with juvenile rheumatoid arthritis. *Semin. Arthritis Rheum.* 23(10):34–46.

32. Manners, P.J. and B.M. Ansell. 1986. Slow-acting antirheumatic drug use in systemic onset juvenile chronic arthritis. *Pediatr.* 77:99–103.

33. Grom, A.A. and M. Passo. 1996. Macrophage activation syndrome in systemic juvenile rheumatoid arthritis (editorial). *J. Pediatr.* 129:630–632.

34. Cronstein, B.N., D. Naime, and E. Ostad. 1993. The antiinflammatory mechanism of methotrexate. Increased adenosine release at inflamed sites diminishes leukocyte accumulation in an in vivo model of inflammation. *J. Clin. Invest.* 92(6):2675–2682.

35. Genestier, L., R. Paillot, S. Fournel, C. Ferraro, P. Miossec, and J.P. Revillard. 1998. Immunosup-pressive properties of methotrexate: apoptosis and clonal deletion of activated peripheral T cells. *J. Clin. Invest.* 102(2):322–328.

36. Hunt, P.G., C.D. Rose, G. McIlvain-Simpson, and S. Tejani. 1997. The effects of daily intake of folic acid on the efficacy of methotrexate therapy in children with Juvenile Rheumatoid Arthritis. A controlled study. *J. Rheumatol.* 24(11):2230–2232.

37. Falcini, F., G. Taccetti, M. Ermini, S. Trapani, A. Calzolari, A. Franchi, and M.M. Cerinic. 1997. Methotrexate-associated appearance and rapid progression of rheumatoid nodules in systemic-onset Juvenile Rheumatoid Arthritis. *Arthritis Rheum.* 40(1):175–178.

38. Wallace, C.A. 1998. The use of methotrexate in childhood rheumatic diseases. *Arthritis Rheum.* 41(3):381–391.

39. Cronstein, B.N. 1996. Molecular therapeutics methotrexate and its mechanism of action. *Arthritis Rheum.* 39(12):167-A–167-G.

40. Giannini, E.H., E.J. Brewer, N. Kuzmina, A. Shaikov, A. Maximov, I. Vorontsov, et al. 1992. Methotrexate in resistant Juvenile Rheumatoid Arthritis. *NEJM.* 326:1043–1049.

41. Ravelli, A., S. Viola, B. Ramenghi, G. Beluffi, L.A. Zonta., and A. Martini. 1998. Radiologic progression in patients with juvenile chronic arthritis treated with methotrexate. *J. Pediatr.* 133(2):262–265,

42. Harel, L., L. Wagner-Weiner, A.K. Poznanski, C.H. Spencer, E. Ekwo, and D.B. Magilavy. 1993. Effects of methotrexate on radiologic progression in juvenile rheumatoid arthritis. *Arthritis Rheum.* 36:1370–1374.

43. Ravelli, A., S. Viola, B. Ramenghi, G. Di Fuccia., N. Ruperto, L. Zonta., and A. Martini. 1995. Evaluation of response to methotrexate by a functional index in Juvenile Chronic Arthritis. *Clin. Rheumatol.* 14(3):322–326.

44. Martini, A., A. Ravelli, S. Viola, and R.G. Burgio. 1991. Methotrexate hepatotoxic effects in children with juvenile rheumatoid arthritis (Editorial correspondence). *J. Pediatr.* 119(2):333–334.

45. Cron, R.Q., D.D. Sherry, and C.A. Wallace. 1998. Methotrexate-induced hypersensitivity pneumonitis in a child with juvenile rheumatoid arthritis. *J. Pediatr.* 132(5):901–902.

46. Kugathasan, S., A.J. Newman, B.B. Dahms, and J.T. Boyle. 1996. Liver biopsy findings in patients with juvenile rheumatoid arthritis receiving long-term, weekly methotrexate therapy. *J. Pediatr.* 128(1):149–151.

47. Hashkes, P.J., W.F. Balistreti, K.E. Bove, E.T. Ballard, and M.H. Passo. 1999. The relationship of hepatotoxic risk factors and liver histology in methotrexate therapy for juvenile rheumatoid arthritis. *J. Pediatr.* 134(1):48–52.

48. Ravelli, A., S. Viola, B. Ramenghi, A. Aramini, N. Ruperto, and A. Martini. 1995. Frequency of relapse after discontinuation of methotrexate therapy for clinical remission in Juvenile Rheumatoid Arthritis. *J. Rheumatol.* 22(8):1574–1576.

49. Gottlieb, B.S., G.F. Keenan, T. Lu, and N.T. Ilowite. 1997. Discontinuation of methotrexte treatment in Juvenile Rheumatoid Arthritis. *Pediatr.* 100(6):994–997.

50. Kotaniemi, K. 1998. Late onset uveitis in juvenile-type chronic polyarthritis controlled with prednisolone, cyclosporin A and methotrexate. *Clin. Exp. Rheumatol.* 16:469–471.

51. Weiss, A.H., C.A. Wallace, and D.D. Sherry. 1998. Methotrexate for resistant chronic uveitis in children with juvenile rheumatoid arthritis. *J. Pediatr.* 133(2):266–268.

52. Wallace, C.A. and D.D. Sherry. 1995. A Practical approach to avoidance of methotrexate toxicity (Editorial). *J. Rheumatol.* 22(6):1009–1012.

53. Olsen, N.J., V. Strand, and J.M. Kremer. 1999. Leflunomide for the treatment of Rheumatoid Arthritis. *Bull. Rheum. Dis.* 48(8):1–4.

54. Smolen, J.S., J.R. Kalden, D.L. Scott, B. Rozman, R.K. Kvien, A. Larsen, et al., and the European Leflunomide Study Group. 1999. Efficacy and safety of leflunomide compared with placebo and sulphasalazine in active rheumatoid arthritis: a double-blind, randomized, multicentre trial. *Lancet* 353(9149):259–266.

55. Weinblatt, M.E., J.M. Kremer, J.S. Coblyn, A.L. Maier, S.M. Helfgott, M. Morrell, et al. 1999. Pharmacokinetics, safety, and efficacy of combination treatment with methotrexate and leflunomide in patients with active rheumatoid arthritis. *Arthritis Rheum.* 42(7):1322–28.

56. Cassidy, J.T. 1999. Medical management of children with Juvenile Rheumatoid Arthritis. *Drugs* 58(5):831–850.

57. Toovey, S., E. Hudson, W.F. Hendry, and A.J. Levi. 1981. Sulphasalazine and male infertility: reversibility and possible mechanism. *Gut* 22(6):445–51.

58. Fuchs, H.A. 1997. Use of sulfasalazine in rheumatic diseases. *Bull. Rheum. Dis.* 46(7):3–4.

59. Varbanova, B.B. and E.D. Dyankov. 1999. Sulphasalazine an alternative drug for second-line treatment of juvenile chronic arthritis. *RheumaDerm.* 331–336.

60. Huppertz, H.-I., A. Tschammler, A. Horwitz, and K.O. Schwab. 1995. Intraarticular corticosteroids for chronic arthritis in children: efficacy and effects on cartilage and growth. *J. Pediatr.* 127(2):317–321.

61. Padeh, S. and J.H. Passwell. 1998. Intraarticular corticosteroid injection in the management of children with chronic arthritis. *Arthritis Rheum.* 41(7):1210–1214.

62. Sherry, D.D., L.D. Stein, A.M. Reed, L.E. Schanberg, and D.W. Kredich. 1999. Prevention of leg length discrepancy in young children with pauciarticular Juvenile Rheumatoid Arthritis by treatment with intraarticular steroids. *Arthritis Rheum.* 42(11):2330–2334.

63. Adegajo, A.O. and M.A. Hall. 1998. The use of intravenous pulsed methylprednisolone in the treatment of systemic-onset juvenile chronic arthritis. *Br. J. Rheumatol.* 37(11):1240–1242.

64. Picco, P., M. Gattorno, A. Buoncompagni, V. Pistoia, and C. Borrone. 1996. 6-methyllprednisolone 'Mini-pulses': a new modality of glucocorticoid treatment in systemic onset juvenile chronic arthritis. *Scand. J. Rheumatol.* 25(1):24–27.

65. Jones, R.E. and L.W. Moreland. 1999. Tumor necrosis factor inhibitors for Rheumatoid Arthritis. *Bull. Rheum. Dis.* 48(3):1–4.

66. Moreland, L.W. 1999. Inhibitors of tumor necrosis factor: new treatment options for rheumatoid arthritis. *Clev. Clin. J. Med.* 66(6):367–373.

67. Moreland, L.W. 1999. Inhibitors of tumor necrosis factor for Rheumatoid Arthritis. *J. Rheumatol.* 26 (Suppl. 57):7–15.

68. Moreland, L.W., S.W. Baumgartner, M.H. Schiff, E.A. Tindall, R.M. Fleischmann, A.L. Weaver, et al. 1997. Treatment of rheumatoid arthritis with a recombinant human tumor necrosis factor recetor (p75)-Fc fusion protein. *NEJM* 337:141–147.

69. Beutler, B.A. 1999. The role of tumor necrosis factor in health and disease. *J. Rheumatol.* 26 (Suppl. 57):16–21.

70. Lovell, D.J., E.H. Giannini, J.B. Whitmore, L. Soffes, and B.K. Finck. 1998. Safety and efficacy of tumor necrosis factor receptor P75 FC fusion protein (TNFR:FC; Enbrel™) in polyarticular course Juvenile Rheumatoid Arthritis. *Arthritis Rheum.* 41:S130 (Abstract).

71. Lovell, D.J., E.H. Giannini, A. Reiff, G.D. Cawkwell, E.D. Silverman, J.J. Nocton, et al. 2000. Etanercept in children with polyarticular juvenile rheumatoid arthritis. Pediatric Rheumatology Collaborative Study Group. *NEJM* 16;342(11):763–769.

72. Uziel, Y., R.M. Laxer, R. Schneider, and E.D. Silverman. 1996. Intravenous immunoglobulin therapy in systemic onset Juvenile Rheumatoid Arthritis: a follow-up study. *J. Rheumatol.* 23(5):910–918.

73. Prieur, A.M. 1996. Intravenous immunoglobulins in still's disease: still controversial, still unproven (Editorial). *J. Rheumatol.* 23(5):797–799.

74. Giannini, E.H., D.J. Lovell, E.D. Silverman, R.P. Sundel, B.L. Tague, and N. Ruperto. 1996. Intravenous immunoglobulin in the treatment of polyarticular Juvenile Rheumatoid Arthritis: a phase I/II Study. *J. Rheumatol.* 23(5):919–924.

75. Savolainen, H.A., H. Kautiainen, H. Isomaki, K. Aho, and P. Verronen. 1997. Azathioprine in patients with Juvenile Chronic Arthritis: a longterm follow-up study. *J. Rheumatol.* 24(12):2444–2450.

76. Wallace, C.A. and D.D. Sherry. 1997. Trial of intravenous pulse cyclophosphamide and methylprednisolone in the treatment of severe systemic-onset Juvenile Rheumatoid Arthritis. *Arthritis Rheum.* 40(10):1852–1855.

77. Reiff, A., D.J. Rawlings, B. Shaham, E. Franke, L. Richardson, I.S. Szer, and B.H. Bernstein. 1997. Preliminary evidence for cyclosporin A as an alternative in the treatment of recalcitrant Juvenile Rheumatoid Arthritis and Juvenile Dermatomyositis. *J. Rheumatol.* 24(12):2436–2443.

78. Goldstein, S.L. 2000. Update on mycophenolate mofetil. *Pediatr. Infect. Dis.* 19(1):73–75.

79. Glicklich, D. and A. Acharya. 1998. Mycophenolate mofetil therapy for lupus nephritis refractory to intravenous cyclophosphamide. *Am. J. Kidney Dis.* 32(2):318–322.

80. Goldblum, R. 1993. Therapy of rheumatoid arthritis with mycophenolate mofetil. *Clin. Exp. Rheumatol.* (Suppl.) 8:S117–S119.

81. Golub, L.M., N.S. Ramamurthy, T.F. McNamara, B. Gomes, M. Wolff, A. Cianco, et al. 1984. Tetracycline inhibit tissue collagenase activity. *J. Periodont. Res.* 19:651–695.

82. Greenwald, R.A., L.M. Golub, B. Lavietes, N.S. Ramamurthy, B. Gruber, R.S. Laskin, and T.F. McNamara. 1987. Tetracyclines inhibit human synovial collagenase in vivo and in vitro. *J. Rheumatol.* 14: 28–32.

83. Akin, E., L.C. Miller, and L.B. Tucker. 1998. Minocycline-induced lupus in adolescents. *Pediatr.* 101(5):926–928.

84. Knights, S.E., M.J. Leandro, M.A. Khamashta, and G.R. Hughes. 1998. Minocycline-induced arthritis. *Clin. Exp. Rheumatol.* 16(5):587–590.

85. Alarcon, G.S. and A.A. Bartolucci. 2000. Radiographic assessment of disease progression in Rheumatoid Arthritis patients treated with methotrexate or minocycline. *J. Rheumatol.* 27(2):530–534.

86. O'Dell, J.R., C.E. Haire, W. Palmer, W. Drymalski, S. Wees, K. Blakely, et al. 1997. Treatment of early Rheumatoid Arthritis with minocycline or placebo. *Arthritis Rheum.* 40(5):842–848.

87. Wulffraat, N., A. van Royen, M. Bierings, J. Vossen, and W. Kuis. 1999. Autologous haemo-poietic stem-cell transplantation in four patients with refractory juvenile chronic arthritis. *Lancet* 353(9152):550–553.

88. Quartier, P., A.-M. Prieur, and A. Fischer. Correspondence re: haemopoietic stem-cell transplanta-tion for juvenile chronic arthritis. *Lancet* 353(9167):1885–1886

89. Cron, R.Q., S. Sharma, and D.D. Sherry. 1999. Current treatment by United States and Canadian pediatric rheumatologists. *J. Rheumatol.* 26(9):2036–2038.

90. Weinblatt, M.E., J.M. Kremer, A.D. Bankhurst, K.J. Bulpitt, R.M. Fleischmann, R.I. Fox, et al. 1999. A trial of etanercept, a recombinant rumor necrosis factor receptor:Fc fusion protein, in patients with Rheumatoid Arthritis Receiving methotrexate. *NEJM* 34(4):253–259.

91. Section on Rheumatology and Section on Ophthalmology, American Academy of Pediatrics. 1993. Guidelines for ophthalmologic examinations in children with Juvenile Rheumatoid Arthritis (RE9320). *Pediatr.* 92(2):295–296.

92. Grom, A.A. and M. Passo. 1996. Macrophage activation syndrome in systemic juvenile rheumatoid arthritis. Editorial. *J. Pediatr.* 129(5):630–632.

93. Hirst, W.J., D.M. Laayton, S. Singh, G. Mieli-Vergani, J.M. Chessells, S. Strovel, and J. Pritchard. 1994. Haemophagocytic lymphohistiocytosis: experience at two U.K. centres. *Br. J. Haematol.* 88(4):731–739.

94. Stephan, J.L., J. Zeller, H.P. Hervelin, J.M. Dayer, and A.M. Prieur. 1993. Macrophage activation syndrome and rheumatic disease in childhood: a report of four new cases. *Clin. Exp. Rheumatol.* 11(4):451–456.

95. Ravelli, A., F. De Benedetti, S. Viola, and A. Martini. 1996. Macrophage activation syndrome in systemic juvenile rheumatoid arthritis successfully treated with cyclosporine. *J. Pediatr.* 128(2): 275–278.

96. Mouy, R., J.-L. Stephan, P. Pillet, E. Haddad, P. Hubert, and A.M. Prieur. 1996. Efficacy of cyclosporine A in the treatment of macrophage activation syndrome in juvenile rheumatoid arthritis: report of five cases. *J. Pediatr.* 129:750–754.

26 Treatment of Inflammatory Myopathies

William R. Gilliland

CONTENTS

INTRODUCTION

Idiopathic inflammatory myopathies (IIM) are chronic, acquired inflammatory diseases of muscle. Clinically, patients present with symmetric proximal muscle weakness. However, the weakness may also be more generalized and involve the neck, back, diaphragm, and pharyngeal musculature. In addition, other nonspecific symptoms including muscle pain, low-grade fevers, arthritis, Raynaud's phenomenon, and fatigue may be present. When the muscle weakness is accompanied by specific skin findings (Gottron's papules, Gottron's rash, and heliotrope), it is referred to as dermatomyositis.

Classification of the various subtypes of IIM is based on clinical, histologic, and serologic data. The most useful criteria for diagnosing polymyositis/dermatomyositis are a recent modification of Bohan and Peter's criteria (Table 1) *(1,2)*.

It should be emphasized that many diseases can mimic the inflammatory myopathies. The differential diagnosis of disorders that cause generalized muscle weakness is extensive and includes a number of metabolic, viral, bacterial, parasitic, toxic, neuromuscular, endocrine, and systemic disorders. When these other causes of muscle weakness and pain are ruled out and the patient has the appropriate clinical, laboratory, and histologic findings, only then can an idiopathic inflammatory myopathy be diagnosed.

From: *Modern Therapeutics in Rheumatic Diseases*
Edited by: G. C. Tsokos, et al. © Humana Press, Inc., Totowa, NJ

Table 1
Criteria for the Diagnosis of Idiopathic Inflammatory Myopathy (IIM)

1. Symmetric weakness, usually progressive, of the limb-girdle muscles.
2. Muscle biopsy evidence of myositis
   - Necrosis of type I and type II muscle fibers
   - Phagocytosis
   - Degeneration and regeneration of myofibers with variation in myofiber size
   - Endomysial, perimysial, perivascular, or interstitial mononuclear cells
3. Elevation of serum levels of muscle-associated enzymes
   - Creatine kinase
   - Aldolase
   - Lactate dehydrogenase
   - Transaminases (ALT/SGPT and AST/SGOT)
4. Electromyographic triad of myopathy
   - Short, small, low-amplitude polyphasic motor unit potentials
   - Fibrillation potentials, even at rest
   - Bizarre high-frequency repetitive discharges
5. Characteristic rashes of dermatomyositis
   - Heliotrope rash
   - Gottron's papules
   - Gottron's sign

Definite IIM = 4 of the above criteria 1–4; or 4 of the above (including the rash) for dermatomyositis
Probable IIM = 3 of the above criteria 1–4; or 3 of the above (including the rash) for dermatomyositis
Possible IIM = 2 of the above criteria I–4; or 2 of the above (including the rash) for dermatomyositis

---

One of the first attempts to try to categorize this group of disorders based on clinical and pathological features was by Bohan and Peter *(1)*. In this landmark article, they not only suggested diagnostic criteria, but also categorized patients with myositis into various subsets: polymyositis, dermatomyositis, polymyositis and dermatomyositis with neoplasia, childhood dermatomyositis and polymyositis with vasculitis, and the overlap syndromes *(1)*. In 1971, inclusion body myositis was first described *(3)*. Plotz later coined the term "idiopathic inflammatory myopathies" to include those patients who after a thorough investigation did not have another recognizable cause for their myositis *(4)*.

According to his terminology, the idiopathic inflammatory myopathies include polymyositis, dermatomyositis, cancer-associated myositis, connective tissue-associated myositis, juvenile dermatomyositis, and inclusion body myositis.

More recently, the recognition of newer myositis-specific antibodies (MSAs) have provided clinicians with additional information about classifying and predicting clinical features and therapeutic response of myositis patients. The three most commonly recognized MSAs are various antisynthetases (i.e., Jo-1), anti-Mi-2, and anti-signal recognition particle (SRP). Love and colleagues description of the clinical features and prognosis associated with these serologic tests have helped clinicians design individualized treatment plans *(5)*.

Table 2
Poor Prognostic Factors in IIM

Based on Demographics:
  Black race (vs white)
  Old (vs young)
  Female gender (vs male)
Based on Sign-Symptom Complex:
  Fever
  Severe myositis
  Dysphagia
  Pulmonary involvement
  Cardiac involvement
  Delay to diagnosis and therapy
  Failure to induce a complete remission
Based on Clinicopathologic Group:
  Polymyositis vs dermatomyositis
  Cancer-associated myositis
  Inclusion body myositis
Based on Serologic Group:
  Antisynthetase autoantibodies
  Anti-SRP autoantibodies

Polymyositis/dermatomyositis are not common disorders. Although they are being recognized more frequently, the estimated incidence in the United States is 5–10 cases per million *(6)*. Unfortunately, they can cause significant morbidity and disability if not properly recognized and treated aggressively.

Proper management of this heterogeneous group of disorders can be difficult and requires an individualized plan that takes into account the clinical presentation, other extramuscular features, and consideration of more aggressive therapy in patients with poor prognostic features (Table 2) *(7)*. Although this chapter will primarily focus on the historical as well as current pharmacologic treatment of these diseases, it will initially discuss the role of physical therapy and later address treatment options for special categories of patients and extra-muscular muscle features.

ASSESSING DISEASE ACTIVITY

Before discussing the various options for treating this heterogeneous group of disorders, it is important to review the ways to assess disease activity. Evaluation of the effect of therapy can be difficult. Many of the instruments used are not readily available to clinicians, so most physicians rely on muscle-associated enzyme tests and manual muscle testing. In general, traditional evaluation methods fall into four categories: serum tests of muscle-associated enzymes, muscle-strength testing, functional assessments, and pulmonary-function testing.

The first group, serum biochemical testing, is used most commonly to follow patients with IIM. According to diagnostic criteria, these tests include the following skeletal muscle-associated enzymes: creatine kinase (CK), aldolase, serum glutamate oxaloacetate (SGOT) and pyruvate (SGPT) transaminases, and lactate dehydrogenase *(1)*. These serum markers of muscle damage correlate with inflammation seen on biopsy *(8)*. In another study of 105 patients with polymyositis or dermatomyositis, Tymm and colleagues found that serum concentration of CK, aspartate aminotransferase (AST), and alanine transferase (ALT) correlated well with muscle weakness, electromyography (EMG) abnormalities, and muscle biopsies *(9)*. Serum myoglobin *(10)*, interleukin-2 (IL-2) receptors *(11)*, and serum von Willebrand factor (vWF) *(12)* may also helpful in assessing disease activity, but may not offer any additional information than that provided by other more readily available tests.

Although muscle-associated enzymes should be used to monitor treatment response, the degree of muscle-associated enzyme elevation may not always reflect disease activity. It is also important to recognize that muscle-associated enzymes may improve or even normalize before the patient or physician notes clinical improvement. The improvement in muscle strength may lag behind improvement in muscle-associated enzymes by 3–8 wk *(13)*. In addition, some studies suggest that individuals may have discordant elevations in only certain muscle-associated enzymes (i.e., the CK may be normal and the myoglobin elevated, or vice versa) *(10)*.

Muscle strength testing is also used frequently to assess clinical response to therapy. Typically clinicians use an arbitrary scale ranging from 0 (absent: no muscle contraction) to 5 (normal: movement against gravity with full resistance). Unless the same examiner does serial testing, there is much subjectivity. Other more sophisticated methods are not widely available, but include hand-held instruments such as dynamometers. These techniques are also dependent on a standardized approach and vary from examiner to examiner *(14)*.

Functional testing generally falls into two categories. The first includes ability to do normal daily activities such as the ability to arise from a chair without the use of their arms, get up from a squatting position, climb stairs, or comb their hair. Time tests measure the time it takes to do a certain task (i.e., time it takes to walk 30 ft).

In patients with suspected progressive diaphragmatic weakness or other pulmonary manifestations, it often is helpful to perform pulmonary function testing such as forced vital capacities, maximum inspiratory pressures, and maximum expiratory pressures.

More recently, multicenter studies have found the use of instruments such as the Childhood Health Assessment Questionnaire (CHAQ) *(15,16)* and the Childhood Myositis Assessment Scale (CMAS) *(17)* to be valid and reliable tools. Owing to the invasive nature of biopsies and EMGs, they are not generally used to assess short-term changes in clinical activity.

INITIAL THERAPY

General Considerations

After the proper diagnosis is established, patient education plays an important role in the treatment of patient with IIM. The patient should be provided with information concerning the diagnosis, symptoms, course, and treatment of these myopathies. Useful patient information about myositis and various medications used to treat them can be obtained from the Arthritis Foundation at www.arthritis.org.

Physical Therapy and Rehabilitation

The primary goals in the management of IIM are to prevent muscle atrophy, prevent contractures, and most importantly maintain muscle strength and function. Physical and occupational therapy are important adjuvants to the pharmacotherapy. However, the optimal use of these modalities is not well-known.

Rehabilitation programs should be tailored to the individual based on issues such as the stage of the disease, type of myositis, degree of weakness, patient's age, and patient's functional status. The plan is devised to gradually improve the patient's strength and functional status. The graduated approach starts with patient education, stretching, massage, and passive range of motion exercises during the acute phase. In the recovery stage (when the patient has movement against gravity), active range of motion and isometric exercises may be added. Finally in the late recovery phase, isotonic exercises in a pool or on land are added *(18)*.

Corticosteroids

Despite the fact that no randomized controlled study demonstrates efficacy, the cornerstone of therapy remains corticosteroids. A retrospective analysis of 289 patients that presented to the Mayo Clinic demonstrated that those patients treated with high-dose (greater than 50 mg/d) prednisone had less morbidity than those treated with no or low-dose (less than 50 mg/d) prednisone *(19)*. In another study investigating the efficacy of corticosteroids in children, those treated with prednisone had both a shorter hospitalization time and period of acute illness *(20)*. Because of their potent anti-inflammatory and immunosuppressive effects, corticosteroids should be administered early in the course of disease. However, the proper dose and duration of corticosteroid therapy is not known.

Initial therapy in adult dermatomyositis/polymyositis range from 40–60 mg/d of prednisone *(21)* to 1 mg/kg/d of prednisone *(22)*. Both of these articles suggest that the dosage be divided and eventually consolidated. According to these authors, the initial high doses of prednisone should be continued until the CK normalizes *(21)* or clinical improvement *(22)*. There is no clear consensus about the endpoint or tapering schedule of corticosteroids *(23)*. After the acute phase of illness, everyone advocates a reduction in the corticosteroid dose. However, no studies have addressed the proper way to taper the steroid dose or when to stop therapy with corticosteroids. One scheme recommends tapering to a maintenance dose of 5–10 mg/d of prednisone in 6–8 mo after initiation of therapy and does not consider stopping it until the disease has been in remission for at least a year *(24)*.

The treatment of patients with IIM should be individualized *(2)*. Although the initial dose should be greater or equal to 1 mg/kg/d, the reduction in dose should be based on the presence of individual poor prognostic factors (Table 2; *7)* and the risk factors for corticosteroid use *(2)*. In order to minimize a flare of the myositis, one should average "about 10 mg/mo or 25% of the existing dose per month, whichever is less, from the reduction until such a time that the maintenance dose is achieved" *(2)*. The implication is that in those individuals with poor prognostic factors, the corticosteroid dose may need to be tapered more slowly.

Only a few studies have addressed the use of intravenous (IV) corticosteroids for the treatment of idiopathic inflammatory myopathies. A small case series of seven children with dermatomyositis reported that three of the children achieved a complete remission and required no further oral corticosteroid therapy after being treated with pulse methylprednisolone *(25)*. Conversely, a retrospective study of seven children treated solely with pulse methylprednisolone administered weekly for three doses concluded that there was no benefit and a potential for deterioration of muscle strength *(26)*. Although little is written about the use of pulse IV corticosteroids in adults, in practice I have used it in individuals with profound peripheral muscle, dysphagia, or respiratory weakness. The theoretic benefits of pulse corticosteroids are twofold: more rapid control of muscle inflammation and the potential for less need for corticosteroids in the future.

Even less is known about the efficacy of alternate-day corticosteroids. It has been recommended therapy be started with 100 mg/d (or 1 mg/kg/d) and tapered to 80–100 mg every other day over a 10-wk period. The "off day" dose can be reduced by 10 mg/wk *(27)*. The obvious advantage to this regimen is that it may lessen the long-term effects of daily corticosteroids.

In certain subsets of patients, the required dose of prednisone may be lower than 1 mg/kg. Patients with polymyositis associated with other connective-tissue disorders may require lower doses of corticosteroids for a shorter period of time. Patients with dermatomyositis sine myositis may not need corticosteroid therapy at all *(28)*.

The use of corticosteroids is fraught with many side effects. Most notable are complications related to osteoporosis: vertebral fractures, hip fractures, and other long-bone fractures. Physicians should consider the use of medications to prevent osteoporosis such as calcium, vitamin D, and estrogen-replacement therapy. In addition, in patients who have multiple poor prognostic signs and who are anticipated to be on corticosteroids of greater than 6 mo, one should strongly consider the use of a bisphosphonate such as alendronate. Bisphosphonates increase the bone density in patients receiving corticosteroids *(29)*.

In addition, other side effects include weight gain, skin atrophy, hypertension, premature atherosclerosis, virilization, avascular necrosis, hyperglycemia, steroid myopathy, and an increased susceptibility to infections. In children, corticosteroids may also cause growth retardation.

THERAPY FOR STEROID-RESISTANT DISEASE

Although some patients will have a complete response to corticosteroid therapy, many will not. Bohan and Peter defined those patients receiving 60 mg of prednisone daily for 3–4 mo with no response as being "steroid resistant" *(1)*. They did not provide information about how frequently steroid resistance occurred. Others have suggested that it is approx 20% *(30,31)*. However, a retrospective study from the National Institutes of Health (NIH) found only 25% of patient to have a complete remission and 61% to have a partial response *(32)*. The higher percentages obviously may represent a referral bias of more severe disease at the NIH.

When there is not an adequate response to corticosteroid therapy, it is important to review the clinical material and assure that the diagnosis is correct. Also consider the possibility of underlying malignancy or noncompliance with medical regimen.

Another common problem after the patient has been on corticosteroids for several months is differentiating the symptoms from a steroid myopathy. Although there may be some clinical clues that help distinguish the two diseases, it ultimately may require a repeat biopsy.

Many medications have been tried as second-line agents. The choice of medication is largely empiric and frequently based on physician and institutional preference. Little comparative data with these agents exist. At NIH, aggressive therapy with these second-line agents may be started as soon as the diagnosis is made *(33)*. This is in part to improve the patient's functional outcomes but also to use these agents as "steroid-sparing" agents. Miller also advocates using these agents once the diagnosis is established in those patients with poor prognostic markers *(2)*. Although this is not discussed much in the literature, many rheumatologists in the community are adopting similar aggressive therapy.

Methotrexate

Methotrexate (MTX) is probably the most widely used second-line agent, even though there are no controlled clinical studies of its use. It is an inhibitor of dihydrofolate reductase and has been used in the treatment of rheumatoid arthritis (RA) and psoriatic arthritis since at least 1951 *(34)*. Because of the familiarity of rheumatologists using this agent and the its ease in administration, it is often the first choice of many physicians.

In early studies, it was administered intravenously. Several case reports suggested the use of MTX in the treatment of resistant myositis *(35,36)*. In a larger case series of 25 patients with steroid-resistant or intolerant disease, 88% had improved strength and 43% were able to reduce the corticosteroid dose. The initial dose used in this study was 10–15 mg IV that was increased weekly by 0.5–0.8 mg/kg and administered every 5–7 d *(37)*. Intravenous MTX has also been used successfully in children with dermatomyositis *(38)*. MTX is not only helpful in controlling the muscle inflammation, but also has been shown to improve the dermatologic features as well *(39)*.

Because many rheumatologists are familiar with using oral MTX in the management of RA, most initiate therapy using oral doses ranging from 7.5–15 mg weekly. The dose can then be increased at doses of 2.5 mg increments to a maximum dose of 30–40 mg/wk *(40)* at 6–8-wk intervals. However because of questions concerning adequate absorption and because of gastrointestinal (GI) intolerance, many choose to administer MTX by subcutaneous injections when using higher doses. Although some patients with RA are treated with intramuscular MTX, intramuscular injections should not be used in patients with inflammatory muscle disease because of their potential to increase muscle-associated enzymes *(41)*.

Common side effects include skin rash, oral ulcerations, stomatitis, fever, GI symptoms (diarrhea, cramping, or vomiting), hair loss, headaches, and cognitive dysfunction *(42)*, which occur more frequently in patients with inflammatory myositis than in RA *(43)*. Hepatotoxicity is generally associated with chronic use of MTX. The recommended schedule for blood testing and other monitoring is frequently adapted from guidelines offered for MTX use in RA *(44)*. MTX pneumonitis may also be seen in patients with polymyositis. It may be difficult to differentiate this from pulmonary manifestations of polymyositis, especially in individuals who are anti-Jo1 positive. Although initially thought to have little oncogenic potential, low-dose MTX has been associated with Epstein-Barr virus (EBV)-associated non-Hodgkin's lymphoma in RA *(45)* and non-Hodgkin's lymphoma in dermatomyositis *(46,47)*.

Azathioprine

Along with MTX, azathioprine is the other commonly used "first-line" agent for steroid-resistant patients. It is a purine analog that is converted in the liver to mercaptopurine, the active metabolite. Although the precise mechanism is not known, azathioprine inhibits DNA and RNA synthesis in lymphocytes. It has both cytotoxic and immunosuppressive properties.

In one of the few controlled, randomized trials of any therapeutic agents in poly-myositis, 16 patients were treated with 60 mg of prednisone plus either azathioprine (2 mg/kg) or placebo for 3 mo with no improvement in terms of muscle-enzyme levels, muscle strength, or histiopathologic features *(48)*. The failure of this study may be owing to the fact that azathioprine may not be seen at 3 mo. Yet, when prednisone and azathioprine are used in combination for longer periods of time, some benefits may be seen *(49)*.

Azathioprine is administered orally in the dose of 2 mg/kg/d *(49)* or approx 100–200 mg/d *(21)*. Although it is usually well-tolerated, a small number of patients may exhibit an idiosyncratic reaction manifested by fevers, vomiting, rash, and abdominal pain. More worrisome long-term side effects include a drug-induced hepatotoxicity, leukopenia, macrocytosis, thrombocytopenia, and an increased risk of lymphoma. Liver associated enzymes and complete blood counts should be monitored every 1–2 mo.

Cyclophosphamide

Cyclophosphamide is an alkylating agent used to treat other systemic inflammatory diseases such as systemic lupus erythematosus (SLE), RA, and Wegener's granulomatosus (WG), and other vasculitides. Its cytotoxicity is secondary to its ability to alkylate various cellular constituents especially affecting lymphoid cells and subsequently leading to immunosuppression *(50)*. In clinical practice, it is used less frequently than MTX and azathioprine in part because the clinical data that exists about its use is not as favorable and the fear of long-term risk for lymphoid malignancies, susceptibility to infection, and other serious side effects.

Cyclophosphamide alone may not be useful in controlling the inflammatory aspects of myositis, but may be useful when used with corticosteroids *(51)*. Several studies have reported some beneficial effects when patients were treated with prednisone and monthly intravenous cyclophosphamide (doses ranging from 750–1357 mg/m^2) *(52–54)*. Cyclophosphamide has been effective in the treatment of lung disease secondary to polymyositis *(55,56)*. Another case report demonstrated the successful treatment of interstitial pneumonia secondary to dermatomyositis with intravenous cyclophosphamide in combination with cyclosporine and prednisone *(57)*.

Cyclophosphamide can also be administered orally in daily doses (2–2.5 mg/kg) or intravenously on weekly to monthly doses. Close monitoring of the complete blood count is necessary to avoid complications related to leukopenia, thrombocytopenia, and anemia. As mentioned previously, although they may be effective in treating rheumatic disorders, the use of alkylating agents is limited by their potential side effects.

Short-term adverse effects of alkylating agents include hematologic, GI, infectious, urologic, pulmonary, and dermatologic complications *(51)*. Other potential long-term concerns include the increased risk of bladder and hematologic malignancies, male infertility, and ovarian failure.

Chlorambucil

Chlorambucil, another alkylating agent, has also been used to treat various rheumatic disorders in addition to hematologic and malignant diseases. However, it has not been used as frequently as cyclophosphamide and little is written about its use in treating inflammatory myopathies. In a recent case series of five patients with dermatomyositis that had failed prior treatment with immunosuppressive agents (azathioprine and/or methotrexate), beneficial results were noted within 4–6 mo in all patients. All were treated with oral chlorambucil (4 mg/d) and other immunosuppressive agents (except prednisone) were discontinued. In four patients, treatment was continued for 13–30 mo at which time remission was attained. One patient remained on chlorambucil with persistent disease *(58)*.

As with cyclophosphamide, careful monitoring of blood cell counts is mandatory. Potential adverse effects are similar to cyclophosphamide. It should be noted that the Food and Drug Administration (FDA) has not approved any alkylating agent for the treatment of rheumatic diseases, so all patients should give informed consent prior to their use.

Cyclosporine

Cyclosporine inhibits the activation and proliferation of T cells, lymphokine (IL-2, IL-3, IL-4, IL-5, and γ-interferon [IFN-γ]) release, and antigen presentation. Clinically, it is used most frequently in organ transplantation, but has also been used to treat autoimmune disorders such as graft vs host disease (GVHD), Behcet's disease, uveitis, and Crohn's disease *(59)*.

As with many of the other drugs discussed previously, there have been no large studies using cyclosporine to treat idiopathic inflammatory myopathies. Interestingly, much of the experience using cyclosporine to treat polymyositis is in children. An early case report described a 15-yr-old girl with dermatomyositis who had failed treatment with azathioprine and methylprednisolone and then noted improvement in function and muscle enzymes after starting on cyclosporine (3 mg/kg/d) *(60)*. Several more recent case series also suggest cyclosporine may play a role in the treatment of juvenile dermatomyositis. In a case series of 14 children who had ongoing active disease with only partial responses to prior therapy with corticosteroids and other immunosuppressive agents, cyclosporine (2.5–7.5 mg/kg/d) was found to be effective and safe *(61)*. In another small retrospective case series of 6 children with refractory dermatomyositis, treatment with cyclosporine (5–6 mg/kg/d) led to clinical improvement and a reduction or discontinuation of corticosteroids in all patients. (It should also be noted that three relapsed after discontinuation of cyclosporine, but recovered after it was reinitiated *[62]*) Less information exists about the treatment of adults with cyclosporine, but it has been shown to be effective with the usual dose being 5–10 mg/kg/d and adjusted based on clinical effects, side effects, and cyclosporine levels *(63–65)*.

A recent randomized study compared patients receiving methotrexate plus prednisone and cyclosporine plus prednisone. In this study of 36 patients with active polymyositis or dermatomyositis, significant improvement was noted in both groups in terms of functional muscle testing, clinical assessment, global patient's assessment, and muscle magnetic resonance imaging (MRI). Interestingly in the MTX-treated group, the CK tended to improve sooner than in the cyclosporine group *(66)*.

Although cyclosporine may be considered as an alternative therapy, especially when other treatments have failed, its side-effect profile limits its use. Minor side effects include hirsutism, nausea, headache, thrombocytopenia, anemia, and gum hypertrophy. More serious side effects include hypertension, renal failure, and an increased risk for lymphoproliferative malignancy.

Intravenous Immune Gamma Globulin

Although intravenous immunoglobulin (IVIG) was initially used for treatment of primary and secondary immunodeficiencies, it is now being used to treat neurologic (i.e., myasthenia gravis and Guillain-Barre), hematologic (i.e., idiopathic thrombocytopenic purpura), infectious (i.e., sepsis), dermatologic (i.e., pemphigus), and systemic inflammatory diseases (i.e., Kawasaki's). Given the suspected role of immune-mediated mechanisms in the pathogenesis of these diseases and in inflammatory myopathies, IVIG has also been used to treat IIM as well.

Roifman initially described the successful use of IVIG to treat a 15-yr-old girl who had previously failed traditional therapies: corticosteroids, MTX, and cyclophosphamide *(67)*. Several years later in an uncontrolled study, 14 patients with "chronic, refractory" polymyositis and 6 patients with dermatomyositis with IVIG after failing "traditional therapy" were treated with IVIG and average of 4 mo (1–12 mo) with all patients receiving 1 g/kg for 2 d or 0.4 g/kg for 5 d each month. Muscle strength and muscle enzymes improved in significantly in 75% of these patients, but long-term follow-up was not provided *(68)*.

More recently, Dalakas and colleagues conducted the only double-blind, placebo-controlled study using IVIG in IIM. He enrolled 15 patients ranging from 18–55 yr of age with "treatment-resistant" dermatomyositis. The patients were randomized to receive either a monthly infusion of IVIG (2 g/kg) or placebo for 3 mo. (They also continued to receive corticosteroids.) In addition, an option to cross-over to the other therapy was also offered the patients. Clinical outcomes included strength assessment, rash, and neuromuscular symptoms. In addition, biopsies were repeated in all patients. In total 12 patients received IVIG (8 patients from the initial randomization and 4 crossover patients), 9 of these patients showed major improvement in functional disability as well as in muscle strength and neuromuscular scores. Of the 11 patients in the placebo group, 8 had either a worsening or no change in their condition and 3 had a mild improvement in their condition. Histologic improvement was also noted on biopsies *(69)*.

In regards to the use of IVIG, many questions have yet to be answered, including the optimal time to use this therapy and the optimal duration. In clinical practice, IVIG is generally used in patients who have failed other agents. This may be partially owing to the expense of the drug and concern about adverse effects (headaches, chills, fevers, aseptic meningitis, thromboembolic events, transmission of infectious diseases, and anaphylactic reactions). Guidelines for administration of IVIG vary, but in adults the total IVIG dosage is 2 g/kg that can be divided and given over 1–5 d *(70)*. Total duration of therapy also varies and is largely dependent on patient improvement.

Plasmapheresis

Excitement about the possibility of plasmapheresis being used to treat inflammatory myopathies stems from an early uncontrolled study of 33 patients. All patients were treated with plasmapheresis and prednisone in addition to continuing cytotoxic therapy with either cyclophosphamide or chlorambucil. Improvement was noted in 32 patients in regards to muscle testing, forced vital capacity, EMG findings, CPKs, and muscle biopsy *(71)*. Skeptics suggested that the improvement could be due to the effects of other cytotoxic therapy. However a more recent retrospective study of 21 patients treated with plasma exchange also demonstrated a 71% response rate *(72)*.

In one of the few double-blinded, controlled studies of therapy in polymyositis, Miller and colleagues *(73)* randomly assigned 39 patients with polymyositis or dermatomyositis into three groups. The first group was treated with plasma exchange (replacement of one volume of plasma with 5% albumin in saline), the second group with leukopheresis (removal of $5–10 \times 109$ lymphocytes), and the third group with sham apheresis. Twelve treatments were given over a 1-mo period while the patients' prednisone dose remained constant. No other immunosuppressive agents were allowed. Outcome measurements included muscle strength, functional capacity, and serum muscle-associated enzymes. While 3 patients in each group of 13 patients had improvement in strength and functional capacity, no significant differences were noted in any of the three treatment arms in terms of final muscle strength or functional capacity *(73)*.

Theoretically, such therapies could remove cytokines, immunoglobulins, and lymphocytes from the peripheral circulation, thereby affecting the systemic inflammatory response in inflammatory myopathies. Immunologic studies of patients with polymyositis treated with apheresis demonstrated a decrease in serum IgG, natural killer (NK) lymphocytes, B cells, and T cells. In addition, maturation of CD4+ T cells also increased, leading the authors to speculate that the maturation of these cells may downregulate the inflammatory process *(71)*. The most severe adverse effects in Miller's study were the requirement of a central venous catheter (23%), major vasovagal episodes (8%), and clinically important citrate reactions (5%) *(73)*.

Irradiation

The use of ionizing radiation to treat patients with severe life-threatening disease was first reported by Engel *(74)*. Some clinicians have used whole-body, low-dose irradiation administered over a 5-wk period *(75,76)*, whereas others have used total lymphoid irradiation with higher-dose irradiation also delivered over a 5–6 wk period *(77)*. The use of irradiation is limited by multiple, serious side effects including pancytopenia, increased risk of malignancy, and death. Therefore, it should only be considered in patients who have severe incapacitating disease who have failed to respond to conventional therapy.

Combined Therapy

In a sense when corticosteroids are used in combination with other immunosuppressive or cytotoxic agents, it may be considered to be "combined therapy." However most clinicians reserve the term "combined therapy" to mean combining two or more immunosuppressive and/or cytotoxic agents. Clinical data using these combinations of two or more immunosuppressive and/or cytotoxic agents is scant. Most of the information is from case reports or small case series. The combination of MTX and cyclosporine A has successfully been used to treat a woman with myositis unresponsive to pulse corticosteroid therapy and the combination of azathioprine and MTX *(78)*. As mentioned previously, pulse cyclophosphamide and cyclosporine were used successfully to treat an interstitial pneumonia associated with dermatomyositis *(57)*. In one of the few randomized, controlled studies of therapies in myositis, the combination of oral MTX and daily azathioprine was compared with intravenous MTX in a crossover design. Of the 30 patients with "refractory disease," 12 patients improved while on the combination of MTX and azathioprine *(79)*.

TREATMENT OF MISCELLANEOUS MANIFESTATIONS

Skin Manifestations

The cutaneous manifestations of dermatomyositis may or may not improve with therapy aimed at treating the muscle inflammation. Sunscreen, avoidance of sun, and topical corticosteroids may be helpful in treating these manifestations, although there is little clinical information about their use.

In addition, antimalarial agents such as chloroquine, hydroxychlorquine, and quinacrine may also be useful in treating the cutaneous manifestations. Patients may respond to hydroxychloroquine with resolution of the skin manifestations. In addition, although hydroxychloroquine did not seem to be beneficial in treating the muscle disease, it may help decrease the prednisone dose *(80)*.

Joint Manifestations

In addition to muscle weakness and/or pain, patients with IIM may also develop an inflammatory arthritis. The arthritis associated with IIM is usually a nonerosive and affects the small joints of the hands and wrists. In the Jo-1 associated myopathies, it may be especially troubling and even deforming. Nonsteroidal anti-inflammatory agents and low-dose prednisone are often helpful in treating these symptoms; although occasionally disease-modifying agents may be required like those used to treat RA.

Calcinosis

Subcutaneous calcifications are a late manifestation of chronic disease, especially in juvenile dermatomyositis. Calcinosis often occurs in areas of repeated trauma (elbows, fingers, buttocks, and so on). Secondary infections and persistent drainage may complicate these lesions. Some may require surgical removal. Unfortunately, there is no good therapy to treat these lesions. Clinicians have used agents such as probenecid, colchicine, and warfarin with little success.

Raynaud's Phenomenon

Raynaud's phenomenon can be seen in any patient with IIM, however, it is more common in patients with Jo-1 antibodies. Much like Raynaud's in association with systemic lupus erythematosus (SLE) or scleroderma, it generally will respond to the avoidance of cold or by using calcium-channel blockers.

Lungs and Heart

Pulmonary and cardiac problems associated with IIM are serious problems. Shortness of breath may be owing to alveolitis, respiratory muscle weakness, chronic aspiration secondary to pharyngeal muscle involvement, pulmonary fibrosis, or congestive heart failure. Cardiac conduction abnormalities may also be present. Pulmonary involvement may respond to corticosteroids, MTX, azathioprine, or cyclophosphamide. Involvement of the cardiac muscle should be treated aggressively with agents designed to treat the underlying myositis. Adjuvant therapy may require the use of diuretics, antiarrythmics, and inotropic agents such as digoxin.

GI Tract

Involvement of the pharyngeal muscles may cause dyspepsia, dysphagia, dysphonia, and/or aspiration. Dyspepsia generally will respond to antacids, H_2 blockers, or proton-pump inhibitors. It is also important in patients with severe dysphagia or dysphonia to educate the patient in how to prevent aspiration by having them always eat in an upright position until their food has been digested and to elevate the head of the bed when they are sleeping.

SELECTED PATIENT SUBSETS: TREATMENT ISSUES

Pregnancy

Little clinical information exists about polymyositis and pregnancy. Fetal demise has been reported to be as high as 33% in all pregnancies and up to 50% of women with active disease (81,82). In another study that investigated the risk of exacerbation of the polymyositis/dermatomyositis in 18 pregnant women, Gutierrez and colleagues reported that several women had an exacerbation of their disease during pregnancy (83). A case report described the successful treatment of one pregnant woman with prednisolone (0.3 mg/kg/d) (84). It should be noted that of the medications discussed in the previous sections, only corticosteroids are assigned an FDA risk to the fetus of category B (no evidence of risk in humans). Cyclosporine has an FDA risk of C (risk cannot be ruled out). Azathioprine, chlorambucil, and cyclophosphamide are assigned an FDA risk of D (positive evidence of risk, potential benefits may outweigh the potential risk). MTX has an FDA risk of X (contraindicated in pregnancy) (85). Therefore if the disease requires therapy during pregnancy, no medications other than corticosteroids should be used to control the disease if possible. Other medications are considered to have some risk to the fetus.

Malignancy

Although myositis has been associated with many malignancies, the most common sites in men tend to be the lung and GI tract and in women tend to be the breast and ovary (86). This association is stronger in patients older that the age of 50. A two level search for a malignancy has been recommended. The first level includes a chest radiograph, stool for occult blood, liver-function profile, prostate specific antigen (PSA) in men and mammography, CA-125 testing, and a complete pelvic examination in women. The second level of testing is dependent on the history and physical examination as well as the first level of testing and includes complete barium studies of the GI tracts (or endoscopy and colonoscopy), abdominal and chest CT scans, and pelvic culdoscopy *(87)*. In terms of treatment of the myositis associated with malignancy, it is important to treat the underlying malignancy in addition to the myositis. Although the myositis may respond to therapy aimed at treating the underlying malignancy, it may also require therapy aimed specifically at the muscle inflammation.

Inclusion Body Myositis

Inclusion body myositis (IBM) represents a form of myositis that may lead to slowly progressive, disabling myositis. It commonly affects distal musculature and more commonly affects males. The characteristic histologic feature is cytoplasmic vacuoles on biopsy of skeletal muscle.

Unfortunately, another common feature of IBM is that it is generally thought to be refractory to traditional therapies. However, a retrospective study at the NIH challenges that idea and suggests that corticosteroids and other "traditional" immunosuppressive agents may stabilize or slow down the progressions of the disease *(88)*. Regardless of the lack of evidence, many physicians will try to treat these patients with prednisone and other agents.

Intravenous immunoglobulin (IVIG) may play a role in the treatment of IBM. Two double-blinded, placebo-controlled, crossover studies demonstrate mild or no improvement depending on the outcome measured. Nineteen patients were randomized in the first study and received either monthly infusions of 2 g/kg IVIG or placebo. Patients were then crossed over to the alternate arm after a brief washout phase. Although 28% of the patients demonstrated "functionally important improvement" on IVIG, the improvement was not statistically significant *(89)*. The second study had a similar design and enrolled 22 patients. The authors noted an 11% improvement in clinical symptoms and reported a trend toward improvement on other parameters as well *(90)*. No long-term studies have been performed using IVIG in IBM. Given the cost of IVIG, it is hard to justify its use in all patients with IBM.

As in other patients with IIM, physical therapy can improve muscle strength in patients with IBM. A recent study at the NIH suggests that patients with IBM can tolerate a progressive resistance strength-training program with no evidence of muscle injury *(91)*.

Juvenile Dermatomyositis

As in adult disease, corticosteroids are also used as the initial therapy in juvenile dermatomyositis. Typically, corticosteroids in higher doses than used in adults are used for the initial therapy. Sullivan recommends starting prednisone at the dose of 2 mg/kg/d in four divided doses for at least 1 mo. If there is a good clinical response or decrease in muscle-associated enzymes, then the corticosteroids are decreased to 1 mg/kg/d in divided doses *(22)*. Thereafter, the taper is based on symptoms, clinical examination, and muscle enzymes. As in adults, improvement in strength may lag behind improvement in muscle-enzyme testing. High-dose corticosteroids in children are fraught with the same complications as in adults. However, growth retardation is an additional concern.

Table 3
Doses of Immunosuppressive Agents in Childhood Dermatomyositis

Methotrexate: 0.35–0.65 mg/kg/wk
Cyclosporine: 2.5–7.5 mg/kg/d
Cyclophosphamide: 1 mg/kg/d orally or 500–750 $mg/m^2/mo$
Azathioprine: 1–3 mg/kg/d

In children who are not controlled with corticosteroids, similar therapeutic options are used. Immunosuppressive agents such as MTX, cyclosporine, cyclophosphamide, and azathioprine have all been used with success. Dosages of these agents for children are listed in Table 3 *(92)*. Although IVIG therapy is also controversial in children, Lang reported a case series of five steroid-dependent or steroid-resistant children who responded to IVIG (2 mg/kg over 2 d) *(93)*. Cassidy and Petty suggest that it may be particularly useful in children with early, presumably severe disease *(92)*.

CONCLUSION

Successful treatment of the idiopathic inflammatory myopathies remains challenging even to the most experienced clinicians. Although most patients with IIM respond to initial therapy with corticosteroids, many will require other agents. Of the immunosuppressive and cytotoxic agents used, MTX and azathioprine are the most commonly used "second-line" agents. The role of IVIG in the treatment of IIM remains unclear.

REFERENCES

1. Bohan, A. and J.B. Peter. 1975. Polymyositis and dermatomyositis (parts 1 and 2). *N. Engl. J. Med.* 292(7):344–347, 403–407.
2. Miller, F. 1997. Inflammatory myopathies: polymyositis, dermatomyositis, and related condition. *In* Arthritis and Allied Conditions: A Textbook of Rheumatology. WJ Koopman, editor. Williams and Wilkens, Baltimore. 1407–1431.
3. Yunis, E.J. and F.J. Samaha. 1971. Inclusion body myositis. *Lab. Invest.* 25:240–248.
4. Plotz, P., M. Dalakas, R.L. Leff, L.A. Love, F.W. Miller, and M.E. Cronin. 1989. Current concepts in the idiopathic inflammatory myopathies: polymyositis, dermatomyositis, and related disorders. *Ann. Intern. Med.* 111:143–157.
5. Love, L.A., R.L. Leff, D.D. Fraser, I.N. Targoff, M. Dalakas, P.H. Plotz, and F.W. Miller. 1991. A new approach to the classification of idiopathic inflammatory myopathy: myositis-specific autoantibodies define useful homogenous patient groups. *Medicine* (Baltimore) 70(6):360–374.
6. Oddis, C.V., C.G. Conte, V.D. Steen, and T.A. Medsger, Jr. 1990. Incidence of polymyositis-dermatomyositis: a 20-year study of hospital diagnosed cases in Allegheny County, PA 1963–1982. *J. Rheumatol.* 17(10):1329–1334.
7. Miller, F.W. 1994. Classification and prognosis of inflammatory muscle disease. *Rheum. Dis. Clin. North Amer.* 20(4):811–826.
8. Hood, D., F. Van Lente, and M. Estes. 1991. Serum enzyme alterations in chronic muscle disease: a biopsy-based diagnostic assessment. *Am. J. Clin. Pathol.* 95(3):402–7.
9. Tymms, K.E., E.M. Beller, J. Webb, L. Schrieber, and W.W. Buchanan. 1990. Correlation between tests of muscle involvement and clinical muscle weakness in polymyositis and dermatomyositis. *Clin. Rheumatol.* 9(4):523–9.
10. Lovece, S. and L.J. Kagen. 1993. Sensitive rapid detection of myoglobin in serum of patients with myopathy by immunoturbidimetric assay. *J. Rheumatol.* 20(8):1331–1334.
11. Wolf, R.E. and B.A. Baethge. 1990. Interleukin-1 alpha, interleukin-2, and soluble interleukin-2 receptors in polymyositis. *Arthritis. Rheum.* 33(7):1007–1014.

12. Guzman, J., R.E. Petty, and P.N. Malleson. 1994. Monitoring disease activity in juvenile dermatomyositis: the role of von Willebrand factor and muscle enzymes. *J. Rheumatol.* 21(4):739–743.

13. Kroll, M., J. Otis, and L. Kagen. 1986. Serum enzyme, myoglobin and muscle strength relationships in polymyositis and dermatomyositis. *J. Rheumatol.* 13(2):349–355.

14. Moxley, R.T. 3rd. 1994. Evaluation of neuromuscular function in inflammatory myopathy. *Rheum. Dis. Clin. North Am.* 20(4):827–843.

15. Feldman, B.M., A. Ayling-Campos, L. Luy, D. Stevens, E.D. Silverman, and R.M. Laxer. 1995. Measuring disability in juvenile dermatomyositis: validity of the childhood health assessment questionnaire. *J. Rheumatol.* 22(2):326–331.

16. Huber, A.M., B. Lang, C.M. LeBlanc, N. Birdi, R.K. Boaria, P. Malleson, et al. 2000. Medium- and long-term functional outcomes in a multicenter cohort of children with juvenile dermatomyositis. *Arthritis Rheum.* 43(3):541–549.

17. Lovell, D.J., C.B. Lindsley, R.M. Rennebohm, S.H. Ballinger, S.L. Bowyer, E.H. Giannini, et al. 1999. Development of a validated disease activity and damage indices for the juvenile idiopathic inflammatory myopathies. II. The Childhood Myositis Assessment Scale (CMAS): a quantitative tool for the evaluation of muscle function. The Juvenile Dermatomyositis Disease Activity Collaborative Study Group. *Arthrtitis Rheum.* 42(10):2213–2219.

18. Hicks, J.E. 1998. Role of rehabilitation in the management of myopathies. *Curr. Opin. Rheumatol.* 10(6):548–555.

19. Winkelmann, R.K., D.W. Mulder, E.H. Lambert, F.M. Howard, Jr., G.R. Diessner. 1968. Course of dermatomyositis-polymyositis: comparison of untreated and cortisone-treated patients. *Mayo Clin. Proc.* 43:546–556.

20. Rose, A.L. Childhood polymyositis. 1974. A follow-up study with special reference to treatment with corticosteroids. *Am. J. Dis. Child* 127(4):518–522.

21. Oddis, C.V. and T.A. Medsger. 1989. Current management of polymyositis and dermatomyositis. *Drugs* 37:382–390.

22. Sullivan, D.B., J.T. Cassidy, and R.E. Petty. 1972. Prognosis in childhood dermatomyositis. *J. Pediatr.* 80:555–563.

23. Boyd, A.S. and K.H. Neldner. 1994. Therapeutic options in dermatomyositis/polymyositis. *Int. J. Dermatol.* 33(4):240–250.

24. Oddis, C.V. 1994. Therapy of the inflammatory myopathy. *Rheum. Dis. Clin. North Amer.* 20:899–918.

25. Laxer, R.M., L.D. Stein, and R.E. Petty. 1987. Intravenous pulse methylprednisolone treatment of juvenile dermatomyositis. *Arthritis Rheum.* 30(3):328–334.

26. Lang, B. and J. Dooley. 1996. Failure of pulse methylprednisolone treatment in juvenile dermatomyositis. *J. Pediatr.* 128(3):429–432.

27. Dalakas, M.C. 1994. Current treatment of the inflammatory myopathies. *Curr. Opin. Rheumatol.* 6(6):595–601.

28. Cosnes, A., F. Amaudric, R. Gherardi, J. Verroust, J. Wechsler, J. Revuz, and J.C. Roujeau. 1995. Dermatomyositis without muscle weakness: long-term follow-up of 12 patients without systemic corticosteroids. *Arch. Dermatol.* 131:1381–1385.

29. Saag, K.G., R. Emkey, T.J. Schnitzer, J.P. Brown, F. Hawkins, S. Goemaere, et al. 1998. Alendronate for the prevention and treatment of glucocorticoid-induced osteoporosis. Glucocorticoid-Induced Osteoporosis Intervention Study Group. *N. Engl. J. Med.* 339(5):292–299.

30. Pearson, C.M. 1963. Patterns of polymyositis and their response to treatment. *Ann. Intern. Med.* 59:827–838.

31. Mastaglia, F.L., B.A. Phillips, and P. Zilko. 1997. Treatment of inflammatory myopathies. *Muscle Nerve* 20(6):651–664.

32. Joffe, M.M., L.A. Love, R.L. Leff, D.D. Fraser, I.N. Targoff, J.E. Hicks, et al. 1993. Drug therapy of the idiopathic inflammatory myopathies: predictors of response to prednisone, azathioprine, and methotrexate and a comparison of their efficacy. *Am. J. Med.* 94(4):379–387.

33. Adams, E.M. and P.H. Plotz. 1995. The treatment of myositis. How to approach resistant disease. *Rheum. Dis. Clin. North Am.* 21(1):179–202.

34. Gubner, R., S. August, and V. Ginsberg. 1951. Therapeutic suppression of tissue reactivity. II. Effect of aminopterin in rheumatoid arthritis and psoriasis. *Am. J. Med. Sci.* 221:176–182.

35. Malaviya, A.N., A. Many, and R.S. Schwartz. 1968. Treatment of dermatomyositis with methotrexate. *Lancet* 2(7566):485–488.

36. Sokoloff, M.C., L.S. Goldberg, and C.M. Pearson. 1971. Treatment of corticosteroid-resistant polymyositis with methotrexate. *Lancet* 1(7688):14–16.

37. Metzger, A.L., A. Bohan, L.S. Goldberg, R. Bluestone, and C.M. Pearson. 1974. Polymyositis and dermatomyositis: combined methotrexate and corticosteroid therapy. *Ann. Intern. Med.* 81(2):182–189.

38. Jacobs, J.C. 1977. Methotrexate and azathioprine treatment of childhood dermatomyositis. *Pediatrics* 59(2):212–218.

39. Kasteler, J.S. and J.P. Callen. 1997. Low-dose methotrexate administered weekly is an effective corticosteroid-sparing agent for the treatment of the cutaneous manifestations of dermatomyositis. *J. Am. Acad. Dermatol.* 36(1):67–71.

40. Oddis, C.V. 1991. Therapy for myositis. *Curr. Opin. Rheumatol.* 3(6):919–924.

41. Kaye, S.A. and D.A. Isenberg. 1994. Treatment of polymyositis and dermatomyositis. *Br. J. Hosp. Med.* 52(9):463–468.

42. Rooney, T.W. and D.E. Furst. 1993. Methotrexate, in Arthritis and Allied Conditions: A Textbook of Rheumatology. McCarty and Koopman, editors. Lea and Febiger, Philadelphia. 621–637.

43. Zieglschmid-Adams, M.E., A.G. Pandya, S.B. Cohen, and R.D. Sontheimer. 1995. Treatment of dermatomyositis with methotrexate. *J. Am. Acad. Dermatol.* 32(5Pt1):754–757.

44. Kremer, J.M., G.S. Alarcon, R.W. Lightfoot, Jr., R.F. Wilkens, D.E. Furst, H.J. Williams, et al. 1994. Methotrexate for rheumatoid arthritis: suggested guidelines for monitoring liver toxicity. *Arthritis Rheum.* 37(3):316–328.

45. Shiroky, J.B. and M.M. Newkirk. 1993. Reversible lymphomas. *N. Engl. J. Med.* 329(22): 1657–1658.

46. Bittar, B. and C.D. Rose. 1995. Early development of Hodgkin's lymphoma in association with the use of methotrexate for the treatment of dermatomyositis. *Ann. Rheum. Dis.* 54(7):607–608.

47. Kamel, O.W., M. van de Rijn, L.M. Weiss, G.J. Del Zoppo, P.K. Hench, B.A. Robbins, et al. 1993. Brief report: reversible lymphomas associated with Epstein-Barr virus occurring during methotrexate therapy for rheumatoid arthritis and dermatomyositis. *New Engl. J. Med.* 328(18):1317–1321.

48. Bunch, T.W., J.W. Worthington, J.J. Combs, D.M. Ilstrup, and A.G. Engel. 1980. Azathioprine with prednisone for polymyositis. A controlled clinical trial. *Arthritis Rheum.* 55(3):365–369.

49. Bunch, T.W. 1981. Prednisone and azathioprine for polymyositis: long-term followup. *Arthritis Rheum.* 24(1):45–48.

50. Kawabata, T.T., M.Y. Chapman, D.H. Kim, W.D. Stevens, and M.P. Holapple. 1990. Mechanisms of in vitro immunosuppression by hepatocyte-generated cyclophosphamide metabolites and 4-hydroperoxycyclophosphamide. *Biochem. Pharmacol.* 40(5):927–935.

51. Fries, J.F., G.C. Sharp, H.O. McDevitt, and H.R. Holman. 1973. Cyclophosphamide therapy in systemic lupus erythematosus and polymyositis. *Arthritis Rheum.* 16(2):154–162.

52. Cronin, M.E., F.W. Miller, J.E. Hicks, et al. 1989. Failure of intravenous cyclophosphamide therapy in refractory idiopathic polymyositis. *J. Rheumatol.* 16:1225–1228.

53. Bombardieri, S., G.R. Hughes, R. Neri, P. Del Bravo, and L. Del Bono. 1989. Cyclophosphamide in severe polymyositis. *Lancet* 1(8647):1138–1139.

54. Haga, H.J., D.P. D'Cruz, R. Asherson, and G.R. Hughes. 1992. Short term effects of intravenous pulses of cyclophosphamide in the treatment of connective tissue disease crisis. *Ann. Rheum. Dis.* 51(7):885–888.

55. Schnabel, A., M. Reuter, and W.L. Gross. 1998. Intravenous pulse cyclophosphamide in the treatment of interstitial lung disease due to collagen vascular disease. *Arthritis Rheum.* 41(7):1215–1220.

56. Al-Janadi, M., C.D. Smith, and J. Karsh. 1989. Cyclophosphamide treatment for interstitial pulmonary fibrosis in polymyositis/dermatomyositis. *J. Rheum.* 16:1592–1596.

57. Tanaka, F., T. Origuchi, K. Migita, M. Tominaga, A. Kawakami, Y. Kawabe, and K. Eguchi. 2000. Successful combined therapy of cyclophosphamide and cyclosporine for acute exacerbated interstitial pneumonia associated with dermatomyositis. *Intern. Med.* 39(5):428–430.

58. Sinoway, P.A., C.L. Davidson, and J.P. Callen. Chlorambucil. 1993. An effective corticosteroid-sparing agent for patients with recalcitrant dermatomyositis. *Arthritis Rheum.* 36(3):319–324.

59. Faulds, D., K.L. Goa, and P. Benfield. Cyclosporin. 1992. A review of its pharmacodynamic and pharmacokinetic properties, and therapeutic use in immunoregulatory disorders. *Drugs* 45(6):953–1040.

60. Zabel, P., G. Leimenstoll, and W.L. Gross. 1984. Cyclosporin for acute dermatomyositis. *Lancet* 1(8372):343.

61. Heckmatt, J., N. Hasson, C. Saunders, N. Thompson, A.M. Peters, G. Cambridge, et al. 1989. Cyclosporin in juvenile dermatomyositis. *Lancet* 1(8646):1063–1066.

62. Zeller, V., P. Cohen, A.M. Prieur, and L. Guillevin. 1996. Cyclosporin a therapy in refractory juvenile dermatomyositis. Experience and longterm followup in 6 cases. *J. Rheumatol.* 23(8):1424–1427.

63. Grau, J.M., C. Herrero, J. Casademont, J. Fernandez-Sola, and A. Urbano-Marquez. Cyclosporine A as the first choice therapy for dermatomyositis. 1994. *J. Rheumatol.* 21(2):381–382.

64. Lueck, C.J., P. Trend, and M. Swash. 1991. Cyclosporin in the management of polymyositis and dermatomyositis. *J. Neurol. Neurosurg. Psychiatry* 54(11):1007–1008.

65. Mehregan, D.R. and W.P. Su. 1993. Cyclosporine treatment for dermatomyositis/polymyositis. *Cutis* 51(1):59–61.

66. Vencovsky, J., K. Jarosova, S. Machacek, J. Studynkova, J. Kafkova, J. Bartunkova, et al. 2000. Cyclosporine A versus methotrexate in the treatment of polymyositis and dermatomyositis. *Scand. J. Rheumatol.* 29(2):95–102.

67. Roifman, C.M., F.M. Schaffer, S.E. Wachsmuth, G. Murphy, and E.W. Gelfand. 1987. Reversal of chronic polymyositis following intravenous immune serum globulin therapy. *JAMA* 258(4):513–315.

68. Cherin, P., S. Herson, B. Wechsler, J.C. Piette, O. Bletry, A. Coutellier, et al. 1991. Efficacy of intravenous gammaglobulin therapy in chronic refractory polymyositis and dermatomyositis: an open study with 20 adult patients. *Am. J. Med.* 91(2):162–168.

69. Dalakas, M.C., I. Illa, J.M. Dambrosia, S.A. Soueidan, D.P. Stein, C. Otero, et al. 1993. A controlled trial of high-dose intravenous immune globulin infusions as treatment for dermatomyositis. *N. Engl. J. Med.* 329(27):1993–2000.

70. Boyd, A.S. and K.H. Neldner. 1994. Therapeutic options in dermatomyositis/polymyositis. *Int. J. Dermatol.* 33(4):240–250.

71. Dau, P.C. 1981. Plasmapheresis in idiopathic inflammatory myopathy. Experience with 35 patients. *Arch. Neurol.* 38(9):553–560.

72. Lok, C., S. Herson, J.C. Roujeau, et. al. 1989. Plasma exchange in dermatomyositis. A retrospective study of 21 cases. *Ann. Dermatol. Venereol.* 116:219–224.

73. Miller, F.W., S.F. Leitman, M.E. Cronin, J.E. Hicks, R.L. Leff, R. Wesley, et al. 1992. Controlled trial of plasma exchange and leukapheresis in polymyositis and dermatomyositis. *N. Engl. J. Med.* 326(21):1380–1384.

74. Engel, W.K., A.S. Lichter, and A.P. Galdi. 1981. Polymyositis: remarkable response to total body irradiation. *Lancet* 1(8221):658.

75. Kelly, J.J., H. Madoc-Jones, L.S. Adelman, P.L. Andres, and T.L. Munsat. 1988. Response to total body irradiation in dermatomyositis. *Muscle Nerve* 11(2):120–123.

76. Morgan, S.H., R.M. Bernstein, J. Coppen, K.E. Halnan, and G.R. Hughes. 1985. Total body irradiation and the course of polymyositis. *Arthritis Rheum.* 28(7):831–835.

77. Rosenberg, N.L. and S.P. Rangel. 1988. Adult polymyositis and dermatomyositis, in Inflammatory Diseases of Muscle. Mastalgia FL, editor. Blackwell Scientific Publications, Oxford, 87–106.

78. Mitsunaka, H., M. Tokuda, T. Hiraishi, H. Dobashi, and J. Takahara. 2000. Combined use of cyclosporine A and methotrexate in refractory polymyositis. *Scand. J. Rheumatol.* 29(3):192–194.

79. Villalba, L., J.E. Hicks, E.M. Adams, J.B. Sherman, M.F. Gourley, R.L. Leff, et al. 1998. Treatment of refractory myositis. A randomized crossover study of two new cytotoxic regimens. *Arthritis Rheum.* 41(3):392–399.

80. Woo, T.Y., J.P. Callen, J.J. Voorhees, D.R. Bickers, R. Hanno, and C. Hawkins. 1984. Cutaneous lesions of dermatomyositis are improved by hydroxychloroquine. *J. Am. Acad. Dermatol.* 10:592–600.

81. England, M.J., T. Perlmann, and Y. Veriava. 1986. Dermatomyositis in pregnancy. *J. Reprod. Med.* 31(7):633–636.

82. King, C.R. and S. Chow. 1985. Dermatomyositis and pregnancy. *Obstet. Gynecol.* 66(4): 589–592.

83. Gutierrez, G., R. Dagnino, and G. Mintz. 1984. Polymyositis/dermatomyositis and pregnancy. *Arthritis Rheum.* 27(3):291–294.

84. Ishii, N., H. Ono, T. Kawaguchi, and H. Nakajima. 1991. Dermatomyositis and pregnancy. Case report and review of the literature. *Dermatologica* 83(2):146–149.

85. Ramsey-Goldman, R. and E. Schilling. 1997. Immunosuppressive drug use during pregnancy. *Rheum. Dis. Clin. North Amer.* 23(1):149–168.

86. Barnes, B.E. 1976. Dermatomyositis and malignancy: a review of the literature. *Ann. Intern. Med.* 84:68–76.

87. Olsen, N. 1998. Polymyositis and malignancy, in Rheumatology. Klippel and Dieppe, editors. Mosby, London. 7.16.6–7.16.9.

88. Leff, R., F.W. Miller, J.E. Hicks, D.D. Fraser, and P.H. Plotz. 1993. The treatment of inclusion body myositis (IBM): a retrospective review and a randomized, prospective trial of immunosuppressive therapy. *Medicine* (Baltimore) 72(4):225–235.

89. Dalakas, M.C., B. Sonies, J. Dambrosia, E. Sekul, E. Cupler, and K. Sivakumar. 1997. Treatment of inclusion-body myositis with IVIg: a double-blind, placebo-controlled study. *Neurology* 48(3):712–716.

90. Walter, M.C., H. Lochmuller, M. Toepfer, B. Schlotter, P. Reilich, M. Schroder, et al. 2000. High-dose immunoglobulin therapy in sporadic inclusion body myositis: a double-blind, placebo-controlled study. *J. Neurol.* 247(1):22–28.

91. Spector, S.A., J.T. Lemmer, B.M. Koffman, T.A. Fleisher, I.M. Feuerstein, B.F. Hurley, and M.C. Dalakas. 1997. Safety and efficacy of strength training in patients with sporadic inclusion body myositis. *Muscle Nerve* 20(10):1242–1248.

92. Cassidy, J.T. and R.E. Petty. 1995. Juvenile dermatomyositis, in Textbook of Pediatric Rheumatology. J.T. Cassidy and R.E. Petty, editors. W.B. Saunders Company, Philadelphia. 323–364.

93. Lang, B.A., R.M. Laxer, G. Murphy, E.D. Silverman, and C.M. Roifman. 1991. Treatment of dermatomyositis with intravenous gammaglobulin. *Am. J. Med.* 91(2):169–172.

27 Psoriatic Arthritis

Dimitrios T. Boumpas and Gabor G. Illei

INTRODUCTION

An inflammatory arthritis involving both the axial and the peripheral skeleton develops in some 5–25% of patients with psoriasis. The disease is heterogeneous with features of the spondyloarthropathies predominating in some patients while resembling rheumatoid arthritis (RA) in other patients *(1)*. Psoriatic arthritis provides an ideal disease model to investigate the bioactivities of potentially therapeutic biologic agents at multiple sites of tissue inflammation that are easily accessible for clinical and pathological assessment.

PATHOGENESIS

The etiology of both psoriasis and psoriatic arthritis are not known. Genetic, environmental, and immunologic factors appear to influence the susceptibility to disease and its expression *(1)*. The pattern of inheritance is suggestive of a polygenic influence with ubiquitous genetic and environmental factors contributing to phenotype diversity. Formal twins studies have not been undertaken in patients with psoriatic arthritis, and thus the relative importance of genetic and environmental factors is not known. Family studies suggest an approx 50-fold increased risk of psoriatic arthritis in first-degree relatives of patients with the disease. An important role for class I human leukocyte antigens (HLA) in the pathogenesis of psoriatic arthritis is supported by data derived from the HLA-B27 transgenic rat model where psoriasiform skin and nail lesions have been observed *(2)*. Of interest, these lesions develop in animals grown in germ-free

From: *Modern Therapeutics in Rheumatic Diseases*
Edited by: G. C. Tsokos, et al. © Humana Press, Inc., Totowa, NJ

environments in whom gut or joint involvement does not occur. Psoriasis and psoriatic arthritis are associated with certain HLA alleles, mainly with class I antigens. Thus, HLA class I antigens B13, B16 (B38/B39), B17 and Cw6 have been related to psoriasis with or without arthritis *(1)*. Trauma, infection, drugs, and certain biologic agents may result in psoriasis—probably through different mechanisms—suggesting that this phenotype may be the final pathway of a number of triggers.

The histopathologic changes in the skin and the synovium are remarkably similar with activation and expansion of tissue-specific cell subsets (keratinocytes and synoviocytes), accumulation of inflammatory cells (T cells, B cells, macrophages, and neutrophils), and angiogenesis. Recent studies using magnetic resonance imaging (MRI) have highlighted the importance of enthesitis as a key feature of the disease *(3)*. T cells play an important pathogenic role in the skin and joint manifestations of psoriatic arthritis as evidenced by findings of T-cell activation with skewing of T-cell receptors (TCR) receptor repertoire and commensurate with an ongoing T-helper 1 (Th1) phenotype; induction of psoriatic skin lesions in uninvolved skin transferred onto severe combined immunodeficiency (SCID) mice after injection of autologous blood-derived immunocytes from patients with psoriasis; development of psoriasiform skin lesions in SCID mice reconstituted with minor HLA mismatched naïve CD4+ T cells; and improvement of psoriasis following T-cell directed therapies such as cyclosporine, interleukin-2 (IL-2) fusion toxins, and the inhibitor of T-cell costimulation CTLA4Ig *(4–8)*. In addition to CD4 T-cells, an important role for CD8 T cells is favored by the association of the disease with class I MHC antigens and the observed association of HIV-1 infection with an explosive onset of psoriasis and psoriatic arthritis *(9)*.

The cytokine network in the psoriatic skin and synovium is dominated by the monocyte-derived cytokines tumor necrosis factor-α TNF-α), IL-1α, IL-1β, IL-6, IL-15, and IL-10. Compared to rheumatoid synovium, the TNF-α: IL-10 ratio in psoriatic arthritis patients is elevated suggesting that a relative deficiency IL-10 may play a significant role in psoriatic arthritis *(10)*. Cytokines such as IL-15 may play an important role in the pathogenesis of psoriatic skin lesions by inhibiting keratinocyte apoptosis and promoting keratinocyte accumulation *(11)*. Evidence for endothelial-cell activation and enhanced adhesion-molecule expression coupled with increased metalloproteinase and pro-angiogenic activity (the latter mediated through vascular endothelial growth factor [VEGF], basic fibroblast growth factor [bFGF], and αVβ3 integrin expression) has also been reported in both cutaneous and synovial lesions *(12–14)*.

TREATMENT

Therapy for psoriatic arthritis has largely been based in clinical experience in RA and psoriasis, without corroborating evidence from studies in patients with psoriatic arthritis.

Skin Disease

The initial treatment for stable plaque psoriasis is topical. However, topical therapy may be impractical for patients with extensive psoriasis (more than 20% involvement) and systemic therapy may be indicated at the onset *(15)*. Topical treatment includes emollients and keratolytic agents alone or in combination with anthralin, corticosteroids, vitamin D derivatives such as calcipotriene, and topical retinoids. Patients with extensive skin disease may benefit from photochemotherapy (PUVA therapy) (psoralen followed 2 h later with ultraviolet A [UVA] radiation) *(15)*.

Joint Disease

The general principles of managing patients with RA and the spondyloarthropathies also apply to patients with psoriatic arthritis *(1)*. For patients whose response to nonsteroidal anti-inflammatory drugs (NSAIDs) is inadequate and patients with progressive, erosive, polyarticular disease or patients with oligoarticular disease involving large joints that does not respond to local corticosteroid injections, disease-modifying drugs (DMARDs) should be initiated as early as possible. Methotrexate (MTX) is effective for both the skin disease and peripheral arthritis in patients with oligo- or polyarticular disease *(16)*. In general, dosage and monitoring are the same as for patients with RA. Sulfasalazine (2–3 g/d) is helpful for peripheral arthritis *(17,18)* but not for axial disease *(19)*. PUVA therapy is effective for both skin and joint disease, but only in nonspondylitic disease *(20)*, and may be especially helpful for patients with extensive skin involvement. Antimalarials, gold, azathioprine, cyclosporine, mycophenolate mofetil, leflunomide, etretinate, and calcitriol may also be effective based on small, open-label, uncontrolled trials *(1)*. Azathioprine, cyclosporine, mycophenolate mofetil, leflunomide, etretinate, and calcitriol are likely to improve both skin and joint disease *(1,21)*. Etretinate should probably be avoided in patients with axial disease because spinal ligamentous calcification is associated with long-term use. Corticosteroids can be used safely in low doses, either in combination with DMARDs or as bridge therapy while waiting for onset of action of DMARDs. Reports of generalized pustular psoriasis upon tapering of corticosteroids used in high doses for the treatment of psoriasis—albeit rare—dictate caution, especially in patients with extensive skin disease.

In patients with aggressive, destructive disease who have an inadequate response to single-agent combination therapy (i.e., MTX with sulfasalasine, cyclosporine, or leflunomide) may be considered *(22)*. However, these modalities are not uniformly effective and toxicity is a limiting factor. Studies evaluating the role of biologic therapies are in progress and will be reviewed next.

CYTOKINE-TARGETED THERAPIES

Neutralization of TNF-α

TNF-α induces inflammatory effects by acting directly on multiple target tissues and indirectly by inducing other proinflammatory cytokines such as IL-1, IL-6, and IL-8. TNF-α potentiates lymphocyte activation and facilitates their recruitment to sites of inflammation by inducing expression of adhesion molecules, chemokines, and angiogenesis. TNF-α neutralization has been achieved in humans using monoclonal antibodies (MAbs) or genetically engineered sTNFR. Etanercept, a genetically engineered TNFR, has demonstrated efficacy in the treatment of RA *(23)*. Because TNF-α is elevated in joints and the skin of psoriatic arthritis patients *(10)*, etanercept was evaluated in a randomized double-blind, placebo-controlled, 12-wk study *(24)*. In this study, etanercept (25 mg twice-weekly subcutaneous injections) or placebo were administered in 60 patients with psoriatic arthritis (median baseline tender joint count ≥19; median swollen joint count ≥14; psoriasis activity and severity index [PASI] ≥6.0).

Eighty-seven (87%) of etanercept-treated patients met response criteria for psoriatic arthritis compared to 23% of placebo-treated patients ($p < 0.001$). The ACR20 and ACR50 response criteria for RA were achieved by 73% and 50% of the etanercept-treated patients compared to 13% and 3%, respectively, in the placebo-treated patients ($p < 0.001$). Of the 38 patients who where evaluable for psoriasis (involvement of equal or more than 3% of body surface), 26% of etanercept-treated patients achieved a 75% improvement in the PASI, compared to 0% in the placebo treated patients ($p = 0.015$). Etanercept was well-tolerated with no patient developing infections requiring hospitalization of intravenous antibodies.

ANTI-INFLAMMATORY CYTOKINES

Interleukin 10

Studies in animals with genetic deletion of the *IL-10* gene have demonstrated the essential role of IL-10 in preventing exaggerated Th1 inflammatory responses to a variety of stimuli *(25)*. IL-10 suppresses Th1 cytokines such as TNF-α and IL-12 modulates monocyte and endothelial-cell activation, and inhibits metalloproteinase and angiogenic activity *(25–31)*. Clinical phase I/II studies in normal volunteers and patients with Crohn's disease suggest that recombinant IL-10 may downregulate inflammatory responses ex vivo and decrease disease activity *(32–34)*. A phase I/II placebo-controlled study in 29 patients with polyarticular psoriatic arthritis receiving daily IL-10 subcutaneously for 28 d showed improvement in the skin disease (>30% improvement in PASI score) in 75% of patients receiving 10 µg/kg/d of IL-10 vs 10% in the placebo group *(35)*. No clinically significant changes were observed in joint-disease activity; however, the study was not adequately powered to address efficacy. "Type 1" but not "type 2" T-cell cytokine production in vitro was suppressed in IL-10 compared with placebo recipients. Monokine production was reduced after treatment, whereas serum sTNFR levels were elevated, indicating suppression of monocyte function. T-cell and macrophage infiltration and P-selectin expression in synovial tissues were decreased. Of interest, angiogenesis was modulated as indicated by suppressed synovial enhancement on MRI and reduced αvβ3 integrin expression on vWF+ vessels. IL-10 was well-tolerated with only minor adverse effects. Longer duration of treatment or combination therapy with other agents such as MTX may enhance its therapeutic effects.

Interleukin 11

In addition to its thrombocytopoietic effects, IL-11, a multifunctional cytokine, has been shown to have also inflammatory and musculoskeletal protective effects. IL-11 reduces proinflammatory cytokine production by upregulating the expression of the inhibitor of NF-κB, IκB and inhibits type 1 T-cell responses *(36,37)*. Treatment with rhIL-11 reduces disease activity in animal models of inflammatory diseases *(38,39)*. Phase I/II studies are in progress in patients with active Crohn's disease, psoriasis, and RA with early results suggesting a potential benefit for patients with Crohn's disease and psoriasis *(40,41)*. In a phase I, open-label, dose-escalation clinical trial in 12 patients with psoriasis, 7 of 12 patients responded to rhIL-11 treatment. Amelioration of disease was associated with decreased expression of products of disease-related genes such as

K16, iNOS (nitric oxide synthase), interferon-γ (IFN-γ), IL-12, TNF-α, IL-1β, and CD8, and with increased expression of endogenous IL-11.

INHIBITION OF T-CELL COSTIMULATION

CTLA4Ig

The soluble chimeric protein CTLA4Ig inhibits costimulatory signals essential for T-cell activation and has been shown to ameliorate disease activity in a variety of animal models of autoimmunity *(42–43)*. Forty-three patients with psoriasis vulgaris received four infusions of CTLA4Ig. Almost 50% (46%) of the patients achieved a 50% or greater sustained improvement (especially those in the highest doses). Improvement was associated with reduction in skin-infiltrating T cells, altered antibody responses to T-cell-dependent neoantigens but no evidence of induction of T-cell tolerance to these antigens *(8)*.

CURRENT RECOMMENDATIONS

Modern therapy for psoriatic arthritis is at a state of evolution. The marked heterogeneity of the disease and the low prevalence of the disease (approx 10-fold lower than in RA) have hampered thus far efforts to conduct large, controlled clinical trials and most available modalities are derived from clinical experience in RA. Results from anti-TNF therapy are certainly exciting and represent a major breakthrough in the treatment of moderate to severe psoriatic arthritis. In addition to its significant effects in RA, early experience from anti-TNF therapy suggests that may also be of benefit in spondyloarthropathies such as the ankylosing spondylitis *(44)*, a feature especially attractive for a disease in which axial involvement is common and notoriously difficult to treat. Early data from other biologic therapies (IL-10, IL-11, CTLA4Ig) suggest that these agents are probably not likely to be of substantial clinical value when used alone, but they hold promise in combination protocols with conventional agents such as MTX. Agents targeting other pathways such as NF-κB, IL-15, and angiogenesis inhibitors such as anti-αvβ3 *(45)* are in the early stages of clinical evaluation. For the time being and until questions about the long-term efficacy and toxicity of biologic therapies have been resolved, these agents should probably be reserved for patients with severe disease, refractory to combination treatment with conventional DMARDS.

REFERENCES

1. Boumpas, D.T., G.G. Illei, and I.O. Tassiulas. Psoriatic arthritis, in Primer on the Rheumatic diseases, 12th edition, J.H. Klippel, C.W. Weyand, L.J. Crofford, J.H. Stone, editors. Arthritis Foundation, Atlanta, in press.

2. Hammer, R.E., S.D. Maika, J.A. Richardson, J.P. Tang, and J.D. Taurog. 1990. Spontaneous inflammatory disease in transgenic rats expressing HLA-B27 and human β2m: an animal model of HLA-B27-associated human disorders. *Cell* 63:1099–1112.

3. McGonagle, D., P.G. Conaghan, and P. Emery. 1999. Psoriatic arthritis: a unified concept twenty years on. *Arthritis Rheum.* 6:1080–1086.

4. Tassiulas, I., S. Duncan, M. Centola, A. Theofilopoulos, and D.T. Boumpas. 1999. Clonal characteristics of T cell infiltrates in skin and synovium of patients with psoriatic arthritis. *Human Immunol.* 60:479–491.

5. Wrone-Smith, T. and B.J. Nickoloff. 1997: Dermal injection of immunocytes induces psoriasis. *J. Clin. Invest.* 98:1878–1987

6. Schon, M.P., M. Detmar, and C.M. Parker. 1997. Murine psoriasis-like disorder induced by naïve CD4+ T cells. *Nature* (Medicine) 3:183–188.

7. Gottlieb, S.L., P. Gilleaudeau, R. Johnson, L. Estes, T.G. Woodworth, A.B. Gottlieb, and J.G. Kreuger. 1995. Response of psoriasis to a lymphocyte selective toxin (DAB389 IL-2) suggests a primary immune but not keratinocyte, pathogenic basis. *Nature* (Medicine) 1:442–447.

8. Abrams, J.R., M.G. Lebwohl, C.A. Guzzo, B.V. Jegasothy, M.T. Goldfarb, B.S. Goffe, et al. 1999. CTLA4Ig-mediated blockade of T-cell costimulation in patients with psoriasis vulgaris. *J. Clin. Invest.* 103:1243–1252.

9. Calabrese, L.H. 1933. Human immunodeficiency virus (HIV) infection and arthritis. *Rheum. Dis. Clin. North Am.* 19:477–488.

10. Danning, C.L., G.G. Illei, C. Hitchon, M.R. Greer, D.T. Boumpas, and I.B. McInnes. 2000. Macrophage-derived cytokine and nuclear factor κB p65 expression in synovial membrane and skin of patients with psoriatic arthritis. *Arthritis Rheum.* 43:1244–1256.

11. Ruckert, R., K. Asadullah, M. Seifert, V.M. Budagian, R. Arnold, C. Trombotto, et al. 2000. Inhibition of keratinocyte apoptosis by IL-15: a new parameter in the pathogenesis of psoriasis, *J. Immunol.* 165:2240–2250.

12. Detmar, M., L.F. Brown, K.P. Claffey, K.T. Yeo, O. Kocher, R.W. Jackson, et al. 1994. Overexpression of vascular permeability factor/vascular endothelial growth factor and its receptors in psoriasis. *J. Exp. Med.* 180:1141–1146.

13. Danning, C.L., G.G. Illei, E. Lee, D.T. Boumpas, and I.B. McInnes. 1988. αvβ3 integrin expression in psoriatic arthritis (PsA) synovial membrane. *Arthritis Rheum.* 41: S333.

14. Hitchon, C.A., C.L. Danning. G.G. Illei, J. Lee, H.S. El-Gabalawy, and D.T. Boumpas. 1999. Matrix metaloproteinase expression and activity in psoriatic arthritis skin and synovium. *Arthritis Rheum.* 42: S235

15. Greaves, M.W. and G.D. Weinstein. 1995. Treatment of psoriasis. *N. Engl. J. Med.* 332:581–588.

16. Espinoza, L.R., L.Z. Oui, and C.G. Espinoza. 1992. Psoriatic arthritis: clinical response and side effects to methotrexate. *J. Rheumatol.* 16:872–877.

17. Dougados, M., S. vam der Linden, M. Leirisalo-Repo, B. Huitfeldt, R. Juhlin, E. Veys, et al. 1995. Sulfasalazine in the treatment of spondyloarthropathy. A randomized, multicenter, double-blind, placebo-controlled study. *Arthritis Rheum.* 38:618–627.

18. Clegg, D.O., D.J. Reda, E. Mejias, G.W. Cannon, M.H. Weisman, T. Taylor, et al. 1996. Comparison of sulfasalazine and placebo in the treatment of psoriatic arthritis. A Department of Veterans Affairs Cooperative Study. *Arthritis Rheum.* 39:2013–2020.

19. Clegg, D.O., D.J. Reda, and M. Abdellatif. 1999. Comparison of sulfasalazine and placebo for the treatment of axial and peripheral articular manifestations of the seronegative spondylarthropathies: a Department of Veterans Affairs cooperative study. *Arthritis Rheum.* 42:2325–2329.

20. Perlman, S.G., L. Gerber, M. Roberts, T.P. Nigra, and W.F. Barth. 1979. Photochemotherapy and psoriatic arthritis. A prospective study. *Ann. Intern. Med.* 91:717–722.

21. Grundmann-Kollmann, M., F. Ochsendorf, T.M. Zollner, K. Spieth, R. Kaufmann, and M. Podda. 2000. Treatment of chronic plaque-stage psoriasis and psoriatic arthritis with mycophenolate mofetil. *J. Am. Acad. Dermatol.* 142:835–837.

22. Pioro, M.H. and J.M. Cash. 1995. Treatment of refractory psoriatic arthritis. *Rheum. Dis. Clin. North Am.* 21:129–149.

23. Illei, G.G. and P.E. Lipsky. 2000. Novel antigen non-specific approaches to autoimmune/inflammatory diseases. *Curr. Opin. Immunol.* 12:712–718.

24. Mease, P.J., B.S. Goffe, J. Metz, A. Vander-Stoep, B. Finck, and D.J. Burge. 2000. Randomized trial of etanercept (Enbrel) in the treatment of psoriatic arthritis and psoriasis. *Lancet* 356:385–390.

25. Kuhn, R., J. Lohler, D. Rennick, K. Rajewsky, and W. Muller. 1993. Interleukin-10-deficient mice develop chronic enterocolitis. *Cell* 75(2): 263–274.

26. de Waal Malefyt, R., J. Abrams, B. Bennett, C.G. Figdor, and J.E. de Vries. 1991. Interleukin 10 (IL-10) inhibits cytokine synthesis by human monocytes: an autoregulatory role of IL-10 produced by monocytes. *J. Exp. Med.* 174:1209–1220.

27. Groux, H., A. O'Garra, M. Bigler, M. Rouleau, S. Antonenko, J.E. deVries, and M.G. Roncarolo. 1997. A CD4+ T-cell subset inhibits antigen-specific T-cell responses and prevents colitis. *Nature* 389: 737–742.

28. Vora, M., H. Yssel, de J.E. Vries, and M.A. Karasek. 1994. Antigen presentation by human dermal microvascular endothelial cells. Immunoregulatory effect of IFN-gamma and IL-10. *J. Immunol.* 152:5734–5741.

29. Reitamo, S., A. Remitz, K. Tamai, and J. Uitto. 1994. Interleukin-10 modulates type I collagen and matrix metalloprotease gene expression in cultured human skin fibroblasts. *J. Clin. Invest.* 94:2489–2492.

30. Lacraz, S., L.P. Nicod, R. Chicheportiche, H.G. Welgus, and J.M. Dayer. 1995. IL-10 inhibits metalloproteinase and stimulates TIMP-1 production in human mononuclear phagocytes. *J. Clin. Invest.* 96:2304–2310.

31. Walmsley, M., P.D. Katsikis, E. Abney, S. Parry, R.O. Williams, R.N. Maini, and M. Feldmann. 1996. Interleukin-10 inhibition of the progression of established collagen- induced arthritis. *Arthritis Rheum.* 39:495–503.

32. Chernoff, A.E., E.V. Granowitz, L. Shapiro, E. Vannier, G. Lonnemann, J.B. Angel, et al. 1995. A randomized, controlled trial of IL-10 in humans. Inhibition of inflammatory cytokine production and immune responses. *J. Immunol.* 154:5492–5499.

33. Asadullah, K., W. Sterry, K. Stephanek, D. Sasulaitis, M. Leopold, H. Audring, et al. 1998. IL-10 is a key cytokine in psoriasis. Proof of principle by IL-10 therapy: a new therapeutic approach. *J. Clin. Invest.* 101:783–794.

34. Van Deventer, S.D.J., C.O. Elson, and R.N. Fedorak. 1997. Multiple doses of intravenous Interleukin 10 in steroid-refractory Crohn's disease. *Gastroenterology* 113:383–389.

35. McInnes, I.B., G.G. Illei, C.L. Danning, C.H. Yarboro, M. Crane, T. Kuroiwa et al. 1999. Interleukin-10 improves skin disease and modulates endothelial activation and leukocyte effector function in patients with psoriatic arthritis. *J. Immunol.*, in press.

36. Leng, S.X. and J.A. Elias. 1997. Interleukin-11 inhibits macrophage interleukin-12 production. *J. Immunol.* 159:2161–2168.

37. Trepicchio, W.L., L. Wang, M. Bozza, and A.J. Dorner. 1997. IL-11 regulates macrophage effector function through inhibition of nuclear factor-κB. *J. Immunol.* 159:5661–5670.

38. Peterson, R., L. Wang, L. Albert, J.C. Keith, and A.J. Dorner. 1998. Molecular effects of rhIL-11 in the HLA-B27 rat model of inflammatory bowel disease. *Lab. Invest.* 78:1503–1512.

39. Redlich, C.A., X. Gao, S. Rockwell, M. Kelley, and J.A. Elias. 1996. IL-11 enhances survival and decraeses TNF production after radiation-induced thoracic injury. *J. Immunol.* 157:1705–1710.

40. Sands, B.E., S. Bank, C.A. Sninsky, M. Robinson, S. Katz, J.W. Singleton, et al. 1999. Preliminary evaluation of safety and activity of rhIL-11 in patients with active Crohn's disease. *Gastroenterology* 117: 58–64.

41. Trepiccio, W.L., M. Ozawa, I.B. Walters, T. Kikuchi, P. Gilleaudeau, J.L. Bliss, et al. 1999. Interleukin-11 therapy selectively downregulates type I cytokine proinflammatory pathways in psoriasis lesions. *J. Clin. Invest.* 104:1527–1537.

42. Reiser, H. and M.D. Stadecker. 1996. Costimulatory B7 molecules in the pathogenesis of infectious and autoimmune diseases. *N. Engl. J. Med.* 335:1369–1377.

43. Webb, L.M.C., M.J. Walmsley, and M. Feldmann. 1996. Prevention and amelioration of collagen-induced arthritis by blockade of the CD28 co-stimulatory pathway: requirement for both B7-1 and B7-2. *Eur. J. Immunol.* 26:2320–2328.

44. Brandt, J., H. Haibel, D. Cornely, W. Golder, J. Gonzalez, J. Reddig, et al. Succeful treatment of active ankylosing spondylitis with the anti-TNFα monoclonal antibody infliximab. *Arthritis Rheum.* 43:1346–1352

45. Storgard, C.M., D.G. Stupack, A. Jonczyk, S.L. Goodman, R.I. Fox, and D.A. Cheresh. 1999. Decreased angiogenesis and arthritic disease in rabbits treated with an αvβ3 antagonist. *J. Clin. Invest.* 103:47–54.

28

Complement Inhibitors in Rheumatic Diseases

Sherry D. Fleming and George C. Tsokos

CONTENTS

INTRODUCTION

The complement system is composed of over 30 serum and cellular proteins in three distinct pathways and is important in the proinflammatory response to injury and pathogens. The complement pathways converge in the membrane attack complex (MAC), the terminal effector of the system. Because this cascade of proteins results in cell lysis and tissue destruction, the complement system includes multiple regulatory proteins that prevent nonspecific complement activation. Some of these regulatory proteins are cellular receptors for the breakdown products of the components of the system. The understanding of natural regulatory proteins and receptors and their involvement in rheumatic diseases has allowed the design and development of therapeutic interventions that inhibit complement activation and prevent inflammatory tissue damage.

In this chapter we will discuss the role of complement inhibitors, both natural and recombinant-engineered molecules, in rheumatic diseases. We will briefly review the complement system including the regulatory molecules that control complement activation, and the available information of complement-activation inhibitors used in animal models of tissue injury. Finally, we will discuss human trials, in which complement-activation inhibitors have been used, along with future directions.

COMPLEMENT ACTIVATION

Classical Pathway

The classical complement pathway and the subsequent MAC formation constitute the basis of the complement system (reviewed in ref. *1, see* Fig. 1). This pathway begins

From: *Modern Therapeutics in Rheumatic Diseases*
Edited by: G. C. Tsokos, et al. © Humana Press, Inc., Totowa, NJ

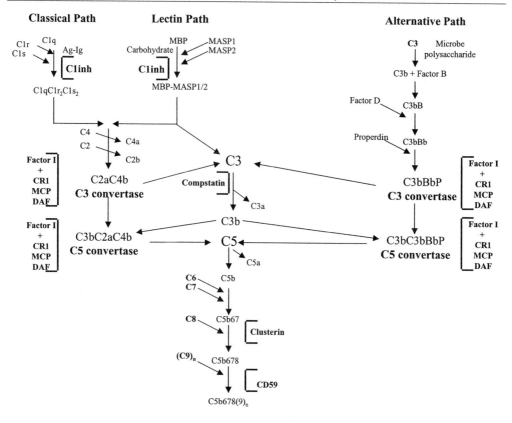

Fig. 1. Overview of the complement system and its inhibitors. The three initiation pathways, classical, lectin, and alternative, converge with C3 cleavage and then again with the cleavage of C5. The formation of C5b is the initiating molecule of the MAC complex. Inhibitors of specific complement components are in brackets ([]). The breakdown products, C4a, C3a, and C5a are potent anaphylotoxins. Adapted with permission from ref. *39*.

with C1q binding to an antigen-IgG or IgM complex through the Fc region, activation of 2 molecules, C1r and C1s, and the formation of the $C1qC1r_2C1s_2$ complex. This activated complex splits both C2 and C4 to form the C3 convertase, C2aC4b. The C3 convertase cleaves C3 generating C3b that binds C2aC4b and becomes C2aC4bC3b, the C5 convertase. This complex severs C5 generating C5b, the initiator of the MAC complex. In addition to generating convertases, the classical pathway produces byproducts, C4b, C5a, and C3a. These byproducts are also immunologically active as anaphylotoxins.

The MAC is the lytic component of the complement system. Unlike the other complement pathways that depend on enzymatic cleavage for activation, the MAC is an assembled complex of C5b, C6, C7, C8, and C9. These proteins can attach to cell membranes or form a soluble complex. When C5 convertase divides C5, C5b remains attached to the convertase on the cell surface. C6 and C7 then bind the complex inducing a conformational change such that the C5b-6-7 complex is released to the fluid phase. If this complex of proteins is not immediately degraded, it will quickly bind tightly to the cell surface without inserting into the membrane. C8 then binds and the complex is inserted into the membrane, causing the cell to leak. After insertion into the membrane, C9 is recruited and multiple C9 proteins polymerized, forming a large pore. This causes cellular lysis and tissue destruction.

Alternative Pathway

The complex polysaccharide moieties on bacterial and other surfaces activate the alternative complement pathway (reviewed in ref. *1*). In this pathway, C3 is activated and C3b is produced by low-level hydrolysis of an internal thioester bond. This spontaneous cleavage is termed "tickover." C3b is fixed on the pathogenic surface and is quickly complexed with Factor B. Factor D cleaves Factor B, forming the alternative pathway C3 convertase, C3bBb. The C3 convertase is stabilized by the addition of Properdin, forming C3bBbP. When this stable C3 convertase enzymatically cleaves additional C3 molecules, another C3b protein is added to the complex forming C3bC3bBbP, a C5 convertase that cleaves C5, producing C5b and initiating MAC formation.

Lectin Pathway

Although called the lectin pathway, only 1 lectin, mannose-binding protein (MBP), is involved (reviewed in ref. *2*). MBP binds to mannose, *N*-acetylglucosamine, fucose, and glucose but not to galactose residues of carbohydrates on bacteria. The lectin pathway may play a role in rheumatoid arthritis (RA) owing to the ability of MBP to recognize the increased levels of exposed agalactosyl-IgG in these patients *(3)*. Complement is activated when MBP is complexed with MBP-associated serine proteases (MASP). Recently, 2 MASPs, MASP1, and MASP2, and a related protein, Map19 have been identified *(4)*. These proteins are enzymatically activated similar to the C1r and C1s proteins. Specifically, MASP2 is similar to C1s and MASP1 is similar to C1r whereas Map19 has unknown properties at this time *(4)*. The MBP/MASP activated complex can then cleave C4 and C2 creating the C3 convertase, C4b2a, and merging with the classical complement pathway.

NATURAL/BIOLOGICAL INHIBITORS OF COMPLEMENT ACTIVATION

Complement is controlled by 10 or more inhibitory proteins found either in the serum or on cell membranes (reviewed in ref. *5*). A deficiency in some of these inhibitory molecules causes increased susceptibility to immune complexes that are found frequently in patients with rheumatic diseases. Without complement inhibitors to prevent continued growth, the lattice of antibody/antigen complexes becomes extremely large and precipitate in organs. In addition, complement coating of the complexes aids phagocytosis of the complexes by binding to surface erythrocyte-complement receptors and trafficking to the liver and spleen.

Because of the similarities of the three pathways, many of the regulatory molecules can inhibit multiple pathways. In addition, because all pathways converge at the formation of the MAC, inhibitors downstream of C5, regulate all forms of complement activation. The primary function of these natural regulatory proteins is to control the C3 and C5 convertases by degrading C3b and C4b. The specific regulatory functions of some of the natural inhibitors are detailed below.

Complement Receptor 1

Complement receptor 1 (CR1; CD35) inhibits the both the C3 and C5 convertases of both classical and alternative pathways. C3 cleavage results in C3b and C3f with C3b undergoing a conformational change that allows it to attach to the surface. With CR1 as a cofactor, factor I cleaves C3b, forming iC3b. The same two proteins can split iC3b, forming C3dg and C3c, all of which remain on the cell surface. To inactivate the classical pathway, CR1 binds to C3b, iC3b, and C4b on the surface of other cells only. In addition, CR1 also dissociates B and Bb from C3b in the alternative pathway convertases. In mice, complement receptor related protein y (Crry) has activities similar to CR1 in humans, inhibiting both C3 and C5 convertases.

Membrane Cofactor Protein

Membrane cofactor protein (MCP; CD46) serves as a cofactor for factor I cleavage of C3b and C4b, inhibiting C3 and C5 convertase. However, it has no activity in dissociating the convertase complexes. MCP is expressed on all cells except red blood cells and is active only on the same cell on which it is expressed. MCP is an alternatively spliced membrane protein with at least four different variants that cleave C4b to various degrees. Most cells express some of each splice variant although there are some differences in kidney. This differential expression within the kidney and the fact that diseased kidneys express high levels of MCP may be useful in designing therapeutic agents for glomerulonephritis.

C1 Inhibitor

C1 inhibitor (C1inh) is found in serum and inhibits both the classical and lectin pathways by covalently binding to soluble C1r and C1s. It does not prevent surface complement activation. However, because there is seven times as much C1inh in the serum as C1, it quickly deactivates the classical pathway. C1inh is also a serine protease inhibitor that prevents MASP activity in the lectin pathway *(4)*.

Decay Accelerating Factor

Decay accelerating factor (DAF; CD55) is a glycosyl-phosphotyidylinositol (GPI)-linked, recyclable protein that can inactivate C3 and C5 convertases of both classical and alternative pathways. Similar to MCP, DAF can only inactivate the complexes that are assembled on the same cell surface that it exists on reviewed in *(6)*; *(7,8)*. DAF has no cofactor activity for factor I. When removed from the cell surface by phosphotidylinositol-specific phosphatases, DAF can also be a soluble complement inhibitor *(9)*.

CD59

CD59 (protectin) is a GPI-linked membrane protein that incorporates into the MAC complex after C5b-8 insert✦ in the cell membrane and inhibits insertion and polymerization of C9. CD59 can be shed from the cell surface such that the soluble form retains its GPI anchor. This allows the protein to be recycled and inserted into the membrane of other cells.

Clusterin blocks MAC formation by preventing C5b-6-7 from binding to the membrane. After C5b-6-7 binds the membrane, clusterin can not inhibit the complex.

Clusterin is found in high concentration in most body fluids and is frequently found in immune complexes of nephritic kidney disease.

ANIMAL STUDIES

Rheumatic diseases are chronic and therefore, therapeutic agents must have different characteristics from those used in the treatment of acute disease. To be useful as drugs, complement regulatory molecules must have a long half-life and not provoke an immune response *(10)*. The most common approaches involve (1) the humanization of monoclonal antibodies (MAbs), (2) the fusion of a natural inhibitor with the Fc portion of IgG to prolong the half-life in the serum, and (3) the designing of chimeric molecules from natural inhibitors. These inhibitors can be planned to include molecules that inhibit complement activation at various points. For example, a chimeric DAF-CD59 inhibitor has been designed that can inhibit in vitro both the C3 convertase and the formation of MAC *(11)*. Also, multimeric membrane inhibitors have been designed, such as multimeric sCR1 *(12)*. However, the multimeric- and chimeric-inhibitor molecules have yet to be studied in animal models before proceeding on to human trials. Finally, a futuristic approach has been considered to design complement-activation inhibitors conjugated to molecules that will direct the inhibitor to an organ site where complement inhibition is desirable and avoid general inhibition of complement activation. For example, conjugation of a complement inhibitor to a cationic IgG will direct it to the kidneys and can be used more effectively in the treatment of glomerulonephritis. Below we discuss animal models of lupus, glomerulonephritis, and RA in which complement-inhibitory molecules have been studied.

Systemic Lupus Erythematosus (SLE)

Female NZB/NZW F_1 mice and MLR/*lpr* mice spontaneously develop lupus-like disease with autoantibody production (anti-DNA) and immune complex-mediated glomerulonephritis. The NZB/NZW F_1 mice primarily produce IgG antibody, develop vasculitis and glomerulonephritis, and die by the age of 12 mo. Wang et al. *(13)* showed that when 18-wk-old NZB/NZW F1 mice were given 1 mg of anti-C5 MAb, 2–3 times/wk for up to 22 wk, the onset of disease was delayed. In addition, the MAb markedly decreased the severity of glomerulonephritis and prolonged survival of the NZB/NZW F1 mice.

Recently, the MRL/lpr mouse was crossed to Factor B deficient mice *(14)*. The MRL/*lpr* B-/- mice did not develop vasculitic skin lesions, had less proteinuria, and had minimal renal pathology. Interestingly, although these mice had similar levels of anti-DNA Ab in their serum, compared to the MRL/*lpr* B+/+ or B+/– mice, they had less serum IgG3 and higher levels of serum C3. These findings suggest that factor B is important in the development of vasculitis and renal disease caused by C3 consumption. Therefore the alternative pathway, and specifically factor B, plays a significant role in the development of lupus-related pathology.

Another approach to prevent lupus-related symptoms is to increase the levels of natural complement inhibitors. In both mice and humans, CR1 has been considered to have a role in preventing immune complex deposition *(15,16)*. Takahashi et al. found that B cells from MRL/*lpr* mice have decreased CR1 expression by 7 wk of age, whereas the onset of lupus symptoms (high levels of autoantibodies and nephritis) did not occur until 12–15 wk of age *(16)*. Taken together, these data demonstrate that complement factors of both alternative and classical pathways modulate autoimmune inflammatory tissue damage and suggest that inhibition of both pathways may have therapeutic benefit. The aforementioned data suggest that therapeutic strategies in the treatment of lupus may include the decrease of either factor B or MAC formation or the increase of CR1.

Autoimmune Glomerulonephritis (GN)

It has been known for many years that complement activation plays a role in the development of GN *(17)*. The availability of genetically manipulated mice has provided the tools to study the role of individual complement components in the process. Study of C1q-deficient mice *(18)* revealed that C1q is important in preventing complement induced damage to the kidney and increased polymorphonuclear (PMN) infiltration, whereas the study of C5 deficient mice has underscored the role of C5 in the development glomerular lesions or inflammatory infiltrates *(19)*. Depletion of clusterin, a natural inhibitor of C5b-9, leads to significantly more glomerular injury in the Heymann nephritis rat model *(20)*. Therefore, in various animal models, inhibition of early complement components or of MAC formation prevents renal damage.

Soluble Crry is the rodent analog of sCR1 and inhibits both classical and alternative pathways. Quigg et al. *(21)* showed that sCrry protects against glomerular injury induced by a nephrotoxic antibody. The protection was seen as a decrease in albuminuria and PMN infiltration without inhibiting the binding of the IgG to the glomeruli. In a rat model of glomerulonephritis, Quigg's group also found that Crry is the critical component in the renal tubular preparation, which is injected to induce nephritis *(22)*. The rat produces antibody to Crry leading to inactivation of the C3 and C5 convertase regulator. This prompts uncontrolled complement activation and C3 deposition in the glomeruli. Thus in rodents, Crry plays a key role in preventing complement-induced injury and suggests that CR1 and/or CR2 may play an equivalent role in humans.

Rheumatoid Arthritis

Complement has been found to play a role in various RA rodent models. Injection of cobra venom factor (CVF; stabilizes the C3 convertase and depletes the animal of C3 for 2–3 d), delays arthritis in a collagen-induced rat arthritis model until the complement system was functional again, that is, 3 d later *(23)*. However, in a different arthritis model (injection of anti-CD59) others found that systemic complement depletion did not improve arthritis and that local depletion was important *(24)*. Specifically, they found that rats receiving sCR1 or C5a receptor antagonist 30 min prior to intra-articular injection of anti-CD59 had as much joint swelling as control animals. In contrast, if sCR1 was intra-articularly injected simultaneously with anti-CD59, the joint-swelling index and inflammation were significantly lower. Both groups have shown that sCR1 given prior to disease onset delayed or prevented the onset of the disease. Intra-articular injection of CD59 (inhibition of MAC complex) in inflamed joints failed to reverse the process *(25)*.

An anti-C5 MAb has been developed that inhibits the cleavage of C5 *(10)*. This prevents the formation of C5b-9 and the generation of the anaphylotoxin C5a. Using a mouse collagen-induced arthritis (CIA) model, Wang et al. *(26)* showed that anti-C5

MAb could not only prevent disease but prevented established disease from spreading to additional joints *(26)*. In addition, anti-C5 MAb treatment decreased the inflammatory response, as indicated by decreased swelling and PMN infiltration *(26)*. In the same model, this group recently found that only 3 of 30 C5-deficient mice developed joint inflammation as compared with 100% of littermate controls *(27)*. In addition, these mice had normal cellular and humoral immune responses. Thus manipulation of complement activation may prove useful in the treatment of arthritis and these studies suggest that arthritis therapeutics should focus on inhibition of MAC formation.

HUMAN STUDIES

Complement is involved in the development of tissue pathology in most of human rheumatic diseases. For example, patients with RA and ankylosing spondylitis have increased soluble MAC complexes in the synovial joints compared with patients with other forms of joint disease *(28,29)*. These studies also showed that both the classical and alternative complement paths are activated. In addition, patients with RA have IgG immune complexes that have terminal *N*-acetyl glucosamine residues that can bind MBP, indicating that the lectin pathway may also be activated *(4)*.

Patients with C1q, C4, and C2 deficiencies develop lupus frequently, suggesting a role of the early complement factors in the establishment and maintenance of tolerance, in which the clearance of immune complexes may play an important role *(30,31)*. On the other hand, immune-complex formation is abundant in lupus patients and the activation of complement pervasive. Immune complexes deposit and cause disease in multiple tissues including the kidneys and the central nervous system (CNS) *(32)*. Activation of complement leads to depletion of complement factors such as C3 and C4 and their low levels represent a measure of active lupus nephritis *(33)*. It is intuitive to develop complement inhibitors that prevent complement-mediated damage without affecting the immune complex clearing function of complement.

As yet, there are very few human studies using complement inhibitors and those that are being performed are in phase I or II trials. Nevertheless, the few phase I trials will be reviewed. Jain et al. *(34)* used a humanized anti-C5 MAb in a phase I study of RA patients and found that the antibody was safe, active for 7–10 d, improved clinical symptoms, and caused significant decrease in C-reactive protein (CRP) levels. This study used the whole antibody, which was engineered to have the mouse binding sites on the framework of a human antibody. A similar antibody, anti-C5-scFv has also been used successfully in phase I trials to prevent complement activation in patients undergoing cardiopulmonary bypass *(35)*. The anti-C5 scFv is a single chain (heavy and light chain) of the humanized Ab used above *(10)*. Recently, Compstatin, a synthethic peptide, has been described that binds to C3 and inhibits both C3a release and MAC formation *(36,37)*. In vitro and ex vivo animal models have shown that Compstatin maybe a useful complement inhibitor for transplantation and cardiopulmonary bypass-related pathology *(36,38)*. The use of peptides in complement inhibition has a number of distinct advantages: they are very specific, small, defined by complement components, and therefore an antibody response is not expected, and may be delivered orally. Ongoing trials in patients with lupus nephritis may reveal their usefulness in complement inhibition in the treatment of lupus nephritis, arthritis, and, it is hoped, other rheumatic diseases.

FUTURE DIRECTIONS

That complement activation is part of the pathogenic process in rheumatic diseases has been known for a long time. The complement-activation processes involves three initiation channels and a common terminal pathway that is responsible for the infliction of cell and organ injury. Complement activation occurs in a precise cascade manner and involves a number naturally occurring inhibitors that safeguard the outright consumption of the complement system. Animal models of arthritis, lupus, and glomerulonephritis have clearly shown, as discussed earlier, that inhibition of complement activation can delay, improve, or reverse the disease pathology. There are a number of important questions that need to be addressed in each human disease in order to choose the most the logical complement inhibitor for therapeutic use. First, to what extent is complement central in disease pathology? Second, which pathway is primarily involved? Third, is general complement inhibition associated with side effects such as suppression of the innate immunity and the appearance of overwhelming infections?

There has been a logical design of complement inhibitors for therapeutic use in human disease. First, MAbs that eliminate or block the activation of complement factors can be humanized by molecular engineering and used in the treatment of disease. As discussed earlier, an anti-C5 antibody is in human trials. Second, natural complement-activation inhibitors such as DAF, CD59, and CR1 can be genetically fused to Fc portion of IgG to prolong half-life. Third, complement inhibitors that act at different stages of the activation cascade can be genetically, recombinately engineered or chemically fused. Such compounds have the potential to act at different phases and bring about more specific and more effective complement inhibition. Fourth, recently, the design of peptide inhibitors that block the interaction of two complement factors or the cleavage of a factor by a protease/activator, such as convertase, at a precise point has emerged as a new promising approach. Compstatin, which was developed by the Lambris lab (36–38), represents such an example because it inhibits complement activation by blocking C3 convertase-mediated cleavage of C3. Fifth, and last, in response to the consideration that the use of complement inhibitors may cause systematic inhibition and unwanted side effects—from the complete lack of complement, such as overwhelming infection—investigators have considered the fusion of complement inhibitors to molecules that will direct it to the site of inflammation. Besides the example of cationic IgG that was discussed earlier, complement inhibitors can be conjugated to selectin ligands that will direct them to sites of increased selectin expression, i.e., inflammation or delivered via targeted liposomes to a specific location where the inhibitor is released in a concentrated region.

REFERENCES

1. Holers, V.M. 2000. Complement, in Current Molecular Medicine: Principles of Molecular Rheumatology. G. C. Tsokos, editor. Humana Press, Totowa, NJ, pp. 1–269.

2. Matsushita, M. 1996. The lectin pathway of the complement system. *Microbiol. Immunol.* 40:887–893.

3. Malhotra, R., M.R. Wormald, P.M. Rudd, P.B. Fischer, R.A. Dwek, and R.B. Sim. 1995. Glycosylation changes of IgG associated with rheumatoid arthritis can activate complement via the mannose-binding protein. *Nature Medicine* 1:237–243.

4. Wong, N.K.H., M. Kojima, J. Dobo, G. Ambrus, and R.B. Sim. 1999. Activities of the MBL-associated serine proteases (MASPs) and their regulation by natural inhibitors. *Mol. Immunol.* 36:853–861.

5. Morgan, B.P. 1994. Clinical complementology: recent progress and future trends. *Eur. J. Clin. Invest.* 24:219–228.

6. Makrides, S.C. 1998. Therapeutic inhibition of the complement system. *Pharmacol. Rev.* 50: 59–87.

7. Medof, M.E., T. Kinoshita, and V. Nussenzweig. 1984. Inhibition of complement activation on the surface of cells after incorporation of decay-accelerating factor (DAF) into their membranes. *J. Exp. Med.* 160:1558–1578.

8. Kinoshita, T., M.E. Medof, and V. Nussenzweig. 1986. Endogenous association of decay-accelerating factor (DAF) with C4b and C3b on cell membranes. *J. Immunol.* 136:3390–3395.

9. Christiansen, D., J. Milland, B.R. Thorley, I.F. McKenzie, and B.E. Loveland. 1996. A functional analysis of recombinant soluble CD46 in vivo and a comparison with recombinant soluble forms of CD55 and CD35 in vitro. *Eur. J. Immunol.* 26:578–585.

10. Thomas, T.C., S.A. Rollins, R.P. Rother, M.A. Giannoni, S.L. Hartman, E.A. Elliott, et al. 1996. Inhibition of complement activity by humanized anti-C5 antibody and single-chain Fv. *Mol. Immunol.* 33: 1389–1401.

11. Fodor, W.L., S.A. Rollins, E.R. Guilmette, E. Setter, and S.P. Squinto. 1995. A novel bifunctional chimeric complement inhibitor that regulates C3 convertase and formation of the membrane attack complex. *J. Immunol.* 155:4135–4138.

12. Oudin, S., M.T. Libyh, D. Goossens, X. Dervillez, F. Philbert, B. Reveil, et al. 2000. A soluble recombinant multimeric anti-Rh(D) single-chain Fv/CR1 molecule restores the immune complex binding ability of CR1-deficient erythrocytes. *J. Immunol.* 164:1505–1513.

13. Wang, Y., Q. Hu, J.A. Madri, S.A. Rollins, A. Chodera, and L.A. Matis. 1996. Amelioration of lupus-like autoimmune disease in NZB/W F_1 mice after treatment with a blocking monoclonal antibody specific for complement component C5. *Proc. Natl. Acad. Sci. USA* 93:8563–8568.

14. Watanabe, H., G. Garnier, A. Circolo, R.A. Wetsel, P. Ruiz, V.M. Holers, et al. 2000. Modulation of renal disease in MRL/lpr mice genetically deficient in the alternative complement pathway factor B. *J. Immunol.* 164:786–794.

15. Birmingham, D.J. 1999. Type one complement receptor and human SLE, in Lupus: Molecular and Cellular Pathogenesis. G. M. Kammer and G. C. Tsokos, editors. Humana Press, Totowa, NJ, pp. 541–556.

16. Takahashi, K., Y. Kozono, T.J. Waldschmidt, D. Berthiaume, R.J. Quigg, A. Baron, and V.M. Holers. 1997. Mouse complement receptors type 1 (CR1;CD35) and type 2 (CR2; CD21). Expression on normal B cell subpopulations and decreased levels during development of autoimmunity in MRL/lpr mice. *J. Immunol.* 159:1557–1569.

17. Unanue, E. and F.J. Dixon. 1964. Experiemental glomerulonephritis. IV. Participation of complement in nephrotoxic nephritis. *J. Exp. Med.* 119:965–982.

18. Mitchell, D.A., P.R. Taylor, H.T. Cook, J. Moss, A. Bygrave, M.J. Walport, and M. Botto. 1999. C1q protects against the development of glomerulonephritis independently of C3 activation. *J. Immunol.* 162: 5676–5679.

19. Falk, R.J. and J.C. Jennette. 1986. Immune complex induced glomerular lesions in C5 sufficient and deficient mice. *Kidney Int.* 30:678–686.

20. Saunders, J.R., a. Aminian, J.L. McRae, K.A. O'Farrell, W.R. Adam, and B.F. Murphy. (1994) Clusterin depletion enhances immune glomerular injury in the isolated perfused kidney. *Kidney Int.* 45: 817–827.

21. Quigg, R.J., C. He, A. Lim, D. Berthiaume, J.J. Alexander, D. Kraus, and V.M. Holers. 1998. Transgenic mice overexpressing the complement inhibitor Crry as a soluble protein are protected from antibody-induced glomerular injury. *J. Exp. Med.* 188:1321–1331.

22. Schiller, B., C. He, D.J. Salant, A. Lim, J.J. Alexander, and R.J. Quigg. 1998. Inhibition of complement regulation is key to the pathogenesis of active heymann nephritis. *J. Exp. Med.* 188:1353–1358.

23. Goodfellow, R.M., A.S. Williams, J.L. Levin, B.D. Williams, and B.P. Morgan. 2000. Soluble complement receptor one (sCR1) inhibits the development and progression of rat collagen-induced arthritis. *Clin. Exp. Immunol.* 119:210–216.

24. Mizuno, M., K. Nishikawa, B.P. Morgan, and S. Matsuo. 2000. Comparison of the suppressive effects of soluble CR1 and C5a receptor antagonist in acute arthritis induced in rats by blocking of CD59. *Clin. Exp. Immunol.* 119:368–375.

25. Morgan, B.P. 1999. Regulation of the complement membrane attack pathway. *Crit. Rev. Immunol.* 19: 173–198.

26. Wang, Y., S.A. Rollins, J.A. Madri, and L.A. Matis. 1995. Anti-C5 monoclonal antibody therapy prevents collagen-induced arthritis and ameliorates established disease. *Proc. Natl. Acad. Sci. USA* 92:8955–8959.

27. Wang, Y., J. Kristan, L. Hao, C.S. Lenkoski, Y. Shen, and L.A. Matis. 2000. A role for complement in antibody-mediated inflammation: C5-deficient DBA/1 mice are resistant to collagen-induced arthritis. *J. Immunol.* 164:4340–4347.

28. Brodeur, J.P., S. Ruddy, L.B. Schwartz, and G. Moxley. 1991. Synovial fluid levels of complement SC5b-9 and fragment Bb are elevated in patients with rheumatoid arthritis. *Arthritis Rheum.* 34:1531–1537.

29. Rumfeld, W.R., B.P. Morgan, and A.K. Campbell. 1986. The ninth complement component in rheumatoid arthritis, Behcet's disease and other rheumatic diseases. *Br. J. Rheumat.* 25:266–270.

30. Atkinson, J.P. and J.A. Schifferli. 1999. Complement system and systemic lupus erythematosus. *In* Lupus: Molecular and Cellular Pathogenesis. G. M. Kammer and G. C. Tsokos, editors. Humana Press, Totowa, NJ. 529–540.

31. Navratil, J.S., L.C. Korb, and J.M. Ahearn. 1999. Systemic lupus erythematosus and complement deficiency: clues to a novel role for the classical complement pahtway in the maintenance of immune tolerance. *Immunopharmacology* 42:47–52.

32. Wener, M.H. 1999. Immune complexes and autoantibodies to C1q, in Lupus: Molecular and Cellular Pathogenesis. G. M. Kammer and G. C. Tsokos, editors. Humana Press, Totowa, NJ, pp. 574–598.

33. Pillemer, S.R., H.A. Austin, G.C. Tsokos, and J.E. Balow. 1988. Lupus nephritis: association between serology and renal biopsy measures. *J. Rheumatol.* 15:284–288.

34. Jain, R.I., L.W. Moreland, J.R. Caldwell, S.A. Rollins, and C.F. Mojcik. 1999. A single dose, placebo controlled, double blind phase I study of the humanized anti-C5 antibody h5G1.1 in patients with rheumatoid arthritis. *Arthritis Rheum.* 42:S77.

35. Fitch, J.C.K., S. Rollins, L. Matis, B. Alford, S. Aranki, C.D. Collard, et al. 1999. Pharmacology and biological efficacy of a recombinant, humanized, single-chain antibody C5 complement inhibitor in patients undergoing coronary artery bygass graft surgery with cardiopulmonary bypass. *Circulation* 100:2499–2506.

36. Nilsson, B., R. Larsson, J. Hong, G. Elgue, K.N. Ekdahl, A. Sahu, and J.D. Lambris. 1998. Compstatin inhibits complement and cellular activation in whole blood in two models of extracorporeal circulation. *Blood* 92:1661–1667.

37. Morikis, D., N. Assa-Munt, A. Sahu, and J.D. Lambris. 1998. Solution structure of Compstatin, a potent complement inhibitor. *Protein Sci.* 7:619–627.

38. Fiane, A.E., T.E. Mollens, V. Videm, T. Hovig, K. Hogasen, O.J. Mellbye, et al. 1999. Compstatin, a peptide inhibitor of C3, prolongs survival of ex vivo perfused pig xenografts. *Xenotransplantation* 6:52–65.

39. Makrides, S.C. 2000. Complement inhibitors, in Current Molecular Medicine: Principles of Molecular Rheumatology. G.C. Tsokos, editor. Humana Press, Totowa, NJ, pp. 465–476.

29 Hematopoietic Stem Cell Transplantation of Autoimmune Disease

Richard K. Burt and Ann E. Traynor

CONTENTS

INTRODUCTION

An autoimmune etiology is proven if adoptive transfer of lymphocytes or antibody that recognizes a self-epitope(s) causes disease *(1)*. However, adoptive transfer of disease has been infrequently demonstrated for suspected autoimmune disorders. An exception is Idiopathic Thrombocytopenic Purpura (ITP). In 1951, an American physician (William Harrington) injected plasma containing antibodies to platelets from a patient with ITP into himself, resulting in transient thrombocytopenia *(2)*. Again, in the 1950s, an Italian physician (Marmont) injected 300–500cc of plasma from patients with lupus nephritis into normal volunteers *(3)*. These patients developed circulating Lupus Erythematosus (LE) cells, but no other manifestations of lupus, although repeated injections were not administered. Rarely, a patient undergoing transplant for a malignant disease has developed an autoimmune disease from the infused donor cells. Type I diabetes mellitus was transferred from a donor to a human leukocyte antigen (HLA)-matched sibling recipient by bone marrow transplantation *(4)*. Other evidence for an autoimmune pathogenesis is detection of auto-reactive antibodies and/or lymphocytes. However, the self-epitope towards which the autoimmune response is directed is usually unknown, and whether antibodies such as rheumatoid arthritis (RA)-associated rheumatoid factor (RF) or scleroderma-associated SCL-70 are disease causing or epiphenomena remains unclear.

From: *Modern Therapeutics in Rheumatic Diseases*
Edited by: G. C. Tsokos, et al. © Humana Press, Inc., Totowa, NJ

Indirect evidence for an autoimmune pathogenesis is response to immune suppressive medications. For a severe autoimmune disease that fails standard treatment, dose intensification of immune suppression has been suggested as a new therapy. Depending on the immune-suppressive regimen, hematopoietic stem cells may have to be infused to prevent prolonged or permanent marrow aplasia. Three clinical options are available: (1) intense immune suppression without hematopoietic stem cell support, (2) intense immune suppression with autologous hematopoietic stem cell support, or (3) allogeneic hematopoietic stem cell transplantation. Intense immune-suppressive regimens with or without stem cell reinfusion may, even if not curative, help clarify the pathogenesis of a disease assumed to be autoimmune.

PATHOGENIC MECHANISMS THAT RATIONALIZE THE USE OF THE NEW TREATMENT

To rationalize or justify this approach, one must first understand how an autoimmune disease arises. This question is best investigated via animal models of autoimmunity. There are two basic manners by which animals develop an autoimmune-like disease: (1) environmental exposure, i.e., immunization or infection, and (2) spontaneous onset without specific environmental triggers.

Experimental autoimmune encephalomyelitis (EAE) is an animal model of multiple sclerosis (MS) *(5)*. EAE is an inflammatory demyelinating disease confined to the central nervous system (CNS). EAE does not occur spontaneously but may be induced in virtually any mammal (mice, rats, guinea pigs, monkeys, humans) by immunization with myelin protein. Therefore, lymphocytes with myelin-reactive repertoires circulate in the periphery but are anergic or tolerant to self. Two of the most common proteins in myelin are proteolipid protein (PLP) and myelin basic protein (MBP). Injection of either of these proteins (or immunogenic peptide fragments from these proteins) does not cause disease unless accompanied by an adjuvant. An adjuvant is an immune stimulant (e.g., Freund's adjuvant) that causes upregulation of costimulatory and adhesion molecules on antigen-presenting cells (APCs). Presentation of myelin peptides simultaneous with costimulatory molecules is required to break peripheral tolerance, resulting in immune-mediated myelin injury. Therefore, self peptides or epitopes when presented in a proinflammatory environment may trigger an autoimmune disease.

Theiler's murine encephalomyelitis virus (TMEV)-induced demyelinating disease is a viral-induced disease that is clinically and histologically similar to MS *(6)*. TMEV is a picornavirus (small RNA virus) whose natural route of infection is oral ingestion. The immune system determines susceptibility to disease *(7,8)*. Resistant strains of mice clear virus within 2 wk of infection and do not develop a demyelinating sequela. In susceptible strains, infection is never cleared and the initial gray-matter infection progresses to a chronic demyelinating white-matter disease *(9)*. With transition from a neuronal gray-matter to a demyelinating white-matter disease (approx 40 d after infection), lymphocytes begin to proliferate to myelin epitopes. This immune responsiveness to myelin epitopes occurs in the same ordered temporal manner as seen in EAE *(10)*. How does a viral infection initiate a chronic autoimmune demyelinating disease? Two hypothesis are: (1) epitope mimicry and (2) viral adjuvant. Similarity or mimicry between viral and self (myelin) proteins could result in immune-mediated attack initiated against TMEV subsequently being directed against myelin. Alternatively, attempts to clear virus may result in activation of macrophages causing phagocytosis and representation of myelin peptides with costimulatory molecules leading to breakdown in self-tolerance. In this scenario, the virus acts as a local immune adjuvant similar to Freund's adjuvant in EAE.

In both EAE- and TMEV-induced immune-mediated demyelination, peripheral tolerance is broken by a defined environmental exposure. In contrast, some autoimmune diseases occur spontaneous of any environmental event and appear to be preordained by inherited genetic loci. Mouse models of spontaneous lupus-like diseases are examples of preordained stem cell defects. The Murthy Roth laboratory lymphoproliferative (MRL/lpr) mouse develops a spontaneous lymphoproliferative disorder accompanied by lupus-like manifestations, including nephritis and anti-double DNA stranded (anti-ds DNA) antibody *(11)*. MRL/lpr mice have a genetic defect in apoptosis owing to deficient Fas-protein expression, allowing outgrowth of autoreactive clones *(12)*. New Zealand Black/New Zealand White (NZB/NZW) mice are another spontaneous-onset mouse model of lupus. In NZB/NZW mice, lupus like phenomena appear to be inherited through multiple genetic loci, which result in hyper-reactivity to environmental stimuli *(13)*.

Unlike highly inbred strains of mice, the genetic and/or environmental dependence of human autoimmune diseases is poorly understood. If a disease is due to environmentally induced loss of self-tolerance, then attempted immune ablative high-dose chemotherapy with autologous stem cell support may induce long-term remissions. If the disease is genetically predetermined, then an allogeneic transplant using stem cells from a normal person may be required to cure disease.

REVIEW OF ANIMAL DATA

The outcome of hematopoietic stem cell transplantation in animal models of MS (EAE and TMEV) and lupus (MRL/lpr, NZB/NZW) are informative for anticipating outcome and design of human trials.

Experimental Autoimmune Encephalomyelitis (EAE)

The natural course of EAE in Swiss Jackson Lab/Jackson (SJL/J) mice is relapsing and remitting. Events initiating remission and relapse are incompletely understood. However, immune ablation with total-body irradiation followed by syngeneic hematopoietic stem cell transplantation (to prevent lethal marrow failure) induces durable remission of disease *(14,15)*.

One of the most potent disease-causing myelin peptides is segment 139-151 of proteolipid protein (PLP 139-151). Lymphocytes from a normal or nonimmunized SJL/J mouse do not react (i.e., proliferate) to myelin peptides such as PLP 139-151. Lymphocytes from mice with EAE have a strong proliferative response when exposed to PLP 139-151. Because attempts at immune ablation and hematopoietic stem cell transplantation from syngeneic normal donors induces disease remission, it was assumed that the post-transplant immune system would be similar to the donor, i.e., unresponsive to PLP 139-151. However, despite clinical remission, the post-transplant immune system remained responsive to PLP 139-151, similar to mice with EAE *(15)*.

Transplant failed to induce anergy (i.e., unresponsiveness) to myelin epitopes despite clinical remission. Therefore, clinical disease activity does not necessarily correlate with reactivity (i.e., proliferation) to myelin epitopes. This may be explained by three possibilites: (1) post-transplant lymphocytes may proliferate to myelin but have impaired effector function, (2) post-transplant lymphocytes may proliferate to myelin but instead of causing disease may have a regulatory function that inhibits disease, or (3) post-transplant disease causing lymphocytes may be unable to traffic into the CNS.

Little data exists concerning dissociation of proliferative from effector function, although alterations in adhesion or homing molecules (such as integrins or selectins) could prevent reactive lymphocytes from infiltrating into their target organ (CNS) (16). In EAE, data exists for cells with a suppressor phenotype. The clinical course suggests auto-regulation. In SJL/J mice, EAE has a cyclic nature and undergoes spontaneous remission. In some animals such as the Lewis rat, the disease is monophasic. Following remission, Lewis rats are resistant to reinduction of disease (17).

T-helper cells (Th) that transfer disease are obtained by ex vivo culture of draining lymph nodes from actively immunized animals with myelin peptide(s). In the Lewis rat, suppressor cells (Ts) may be selected (instead of disease causing Th cells) by addition of cyclosporine A to the ex vivo culture conditions (18). If myelin specific Th cells are admixed with myelin specific Ts cells, adoptive transfer of disease is prevented. These suppressor cells are autoantigen (i.e., myelin)-specific (18).

Besides regulator cells directed against the autoantigen, disease inhibiting cells may develop against disease causing Th cells (19). Culturing T cells from spleens of post-EAE Lewis rats with an irradiated EAE disease causing Th cell line in the absence of myelin antigens will generate Ts cells (19). These Ts cells are cytotoxic to T-cell receptor (TCR) idiotype repertoires unique to EAE causing Th cells.

Knockout and transgenic mice also provide evidence for suppressor cells that regulate EAE in vivo (20). Transgenic mice expressing a rearranged TCR for MBP may develop spontaneous EAE, but in a germ-free environment the occurrence is low (21). In contrast, 100% of MBP TCR transgenic mice with coexistent recombinase-activating gene (RAG) disruption develop EAE (22). Immunoglobulins as well as TCRs are generated by recombination of variable (V), diversity (D), and joining (J) DNA genes. RAG genes are required for V(D)J recombination and are essential for lymphocyte development. MBP TCR transgenic mice generally do not develop EAE unless the immune system is unable to develop new repertoires (RAG knockout). This implies that the immune system is capable of generating suppressor or regulator lymphocytes that inhibit MBP-specific, disease-causing T cells (23).

Several clinical lessons may be learned from hematopoietic stem cell transplantation of EAE. An environmentally induced but noninfectious autoimmune disease may enter durable remission after intense immunosuppression and syngeneic hematopoietic stem cell support. However, the post-transplant immune system is fundamentally altered compared to a normal animal. Mechanisms of post-transplant remission are unknown. Further work is needed in EAE to determine if regulatory cells contribute to post-transplant remission. If regulatory cells are involved, every disease causing cell may not have to be eliminated, and the toxicity of intense conditioning regimens could be avoided. In clinical trials most investigators have focused on maximal lymphocyte depletion of the autologous hematopoietic stem cell graft. Intensive purging of lymphocytes from the autologous stem cell graft could alter post-transplant regulatory cell frequency *(24)*.

TMEV-Induced Demyelinating Disease

TMEV is a small RNA virus causing a demyelinating disease confined to the CNS that clinically and histologically mimics primary progressive MS *(6,25,26)*. TMEV is cidal to neurons in culture. In vivo, the response to infection varies by murine strain. In some strains, infection is cleared within 2 wk without permanent sequela. In immune-compromised mice, infection results in high mortality from uncontrolled viral replication *(27)*. In immune-competent but susceptible strains, the initial gray-matter infection is substituted by an immune-mediated chronic demyelination of white-matter *(6)*.

SJL/J mice are susceptible to TMEV-induced demyelination. Syngeneic transplantation of SJL/J mice with marrow from a normal donor results in early mortality from viral hyperinfection of the CNS *(28)*. In contrast, allogeneic transplantation from a resistant strain that was previously immunized with TMEV is capable of curing TMEV-induced disease in SJL/J mice *(28)*. The TMEV-induced demyelination model would predict that if an infectious agent initiates an autoimmune disease, hematopoietic stem cell transplantation may be lethal unless accompanied by adoptive immunotherapy directed towards the infectious agent. This would apply only if the infectious agent is still present at the time of transplant.

MRL/lpr and NZB/NZW Mice

MRL/lpr and NZB/NZW mice develop a lupus-like autoimmune disease without a known specific environmental trigger. As mentioned earlier, for MRL/lpr mice, a defective *Fas* gene prevents appropriate apoptosis of autoreactive lymphocytes *(12)*. For NZB/NZW mice, multiple alleles increase the probability of disease but none is absolutely essential for disease onset *(29–34)*. Multiple systemic lupus erythematosis (SLE) prone alleles have been discovered such as *Sle1* on chromosome 1 *(32)*, *Sle2* on chromosome 4 *(33)*, *Sle3* on chromosome 7 *(30)*, and the MHC complex. The *Sle* loci appear to be involved in T- and/or B-cell antigen hyper-reactivity *(29–34)*.

Lupus-prone mice have been cured by an allogeneic transplant from a nondisease susceptible strain *(35,36)*. In contrast, MRL/lpr mice had initial improvement, but then relapsed after an autologous transplant *(37)*. The clinical implication of these lupus-like diseases is that some autoimmune diseases may be genetically preordained. An autologous transplant would be anticipated to only cause transient improvement and an allogeneic transplant would be required for cure.

REVIEW OF CLINICAL TRIALS

Compared to autologous transplantation, allogeneic stem cell transplants are associated with an increased morbidity and mortality owing predominately to graft-vs-host disease (GVHD). Consequently, clinical trials of hematopoietic stem cell transplantation for autoimmune diseases have focused on reinfusion of autologous stem cells. Early published data suggests that different autoimmune diseases appear to behave differently to hematopoietic stem cell transplantation. As a rule, those autoimmune diseases that generally respond best to standard immune-suppressive therapy also seem to have the best response to dose-intense immune suppression and autologous HSCT.

To comprehend the following discussion, one must understand the stages or phases of clinical trials. A phase I trial is a small pilot study designed to monitor toxicity, although data is collected on efficacy to determine if a phase II trial is appropriate. A phase II trial is designed with larger number of patients to evaluate efficacy, although a well-designed phase II trial will also attempt to determine mechanism(s) of action. A phase III trial is a prospective randomized and often blinded study to determine if the treatment is better than currently accepted standard care. New treatment concepts such as hematopoietic transplantation of autoimmune diseases begin as phase I trials.

Systemic Lupus Erythematosus (SLE)

The clinical presentation of lupus is heterogeneous *(38,49)*. A patient need only meet 4 of 11 criteria (either simultaneously or sequentially) to have a diagnosis of SLE *(40)*. The criteria for SLE are malar rash, discoid rash, oral ulcers, arthritis, serositis, renal disease (proteinuria or cellular casts), neurologic disease (seizures or psychosis), hematologic disease (autoimmune hemolytic anemia, leukopenia, lymphopenia, thrombocytopenia), positive anti-nuclear antibodies (ANA), or immunologic disorder (LE cells, anti-double-stranded DNA, anti-Sm, false-positive syphilis VDRL test). The protean clinical presentation and disease course associated with SLE are manifestations of systemic T- and B-cell immune hyper-reactivity.

As a rule of thumb, the mortality from SLE is 1%/yr *(41–51)*. The worst prognostic indicator is persistently active disease, especially involvement of visceral organs such as nephritis, pneumonitis, or cerebritis. A subset of patients have persistently active SLE despite immune-suppressive therapy including corticosteroids and monthly pulse cyclophosphamide (500–1000 mg/m^2). For patients with visceral involvement who fail pulse cyclophosphamide and cortiosteroids, intense immune suppression with or without autologous hematopoietic stem cell support is an option.

Anecdotal case reports of patients with SLE who underwent hematopoietic stem cell transplantation for another indication (malignancy or aplastic anemia) suggest that durable remissions may be obtained by either autologous or allogeneic hematopoietic stem cell transplants (Table 1) *(52–56)*. Five cases have been reported in the literature (4 autologous, 1 allogeneic). One patient had a clinical relapse 1 yr after transplant *(56)*. One patient developed ITP 3 yr post-transplant, although the criteria for SLE were not met *(55)*. Three patients have maintained clinical remission for 30 mo, 34 mo, and 15 yr, respectively *(52–54)*.

Five patients with no other indication except SLE have undergone autologous transplantation (Table 2) *(57–61)*. Unlike transplant for patients with a hematologic disease and coincidental SLE, the autograft was partially purged of lymphocytes prior to infusion. Purging was performed based on the unproven assumption that potential disease causing lymphocytes should be removed before the graft is infused. To date, the longest follow-up is between 3–4 yr and patients remain without clinical evidence of disease. Serologic remissions are also common although an intermittent and sometimes transiently positive ANA may recur.

SLE is responsive to cyclophosphamide. Both oral and intravenous (iv) pulse cyclophosphamide are standard therapies for SLE. Most SLE transplant regimens are,

Table 1
Hematopoietic Stem Cell Transplantation in Patients with a Malignancy or Aplastic Anemia and Coincidental SLE

Type of transplant /ref.	Number of patients/indication for transplant	SLE manifestations	Outcome of transplant on SLE
Autologous PBSC (unmanipulated) (52)	1/Hodgkin's lymphoma	Serositis, polyarthritis, mucocutaneous features, nephrotic syndrome, ANA, anti-ds DNA	Complete clinical and serolgic remission of SLE at last follow-up (34 mo)
Allogeneic BMT (unmanipulated) (53)	1/Aplastic anemia	Malar rash, discoid lesions, photosensitivity, oral ulcers, arthritis ANA, anti-ds DNA, anti-Sm, anti-RNP, hypocomplementemia	Complete clinical remission for more than 15 yr. Serologic remission except for low ANA titer (1:80)
Autologous BMT (unmanipulated) (54)	1/CML	Photosensitivity, arthralgia, serositis, ANA, nephrotic syndrome, ulcers, hypocomplementemia	Complete clinical and serologic remission at last follow-up (30 mo)
Autologous BMT (unmanipulated) (55)	1/High-grade non-Hodgkin's lymphoma	Discoid lesions, arthralgias, AIHA, ANA, anti-ds DNA, anti-RNP	Complete clinical and serologic remission for 3 yr, then new-onset ITP
Autologous PBSC (unmanipulated) (56)	1/High-grade non-Hodgkin's lymphoma	Arthralgias, discoid rash, malar rash, photosensitivity, oral ulcers, cytopenias, ANA, anti-ds DNA	Clinical remission but relapse at d 352 post-transplant, never obtained serologic remission

Table 2
Clinical Trials of Autologous Hematopoietic Stem Cell Transplant for SLE

Author/City/ref.	Type of transplant	Number of patients/conditioning	Results
Marmont/ Genova, Italy (61)	Autologous lymphocyte-depleted marrow	1/Thiotepa/cyclophosphamide	Clinical remission for over 3 yr
Burt/Chicago, IL (59,60)	Autologous lymphocyte-depleted PBSC	2/Cyclophosphamide/ antithymocyte globulin/ corticosteroids	Clinical remission for over 3 yr
Fouilland/Paris, France (57)	Autologous lymphocyte-depleted PBSC	1/BEAM (carmustine, etoposide, cytosine arabinoside, melphalan)	Clinical remission for 1 yr
Musso/Palmero, Italy (58)	Autologous lymphocyte-depleted PBSC	1/cyclophosphamide/antithymocyte globulin/corticosteroids	At 8 mo post-transplant low ANA titer and low coombs-positive, but anti-ds DNA-negative and anti-cardiolipin antibody-negative

therefore, based on dose intensification of cyclophosphamide, given by itself or in combination with other agents. Cardiac dysfunction is the dose-limiting toxicity of cyclophosphamide and occurs at doses over 240 mg/kg. For this reason, transplant doses of cyclophosphamide do not exceed 200 mg/kg. This dose of cyclophosphamide is not myeloablative and if other myelosuppressive agents are not included in the conditioning regimen, neutropenia will recover around 15 d after transplant *(62)*. If stem cells are infused, neutrophil recovery occurs by d 10. Selection of patients may be important in determining whether stem cells should be infused. Previously untreated patients are more likely to tolerate prolonged neutropenia. Heavily pretreated and immune-suppressed candidates on high doses of corticosteroids, however, are at a high risk of opportunistic infection during the neutropenic interval and stem cell support may be indicated to decrease neutropenic duration and risk of infectious complications.

Current data suggests that SLE is highly responsive to dose-intense, immune-suppression and autologous hematopoietic stem cell support with clinical and drug-free remissions exceeding 3 yr *(57–61)*. The superiority of one conditioning regimen over another has not yet been established, although one of the least toxic regimens (high-dose cyclophosphamide and anti-thymocyte globulin) has demonstrated remissions similar to more intense multi-agent conditioning regimens. Therefore, phase II/III trials using cyclophosphamide, anti-thymocyte globulin, and lymphocyte-depleted autologous stem cell support are currently being planned.

Rheumatoid Arthritis (RA)

RA is an inflammatory disease that primarily affects the joint synovial membrane *(63)*. RA is a common disease affecting approx 1% of the North American population *(64)*. Patients with a large number of involved joints or marked limitations in daily activities have a 5-yr mortality of 20–70% *(65–70)*. In high-risk patients who fail immune suppressive medications (e.g., corticosteroids, methotrexate [MTX], D-penicillamine, gold, hydroxychloroquine) and TNF inhibitors, hematopoietic stem cell transplantation may be considered.

Several patients undergoing allogeneic transplant for a hematologic disease and coincidental RA have been reported in the literature (Table 3) *(71–76)*. The most common indication for transplant was aplastic anemia arising as a complication of medical therapy (e.g., gold salts). A total of 8 patients with RA have undergone allogeneic transplant for aplastic anemia. As early as 1977, the outcome of allogeneic transplantation in four patients with RA and gold-induced marrow aplasia was reported. Three patients died early from transplant complications. The one surviving patient was without evidence of RA for 2 yr of follow-up. In other reports, two patients maintained clinical and serologic remissions for over 6 and 8 yr, respectively. In two patients RA recurred after 2 yr. One patient was determined by polymerase chain reaction (PCR) for variable number of tandem repeats (VNTR) to be a full chimera. Although the serologic (rheumatoid factor; RF) status of the donor was not reported, apparently 100% donor engraftment does not necessarily preclude recurrence of RA.

Patients with RA have been reported to have an increased risk of developing lymphomas possibly owing to medications or the disease itself *(77–84)*. Consequently, three patients underwent transplant for lymphoma who had coexistent RA. Because lymphomas are often treated by autologous HSCT, all patients had autologous transplants.

Table 3
Hematopoietic Stem Cell Transplantation in Patients with a Malignancy or Aplastic Anemia and Coincidental RA

Type of transplant /ref.	Number of patients/ indication for transplant	Outcome of transplant on RA
Autologous marrow (unmanipulated)(71)	1/Lymphoma	RA relapsed after 20 mo of sustained remission
Autologous marrow (unmanipulated)(72)	1/Lymphoma	RA and Sjogren's in complete remission at last follow-up (19 mo)
Autologous peripheral blood (unmanipulated) (56)	1/Lymphoma	Slight post-transplant improvement in RA, then flare-up 4 mo after transplant
Allogeneic marrow (unmanipulated) (76)	1/Aplastic anemia	RA relapse after 2 yr: VNTR revealed full donor chimerism
Allogeneic marrow (unmanipulated) (73)	4/Aplastic anemia	1 patient died 93 d after transplant from CMV-RF remained positive
		1 patient alive 2 yr after transplant without evidence of RA and RF-negative
		1 patient died d 75 after transplant from graft failure, no evidence of RA
		1 patient died d 58 after transplant from CMV, no evidence of RA
Allogeneic marrow (unmanipulated) (74)	2/Aplastic anemia	RA in complete remission for 6 and 8 yr, respectively
Allogeneic marrow (unmanipulated) (75)	1/Aplastic anemia	RA in complete remission for 2 yr, then clinical and serologic relapse

Table 4
Clinical Trials of Autologous and Syngeneic Hematopoietic Stem Cell Transplant for RA

Author/city/ref.	Number of patients/conditioning	Results
Burt/Chicago, IL (85)	4/200 mg/kg Cyclophosphamide/ATG/Methylprednisolone[a]	All patients improved, two relapsed
Joske/Nedlands, Western Australia (86)	1/200 mg/kg Cyclophosphamide	Improved from wheel-chair bound to ambulating
Snowden/Leeds, UK (87)	Cohort I: 4 patients, 100 mg/kg cyclophosphamide	Cohort I: transient response for 1–2 mo
	Cohort II: 4 patients, 200 mg/kg cyclophosphamide	Cohort II: substantial improvement for 17–19 mo
Durez/Brussels, Belgium (88)	1/Busulfan/cyclophosphamide	Medication-free complete remission for 10 mo of follow-up
McColl/Victoris, Australia (89)	1/cyclophosphamide/ATG (syngeneic)	Clinical remission for 24 mo

[a]One patient also received low-dose (400cGy) TBI.

One patient had only a partial improvement and disease flared by 4 mo after transplant. In the other two patients, autologous transplantation induced remission of RA for 19 and 20 mo, respectively, although again one patient relapsed.

Several centers have initiated phase I trials of autologous HSCT for RA (Table 4) *(85–89)*. In general, remissions occur rapidly, but a durable, complete remission is rare and relapse is common. The duration of improvement (ACR50 or ACR70) is unknown but may exceed 2 yr. Despite improvement, most patients do not become drug-free. Post-transplant disease is, however, easier to control with fewer medications. In a cyclophosphamide dose-escalation study the cohort receiving the lowest dose (100 mg/kg) all relapsed within a few months, whereas the cohort at the highest dose (200 mg/kg) had sustained improvements for 17–19 mo *(87)*. This implies a conditioning-regimen dose-response effect. Because almost all centers used nonmyeloablative cyclophosphamide or cyclophosphamide and anti-thymocyte conditioning regimens, the next advance to improve remission duration or attempt durable complete remission is autologous transplantation using a more intense myeloablative regimen. The current phase I studies were performed safely. However, phase I studies utilizing more intense conditioning regimens may be necessary before designing phase II/III trials.

Multiple Sclerosis (MS)

MS is an immune-mediated inflammatory demyelinating disease confined to the CNS *(90,91)*. It is a common disease, with a North American prevalence of 1 in 2000 *(92)*. The natural course is variable *(93,94)*. At onset, 15% are primary progressive and 85% are relapsing-remitting in which neurologic impairments are temporary. After 10 yr, 50% of relapsing-remitting patients have become secondary progressive, meaning that neurologic dysfunction is permanent and progressive. Mean time to a Kurtzke disability of 6.0 (cane, crutch, or brace required to walk 100) is 10 yr for both primary and secondary progressive disease *(95)*. Behavior of disease within the first 2 yr of onset correlates with 10-yr morbidity and mortality *(96)*. A retrospective analysis by Weinshenker et al. reported that the more frequent the relapses, the shorter the relapse interval, and the more rapid the accumulation of neurologic deficits within the first 2 yr of diagnosis, the higher the 10-yr morbidity *(96)*. For MS patients, survival correlates with functional disability. The more disabled the patient, the worse the mortality.

The results of hematopoietic transplantation in two patients with CML and coincidental MS have been reported (Table 5) *(97,98)*. Both patients received a chemotherapy only (busulfan/cyclophosphamide) regimen. Both underwent transplant safely. One received an autograft with a short post-transplant follow-up *(97)*. The other received an allograft with neurologic improvement and no clinical or magnetic resonance imaging (MRI) evidence of disease activity for 1 yr post-transplant *(98)*.

Three centers have reported on phase I studies of autologous HSCT for secondary and primary progressive MS (Table 6) *(99–101)*. The two European centers used BEAM (carmustine, etoposide, cytosine arabinoside, melphalan), a standard lymphoma-conditioning regimen *(100,101)*. The hallmark of lymphomas is clonality. Although MS is not a lymphoma, oligoclonality is present in both B and T cells. B-cell restriction is manifest by oligoclonal bands in cerebrospinal fluid (CSF) fluid. TCR repertoire skewing is present within plaques. Therefore, a proven and relatively safe lymphoma-transplant regimen is a reasonable consideration for patients with MS.

Table 5
Hematopoietic Stem Cell Transplantation in Patients with a Malignancy and Coincidental MS

Type of transplant/ref.	Number of patients/indication for transplant	Outcome of transplant on MS
Autologous marrow (unmanipulated) (97)	1/CML	Follow-up short, but no disease exacerbation or neurotoxicity from transplant. Post-transplant MRI without evidence of disease activity
Allogeneic marrow (unmanipulated) (98)	1/CML	Neurologically improved without disease exacerbation for the 12 mo of follow-up

Table 6
Clinical Trials of Autologous Hematopoietic Stem Cell Transplant for MS

Author/city/ref.	Number of patients/conditioning	Results
Fassas/Thessaloniki, Greece (100)	15/BEAM (carmustine, etoposide, cytosine arabinoside, melphalan)	EDSS improved in 7 patients, unchanged in 7 patients, and deteriorated in 1 patient
Burt/Chicago, IL (56,99)	6/120 mg/kg cyclophosphamide/1200 cGy TBI	Stable for over 3 yr
Kozak/Prague, Czech Republic (101)	8/BEAM (carmustine, etoposide, cytosine arabinoside, melphalan)	1 patient improved on EDSS, 1 patient deteriorated, 6 patients stabilized

The North American center used a regimen of cyclophosphamide, corticosteroids, and total-body irradiation *(99)*. The conditioning agents were selected in order to maximize immunosuppression. Total-body irradiation was combined with cyclophosphamide and corticosteroids because radiation could penetrate to lymphocytes sequestered within the CNS without regard for permeability of the blood brain barrier (BBB). To minimize toxicity, TBI was given in AP/PA position with 50% lung and 30% kidney and right lobe of the liver-transmission blocks.

These phase I studies demonstrated that hematopoietic stem cell transplants may be done safely in patients with MS. The studies are limited owing to the small number of patients and unblinded and nonrandomized nature of phase I trials. We know nothing about the transplant outcome according to disease type (primary progressive or secondary progressive), neurologic disability (low or high disability score), patient age, or other factors.

Candidates for these initial studies in which safety was the primary endpoint also had severe neurologic disabilities. In these candidates, even if immune destruction of myelin is "cured," it is unlikely that any prior neurologic impairment would improve and it is also possible that independent of immune-mediated damage, neurologic deterioration may continue to progress.

Previously, it was assumed that MS affects myelin produced by oligodendrocytes and spares axons. Recently, axonal transection has been identified in both active acute and chronic inactive lesions *(102)*. Axonal injury could result from immunologic assault directed at axons, bystander axonal injury from inflammatory cytokines, and/or demyelination itself. Hematopoietic transplantation is designed to arrest immune-mediated injury and dampen inflammatory cytokines. However, axonal degeneration may continue if remyelination does not occur. Oligodendrocytes and myelin provide growth signals to axons *(103–105)*. Besides providing insulation for neural conduction, oligodendrocytes may function as supporting stromal cells necessary to maintain axonal integrity. Myelin may protect neurons from "death by murder" by insulating the axons from toxin (free radical, cytokine) exposure, as well as protect neurons from "death by neglect" by providing growth stimulating factors. If hematopoietic transplantation is to have a significant impact on MS, phase II/III trials may need to target candidates with early disease before lesion burden accumulates.

Scleroderma

Scleroderma is a disease whose etiology is unknown. It may be treated with multiple agents (azathioprine, cyclophosphamide, chlorambucil, cyclosporine, anti-thymocyte globulin, photopheresis, cholchicine, and D-penicillamine) *(106,107)*, but no therapy has proven efficacious in randomized prospective trials. Unlike SLE, RA, and MS, scleroderma is relatively rare (19 cases per million/yr) *(108)*. Mortality is increased for diffuse cutaneous scleroderma (skin sclerosis distal and proximal to elbows and knees), poor performance status (assessed by the Health Assessment Questionaire [HAQ]), or visceral involvement (renal, pulmonary, or cardiac) *(109–121)*. For diffuse scleroderma, mortality may be as high as 20% at 2 yr and 35% at 5 yr *(120)*. Mortality increases for a DLCO < 70% *(121)*. Five-year mortality is 75% for patients with a DLCO < 40% *(121)*. The cause of death is generally cardiopulmonary (e.g., pulmonary hypertension, pulmonary fibrosis, pneumonia, myocardial infarct). Such high-risk patients may be considered candidates for hematopoietic stem cell transplantation especially if identified before manifesting significant organ deterioration.

Although the etiology of scleroderma is unknown, chronic GVHD (cGVHD) has similar clinical features implying that scleroderma may also have an immune-mediated pathogenesis. Chronic GVHD is an immune-mediated disease caused by lymphocte chimerism following allogeneic hematopoietic stem cell transplantation. Allogeneic microchimerism has been reported in scleroderma. Y-chromosome specific sequences have been detected by polymerase chain reaction (PCR) in the peripheral blood of female scleroderma patients who had given birth to sons (122). Microchimerism may arise in women who have never been pregnant, or in men owing to blood transfusions or from their mother owing to transplacental trafficking of maternal cells during fetal development. It is conceivable that scleroderma in fact arises from allogeneic immune-mediated microchimerism, i.e., cGVHD. This pathogenesis remains uncertain because immune microchimerism may also be found in healthy individuals.

Hematopoietic stem cell transplantation is being offered as a treatment for scleroderma on the assumption that at least part of its pathogenesis is immune-mediated by either autologous or allogeneic lymphocytes. Dose-intense immune suppression and hematopoietic stem cell transplantation by taking immune-mediated therapy to an extreme will help elucidate whether scleroderma is immune-mediated. Two patients from two centers have undergone autologous HSCT (Table 7) (123,124). Disease has improved, at least short term, in both patients.

SIDE EFFECTS AND PRECAUTIONS

While early reports in patients with refractory disease seem promising, follow-up is brief and duration of remission is unknown. Affirmation of efficacy will require carefully designed phase III trials, comparing transplantation to standard care. Because autoimmune diseases vary in response to immune-based therapies, it is reasonable to assume that their post-transplant outcomes will also vary. Different diseases may require different approaches: intense but nonmyeloablative immune suppression, or myeloablation with autologous stem cell transplantation vs allogeneic stem cell transplantation. Disease stage may also affect transplant outcome. Accumulated deficits may be irreversible or even progressive because late degenerative events may be preordained by early immune-mediated injury.

An interim analysis of European cases revealed a mortality of approx 8.0% for autologous transplantation of autoimmune disease, mandating careful selection of patients (125). Some diseases such as scleroderma may have a higher regimen related mortality. Some conditioning agents such as total-body irradiation may be especially toxic for some diseases such as pulmonary scleroderma. Proper design of patient eligibility and transplant regimen requires understanding of the pathogenesis and prognosis of each autoimmune subset which is currently incompletely understood. Several questions remain unanswered: Can cytokine (e.g., granulocyte-colony stimulating factor [G-CSF]) mobilization cause a flare of disease? Are other mobilization methods such as combined cyclophosphamide and G-CSF safer? Does lymphocyte depletion of an autologous graft affect relapse rate or post-transplant opportunistic infections? What is the optimal conditioning regimen? How durable are remissions? What is the role of allogeneic hematopoietic transplantation in autoimmune diseases?

Table 7
Clinical Trials of Autologous Hematopoietic Stem Cell Transplant for Scleroderma

Author/city/ref.	Number of patients/ conditioning	Results
Martini/Pavia, Italy (121)	1/Cyclophosphamide and CAMPATH-1G	Resolution of exertional dyspnea and alveolitis, improved skin score, height, and well-being for 2 yr of follow-up
Tyndall/ Basel, Switzerland (122)	1/Cyclophosphamide	Subjective and objective improvements 6 mo after transplantation

CONCLUSION

Treatment of autoimmune disorders by hematopoietic stem cell transplantation is a rapidly expanding field. Early reports suggest that remission or improvement may occur following autologous HSCT. Further studies should focus on defining the mechanism of remission. The immune system may be fundamentally unaltered and an autologous transplant may be nothing more than dose-intense immunosuppression. Disease-mediating effector cells may be entirely destroyed. Alternatively, pretransplant disease causing cells may persist, but an autologous transplant may shift the balance between immunity and tolerance. This may arise by augmenting autoregulatory mechanisms such as: clonal exhaustion, veto cells, suppressor cells, immune indifference, idiotypic T- or B-cell networks, inhibitory cytokines, changes in receptor avidity, or changes in T- or B-cell repertoire or function.

A second fundamental question is if relapse occurs, does it arise from the stem cell compartment or lymphocytes that survived the conditioning regimen? Scenarios can be imagined where lymphocytes that survived the conditioning regimen expand in the periphery and display abnormalities consistent with an autoimmune disease, while lymphocytes that arise from the stem cell compartment do not display these abnormalities or are actually autoregulatory and inhibit the autoimmune phenotype. The phenotype and characteristics of lymphocytes that arise from reinfused stem cells may be determined by gene marking of infused stem cells *(126)*.

Understanding the mechanisms of remission and whether stem cells are the source of disease recurrence, and elucidating the optimal but least toxic conditioning regimen are essential to properly designed prospective randomized (phase III) studies.

REFERENCES

1. Rose, N.R. and C. Bona. 1993. Defining criteria for autoimmune diseases (Witebsky's postulates revisited). *Immunol. Today* 14(9):426–429.

2. Harrington, W.J., V. Minnich, J.W., Hollingsworth, et al. 1951. Demonstration of a thrombocytopenic factor in the blood of patients with thrombocytopenic purpura. *J. Lab. Clin. Med.* 38:1.

3. Marmont, A.M. 1965. The transfusion of active LE plasma into nonlupus recipients, with a note on the LE-like cell. *Ann. NY Acad. Sci.* 124(2):838–851.

4. Lampeter, E.F., M. Homberg, K. Quabeck, U.W. Schaefer, P. Wernet, J. Bertrams, et al. 1993. Transfer of insulin-dependent diabetes between HLA-identical siblings by bone marrow transplantation [see comments]. *Lancet* 341(8855):1243–1244.

5. Brocke, S., K. Gijbels, and L. Steinman. 1994. Experimental autoimmune encephalomyelitis in the mouse. *In* Autoimmune Disease Models: A Guidebook. I.R. Cohen and A. Miller, editors. Academic Press, San Diego, CA. 1.

6. Lipton, H.L. 1975. Theiler's virus infection in mice: an unusual biphasic disease process leading to demyelination. *Infect. Immun.* 11:1147.

7. Miller, S.D. and S.J. Gerety. 1990. Immunologic aspects of Theiler's murine encephalomyelitis virus (TMEV)-induced demyelinating disease. *Semin. Virol.* 1:263.

8. Rodriguez, M., J. Leibowitz, and C.S. David. 1986. Susceptibility to Theiler's virus-induced demyelination. Mapping of the gene within the H-2D region. *J. Exp. Med.* 163:620.

9. Lipton, H.L., J. Kratochvil, P. Sethi, and M.C. Dal Canto. 1984. Theiler's virus antigen detected in mouse spinal cord 2 1/2 years after infection. *Neurology* 34:1117.

10. Miller, S.D., C.L. Vanderlugt, W.S. Begolka, W. Pao, R.L. Yauch, K.L. Neville, et al. 1997. Persistent infection with Theiler's virus leads to CNS autoimmunity via epitope spreading. *Nature Med.* 3:1133.

11. Murphy, E.D. and J.B. Roths. 1976. A single gene for massive lymphoproliferation with immune complex disease in a new mouse strain MRL. Proceedings of the 16th International Congress in Hematology. *Amsterdam Excerpta Med.* 69–80.

12. Drappa, J., N. Brot, and K.B. Elkon. 1993. The Fas protein is expressed at high levels on CD4+CD8+ thymocytes and activated mature lymphocytes in normal mice but not in the lupus-prone strain, MRL lpr/lpr. *Proc. Natl. Acad. Sci. USA* 90(21):10,340–10,344.

13. Kono, D.H., R.W. Burlingame, D.G. Owens, A. Kuramochi, R.S. Balderas, D. Balomenos, and A.N. Theofilopoulos. 1994. Lupus susceptibility loci in New Zealand mice. *Proc. Natl. Acad. Sci. USA* 91:10,168–10,172.

14. Karussis, D.M., U. Vourka-Karussis, and D. Lehmann. 1993. Prevention and reversal of adoptively transferred, chronic relapsing experimental autoimmune encephalomyelitis with a single high dose cytoreductive treatment followed by syngeneic bone marrow transplantation. *J. Clin. Invest.* 92:765.

15. Burt, R.K., J. Padilla, W. Smith-Begolka, M.C. Dal Canto, and S.D. Miller. 1998. Effect of disease stage on clinical outcome after syngeneic bone marrow transplantation for relapsing experimental autoimmune encephalomyelitis. *Blood* 91:2609–2616.

16. Baron, J.L., J.A. Madri, N.H. Ruddle, G. Hashim, and C.A. Janeway, Jr. 1993. Surface expression of [alpha] 4 integrin by CD4 T cells is required for their entry into brain parenchyma. *J. Exp. Med.* 177:57–68.

17. Willenborg, D.O. 1979. Experimental allergic encephalomyelitis in the Lewis rat: Studies on the mechanism of recovery from disease and acquired resistance to reinduction. *J. Immunol.* 123(3):1145–50.

18. Ellerman, K.E, J.M. Powers, and S.W. Brostoff. 1988. A suppressor T-lymphocyte cell line for autoimmune encephalomyelitis. *Nature* 331(6153):265–267.

19. Sun, D., Y. Qin, J. Chluba, J.T. Epplen, and H. Wekerle. 1988. Suppression of experimentally induced autoimmune encephalomyelitis by cytolytic T-T cell interactions. *Nature* 332(6167):843–845.

20. Wong, F.S., B.N. Dittel, and C.A. Janeway, Jr. 1999. Transgenes and knockout mutations in animal models of type 1 diabetes and multiple sclerosis. *Immunolog. Rev.* 169:93–104.

21. Goverman, J., A. Woods, L. Larson, L.P. Weiner, L. Hood, and D.M. Zaller. 1993. Transgenic mice that express a myelin basic protein-specific T cell receptor develop spontaneous autoimmunity. *Cell* 72:551–560.

22. Lafaille, J.J., K. Nagashima, M. Katsuki, and S. Tonegawa. 1994. High incidence of spontaneous autoimmune encephalomyelitis in immunodeficient anti-myelin basic protein T cell receptor transgenic mice. *Cell* 78:399–408.

23. Van de Keere, F. and S. Tonegawa. 1998. CD4+ T cells prevent spontaneous experimental autoimmune encephalomyelitis in anti-myelin basic protein T cell receptor transgenic mice. *J. Exp. Med.* 188:1875–1882.

24. Sugiura, K., S. Pahwa, Y. Yamamoto, K. Borisov, R. Pahwa, R.P. Nelson. Jr., et al. 1998. Characterization of natural suppressor cells in human bone marrow. *Stem Cells* 16(2):99–106.

25. Lipton, H.L. and A. Friedmann. 1980. Purification of Theiler's murine encephalomyelitis virus and analysis of the structural virion polypeptides: correlation of the polypeptide profile with virulence. *J. Virol.* 33:1165.

26. Rodriguez, M., L.R. Pease, and C.S. David. 1986. Immune-mediated injury of virus-infected oligodendrocytes: A model of multiple sclerosis. *Immunol. Today* 7:359.

27. Lipton, H.L. and M.C. Dal Canto. 1976. Theiler's virus-induced demyelination: prevention by immunosuppression. *Science* 192:62.

28. Burt, R.K., J. Padilla, M.C. Dal Canto, and S.D. Miller. 1999. Viral hyperinfection of the central nervous system and high mortality after hematopoietic stem cell transplantation for treatment of Theiler's murine encephalomyelitis virus-induced demyelinating disease. *Blood* 94:2915–2922.

29. Mohan, C., L. Morel, P. Yang, H. Watanabe, B. Croker, G. Gilkeson, and E.K. Wakeland. 1999. Genetic dissection of lupus pathogenesis: a recipe for nephrophilic autoantibodies. *J. Clin. Invest.* 103(12):1685–1695.

30. Mohan, C., Y. Yu, L. Morel, P. Yang, and E.K. Wakeland. 1999. Genetic dissection of Sle pathogenesis: Sle3 on murine chromosome 7 impacts T cell activation, differentiation, and cell death. *J. Immunol.* 162(11):6492–502.

31. Sobel, E.S., C. Mohan, L. Morel, J. Schiffenbauer, and E.K. Wakeland. 1999. Genetic dissection of SLE pathogenesis: adoptive transfer of Sle1 mediates the loss of tolerance by bone marrow-derived B cells. *J. Immunol.* 162(4):2415–2421.

32. Mohan, C., E. Alas, L. Morel, P. Yang, and E.K. Wakeland. 1998. Genetic dissection of SLE pathogenesis. Sle1 on murine chromosome 1 leads to a selective loss of tolerance to H2A/H2B/DNA subnucleosomes. *J. Clin. Invest.* 101(6):1362–72.

33. Mohan, C., L. Morel, P. Yang, and E.K. Wakeland. 1997. Genetic dissection of systemic lupus erythematosus pathogenesis: Sle2 on murine chromosome 4 leads to B cell hyperactivity. *J. Immunol.* 159(1):454–465.

34. Wakeland, E.K., L. Morel, C. Mohan, and M. Yui. 1997. Genetic dissection of lupus nephritis in murine models of SLE. [Review] [53 refs] *J. Clin. Immunol.* 17(4):272–281.

35. Wang, B., Y. Yamamoto, N.S. El-Badri, and R.A. Good. 1999. Effective treatment of autoimmune disease and progressive renal disease by mixed bone-marrow transplantation that establishes a stable mixed chimerism in BXSB recipient mice. *Proc. Natl. Acad. Sci. USA* 96(6):3012–6.

36. Wang, B.Y., Cherry, N.S. El-Badri, and R.A. Good. 1997. Prevention of development of autoimmune disease in BXSB mice by mixed bone marrow transplantation. *Proc. Natl. Acad. Sci. USA* 94(22):12,065–12,069.

37. Karussis, D.M., U. Vourka-Karussis, D. Lehmann, O. Abramsky, A. Ben-Nun, and S. Slavin. 1995. Immunomodulation of autoimmunity in MRL/lpr mice with syngeneic bone marrow transplantation (SBMT). *Clin. Exp. Immunol.* 100(1):111–117.

38. Boumpas, D.T., H.A. Austin III, B.J. Fessler, J.E. Balow, J.H. Klippel, and M.D. Lockshin. 1995. Systemic lupus erythematosus: emerging concepts. Part 1. Renal, neuropsychiatric, cardiovascular, pulmonary, and hematologic disease. *Ann. Intern. Med.* 122:940–950.

39. Boumpas, D.T., B.J. Fessler, H.A. Austin III, J.E. Balow, J.H. Klippel, and M.D. Lockshin. 1995. Systemic lupus erythematosus: emerging concepts. Part 2. Dermatologic and joint disease, the antiphospholipid antibody syndrome, pregnancy and hormonal therapy, morbidity and mortality, and pathogenesis. *Ann. Intern. Med.* 123:42–53.

40. Tan, E.M., A.S. Cohen, J.F. Fries, A.T. Masi, D.J. McShane, N.F. Rothfield, et al. 1982. The 1982 revised criteria for the classification of systemic lupus erythematosus. *Arthritis Rheum.* 25(11):1271–1277.

41. Urowitz, M.B. and D.D. Gladman. 1999. Evolving spectrum of mortality and morbidity in SLE [editorial]. *Lupus* 8(4):253–255

42. Cervera, R., M.A. Khamashta, J. Font, G.D. Sebastiani, A. Gil, P. Lavilla, et al. 1999. Morbidity and mortality in systemic lupus erythematosus during a 5-year period. A multicenter prospective study of 1,000 patients. European Working Party on Systemic Lupus Erythematosus. *Medicine* 78(3):167–175.

43. Jacobsen, S., J. Petersen, S. Ullman, P. Junker, A. Voss, J.M. Rasmussen, et al. 1999. Mortality and causes of death of 513 Danish patients with systemic lupus erythematosus. *Scand. J. Rheumatol.* 28(2):75–80.

44. Uramoto, K.M., C.J. Michet Jr, J. Thumboo, J. Sunku, W.M. O'Fallon, and S.E. Gabriel. 1999. Trends in the incidence and mortality of systemic lupus erythematosus, 1950–1992. *Arthritis Rheum.* 42(1):46–50.

45. Blanco, F.J., J.J. Gomez-Reino, J. de la Mata, A. Corrales, V. Rodriguez-Valverde, J.C. Rosas, et al. 1998. Survival analysis of 306 European Spanish patients with systemic lupus erythematosus. *Lupus* 7(3):159–163.

46. Urowitz, M.B., D.D. Gladman, M. Abu-Shakra, and V.T. Farewell. 1997. Mortality studies in systemic lupus erythematosus. Results from a single center. III. Improved survival over 24 years. *J. Rheumatol.* 24(6):1061–1065.

47. Kim, W.U., S.I. Kim, W.H. Yoo, J.H. Park, J.K. Min, S.C. Kim, et al. 1999. Adult respiratory distress syndrome in systemic lupus erythematosus: causes and prognostic factors: a single center, retrospective study. *Lupus* 8(7):552–557.

48. Ward, M.M., E. Pyun, and S. Studenski. 1996. Mortality risks associated with specific clinical manifestations of systemic lupus erythematosus. *Arch. Int. Med.* 156(12):1337–1344.

49. Abu-Shakra, M., M.B. Urowitz, D.D. Gladman, and J. Gough. 1995. Mortality studies in systemic lupus erythematosus. Results from a single center I. Causes of death. *J. Rheumatol.* 22(7): 1259–1264.

50. Abu-Shakra, M., M.B. Urowitz, D.D. Gladman, and J. Gough. 1995. Mortality studies in systemic lupus erythematosus. Results from a single center. II. Predictor variables for mortality. *J. Rheumatol.* 22(7):1265–1270.

51. Ward, M.M., E. Pyun, and S. Studenski. 1995. Causes of death in systemic lupus erythematosus. Long-term followup of an inception cohort. *Arthritis Rheum.* 38(10):1492–1499.

52. Schachna, L., P.F. Ryan, and A.P. Schwarer. 1998. Malignancy-associated remission of systemic lupus erythematosus maintained by autologous peripheral blood stem cell transplantation. *Arthritis Rheum.* 41(12):2271–2272.

53. Gur-Lavi, M. 1999. Long-term remission with allogenic bone marrow transplantation in systemic lupus erythematosus. *Arthritis Rheum.* 42(8):1777.

54. Meloni, G., S. Capria, M. Vignetti, F. Mandelli, and V. Modena. 1997. Blast crisis of chronic myelogenous leukemia in long-lasting systemic lupus erythematosus: regression of both diseases after autologous bone marrow transplantation [letter; comment]. *Blood.* 89(12):4659.

55. Snowden, J.A., W.N. Patton, J.L. O'Donnell, E.E. Hannah, and D.N. Hart. 1997. Prolonged remission of longstanding systemic lupus erythematosus after autologous bone marrow transplant for non-Hodgkin's lymphoma. *Bone Marrow Transplant.* 19(12):1247–1250.

56. Euler, H.H., A.M. Marmont, A. Bacigalupo, S. Fastenrath, P. Dreger, M. Hoffknecht, et al. 1996. Early recurrence or persistence of autoimmune diseases after unmanipulated autologous stem cell transplantation [see comments]. *Blood* 88(9):3621–3625.

57. Fouillard, L., N.C. Gorin, J.P. Laporte, A. Leon, J.F. Brantus, and P. Miossec. 1999. Control of severe systemic lupus erythematosus after high-dose immunusuppressive therapy and transplantation of CD34+ purified autologous stem cells from peripheral blood. *Lupus* 8(4):320–323.

58. Musso, M., F. Porretto, A. Crescimanno, F. Bondi, V. Polizzi, R. Scalone, and G. Mariani. 1998. Autologous peripheral blood stem and progenitor (CD34+) cell transplantation for systemic lupus erythematosus complicated by Evans syndrome. *Lupus* 7(7):492–494.

59. Burt, R.K., A.E. Traynor, R. Pope, J. Schroeder, B. Cohen, K.H. Karlin, et al. 1998. Treatment of autoimmune disease by intense immunosuppressive conditioning and autologous hematopoietic stem cell transplantation. *Blood* 92(10):3505–3514.

60. Burt, R.K., A. Traynor, and R. Ramsey-Goldman. 1997. Hematopoietic stem cell transplantation for systemic lupus erythematosus *N. Engl. J. Med.* 337(24):1777–1778.

61. Marmont, A.M., M.T. van Lint, F. Gualandi, and A. Bacigalupo. 1997. Autologous marrow stem cell transplantation for severe systemic lupus erythematosus of long duration. *Lupus* 6(6):545–548.

62. Brodsky, R.A., M. Petri, B.D. Smith, J. Steifter, J.L. Spivak, M. Styler, et al. 1998. Immunablative high dose cyclophosphamide without stem cell rescue for refractory severe autoimmune disease. *Ann. Intern. Med.* 129:1031–1035.

63. Arnett, F.C., S.M. Edworthy, D.A. Bloch, D.J. McShane, J.F. Fries, N.S. Cooper, et al. 1988. The American Rheumatism Association 1987 revised criteria for the classification of rheumatoid arthritis. *Arthritis Rheum.* 31:315–324.

64. Abdel-Nasser, A.M., J.J. Rasker, and H.A. Valkenburg. 1997. Epidemiological and clinical aspects relating to the variability of rheumatoid arthritis. *Semin. Arthritis Rheum.* 27(2):123–140.

65. Callahan, L.F. and T. Pincus. 1995. Mortality in the rheumatic diseases. *Arthritis Care Res.* 8(4):229–241.

66. Pincus, T., R.H. Brooks, and L.F. Callahan. 1994. Prediction of long-term mortality in patients with rheumatoid arthritis according to simple questionnaire and joint count measures. *Ann. Int. Med.* 120(1):26–34.

67. Mitchell, D.M., P.W. Spitz, D.Y. Young, D.A. Bloch, D.J. McShane, and J.F. Fries. 1986. Survival, prognosis, and causes of death in rheumatoid arthritis. *Arthritis Rheum.* 29:706–714.

68. Leigh, J.P. and J.F. Fries. 1991. Mortality predictors among 263 patients with rheumatoid arthritis. *J. Rheumatol.* 18:1307–1312.

69. Pincus, T., L.F. Callahan, and W.K. Vaughn. 1987. Questionnaire, walking time and button test measures of functional capacity as predictive markers for mortality in rheumatoid arthritis. *J. Rheumatol.* 14:240–51.

70. Cobb, S., F. Anderson, and W. Bauer. 1953. Length of life and cause of death in rheumatoid arthritis. *N. Engl. J. Med.* 249:553–556.

71. Cooley, H.M., J.A. Snowden, A.P. Grigg, and I.P. Wicks. 1997. Outcome of rheumatoid arthritis and psoriasis following autologous stem cell transplantation for hematologic malignancy. *Arthritis Rheum.* 40(9):1712–5.

72. Jondeau, K., C. Job-Deslandre, D. Bouscary, N. Khanlou, C.J. Menkes, and F. Dreyfus. 1997. Remission of nonerosive polyarthritis associated with Sjogren's syndrome after autologous hematopoietic stem cell transplantation for lymphoma. *J. Rheumatol.* 24(12):2466–2468.

73. Baldwin, J.L., R. Storb, E.D. Thomas, and M. Mannik. 1977. Bone marrow transplantation in patients with gold-induced marrow aplasia. *Arthritis Rheum.* 20(5):1043–1048.

74. Lowenthal, R.M., M.L. Cohen, K. Atkinson, and J.C. Biggs. 1993. Apparent cure of rheumatoid arthritis by bone marrow transplantation. *J. Rheumatol.* 20(1):137–140.

75. Jacobs, P., M.D. Vincent, and R.W. Martell. 1986. Prolonged remission of severe refractory rheumatoid arthritis following allogeneic bone marrow transplantation for drug-induced aplastic anaemia. *Bone Marrow Transplant.* 1(2):237–239.

76. McKendry, R.J., L. Huebsch, and B. Leclair. 1996. Progression of rheumatoid arthritis following bone marrow transplantation. A case report with a 13-year followup. *Arthritis Rheum.* 39(7):1246–1253.

77. Sibilia, J., F. Liote, and X. Mariette. 1998. Lymphoproliferative disorders in rheumatoid arthritis patients on low-dose methotrexate. *Revue Du Rhumatisme*, English Edition. 65(4):267–273.

78. Georgescu, L. and S.A. Paget. 1999. Lymphoma in patients with rheumatoid arthritis: what is the evidence of a link with methotrexate? *Drug Safety* 20(6):475–487.

79. Baecklund, E., A. Ekbom, P. Sparen, N. Feltelius, and L. Klareskog. 1998. Disease activity and risk of lymphoma in patients with rheumatoid arthritis: nested case-control study. *BMJ* 317(7152):180–181.

80. Prior, P., D.P.M. Symmons, C.F. Hawkins, D.L. Scott, and R. Brown. 1984. Cancer morbidity in rheumatoid arthritis. *Ann. Rheum. Dis.* 43:128–131.

81. Myllykangas-Luosujarvi, R., K. Aho, and H. Isomaki. 1995. Mortality from cancer in patients with rheumatoid arthritis. *Scand. J. Rheumatol.* 24:76–78.

82. Gridley, G., J.K. McLaughlin, A. Ekbom, L. Klareskog, H.O. Adami, D.G. Hacker, et al. 1993. Incidence of cancer among patients with rheumatoid arthritis. *J. Natl. Cancer Inst.* 85:307–311.

83. Symmons, D.P.M. 1985. Neoplasms of the immune system in rheumatoid arthritis. *Am. J. Med.* 78:22–28.

84. Silman, A.J., J. Petrie, B. Hazleman, and S.J.W. Evans. 1988. Lymphoproliferative cancer and other malignancy in patients with rheumatoid arthritis treated with azathioprine: a 20 year follow up study. *Ann. Rheum. Dis.* 47:988–992.

85. Burt, R.K., C. Georganas, J. Schroeder, A. Traynor, J. Stefka, F. Schuening, et al. 1999. Autologous hematopoietic stem cell transplantation in refractory rheumatoid arthritis: sustained response in two of four patients. *Arthritis Rheum.* 42(11):2281–2285.

86. Joske, D.J., D.T. Ma, D.R. Langlands, and E.T. Owen. 1997. Autologous bone-marrow transplantation for rheumatoid arthritis *Lancet* 350(9074):337–338.

87. Snowden, J.A., J.C. Biggs, S.T. Milliken, A. Fuller, and P.M. Brooks. 1999. A phase I/II dose escalation study of intensified cyclophosphamide and autologous blood stem cell rescue in severe, active rheumatoid arthritis. *Arthritis Rheum.* 42(11):2286–2292.

88. Durez, P., M. Toungouz, L. Schandene, M. Lambermont, and M. Goldman. 1998. Remission and immune reconstitution after T-cell-depleted stem cell transplantation for rheumatoid arthritis. *Lancet* 352(9131):881.

89. McColl, G., H. Kohsaka, J. Szer, and I. Wicks. 1999. High-dose chemotherapy and syngeneic hemopoietic stem cell transplantation for severe, seronegative rheumatoid arthritis. *Ann. Int. Med.* 131(7):507–509.

90. Steinman, L. 1996. Multiple sclerosis: a coordinated immunological attack against myelin in the central nervous system. *Cell* 85:299–302.

91. Martin, R. and H.F. McFarland. 1995. Immunological aspects of experimental allergic encephalomyelitis and multiple sclerosis. *Crit. Rev. Clin. Lab. Sci.* 32:121–182.

92. Kurtzke, J.F. 1975. A reassessment of the distribution of multiple sclerosis. Part one. *Acta Neurolog. Scand.* 51(2):110–136.

93. Wingerchuk, D.M. and B.G. Weinshenker. 1999. The natural history of multiple sclerosis: implications for trial design. *Curr. Opin. Neurol.* 12(3):345–349.

94. Weinshenker, B.G. 1998. The natural history of multiple sclerosis: update 1998. *Semin. Neurol.* 18(3):301–307.

95. Andersson, P.B., E. Waubant, L. Gee, and D.E. Goodkin. 1999. Multiple sclerosis that is progressive from the time of onset: clinical characteristics and progression of disability. *Arch. Neurol.* 56(9):1138–1142.

96. Weinshenker, B.G., G.P. Rice, J.H. Noseworthy, W. Carriere, J. Baskerville, and G.C. Ebers. 1991. The natural history of multiple sclerosis: a geographically based study. 3. Multivariate analysis of predictive factors and models of outcome. *Brain* 114 (Pt 2):1045–1056.

97. Meloni, G., S. Capria, M. Salvetti, I. Cordone, M. Mancini, and F. Mandelli. 1999. Autologous peripheral blood stem cell transplantation in a patient with multiple sclerosis and concomitant Ph+ acute leukemia [letter]. *Haematologica* 84(7):665–667.

98. McAllister, L.D., P.G. Beatty, and J. Rose. 1997. Allogeneic bone marrow transplant for chronic myelogenous leukemia in a patient with multiple sclerosis. *Bone Marrow Transplant.* 19(4): 395–397.

99. Burt, R.K., A.E. Traynor, B. Cohen, K.H. Karlin, F.A. Davis, D. Stefoski, et al. 1998. T cell-depleted autologous hematopoietic stem cell transplantation for multiple sclerosis: report on the first three patients. *Bone Marrow Transplant.* 21(6):537–541.

100. Fassas, A., A. Anagnostopoulos, A. Kazis, K. Kapinas, I. Sakellari, V. Kimiskidis, and A. Tsompanakou. 1997. Peripheral blood stem cell transplantation in the treatment of progressive multiple sclerosis: first results of a pilot study. *Bone Marrow Transplant.* 20(8):631–638.

101. Kozak, T., E. Havrdova, J. Pit'ha, E. Gregora, R. Pylik, J. Maaloufova, et al. 2000. High dose immunosuppressive therapy with PBPC support in the treatment of poor risk multiple sclerosis. *Bone Marrow Transplant.* 25, 525–531.

102. Trapp, B.D., J. Peterson, R.M. Ransohoff, R. Rudick, S. Mork, and L. Bo. 1998. Axonal transection in the lesions of multiple sclerosis [see comments]. *N. Engl. J. Med.* 338(5):278–285.

103. Windebank, A.J., P. Wood, R.P. Bunge, and P.J. Dyck. 1985. Myelination determines the caliber of dorsal root ganglion neurons in culture. *J. Neurosci.* 5:1563–1569.

104. Sanchez, I., L. Hassinger, P.A. Paskevich, H.D. Shine, and R.A. Nixon. 1996. Oligodendroglia regulate the regional expansion of axon caliber and local accumulation of neurofilaments during development independently of myelin formation. *J. Neurosci.* 16:5095–5105.

105. Fruttiger, M., D. Montag, M. Schachner, and R. Martini. 1995. Crucial role for the myelin-associated glycoprotein in the maintenance of axon-myelin integrity. *Eur. J. Neurosci.* 7:511–515.

106. Herrick, A.L. 1998. Advances in treatment of systemic sclerosis. *Lancet* 352(9144):1874–1875.

107. Rose, N.R. and N. Leskovsek. 1998. Scleroderma: immunopathogenesis and treatment. *Immunol. Today* 19(11):499–501.

108. Mayes, M.D. 1997. Epidemiology of systemic sclerosis and related diseases. *Curr. Opin. Rheumatol.* 9(6):557–561.

109. Ho, M. and J. Belch. 1999. Causes of mortality in systemic sclerosis. *Rheumatology* 38(3): 283–284.

110. Englert, H., J. Small-McMahon, K. Davis, H. O'Connor, P. Chambers, and P. Brooks. 1999. Systemic sclerosis prevalence and mortality in Sydney 1974–88. *Austr. NZ J. Med.* 29(1):42–50.

111. Poole, J.L. and V.D. Steen. 1991. The use of the Health Assessment Questionnaire (HAQ) to determine physical disability in systemic sclerosis. *Arthritis Care Res.* 4:27–31.

112. Bryan, C., Y. Howard, P. Brennan, C. Black, and A. Silman. 1996. Survival following the onset of scleroderma: results from a retrospective inception cohort study of the UK patient population. *Br. J. Rheumatol.* 35(11):1122–1126.

113. Silman, A.J. 1997. Scleroderma: demographics and survival. *J. Rheumatol.* (Suppl.) 48:58–61.

114. Godeau, B., E. Mortier, P.M. Roy, S. Chevret, G. Bouachour, B. Schlemmer, et al. 1997. Short and longterm outcomes for patients with systemic rheumatic diseases admitted to intensive care units: a prognostic study of 181 patients. *J. Rheumatol.* 24(7):1317–1323.

115. Nagy, Z. and L. Czirjak. 1997. Predictors of survival in 171 patients with systemic sclerosis (scleroderma). *Clin. Rheumatol.* 16(5):454–460.

116. Steen, V.D. and T.A. Medsger Jr. 1997. The value of the Health Assessment Questionnaire and special patient-generated scales to demonstrate change in systemic sclerosis patients over time. *Arthritis Rheum.* 40(11):1984–1991.

117. Simeon, C.P., L. Armadans, V. Fonollosa, M. Vilardell, J. Candell, C. Tolosa, et al. 1997. Survival prognostic factors and markers of morbidity in Spanish patients with systemic sclerosis. *Ann. Rheum. Dis.* 56(12):723–728.

118. Jacobsen, S., P. Halberg, and S. Ullman. 1998. Mortality and causes of death of 344 Danish patients with systemic sclerosis (scleroderma). *Br. J. Rheumatol.* 37(7):750–755.

119. Hesselstrand, R., A. Scheja, and A. Akesson. 1998. Mortality and causes of death in a Swedish series of systemic sclerosis patients. *Ann. Rheum. Dis.* 57(11):682–686.

120. Bulpitt, K.J., P.J. Clements, P.A. Lachenbruch, H.E. Paulus, J.B. Peter, M.S. Agopian, et al. 1993. Early undifferentiated connective tissue disease: III. Outcome and prognostic indicators in early scleroderma (systemic sclerosis). *Ann. Int. Med.* 118(8):602–609.

121. Clements, P., P. Lachenbruch, J.R. Seibold, et. al. 1995. Ketanserin versus placebo in systemic sclerosis trial: Predictors of long term survival (abst). *Arthritis Rheum.* (Suppl.)38: S335.

122. Nelson, J.L., D.E. Furst, S. Maloney, T. Gooley, P.C. Evans, A. Smith, et al. 1998. Microchimerism and HLA-compatible relationships of pregnancy in scleroderma. *Lancet* 351(9102):559–562.

123. Martini, A., R. Maccario, A. Ravelli, D. Montagna, F. De Benedetti, F. Bonetti, et al. 1999. Marked and sustained improvement two years after autologous stem cell transplantation in a girl with systemic sclerosis. *Arthritis Rheum.* 42(4):807–811.

124. Tyndall, A., C. Black, J. Finke, J. Winkler, R. Mertlesmann, H.H. Peter, and A. Gratwohl. 1997. Treatment of systemic sclerosis with autologous haemopoietic stem cell transplantation *Lancet* 349(9047):254.

125. Tyndall A., et al. 1999. Autologous haematopoietic stem cell transplants for autoimmune diseases-feasibility and transplant related mortality. *Bone Marrow Transplant.* 24:729–734.

126. Burt, R.K., M. Brenner, W. Burns, E. Courier, G. Firestein, B. Hahn, et al. 2000. Gene marked autologous hematopoietic stem cell transplantation of autoimmune disease. *J. Clin. Immunol.* 20(1):1–9.

IV   GENE THERAPY IN RHEUMATIC DISEASES

30 Vectors for Gene Delivery

Sandro Rusconi and Maurizio Ceppi

INTRODUCTION

Gene therapy bases its rationale on the transfer of genetic components (genes or fragments thereof) into somatic cells, with the aim of preventing, correcting, or healing various types of disorders. After this introductory sentence, the reader likely expects us to begin discussing some of the marvellous achievements in setting up the tools that allow this transfer. However, before entering into the intricate details of vectorology, please allow us the following clear-cut statement: *As of today there is no perfect or general vector for gene therapy and there won't be probably any in the foreseeable future.* We hope that with this statement in mind, it will be easier for the readers to understand why there is still such a multitude of seemingly disparate efforts in establishing appropriate vehicles for the gene transfer.

Therefore, the efficacy of gene therapy largely depends on the properties of the chosen "vector" for gene transfer and expression. The reader should be reminded that there is still some ambiguity in the denomination "vector" because this concept can be understood either as the mere *cis*-elements that compose the transferred sequence (that is the nucleic acid sequence arrangement) or as the vehicle/method that is utilized for the transfer of the required gene.

PROBLEMS INFLUENCING VECTOR'S CHOICE

Nucleic Acids as Medicine: Megadaltons Instead of Kilodaltons

In gene therapy, the drug is a segment of either DNA or RNA and this imposes major constraints in the delivery. In conventional pharmacology the drugs are molecules of limited size (hundreds of Daltons) that either freely enter into cells owing to their lipophilic character or are hydrophilic and destined to either act in the extracellular space

From: *Modern Therapeutics in Rheumatic Diseases*
Edited by: G. C. Tsokos, et al. © Humana Press, Inc., Totowa, NJ

or to be imported through specific biological channels. The classical pharmacological drugs are designed to act over a relatively short time and their therapeutic concentration is usually controlled by readministration. A termination of the administration results in a dilution and termination of the pharmacological effects. Nucleic acids do not share many of the aforementioned properties: they have a large molecular size (1 MDa for a segment of 1500 base pairs), are destined to work in the cell nucleus but are neither lipophilic, nor can count on a physiological import system. Once delivered into the nucleus they either integrate and persist for the rest of the cell's life or are maintained episomally for variable amounts of time. Therefore, the usual pharmacological strategies only marginally apply to the delivery of these monstrous molecules. For instance, in order to render them permeable to the cell membrane, one has to either compact them into lipid-containing particles or into viral envelopes or capsids. This means that the units of delivery are no longer single, soluble molecules but relatively large (100–500 nm) and only partially soluble aggregates. This latter aspect makes the work with nucleic acids as medicines very arduous and still poorly reproducible in the complexity of a living organism. To conclude these considerations we will mention that in the jargon of the gene therapists, the transferred gene is also usually referred to as the "transgene." The use of this term will hopefully simplify the reading of the further paragraphs.

Correcting Disorders Derived from Loss-of-Function or Gain-of-Function

Genetic and acquired disorders result from an imbalance of metabolic functions, which are ultimately controlled by the genetic layout of the affected cells. The nature of the delivery vector and the properties of the transgene will largely depend on whether the therapy is aimed at inhibiting or supplementing (or enhancing) metabolic functions. In most monogenic disorders, the phenotype is caused by a single loss-of-function that depending on the hyerarchical position of the affected gene can cause a simple or a very pleiotropic defect. For instance in cystic fibrosis (CF) or in muscle dystrophy (MD), the lack of function of the corresponding genes results in rather circumscribed phenotypes. In this case the therapy shall be aimed at the organs that cause the most debilitating symptoms. Thus, it may be necessary to count on a rather well-targeted delivery of the therapeutic supplemental gene. When trying to correct another monogenic disorder such as lack of factor VIII, the vector does not need to be targeted to the original tissue (the liver), because the corrective factor will be secreted virtually from any targeted tissue.

When trying to compensate loss-of-function disorders, the level of gene transfer will not need to be 100% because in most cases a small percentage of cured cells will exert a corrective function. Therefore there will be lower requirements in terms of efficiency of gene transfer on the chosen vector. For these reasons, monogenic disorders, though relatively rare and unattractive from the marketing point of view, have received a fair amount of attention by academically or industrially based gene therapists. On the other hand, when trying to control disorders derived from gain-of-function such as most hyper-proliferatory diseases (cancers, auto-immune disorders, etc.) it will be more important to reach transfer levels close to 100% or to ensure at least that the transfected cells initiate a feedback control on the still untransfected partners and produce a "bystander effect" *(1,2)*. Thus, the type of vector and the construction of the transgene have to be adapted to this task.

The Choice of cis-*Elements: Constitutive or Regulated Expression*

The first level at which the properties of a vector are defined is the assembly of the regulatory and coding elements. In most of proof-of-principle experiments in which the transgene was a reporter gene, the promoter of choice was taken from the panel of conventionally strong constitutive champions such as the promoter/enhancer of the cytomegalo virus (CMV), the Rous sarcoma virus (RSV), or the simian virus 40 (SV40). These promoters could be also considered for clinically valid therapeutic vectors, although their strength is strongly cell-specific. Therefore, in "second-generation" experiments, we have witnessed the use of tissue-specific promoters, although with erratic results *(3–6)*. In fact, the use of a genuinely tissue-specific control would circumvent the need of precisely targeting the delivery, because the regulation would be brought at the transcriptional level. However, our understanding of tissue specificity of transcription is restricted to relatively short *cis*-acting elements, whereas in chromosomal genes, locus regulation occupies probably relatively extensive sequences *(7,8)*. This is very relevant, because the currently available strategies that ensure long-term expression are based on random integration in the host genome. This random integration is different in each individual transformed cell and leads to unpredictable position effects that influence the expression of the transgene *(4,9–11)*. As learned from conventional transgenic animal models obtained by pronuclear microinjection, in the majority of the cases the transgenes are silenced, and only a fully equipped locus is "protected" from the erratic influence of the flanking regions.

Such large DNA segments are not compatible with the packaging capacity of most current vectors, therefore we are momentarily "condemned" to use surrogate mini-regulatory elements *(12,13)*.

For some disorders, another important goal is the search for bio-sensing, *cis*-regulatory elements that can respond to metabolic status such as hypoxia *(14,15)*, glucose levels *(16)*, and so on, these elements will be indispensable in the assembly of artificial glands that are designed to respond to natural balances of metabolites, thereby producing factors such as insulin or Epo in physiologically relevant and homeostatically controlled amounts.

Finally, an interesting collection of externally controllable \-elements can be found in the literature, such as promoters that can be regulated by insect hormones *(17)*, steroid antagonists *(18–20)*, rapamycin, or tetracycline derivatives *(21,22)*. The advantage of these systems is that the action of the transgene can be pharmacologically regulated. These have been used with variable success in animal models, where the administration of the external drugs was shown to exert the anticipated effects on the gene expression *(18)*. Four parameters are important in these vectors: (1) the magnitude of control; (2) the potential for immunogenicity of the regulatory factor; (3) the crossreaction of the controlling drug with resident metabolism; (4) the half-life of the drug, the regulatory gene product, and the target gene product, which together determine the rapidity of the response. The systems that use vertebrate regulators such as receptor mutants that respond to steroid antagonists have some advantage in their low immunogenicity, but have some disadvantage in potential crossreaction with resident receptors. On the other hand, the immunogenicity of the popular tet-regulatory system, which has a high magnitude of regulation but utilizes a procaryotic regulatory factor, has not yet been fully assessed. This means that so far there is still a lot to optimize in this field and that no perfect system is yet available.

The Three Fundamental Questions in Gene Delivery: Efficiency, Specificity, and Persistence

One gram of tissue contains an average of 1 billion cells and the interstitial passages are rarely larger than 150–200 nm. These numbers should suffice to illustrate the first big problem in gene delivery: efficiency of transfer. To this we should add the nonspecific binding of particles by the extra-cellular matrix and the consequent dilution of active principle. Finally, we should remember that there is no specific import for nucleic acids though the cell membrane and through the nuclear envelope (*see* Nucleic Acids as Medicine and Viral vs Nonviral sections). Therefore, it becomes evident that the best current vehicles are packaging bio-particles that have evolved the capacity to solve many of these problems: the viruses (*see* Viral vs Nonviral, Replication-Defective and Replication-Competent Viruses, and Bio-Weapon 1 sections).

Because it is not always possible to guarantee absolute specificity of gene expression (*see* The Choice of *cis*-Elements section), we have sometimes to delegate the specificity to the delivery particle. To this aim, several strategies have been designed (*see* Bio-Weapon 1/Targeting and Retargeting and Bio-Weapon 2/Targeting and Retargeting sections).

Finally we should consider that when correcting chronic or degenerative disorders, the transgene must persist and be active over a very long time, preferably for indefinite time. This is one of the most difficult tasks. Even if we manage to concoct the best regulatory regions that will prevent gene silencing through random integration in the genome (*see* Integration section), we cannot prevent the transformed cells to be lost by natural shedding such as in rapidly growing epithelia. This forces us to choose among two alternatives: (1) target master stem cells that will be maintained throughout the renewal of the target tissue, and (2) accept the discomfort of periodical readministration of the transgene. With partial exception of the bone marrow, and in spite of the spectacular recent advances in stem cell research, we are not yet able to guarantee the efficient transformation of pluripotent precursors and so far we are forced to consider readministration as inevitable for the long-term correction of most chronic disorders. Readministration brings with itself all the unpredictabilities of the immune reactions, specially but not exclusively when working with viral vectors. Thus, we can affirm that at the state of the art, there is still no single or clear solution to the long-term treatment of chronic conditions.

Efficiency of Transfer and Persistence of Expression: Not Always 100% Required

The former paragraph could lead a pessimist to the conclusion that chronic conditions will never be treatable by gene therapy. The good news come from the fact that for some conditions such as hemophilia *(23)* or CF and many others, a fraction of the natural levels of expression is sufficient to achieve therapeutic effects. When attempting to correct those conditions, it is sufficient to guarantee between 5 and 10% of transformation of the target tissue. Therefore, the corresponding vehicles do not need to sustain a 100% transfer, although the problem of persistence of the transformed cells is still relevant.

On the other hand, there are treatments that require neither high efficiency nor specificity nor persistence of the transfer. On example is DNA-based vaccination *(24,25)*, where a permanent effect is achieved upon transient expression of a transgene. Another spectacular example is the corrections of critical limb ischemia *(26)* where the ectopic and transient expression of naked DNA injected intramuscularly brings about sufficient vascular-endothelial growth factor (VEGF) signal to rescue ischemic tissue. Analogous protocols are currently considered for treatment of other cardiovascular conditions where a short-term treatment can produce long-lasting beneficial effects. These examples should suffice to illustrate the concept that efficiency, specificity, and persistence are not matter of business in all cases of gene-assisted therapy, and this is of encouragement for all those who believe in this type of intervention.

Specificity: Strategies, Satisfactions, and Frustrations

The choice of the physical strategy for delivery determines the requirements to the vehicle. Gene transfer can be achieved ex vivo (for example in bone marrow explants) and in this case, the specificity and immediate immunogenicity (*see* below) of the vector are less relevant. In other protocols, specificity can also be achieved in vivo by local application (inhalation, double-balloon catheter, intramuscular, intratumoral, brain stereotactic injection, etc.). Also in this case, the properties of the gene carrier are focusing on efficiency rather than on specificity, because this latter is defined by the administration protocol. Only in systemic delivery (intravenous injection) the problem of targeting becomes relevant. In the simplest cases, one can exploit the natural tendency of some organs such as liver and kidney to accumulate particulated drugs *(27–30)*. However, these organs are not necessarily the targets in all disorders and this poses some serious problems of readdressing the accumulation of the transgene-bearing vehicle (*see* Bio-Weapon 1/Targeting and Retargeting and Bio-Weapon 2/Targeting and Retargeting sections). The problem is double, because not only does one have to devise specific docking elements on the carrier particles, but one has also to circumvent nonspecific accumulation in the aforementioned organs (*see* one example in ref. *31*).

Integration: To Be or Not To Be? In Either Case You'll Pay a Fee

As noted earlier, a reproducible and efficient method for inserting the transgene into a defined chromosomal location is still lacking. This situation causes two side-problems: gene silencing from position effects (*see* also The Choice of *cis*-Elements section) and random insertional mutagenesis (that will be further commented upon in Safety Considerations section). Therefore there is not yet a satisfactory protocol that ensures indefinite persistence of the transgene without causing the two aforementioned effects. This problem will be solved only when either locus-specific integration can be achieved (as originally hoped with the AAV vectors *[32,33]*) or when self-replicating and segregating artificial chromosomes *(34)* will be available. Until then, when we choose an integrating vector for our preferred protocol, we must be aware that we shall benefit from its potential to make the gene persist, but at the same time to randomly disturb resident functions and to be subject to uncontrollable position effects.

Of course we can choose to utilize a nonintegrating vector such as an RNA virus, an adenovirus *(35)*, or a herpes virus *(36)*. In these cases, the transgene persists for a while but is not co-replicated when the host cell proliferates and is destined to be lost. Therefore, the dilemma is in the choice of accepting the benefits of chromosomal integration and pay the fee of random silencing and insertional mutagenesis, or avoid these latter but paying the fee of nonpermanent transformation.

Viral vs Nonviral: Who Wins?

The nonviral modes of gene transfer include physical, chemical, and biochemical protocols. Among the physical methods direct injection of naked DNA *(37)*, pressure-mediated transfer *(38,39)*, electrically enhanced transfer *(40,41)*, and biolistic bombardment *(42,43)* have showed various degrees of efficiency. The chemicals/biochemical protocols include the use of cationic lipids and different compaction methods and each company or research lab claims to have better results, although it is rare to see direct and extensive cross-comparisons in the published papers. Recently, the biochemical methods in which viral proteins are included to spike liposomes *(33,44–46)* have received increased attention, because they seem to promise enhanced gene transfer coupled to increased targeting. Although we can observe that in cell cultures DNA can be delivered to more than 99% of the cells, only a minor portion (3–10%) will ultimately transiently express the transgene (Rusconi and Ceppi, unpublished results). This discrepancy is owing to the second barrier in gene transfer: the nuclear envelope *(37,47)*. It is hypothesized that the majority of the transfected DNA is degraded in the cytoplasm and is not reaching the nucleus. Among the strategies that have been recently proposed to reinforce this second transfer, we shall mention the attempts to link to the DNA oligopeptides containing nuclear localization sequences *(48,49, and references therein)*. In our laboratory, we are exploring the possibility of using resident nuclear shuttles to favor the import of the transgenes into the target cells. The strategy has been named Steroid-Mediated Gene Delivery (SMGD; Fig. 1) and aims at using intracellular nuclear receptors as ferrying vectors for the transfected DNA. Nuclear receptors such as the steroid receptors have nanomolar affinities for specific ligands and are nucleophilic; therefore, they appear to be excellent candidates for efficient and specific shuttles for macromolecules that display at their surface the cognate ligands. To achieve this, we had to devise strategies to chemically "decorate" the transgene with ligands. So far, we have obtained encouraging results with model compounds interacting with the glucocorticoid receptor (Rebuffat et al., submitted).

SMALL PARADE OF CURRENTLY POPULAR VECTORS

The Simplest Way: Delivering Naked or "Biochemically Dressed" DNA

STRUCTURES AND METHODS

Attempts to deliver naked DNA by direct intramuscular injection have been pioneered by Wolff *(47,50, and references therein)*. The initial encouraging results have prompted a series of emulatory protocols aimed at exploiting this simple delivery system for gene-based vaccination. The mechanism of DNA uptake by muscles is only tentatively explained *(50)*, and has so far precluded the rational design of improvements of the

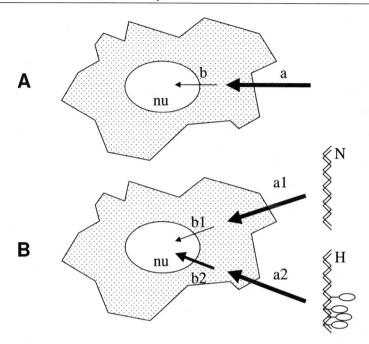

Fig. 1. The two barriers for gene transfer and the principle of SMGD. **(A)** In gene transfer, the genetic material must pass two barriers: the cell membrane (a) and the nuclear envelope (b). Only a small proportion of the transferred nucleic acids undergoes nuclear transfer (compare thin arrow under b and thick arrow under a). **(B)** The concept of steroid-mediated gene delivery. Conventional DNA (N), even if abundantly transfected (thick arrow marked a1) is only poorly translocated into the nucleus (thin arrow marked b1). Ligand-decorated DNA (marked H, where ovals with bar represent covalently linked ligands) is equally well-transfected (a2), but better transported to the nucleus (b2) by the nuclear receptor that binds to the cognate ligand. This approach permits the selective facilitation of nuclear uptake of transgenes. In our laboratory we have proved this concept with model systems involving the glucocorticoid receptor (Rebuffat et al., submitted).

efficiency. In spite of its simplicity, this method has been the first ever bringing clinically relevant results in the treatment of critical limb ischemia with ectopic expression of VEGF *(26)*.

Besides these straightforward but highly empirical approaches, a number of ways to enhance the uptake of DNA has been adapted from the long-standing experience with cell-cultures. This has led to the reformulation of various combinations of liposomes, lipoplexes, and poly-lipoplexes *(51)* and to other sophisticated receptor-ligand mediated internalization systems *(52)*. These efforts have built an important platform of technologies for general and specific gene transfer, although the efficiency of these transfer methods is still several logs inferior to the virally based modes. In general, to achieve anything between 0.1 and few percent of transfected cells, one has to employ a 10exp[4] to 10exp[5] molecules/cell, whereas with viral transfer 1–10 particles/cell can give up to 100% transfer. This poses also the problem of the kinetics of delivery. When added in one bulk, the excess molecules are either lost, degraded or can generate nonspecific immune reactions. Therefore, nonviral transfer usually implies the continuous delivery over a period of time. Recent advances in the design of biodegradable microspheres or encapsulating biopolymers that progressively liberate trapped DNA has shed new perspectives on this strategy *(28,53–56)*. Still, when working with nonviral delivery, one has to deal with the meager efficiency of nuclear transfer of the transfected DNA *(see* above). This problem subsists independently to the delivery method and is one of the reasons of the large ratio (active molecules/cell) that is required to achieve reasonable transformation rates. Finally, there is no specific mechanism for integration into the host genome, and this relegates nonviral transfer to the realm of transient treatments, unless the encouraging results with transposase co-expression will be confirmed *(57)*. For these reasons, transfer of naked DNA is currently only indicated for DNA-based vaccinations, which nevertheless held a phenomenal potential in the prevention of infectious diseases and cancer *(25)*.

TARGETING

The use of microsphere-aided delivery *(see* above) can help in specific augmentation of local concentration of the active molecules, thus providing a sort of topical specificity. Other ways of simple targeting are offered by the body anatomy, which permits molecular treatment of mucosae, epithelia, and so on. When injected systemically, each liposome formulation displays minor differences in the preferences of organ accumulation *(28,30)*. However, the common tendency is that formulations accumulate in liver and kidney and are not able to pass blood-brain barrier *(36,58)*. This natural trend will be an important hurdle in designing specifically targeted formulations. Drastic protocols such as liver by-pass *(31)* are good for a proof-of-principle of how to short-circuit this problem but cannot be clinically implemented in a generalized manner. A major effort has been devoted to the identification of molecular components of the endothelial zip-code system *(59,60)*. Once understood, this tissue-specific marking of the vascular system could provide an elegant system of local accumulation of active particles.

At the cellular level, the best candidates protocols in particle targeting are the ones that exploit affinity of ligands for surface receptors *(52)*. Some important improvements have been achieved by preparing "virosomes" *(33,44)*, in which viral proteins are decorating the surface of liposomes. If proven to be reproducibly infectious and compatible with large-scale preparation, these hybrid particles can pave the way to the generation of "artificial viruses" that may enjoy the advantages of in vitro assembly and avoid some of the disadvantages of biologically assembled viruses *(see* Macromolecular Weapons/Advantages and Disadvantages section).

ADVANTAGES AND DISADVANTAGES

The production of in vitro assembled particles can be better controlled and guaranteed be devoid of adventitious infectious pathogens. Therefore, these formulations are pharmacologically safer than biologically assembled infectious particles. Secondly, there will be less constraints on the size of the transgene, which is a major problem in biologically assembled viral particles *(see* Bio-Weapon 1 section). Furthermore, the composition of synthetic particles can be designed to be devoid of immunogenic elements. Therefore, in vitro formulations containing nucleic acids can be considered suitable for multiple readministrations, a property that is not yet guaranteed with the most popular viral vectors. The lack of immunogenicity should not, however, be overemphasized, because DNA that has been conventionally amplified in bacterial systems (the most convenient basis of molecular large-scale preparation) acquires some intrinsic immunogenicity because of the loss of methylation of CpG-rich sequences *(61–64)* and perhaps also because of some other newly acquired bacterial-methylation patterns *(63)*. Those problems can be theoretically solved, although there is no clear picture of the mid- and long-term reaction of an immune-competent organism subjected to repeated DNA delivery that does not go through the digestive tract.

The major disadvantage of nonviral transfer methods remains obviously the intrinsic low efficiency of transfer. The improvements of the last f–10 yr have increased the transfer rate perhaps by a factor of ten, but there are several logs to catch up with the viral transfer (*see* The Simplest Way/Structures and Methods section). Even more recent advances *(65)* make us believe that nonviral gene transfer may become suitable one day also for situations where transfer efficiency is crucial.

SUITABILITY AND EXAMPLES

Paradoxically to its intrinsic inefficiency, nonviral gene delivery has been the first treatment to demonstrate unequivocal therapeutic value. This occurred in the seminal experiments by the research team of Jeff Isner *(26)*, in which the expression of a provascularizing factor (VEGF) through simple intramuscular injection of a suitable recombinant plasmid has rescued necrotizing limbs already in Phase I trials. We are looking forward to confirmations of these encouraging data in Phase II and Phase III trials, as well as their extension of other treatments in the cardiovascular field. The trials of Victor Dzau and colleagues *(39)* are another success story in nonviral gene-assisted treatment. Artery bypass based on vein grafts currently fails in a high proportion owing to the aberrant growth of the intima, induced by the higher blood pressure in the transplanted vein. The team of Dzau has pretreated the graft with a simple pressure-mediated gene transfer and shown that the transferred genes were able to inhibit the hyper-proliferation of the smooth-muscle cells, thus reducing significantly the occlusion of the graft. The transgenes chosen were either growth-inhibitory genes or decoy-oligonucleotides that transiently titrate transcriptional factors that are essential for the expression of proproliferatory genes.

We conclude this paragraph by mentioning the discovery of the interesting properties of the herpes viral protein VP22 *(66)*. This protein is capable of cell-to-cell transfer and can translocate into cells even when added to the extracellular medium. This property extends to some VP22 chimeric proteins *(67,* and references therein). It appears that this is *(68)* just the tip of the iceberg of several new protein-mediated macro-molecular transfer systems that may solve some of the current problems of nonviral transfer, provided they can be designed to be invisible to the immune system.

Replication-Defective and Replication-Competent Viruses

GENERAL FEATURES OF REPLICATION-DEFECTIVE RECOMBINANT VIRUSES

Viruses have evolved over millions of years to become professional gene-porters. They can exploit the most sophisticated molecular mechanisms to escape immune surveillance, to specifically dock to target tissues, to enter through cell membranes, to resist intracellular degradative enzymes, to deliver nucleic acids to the nucleus, or to organize specialized compartments for genome replication and expression, to integrate into host genome, or to remain latent for several years in host organisms. Therefore, there is no better vehicle that can be envisioned by gene therapists to transfer efficiently the preferred therapeutic gene. Viruses have however a very nasty property: their capsid proteins are mostly immunogenic or toxic and their genetic reprogramming strongly disturbs the cell metabolism and causes diseases of various severity. A better knowledge of the viral genomes has permitted the distinction of segments necessary for the packaging into the capsid from those encoding replicative functions and capsid or envelope components. This has permitted to construct viruses that retain only fragments of their genome and are debilitated in some vital functions. These defective viruses need to be amplified either in specialized packaging cells or in presence of helper viruses that provide *in trans* the missing functions. The situation is different for each virus and it would be too intricate to comment all the sequence geographies, thus I will take the example of the adenovirus to illustrate the steps undertaken to optimize transfer vectors for gene therapy. The adenoviral genome consists of 36 kb of linear DNA with inverted terminal repeats that are indispensable for replication and packaging into the capsid *(35,69)*. The "left" portion (E1/E2 in Fig. 2A) contains the early genes whose expression is indispensable to prepare the conditions for genome replication *(69)*. Other early functions are scattered in other regions and are dispensable for replication. The remaining 80% of the genome is occupied by the late genes, mostly expressed through the major late promoter (MLP; Fig. 2A) and giving rise to variegated proteins through differential splicing. In packaging cells, the "early" portion of the genome could be anchored into the chromosomes and shown to be functioning *in trans*. This permits the growth and assembly of viral genomes whose early segment is either missing or substituted by a transgene of interest (Fig. 2B). This scheme has been maintained in all the viruses of so called first and second generation. Those recombinant viruses have proven invaluable to demonstrate efficient gene transfer in animal models and also in patients *(33,69–71)*. However, the remaining leaky segment encoding late genes confers a significant immunogenic potential to those generation I vectors. Therefore, the expression in immune-competent animals is restricted to few weeks. Several strategies have been proposed to reduce this immunogenicity *(69)*. The best solution so far has been offered by the so-called "gutless" (also called "helper-dependent" or "high-capacity" or "third generation") adeno-vectors. In these constructs, the entire late region is replaced by a neutral DNA segment (Fig. 2C) and the recombinant genome is grown and packaged in presence of a helper virus whose assembly is repressed by various strategies *(69,70)*. After careful purification one can obtain significant titers of the recombinant vectors that are minimally contaminated (approx 10exp[-4]) by the helper virus. Extremely encouraging results have been recently reported with these gutted Adenovectors that were shown to produce a permanent somatic-gene alteration that can persist for several months *(72,73)* even in immunocompetent animals. We are confident that clinical trials involving gutted viruses will confirm the compatibility of these vectors with long-term correction by gene transfer.

PRINCIPLE OF REPLICATION-COMPETENT VIRUSES

Several viruses encode early proteins that interact with tumor suppressors such as *p53* or *retinoblastoma*. By exploiting this situation, some research teams have developed recombinant viruses that maintain a conditional replicative potential whose fulfilment depends on the absence of tumor-suppressor functions. Selective or at least preferential replication has been reported for adenoviruses that retain the *E1B* gene *(74–76)*, for

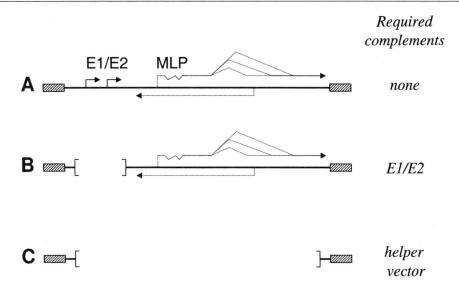

Fig. 2. Genomes of wild type and recombinant adenovectors. **(A)** The genome of wild type adenoviruses (*see* text for refs.) is a linear 36 kb dsDNA flanked by inverted terminal repeats (ITR, hatched boxes) that are necessary for DNA replication and packaging. The indispensable early functions are E1 and E2 that are encoded by a 25% left portion of the genome (*see* E1 and E2). The late functions (capsid protein) are encoded by the remaining part and are mostly transcribed through the major late promoter (MLP) that gives rise to alternatively spliced mRNAs (broken dotted line). The late portion of the genome encodes in the opposite direction the viral DNA polymerase (dotted arrow pointing to left). **(B)** Replication-deficient adenovectors of the first generation are deleted in the early region and can be grown in packaging cells that provide the E1 and E2 functions. The deletion allows the accommodation of up to 8 kb of foreign DNA. **(C)** "Gutless" or "high-capacity" adenovectors retain only the ITR region and can accommodate up to 32 kb of foreign DNA. These recombinant genomes can only be packaged in presence of a helper vector (*see* text).

HSV *(77–80)* and other RNA viruses *(33)*. These viruses are capable of lithic growth in cells that are missing or underexpressing tumor suppressors and this property makes them attractive candidates for tumor treatments, and this has also led to some clinical protocols. Only the future will tell *(81)* whether these expectations are well-placed and whether these oncolytic viruses can be safely used either as stand-alone or as combination-treatment in tumor therapy.

Bio-Weapon 1: DNA Viruses

STRUCTURES AND METHODS

In the preceding paragraphs, we have illustrated the principles behind recombinant adenoviruses. Therefore we will not comment further on these developments. With analogous protocols two other important DNA viral carriers have been designed: the adeno-associated viruses (AAV) and the herpes viruses (HSV). These two are distinguished by diametrically opposite properties. The recombinant AAV particles have a very limited packaging capacity (3.5–4 kb) and integrate the recombinant DNA into the host genome *(32,36,82)*. The intact AAV has the capacity of integrating specifically into a site on chromosome 19, but this property is missing in the emptied recombinant genomes, which integrate randomly, although there is some open controversy on the real extent of their integration *(83)*. In spite of this random integration, the recombinant-AAV constructs seem to be refractory to gene silencing through position effects. this property is currently attributed to the AAV terminal repeats that seem to possess some kind of "insulator" property that renders the intervening sequence rather independent of the integration context *(84)*. The increasingly simple protocols for production of r-AAVs and the extremely low immunogenicity and toxicity of these particles has prompted a large number of investigations of therapeutic gene transfer both preclinical and clinical *(13,23,85–88)*. Therefore, these vectors promise to be a reasonable choice for the permanent transfer of small-sized constructs. The construction of HSV vectors is more laborious but offers several advantages. Particularly interesting is the possibility of generating recombinant genomes of very high capacity (up to 150 kb *[33,36,89]*). This opportunity could permit the transfer of large loci or of multiple regulatory cassettes for precise tuning of gene expression.

Recently, an interesting variation on the theme has emerged: the possibility of combining the advantages of two independent viruses. For instance, hybrid genomes that combine the great infectious capacity of adenovectors and the possibility of integrating the transgene through a surrogate retroviral transposition have been proposed *(32,33,76,82)*. Analogously, hybrid HSV-AAV vectors that combine the large capacity of packaging of HSV and the integration power of AAV have also been proposed *(32,33,36,89)*. These hybrid viral vectors are probably still at their rudimentary stage, but represent exciting developments in a field that would otherwise have stagnated over the intrinsic limitations of each individual carrier.

TARGETING AND RETARGETING

Every virus has a natural tropism that is defined by the host molecular partners required for infection, replication, and packaging. When working with recombinant viruses, the primary factor is represented by the infection mechanism. This is dependent on the match between the cell-surface receptors/coreceptors and the docking sites displayed at the surface of the infectious particle. There are essentially two ways of changing the infectivity tropism: one is to alter the docking proteins (for instance the adeno fibers *[71,76,90,91]*) by adding protein domains that represent ligands for alternative receptors; another consists in preparing Janus-type ligands that on one side interact with the original docking structure and on the other face they provide a new ligand *(90)*. The latter strategy has the advantage of maintaining the same general structure of the vector and is probably preferable to the former strategy, which can alter the properties of the capsid but requires specially engineered packaging cells for the amplification of the recombinant vector. Both strategies have been tried in cellular and animal models, but the success has been so far only moderate, because the new specificity imposed a high price in infectivity. These approaches will require substantial improvement before being suitable for serious clinical trials.

ADVANTAGES AND DISADVANTAGES

The recombinant DNA viruses mentioned above share several advantages. They can be grown at very high titers (between 10exp[9] to 10exp[11] per mL), they have a very stable genome, and they can efficiently infect both proliferating and nonproliferating cells. This latter property is certainly the most attractive for somatic-gene transfer, because many therapies would require the gene transfer in cells that do not proliferate such as neurons, endothelial cells, and so on. Adeno and HSV do not integrate their genome, and this can be considered as both advantageous and disadvantageous. The persistence as unintegrated genomes makes them immune to position effects (good news), but also implies the dilution of the recombinant genome upon proliferation of the infected cells (bad news). The recombinant AAVs combine the capacity of integrating with a partial resistance towards position effects. However, a major disadvantage of AAV is the restricted packaging capacity (at most 4 kb of foreign DNA), whereas r-adenos of the first generation can carry transgenes around 8 kb and "gutted" adeno can accommodate more than 30 kb or HSV episomes can arrange up to 150 kb *(36,89)*. The immunogenic potential of the DNA viruses is different fore each vector, with r-Adenos of the first generation being the most immunogenic and thus suitable only for unique treatments and for treatment of disorders where a certain immune reaction may even be advantageous such as cancer.

SUITABILITY AND EXAMPLES

The literature on preclinical studies with DNA viral vectors is extremely wide and covers all possible disease models from cancer to infectious disorders. However, very few reports bring convincing evidence of potential up-scalability to large animals. For several years, hyper-critical circles used to say that gene therapy has until now "only been good to cure mice." In spite of these sarcastic affirmations, progress in some areas has been rather spectacular. The natural tendency of adenoviruses to accumulate in the liver after systemic administration had prompted a series of interesting trials for the correction of metabolic disorders *(33,69,76)*. Unfortunately, the tragic events linked with one of these trials *(92–96)* has slowed down the experimentation with further improved adenovectors, including gutted adenos. Furthermore, the transduction of recombinant AAV expressing blood-clotting factors has been demonstrated to provide long-term therapeutic benefits in both small and large animal models *(23,33,85,87,88,97)*. Similarly, the use of HSV and gutted adenoviruses in preclinical tests has shown convincing persistence of gene expression in many tissues *(33,87)*. Thus, DNA viruses remain powerful tools for the treatment of both acute and chronic conditions.

Bio-Weapon 2: RNA Viruses

STRUCTURES AND METHODS

RNA viruses tend to have a relatively small and less stable genome compared to DNA viruses. The unstability of RNA genomes is mainly owing to the lack of proofreading in RNA replication and this results in error rates in the range of one mistake in 10,000 nucleotides. Most RNA viruses can only transiently persist within a cell, but the retroviruses can convert their RNA genome into a cDNA, which is transposed into the host genome and thus can be virtually carried indefinitely within the host cell. This latter property has immediately evidenced retroviruses as preferred vectors for gene transfer. The inspiration of the ability of retroviruses to carry foreign genes certainly comes from the early discovery of murine and avian oncogenic retroviruses, which can transduce cellular protooncogenes. The first attempts to construct engineered retroviruses was indeed based on murine retroviruses. The essential *cis*-elements that must be carried along with the engineered genome are the long terminal repeats (LTR), the packaging region, and the primer annealing sequence *(98)*. The genes for the necessary proteins (reverse transcriptase, capsid, and envelope protein) can be transferred to host chromosomes in packaging cells. Once transfected with a plasmid encoding the engineered retroviral backbone, these packaging cells can produce infectious particles at titers around 10exp[6] 10exp[7] *(98)*. The engineering of recombinant lentiviruses is more laborious because several regulatory proteins must be concertedly expressed to allow packaging *(33,36,99)*. Initially, the best system seems to be via co-transfection of *trans*-complementing plasmids *(100)*. The complexity of the procedure is such that it cannot fully exclude the arising of recombinant genomes that are capable of autonomous replication (replication competent particles; RCP). The latent chance of the emergence of these RCPs has certainly strongly hampered the clinical implementation of protocols with lentiviral backbones, and this in spite of the obvious advantage of lentivirus over other retroviruses: their capacity for infecting quiescent cells *(99)*. The recent availability of stable packaging cell lines *(101–103)* may solve the biosafety dilemma.

TARGETING AND RETARGETING

The viral envelope (consisting of host cell membrane spiked by env proteins) can be virtually engineered at will. The currently used winning horse is the VSV env protein *(98)*. Several attempts to engineer the env proteins to change their docking specificities have been reported. These attempts have invariably resulted in lower titers because there is little way to rationally redesign docking surfaces. Given the improvements in recombinant virus handling, we can anticipate that new specificities will be obtained through genetic selection from combinatorial libraries rather than through rational design. Alternatively, changes of tropism can be obtained as for the Adenovirus, by coating a general env-protein with bifunctional ligands that on one hand mask the natural specificity and on the other hand contact alternative docking sites (*see* also Bio-Weapon 1/Targeting and Retargeting section). Unfortunately, it is not guaranteed that all docking sites will be suitable for viral internalization, which is a rather complicated process.

ADVANTAGES AND DISADVANTAGES

The major advantage of retroviral backbones is that they can be assembled free of viral-protein coding genes. This means that after integration a properly engineered provirus will not encode for immunogenic viral proteins, thus guaranteeing a long term survival of the transduced cell. The major advantage of lentiviruses is the capacity of infecting nonproliferating cells (*see* Bio-Weapon 2/Structures and Methods section), a situation that is advantageous for the treatment of differentiated tissues or slowly turning over tissues such as the central nervous system (CNS), endothelium, or bones.

A major disadvantage of retroviruses is the low titer (two to four logs lower than the one of DNA viruses. A standard in vivo therapy may require between 10exp[12] an 10exp[13] infectious particles. For DNA vectors, this means processing volumes of less than 1 L, whereas tens to hundreds of liters may be necessary to obtain the same amount of retroviruses. This situation may become a strong drawback for the industrial preparation of clinical materials. The more subtle disadvantage of retroviruses is the intrinsic low-fidelity of replication. Assuming 1 mutation for every 10 kb, every third copy of a 3 kb transgene sequence will contain at least one mismatch. This can result in the loss of the biological activity in a large fraction of the transduced cells. Finally, as with AAV systems, the random integration into the host genome and the rather limited (about 9 kb) packaging capacity pose problems of long-term maintenance of gene expression (*see* Integration section) and to insertional mutagenesis.

SUITABILITY AND EXAMPLES

The very first bona fide gene-therapy clinical trial (treatment of ADA deficiency *[104]*) was indeed performed with recombinant murine retroviruses. Since then, retroviruses have been used to carry compensatory genes or toxic genes in many clinical protocols. However, none of these attempts appeared to demonstrate significant therapeutic effects. Recently (C. Bordignon, personal communication) it could be demonstrated that the positive outcome was probably obscured by the concomitant treatment with the detoxifying drug PEG-ADA, which prevented the positive selection of transduced cells. The major drawback of recombinant murine retrovirus is their inability to infect quiescent cells, but this property is rescued in the lentiviral systems (*see* Bio-Weapon 2/Structures and Methods section), which have shown to be equally versatile and yet capable of infecting postmitotic cells *(99)*. The improvements in assembly will soon permit to produce recombinant lentiviruses guaranteed free of replication-competent particles, and this will open their option for clinical trials.

Finally, the simplicity of the original murine retroviral system already used in the very first gene therapy attempts by Anderson or Bordignon *(104,105)*, has not discouraged the team of Alain Fischer, that ultimately has brought the very first historical example of permanent radical cure of a genetic disorder by the ex vivo transduction of bone marrow transplants with vectors supplementing the IL-2-receptor gene that is defective in a rare form of severe combined immunodeficiency (SCID) *(87,106)*. The four young patients of Dr. Fischer are the best results that gene therapy has scored within its short adventure, and for the public opinion are more worth than thousands of preclinical "mouse therapies" or reporter assays. Resting on these encouraging indications, gene therapy-based simple viral vectorology may indeed pave the way to several efficacious intermediate clinical applications. Whether or not this strategy will persist in the long term depends only on further improvements, but we can say that, if wisely used, today's vectors already have a significant potential for the treatment of chronic disorders.

Macromolecular Weapons: A Short Click at the www.fantasticoligo.com Site

STRUCTURES AND METHODS

Gene therapy does not require the transfer of full genetic complements to become effective. Small gene fragments, in form of synthetic single-stranded or double-stranded oligonucleotides, can exert a powerful control on gene expression. The most popular form of oligonucleotide-assisted therapy is done with antisense sequences that are destined to block either the maturation or the translation of specific mRNAs. Protocols aimed at tumor control through oligonucleotides that downregulate the production of protoonogenic proteins or anti-apoptotic factors have achieved phase III *(107)*. A further sophistication is the use of oligonucleotides that have a ribozyme function *(108)* and are able to specifically hydrolyze target mRNAs. Also double-stranded "decoy" oligonucleotides that compete with genomic sequences by binding transcription factors have been successfully used in the clinic *(39)*. A further level of sophistication is represented by oligonucleotides that are capable of forming triple-helix structures with specific target sequences. For triplex formation, the only *a priori* requirement for the target sequence is that purines and pyrimidines should be segregated on the two strands (*109,* and references therein). Oligonucleotides capable of repressing or stimulating gene expression have been designed in this manner *(110,111).* Recently, triplex-forming oligos capable of guiding molecules that induce specific repair of target sequences have been proposed *(112).* The major disadvantage of oligonucleotides is their short survival within a cell. Therefore, these protocols imply either continuous supply of the therapeutic oligo or single treatment of acute conditions. Several modifications of the desoxy-ribonucleotide backbone have been proposed to augment the resistance of oligos toward degradative nucleases. The most spectacular modification is probably the so-called peptide-nucleic acid (PNA) backbone, in which the carrier polymer is no longer a phosphate-ribose chain *(113,114,* and references therein). A great advantage of PNA is certainly the lower negative charge of the polymer, which enormously stabilizes either the double- or triple-stranded structures that it can form with target sequences. PNA has been shown to be easy to handle and to permit also accumulation into cellular subcompartments such as mitochondria *(115),* a condition that is not met by other nucleic acid-transfer methods. We are certain that PNA will become the polymer of choice for the locus-specific accumulation of active principles.

Finally, a bizarre family of chimeric oligonucleotides called "chimeroplasts" or "chimeraplasts" has been reported to be capable of inducing specific gene repair at impressing frequency *(112,116–119).* Although the exact mechanism and the prerequisites imposed on the chimeric oligonucleotide structure remain poorly rationalized, the efficiency with which it repairs if single-base pair mutations has reached up to 40% under some circumstances *(117,120).* There is still some controversy about the general applicability of the chimeraplasty, about its real efficiency and safety, and about the number of molecules that must accumulate into a cell to obtain satisfactory frequencies of repair. Also, for a certain time this technology could not be reproduced by research teams independent of the original discoverer. However, recent reports indicate that this technique may have finally worked in several laboratories *(119,120).* If indeed broadly applicable, chimeraplasty may become the method of choice for the treatment of many disorders caused by small genetic defects (single nucleotide mutations). The greatest advantage of this technique is that it promises to be exquisitely site-specific, thus to generate far fewer if any undesired side effects. If chimeraplasty can be ameliorated to achieve close to 100% repair, it may become a technique that reopens the option of germline interventions, with all the bulky complement of ethical problems accompanying this dossier. In fact, taken at face value, chimeraplasty is the only available technology that fully deserves the denomination of "gene therapy" in its strictest sense.

TARGETING

Owing to its principle, oligonucleotide-mediated therapy does not need to be strictly targeted, because it is aimed at precise interactions through base-pairing. However, given the very high costs of oligonucleotides, it will certainly be pharmacologically advantageous if the therapeutic oligos can be specifically delivered or accumulated to target tissues. We envisage that our SMGD protocol (*see* Viral vs Nonviral section) can be also adapted to ameliorate the accumulation of oligonucleotides in a tissue-preferential manner. Local delivery is so far the most popular option, although decoration with specific ligands for internalizing receptors has been very promising, at least with liver-directed therapy with chimeraplasts *(121).*

ADVANTAGES AND DISADVANTAGES

Compared to intact genes, oligonucleotides have molecular sizes of several orders of magnitude smaller (few thousand Daltons). This smaller size renders them more similar to conventional drugs, although they do not easily permeate through cell membranes. A second advantage is that oligonucleotides do not require biosynthetic steps for their preparation, an thus can be more easily formulated under pathogen-free conditions.

The main disadvantage is that oligos tend to be degraded after a relatively short time, implying that the treatment of persisting diseases will require repeated administrations. The chimeraplasts are indeed able to produce a permanent effect, but their current range of correction is limited to single-point mutations.

SUITABILITY AND EXAMPLES

In spite of the limitations mentioned earlier, oligonucleotides have been maintaining their therapeutic promises. After transfer of double-stranded decoy oligonucleotides that titrate transcription factors controlling cell proliferation, Dzau and colleagues have been able to reduce significantly the incidence of intima-growth in vein transplants *(39)*. In this case, the merit of the approach is that the transient treatment is sufficient to bring a permanent effect, because it sustains the nondegenerative adaptation of veins to the higher pressure. We have also already mentioned the spectacular correction rate obtained in rat models of a liver disorder *(117)* with chimeroplasty. Here also, a short treatment permits a long-term therapeutic effect. Several antisense oligo approaches against protooncogenes are now in advanced clinical testing. However, we have to wait for these tests to assess the validity of this approach. Personally, we are quite skeptical about these anti-cancer therapies, especially because they do not offer a priori any bystander effect (*see* Correcting Disorders Derived from Loss-of-Function or Gain-of-Function section) and therefore seem less suitable for tumor eradication.

FINAL HURDLES AND CONCLUSIONS

Immune Response and Readministration

This book focuses on the molecular treatment of a disorder with auto-immune and inflammatory components. In this kind of treatment, it is absolutely imperative that the procedure should not imply reagents or manipulations that could unnecessarily activate the cellular or humoral immune system, be it specific or innate. Therefore, the work with viral vectors of any kind should be considered with substantial caution. Also, nonviral gene transfer could pose several problems when using entire genes, owing to the innate reaction against unmethylated CpG-rich motifs. In general, readministration is almost unavoidable with the current technology and it does not simplify the foreseeable clinical protocols for the treatment of chronic disorders with inflammatory components. Thus, until better control on the short-term and long-term immunogenicity of gene-delivery systems can be obtained, gene therapy cannot be considered as a first priority for this class of disorders, where it could ultimately exacerbate the outcome instead of bringing a therapeutic effect *(122)*. Finally, the immune system also poses a problem when the vectors themselves are clean of any proinflammatory properties. In fact, in some genetic loss-of-functions the resident gene is either deleted or totally nonfunctional. In this cases, the expression of the healthy gene product can lead to tissue rejection because it is detected as a "foreign" antigen by the host immune system *(23,72,123)*. For these cases, tolerization strategies must be devised before considering gene transfer.

Safety Considerations: From RCP to Insertional Mutagenesis

The immune reactions are not our sole hurdle in virally assisted gene transfer. Some capsid proteins, although providing useful functions such as translocation and protection from degratative enzymes, are themselves toxic and can produce adverse reactions. In fact, most biologically assembled viral preparations contain a large excess (between 10 and 100-fold) of nonfunctional viral particles. These particles can contribute significantly to the overall toxicity of the gene transfer procedure. Also we have mentioned that no biological recombinant viral preparation can be a priori guaranteed to be free of adventitious recombinants that have reacquired viral genes sufficient for autonomous replication (the so-called RCPs; *see* Bio-Weapon 2/Structures and Methods section). Even if the incidence of RCP can be reduced to less than one event in 10exp[14], it may pose serious constraints and cause severe costs augmentation to the industrial preparation of clinical materials.

The vectors that currently permit permanent transfer do not have ways of controlling the site of integration of the transgene. Thus, every cellular integration event is in principle an insertional mutagenesis event. At the somatic level, the large amount of insertional mutagenesis has the potential of generating protumorigenic cells by activating protooncogenes. This relegates the use of integrating vectors for the treatment of life-threatening diseases, where the risk of generating a secondary tumor is still acceptable. The random mutagenesis generates another dilemma if the gene delivery vector transforms germ cells. In this case we would have a large number of additional mutations that would be inherited to subsequent generations, and the potential benefit for the treated individual could become a strong disadvantage for his/her progeny. These dilemmas will be solved when we are able to assemble vectors that can permanently deliver transgenes in specific chromosomal locations. Considering the current pace of progress, this goal should not be very far off.

Pulling it all Together

If a pragmatic reader has had the patience to read all the good and bad news about the existing and prospected vectors, he/she may ask: but after all, which vector/delivery is suitable for my goal?

In Table 1, we summarize the suitability of the currently available gene-transfer methods (columns) for different types of treatment. The number of "+" signs indicates qualitatively the suitability of a given combination. We hope that this synopsis may help in the identification of the most appropriate combination.

Outlook: Will Rudimentary Vectorology with all its Troubles Survive the Emerging Challenge of Stem Cell Therapy?

Stem cell research has been booming in the last few months. Primordial cells for almost all the tissues, including the CNS, have been characterized, and the major hope is that the ex vivo cultivation of those may permit tissue regeneration for various treatments *(124,125)*. The most spectacular observation is certainly that some stem cells seem to be capable of *trans*-determination; that is, to give rise to differentiated cells that are

Table 1
Qualitative Assessment of Suitability of Delivery Vehicles

Application	ADV	AAV	HSV	HIV	OLI	PEM	GUN	LIP
Vaccination/prevention	++	(+)	(+)	(+)	–	–	+++	(+)
Acute treatment	++	–	–	–	++	–	–	+
Chronic treatment	–	++	++	+++	(+)	–	–	+
In vivo local delivery	++	++	++	++	++	+	++	+
In vivo systemic delivery	+	+	+	+	+	n	n	+
Ex vivo delivery	++	+	+	+++	++	++	+	++
Single administration	+++	+++	+++	+++	+	+	+	+
Repeated administration	(+)	+	(+)	++	+++	+	+++	+++
Treat loss-of-function	+++	+++	+++	+++	+	++	+	++
Treat gain-of-function	(+)	+	+	+	+++	–	–	+
Gene correction	–	–	–	–	+++	–	–	–

Symbols: ADV, Adenovirus vectors; AAV, adeno-associated virus vectors; HSV, Herpes virus vectors; HIV, lentiviral vectors; OLI, oligonucleotides; PEM, pressure or electroporation-mediated delivery; GUN, biolistic or macroinjection; LIP, lipoplexes or polyplexes. Symbols for suitability: –, not suitable; (+) questionable; +, hardly suitable; ++ , offers several applications; +++, excellent choice; n, does not apply. Most of the indicated degrees of suitability are justified in this chapter.

different from the donor tissue *(105,125,126)*. Many of the claims and reports in this field do not even appear in the peer-reviewed literature, but have been propagated through press releases or news-agency despatches. According to this news, in the foreseeable future, it should be possible to explant bone marrow cells and later reconstruct muscle, nerves, bones, epidermis, and other types of tissues from this original population. The mechanisms that govern the maintenance of the pluripotency and the commitment toward one or another lineage are still obscure, but they are being studied so intensively studied that we can anticipate major breakthroughs within the next few years.

THE WORST AND BEST CASE SCENARIO

Being able to culture stem cells without losing their pluripotency and to then determine their commitment would pave the way to autologous organ reconstruction that could cure an immense number of degenerative disorders. If the disorder has a genetic component, the corresponding correction could be easily achieved with conventional gene transfection ex vivo and corresponding selection of precharacterized recombinant cell clones. This would render obsolete most of the efforts to obtain high-efficiency gene delivery vectors. Those latter would only be required for those cases where a cell therapy is not indicated, such as in acute treatments or corrections of gain-of-function disorders.

Thus, taken at face value, cell therapy has all the hallmarks to become a superior procedure for the treatment of chronic conditions. The worst that could happen is when patents and human ambitions would transform the natural tendency towards a better therapy in a ferocious battle between gene therapists and cell therapists for the best slices of the health market.

The balance of the odds for gene or cell therapy could change drastically if gene correction procedures such as chimeroplasty (*see* Macromolecular Weapons/Structures and Methods section) would confirm their efficacy or if hybrid vectors (*see* Bio-Weapons 1/Structures and Methods section), artificial viruses (*see* The Simplest Way/Targeting section), or coherently integrating vectors (*see* The Choice of *cis*-Elements, Bio-Weapon 1/Advantages and Disadvantages, and Immune Response and Readministration sections) would make it through. If any of those tools would become generally applicable, then gene transfer in vivo would certainly remain competitive, because it implies lower costs, shorter intervention time, and also probably lower invasivity than cell therapy.

A FINAL HOMILY FOR GENE TRANSFER

We have recapitulated the aims and efforts toward developing tools and methods for efficient gene transfer. When taken pessimistically, one could imagine that the few, but highly celebrated, therapeutic achievements are condemned to remain anecdotal, and one wonders why scientists should continue in this direction, which has brought more frustrations than successes. From the point of view of fundamental research, the answer is refreshingly simple. While trying to solve the engineering problem of gene therapy, scientists have rediscovered and partially solved old neglected problems related to cell biology, virology, molecular transport and degradation, cell-surface properties, and so on. Furthermore, the preclinical efforts have produced vectors that are phenomenal tools for fundamental research. Gene transfer vectors are already considered for hit-and-run gene-alteration procedures that will permit temporally and spatially controlled gene knock-out or knock-in in experimental animals, a situation that is laborious to achieve with conventional transgenesis. Furthermore, the gene-transfer vectors open the way to the experimentation with primary cell cultures, which are notoriously refractory to biochemical gene transfer. This will permit the functional study of genes under semi- or fully physiological conditions and a better understanding of the intricate interactions between gene products. Therefore, gene therapy has brought an immense flood of novel knowledge that will substantially accelerate the overall progress in experimental life sciences.

From the clinical/pragmatic point of view, the heroic efforts made in gene therapy must be regarded as necessary steps that have broken the ice and paved the way towards more efficacious molecular therapies. We should not forget that any technological progress, from the airplane to the computer, has started with prototypes that seem almost ridiculous when compared with the today's opportunities. But without these glorious steps, we would still be devoid of such marvelous achievements and would still be gasping for intellectual conjectures about their feasibility instead of enjoying their concrete advantages. So, let's keep going and be proud thereof!

ACKNOWLEDGMENTS

This work has been supported by the Canton of Fribourg and by the Swiss National Science Foundation, program NFP37 'somatic gene therapy' www.unifr.ch/nfp37.

REFERENCES

1. Paillard, F. 1997. Commentary: bystander effects in enzyme/prodrug gene therapy. *Human Gene Ther.* 8:1733–1736.

2. Dilber, M.S. and C.I.E. Smith. 1997. Suicide genes and bystander killing: local and distant effects. *Gene Ther.* 4:273–274.

3. Bennett, J., Y. Zeng, R. Bajwa, L. Klatt, Y. Li, and A.M. Maguire. 1998. Adenovirus-mediated delivery of rhodopsin-promoted bcl-2 results in a delay in photoreceptor cell death in the rd/rd mouse. *Gene Ther.* 5:1156–1164.

4. Boyer, O., J.C. Zhao, J.L. Cohen, D. Depetris, M. Yagello, L. Lejeune, et al. 1997. Position-dependent variegation of a CD4 minigene with targeted expression to mature CD4+ T cells. *J. Immunol.* 159:3383–3390.

5. de Geest, B., L.S. van, M. Lox, D. Collen, and P. Holvoet. 2000. Sustained expression of human apolipoprotein A-I after adenoviral gene transfer in C57BL/6 mice: role of apolipoprotein A-I promoter, apolipoprotein A-I introns, and human apolipoprotein E enhancer. *Human Gene Ther.* 11:101–112.

6. Larochelle, N., H. Lochmüller, J. Zhao, A. Jani, A., P. Hallauer, K. Hastings, et al. 1997. Efficient muscle-specific transgene expression after adenovirus-mediated gene transfer in mice using a 1.35 kb muscle creatine kinase promoter/enhancer. *Gene Ther.* 4:465–472.

7. Grosveld, F. 1999. Activation by locus control regions? *Curr. Opin. Genet. Dev.* 9:152–157.

8. Grosveld, F., B.E. De, N. Dillon, J. Gribnau, E. Milot, T. Trimborn, et al. 1998. The dynamics of globin gene expression and gene therapy vectors. *Ann. NY Acad. Sci.* 850:18–27.

9. Fox, C. and J. Rine. 1996. Influences of the cell cycle on silencing. *Cell* 8:354–357.

10. Paillard, F. 1997. Commentary: Promoter Attenuation in Gene Therapy: Causes and Remedies. *Human Gene Ther.* 8:2009–2010.

11. Ratcliff, F., B. Harrison, and D. Baulcombe. 1997. A similarity between viral defense and gene silencing in plants. *Science* 276:1558–1560.

12. Emery, D.W., H. Chen, Q. Li, and G. Stamatoyannopoulos. 1998. Development of a condensed locus control region cassette and testing in retrovirus vectors for A gamma-globin. *Blood Cells Mol. Dis.* 24:322–339.

13. Inoue, T., H. Yamaza, Y. Sakai, S. Mizuno, M. Ohno, N. Hamasaki, and Y. Fukumaki. 1999. Position-independent human beta-globin gene expression mediated by a recombinant adeno-associated virus vector carrying the chicken beta-globin insulator. *J. Human Genet.* 44:152–162.

14. Dupraz, P., C. Rinsch, W.F. Pralong, E. Rolland, R. Zufferey, D. Trono, and B. Thorens. 1999. Lentivirus-mediated Bcl-2 expression in beta-TC-tet cells improves resistance to hypoxia and cytokine-induced apoptosis while preserving in vitro and in vivo vontrol of insulin secretion. *Gene Ther.* 6:1160–1169.

15. Rinsch, C., E. Regulier, N. Deglon, B. Dalle, Y. Beuzard, Y., and P. Aebischer. 1997. A gene therapy approach to regulated delivery of erythropoietin as a function of oxygen tension [see comments]. *Human Gene Ther.* 8:1881–1889.

16. Simpson, A.M., G.M. Marshall, B.E. Tuch, L. Maxwell, B. Szymanska, J. Tu, et al. 1997. Gene therapy of diabetes: glucose-stimulated insulin secretion in a human hepatoma cell line (HEP G2ins/g). *Gene Ther.* 4:1202–1215.

17. No, D., T.P. Yao, and R.M. Evans. 1996. Ecdysone-inducible gene expression in mammalian cells and transgenic mice. *Proc. Natl. Acad. Sci. USA* 93:3346–3351.

18. Burcin, M.M., G. Schiedner, S. Kochanek, S.Y. Tsai, and B.W. O'Malley. 1999. Adenovirus-mediated regulable target gene expression in vivo. *Proc. Natl. Acad. Sci. USA* 96:355–360.

19. Miller, N. and J. Whelan. 1997. Progress in Transcriptionally Targeted and Regulatable Vectors for Genetic Therapy. *Human Gene Ther.* 8:803–815.

20. McInerney, E.M. and B.S. Katzenellenbogen. 1996. Different regions in activation function-1 of the human estrogen receptor required for antiestrogen- and estradiol-dependent transcription activation. *J. Biol. Chem.* 271:24,172–24,178.

21. Pollock, R. and V.M. Rivera. 1999. Regulation of gene expression with synthetic dimerizers. *Methods Enzymol.* 306:263–281.

22. Bujard, H. 1999. Controlling genes with tetracyclines. *J. Gene Med.* 1:372–374.

23. Kay, M.A., C.S. Manno, M.V. Ragni, P.J. Larson, L.B. Couto, A. McClelland, et al. 2000. Evidence for gene transfer and expression of factor IX in haemophilia B patients treated with an AAV vector [see comments]. *Nature Genet.* 24:257–261.

24. Ulmer, J. and M. Liu. 1999. Delivery systems and ajuvants for DNA vaccines, in The Development of Human Gene Therapy. T. Friedmann, editor. Cold Spring Harbor Laboratory Press, Cold Spring Harbor, NY. 309–330.

25. Restifo, N.P., H. Ying, L. Hwang, and W.W. Leitner. 2000. The promise of nucleic acid vaccines. *Gene Ther.* 7:89–92.

26. Baumgartner, I., A. Pieczek, O. Manor, R. Blair, M. Kearney, K. Walsh, and J.M. Isner. 1998. Constitutive expression of phVEGF165 after intramuscular gene transfer promotes collateral vessel development in patients with critical limb ischemia [see comments]. *Circulation* 97:1114–1123.

27. Dash, P.R., M.L. Read, L.B. Barrett, M.A. Wolfert, and L.W. Seymour. 1999. Factors affecting blood clearance and in vivo distribution of polyelectrolyte complexes for gene delivery. *Gene Ther.* 6:643–650.

28. Lunsford, L., U. McKeever, V. Eckstein, and M.L. Hedley. 1999. Tissue distribution and persistence in mice of plasmid DNA encapsulated in a PLGA-based microsphere delivery vehicle [In Process Citation]. *J. Drug Target* 8:39–50.

29. Reynolds, P., I. Dmitriev, and D. Curiel. 1999. Insertion of an RGD motif into the HI loop of adenovirus fiber protein alters the distribution of transgene expression of the systemically administered vector. *Gene Ther.* 6:1336–1339.

30. Thierry, A.R., P. Rabinovich, B. Peng, L.C. Mahan, J.L. Bryant, and R.C. Gallo. 1997. Characterization of liposome-mediated gene delivery: expression, stability and pharmacokinetics of plasmid DNA. *Gene Ther.* 4:226–237.

31. Ye, X., M. Jerebtsova, and P.E. Ray. 2000. Liver bypass significantly increases the transduction efficiency of recombinant adenoviral vectors in the lung, intestine, and kidney. *Human Gene Ther.* 11:621–627.

32. Schagen, F.H.E., H.J. Rademaker, F.J. Fallaux, and R.C. Hoeben. 2000. Insertion vectors for gene therapy. *Gene Ther.* 7:271–272.

33. Dyer, M.R. and P.L. Herrling. 2000. Progress and potential for gene-based medicines. *Mol. Ther.* 1:213.

34. Ascenzioni, F., P. Donini, and H.J. Lipps. 1997. Mammalian artificial chromosomes: vectors for somatic gene therapy. *Cancer Lett.* 118:135–142.

35. Hitt, M., R.J. Parks, and F.L. Graham. 1999. Structure and genetic organisation of adenovirus vectors, in The Development of Human Gene Therapy. T. Friedmann, editor. Cold Spring Harbor Laboratory Press, Cold Spring Harbor, NY, pp. 61–86.

36. Costantini, L.C., J.C. Bakowska, X.O. Breakfield, and O. Isacson. 2000. Gene therapy in the CNS. *Gene Ther.* 7:93–109.

37. Wolff, J. 1999. Naked DNA gene transfer in mammalian cells, in The Development of Human Gene Therapy. T. Friedmann, editor. Cold Spring Harbor Laboratory Press, Cold Spring Harbor, NY, pp. 279–307.

38. Beardsley, T. 2000. Working under pressure. *Sci. Am.* 282:34.

39. von der Leyen, H.E., R. Braun-Dullaeus, M.J. Mann, L. Zhang, J. Hiebauer, and V.J. Dzau. 1999. A pressure-mediated nonviral method for efficient arterial gene and oligonucleotide transfer. *Human Gene Ther.* 10:2355–2364.

40. Wells, J.M., L.H. Li, A. Sen, G.P. Hahreis, and S.W. Hui. 2000. Electroporation enhanced gene delivery in mammary tumours. *Gene Ther.* 7:541–547.

41. Yanez, R.J. and A.C.G. Porter. 1998. Therapeutic gene targeting. *Gene Ther.* 5:149–159.

42. Mahvi, D. 1997. Phase I/IB study of immunization with autologous tumor cells transfected with the GM-CSF gene by particle-mediated transfer in patients with melanoma or sarcoma. *Human Gene Ther.* 8:875–891.

43. Rakhmilevich, A., K. Janssen, J. Turner, J. Culp, and N.S. Yang. 1997. Cytokine gene therapy of cancer using gene gun technology: superior antitumor activity of interleukin-12. *Human Gene Ther.* 8:1303–1311.

44. Waelti, E. and R. Glück. 1998. Delivery to cancer cells of antisense L-myc oligonucleotides incorporated in fusogenic, cationic-lipid-reconstituted influenza-virus envelopes (cationic virosomes). *Int. J. Cancer* 77:1–6.

45. Saeki, Y., N. Matsumoto, Y. Nakano, M. Mori, K. Awai, and Y. Kaneda. 1997. Development and characterization of cationic liposomes conjugated with HVJ (Sendai Virus): reciprocal effect of cationic lipid for in vitro and in vivo gene tranfer. *Human Gene Ther.* 8:2133–2141.

46. Schoen, P., A. Chonn, P.R. Cullis, J. Wilschut, and P. Scherrer. 1999. Gene transfer mediated by fusion protein hemagglutinin reconstituted in cationic lipid vesicles. *Gene Ther.* 6:823–832.

47. Wolff, J.A. 1997. Naked DNA transport and expression in mammalian cells. *Neuromuscul. Disord.* 7:314–318.

48. Branden, L.J., A.J. Mohamed, A.J., and C.I. Smith. 1999. A peptide nucleic acid-nuclear localization signal fusion that mediates nuclear transport of DNA. *Nature Biotechnol.* 17:784–787.

49. Neves, C., G. Byk, D. Scherman, and P. Wils. 1999. Coupling of a targeting peptide to plasmid DNA by covalent triple helix formation. *FEBS Lett.* 453:41–45.

50. Budker, V., T., B., G., Z., V. Subbotin, A. Loomis, and J. Wolff. 2000. Hypothesis; naked plasmid DNA is taken up by cells in vivo by a receptor-mediated process. *J. Gene Med.* 2:76–88.

51. Felgner, P., O. Zelphati, and X. Liang. 1999. Advances in synthetic gene delivery system technology, in The Development of Human Gene Therapy. T. Friedmann, editor. Cold Spring Harbor Laboratory Press, Cold Spring Harbor, NY. 241–260.

52. Cotten, M. and E. Wagner. 1999. Receptor-mediated gene delivery strategies. In The Development of Human Gene Therapy. T. Friedmann, editor. Cold Spring Harbor Laboratory Press, Cold Spring Harbor, NY, pp. 261–277.

53. Shea, L.D., E. Smiley, J. Bonadio, and D.J. Mooney. 1999. DNA delivery from polymer matrices for tissue engineering [see comments] [published erratum appears in *Nature Biotechnol.* 1999 Aug;17(8):817]. *Nature Biotechnol.* 17:551–554.

54. Roy, K., H.Q. Mao, S.K. Huang, and K.W. Leong. 1999. Oral gene delivery with chitosan—DNA nanoparticles generates immunologic protection in a murine model of peanut allergy [see comments]. *Nature Med.* 5:387–391.

55. Mathiowitz, E., J.S. Jacob, Y.S. Jong, G.P. Carino, D.E. Chickering, P. Chaturvedi, et al. 1997. Biologically erodable microspheres as potential oral drug delivery systems. *Nature 386:410–414.*

56. Hedley, M.L., J. Curley, and R. Urban. 1998. Microspheres containing plasmid-encoded antigens elicit cytotoxic T-cell responses. *Nature Med.* 4:365–368.

57. Izsvak, Z., Z. Ivics and R.H. Plasterk. 2000. Sleeping Beauty, a wide host-range transposon vector for genetic transformation in vertebrates. *J. Mol. Biol.* 302:93–102.

58. Lewis, M.E. 1999. Crossing the blood-brain barrier to central nervous system gene therapy. *Clin. Genet.* 56:10–13.

59. Giancotti, F.G. and R. Ruoslahti. 1999. Integrin signaling. *Science* 285:1028–1032.

60. Folkman, J. 1999. Angiogenic zip code. *Nature Biotech.* 17:749.

61. Hartmann, G. and A.M. Krieg. 1999. CPG DNA and LPS induce distinct patterns of activation in human monocytes. *Gene Ther.* 6:893–903.

62. Krieg, A.M. 2000. Minding the Cs and the Gs. *Mol. Ther.* 1:209.

63. McLachlan, G., B.J. Stevenson, D.J. Davidson, and D.J. Porteous. 2000. Bacterial DNA is implicated in the inflammatory response to delivery of DNA/DOTAP to mouse lungs. *Gene Ther.* 7: 384–392.

64. Paillard, F. 1999. CpG: The double-edged sword. *Human Gene Ther.* 10:2089–2090.

65. Zhang, G., V. Budker, P. Williams, V. Subbotin, and J.A. Wolff. 2001. Efficient expression of naked DNA delivered intraarterially to limb muscles of nonhuman primates. *Hum. Gene. Ther.* 12:427–438.

66. Luft, F.C. 1999. Can VP22 resurrect gene therapy? *J. Mol. Med.* 77:575–576.

67. Elliott, G. and P. O'Hare. 1999. Intercellular trafficking of VP22-GFP fusion proteins. *Gene Ther.* 6:149–151.

68. Xia, H., Q. Mao, and B.L. Davidson. 2001. The HIV Tat protein transduction domain improves the biodistribution of beta-glucuronidase expressed from recombinant viral vectors. *Nat. Biotechnol.* 19:640–644.

69. Wivel, N.A., G.-P. Gao, and J.M. Wilson. 1999. Adenovirus vectors, in The Development of Human Gene Therapy. T. Friedmann, editor. Cold Spring Harbor Laboratory Press, Cold Spring Harbor, NY, pp. 87–110.

70. Amalfitano, A. 1999. Next-generation adenoviral vectors: new and improved. *Gene Ther.* 6:1643–1645.

71. Wickham, T.J. 2000. Targeting adenovirus. *Gene Ther.* 7:110–114.

72. Gallo-Penn, A.M., P.S. Shirley, J.L. Andrews, D.B. Kayda, A.M. Pinkstaff, M. Kaloss, et al. 1999. In vivo evaluation of an adenoviral vector encoding canine factor VIII: high-level, sustained expression in hemophiliac mice. *Human Gene Ther.* 10:1791–1802.

73. Sandig, V., R. Youil, A.J. Bett, L.L. Franlin, M. Oshima, D. Maione, et al. 2000. Optimization of the helper-dependent adenovirus system for production and potency in vivo. *Proc. Natl. Acad. Sci. USA* 97:1002–1007.

74. Heise, C.C., A.M. Williams, S. Xue, M. Propst, and D.H. Kirn. 1999. Intravenous administration of ONYX-015, a selectively replicating adenovirus, induces antitumoral efficacy. *Cancer Res.* 59: 2623–2628.

75. Rogulski, K.R., M.S. Wing, D.L. Paielli, J.D. Gilbert, J.H. Kim, and S.O. Freytag. 2000. Double suicide gene therapy augments the antitumor activity of a replication-competent lytic adenovirus through enhanced cytotoxicity and radiosensitization. *Hum. Gene Ther.* 11:67–76.

76. Reynolds, P.N. and D.T. Curiel. 1999. Strategies to adapt adenoviral vectors to gene therapy applications: targeting and integration, in The Development of Human Gene Therapy. T. Friedmann, editor. Cold Spring Harbor Laboratory Press, Cold Spring Harbor, NY, pp. 111–130.

77. Carew, J.F., D.A. Kooby, M.W. Halterman, H.J. Federoff, and Y. Fong. 1999. Selective infection and cytolysis of human head and neck squamous cell carcinoma with sparing of normal mucosa my a cytotoxic herpes simplex virus type 1 (G207). *Human Gene Ther.* 10:1599–1606.

78. Chase, M., R. Chung, and E.A. Chiocca. 1998. An oncolytic viral mutant that delivers the CYP2B1 transgene and augments cyclophosphamide chemotherapy. *Nature Biotechnol.* 16:444–448.

79. Martiniello-Wilks, R., J. Garcia-Aragon, M. Daja, P. Russell, P., G. Both, P. Molloy, et al. 1998. In vivo gene therapy for prostate cancer: preclinical evaluation of two different enzyme-directed prodrug therapy systems delivered by identical adenovirus vectors. *Human Gene Ther.* 9:1617–1626.

80. Morris, J.C. and O. Wildner. 2000. Therapy of head and neck squamous cell carcinoma with an oncolytic adenovirus expressing HSV-tk. *Mol. Ther.* 1:56–62.

81. Kirn, D. 2001. Clinical research results with dl1520 (Onyx-015), a replication-selective adenovirus for the treatment of cancer: what have we learned? *Gene. Ther.* 8:89–98.

82. Hirata, R.K. and D.W. Russell. 2000. Design and packaging of adeno-associated virus gene targeting vectors [In Process Citation]. *J. Virol.* 74:4612–4620.

83. Nakai, H., S.R. Yant, T.A. Storm, S. Fuess, L. Meuse, and M.A. Kay. 2001. Extrachromosomal recombinant adeno-associated virus vector genomes are primarily responsible for stable liver transduction in vivo. *J. Virol.* 75:6969–6976.

84. Fu, Y., Y. Wang, and S. Evans. 1998. Viral sequences enable efficient and tissue-specific expression of transgenes in Xenopus. *Nature Biotechnol.* 16:253–257.

85. Chao, H., R.J. Samulski, D.A. Bellinger, P. Monahan, T. Nichols, and C.E. Walsh. 1999. Persistent expression of canine factor IX in hemophilia B canines. *Gene Ther.* 6:1695–1704.

86. Monahan, P.E., R.J. Samulski, J. Tazelaar, X. Xiao, T.C. Nichols, D.A. Bellinger, et al. 1998. Direct intramuscular injection with recombinant AAV vectors results in sustained expression in a dog model of hemophilia. *Gene Ther.* 5:40–49.

87. Stephenson, J. 2000. Gene therapy trials show clinical efficacy. *JAMA* 283:589–590.

88. Wang, D., H. Fischer, L. Zhang, P. Fan, R.X. Ding, and J. Dong. 1999. Efficient CFTR expression from AAV vectors packaged with promoters: the second generation. *Gene Ther.* 6:667–675.

89. Fraefel, C., D.R. Jacoby, C. Lage, H. Hilderbrand, J.Y. Chou, F.W. Alt, et al. 1997. Gene transfer into hepatocytes mediated by helper virus-free HSV/AAV hybrid vectors. *Mol. Med.* 3:813–825.

90. Watkins, S.J., V.V. Mesyanzhinov, L.P. Kurochkina, and R.E. Hawkins. 1997. The 'adenobody' approach to viral targeting: specific and enhanced adenoviral gene delivery. *Gene Ther.* 4:1004–1012.

91. Paillard, F. 1999. Dressing up adenoviruses to modify their tropism. *Human Gene Ther.* 10:2575–2576.

92. Brenner, M. 2000. Reports of adenovector 'death' are greatly exaggerated. *Mol Ther.* 1:205.

93. Friedmann, T. 2000. Principles for human gene therapy. *Science* 287:2163–2165.

94. Marshall, E. 1999. Gene therapy death prompts review of adenovirus vector. *Science* 286:2244–2245.

95. Rosenberg, L.E. and A.N. Schechter. 2000. Gene therapist: heal thyself. *Science* 287:1751.

96. Steele, F. 2000. Painful lessons. *Mol. Ther.* 1:iii.

97. Wang, L., T.C. Nichols, M.S. Read, D.A. Bellinger, and I.M. Verma. 2000. Sustained expression of therapeutic levels of factor IX in hemophilia B dogs by AAV-mediated gene therapy in liver. *Mol. Ther.* 1:154–158.

98. Yee, J.-K. 1999. Retroviral vectors, in The Development of Human GeneTherapy. T. Friedmann, editor. Cold Spring Harbor Laboratory Press, Cold Spring Harbor, NY, pp. 21–45.

99. Naldini, L. and I. Verma. 1999. Lentiviral vectors. In The Development of Human Gene Therapy. T. Friedmann, editor. Cold Spring Harbor Laboratory Press, Cold Spring Harbor, NY. 47–60.

100. Dull, T., R. Zufferey, M. Kelly, R.J. Mandel, M. Nguyen, D. Trono, and L. Naldini. 1998. A third-generation lentivirus vector with a conditional packaging system. *J. Virol.* 72:8463–8471.

101. Klages, N., R. Zufferey, and D. Trono. 2000. A stable system for the high-titer production of multiply attenuated lentiviral vectors. *Mol. Ther.* 2:170–176.

102. Xu, K., H. Ma, T.J. McCown, I.M. Verma, and T. Kafri. 2001. Generation of a stable cell line producing high-titer self-inactivating lentiviral vectors. *Mol. Ther.* 3:97–104.

103. Pacchia, A.L., M.E. Adelson, M. Kaul, Y. Ron, and J.P. Dougherty. 2001. An inducible packaging cell system for safe, efficient lentiviral vector production in the absence of HIV-1 accessory proteins. *Virology* 282:77–86.

104. Culver, K.W., W.F. Anderson, and R.M. Blaese. 1991. Lymphocyte gene therapy. *Human Gene Ther.* 2:107–109.

105. Bordignon, C., C. Carlo-Stella, M.P. Colombo, V.A. De, L. Lanata, R.M. Lemoli, et al. 1999. Cell therapy: achievements and perspectives. *Haematologica* 84:1110–1149.

106. Cavazzana-Calvo, M., S. Hacein-Bey, S.B.G. de, F. Gross, E. Yvon, P. Nusbaum, et al. 2000. Gene therapy of human severe combined immunodeficiency (SCID)-X1 disease [see comments]. *Science* 288:669–672.

107. Galderisi, U., A. Cascino, and A. Giordano. 1999. Antisense oligonucleotides as therapeutic agents. *J. Cell Physiol.* 181:251–257.

108. Kruger, M., C. Beger, and F. Wong-Staal. 1999. Use of ribozymes to inhibit gene expression. *Methods Enzymol.* 306:207–225.

109. Kukreti, S., J.S. Sun, D. Loakes, D. Brown, C.H. Nguyen, E. Bisagni, et al. 1998. Triple helices formed at oligopyrimidine . oligopurine sequences with base pair inversions: effect of a triplex-specific ligand on stability and selectivity. *Nucleic Acids Res.* 26:2179–2183.

110. Braun, S., K. Chen, M. Battiwalla, and K. Cornetta. 1997. Gene therapy strategies for leukemia. *Mol. Med. Today* 3:39–46.

111. Faruqi, A., M. Egholm, and P. Glazer. 1998. Peptide nucleic acid-targeted mutagenesis of a chromosomal gene in mouse cells. *Proc. Natl. Acad. Sci. USA* 95:1398–1403.

112. Culver, K.W., W.T. Hsieh, Y. Huyen, V. Chen, J. Liu, Y. Khripine, and A. Khorlin. 1999. Correction of chromosomal point mutations in human cells with bifunctional oligonucleotides. *Nature Biotechnol.* 17:989–993.

113. Uhlmann, E. 1998. Peptide nucleic acids (PNA) and PNA-DNA chimeras: from high binding affinity towards biological function. *Biol. Chem.* 379:1045–1052.

114. Nielsen, P.E. 1999. Peptide nucleic acids as therapeutic agents. *Curr. Opin. Struct. Biol.* 9:353–357.

115. Chinnery, P.F., R.W. Taylor, K. Diekert, R. Lill, D.M. Turnbull, and R.N. Lightowlers. 1999. Peptide nucleic acid delivery to human mitochondria [see comments]. *Gene Ther.* 6:1919–1928.

116. Dr, K. 1998. Chimeraplasty: a gene modification technology employing oligonucleotides. *Human Gene Ther.* 9:2435–2437.

117. Kren, B.T., B. Parashar, P. Bandyopadhyay, N.R. Chowdhury, J.R. Chowdhury, and C.J. Steer. 1999. Correction of the UDP-glucuronosyltransferase gene defect in the gunn rat model of crigler-najjar syndrome type I with a chimeric oligonucleotide. *Proc. Natl. Acad. Sci. USA* 96:10,349–10,354.

118. Gura, T. 1999. Repairing the genome's spelling mistakes. *Science* 285:316–318.

119. Blaese, R.M. 1999. Optimism regarding the use of RNA/DNA hybrids to repair genes at high efficiency. *J. Gene Med.* 1:144–147.

120. Tagalakis, A.D., I.R. Graham, D.R. Riddell, J.G. Dickson, and J.S. Owen. 2001. Gene correction of the apolipoprotein (Apo) E2 phenotype to wild-type ApoE3 by in situ chimeraplasty. *J. Biol. Chem.* 276:13,266–13,230.

121. Kren, B., P. Bandyopadhyay, and C. Steer. 1998. In vivo site-directed mutagenesis of the factor IX gene by chimeric RNA/DNA oligonucleotides. *Nature Med.* 4:285–290.

122. Deng, G.M., I.M. Nilsson, M. Verdrengh, L.V. Collins, and A. Tarkowski. 1999. Intra-articularly localized bacterial DNA containing CpG motifs induces arthritis. *Nat Med.* 5:702–705.

123. Mannucci, P.M., A.R. Zanetti, A. Gringeri, E. Tanzi, M. Morfini, A. Messori, et al. 1989. Long-term immunogenicity of a plasma-derived hepatitis B vaccine in HIV seropositive and HIV seronegative hemophiliacs. *Arch. Intern. Med.* 149:1333–1337.

124. Asahara, T., C. Kalka, and J.M. Isner. 2000. Stem cell therapy and gene transfer for regeneration. *Gene Ther.* 7:451–457.

125. Weissmann, I. 2000. Translating stem and progenitor cell biology to the clinic: barriers and opportunities. *Science* 287:1442–1446.

126. Brenner, M. 1999. Gene transfer and stem cell transplantation, in The Development of Human Gene Therapy. T. Friedmann, editor. Cold Spring Harbor Laboratory Press, Cold Spring Harbor, NY, pp. 459–476.

31

Gene Targeting of Cytokines and the Mitogen-Activated Protein Kinase Pathways in Human Rheumatoid Synovium Using the Severe Combined Immunodeficiency Mouse Model

Jörg Schedel, Thomas Pap, Ulf Müller-Ladner, Renate E. Gay, and Steffen Gay

CONTENTS

INTRODUCTION

Rheumatoid arthritis (RA) is the most common inflammatory joint disease, and frequently accompanied by extra-articular systemic manifestations. Hallmarks of RA are: (1) inflammation of the synovial tissue owing to infiltration of inflammatory cells (T cells, B cells, macrophages); (2) synovial hyperplasia, partly owing to an impaired balance of apoptosis and growth of synovial cells; and (3) pathological immune phenomena. These factors result subsequently in the progressive destruction of cartilage and bone *(1,2)*. Because the etiology of the disease remains unknown, a causal therapy does not exist. The current treatment of patients focuses mainly on antagonizing the inflammatory reaction (nonsteroidal anti-inflammatory drugs; NSAIDs), and suppressing the upregulated immune response (immunosuppressive

From: *Modern Therapeutics in Rheumatic Diseases*
Edited by: G. C. Tsokos, et al. © Humana Press, Inc., Totowa, NJ

drugs, disease-modifying anti-rheumatic drugs; DMARDs) *(3–5)*. However, there is no compelling evidence that any of these agents alter substantially the long-term progression and the outcome of RA, which results in disability and enhances the socio-economic burden. During the past years, progress in molecular biology has led to a better understanding of the pathophysiology underlying RA and has offered new therapeutic options *(6–9)*. Biologic agents *(10,11)* have been developed that act as antagonists of proinflammatory cytokines (e.g., interleukin-1 receptor antagonist [IL-1Ra]) *(12)*, that are soluble receptors of IL-1 (sIL-1R) *(13)* and tumor necrosis factor-α (sTNFR) *(14)*, or that have anti-inflammatory properties (e.g., IL-4, IL-10) *(15,16)*. Although these agents have shown promising results with regard to improvement of disease activity in animal models and some clinical studies, their effects are far from providing the cure for the disease. Importantly, they do not always interfere with disease processes specific for RA but inhibit the inflammatory response un-selectively. Moreover, they still cannot be delivered specifically to the sites of interest (i.e., the affected joints), thus causing systemic side effects, especially when applied for extended periods of time. Among the alternative novel approaches that have been developed, gene transfer is one of the most attractive *(17)*. Originally intended to treat inherited disorders such as cystic fibrosis (CF) or hemophilia, gene therapy has also become an interesting option for noninherited diseases such as RA. Here, gene therapy is used to modulate pathways in the pathogenesis of the disease by specifically overexpressing or inhibiting genes involved in these pathways. During the past years, a variety of different approaches has been studied using both in in vitro systems and animal models *(18)*. Recently, the first clinical trial in RA using an ex vivo gene transfer approach in RA has been completed and is currently being evaluated *(19)*. Thus, expectations have increased to promote gene transfer as a tool for clinical application. However, prior to a broad clinical use of gene therapy, several questions need to be addressed. Among these, the problem of which genes to target and how to deliver these genes for an extended period of time are the most challenging.

PATHOGENESIS OF RHEUMATOID ARTHRITIS

The "T-cell hypothesis" suggests that T lymphocytes are the driving force in initiation and perpetuation of the inflammatory process *(20)*. However, levels of T-cell-derived cytokines are very low in the rheumatoid synovial tissue *(21)*, and controlled clinical trials in RA patients with anti-T-cell monoclonal antibodies (MAbs) (for example anti-CD4 *[22]* and anti-CD5 *[23]*) have only limited effects. Moreover, in animal models, it has been demonstrated that inflammation on one side and cartilage and bone destruction on the other side can occur independently *(24)*. This is supported by the observation that, on a cellular level, synovial fibroblasts have been shown to invade and degrade normal human cartilage in the absence of an inflammatory environment *(25)*.

Apart from infiltrating T cells, the synovium contains macrophage-like (type A synoviocytes) and fibroblast-like cells (type B synoviocytes), and these two populations are predominantly located at sites of invasion into cartilage and bone *(26)*. This has led to the hypothesis that T-cell-independent mechanisms are of importance particularly in the process of joint destruction, and growing interest has focused on the role of synovial fibroblasts in RA *(27)*. Rheumatoid synovial fibroblasts differ morphologically from normal fibroblasts in that they show a large, rounded shape, and have large pale nuclei with prominent nucleoli *(28)*. Furthermore, they exhibit some features of cellular activation such as upregulation of proto-oncogenes *(29)*, altered expression of tumor-suppressor genes *(30,31)*, and anchorage-independent growth *(32,33)*. Increased levels of proto-oncogenes (e.g. c-ras, c-myc, c-fos *[32,33]*) most likely account for the activation of intracellular pathways leading ultimately to the enhanced expression of effector molecules. A particular importance is attributed to c-Fos and c-Jun, which form the transcription factor activator protein-1 (AP-1) as AP-1 has been associated with the expression of disease-related molecules such as matrix metalloproteinases (MMPs) *(34)*.

RA synovial fibroblasts exhibit also an enhanced expression of several adhesion molecules, among them members of the integrin family (e.g., β-1-containing integrins) and the immunoglobulin superfamily (e.g., vascular adhesion molecule [VCAM]-1) *(35–37)*. These surface molecules have been demonstrated to contribute to the accumulation of inflammatory cells within the synovium through interaction with corresponding counter receptors expressed by infiltrating cells (T cells, B cells, macrophages) *(38)* and play a pivotal role in the attachment of synovial cells to cartilage and bone by interacting with ligands in the extracellular matrix *(39)*. Moreover, adhesion molecules are able to interfere with the regulation of cytokine gene expression *(40)*, contribute to the inhibition of apoptosis of T cells *(41)*, are involved in the cell cycle and modulate synthesis of matrix-degrading enzymes *(42)*.

The expression and secretion of matrix-degrading enzymes is another hallmark of RA synovial fibroblasts. MMPs represent a family of structurally and functionally related enzymes responsible for the proteolytic degradation of extracellular matrix (ECM) components such as collagen or aggrecan. Several MMPs have been demonstrated to be expressed in RA synovium including MMP-1 *(43)*, MMP-3 *(44,45)*, MMP-9 *(46)*, and MMP-13 *(47,48)*, and particularly at sites of cartilage and bone invasion *(49)*. Moreover, some of these enzymes have been shown to be capable of destroying cartilage matrix *(50)*. *In situ* studies have also demonstrated the expression of membrane-type metalloproteinases (MT-MMPs) in RA synovial tissue, which contribute both to matrix degradation and activation of other MMPs *(51)*. Most recently, it has been suggested that the expression of MMP-13 and -15 (MT2-MMP) are exclusively associated with RA *(52)* and, thus, may differentiate RA from other arthritic conditions.

Cathepsins are part of a family of cysteine proteases that have also been implicated in the degradation of cartilage matrix in RA; in particular, cathepsins B, K, and L could be found in patients with early arthritis as well as in long-term erosive RA *(32,53,54)*.

A third class of matrix-degrading enyzmes constitute serine proteases, among which plasmin and plasminogen activators appear to be of importance both because of their ability to degrade extracellular matrix proteins and to activate MMPs *(55)*.

The cytokine expression pattern in RA is characterized by a dysbalance between pro- and anti-inflammatory cytokines as well as between their respective naturally inhibitors. Proinflammatory cytokines such as IL-1, IL-6, and tumor necrosis factor (TNF)-α are upregulated in RA *(56)*. They result in a sustained inflammatory reaction within the joint by acting as multipliers inducing the release of other cytokines, chemotactic factors, and prostaglandins. Produced mainly by mononuclear and fibroblast-like cells in the synovium, these cytokines trigger intracellular signaling cascades and activate effector pathways, which result in an enhanced expression of adhesion molecules or matrix-degrading proteases *(57)*. TNF-α is ascribed a pivotal pathogenic role in the formation of hyperplasia, as it stimulates the proliferation of synovial cells and triggers a cascade of secondary mediators leading to the recruitment of inflammatory cells and neo-angiogenesis. IL-1β, on the other hand, induces also inflammatory reactions, the release of enzymes, proliferation of fibroblasts, and tissue destruction. Furthermore, IL-1β shows synergistic effects with TNF-α on further downstream cytokines, e.g., IL-1β could be demonstrated on IL-6 production *(58)*. However, TNF-α and IL-1β appear to be involved in different aspects of RA pathophysiology: TNF-α is believed to be responsible predominantly for the degree of inflammation, whereas IL-1β appears to determine the extent of cartilage and bone degradation *(59)*. Similarly, in rheumatoid synovium, a dysbalance between IL-1β and its naturally occurring inhibitor, IL-1Ra, has been described *(60)*.

Other cytokines, such as IL-4, IL-10, and IL-13, predominantly act as anti-inflammatory molecules. Although these anti-inflammatory cytokines are present in rheumatoid joints, they are not able to antagonize the deleterious effects of proinflammatory cytokines sufficiently *(61)*.

Synovial tissue in RA is characterized by an increased cellularity and by an aggressive behavior of synovial cells invading cartilage and bone. Potential reasons for this observation comprise an enhanced proliferation index and/or a prolonged cellular life-span of synovial cells. Because data convincingly showing an increased proliferation of the synovial cells in vivo are rather spare *(62–64)*, increasing attention has been drawn to apoptosis. In this context, it has been shown that several synovial cells express Fas antigen, and a smaller part of mononuclear cells (MNCs) also express Fas ligand *(65)*. However, despite the abundant expression of Fas/CD95 on the surface of RA fibroblasts, only a very limited number of these cells undergo apoptosis in vivo *(66,67)*. This might be owing to the expression of anti-apoptotic molecules such as bcl-2 or sentrin that, in vivo, outweigh functionally the balance with pro-apoptotic molecules *(67,68)*. Subsequently, synovial lining cells gain an extended life span, which may account for a prolonged expression and secretion of matrix-degrading enzymes at sites of cartilage and bone erosion.

SEVERE COMBINED IMMUNODEFICIENCY (SCID) MOUSE COIMPLANTATION MODEL OF RA

Development of the SCID Mouse Model

To study pathogenetic mechanisms in RA, several animal models have been established *(69)*. However, each of these reflects only certain aspects of the disease, and does not cover the disease process in toto *(70)*. Based on the observation that a synovial cell suspension is able to form a pannus-like structure after implantation into nude mice and to retain the ability to synthesize matrix-degrading enzymes *(71)*, as well as the demonstration that transfer of a functional human immune system into SCID mice is feasible *(72)*, Adams et al. transplanted human RA synovium into SCID mice as a model for the determination of disease activity *(73)*. Owing to a mutation on chromosome 16 that accounts for a defective DNA repair enzyme and a VDJ recombinase-associated defect, SCID mice do not have functional T and B cells and, thus, do not reject implanted human cells *(74)*. In addition, Adams et al. *(73)* showed that RA synovium not only survived but also maintained its biological properties in the SCID mice *(73)*. To study

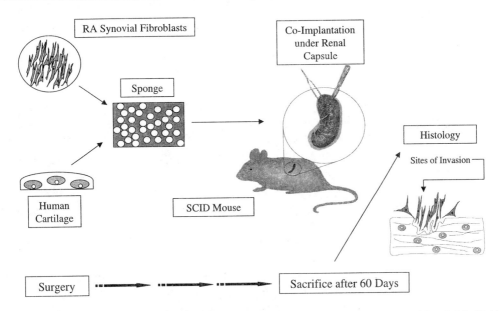

Fig. 1. The severe combined immunodeficiency (SCID) mouse model of rheumatoid arthritis (RA). Using an inert sponge as carrier, RA synovial fibroblasts are coimplanted with human cartilage under the renal capsule of SCID mice. Sixty days after surgery, the mice are sacrificed and the implants removed. Histological analysis revealed deep invasion of RA synovial fibroblasts into the cartilage.

the interaction between rheumatoid synovial cells and cartilage and to explore the cellular basis of joint destruction in RA, the SCID mouse model was further modified in our laboratory *(75)*. In our model *(see also* Fig. 1), human synovial tissue and cartilage were coimplanted into SCID mice and maintained there for more than 300 d. *In situ* hybridization on tissue sections after sacrifice revealed the expression of cathepsin L at sites of cartilage destruction *(75)*, reflecting the situation in the human RA joint.

In a next step, isolated synovial fibroblasts were engrafted into SCID mice specifically to examine the role of T-cell independent mechanisms in RA joint destruction. Using immunohistochemistry and *in situ* hybridization, it could be demonstrated that these fibroblasts invaded the adjacent cartilage while maintaining their transformed-appearing phenotype and expressing VCAM-1, as well as MMPs *(31)* and cathepsin B and L at sites of destruction *(76)*. In contrast, osteoarthritis (OA) as well as normal synovial fibroblasts did not invade and degrade the coimplanted cartilage.

Subsequent studies in the SCID mouse model further characterized the aggressive phenotype of these fibroblasts, and provided novel insights in the underlying pathogenetic mechanisms. As example, the expression of the anti-apoptotic molecule sentrin-1 could be demonstrated at sites of invasion of RA synovium into cartilage, whereas in normal synovial tissues, no sentrin-1 mRNA was detectable *(68)*. Most likely, the expression of sentrin protects RA fibroblasts from apoptosis, and therefore contributes to an enhanced life span especially of the cells located at sites of cartilage destruction *(68)*. Furthermore, the invading synovial fibroblasts did not express the tumor-suppressor gene PTEN, suggesting that the lack of PTEN expression may constitute another characteristic of the activated phenotype of RA fibroblasts *(31)*. Inhibition of the tumor-suppressor p53 by gene transfer using a human papilloma virus-18 (HPV-18) encoding the E6 protein resulted in enhanced invasiveness and cellularity of RA fibroblasts, and also transformed normal synovial fibroblasts into invasive cells. From these data, it was concluded that an impaired function of p53 in RA-SF might contribute to the aggressive behavior of the synovial tissue in RA (77).

Most recently, a new aspect in the cartilage-destruction process emerged when significant differences in the degree of invasion of fibroblasts was seen between fresh and stored cartilage (78). Whereas, as published recently, fibroblast invasion into fresh cartilage was seen, invasion into stored cartilage (24 h before implantation at either 4°C or 37°C) was considerably less intense. Additionally, using a three-dimensional in vitro cartilage-destruction model, a decreased invasion of synovial fibroblasts was observed after administration of a protein-synthesis inhibitor to the chondrocytes. Taking these two results together, it can be hypothesized that chondrocytes in fresh cartilage influence the invasion process of synovial fibroblasts and might directly trigger cartilage destruction by releasing factors that stimulate RA-SF.

In conclusion, RA synovial fibroblasts engrafted into the SCID mice are capable of surviving for an extended period of time while still maintaining their aggressive phenotype. Most importantly, in the absence of inflammatory cells, they attach to and invade deeply into the coimplanted cartilage by synthesis of matrix-degrading enzymes. Thus, this model is an important tool to examine cartilage destruction in RA, and offers the potential to investigate RA fibroblasts and their altered properties. In addition, the SCID mouse model facilitates the examination of novel therapeutic strategies, including gene therapy.

Methods

PREPARATION OF SYNOVIAL FIBROBLASTS AND CARTILAGE

In the SCID mouse model, cultured synovial fibroblasts from patients with RA are coimplanted with normal human cartilage under the renal capsule of these mice. For research use, commercially available SCID mice are obtained from germ-free breeding colonies, and are used for experiments at the age of 6–8 wk. Synovial tissue samples are obtained from patients with RA during synovectomy or arthroplastic surgery. As control, tissue samples from OA patients and from normal individuals (traumatic injury) are used. The synovial tissue is minced and enzymatically digested, and the resulting cell suspension is transferred into cell culture flasks. After testing for mycoplasma contamination and immunocytochemical identification as synovial fibroblasts (CD68–, fibroblast marker +), adhering cells are cultured for 3–6 passages and harvested by trypsinization immediately prior to implantation. Normal cartilage is obtained from patients undergoing trauma surgery or amputations owing to nonarthritic conditions.

IMPLANTATION TECHNIQUE

To coimplant synovial fibroblasts and cartilage slices under the renal capsule of SCID mice, a novel technique was developed in which fibroblasts are inserted into an inert sterile sponge to ensure close contact of cells and cartilage. After desinfection and retroperitoneal incision, the left kidney is mobilized, the capsule opened, and the sponge placed directly under the capsule. Subsequently, the peritoneum and skin are sutured followed by final desinfection.

HISTOLOGICAL EVALUATION

Although it has been shown that synovial fibroblasts can survive within SCID mice up to 300 d, the experimental setting has been standardized to 60 d *(76)*. After sacrificing the mice, the implants together with the adjacent kidney are removed. For histological examination, paraffin-embedded sections are prepared. To examine the integrity of the implant, a primary evaluation is made using hematoxylin-eosin stained tissue sections. Further evaluation comprises both the grade of invasion of fibroblasts into the cartilage as well as the perichondrocytic-cartilage degradation. Subsequently, additional examinations using immunohistochemistry and *in situ* hybridization can be performed.

TRANSDUCTION OF SYNOVIAL FIBROBLASTS

Several approaches have been made to deliver a gene into a target cell (for review, *see [79]* and Chapter 30 in this volume). For the use in the SCID mouse model, retroviral gene transfer into synovial fibroblasts has been efficient, because retroviruses are capable of transducing dividing cells and are stably incorporated into the genome. In our laboratory, we have used the retroviral pLXSN vector that is based on the Moloney murine leukemia virus (MMLV). It contains a multiple cloning site (MCS) downstream of the 5′ LTR promoter, and additionally expresses a Neo^r from the early SV40 promoter. After cloning the respective gene into the MCS, packaging cells expressing the viral envelope are transfected with the respective construct. Retroviral supernatant produced by these cells can transduce synovial fibroblasts via two surface molecules, Pit2 and Pit1. After selection with G418 for 7–10 d, successful and stably transduced SF can be used for experiments and implantation into the SCID mouse.

CURRENT TARGETS IN RHEUMATOID ARTHRITIS USING THE SCID MOUSE MODEL

Other than classical genetic diseases in which a single gene defect accounts for the clinical phenotype, RA is caused by a number of etiologic, mostly unknown, factors such as environmental and genetic susceptibility. Thus, gene transfer shall be used to interfere specifically with a pathogenetic pathway by delivering a potentially therapeutic gene product. In RA, the overall rationale of any therapeutic effort consists in the inhibition of cartilage and bone destruction (Fig. 2). Another argument for this gene transfer is based on the fact that biologics (e.g., IL-1Ra) are proteins with a short half-life and are cleared rapidly from the synovium. In contrast, gene transfer into a target cell might lead to an enhanced production of the respective protein for an extended period of time.

TNF-α appears to be one of the key players in the inflammatory process within the joint. Natural inhibitors of TNF-α exist in form of the soluble receptors p55 and p75 *(80)*. In RA, there appears to be an imbalance between TNF-α and its inhibitors. Thus, it is attractive to upregulate TNF-α receptors and, subsequently, try to reduce the inflammatory response and joint destruction. The clinical data on the effects of a recombinant fusion protein consisting of the soluble TNF receptor (TNFR) p75 linked to the Fc portion of human IgG1 demonstrated a significant improvement of the inflammatory symptoms in patients with refractory RA *(14)*. However, results in the SCID mouse model showed that TNF-αR p55 gene transfer had only a limited effect

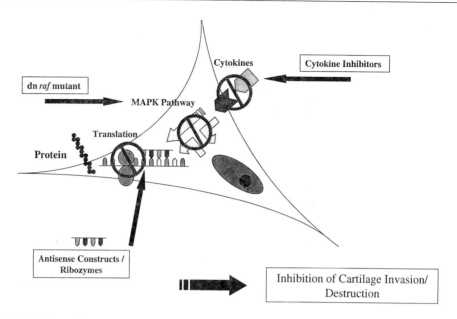

Fig. 2. Inhibition of synovial fibroblast function in RA using gene transfer. To inhibit cartilage invasion, different pathways are targeted: proinflammatory cytokines through delivery of cytokines receptors, cytokine inhibitors, or cytokines with anti-inflammatory properties; the ras-raf-mitogen activated protein kinase (MAPK) pathway through a dominant negative (dn) raf mutant; delivery of anti-sense constructs, which block the protein translation, and ribozymes, which cleave the mRNA of matrix-degrading enyzmes (MMPs, cathepsins).

on inhibition of RA synovial fibroblast invasiveness and cartilage degradation *(81)*. Therefore, it has been concluded that targeting only one pathway might not be sufficient to inhibit both synovial- and cartilage-mediated joint destruction.

In rheumatoid synovial tissue, there exists also an imbalance between IL-1β and its natural inhibitor IL-1 receptor antagonist (IL-1Ra) *(82,83)*. This fact prompted several investigators to modulate the IL-1β effects by increasing IL-1Ra through gene transfer. Using the SCID mouse model, in which retrovirally IL-1Ra transfected synovial fibroblasts had been coimplanted with human normal cartilage, a reduction in the degree of cartilage invasion could not be demonstrated but, on the other hand, IL-1Ra transduction resulted in a significant decrease in the perichondrocytic cartilage destruction *(84)*.

IL-10 reveals both immunostimulatory (B-cell proliferation and differentiation) and anti-inflammatory properties (inhibition of the production of proinflammatory cytokines and chemokines, stimulation of the production of tissue inhibitor of metalloproteinases [TIMP]) *(85)*. Interestingly, the viral homolog of IL-10, vIL-10, which is encoded by Epstein-Barr-virus (EBV), exerts the immunosuppressive effects but lacks immunostimulatory properties. For this reason, vIL-10 has been suggested to be used in gene transfer experiments. In the SCID mouse model, invasion of both vIL-10 and murine IL-10 transfected RA-SF into the coimplanted cartilage was strongly inhibited, whereas no significant effect could be observed with respect to perichondrocytic degradation *(81)*. Similarly, systemic delivery of the vIL-10 gene resulted in the prevention of cartilage invasion by synovial tissue engrafted in the SCID mouse model *(86)*. Moreover, in this experiment, the MMP-3/TIMP-1 balance could be partially restored *(86)*.

As outlined above, synovial fibroblasts exhibit features of transformed-appearing cells, which have been attributed to the enhanced expression of certain proto-oncogenes *(29)*. Further downstream signaling molecules involve members of the ras-raf-mitogen-activated protein kinase (MAPK) pathway *(87)*, which, in turn, has been demonstrated to be activated by IL-1β and TNF-α *(88)*. Accordingly, modulation with signal transduction pathways has become a promising approach in the management of oncologic and inflammatory diseases *(89)*. Thus, it has been shown by inhibition studies with a p38/JNK inhibitor in RA-SF that the IL-1β induced phosphorylation of JNK resulted in an enhanced collagenase mRNA production *(90)*. Conversely, jun D, a member of the jun proto-oncogene family, appears to inhibit fibroblast growth, and, in contrast to c-jun, to antagonize ras-mediated transformation of fibroblasts *(91)*. Intriguingly, transfection of synovial cells with jun D inhibited their proliferation as well as the production of proinflammatory cytokines and MMPs by these cells *(92)*. In our laboratory, a retroviral approach using a dominant negative (dn) raf-1 mutant that encodes a functionally inactive protein by deleting important parts of the gene was performed to investigate the effects on rheumatoid synovial fibroblasts *(93)*. Compared to mock-transduced fibroblasts, dn raf-1 mutants exhibited less invasiveness, but cartilage destruction was still detectable, indicating that raf-independent pathways are involved in the degradation process, which should be targeted as well *(93)*.

Among the agents described in the destruction process in RA, matrix-degrading enzymes such as MMPs, cysteine, and serine proteases are mediating degradation of cartilage and bone directly *(52,54)*. Most recently, an adenoviral-based gene transfer approach has been accomplished targeting the plasmin system in RA *(94)*. Transfection of RA synovial fibroblasts with a cell surface-binding plasmin inhibitor resulted in a significant reduction of cartilage matrix degradation in vitro using a cartilage-like matrix. Moreover, after coimplantation with cartilage in the SCID mouse model, transduced RA-SF exhibited a significantly decreased invasiveness as compared to mock transduced cells. This study supports earlier findings that the plasmin/plasminogen activator system is crucially involved in cartilage destruction. In addition, the data show that targeting matrix-degrading enzymes directly at sites of invasion might be an effective way to inhibit cartilage degradation.

PERSPECTIVES

In line with gene transfer of molecules targeting the plasmin system, MMPs and cathepsins are these enzymes targets in the destruction process. These enzymes are secreted by synovial macrophages and fibroblasts and/or are expressed at the cell surface and have been convincingly shown to degrade extracellular matrix in RA. The direct inhibition of MMPs and cathepsins appears to be attractive because it would circumvent the redundant cytokine network, but still prevent the terminal steps of cartilage degradation. However, the question of whether broad-spectrum inhibitors should be preferred to highly specific inhibitors has not sufficiently been answered. In addition, it is difficult to design inhibitors that exhibit high affinity to the respective enzyme, but still maintain high specificity and efficacy when administered locally or systemically *(95)*. Interestingly, a first report on the efficacy of synthetic MMP inhibitors in an arthritis model indicated that the intra-articular infusion of these MMP inhibitors into rat joints implanted with predigested cartilage slices reduced the proteoglycan and collagen release *(96)*. Apart from these biochemical approaches trying to inhibit degradative enzymes, so far, no gene transfer approach in synovial fibroblasts has been performed. In such an approach, one advantage would be the possibility to modulate the enzyme production directly at sites of invasion. In general, when intending to inhibit the effect of a certain gene using gene transfer technology, two different approaches are possible: antisense constructs, which are supposed to specifically hybridize with its respective messenger RNA in the cytoplasm to prevent the subsequent translation into the protein, and ribozymes, which are capable of cleaving mRNA at specific sites hindering the translation to take place *(97)*. In our laboratory, both approaches are currently under investigation. In vitro data suggest that ribozymes against MMP-1 and cathepsin L indeed decrease their respective mRNA by up to 70% *(98)*. In line with this approach, gene targeting of synovial cells in patients with human T-cell leukemia virus type I (HTLV-I)-associated arthropathy (HAAP) has recently been performed with hammerhead ribozymes cleaving tax/rex mRNA in synoviocytes. This ribozyme gene transfer resulted in the inhibition of synovial cell growth and induction of apoptosis *(99)*.

CONCLUSIONS

In recent years, considerable progress has been achieved in the field of gene transfer. Although gene transfer has just started becoming a tool for gene therapy (*see* Chapter 37), gene transfer trials, so far, have predominantly been undertaken to investigate and modulate pathogenetic pathways and to examine their impact on the disease process. In this respect, the SCID mouse coimplantation model of RA has proven to be an excellent tool to investigate the properties of activated synovial fibroblasts without the influence of inflammatory cells and the cytokine network. With respect to gene transfer, the model allows the examination of fibroblasts after gene transfer and the effects on modulation of cartilage degradation. Using this model, it could be demonstrated that transfer of IL-1Ra, IL-10, and a dn raf mutant was able to decrease fibroblast invasion into cartilage or perichondrocytic degradation. To target more than one mechanism of cartilage degradation, future efforts will, therefore, need to focus on the delivery of combinations of genes *(100,101)*.

REFERENCES

1. Gay, S., R.E. Gay, and W.J. Koopman. 1993. Molecular and cellular mechanisms of joint destruction in rheumatoid arthritis: two cellular mechanisms explain joint destruction? *Ann. Rheum. Dis.* 52 (Suppl. 1):S39–S47.
2. Feldmann, M., F.M. Brennan, and R.N. Maini. 1996. Rheumatoid arthritis. *Cell* 85:307–310.
3. Li, E., P. Brooks, and P.G. Conaghan. 1998. Disease-modifying antirheumatic drugs. *Curr. Opin. Rheumatol.* 10:159–168.
4. Spangler, R.S. 1996. Cyclooxygenase 1 and 2 in rheumatic disease: implications for nonsteroidal anti-inflammatory drug therapy. *Semin. Arthritis Rheum.* 26:435–446.
5. Moreland, L.W., L.W.J. Heck, and W.J. Koopman. 1997. Biologic agents for treating rheumatoid arthritis. Concepts and progress. *Arthritis Rheum.* 40:397–409.
6. Müller-Ladner, U., R.E. Gay, and S. Gay. 1997. Cellular pathways of joint destruction. *Curr. Opin. Rheumatol.* 9:213–220.
7. Müller-Ladner, U., R.E. Gay, and S. Gay. 1998. Molecular biology of cartilage and bone destruction. *Curr. Opin. Rheumatol.* 10:212–219.

8. Panayi, G.S. 1995. The pathogenesis of rheumatoid arthritis and the development of therapeutic strategies for the clinical investigation of biologics. *Agents Actions* (Suppl. 47):1–21.

9. Weyand, C.M. and J.J. Goronzy. 1997. The molecular basis of rheumatoid arthritis. *J. Mol. Med.* 75:772–785.

10. Lorenz, H.M. and J.R. Kalden. 1999. Biologic agents in the treatment of inflammatory rheumatic diseases. *Curr. Opin. Rheumatol.* 11:179–184.

11. Sander, O. and R. Rau. 1998. Clinical trials on biologics in rheumatoid arthritis. *Int. J. Clin. Pharmacol. Ther.* 36:621–624.

12. Gabay, C. and W.P. Arend. 1998. Treatment of rheumatoid arthritis with IL-1 inhibitors. *Springer Semin. Immunopathol.* 20:229–246.

13. Drevlow, B.E., R. Lovis, M.A. Haag, J.M. Sinacore, C. Jacobs, C. Blosche, et al. 1996. Recombinant human interleukin-1 receptor type I in the treatment of patients with active rheumatoid arthritis. *Arthritis Rheum.* 39:257–265.

14. Moreland, L.W., S.W. Baumgartner, M.H. Schiff, E.A. Tindall, R.M. Fleischmann, A.L. Weaver, et al. 1997. Treatment of rheumatoid arthritis with a recombinant human tumor necrosis factor receptor (p75)-Fc fusion protein. *N. Engl. J. Med.* 337:141–147.

15. Chomarat, P. and J. Banchereau. 1997. An update on interleukin-4 and its receptor. *Eur. Cytokine Netw.* 8:333–344.

16. Ho, A.S. and K.W. Moore. 1994. Interleukin-10 and its receptor. *Ther. Immunol.* 1:173–185.

17. Robbins, P.D., C.H. Evans, and Y. Chernajovsky. 1998. Gene therapy for rheumatoid arthritis. *Springer Semin. Immunopathol.* 20:197–209.

18. Evans, C.H. and P.D. Robbins. 1996. Pathways to gene therapy in rheumatoid arthritis. *Curr. Opin. Rheumatol.* 8:230–234.

19. Evans, C.H., P.D. Robbins, S.C. Ghivizzani, J.H. Herndon, R. Kang, A.B. Bahnson, et al. 1996. Clinical trial to assess the safety, feasibility, and efficacy of transferring a potentially anti-arthritic cytokine gene to human joints with rheumatoid arthritis. *Human Gene Ther.* 7:1261–1280.

20. Weyand, C.M. and J.J. Goronzy. 1999. T-cell responses in rheumatoid arthritis: systemic abnormalities-local disease. *Curr. Opin. Rheumatol.* 11:210–217.

21. Smeets, T.J., R.J. Dolhain, A.M. Miltenburg, R. de Kuiper, F.C. Breedveld, and P.P. Tak. 1998. Poor expression of T cell-derived cytokines and activation and proliferation markers in early rheumatoid synovial tissue. *Clin. Immunol. Immunopathol.* 88:84–90.

22. van der Lubbe, P.A., B.A. Dijkmans, H.M. Markusse, U. Nässander, and F.C. Breedveld. 1995. A randomized, double-blind, placebo-controlled study of CD4 monoclonal antibody therapy in early rheumatoid arthritis. *Arthritis Rheum.* 38:1097–1106.

23. Olsen, N.J., R.H. Brooks, J.J. Cush, P.E. Lipsky, E.W. St Clair, E.L. Matteson, et al. 1996. A double-blind, placebo-controlled study of anti-CD5 immunoconjugate in patients with rheumatoid arthritis. The Xoma RA Investigator Group. *Arthritis Rheum.* 39:1102–1108.

24. van den Berg, W.B. 1998. Joint inflammation and cartilage destruction may occur uncoupled. *Springer Semin. Immunopathol.* 20:149–164.

25. Müller-Ladner, U., J. Kriegsmann, B.N. Franklin, S. Matsumoto, T. Geiler, R.E. Gay, and S. Gay. 1996. Synovial fibroblasts of patients with rheumatoid arthritis attach to and invade normal human cartilage when engrafted into SCID mice. *Am. J. Pathol.* 149:1607–1615.

26. Bresnihan, B. 1999. Pathogenesis of joint damage in rheumatoid arthritis. *J. Rheumatol.* 26:717–719.

27. Firestein, G.S. 1996. Invasive fibroblast-like synoviocytes in rheumatoid arthritis. Passive responders or transformed aggressors? *Arthritis Rheum.* 39:1781–1790.

28. Fassbender, H.G. 1983. Histomorphological basis of articular cartilage destruction in rheumatoid arthritis. *Coll. Relat. Res.* 3:141–155.

29. Müller-Ladner, U., J. Kriegsmann, R.E. Gay, and S. Gay. 1995. Oncogenes in rheumatoid arthritis. *Rheum. Dis. Clin. North Am.* 21:675–690.

30. Firestein, G.S., F. Echeverri, M. Yeo, N.J. Zvaifler, and D.R. Green. 1997. Somatic mutations in the p53 tumor suppressor gene in rheumatoid arthritis synovium. *Proc. Natl. Acad. Sci. USA* 94:10,895–10,900.

31. Pap, T., J.K. Franz, K.M. Hummel, E. Jeisy, R.E. Gay, and S. Gay. 2000. Activation of synovial fibroblasts in rheumatoid arthritis: lack of expression of the tumour suppressor PTEN at sites of invasive growth and destruction. *Arthritis Res.* 59–64.

32. Trabandt, A., W.K. Aicher, R.E. Gay, V.P. Sukhatme, M. Nilson-Hamilton, R.T. Hamilton, et al. 1990. Expression of the collagenolytic and Ras-induced cysteine proteinase cathepsin L and proliferation-associated oncogenes in synovial cells of MRL/I mice and patients with rheumatoid arthritis. *Matrix* 10:349–361.

33. Qu, Z., C.H. Garcia, L.M. O'Rourke, S.R. Planck, M. Kohli, and J.T. Rosenbaum. 1994. Local proliferation of fibroblast-like synoviocytes contributes to synovial hyperplasia. Results of proliferating cell nuclear antigen/cyclin, c-myc, and nucleolar organizer region staining. *Arthritis Rheum.* 37:212–220.

34. Han, Z., D.L. Boyle, A.M. Manning, and G.S. Firestein. 1998. AP-1 and NF-kappaB regulation in rheumatoid arthritis and murine collagen-induced arthritis. *Autoimmunity* 28:197–208.

35. el Gabalawy, H. and J. Wilkins. 1993. Beta 1 (CD29) integrin expression in rheumatoid synovial membranes: an immunohistologic study of distribution patterns. *J. Rheumatol.* 20:231–237.

36. Rinaldi, N., D. Weis, B. Brado, M. Schwarz-Eywill, M. Lukoschek, A. Pezzutto, et al. 1997. Differential expression and functional behaviour of the alpha v and beta 3 integrin subunits in cytokine stimulated fibroblast-like cells derived from synovial tissue of rheumatoid arthritis and osteoarthritis in vitro. *Ann. Rheum. Dis.* 56:729–736.

37. Postigo, A.A., R. Garcia-Vicuna, A. Laffon, and F. Sanchez-Madrid. 1993. The role of adhesion molecules in the pathogenesis of rheumatoid arthritis. *Autoimmunity* 16:69–76.

38. Haskard, D.O. 1995. Cell adhesion molecules in rheumatoid arthritis. *Curr. Opin. Rheumatol.* 7:229–234.

39. Rinaldi, N., M. Schwarz-Eywill, D. Weis, P. Leppelmann-Jansen, M. Lukoschek, U. Keilholz, and T.F. Barth. 1997. Increased expression of integrins on fibroblast-like synoviocytes from rheumatoid arthritis in vitro correlates with enhanced binding to extracellular matrix proteins. *Ann. Rheum. Dis.* 56:45–51.

40. Miyake, S., H. Yagita, T. Maruyama, H. Hashimoto, N. Miyasaka, and K. Okumura. 1993. Beta 1 integrin-mediated interaction with extracellular matrix proteins regulates cytokine gene expression in synovial fluid cells of rheumatoid arthritis patients. *J. Exp. Med.* 177:863–868.

41. Salmon, M., D. Scheel-Toellner, A.P. Huissoon, D. Pilling, N. Shamsadeen, H. Hyde, et al. 1997. Inhibition of T cell apoptosis in the rheumatoid synovium. *J. Clin. Invest.* 99:439–446.

42. Sarkissian, M. and R. Lafyatis. 1999. Integrin engagement regulates proliferation and collagenase expression of rheumatoid synovial fibroblasts. *J. Immunol.* 162:1772–1779.

43. Maeda, S., T. Sawai, M. Uzuki, Y. Takahashi, H. Omoto, M. Seki, and M. Sakurai. 1995. Determination of interstitial collagenase (MMP-1) in patients with rheumatoid arthritis. *Ann. Rheum. Dis.* 54:970–975.

44. Okada, Y., N. Takeuchi, K. Tomita, I. Nakanishi, and H. Nagase. 1989. Immunolocalization of matrix metalloproteinase 3 (stromelysin) in rheumatoid synovioblasts (B cells): correlation with rheumatoid arthritis. *Ann. Rheum. Dis.* 48:645–653.

45. Firestein, G.S. and M.M. Paine. 1992. Stromelysin and tissue inhibitor of metalloproteinases gene expression in rheumatoid arthritis synovium. *Am. J. Pathol.* 140:1309–1314.

46. Ahrens, D., A.E. Koch, R.M. Pope, M. Stein-Picarella, and M.J. Niedbala. 1996. Expression of matrix metalloproteinase 9 (96-kd gelatinase B) in human rheumatoid arthritis. *Arthritis Rheum.* 39:1576–1587.

47. Lindy, O., Y.T. Konttinen, T. Sorsa, Y. Ding, S. Santavirta, A. Ceponis, and C. López-Otín. 1997. Matrix metalloproteinase 13 (collagenase 3) in human rheumatoid synovium. *Arthritis Rheum.* 40:1391–1399.

48. Westhoff, C.S., D. Freudiger, P. Petrow, C. Seyfert, J. Zacher, J. Kriegsmann, et al. 1999. Characterization of collagenase 3 (matrix metalloproteinase 13) messenger RNA expression in the synovial membrane and synovial fibroblasts of patients with rheumatoid arthritis. *Arthritis Rheum.* 42:1517–1527.

49. Petrow, P., K.M. Hummel, J.K. Franz, J. Kriegsmann, U. Müller-Ladner, R.E. Gay, and S. Gay. 1997. In situ detection of MMP-13 messenger RNA in the synovial membrane and cartilage-pannus junction in rheumatoid arthritis. *Arthritis Rheum.* 9(Suppl.):S336 (Abstract).

50. Okada, Y., H. Nagase, and E.D. Jr. Harris. 1987. Matrix metalloproteinases 1, 2 and 3 from rheumatoid synovial cells are sufficient to destroy joints. *J. Rheumatol.* 14:41–42.

51. Pap, T., Y. Shigeyama, S. Kuchen, J.K. Fernihough, B.R. Simmen, R.E. Gay, M. Billingham, and S. Gay. 2000. Differential expression pattern of membrane-type matrix metalloproteinases in rheumatoid arthritis (RA) synovium. *Arthritis Rheum.* 43:1226–1232.

52. Konttinen, Y.T., M. Ainola, H. Valleala, J. Ma, H. Ida, J. Mandelin, et al. 1999. Analysis of 16 different matrix metalloproteinases (MMP-1 to MMP-20) in the synovial membrane: different profiles in trauma and rheumatoid arthritis. *Ann. Rheum. Dis.* 58:691–697.

53. Cunnane, G., O. FitzGerald, K.M. Hummel, R.E. Gay, S. Gay, and B. Bresnihan. 1999. Collagenase, cathepsin B and cathepsin L gene expression in the synovial membrane of patients with early inflammatory arthritis. *Rheumatology* 38:34–42.

54. Hummel, K.M., P.K. Petrow, J.K. Franz, U. Müller-Ladner, W.K. Aicher, R.E. Gay, et al. 1998. Cysteine proteinase cathepsin K mRNA is expressed in synovium of patients with rheumatoid arthritis and is detected at sites of synovial bone destruction. *J. Rheumatol.* 25:1887–1894.

55. Werb, Z., C.L. Mainardi, C.A. Vater, and E.D.J. Harris. 1977. Endogenous activiation of latent collagenase by rheumatoid synovial cells. Evidence for a role of plasminogen activator. *N. Engl. J. Med.* 296:1017–1023.

56. Feldmann, M., F.M. Brennan, and R.N. Maini. 1996. Role of cytokines in rheumatoid arthritis. *Annu. Rev. Immunol.* 14:397–440.

57. Migita, K., K. Eguchi, Y. Kawabe, Y. Ichinose, T. Tsukada, T. Aoyagi, et al. 1996. TNF-alpha-mediated expression of membrane-type matrix metalloproteinase in rheumatoid synovial fibroblasts. *Immunology* 89:553–557.

58. Harigai, M., M. Hara, A. Kitani, K. Norioka, T. Hirose, W. Hirose, et al. 1991. Interleukin 1 and tumor necrosis factor-alpha synergistically increase the production of interleukin 6 in human synovial fibroblast. *J. Clin. Lab. Immunol.* 34:107–113.

59. Arend, W.P. and J.M. Dayer. 1995. Inhibition of the production and effects of interleukin-1 and tumor necrosis factor alpha in rheumatoid arthritis. *Arthritis Rheum.* 38:151–160.

60. Chomarat, P., E. Vannier, J. Dechanet, M.C. Rissoan, J. Banchereau, C.A. Dinarello, and P. Miossec. 1995. Balance of IL-1 receptor antagonist/IL-1 beta in rheumatoid synovium and its regulation by IL-4 and IL-10. *J. Immunol.* 154:1432–1439.

61. Isomäki, P., R. Luukkainen, P. Toivanen, and J. Punnonen. 1996. The presence of interleukin-13 in rheumatoid synovium and its antiinflammatory effects on synovial fluid macrophages from patients with rheumatoid arthritis. *Arthritis Rheum.* 39:1693–1702.

62. Ceponis, A., Y.T. Konttinen, S. Imai, M. Tamulaitiene, T.F. Li, J.W. Xu, et al. 1998. Synovial lining, endothelial and inflammatory mononuclear cell proliferation in synovial membranes in psoriatic and reactive arthritis: a comparative quantitative morphometric study. *Br. J. Rheumatol.* 37:170–178.

63. Schaser, K., R.W. Kinne, H. Beil, B. Kladny, and H. Stöss. 1996. Proliferation of T-cells, macrophages, neutrophilic granulocytes and fibroblast-like cells in the synovial membrane of patients with rheumatoid arthritis. *Verh. Dtsch. Ges. Pathol.* 80:276–280.

64. Mohr, W., N. Hummler, B. Pelster, and D. Wessinghage. 1986. Proliferation of pannus tissue cells in rheumatoid arthritis. *Rheumatol. Int.* 6:127–132.

65. Asahara, H., T. Hasumuna, T. Kobata, H. Yagita, K. Okumura, H. Inoue, et al. 1996. Expression of Fas antigen and Fas ligand in the rheumatoid synovial tissue. *Clin. Immunol. Immunopathol.* 81:27–34.

66. Sugiyama, M., T. Tsukazaki, A. Yonekura, S. Matsuzaki, S. Yamashita, and K. Iwasaki. 1996. Localisation of apoptosis and expression of apoptosis related proteins in the synovium of patients with rheumatoid arthritis. *Ann. Rheum. Dis.* 55:442–449.

67. Matsumoto, S., U. Müller-Ladner, R.E. Gay, K. Nishioka, and S. Gay. 1996. Ultrastructural demonstration of apoptosis, Fas and Bcl-2 expression of rheumatoid synovial fibroblasts. *J. Rheumatol.* 23:1345–1352.

68. Franz, J.K., T. Pap, K.M. Hummel, M. Nawrath, W.K. Aicher, Y. Shigeyama, et al. 2000. Expression of sentrin, a novel antiapoptotic molecule, at sites of synovial invasion in rheumatoid arthritis. *Arthritis Rheum.* 43:599–607.

69. O'Sullivan, F.X., R.E. Gay, and S. Gay. 1995. Spontaneous arthritis models, in Mechanisms and Models in Rheumatoid Arthritis. B. Henderson, J.C.W. Edwards, and E.R. Pettipher, editors. Academic Press, London, pp. 471–483.

70. Kaklamanis, P.M. 1992. Experimental animal models resembling rheumatoid arthritis. *Clin. Rheumatol.* 11:41–47.

71. Brinckerhoff, C.E. and E.D.J. Harris. 1981. Survival of rheumatoid synovium implanted into nude mice. *Am. J. Pathol.* 103:411–419.

72. Mosier, D.E., R.J. Gulizia, S.M. Baird, and D.B. Wilson. 1988. Transfer of a functional human immune system to mice with severe combined immunodeficiency. *Nature* 335:256–259.

73. Adams, C.D., T. Zhou, and J.D. Mountz. 1990. Transplantation of human rheumatoid synovium into a SCID mouse as a model for disease activity. *Arthritis Rheum.* 33:S120 (Abstract).

74. Vladutiu, A.O. 1993. The severe combined immunodeficient (SCID) mouse as a model for the study of autoimmune diseases. *Clin. Exp. Immunol.* 93:1–8.

75. Geiler, T., J. Kriegsmann, G.M. Keyszer, R.E. Gay, and S. Gay. 1994. A new model for rheumatoid arthritis generated by engraftment of rheumatoid synovial tissue and normal human cartilage into SCID mice. *Arthritis Rheum.* 37:1664–1671.

76. Müller-Ladner, U., J. Kriegsmann, B.N. Franklin, S. Matsumoto, T. Geiler, R.E. Gay, and S. Gay. 1996. Synovial fibroblasts of patients with rheumatoid arthritis attach to and invade normal human cartilage when engrafted into SCID mice. *Am. J. Pathol.* 149:1607–1615.

77. Pap, T., K.R. Aupperle, R.E. Gay, G.S. Firestein, and S. Gay. 2001. Invasiveness of synovial fibroblasts is regulated by p53 in the SCID mouse in vivo model of cartilage invasion. *Arthritis Rheum.* 44:676–681.

78. Pap, T., W.H. van der Laan, K.R. Aupperle, R.E. Gay, J.H. Verheijen, G.S. Firestein, et al. 2000. Modulation of fibroblast-mediated cartilage degradation by articular chondrocytes in rheumatoid arthritis. *Arthritis Rheum.* 43:2531–2536.

79. Kang, R., P.D. Robbins, and C.H. Evans. 1997. Methods for gene transfer to synovium, in Gene therapy protocols. P.D. Robbins, editor. Humana Press, Inc., Totowa, NJ, pp. 357–368.

80. Camussi, G. and E. Lupia. 1998. The future role of anti-tumour necrosis factor (TNF) products in the treatment of rheumatoid arthritis. *Drugs* 55:613–620.

81. Müller-Ladner, U., C.H. Evans, B.N. Franklin, C.R. Roberts, R.E. Gay, P.D. Robbins, and S. Gay. 1999. Gene transfer of cytokine inhibitors into human synovial fibroblasts in the SCID mouse model. *Arthritis Rheum.* 42:490–497.

82. Chikanza, I.C., P. Roux-Lombard, J.M. Dayer, and G.S. Panayi. 1995. Dysregulation of the in vivo production of interleukin-1 receptor antagonist in patients with rheumatoid arthritis. Pathogenetic implications. *Arthritis Rheum.* 38:642–648.

83. Firestein, G.S., D.L. Boyle, C. Yu, M.M. Paine, T.D. Whisenand, N.J. Zvaifler, and W.P. Arend. 1994. Synovial interleukin-1 receptor antagonist and interleukin-1 balance in rheumatoid arthritis. *Arthritis Rheum.* 37:644–652.

84. Müller-Ladner, U., C.R. Roberts, B.N. Franklin, R.E. Gay, P.D. Robbins, C.H. Evans, and S. Gay. 1997. Human IL-1Ra gene transfer into human synovial fibroblasts is chondroprotective. *J. Immunol.* 158:3492–3498.

85. Keystone, E., J. Wherry, and P. Grint. 1998. IL-10 as a therapeutic strategy in the treatment of rheumatoid arthritis. *Rheum. Dis. Clin. North Am.* 24:629–639.

86. Jorgensen, C., F. Apparailly, F. Canovas, C. Verwaerde, C. Auriault, C. Jacquet, and J. Sany. 1999. Systemic viral interleukin-10 gene delivery prevents cartilage invasion by human rheumatoid synovial tissue engrafted in SCID mice. *Arthritis Rheum.* 42:678–685.

87. Garrington, T.P. and G.L. Johnson. 1999. Organization and regulation of mitogen-activated protein kinase signaling pathways. *Curr. Opin. Cell Biol.* 11:211–218.

88. Saklatvala, J., J. Dean, and A. Finch. 1999. Protein kinase cascades in intracellular signalling by interleukin-I and tumour necrosis factor. *Biochem. Soc. Symp.* 64:63–77.

89. Levitzki, A. 1994. Signal-transduction therapy. A novel approach to disease management. *Eur. J. Biochem.* 226:1–13.

90. Han, Z., D.L. Boyle, K.R. Aupperle, B. Bennett, A.M. Manning, and G.S. Firestein. 1999. Jun N-terminal kinase in rheumatoid arthritis. *J. Pharmacol. Exp. Ther.* 291:124–130.

91. Deckhut, A.M., W. Allan, A. McMickle, M. Eichelberger, M.A. Blackman, P.C. Doherty, and D.L. Woodland. 1993. Prominent usage of V beta 8.3 T cells in the H-2Db-restricted response to an influenza A virus nucleoprotein epitope. *J. Immunol.* 151:2658–2666.

92. Wakisaka, S., N. Suzuki, N. Saito, T. Ochi, and T. Sakane. 1998. Possible correction of abnormal rheumatoid arthritis synovial cell function by jun D transfection in vitro. *Arthritis Rheum.* 41:470–481.

93. Nawrath, M., KM. Hummel, T. Pap, U. Müller-Ladner, R.E. Gay, K. Moelling, and S. Gay. 1998. Effect of dominant negative mutants of raf-1 and c-myc on rheumatoid arthritis synovial fibroblasts in the SCID mouse model. *Arthritis Rheum.* 41:S95 (Abstract).

94. van der Laan, W.H., T. Pap, H.K. Ronday, J.M. Grimbergen, L.G.M. Huisman, J.M. TeKoppele, et al. 2000. Cartilage degradation and invasion by rheumatoid synovial fibroblasts is inhibited by gene transfer of a cell surface-targeted plasmin inhibitor. *Arthritis Rheum.* 43:1710–1718.

95. Vincenti, M.P., I.M. Clark, and C.E. Brinckerhoff. 1994. Using inhibitors of metalloproteinases to treat arthritis. Easier said than done? *Arthritis Rheum.* 37:1115–1126.

96. Karran, E.H., T.J. Young, R.E. Markwell, and G.P. Harper. 1995. In vivo model of cartilage degradation: effects of a matrix metalloproteinase inhibitor. *Ann. Rheum. Dis.* 54:662–669.

97. Arndt, G.M. and G.H. Rank. 1997. Colocalization of antisense RNAs and ribozymes with their target mRNAs. *Genome* 40:785–797.

98. Pap, T., J. Schedel, U. Müller-Laduer, R.E. Gay, W. Zacharias, and S. Gay. 2001. Delivery of antisense constructs and ribozymes to inhibit cartilage destruction in the SCID mouse model of RA. *Arthritis Res.* 3(Suppl. 1):A1.

99. Kitajima, I., N. Hanyu, K. Kawahara, Y. Soejima, T. Kubo, R. Yamada, et al. 1997. Ribozyme-based gene cleavage approach to chronic arthritis associated with human T cell leukemia virus type I: induction of apoptosis in synoviocytes by ablation of HTLV-I tax protein. *Arthritis Rheum.* 40:2118–2127.

100. Jorgensen, C. and S. Gay. 1998. Gene therapy in osteoarticular diseases: where are we? *Immunol. Today* 19:387–391.

101. Pap, T., R.E. Gay and S. Gay. 2000. Gene transfer: from concept to therapy. *Curr. Opin. Rheumatol.* 12:205–210.

32

Retroviral Transduction of Antigen-Specific CD4+ T Cells for Local Delivery of Regulatory Molecules

Gina L. Costa and C. Garrison Fathman

CONTENTS

INTRODUCTION

Rheumatoid arthritis (RA) is an autoimmune disorder that represents inappropriate immune responses directed at joint-specific self-tissue. The clinical manifestations of RA are persistent and chronic in nature and mechanisms that contribute to the immune dysregulation in rheumatoid disorders remains unclear. However, a number of studies report that T cells play a central role in the initiation as well as the perpetuation of this organ-specific disease. Because CD4+ T cells are important mediators in the autoimmune pathogenesis of RA, they would be ideal candidates for cell-based gene therapy. The number of antigen-specific T cells in a single autoimmune lesion may be quite low. Therefore, successful site-targeted gene therapy would require selected transduction of a small number of autoantigen-specific T cells. This chapter will outline the potential for retroviral-mediated transduction of CD4+ T cells ex vivo for the treatment of organ-specific autoimmunity.

BACKGROUND

RA is a chronic multifactorial autoimmune disorder that degrades the body's joint tissue. In the United States alone, autoimmune disorders and rheumatic conditions affect

From: *Modern Therapeutics in Rheumatic Diseases*
Edited by: G. C. Tsokos, et al. © Humana Press, Inc., Totowa, NJ

approx 15% of the population and pose a disease burden close to $65 billion. Prescription sales of the various drugs used to control rheumatoid disease are in excess of $4 billion and have been postulated to grow 11% annually (1). Autoimmune disorders are among the most expansive diseases faced by society today and are therefore the focus of a tremendous amount of research for both acute and long-term treatments.

Historically, effective therapies for reducing inflammation in rheumatic conditions include broad spectrum anti-inflammatory agents, such as glucocorticoids, and nonsteriodal anti-inflammatory drugs (NSAIDs) that inhibit cyclooxygenase (COX) enzymes (2–4). However, there is concern about the true efficacy and tolerance profiles of these drugs following long-term use. More recent therapies result from advances in molecular biology. These techniques have enabled researchers to decipher autoantigens involved in autoimmune disorders, identifying the potential molecular triggers of disease exacerbation.

ROLE OF CD4+ T CELLS IN ORGAN-SPECIFIC AUTOIMMUNITY

A complete understanding of the immunopathogensis of autoimmune diseases and rheumatoid conditions is slowly evolving. The precise role of B cells, antigen-presenting cells (APCs), and T cells in both innate and acquired immunity during rheumatoid disorders is unclear; however, it has become increasingly evident that CD4+ T cells play a central role in the initiation as well as in the perpetuation of organ-specific autoimmunity (5). Studies aimed at elucidating mechanisms of human autoimmune disease are hindered by the difficulty in obtaining organ-infiltrating T cells (6–9). However, in animal models of autoimmune disease, there is direct evidence demonstrating CD4+ T cells as mediators of organ-specific autoimmune disorders. For example, disease can be transferred to naïve syngeneic recipients using CD4+ antigen-specific T cells (10–14). The pathogenic CD4+ T cell exhibits a T helper type 1 (Th1) phenotype characterized by heightened expression levels of type 1 cytokines that include interferon-γ (IFN-γ), interleukin-2 (IL-2), IL-6, and tumor necrosis factor (TNF) (15–20). These Th1 cells represent a T-cell subset with a proinflammatory potential and exhibit effector functions important in perpetuating damaging inflammatory cellular immune responses. Systemic administration of Th2 "regulatory" cytokines, such as IL-4, IL-10, and transforming growth factor-β (TGF-β), which serve to counter the effects of proinflammatory cytokines, has previously been shown to ameliorate autoimmune dysfunction (21–23). However systemic cytokine delivery also induces toxic side effects and global immunosuppression that can lead to increased risk for infections and malignancies (24). Therefore, local delivery of trans-acting immunoregulatory (Th2 type) cytokines to inflammatory disease lesions would be a preferable approach to treating organ-specific autoimmune dysfunction.

REGULATORY CYTOKINES FOR TREATMENT OF RA

A number of regulatory cytokines have been citied for having therapeutic potential in the treatment of proinflammatory rheumatoid disorders (see Table 1). Several studies have demonstrated the development of Th2 autoantigen-specific T cells in the recovery phase of RA, suggesting that Th2 cytokines may be important for disease amelioration

Table 1
**Selected Regulatory Proteins for Potential Application
of Gene Therapy in Rheumatoid Disease**

Protein[a]	Size (bp)[b]	Source[c]	Immunoregulatory function
IL-10	536	Mono, MØ, Th2 activated B	Inhibits Th1 Promotes Th2 Inhibits MØ cytokine release
IL-4	447	Th2, NK1.1	Th2 growth factor Inhibits MØ activation Activates B Promotes Th2
IL-1RA	1000	Mono, MØ, N	Antagonist for IL-1 receptor Blocks IL-1 signaling Inhibits Th1
MDC	300	DC, B, MØ activated: Monon, NK, Th2	Attracts Th2
sTNFR[d]	1400	(activated MØ, Th1, NK, CTL)	Binds secreted TNF Inhibits Th1
Latent TGF-β	1672	Mono, MØ, B, Th2	Inhibits MØ activation Immunosuppression action Promotes Th2
IL-12p40	1000	Mono, MØ, B, NK, activated Th1	Forms p40 homodimer Blocks IL-12R signaling Inhibits IFN-γ production Inhibits Th1

[a]Regulatory proteins are represented as cytokines, chemokines, receptor antagonists, and soluble receptors.
[b]cDNA length in nucleotide base pairs of the open reading frame.
[c]Immune cell subset responsible for regulatory protein expression in vivo. Cell abbreviations: Mono, monocyte; MØ, macrophage; DC, dendritic cell; B, B cell; N, neutrophil; CTL, CD8+ cytotoxic T cell; NK, natural killer cell; NK1.1, natural killer 1.1 cell; CD4+T, CD4+T cell; Th1, CD4+T helper 1; Th2, CD4+T helper 2.
[d]Soluble TNFR as a recombinant molecule. Cells that express TNF cited parenthetically.

(25–32). These studies have postulated that disease recovery may represent a restoration of a more balanced Th1/Th2 profile that results in disease suppression. Exactly how an optimal balance of type 1 and type 2 cytokine homeostasis is achieved within a pathogenic lesion is still under question. The skewing of autoantigen-reactive T-cell cytokine profiles may occur through bystander effects from exogenously administered regulatory proteins acting on circulating CD4+ T cells in the periphery *(21,33–35).* The use of altered peptide ligands (APLs) or oral-tolerance protocols in animal models of autoimmunity have also been demonstrated to act to on circulating CD4+ T cells and induce a Th1 cell to shift to a type 2 phenotype *(36–42).* Therefore, local delivery of regulatory proteins to restore immune homeostasis may prove efficacious in the treatment of rheumatoid lesions.

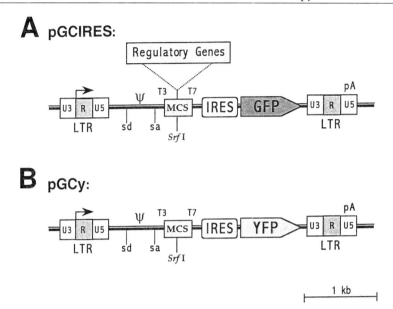

Fig. 1. Schematic diagram of MMLV-based pGC bicistronic retroviral vectors. **(A)** pGCIRES (6691 bp), retroviral vector containing the MMLV-MFG retroviral packaging signal (φ) and 5′ and 3′ LTRs; a *Srf*I-containing multiple cloning site (MCS) flanked with the T3 and T7 oligonucleotide primer sites for the cloning and sequencing of regulatory genes; the encephalomyocarditis virus internal ribosome entry site (IRES); and a mammalian codon-enriched GFP variant; or **(B)** YFP variant, termed pGCy. Arrow indicates transcriptional start site and direction of transcription.

RETROVIRAL TRANSDUCTION

Overview of Retroviral Transduction Procedures

Local expression of regulatory proteins could be directed to inflamed lesions by transducing autoantigen-specific CD4+ T cells to deliver immunomodulatory proteins through techniques of gene therapy. Gene therapy involves the insertion and expression of foreign DNA in a host cell. To date, utilization of viral vectors is the most efficient way to introduce genes into cells by the process of transduction. Many vectors exist, each with advantages and disadvantages *(43,44)*. The murine oncoretroviruses, which include the Moloney murine leukemia virus (MMLV), are widely studied and utilized for gene transfer in murine models, as well as in human studies.

The MMLV genome consists of two long terminal repeats (LTRs), which contain promoter and enhancer elements important for the synthesis and transcription of viral genes. In a conventional retrovirus, LTRs flank the *gag, pol*, and *env* genes and promote expression of essential viral structural proteins, including envelope glycoproteins, which confer the "host range" or tropism of the virus. The ecotropic envelope gene product allows infection of murine cells, whereas amphotropic envelope gene products allow infection of both murine and human cells *(45)*. The packaging signal, psi (φ), lies 3′ to the 5′ LTR and is necessary for the packaging of viral genomes.

The application of gene therapy using retroviruses involves the use of cell lines that have been designed for stable expression, *in trans*, of the *gag, pol*, and *env* genes to allow production of intact virions. A frequently used cell line for retrovirus production is the

A pGC2g:

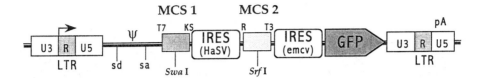

B pGC2y:

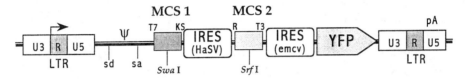

Fig. 2. Schematic diagram of second generation MMLV-based pGC2 tricistronic retroviral vectors. **(A)** pGC2g (7344-bp), retroviral vector containing the MMLV-MFG retroviral packaging signal (ϕ) and 5′ and 3′ LTRs; a SwaI-containing multiple-cloning site (MCS 1) flanked with the T7 and KS oligonucleotide primer sites; the Harvey Sarcoma virus IRES (IRES [HaSV]), a SrfI-containing multiple cloning site (MCS 2) flanked with the reverse (R) and T3 oligonucleotide primer sites; the encephalomyocarditis virus IRES (IRES [emcv]); and a mammalian codon-enriched GFP variant; or **(B)** YFP variant, termed pGC2y. Arrows indicate transcriptional start site and direction of transcription.

Phoenix packaging-cell line, established by Nolan *(46)*. DNA vectors, which contain two retroviral LTRs flanking the internal region encoding the ϕ site and the gene(s) of interest, are transfected into the packaging-cell line. A second open reading frame can be incorporated for the expression of additional genes by including an internal ribosome entry site (IRES). IRES elements allow independent genes to be translated from a single polycistronic mRNA transcript *(47)*. Because translation of each protein is from the same transcript, upstream and downstream gene products are made in approximately equivalent amounts *(48)*. Reporter proteins such as green fluorescent protein (GFP) and/or yellow fluorescent protein (YFP) can be used to identify cells and provide an indirect measurement of the upstream gene expression. Schematic representation of the pGCIRES vectors are outlined in Figs. 1 and 2. The pGCIRES vectors are MMLV-based IRES-containing retroviral vectors with different reporter proteins (Fig. 1). Second-generation retroviral vectors, termed pGC2IRES, contain two unique IRES elements and allow for tricistronic gene expression with either GFP or YFP reporter expression (Fig. 2). Following transfection of the retroviral vector into the packaging-cell line, viral RNA transcripts containing the ϕ packaging signal will be preferentially incorporated into the virions. Because retroviral vectors lack the *gag*, *pol*, and *env* viral genes, the recombinant retroviral particles produced are replication-defective and capable of infecting only one target cell without further propagation of virus. Therefore, once the viral vector is inserted into the packaging cell line, the system can be used to retrieve replication-defective, infection-competent virus particles for transduction of a target-cell population.

Combinatorial Vector Design and Application

Construction of retroviral vectors engineered to express fluorescent proteins to serve as markers for transduction has become common practice. Fluorescent proteins, such as GFP, allow direct visualization of proteins in living cells without the need for substrate addition or cellular manipulation *(49)*. Although blue forms of fluorescent proteins such as the blue-shifted variant of GFP (BFP) and the red fluorescent protein (RFP) are available for use as reporter markers, these blue variants require excitation in the UV range and can therefore cause DNA damage to living cells *(50,51)*. Recently, GFP has been mutagenized to give rise to a "yellow" form, YFP, which has the intrinsic brightness and stability of GFP, and excites with visible light. Although the excitation of YFP is the same as GFP (488 nm), the emission of YFP is "red-shifted" (600 nm) with respect to GFP (509 nm) and therefore allows separation of the two spectra *(52,53)*.

In addition to multiple reporter proteins, retroviral vectors can be engineered to contain T-cell-specific promoters. Although retroviral LTRs contain strong constitutive promoters, such uncontrolled expression is not always desired. Therefore, self-inactivating (SIN) vectors were generated to contain inactivating deletions in the 3′ LTR promoter region that effectively destroy the endogenous retroviral-promoter activity following integration into a host genome *(54)*. T-cell-specific promoters such as the minimal IL-2 promoter or the nuclear factor of activated T cells (NF-AT) promoter can then be inserted between the φ packaging sequence and the open reading frame of cloned gene(s) to allow for expression of the transduced gene product only upon activation of the CD4+ T cell *(55,56)*.

Transduction of Antigen-Specific CD4+ T Cells

A consistent drawback to retroviral-mediated gene therapy has been the inability to transduce nondividing cells by retroviruses. However, antigen-reactive CD4+ T cells will proliferate upon exposure to antigen and are thereby suitable for retroviral transduction. In most cell-mediated autoimmune diseases, inflammatory Th1 type T cells reside in the inflamed lesions. Therefore, transduction of this population would provide targeted delivery of regulatory (or therapeutic) proteins by autoantigen-specific T cells that can traffic to autoimmune lesions and regulate the inflammatory cytokines. To achieve this goal, a robust system of retroviral transduction that would transduce autoantigen-responsive CD4+ T cells was established *(48)*.

For applications of T-cell-based gene therapy, it was necessary to limit retroviral transduction to antigen-specific CD4+ T-cell populations, and for transgene expression to be stable over time. Because oncoretroviruses have the ability to infect dividing cells, polyclonal activation has generally been used as a means to induce proliferation. However, polyclonal activation prior to retroviral infection, provided only a transient and nonspecific transduction of multiple murine lymphoid-cell lineages that included B cells, GR1+ cells, CD8+ T cells, and CD4+ T cells *(48)*. Therefore, to establish optimal retroviral-transduction conditions, specific for autoreactive CD4+ T cells, TCR transgenic mice containing a large population of CD4+ T cells specific for the myelin basic protein (MBP) autoantigen (NAc1-11) were utilized. Splenocytes from either MBP-TCR transgenic mice (H-2^u) or nontransgenic PL/J mice (H-2^u) were stimulated in vitro with the MBP peptide and assessed for the ability of our retroviral vectors to specifically target antigen-activated CD4+ T cells. The results confirmed that upon

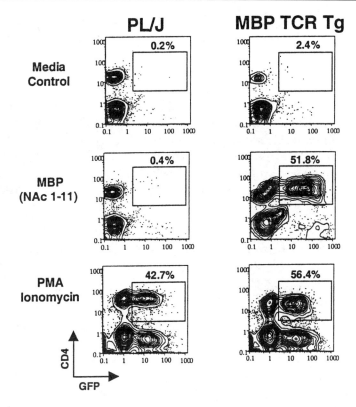

Fig. 3. Preferential transduction of autoantigen-reactive CD4+ T cells. Splenocytes from MBP TCR transgenic mice (MBP TCR Tg) or nontransgenic PL/J mice (PL/J) were cultured in vitro with 5 µg/mL (MBP NAc 1-11), 50 ng/mL PMA, and 1 µM ionomycin (PMA/Ionomycin), or with media alone (Media Control). At 24 h post-stimulation, splenocytes were infected with pGCIRES recombinant retrovirus. At 48 h postinfection, transduced splenocyte populations were stained using antiCD4-PE and analyzed by flow cytometery for expression of GFP. Gated regions (boxed outlines) represent transduction efficiencies (% infected) of CD4+ T cells from the total CD4+ cell population. Adapted with permission from ref. *48*.

stimulation with specific antigen, only antigen-reactive CD4+ T cells were transduced with retrovirus (Fig. 3). Previous barriers in the application of gene therapy to mouse models of autoimmune diseases have included low proviral integration frequency in immune cells, proviral promoter shutdown, and inadequate isolation and expansion of transduced immunoregulatory cells. However, subsequent experimentation demonstrated that the transduced CD4+ T cells could be efficiently expanded in vitro by restimulation at 7–10-d intervals with specific peptide and irradiated APC. Transgene expression appeared to follow the activation profile of the T cell as evidenced by peak transgene expression 2–3 d following each round of restimulation. Additionally, retroviral transduction of recombinant transgenes did not alter the cytokine profile or the cell-surface phenotype of resting and/or activated CD4+ T cells (G. L. Costa, unpublished observations).

An inherent problem of retroviral transduction is that the transduced populations are heterogenous and contain random integration(s) of provirus and thus relatively random expression of the integrated gene product. For use in gene therapy, a regulated and quantifiable gene product is desired. One of these issues was solved by demonstrating that expression of the marker protein (GFP or YFP) exhibited a linear correlation with upstream gene expression. Thus, using this system, it is possible to select the quantity of "regulatory" protein delivered by the transduced T cells based on GFP or YFP expression. Previous retroviral-mediated delivery systems have used antibiotic- or drug-resistance to select transduced cells *(57)*. However, a drawback of drug selection has been the inability to select populations of tranduced cells for multiple (or certainly optimal) therapeutic doses of regulatory proteins. Using IRES-containing retroviral vectors for transduction of antigen-specific CD4+ T cells will allow expression of the marker protein(s) (i.e., GFP and/or YFP), to select for multiple dose or optimal drug delivery.

Targeting Rare Populations of Autoantigen-Reactive CD4+ T Cells for Transduction

Antigen-specific CD4+ T cells normally exist at very low frequency in naïve as well as in memory T cell pools. Limiting dilution studies have established the frequency of antigen-specific T cells in a naïve animal's lymph node at approx 1 in 50,000–300,000 *(58,59)*. Only upon restimulation with specific antigen in vivo do CD4+ T cells undergo extensive expansion that results in an increase in cell number of 150-fold. In model systems defining T-cell reactivity in actively primed and rechallenged mice, it has been found that frequencies of antigen-reactive T cells are 1 in 5000 *(60)*. Application of retroviral transduction of autoantigen reactive CD4+ T cells in gene therapy of autoimmunity must include systems capable of targeting these rare populations of antigen-activated T cells.

As a model system for targeting antigen-responsive cells in vivo, we have used the DBA/2 CD4+ T-cell response to the antigen, sperm-whale myoglobin (SWM) *(61)*. In this system, it was demonstrated that the T cells with upregulated cell surface expression of CD4 (CD4^{high}) contained the proliferating, antigen-reactive T cells. Upon retroviral infection of antigen-reactivated cultures, we found that the majority of the transduced cells were indeed CD4^{high} T cells *(48)*. To confirm that only CD4^{high} T cells (representing the antigen-reactive T cells) were transduced following retroviral infection, flow cytometry was used to sort murine T-cell populations based on levels of CD4 surface expression. Isolation of the CD4^{high} and CD4^{normal} populations demonstrated that retroviral infection of the CD4^{high} T cells resulted in enhanced transduction efficiency over the CD4^{normal} T cells. The CD4^{normal} (nonantigen reactive) were not transduced above background.

Because retroviruses integrate the chromosomal DNA of actively dividing cells, we have used cell cycle analysis to demonstrate a correlation between CD4+ T cells traversing mitosis and retroviral transduction *(48)*. Only the CD4^{high} T-cell population, containing the antigen-activated CD4+ T cells cycling through G2/M and M, were transduced. Enhancing cell cycling by addition of the T-cell growth factor, IL-2, to antigen-activated CD4+ T-cell cultures resulted in an increase in antigen-reactive cell transduction. Antigen-stimulated CD4^{high} T cells, supplemented with exogenous IL-2, exhibited a dramatic enrichment of cells cycling through mitosis. Although IL-2 was necessary for the optimization of transduction in antigen-stimulated CD4+ T cells, exogenously added IL-2, in the absence of specific antigen, did not support efficient transduction of CD4+ T cells. These studies demonstrated that the CD4^{high} phenotype can be used as a marker of antigen reactivity in T cells and that transduction is efficient, but limited to, antigen-reactive CD4^{high} T cells in transit through the M phase at the time of infection. Thus, proliferating, antigen-specific cells can be targeted by infection with retrovirus and isolated by expression of the GFP marker protein. Preliminary studies were therefore initiated to capture rare antigen-specific CD4+ T cells directly from primed mice, in the absence of in vitro activation.

To evaluate the kinetics of antigen-specific T-cell responses to conventional, nontrangenic antigens in vivo, draining lymph-node cells from SWM-immunized mice were harvested and stained for CD4 and the SWM-specific TCR (Vβ8) expression. Limiting dilution analysis (LDA) established the precursor frequency of both CD4^{high}/Vβ8+ and CD4^{high}/Vβ8– T-cell populations at each selected time point (62). Upon evaluating the CD4^{high}/Vβ8+ population, the total number of antigen-specific T cells present in the draining lymph node was estimated from the calculated precursor frequencies and the absolute number in the node. The antigen-specific precursor frequency of the CD4^{high}/Vβ8+ at d 3 after primary immunization (1/3150) was near a baseline level at 33 antigen-specific T cells in the immunized lymph node. In the next 3 d, the number of antigen-specific T cells in the CD4^{high}/Vβ8+ population increased rapidly to reach a maximum at d 6 (1/38) with over 4400 CD4^{high}/Vβ8+ T cells in the draining lymph node, corresponding to a 136-fold expansion in the number of antigen-specific CD4^{high}/Vβ8+ T cells from d 3. The number of antigen-specific T cells decreased threefold by d 8 (1/65) and by d 28 (1/405), only 5% of the peak antigen-specific CD4+ T-cell number were still present. This LDA data provided a priori estimation of the number of antigen-specific present in a draining lymph node following primary immunization. It was then necessary to determine whether retroviral infection ex vivo could be used to "capture" the rare populations of antigen-reactive CD4+ T cells residing in the lymph node in vivo.

As in the LDA experiments, draining lymph-node cells or splenocytes from SWM-immunized mice were harvested and immediately exposed to recombinant retrovirus and exogenous IL-2, to induce T-cell cycling and to facilitate retroviral integration following antigen priming in vivo. Data presented in Fig. 4 is preliminary evidence that retroviral transduction can be used to target in vivo-activated, antigen-reactive CD4+ T cells. The percentage of transduced cells from the lymph node, as marked by the YFP reporter protein, correlated with the LDA frequency of antigen-specific CD4^{high}/Vβ8+ cells found to exist in lymph node cells following primary immunization with SWM peptide. No observable transduction patterns were noted in splenocytes taken at the same time points.

As determined by the lack of retroviral transduction and subsequent YFP expression in CD4+ T cells, there was no evidence of antigen-reactive cells in the lymph node at 1 or 3 d following primary immunization. However, on d 5 postimmunization, there was both an enhancement of CD4^{high} T cells and a concomitant increase in YFP expression, indicative of retroviral transduction. Strikingly, the frequency of transduced CD4+ T cells on d 5 was 2.77%, which correlated with the LDA frequency (1/38) of antigen-specific CD4+ T cells found to exist in the lymph node on d 6. CD4+ T-cell transduction was reduced on d 6 (0.96%), although a prominent YFP expression profile was exhibited by CD4+ T cells, indicative of antigen-reactive CD4+ T cells that resided within the

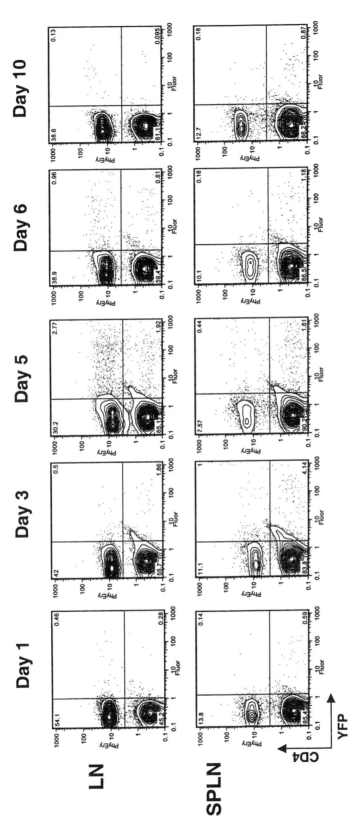

Fig. 4. Capturing rare populations of antigen-reactive CD4+ T lymphocytes activated in *vivo* using retroviral transduction. Draining inguinal lymph node cells (LN) or spleen cells (SPLN) from DBA/2 mice following primary immunization with SWM peptide 110–121 were harvested on days indicated and exposed to recombinant retrovirus containing the pGCγ retroviral vector (*see also* Fig. 1). At 48 h postinfection, cells were stained with CD4-PE and analyzed by flow cytometry using YFP expression as a marker of retroviral transduction. Percentages represent frequency of cells within each quadrant (G. L. Costa, unpublished observations).

lymph node. Again, this reduction correlated with the reduced LDA frequency that followed peak CD4+ T-cell frequencies on d 6. Retroviral transduction as exhibited by YFP expression was back to baseline levels by d 10 and again correlated with the LDA data and most likely represented T-cell emigration from the lymph node following antigen priming. Although these studies are preliminary, future studies to determine optimal targeting of antigen-reactive CD4+ T cells in vivo coupled with functional analyses of the captured transductants will be informative.

Taken together, the application of retroviral transduction coupled with exogenously added IL-2, which serves to both facilitate retroviral transduction and to expand target antigen-activated T cells, should prove beneficial when attempting to isolate rare populations of autoreactive cells with unknown antigen(s) specificity, as in autoimmune disorders such as RA.

CONCLUSION

The use of a replication-defective virus poses a critical safety issue because the presence of replication-competent virus could become a potential health risk, most notably by an increased risk of proviral insertional mutagenesis. Hence, prior to reinfusion of transduced cells, rigorous safety issues must be undertaken to ensure the absence of replication-competent retroviruses. To date, over 3000 patients have received genetically engineered cells for various tissue disease states. The majority of human gene-therapy protocols utilize replication-incompetent retroviruses owing to the fact that the retroviral-mediated gene transfer process is relatively well-understood, particularly for the murine retroviruses, and safety has been rigorously studied *(63–66)*.

Advancements in vector design and application hold great promise for future applications in retroviral-mediated therapy. Animal models of organ-specific autoimmune disease will benefit from use of the distinguishable forms of fluorescent proteins that allow the study of multiple populations of transduced cells simultaneously. Human gene therapy will benefit from the regulatable vector systems that afford stringent and specific release of therapeutic molecules.

In this review, we address the idea of using CD4+ T cells, which have been demonstrated as central mediators in the perpetuation pathogenesis of autoimmunity, for the local delivery of immunoregulatory molecules in retroviral-mediated gene therapy. Retroviral transduction of CD4+ T cells can be used to preferentially target antigen-specific cells. Moreover, it may be possible to capture rare populations of CD4+ T cells of unknown autoantigen specificity following activation in vivo by retroviral transduction ex vivo. Owing to the intrinsic homing capabilities of CD4+ T cells, the transduced T cell would offer the potential for local delivery of therapeutic molecules, thus reducing the inherent toxicities associated with systemic administration.

Although a complete mechanistic understanding of autoimmunity remains elusive, gene therapy offers a platform by which to study the effects of various immunomodulatory proteins on disease pathogenesis. Retroviral-mediated gene therapy in CD4+ T cells coupled with the advent of novel recombinant molecules and optimal use of therapeutic antagonists will undoubtedly be informative in characterizing the underlying immune mechanisms in organ-specific diseases, and may potentially lead to new therapeutic options for treating human autoimmune diseases.

ACKNOWLEDGMENTS

The authors would like to thank Drs. Jacqueline Benson and Anthony Slavin for helpful discussions and critical review of this manuscript. This work was supported by a Molecular and Cellular Immunobiology NIH Grant 5T32-AI-07290 (GLC) and in part by NIH grants AI 39646, AI 36535, and NIH Contract NO1-AR-6-2227 (CGF).

REFERENCES

1. Persidis, A. 1999. Arthritis drug discovery. *Nature Biotechnol.* 17:726–728.

2. Kirwan, J.R., G. Balint, and B. Szebenyi. 1999. Anniversary: 50 years of glucocorticoid treatment in rheumatoid arthritis. *Rheumatology (Oxford).* 38:100–102.

3. Geis, G.S. 1999. Update on clinical developments with celecoxib, a new specific COX-2 inhibitor: what can we expect? *J. Rheumatol.* 26(Suppl.56):31–36.

4. Mandell, B.F. 1999. COX 2-selective NSAIDs: biology, promises, and concerns. *Cleve. Clin. J. Med.* 66:285–292.

5. Liblau, R.S., S.M. Singer, and H.O. McDevitt. 1995. Th1 and Th2 CD4+ T cells in the pathogenesis of organ-specific autoimmune diseases. *Immunol. Today.* 16:34–38.

6. Miltenburg, A.M., J.M. van Laar, R. de Kuiper, M.R. Daha, and F.C. Breedveld. 1992. T cells cloned from human rheumatoid synovial membrane functionally represent the Th1 subset. *Scand. J. Immunol.* 35:603–610.

7. Almawi, W.Y., O.K. Melemedjian, and M.J. Rieder. 1999. An alternate mechanism of glucocorticoid anti-proliferative effect: promotion of a Th2 cytokine-secreting profile. *Clin. Transplant.* 13:365–374.

8. Calabresi, P.A., L.R. Tranquill, H.F. McFarland, and E.P. Cowan. 1998. Cytokine gene expression in cells derived from CSF of multiple sclerosis patients. *J. Neuroimmunol.* 89:198–205.

9. Skapenko, A., J. Wendler, P.E. Lipsky, J.R. Kalden, and H. Schulze-Koops. 1999. Altered memory T cell differentiation in patients with early rheumatoid arthritis. *J. Immunol.* 163:491–499.

10. Kakimoto, K., M. Katsuki, T. Hirofuji, H. Iwata, and T. Koga. 1988. Isolation of T cell line capable of protecting mice against collagen-induced arthritis. *J. Immunol.* 140:78–83.

11. Linington, C., B. Engelhardt, G. Kapocs, and H. Lassman. 1992. Induction of persistently demyelinated lesions in the rat following the repeated adoptive transfer of encephalitogenic T cells and demyelinating antibody. *J. Neuroimmunol.* 40:219–224.

12. Sobel, R.A. and V.K. Kuchroo. 1992. The immunopathology of acute experimental allergic encephalomyelitis induced with myelin proteolipid protein. T cell receptors in inflammatory lesions. *J. Immunol.* 149:1444–1451.

13. McRae, B.L., M.K. Kennedy, L.J. Tan, M.C. Dal Canto, K.S. Picha, and S.D. Miller. 1992. Induction of active and adoptive relapsing experimental autoimmune encephalomyelitis (EAE) using an encephalitogenic epitope of proteolipid protein. *J. Neuroimmunol.* 38:229–240.

14. Suzuki, N., A. Nakajima, S. Yoshino, K. Matsushima, H. Yagita, and K. Okumura. 1999. Selective accumulation of CCR5+ T lymphocytes into inflamed joints of rheumatoid arthritis. *Int. Immunol.* 11:553–559.

15. Kutukculer, N., S. Caglayan, and F. Aydogdu. 1998. Study of pro-inflammatory (TNF-alpha, IL-1alpha, IL-6) and T-cell-derived (IL-2, IL-4) cytokines in plasma and synovial fluid of patients with juvenile chronic arthritis: correlations with clinical and laboratory parameters. *Clin. Rheumatol.* 17:288–292.

16. Lafaille, J.J. 1998. The role of helper T cell subsets in autoimmune diseases. *Cytokine Growth Factor Rev.* 9:139–151.

17. Dudler, J. and A.K. So. 1998. T cells and related cytokines [see comments]. *Curr. Opin. Rheumatol.* 10:207–211.

18. Ohshima, S., Y. Saeki, T. Mima, M. Sasai, K. Nishioka, S. Nomura, et al. 1998. Interleukin 6 plays a key role in the development of antigen-induced arthritis. *Proc. Natl. Acad. Sci. USA* 95:8222–8226.

19. Gross, D.M., A.C. Steere, and B.T. Huber. 1998. T helper 1 response is dominant and localized to the synovial fluid in patients with Lyme arthritis. *J. Immunol.* 160:1022–1028.

20. Dolhain, R.J., A.N. van der Heiden, N.T. ter Haar, F.C. Breedveld, and A.M. Miltenberg. 1996. Shift toward T lymphocytes with a T helper 1 cytokine-secretion profile in the joints of patients with rheumatoid arthritis. *Arthritis Rheum.* 39:1961–1969.

21. Horsfall, A.C., D.M. Butler, L. Marinova, P.J. Warden, R.O. Williams, R.N. Maini, and M. Feldmann. 1997. Suppression of collagen-induced arthritis by continuous administration of IL-4. *J. Immunol.* 159:5687–5696.

22. Racke, M.K., A. Bonomo, D.E. Scott, B. Cannella, A. Levine, C.S. Raine, et al. 1994. Cytokine-induced immune deviation as a therapy for inflammatory autoimmune disease. *J. Exp. Med.* 180: 1961–1966.

23. Tominaga, Y., M. Nagata, H. Yasuda, N. Okamoto, K. Arisawa, H. Moriyama, et al. 1998. Administration of IL-4 prevents autoimmune diabetes but enhances pancreatic insulitis in NOD mice. *Clin. Immunol. Immunopathol.* 86:209–218.

24. Feldmann, M., F.M. Brennan, and R. Maini. 1998. Cytokines in autoimmune disorders. *Int. Rev. Immunol.* 17:217–228.

25. Canete, J.D., S.E. Martinez, J. Farres, R. Sanmarti, M. Blay, A. Gomez, et al. 2000. Differential Th1/Th2 cytokine patterns in chronic arthritis: interferon gamma is highly expressed in synovium of rheumatoid arthritis compared with seronegative spondyloarthropathies. *Ann. Rheum. Dis.* 59:263–268.

26. Yin, Z., S. Siegert, L. Neure, M. Grolms, L. Liu, U. Eggens, et al. 1999. The elevated ratio of interferon gamma-/interleukin-4-positive T cells found in synovial fluid and synovial membrane of rheumatoid arthritis patients can be changed by interleukin-4 but not by interleukin-10 or transforming growth factor beta. *Rheumatology (Oxford)* 38:1058–1067.

27. Pearson, C.I. and H.O. McDevitt. 1999. Redirecting Th1 and Th2 responses in autoimmune disease. *Curr. Top. Microbiol. Immunol.* 238:79–122.

28. Muller, B., U. Gimsa, N.A. Mitchison, A. Radbruch, J. Sieper, and Z. Yin. 1998. Modulating the Th1/Th2 balance in inflammatory arthritis. *Springer Semin. Immunopathol.* 20:181–196.

29. Constantin, A., P. Loubet-Lescoulie, N. Lambert, B. Yassine-Diab, M. Abbal, B. Mazieres, et al. 1998. Antiinflammatory and immunoregulatory action of methotrexate in the treatment of rheumatoid arthritis: evidence of increased interleukin-4 and interleukin-10 gene expression demonstrated in vitro by competitive reverse transcriptase-polymerase chain reaction. *Arthritis Rheum.* 41:48–57.

30. Yin, Z., J. Braun, L. Neure, P. Wu, L. Liu, U. Eggens, and J. Sieper. 1997. Crucial role of interleukin-10/interleukin-12 balance in the regulation of the type 2 T helper cytokine response in reactive arthritis. *Arthritis Rheum.* 40:1788–1797.

31. Chu, C.Q. and M. Londei. 1996. Induction of Th2 cytokines and control of collagen-induced arthritis by nondepleting anti-CD4 Abs. *J. Immunol.* 157:2685–2689.

32. van Roon, J.A., C.M. Verhoef, J.L. van Roy, F.H. Gmelig-Meyling, O. Huber-Bruning, F.P. Lafeber, and J.W. Bijlsma. 1997. Decrease in peripheral type 1 over type 2 T cell cytokine production in patients with rheumatoid arthritis correlates with an increase in severity of disease. *Ann. Rheum. Dis.* 56:656–660.

33. Boyle, D.L., K.H. Nguyen, S. Zhuang, Y. Shi, J.E. McCormack, S. Chada, and G.S. Firestein. 1999. Intra-articular IL-4 gene therapy in arthritis: anti-inflammatory effect and enhanced th2activity. *Gene Ther.* 6:1911–1918.

34. Lechman, E.R., D. Jaffurs, S.C. Ghivizzani, A. Gambotto, I. Kovesdi, Z. Mi, et al. 1999. Direct adenoviral gene transfer of viral IL-10 to rabbit knees with experimental arthritis ameliorates disease in both injected and contralateral control knees. *J. Immunol.* 163:2202–2208.

35. Bessis, N., G. Ghiocchia, G. Kollias, A. Minty, C. Fournier, D. Fradelizi, and M.C. Boissier. 1998. Modulation of proinflammatory cytokine production in tumour necrosis factor-alpha (TNF-alpha)-transgenic mice by treatment with cells engineered to secrete IL-4, IL-10 or IL-13. *Clin. Exp. Immunol.* 111:391–396.

36. Constant, S.L. and K. Bottomly. 1997. Induction of Th1 and Th2 CD4+ T cell responses: the alternative approaches. *Annu. Rev. Immunol.* 15:297–322.

37. Tao, X., C. Grant, S. Constant, and K. Bottomly. 1997. Induction of IL-4-producing CD4+ T cells by antigenic peptides altered for TCR binding. *J. Immunol.* 158:4237–4244.

38. Pfeiffer, C., J. Stein, S. Southwood, H. Ketelaar, A. Sette, and K. Bottomly. 1995. Altered peptide ligands can control CD4 T lymphocyte differentiation in vivo. *J. Exp. Med.* 181:1569–1574.

39. Benson, J.M. and C.C. Whitacre. 1997. The role of clonal deletion and anergy in oral tolerance. *Res. Immunol.* 148:533–541.

40. Faria, A.M. and H.L. Weiner. 1999. Oral tolerance: mechanisms and therapeutic applications. *Adv. Immunol.* 73:153–264.

41. Bitar, D.M. and C.C. Whitacre. 1988. Suppression of experimental autoimmune encephalomyelitis by the oral administration of myelin basic protein. *Cell Immunol.* 112:364–370.

42. Higgins, P.J. and H.L. Weiner. 1988. Suppression of experimental autoimmune encephalomyelitis by oral administration of myelin basic protein and its fragments. *J. Immunol.* 140:440–445.

43. Crystal, R.G. 1995. Transfer of genes to humans: early lessons and obstacles to success. *Science* 270:404–410.

44. Mulligan, R.C. 1993. The basic science of gene therapy. *Science* 260:926–932.

45. Battini, J.L., J.M. Heard, and O. Danos. 1992. Receptor choice determinants in the envelope glycoproteins of amphotropic, xenotropic, and polytropic murine leukemia viruses. *J. Virol.* 66:1468–1475.

46. Pear, W.S., G.P. Nolan, M.L. Scott, and D. Baltimore. 1993. Production of high-titer helper-free retroviruses by transient transfection. *Proc. Natl. Acad. Sci. USA* 90:8392–8396.

47. Sugimoto, Y., I. Aksentijevich, M.M. Gottesman, and I. Pastan. 1994. Efficient expression of drug-selectable genes in retroviral vectors under control of an internal ribosome entry site. *Biotechnology (NY)* 12:694–698.

48. Costa, G.L., J.M. Benson, C.M. Seroogy, P. Achacoso, C.G. Fathman, and G.P. Nolan. 2000. Targeting rare populations of murine antigen-specific T lymphocytes by retroviral transduction for potential application in gene therapy for autoimmune disease. *J. Immunol.* 164:3581–3590.

49. Chalfie, M., Y. Tu, G. Euskirchen, W.W. Ward, and D.C. Prasher. 1994. Green fluorescent protein as a marker for gene expression. *Science* 263:802–805.

50. Heim, R. and R.Y. Tsien. 1996. Engineering green fluorescent protein for improved brightness, longer wavelengths and fluorescence resonance energy transfer. *Curr. Biol.* 6:178–182.

51. Wildt, S. and U. Deuschle. 1999. cobA, a red fluorescent transcriptional reporter for Escherichia coli, yeast, and mammalian cells. *Nature Biotechnol.* 17:1175–1178.

52. Baumann, C.T., C.S. Lim, and G.L. Hager. 1998. Simultaneous visualization of the yellow and green forms of the green fluorescent protein in living cells. *J. Histochem. Cytochem.* 46:1073–1076.

53. Lybarger, L., D. Dempsey, G.H. Patterson, D.W. Piston, S.R. Kain, and R. Chervenak. 1998. Dual-color flow cytometric detection of fluorescent proteins using single-laser (488-nm) excitation. *Cytometry* 31:147–152.

54. Yu, S.F., T. von Ruden, P.W. Kantoff, C. Garber, M. Seiberg, U. Ruther, et al. 1986. Self-inactivating retroviral vectors designed for transfer of whole genes into mammalian cells. *Proc. Natl. Acad. Sci. USA* 83:3194–3198.

55. Tsatsanis, C., C. Patriotis, and P.N. Tsichlis. 1998. Tpl-2 induces IL-2 expression in T-cell lines by triggering multiple signaling pathways that activate NFAT and NF-kappaB. *Oncogene* 17:2609–2618.

56. Ward, S.B., G. Hernandez-Hoyos, F. Chen, M. Waterman, R. Reeves, and E.V. Rothenberg. 1998. Chromatin remodeling of the interleukin-2 gene: distinct alterations in the proximal versus distal enhancer regions. *Nucleic Acids Res.* 26:2923–2934.

57. Flugel, A., M. Willem, T. Berkowicz, and H. Wekerle. 1999. Gene transfer into CD4+ T lymphocytes: green fluorescent protein-engineered, encephalitogenic T cells illuminate brain autoimmune responses. *Nature Med.* 5:843–847.

58. Ford, D. and D. Burger. 1983. Precursor frequency of antigen-specific T cells: effects of sensitization in vivo and in vitro. *Cell Immunol.* 79:334–344.

59. Gebel, H.M., J.R. Scott, C.A. Parvin, and G.E. Rodey. 1983. In vitro immunization to KLH. II. Limiting dilution analysis of antigen-reactive cells in primary and secondary culture. *J. Immunol.* 130:29–32.

60. Kojima, M., K.B. Cease, G.K. Buckenmeyer, and J.A. Berzofsky. 1988. Limiting dilution comparison of the repertoires of high and low responder MHC-restricted T cells. *J. Exp. Med.* 167:1100–1113.

61. Ridgway, W., M. Fasso, and C.G. Fathman. 1998. Following antigen challenge, T cells up-regulate cell surface expression of CD4 in vitro and in vivo. *J. Immunol.* 161:714–720.

62. Fasso, M., N. Anandasabapathy, F. Crawford, J. Kappler, C.G. Fathaman, and W. Ridgeway. 2000. TCR-mediated repertoire selection and loss of TCR Vβ diversity during the initiation of an immune response *in vivo. J. Exp. Med.* 192:1719–1730.

63. Anderson, W.F., G.J. McGarrity, and R.C. Moen. 1993. Report to the NIH Recombinant DNA Advisory Committee on murine replication-competent retrovirus (RCR) assays (February 17, 1993). *Human Gene Ther.* 4:311–321.

64. Anderson, W.F. 1998. Human gene therapy. *Nature* 392:25–30.

65. Kohn, D.B. 1996. Gene therapy for hematopoietic and immune disorders. *Bone Marrow Transplant.* 18(Suppl.3):S55–S58.

66. Miller, A.D. 1992. Human gene therapy comes of age. *Nature* 357:455–460.

33

Gene Transfer to Lymphocytes Targeting Cartilaginous Collagen Type II

Alexander E. Annenkov and Yuti Chernajovsky

INTRODUCTION

The growing knowledge of molecular events promoting or inhibiting inflammatory reaction enables identification of novel means for therapeutic intervention in rheumatoid arthritis (RA). The intensity of inflammation and extent of tissue destruction in rheumatoid joints depends on the balance between various proteins that are synthesized at the site of inflammation by activated resident and blood-borne inflammatory cells and secreted or expressed on their surface. Some of these proteins play a key role in initiation and perpetuation of synovial inflammation because their blockade with specific antibodies or soluble receptors has a therapeutic effect in arthritis. They include the proinflammatory cytokines tumor necrosis factor-α (TNF-α) and interleukin-1 (IL-1), T-cell costimulatory receptors CD80 or CD86, and activated complement components *(1–8)*. On the other hand, some of the proteins produced in the course of inflammation have anti-inflammatory effect because they inhibit activation, proliferation, or survival of inflammatory cells. Some of them, such as cytokines interferon-β (IFN-β), IL-4, IL-10, and transforming growth factor β_1 (TGF-β_1) *(9–12)*, or the mediator of apoptosis galectin 1 *(13)*, can inhibit arthritis. These pro- and anti-inflammatory proteins are candidate therapeutic targets in RA. Indeed, novel therapies inhibiting TNF-α *(14)* and IL-1 *(15,16)* have progressed to clinical trials and demonstrated a therapeutic effect in humans.

From: *Modern Therapeutics in Rheumatic Diseases*
Edited by: G. C. Tsokos, et al. © Humana Press, Inc., Totowa, NJ

We aim to develop a gene therapy approach for RA in which genes encoding therapeutic proteins are expressed locally at sites of disease. As cell-mediated immune response to autoantigens plays an important role in the pathogenesis of RA, cells of the immune system may have the potential to deliver therapeutic protein genes to those sites. Although in most cases, selective genetic modification of cells in vivo cannot be achieved by current gene transfer protocols, in vitro cultured primary cells, including some populations of white blood cells, can be transduced with high efficiency. After genetic modification ex vivo these cells can be returned to the host circulation. Indeed, populations of white blood cells are heterogeneous in their properties and only some of them may have tropism to peripheral inflammatory sites and draining lymphnodes. As arthritogenic CD4+ T lymphocytes specific to some ill-defined autoantigens in the joints do migrate to the sites of disease, they might have the capacity to carry therapeutic gene proteins to those sites. This hypothesis has been tested in experimental autoimmune diseases, such as collagen-induced arthritis (CIA) *(7,17,18)*, insulin-dependent diabetes mellitus (IDDM) *(19)*, experimental allergic encephalomyelitis (EAE) *(20,21)*, and peripheral neuritis *(22)*. In these experiments, pathogenic lymphocytes specific to a known autoantigen, for instance, type II collagen in CIA, were stimulated with the autoantigen in vitro and transduced with a gene encoding an anti-inflammatory protein. Upon adoptive transfer into recipients with an autoimmune disease, the engineered cells exerted a therapeutic effect.

Isolating autoantigen-specific T lymphocytes from RA patients in order to genetically modify them in vitro and use as gene carriers is unlikely to be possible. Although there are several autoantigens implicated in the pathogenesis of RA *(23,24)*, none of them elicits a significant proliferative response in T lymphocytes isolated from patients. Therefore, instead of using autoantigen-specific lymphocytes as gene carriers for gene therapy of RA, we proposed to use to this goal lymphocytes engineered to recognize type II collagen (CII), a protein whose expression is confined to the extracellular matrix of articular cartilage. To confer on lymphocytes an MHC-nonrestricted specificity to CII, we transduced them with a chimeric cell surface protein consisting of the single-chain Fv domain (scFv) of the anti-CII MAb C2 *(25)* and a signaling domain. The latter was represented by the FcεRI signaling γ subunit or T-cell receptor signaling ζ subunit (TCRζ). Upon binding CII, these chimeric receptors mediate in T lymphocytes a physiological response, which resembles the response elicited by antigenic stimulation. Our prediction is that upon stimulation with CII in rheumatoid joints, such engineered lymphocytes could arrest their migration, driven by forces normally mediating migration arrest of antigenically stimulated T lymphocytes. Therapeutic T lymphocytes could be engineered using bicistronic retroviral vectors containing the gene of such chimeric protein together with the gene of an anti-inflammatory protein.

MECHANISM OF T LYMPHOCYTE MIGRATION
THROUGH INFLAMMATORY LESIONS

Increase in T Lymphocyte Migration on the Onset of Inflammation

Post-thymic CD4+ T lymphocytes continuously recirculate between blood and lymph *(26)*. Naïve CD4+ T lymphocytes predominantly migrate into peripheral lymphnodes directly from blood through high-endothelium venules (HEV) *(27)*. Their access to peripheral tissues is restricted, presumably owing to their high dependency on costimulatory signals for full activation *(28–32)*. These signals are fully provided to naïve CD4$^+$ T lymphocytes during priming with an antigen in lymphnodes, but may be deficient in peripheral tissues. Because costimulation requirements of CD4$^+$ T lymphocytes decrease after priming with the antigen, effector and memory CD4$^+$ T lymphocytes can migrate from blood into tissue interstitium without undergoing apoptosis owing to inadequate costimulation. From peripheral tissues, they are delivered to lymphnodes by prenodal lymph *(33)*. Direct entry of effector and memory CD4$^+$ T lymphocytes into lymphnodes from circulation through HEV is also possible *(34,35)*.

The content of CD4$^+$ T lymphocytes in noninflamed tissue is very low. For instance, there are approx 2×10^5 lymphocytes per 1 g of normal skin *(36)*. As demonstrated by analysis of tissue sections and experiments where lymphocytes were labeled ex vivo with a radioactive tracer, such as ^{111}In, and their distribution in different tissues was determined in vivo, on the onset of DTH or some other types of inflammation, the number of CD4$^+$ T lymphocytes in tissue interstitium increases 20–30-fold *(37)*.

CD4$^+$ T lymphocytes infiltrate RA synovium, and in a proportion of cases, they are included in structures resembling germinal centers *(38)*. Activation of CD4$^+$ T lymphocytes specific to joint autoantigens presented by dendritic cells or autoantigen specific B lymphocytes appears to play an important role in the initiation and perpetuation of RA, as suggested by association of the disease with particular HLA haplotypes and its attenuation resulting from deletion or functional inhibition of CD4$^+$ T lymphocytes *(39–42)*.

Retention vs Increased Passage

When the number of migrating T lymphocytes is assessed histologically or by measuring radioactivity of tissue samples after injection of labeled cells, it is impossible to conclude whether visible accumulation of lymphocytes at an inflammatory site results from their retardation or simply reflects their increased passage through the site. This question has been addressed in a series of trafficking studies where in vitro labeled cells were injected in vivo and their appearance in blood, prenodal and postnodal lymph was monitored *(36,37,43)*. These studies demonstrated that lymphocyte throughput does increase at an inflammatory site, but there is no significant retention of lymphocytes, at least when these lymphocytes do not have specificity to antigenic peptides presented at the inflammatory site.

What effect has the activation state and antigenic specificity of T lymphocytes on their capacity to migrate into tissues? This question has been extensively studied on animal models of autoimmune and virus-induced inflammation of the central nervous system (CNS). As first suggested by Wekerle et al. in 1986 *(44)*, the capacity of T lymphocytes to penetrate the intact blood-brain barrier and infiltrate noninflamed parenchyma of the CNS depends on no other parameter than their activation state. It is unassociated with the MHC compatibility between the migrating T lymphocytes and the host, or with the presence in the CNS of the antigenic peptides that these cells are seeking, or with their pathogenic potential (reviewed in ref. *45)*. T lymphocytes activated by exposing them to antigen *(46,47)* or mitogenic lectins *(48–50)* prior to infusion migrate into the CNS. T lymphocytes of both CD4$^+$ and CD8$^+$ phenotypes first appear in the CNS parenchyma few hours following their introduction in the circulation and reach maximum concentration in that tissue 9–12 h after administration *(49)*. However, there is a striking difference in the trafficking pattern between T lymphocytes that can find their cognate antigenic peptides upon migration into the CNS parenchyma and T lymphocytes that do not find their antigens in the CNS. T lymphocytes specific to neural tissue antigens, such as MBP, or viral antigens presented in the CNS arrest their migration, accumulate in the interstitium, and, provided they have an appropriate phenotype, such as Th1, cause demyelinating disease. By contrast, those cells which have no specificity to tissue or viral antigens in the CNS, or cannot recognize the antigen in the context of the host's MHC, disappear from the CNS parenchyma 24 h after their infusion in the circulation. Therefore, the entry of CD4[+] T lymphocytes in the tissue interstitium is random, but their retention and commitment to inflammation is dictated by antigen recognition (48–52).

This hypothesis explains some experimental data obtained in the adoptive EAE model. In this model, pathogenic CD4[+] T lymphocytes specific to myelin antigens can induce demyelinating autoimmune diseases upon transfer into susceptible recipients only if they are activated with the antigen prior to infusion into the host's circulation (47). A possible reason why nonactivated lymphocytes cannot transfer disease is their inability to migrate into the CNS parenchyma. It appears that migration of T lymphocytes in other tissues also increases as a result of antigenic stimulation, because, in similarity to EAE, activated state of pathogenic CD4[+] T lymphocytes specific to appropriate tissue antigens is essential for their capacity to transfer disease in other adoptive models of autoimmunity, such as CIA (53) or IDDM (54,55).

Thus, when T lymphocytes migrate in the interstitial milieu they sample surrounding cells for expression of their cognate antigenic peptide/MHC complex. As a result of the TCR/CD3-mediated stimulation, which they receive upon encountering this complex, they arrest migration and proliferate. This leads to what phenotypically looks as a selective accumulation of antigen-specific CD4[+] T lymphocytes at peripheral sites of inflammation and in lymphoid organs.

What Phenotypic Features of Antigen-Stimulated T Lymphocyte Mediate Their Migration Arrest?

To some extent, cessation of T-lymphocyte migration results from their attachment to the APC expressing the antigenic peptide/MHC complex. The density of cognate complexes on the surface of APC is low, so is the TCR ligand-binding affinity. However, the interaction between the T lymphocyte and APC, is stabilized by binding of some lymphocyte cell surface molecules to their ligands expressed on APC (56,57). The most important lymphocyte receptor stabilizing this interaction is the member of the integrin superfamily LFA-1 ($\alpha_L\beta_2$). Its capacity to bind its ligands, the immunoglobulin superfamily member ICAM-1 expressed on APC, increases following antigenic stimulation of T lymphocytes.

By increasing ligand-binding affinity of LFA-1, antigenic stimulation delivers a stop signal to T lymphocytes, as suggested by the observation that TCR transgenic lymphocytes crawl on the ICAM-1-coated surface but stop upon interaction with their cognate antigenic peptide/MHC complex (58). Naïve CD4[+] lymphocytes can be immobilized by formation of stable conjugates with APC for at least 20 h, because this is the duration of antigenic stimulation that they require to be committed to proliferation (59). Effector T lymphocytes, however, require antigenic stimulation for only 1 h to become fully committed to proliferation, and, in fact, undergo activation-induced cell death if this stimulation lasts longer (59). This suggests that, in addition to conjugation with APC, some other mechanisms are responsible for migration arrest of T lymphocytes, at least those of effector phenotype.

When T lymphocytes receive antigenic stimulation in the tissue interstitium, they upregulate expression and ligand-binding affinity of a variety of adhesion receptors. These receptors can mediate binding of T lymphocytes to extracellular matrix (ECM), to basal membranes, and to those resident and blood-borne inflammatory cells that do not present their cognate antigens. In addition to LFA-1, activated T lymphocytes upregulate VLA-4 ($\alpha_4\beta_1$) and VLA-5 ($\alpha_5\beta_1$), integrin receptors for the major ECM protein fibronectin. VLA-4 also binds another ligand, VCAM-1, which is expressed on the surface of endothelial cells and some cells within the interstitium of inflamed tissue. In addition to the direct effect of antigenic stimulation, upregulation of adhesion receptors in activated T lymphocytes can be induced by their major growth factor IL-2. Thus, IL-2 stimulates adhesion of T lymphocytes to the basement-membrane protein laminin, and ECM proteins fibronectin and type IV collagen *(60,61)*, and upregulates the activity of LFA-1 *(62)*. Cytokine stimulation of resident fibroblasts at the site of inflammation in various tissues, such as dermis, synovium, or lung induces expression of ICAM-1 and VCAM-1, hence providing ligands for the adhesion receptors of T lymphocytes *(63–67)*. Adhesion to extracellular matrix, basement membranes or cells perhaps accounts for the retention of T lymphocytes at the site where they receive antigenic stimulation.

TARGETING T LYMPHOCYTES TO RHEUMATOID JOINTS

CII-Specific Chimeric Receptors for Targeting T Lymphocytes to Rheumatoid Joints

Although exact molecular events involved in cessation of T lymphocytes migration following antigenic stimulation are not completely understood, it is clear that migration arrest is an essential property of antigenically stimulated T lymphocyte. In order to enable T lymphocytes to arrest migration in the tissue affected by autoimmune inflammation, it might be sufficient to introduce into them an engineered cell surface protein that can recognize a target tissue-specific antigen and initiate signaling events normally initiated by TCR ligation. If these cells are also modified to secrete a protein that can inhibit inflammation, they might be able to deliver this protein into sites of disease, hence providing an anti-inflammatory therapy.

To engineer T lymphocytes capable of arresting their migration in rheumatoid joints, we built chimeric cell surface receptors that are similar to ones used for targeting CTL to tumor cells in early studies *(68,69)*. The ectodomains of the prototype receptors used in these studies were represented by single chain Fv domains (scFv) of MAbs recognizing tumor-specific antigens. Their cytoplasmic domains contains immunoreceptor tyrosine-based activation motif (ITAM) *(70)*, a consensus motif of the TCR signaling proteins and FcR signaling γ subunit, which enables these proteins to function as surrogate TCRs. CTL engineered to express such chimeric receptor selectively killed target cells expressing the antigen recognized by the ectodomain of the chimera, hence demonstrating functional competence of the engineered protein.

CII is an ECM protein. As this type of collagen is specific for articular cartilage, we decided to use it as a target protein for directing T lymphocytes to rheumatoid joints. To engineer such lymphocytes, we produced chimeric cell surface receptors scC2Fv/γ, scC2Fv/γIC⁻, and scC2Fv/CD8/ζ that can bind CII and, if expressed in T lymphocytes, induce activation of the TCR signaling pathway *(71,72)*. These receptors have identical CII-binding ectodomains represented by the scFv domain of the anti-CII MAb C2 *(25)*, therefore, they confer on T lymphocytes a MHC-independent specificity to CII. The MAb C2 was selected for the purpose because it has a high antigen-binding affinity and can recognize CII *in situ*, as demonstrated by its capacity to induce synovitis upon injection in mice *(25)*.

The transmembrane and cytoplasmic domains of the chimeric protein scC2Fv/γ are corresponding domains of the FcR signaling γ subunit. The chimeric protein scC2Fv/γIC⁻ is derived from scC2Fv/γ by truncating its cytoplasmic domain so that it did not contain ITAM. When scC2Fv/γ or scC2Fv/γIC⁻ are expressed in cells, they form covalently bound homodimers. In T lymphocytes, they also form covalently bound heterodimers with endogenous TCRζ. T-cell hybridomas transduced with scC2Fv/γ or scC2Fv/γIC⁻ may express either predominantly homodimers of the chimeric receptors, or predominantly heterodimers of the receptor and endogenous TCRζ *(71)*. The third receptor, scC2Fv/CD8/ζ, contains the transmembrane and cytoplasmic domains of TCRζ. In addition, it has the hinge region of CD8α between the MAb C2 scFv and its TCRζ-derived portion. This chimeric protein forms only homodimers and does not associate with endogenous signaling subunits of the TCR/CD3 complex when expressed in T lymphocytes *(72)*.

We generated a variety of T-cell hybridomas expressing different forms of the scFvC2 chimeras on the cell surface (Fig. 1). As expected, T-cell hybridomas expressing predominantly homodimers of the ITAM-less chimera scC2Fv/γIC⁻ were unresponsive to CII. Other forms of the chimeric receptors contained from 2 (scC2Fv/γ homodimers) to 6 (scC2Fv/CD8/ζ homodimers) copies of ITAM per receptor and were functionally competent, as demonstrated by the capacity of chimeric receptor-transduced T-cell hybridomas to secrete IL-2 in response to stimulation with CII.

On the basis of the number of ligand binding sites per receptor, these various forms of scC2Fv chimeras can be divided into two categories: divalent receptors, which include scC2Fv/CD8/ζ and homodimers of scC2Fv/γ or scC2Fv/γIC⁻; and monovalent receptors, which include heterodimers of scC2Fv/γ or scC2Fv/γIC⁻ with endogenous TCRζ. All T-cell hybridomas expressing functionally competent forms of the chimera produced IL-2 in response to stimulation with CII immobilized on the plastic surface, but only those hybridoma cells that expressed divalent forms of the chimera, that is homodimers of scC2Fv/γ or scC2Fv/CD8/ζ, could also respond to native CII added to culture medium. Thus, divalent chimeric receptors had lower crosslinking requirements for activation than monovalent ones. Increasing the number of ITAM per receptor, however, did not reduce crosslinking requirements. The difference between different scC2Fv chimeras in crosslinking requirements may be important for their application because in rheumatoid joints, owing to the inflammation-mediated degradation of cartilage, CII can be present in a soluble form. As the scC2Fv chimeric receptors have different cross-linking requirements, they may differ in the capacity to initiate the stop signal-mediating migration arrest of T lymphocytes.

Engineering Therapeutic T Lymphocytes

To engineer T cells expressing scC2Fv chimeras, we used supernatants of a packaging-cell line transfected with the gene of interest in retroviral vectors. This gene transfer

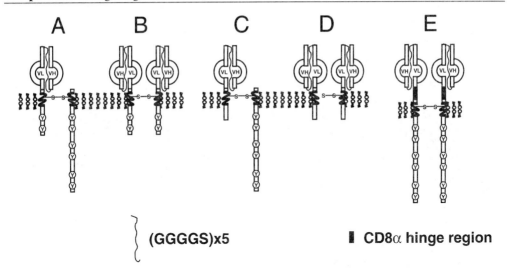

Fig. 1. Different forms of scC2Fv chimeric receptors expressed in T lymphocytes. (**A**) Heterodimers of scC2Fv/γ and endogenous TCRζ. (**B**) Homodimers of *scC2Fv/γ.* (**C**) Heterodimers of scC2Fv/γIC⁻ and endogenous TCRζ. (**D**) Homodimers of scC2Fv/γIC⁻. (**E**) Homodimers of scC2Fv/CD8/ζ.

protocol has been of low efficiency in our hands up until recently, allowing only for 5% level of a chimera gene expression in primary mouse T lymphocytes. This, however, was sufficient to detect proliferation and cytokine production in transduced primary T lymphocytes in response to stimulation with CII. In these studies, normal mouse T lymphocytes were stimulated with Concanavalin A (ConA) in vitro, or T lymphocytes from Keyhole Limpets Hemocyanin (KLH)-immunized DBA/1 mice were reactivated with KLH in vitro to induce cell proliferation and facilitate retrovirus-mediated gene transfer into them. On the whole, the studies on engineered primary lymphocytes confirmed the results obtained on T-cell hybridomas, suggesting that the chimeric receptors are functionally competent. However, they also imply that T lymphocytes activated through the chimeric receptors and through endogenous TCR may be phenotypically different. Thus, KLH-specific CD4⁺ T lymphocytes produced IFN-γ and IL-4 when stimulated with KLH, but when they were transduced with scC2Fv/CD8/ζ and stimulated with CII they produced only IFN-γ (Annenkov and Chernajovsky, submitted).

The increased efficiency of retrovirus-mediated gene transfer into primary lymphocytes that we have achieved recently (35%) will facilitate further studies on scC2Fv chimera-transduced T lymphocytes. They will directly address the question whether T lymphocytes expressing chimeric receptors can deliver anti-inflammatory protein genes to inflamed joints. To this end, we built bi-cistronic genetic constructs containing soluble dimeric TNF receptor (sdTNFR) *(73)* followed by an IRES with either scC2Fv/γ or scC2Fv/CD8/ζ. The control vector in this series of bicistronic constructs contains EGFP instead of a chimeric receptor. As demonstrated in our early report, sdTNFR proved therapeutically efficient when its gene product was delivered by arthritogenic antigen-specific lymphocytes into inflamed joints in CIA in mice *(74)*. A hypothetical mechanism that could lead to migration arrest of scC2Fv chimera-expressing T lymphocytes in rheumatoid joints is represented in Fig. 2.

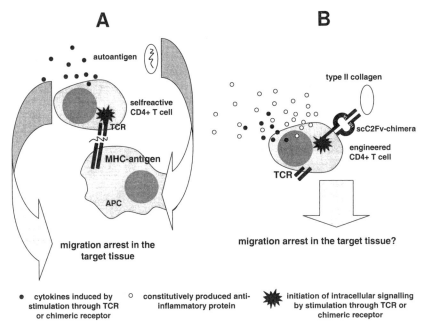

A

autoantigen

selfreactive
CD4+ T cell

TCR

MHC-antigen

APC

migration arrest in the
target tissue

B

type II collagen

scC2Fv-chimera

engineered
CD4+ T cell

TCR

migration arrest in the target tissue?

● cytokines induced by
stimulation through TCR
or chimeric receptor

○ constitutively produced anti-
inflammatory protein

✺ initiation of intracellular signalling
by stimulation through TCR or
chimeric receptor

Fig. 2. Migration arrest of self-antigen specific T lymphocyte and engineered scC2Fv chimera-expressing T lymphocytes in target tissue. **(A)** CD4[+] T lymphocytes specific to self-antigens in synovium arrive in rheumatoid joints where they receive antigenic stimulation. Following this stimulation they arrest migration, proliferate, and produce cytokines perpetuating inflammatory reaction. **(B)** Engineered CD4[+] T lymphocytes expressing a scC2Fv chimeric receptor and constitutively producing an anti-inflammatory protein (sdTNFR, IL-4, IL-10, or TGF-β_1) arrive in rheumatoid joints where they receive stimulation with CII. Following this stimulation they arrest migration, proliferate, and produce cytokines. Some of these induced cytokines can be pro-inflammatory. However, their effect is likely to be overcome by the constitutive secretion of the therapeutic protein from the genetically engineered cells.

Obviously, properties of a T lymphocyte subset used for engineering therapeutic cells have to be considered. By definition, these T lymphocytes will be of activated phenotype, because in order to facilitate transduction with a retroviral vector, they must be activated to proliferate. Because activated T lymphocytes preferentially migrate to peripheral inflammatory sites, they are likely to enable efficient delivery of therapeutic protein genes into inflamed synovium. Another advantage of using activated T lymphocytes is their relative independence of costimulatory signals for activation through TCR. This consideration is important because scC2Fv chimeric receptor-transduced T lymphocytes, which do not require APC for stimulation with CII, may receive this stimulation in the absence of costimulatory signals. A possible drawback of using activated T lymphocytes is their short life-span. These cells are likely to undergo apoptosis at inflammatory sites within a few days after introduction into the circulation. These effector cells, however, may give rise to memory T lymphocytes *(75)*, which persist for a considerably longer period of time *(76)* and may be able to maintain a population of therapeutic cells in the patient.

CD4[+] T lymphocyte subset producing IFN-γ (Th1) is implicated in cell-mediated immune reactions and thought to play a pathogenic role in RA and its animal model

CIA. CIA can be inhibited by some of the cytokines produced by Th2 and Th3 subsets, such as IL-4, IL-10, and TGF-β1. This allows for the suggestion that even without simultaneous transduction with a therapeutic protein gene, lymphocytes of a regulatory Th2 or Th3 subset expressing a scC2Fv chimeric receptor might be able to mediate an anti-inflammatory effect upon stimulation with CII in rheumatoid joints. Indeed, this possibility is not supported by our in vitro study demonstrating that one of the potentially therapeutic cytokines IL-4 is not produced by scC2Fv/CD8/ζ-expressing T lymphocytes stimulated with CII (Annenkov and Chernajovsky, submitted). These data, however, are far from conclusive, and further studies are required to answer the question of which cytokines can by induced by stimulation of T lymphocytes through the scC2Fv chimeras. When more information on signaling pathways involved in induction of different cytokines upon T-lymphocyte activation is available, it will perhaps be possible to design a CII-specific chimeric receptor inducing a desirable cytokine profile in transduced T lymphocyte. At the moment it appears that Th1 cells engineered with anti-inflammatory genes or, as we postulated, with bicistronic vectors expressing chimeric receptors, are an appropriate alternative.

Indeed, in addition to proliferation and migration arrest, activation of the engineered CII-targeted T lymphocytes in rheumatoid joints could result in production of proinflammatory cytokines. In confirmation to this suggestion, we observed arthritis in a mouse injected with CD4$^+$ T lymphocytes expressing scC2Fv/CD8/ζ without the gene of an anti-inflammatory protein (Annenkov and Chernajovsky, unpublished). The carrier lymphocytes, however, will always express the second gene encoding an anti-inflammatory protein in addition to the gene of a scC2Fv chimeric protein. This is likely to reduce the possibility that these cells will augment articular inflammation, because constitutive production of an anti-inflammatory cytokine from the gene introduced into potentially pathogenic CD4$^+$ T lymphocytes seems to overcome their proinflammatory properties mediated by transient production of proinflammatory cytokines induced by antigenic stimulation *(7,17,19–22,77)*. In addition, the potential proinflammatory effect of the therapeutic gene carriers themselves can perhaps be reduced if these carriers are engineered from T lymphocytes, which are unable to produce proinflammatory cytokines, such as Th2 cells.

SIDE EFFECTS AND PRECAUTIONS

How likely is it that the engineered T lymphocytes expressing scC2Fv chimeras could target compartments outside sites of disease, which include articular cartilage of unaffected joints and some extrarticular tissues where CII is present, such as the intervertebral disc, eye, and costal cartilage? It appears that normal cartilage is inaccessible to CD4$^+$ T lymphocytes or other blood-borne cells, because it lacks vascularization. On the contrary, in rheumatoid joints blood-borne cells can get access to the articular cartilage through the invasive front of hyperplastic synovial tissue (pannus). We expect that the difference in the accessibility for T lymphocytes between normal and inflammation-affected cartilage mediated by different cytokine and chemokine milieu will be an important factor contributing to the selectivity of engineered T-lymphocyte accumulation at inflammatory sites. In addition, the proinflammatory potential of these cells might be outbalanced by the therapeutic gene product, or

T lymphocytes unable to promote cell-mediated immune reactions can be used for generating therapeutic cells.

Because CII specific therapeutic T lymphocytes will be generated from cells of normal TCR repertoire, there is a possibility that this procedure could alter reactivity of the immune system, resulting in weakening defense responses or induction of allergic reactions. This, however, seems to be unlikely because the capacity of engineered T lymphocytes to respond to their cognate antigens is reproducibly and profoundly inhibited upon transduction with scC2Fv chimeric receptors, as we observed in T-cell hybridomas *(71,72)*.

CONCLUSIONS

On the basis of the concept that CD4+ T lymphocytes arrest migration in lymphoid organs and peripheral tissues where they receive antigenic stimulation, we are developing an experimental therapeutic system that might allow for targeting rheumatoid joints with CD4+ T lymphocytes producing anti-inflammatory proteins. To this end we built chimeric cell surface receptors combining the capacity to recognize unprocessed CII without presentation by MHC molecules and the capacity to elicit TCR-like signaling in T lymphocytes. These chimeric proteins form homodimers and some of them form heterodimers with endogenous TCRζ in T lymphocytes. Different forms of them differ in the number of CII binding sites and ITAMs per receptor. They have different crosslinking requirements for activation correlating with their valency but not with the ITAM content. Primary mouse CD4+ T lymphocytes transduced with the chimeric receptors proliferate and produce cytokines in response to stimulation with CII. The function of the chimeric receptors in T lymphocytes is similar, but not identical, to that of the endogenous TCR. When transduced with a chimeric receptor gene without an anti-inflammatory protein gene, the engineered T lymphocytes appear to possess an arthritogenic potential, suggesting that they have tropism to the joints. To facilitate studies on the properties of engineered CII-target T lymphocytes in vitro and in experimental therapy of CIA, the scC2Fv chimeric receptors were expressed in bicistronic retroviral vectors together with sdTNFR, a TNF inhibitor shown to be therapeutically effective even when expressed in pathogenic Th1 cells.

REFERENCES

1. Maini, R.N., F.M. Brennan, R. Williams, C.Q. Chu, A.P. Cope, D. Gibbons, et al. 1993. TNF-alpha in rheumatoid arthritis and prospects of anti-TNF therapy. *Clin. Exp. Rheumatol.* 11:S173–S175.

2. Feldmann, M., F.M. Brennan, M.J. Elliott, R.O. Williams, and R.N. Maini. 1995. TNF alpha is an effective therapeutic target for rheumatoid arthritis. *Ann. NY Acad. Sci.* 766:272–278.

3. Williams, R.O., J. Ghrayeb, M. Feldmann, and R.N. Maini. 1995. Successful therapy of collagen-induced arthritis with TNF receptor-IgG fusion protein and combination with anti-CD4. *Immunology* 84: 433–439.

4. Walmsley, M., P.D. Katsikis, E. Abney, S. Parry, R.O. Williams, R.N. Maini, and M. Feldmann. 1996. Interleukin-10 inhibition of the progression of established collagen-induced arthritis. *Arth. Rheum.* 39:495–503.

5. Ghivizzani, S.C., E.R. Lechman, C. Tio, K.M. Mule, S. Chada, J.E. McCormack, et al. 1997. Direct retrovirus-mediated gene transfer to the synovium of the rabbit knee: implications for arthritis gene therapy. *Gene Ther.* 4:977–982.

6. Gabay, C. and W.P. Arend. 1998. Treatment of rheumatoid arthritis with IL-1 inhibitors. *Springer Semin. Immunopathol.* 20:229–246.

7. Mageed, R.A., G. Adams, D. Woodrow, O.L. Podhajcer, and Y. Chernajovsky. 1998. Prevention of collagen-induced arthritis by gene delivery of soluble p75 tumour necrosis factor receptor. *Gene Ther.* 5:1584–1592.

8. Goodfellow, R.M., A.S. Williams, J.L. Levin, B.D. Williams, and B.P. Morgan. 2000. Soluble complement receptor one (sCR1) inhibits the development and progression of rat collagen-induced arthritis. *Clin. Exp. Immunol.* 119:210–216.

9. Kuruvilla, A.P., R. Shah, G.M. Hochwald, H.D. Liggitt, M.A. Palladino, and G.J. Thorbecke. 1991. Protective effect of transforming growth factor beta 1 on experimental autoimmune diseases in mice. *Proc. Natl. Acad. Sci. USA* 88:2918–2921.

10. Horsfall, A.C., D.M. Butler, L. Marinova, P.J. Warden, R.O. Williams, R.N. Maini, and M. Feldmann. 1997. Suppression of collagen-induced arthritis by continuous administration of IL-4. *J. Immunol.* 159:5687–5696.

11. Keystone, E., J. Wherry, and P. Grint. 1998. IL-10 as a therapeutic strategy in the treatment of rheumatoid arthritis. *Rheum. Dis. Clin. North Am.* 24:629–639.

12. Triantaphyllopoulos, K.A., R.O. Williams, H. Tailor, and Y. Chernajovsky. 1999. Amelioration of collagen-induced arthritis and suppression of interferon-gamma, interleukin-12, and tumor necrosis factor alpha production by interferon-beta gene therapy. *Arth. Rheum.* 42:90–99.

13. Rabinovich, G.A., G. Daly, H. Dreja, H. Tailor, C.M. Riera, J. Hirabayashi, and Y. Chernajovsky. 1999. Recombinant galectin-1 and its genetic delivery suppress collagen-induced arthritis via T cell apoptosis. *J. Exp. Med.* 190:385–398.

14. Elliott, M.J., R.N. Maini, M. Feldmann, A. Long-Fox, P. Charles, H. Bijl, and J.N. Woody. 1994. Repeated therapy with monoclonal antibody to tumour necrosis factor alpha (cA2) in patients with rheumatoid arthritis. *Lancet.* 344:1125–1127.

15. Campion, G.V. 1994. The prospect for cytokine based therapeutic strategies in rheumatoid arthritis [see comments]. *Ann. Rheum. Dis.* 53:485–487.

16. Drevlow, B.E., R. Lovis, M.A. Haag, J.M. Sinacore, C. Jacobs, C. Blosche, et al. 1996. Recombinant human interleukin-1 receptor type I in the treatment of patients with active rheumatoid arthritis. *Arth. Rheum.* 39:257–265.

17. Chernajovsky, Y., G. Adams, O.L. Podhajcer, G.M. Mueller, P.D. Robbins, and M. Feldmann. 1995. Inhibition of transfer of collagen-induced arthritis into SCID mice by *ex vivo* infection of spleen cells with retroviruses expressing soluble tumor necrosis factor receptor. *Gene Ther.* 2:731–735.

18. Chernajovsky, Y., G. Adams, K. Triantaphyllopoulos, M.F. Ledda, and O.L. Podhajcer. 1997. Pathogenic lymphoid cells engineered to express TGF β1 ameliorate desease in a collagen-induced arthritis model. *Gene Ther.* 4:553–559.

19. Moritani, M., K. Yoshimoto, S. Li, M. Kondo, H. Iwahana, T. Yamaoka, et al. 1996. Prevention of adoptively transferred diabetes in nonobese diabetic mice with IL-10-transduced islet-specific Th1 lymphocytes. *J. Clin. Invest.* 98:1851–1859.

20. Mathisen, P.M., M. Yu, J.M. Johnson, J.A. Drazba, and V.K. Tuohy. 1997. Treatment of experimental autoimmune encephalomyelitis with genetically modified memory T cells. *J. Exp. Med.* 186:159–164.

21. Shaw, M.K., J.B. Lorens, A. Dhawan, R. DalCanto, H.Y. Tse, A.B. Tran, et al. 1997. Local delivery of interleukin 4 by retrovirus-transduced T lymphocytes ameliorates experimental autoimmune encephalomyelitis. *J. Exp. Med.* 185:1711–1714.

22. Kramer, R., Y. Zhang, J. Gehrmann, R. Gold, H. Thoenen, and H. Wekerle. 1995. Gene transfer through the blood-nerve barrier: NGF-engineered neuritogenic T lymphocytes attenuate experimental autoimmune neuritis. *Nature Med.* 1:1162–1166.

23. Cope, A.P. and G. Sonderstrup. 1998. Evaluating candidate autoantigens in rheumatoid arthritis. *Springer Semin. Immunopathol.* 20:23–39.

24. Blass, S., F. Schumann, N.A. Hain, J.M. Engel, B. Stuhlmuller, and G.R. Burmester. 1999. p205 is a major target of autoreactive T cells in rheumatoid arthritis. *Arthritis Rheum.* 42:971–980.

25. Holmdahl, R., K. Rubin, L. Klareskog, E. Larsson, and H. Wigzell. 1986. Characterisation of the antibody response in mice with type II collagen-induced arthritis, using monoclonal ant-type II collagen antibodies. *Arthritis Rheum.* 29:400–410.

26. Picker, L.J. and E.C. Butcher. 1992. Physiological and molecular mechanisms of lymphocyte homing. *Ann. Rev. Immunol.* 10:561–591.

27. Gowans, J.L. and E.J. Knight. 1964. The route of recirculation of lymphocytes in the rat. *Proc. R. Soc. London Biol.* 159:257–282.

28. Croft, M., D.D. Duncan, and S.L. Swain. 1992. Response of naive antigen-specific CD4+ T cells in vitro: characteristics and antigen-presenting cell requirements. *J. Exp. Med.* 176:1431–1437.

29. Damle, N.K., K. Klussman, P.S. Linsley, and A. Aruffo. 1992. Differential costimulatory effects of adhesion molecules B7, ICAM-1, LFA-3, and VCAM-1 on resting and antigen-primed CD4+ T lymphocytes. *J. Immunol.* 148:1985–1992.

30. Semnani, R.T., T.B. Nutman, P. Hochman, S. Shaw, and G.A. van Seventer. 1994. Costimulation by purified intercellular adhesion molecule 1 and lymphocyte function-associated antigen 3 induces distinct proliferation, cytokine and cell surface antigen profiles in human "naive" and "memory" CD4+ T cells. *J. Exp. Med.* 180:2125–2135.

31. Croft, M. and C. Dubey. 1997. Accessory molecule and costimulation requirements for CD4 T cell response. *Crit. Rev. Immunol.* 17:89–118.

32. Woodside, D.G., D.A. Long, and B.W. McIntyre. 1999. Intracellular analysis of interleukin-2 induction provides direct evidence at the single cell level of differential coactivation requirements for CD45RA+ and CD45RO+ T cell subsets. *J. Interferon Cytokine Res.* 19:769–779.

33. Mackay, C.R., W.L. Marston, and L. Dudler. 1990. Naive and memory T cells show distinct pathways of lymphocyte recirculation. *J. Exp. Med.* 171:801–817.

34. Tietz, W. and A. Hamann. 1997. The migratory behavior of murine CD4+ cells of memory phenotype. *Eur. J. Immunol.* 27:2225–2232.

35. Westermann, J., U. Geismar, A. Sponholz, U. Bode, S.M. Sparshott, and E.B. Bell. 1997. CD4+ T cells of both the naive and the memory phenotype enter rat lymph nodes and Peyer's patches via high endothelial venules: within the tissue their migratory behavior differs. *Eur. J. Immunol.* 27:3174–3181.

36. Seabrook, T., B. Au, J. Dickstein, X. Zhang, B. Ristevski, and J.B. Hay. 1999. The traffic of resting lymphocytes through delayed hypersensitivity and chronic inflammatory lesions: a dynamic equilibrium. *Semin. Immunol.* 11:115–123.

37. Borgs, P. and J.B. Hay. 1986. A quantitative lymphocyte localization assay. *J. Leukoc. Biol.* 39:333–342.

38. Cush, J.J. and P.E. Lipsky. 1991. Cellular basis for rheumatoid inflammation. *Clin. Orthoped.* 265:9–22.

39. Goronzy, J.J. and C.M. Weyand. 1995. T cells in rheumatoid arthritis. Paradigms and facts. *Rheum. Dis. Clin. North Am.* 21:655–674.

40. Salmon, M. and J.S. Gaston. 1995. The role of T-lymphocytes in rheumatoid arthritis. *Br. Med. Bull.* 51:332–345.

41. Weyand, C.M. and J.J. Goronzy. 1997. Pathogenesis of rheumatoid arthritis. *Med. Clin. North Am. 81:29–55.*

42. Thomas, R., K.P. MacDonald, A.R. Pettit, L.L. Cavanagh, J. Padmanabha, and S. Zehntner. 1999. Dendritic cells and the pathogenesis of rheumatoid arthritis. *J. Leukoc. Biol.* 66:286–292.

43. Issekutz, T.B., G.W. Chin, and J.B. Hay. 1981. Lymphocyte traffic through chronic inflammatory lesions: differential migration versus differential retention. *Clin. Exp. Immunol.* 45:604–614.

44. Wekerle, H., G. Linnington, H. Lassmann, and R. Meyermann. 1986. Cellular immune reactivity within the CNS. *Trends Neurosci.* 9:271–277.

45. Hickey, W.F. 1999. Leukocyte traffic in the central nervous system: the participants and their roles. *Semin. Immunol.* 11:125–137.

46. Holda, J.H., A.M. Welch, and R.H. Swanborg. 1980. Autoimmune effector cells. I. Transfer of experimental encephalomyelitis with lymphoid cells cultured with antigen. *Eur. J. Immunol.* 10:657–659.

47. Panitch, H.S. and C. Ciccone. 1981. Adoptive transfer of experimental allergic encephalomyelitis: requirement for macrophages in activation of spleen cells in vitro by concanavalin A or myelin basic protein. *Cell. Immunol.* 60:24–33.

48. Takenaka, A., H. Minagawa, K. Kaneko, R. Mori, and Y. Itoyama. 1986. Adoptive transfer of experimental allergic encephalomyelitis with lectin-activated spleen cells. Part 2. Studies on T cell subsets and interleukin 2 production. *J. Neurol. Sci.* 72:337–345.

49. Hickey, W.F., B.L. Hsu, and H. Kimura. 1991. T-lymphocyte entry into the central nervous system. *J. Neurosci. Res.* 28:254–260.

50. Ludowyk, P.A., D.O. Willenborg, and C.R. Parish. 1992. Selective localisation of neuro-specific T lymphocytes in the central nervous system. *J. Neuroimmunol.* 37:237–250.

51. Irani, D.N. and D.E. Griffin. 1996. Regulation of lymphocyte homing into the brain during viral encephalitis at various stages of infection. *J. Immunol.* 156:3850–3857.

52. Neumann, H. and H. Wekerle. 1998. Neuronal control of the immune response in the central nervous system: linking brain immunity to neurodegeneration. *J. Neuropathol. Exp. Neurol.* 57:1–9.

53. Williams, R.O., Z.C. Plater, D.G. Williams, and R.N. Maini. 1992. Successful transfer of collagen-induced arthritis to severe combined immunodeficient (SCID) mice. *Clin. Exp. Immunol.* 88:455–460.

54. Like, A.A., E.J. Weringer, A. Holdash, P. McGill, D. Atkinson, and A.A. Rossini. 1985. Adoptive transfer of autoimmune diabetes mellitus in biobreeding/Worcester (BB/W) inbred and hybrid rats. *J. Immunol.* 134:1583–1587.

55. Logothetopoulos, J., K. Shumak, and D. Bailey. 1988. Prevention of spontaneous but not of adoptively transferred diabetes by injection of neonatal BB/hooded hybrid rats with splenocytes or concanavalin A blasts from diabetes-free strains. *Diabetes* 37:1009–1014.

56. Wulfing, C. and Davis, M.M. 1998. A receptor/cytoskeletal movement triggered by costimulation during T cell activation. *Science* 282:2266–2269.

57. Dustin, M.L. and A.S. Shaw. 1999. Costimulation: building an immunological synapse [comment]. *Science* 283:649–650.

58. Dustin, M.L., S.K. Bromley, Z. Kan, D.A. Peterson, and E.R. Unanue. 1997. Antigen receptor engagement delivers a stop signal to migrating T lymphocytes. *Proc. Natl. Acad. Sci. USA* 94:3909–3913.

59. Iezzi, G., K. Karjalainen, and A. Lanzavecchia. 1998. The duration of antigenic stimulation determines the fate of naive and effector T cells. *Immunity* 8:89–95.

60. Ariel, A., E.J. Yavin, R. Hershkoviz, A. Avron, Franitza, S., I. Hardan, et al. 1998. IL-2 induces T cell adherence to extracellular matrix: inhibition of adherence and migration by IL-2 peptides generated by leukocyte elastase. *J. Immunol.* 161:2465–2472.

61. Olive, D. and C. Cerdan. 1999. CD28 co-stimulation results in down-regulation of lymphotactin expression in human CD4(+) but not CD8(+) T cells via an IL-2-dependent mechanism. *Eur. J. Immunol.* 29:2443–2453.

62. Nielsen, M., A. Svejgaard, S. Skov, P. Dobson, K. Bendtzen, C. Geisler, and N. Odum. 1996. IL-2 induces beta2-integrin adhesion via a wortmannin/LY294002- sensitive, rapamycin-resistant pathway. Phosphorylation of a 125- kilodalton protein correlates with induction of adhesion, but not mitogenesis. *J. Immunol.* 157:5350–5358.

63. Meng, H., M.J. Marchese, J.A. Garlick, A. Jelaska, J.H. Korn, J. Gailit, et al. 1995. Mast cells induce T-cell adhesion to human fibroblasts by regulating intercellular adhesion molecule-1 and vascular cell adhesion molecule-1 expression. *J. Invest. Dermatol.* 105:789–796.

64. Gao, J.X. and A.C. Issekutz. 1996. Expression of VCAM-1 and VLA-4 dependent T-lymphocyte adhesion to dermal fibroblasts stimulated with proinflammatory cytokines. *Immunology* 89:375–383.

65. Tessier, P.A., P. Cattaruzzi, and S.R. McColl. 1996. Inhibition of lymphocyte adhesion to cytokine-activated synovial fibroblasts by glucocorticoids involves the attenuation of vascular cell adhesion molecule 1 and intercellular adhesion molecule 1 gene expression. *Arthritis Rheum.* 39:226–234.

66. Kaneko, M., H. Inoue, H., R. Nakazawa, N. Azuma, M. Suzuki, S. Yamauchi, et al. 1998. Pirfenidone induces intercellular adhesion molecule-1 (ICAM-1) down-regulation on cultured human synovial fibroblasts. *Clin. Exp. Immunol.* 113:72–76.

67. Musso, A., T.P. Condon, G.A. West, C. De La Motte, S.A. Strong, A.D. Levine, et al. 1999. Regulation of ICAM-1-mediated fibroblast-T cell reciprocal interaction: implications for modulation of gut inflammation. *Gastroenterology* 117:546–556.

68. Eshhar, Z., T. Waks, G. Gross, and D.G. Schindler. 1993. Specific activation and targeting of cytotoxic lymphocytes through chimeric single chains consisting of antibody binding domains and the γ or ζ subunits of the immunoglobulin and T-cell receptors. *Proc. Natl. Acad. Sci. USA* 90:720–724.

69. Weijtens, M.E.M., R.A. Willemsen, D. Valerio, K. Stam, and R.L.H. Bolhius. 1996. Single chain Ig/γ gene-redirected human T lymphocytes produce cytokines, specifically lyse tumor cells, and recycle lytic capacity. *J. Immunol.* 157:836–843.

70. Reth, M. 1989. Antigen receptor tail clue. *Nature* 338:383–384.

71. Annenkov, A.E., S.P. Moyes, Z. Eshhar, R.A. Mageed, and Y. Chernajovsky. 1998. Loss of original antigenic specificity in T cell hybridomas transduced with a chimeric receptor containing single-chain Fv of an anti-collagen antibody and Fc epsilonRI-signaling gamma subunit. *J. Immunol.* 161:6604–6613.

72. Annenkov, A. and Y. Chernajovsky. 2000. Engineering mouse T lymphocytes specific to type II collagen by transduction with a chimeric receptor consisting of a single chain Fv and TCRζ. *Gene Ther.* 7:714–722.

73. Neve, R., M. Kissonerghis, J. Clark, M. Feldmann, and Y. Chernajovsky. 1996. Expression of an efficient small molecular weight tumour necrosis factor/lymphotoxin antagonist. *Cytokine* 8:365–370.

74. Chernajovsky, Y. 1999. Systemic gene therapy for arthritis, in Drugs of Today, vol. 35. C. Evans and P.D. Robbins, editors. Prous Science, Barcelona, pp. 361–377.

75. Lee, W.T. and W.J. Pelletier. 1998. Visualizing memory phenotype development after in vitro stimulation of CD4(+) T cells. *Cell. Immunol.* 188:1–11.

76. Bruno, L., B.H. von, and J. Kirberg. 1996. Cell division in the compartment of naive and memory T lymphocytes. *Eur. J. Immunol.* 26:3179–3184.

77. Chernajovsky, Y., A. Annenkov, C. Herman, K. Triantaphyllopoulos, D. Gould, H. Dreja, et al. 1998. Gene therapy for rheumatoid arthritis. Theoretical considerations. *Drugs Aging* 12:29–41.

34   Gene Therapy in Murine Arthritis

Cytokine-Directed Targeting

Wim B. van den Berg and Fons A. J. van de Loo

CONTENTS

INTRODUCTION

Local gene therapy offers the potential advantage of confined and prolonged overexpression of inhibitors at defined sites *(1–5)*. As such, it provides a challenging alternative for cytokine-directed targeting in chronic arthritides, where systemic administration of neutralizing antibodies and engineered soluble receptors is now accepted as a promising therapeutic modality. It was recently demonstrated that the cytokines tumor necrosis factor (TNF) and interleukin-1 (IL-1) play a key role in the process of chronic arthritis and concomitant cartilage and bone destruction. Suppression of TNF and IL-1 yielded relief of symptoms and reduced joint destruction in rheumatoid arthritis (RA) patients. However, these cytokines also have a significant role in host-defense mechanisms, for instance, in control of infections and tumor growth, implying that it remains a general risk to reduce TNF and IL-1 by systemic treatment for prolonged periods of time.

In the following chapter, attention will be focused on local gene therapy in murine models of arthritis, with particular emphasis on cytokines. Apart from effects in the injected joint, it is becoming more and more clear that local treatment also affects arthritis in nearby joints. This is an intriguing, general finding, which may enlarge the therapeutic applicability of gene transfer in human arthritis.

From: *Modern Therapeutics in Rheumatic Diseases*
Edited by: G. C. Tsokos, et al. © Humana Press, Inc., Totowa, NJ

PROINFLAMMATORY CYTOKINES: TNF AND IL-1

It has long been recognized that TNF and IL-1 play a major role in arthritis; TNF is considered a potent proinflammatory mediator, whereas IL-1 is a pivotal mediator in cartilage destruction. The relevance of both cytokines in arthritis emerged from in vitro culture studies and subsequent in vivo analysis. First, the potential arthritogenicity was demonstrated by intra-articular injection of recombinant forms of TNF and IL-1 in the knee joint of a range of experimental animals, including mice, rats, and rabbits. This showed that these cytokines can induce an arthritis with concomitant joint destruction. IL-1 appeared more potent as compared to TNF, but synergy was also noted. Next, studies with neutralizing antibodies and soluble receptors of TNF and IL-1 were performed in experimental models of arthritis in mice and rabbits and the efficacy demonstrated the crucial role of these cytokines in arthritis. Meanwhile, transgenic mice were made that overexpressed human TNF. These animals developed full signs of chronic destructive arthritis. Intriguingly, this TNF transgenic arthritis could be completely blocked with antibodies against the IL-1 receptor, implying that IL-1 is the pivotal downstream mediator in this model *(6)*. It also identifies that TNF alone is not harmful to the joint. More recent animal model studies demonstrated that IL-1 production can occur in inflamed synovial tissue, independent of TNF, in a range of arthritic processes. This includes direct macrophage activation with bacterial stimuli, T-cell driven processes against protein (auto)antigens and immune complex-mediated synovial activation, in particular *(7–9)*.

Although the historic picture clearly underlines IL-1 as a major therapeutic target, most clinical studies were focused on blockade of TNF. The relative lack of interest in IL-1 was further strengthened by the limited efficacy of IL-1 soluble receptor and IL-1 receptor antagonist in first clinical trials in RA patients, in sharp contrast to the promising effects of anti-TNF antibodies and engineered TNF receptors. However, it appeared that the initial choice of the soluble IL-1 type I receptor for therapeutic studies was unfortunate. This receptor has high affinity for IL-1Ra (receptor antagonist), the natural inhibitor of IL-1 activity, and its therapeutic application is seriously hampered by scavenging of endogenous IL-1Ra. Upcoming studies now focus on potential application of the decoy type II receptor, which lacks high affinity for IL-1Ra, but still binds IL-1.

The other option, usage of IL-1Ra itself as an inhibitor, remains a moot point. Although the approach is straightforward, the efficacy is hampered by the poor pharmacokinetics of the small molecule and the need to occupy fully IL-1 receptors on the cell surface for prolonged periods of time. IL-1 exerts full activation of responder cells upon activation of only 2% of the IL-1 receptors and cells then remain activated for days. In vitro studies revealed that IL-1 blocking could be obtained with 100–1000-fold excess of IL-1Ra over IL-1, making in vivo application a though job. This made IL-1Ra an obvious choice for first attempts of local overexpression by gene therapy.

IL-1Ra Gene Therapy in Collagen Arthritis

Studies with neutralizing anti-IL-1 antibodies identified autoimmune collagen-induced arthritis (CIA) in the mouse as a highly IL-1 dependent model *(10)*. First studies with IL-1Ra as a therapeutic modality in this model made it clear that arthritis could not be suppressed by repeated IL-1Ra dosing with twice-daily injections, but that arthritis was fully controled by sustained application of IL-1Ra by Alzet minipumps *(11)*. This again underlined the need of continued high dosages of the inhibitor.

To obtain local overexpression of IL-1Ra, we followed the approach introduced by Evans and Robbins *(1)*, using retroviral gene constructs and in vitro transfection of cells. Retroviral vectors containing the IL-1Ra construct were incubated with fibroblast cell lines and clones producing high amounts of IL-1Ra were selected by limiting dilution.

Two hundred thousand cells of an IL-1Ra producing line were injected into the knee joint of mice, shortly before expected onset of CIA. This treatment markedly ameliorated the onset and severity of CIA in that joint, whereas control cells, transduced with an empty virus, were ineffective *(12)*. Detailed analysis revealed that IL-1Ra-producing cells lined up along the synovial-lining cells upon intra-articular injection, and remained at this site for at least 14 d. Immunohistochemistry identified prolonged IL-1Ra production by these cells.

Apart from suppression of joint inflammation, local overexpression of IL-1Ra also normalized the synthetic function of the chondrocytes in articular cartilage. Joint inflammation has a profound suppressive effect on chondrocyte proteoglycan synthesis and this lack of matrix formation contributes to net cartilage damage during joint inflammation. Earlier studies with neutralizing antibodies identified IL-1 as the crucial mediator of this inhibition and the studies with the IL-1Ra gene transfer further substantiated this crucial role of IL-1 in cartilage destruction.

IMPACT OF IL-1RA OVEREXPRESSION ON NEARBY JOINTS

CIA is an autoimmune polyarthritis model, showing first macroscopic signs of arthritis in the paws. Upon analysis of the knee joints, expression of arthritis was also often noted at those sites. The level of expression between knees and ankles is generally correlated in this arthritis model, although the degree of correlation, in terms of incidence and severity, can vary in repeat experiments. It is an intriguing finding that nonspecific inflammation at the site is a sufficient trigger to generate expression of smouldering autoimmune arthritis in such a joint, whereas systemic inflammation enhances overall expression in multiple joints *(13)*.

Spreading of arthritis appeared cytokine-dependent, because anti-IL-1 antibodies and anti-TNF antibodies in particular were efficient in reduction of spreading. When retrovirally transduced cells are injected in a knee joint of collagen type II immunized mice, this provokes sufficient inflammation to trigger enhanced expression of CIA in that joint and, when severe enough, also in the ipsilateral paw. When these cells produce sufficient IL-1Ra, it not only suppresses joint inflammation in the knee joint, but also in the nearby paw (Fig. 1) and this suppression was of the same order of magnitude. Arthritis in joints of contralateral knee or ankle was unaffected.

In theory, there are a number of possible mechanisms for this effect. The most obvious one is the local generation of TNF and IL-1 in the control, arthritic joint where spreading of these mediators to the ipsilateral joint provokes arthritis. Local suppression/scavenging of IL-1 in the knee joint by overproduced IL-1Ra prevents this flux and arrests expression at the ipsilateral site. In addition, IL-1Ra produced in the knee and diffusing to the nearby ankle may contribute to this phenomenon. Traffic of the injected fibroblasts to the nearby paw is less likely.

Arthritis in knee and paw

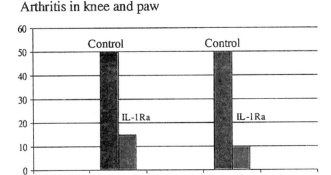

Fig. 1. Effect of retroviral IL-1Ra, injected in the knee, on CIA in that knee, and the ipsilateral paw. Note the remarkable suppression by local treatment in the knee on spreading of arthritis to remote sites.

IL-1-DIRECTED GENE THERAPY IN OTHER MODEL SYSTEMS

An elegant way to prove the usefulness of IL-1Ra gene transfer in the human situation is the use of grafting of human cells in SCID mice. Using the technique of combination of RA synovial fibroblasts with coimplanted cartilage, it was shown that retroviral IL-1Ra transduction of the fibroblasts prevented progressive, chondrocyte-mediated cartilage degradation *(14)*.

Apart from studies in mice, anti-arthritic efficacy of an adenoviral gene construct encoding the IL-1 type I receptor-IgG fusion protein was shown in the knee of rabbits with antigen-induced arthritis. Efficacy was improved when treatment was combined with a gene encoding a TNF-soluble type I receptor protein. Interestingly, anti-arthritic effects were also seen in the contralateral knee, receiving only a marker gene *(15)*. Final studies to be mentioned here regards our recent studies with adenoviral vectors with IL-1Ra, confirming efficacy in CIA, the efficacy of an adeno-associated viral vector delivering IL-1Ra in LPS induced inflammation in the knee of the rat *(16)*; and the systemic treatment by engraftment of hIL-1RII transfected human keratinocytes in the back of mice with CIA *(17)*.

GENERAL CONCLUSIONS ON IL-1-DIRECTED GENE THERAPY

The aforementioned studies proved the feasability of therapeutic gene therapy in small joints, with a promising protective effect on nearby joints. Provided the existence of some interrelationship between arthritis in nearby joints in RA patients, this will ease application in human, where it might prove sufficient to treat only the larger joints. First clinical studies in a limited number of RA patients, shortly before expected joint replacement, provided insight that the procedure is doable in patients and yields consistent expression of IL-1Ra in the synovial tissue *(1)*.

TNF-Directed Gene Therapy

Compared to the overwhelming interest in TNF as a therapeutic target in RA, surprisingly little has been done on TNF-directed gene therapy. This might be linked to paradoxical effects noted. When an adenoviral gene delivery of a dimeric chimeric human p55TNFR-IgG fusion protein was given iv to mice with CIA, it was found that it ameliorated arthritis in the first week. However, a rebound to greater inflammation was observed at later time-points, despite high levels of the TNFR fusion protein, probably related to an increase in anti-collagen type II antibodies *(18)*. The lack of effect of anti-TNF treatment in established CIA is in line with observations with neutralizing antibodies in this model *(11)*, but the increase in auto-immune antibodies identifies a risk of prolonged and effective TNF neutralization.

Local treatment with adenoviral p55 TNFR-IgG fusion protein in the knee joint of rats with CIA failed to show a beneficial effect, although systemic treatment was effective *(19)*. The lack of a local effect might be linked to viral inflammation, but it can also be argued that anti-TNF treatment exerts its effect mainly at other sites, such as the lymphoid system. An elegant approach showing the great efficacy of TNF blocking in T-cell activation was followed by the group of Chernajovsky *(20)*. Ex vivo infection of splenocytes from arthritic DBA/1 mice with a retroviral vector encoding a p75 TNFR prevents the transfer of arthritis to recipient SCID mice. It identifies that gene transfer manipulation of the immune system with TNF inhibitors can ameliorate arthritis.

MODULATORY CYTOKINES: IL-10 AND IL-4

Apart from control by overexpression of cytokine inhibitors, additional control of arthritic and destructive processes by local overexpression of modulatory cytokines is an obvious alternative *(21,22)*. Both IL-10 and IL-4 are known as inhibitors of TNF and IL-1 production by synovial cells. Moreover, they suppress Th1-driven processes. Additional relief may be expected from upregulation of inhibitors, such as IL-1Ra, IL-1, and TNF soluble receptors and tissue inhibitor of metalloproteinases (TIMP) by synovial cells or articular chondrocytes.

As compared to blocking of IL-1, the therapeutic treatment with IL-4 and IL-10 is well-suited to a local approach. These cytokines are considered protective in Th1-driven joint inflammation, but are pathogenic in Th2 driven inflammation at other sites, as is the case in allergic lung diseases. Moreover, it is expected that systemic IL-4 and IL-10 may skew immune responses in lymphoid organs to multiple antigens in an uncontroled fashion.

Adenoviral IL-10 and Arthritis

In contrast to retroviral vectors, which only infect proliferating cells, adenoviral vectors can infect almost all cells and an intermediate step, to enrich for transduced cells in vitro is not needed. Interestingly, direct injection of adenoviral gene constructs in the joint space results in almost selective infection of the synovial lining cells, which form the first cell layer encountered, with scant positivity in deeper layers. Topographically, this creates a situation much like the condition after local injection in the knee joint of cells, transduced in vitro, because the transferred cells associate along the lining cells. Dependent on the dosage of adenoviral construct, high levels of gene expression could be achieved with a single injection, with the limitation that high dose of virus creates some inflammation by itself. The level of expression of IL-10 is high in the first days, but markedly decreases thereafter (Fig. 2).

Intraarticular IL-10 production

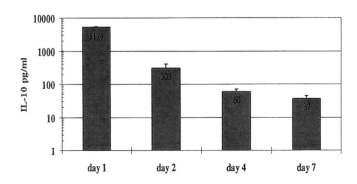

Intraarticular IL-4 production

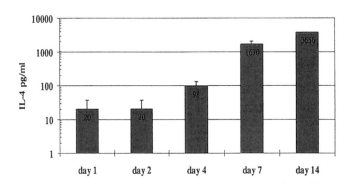

Fig. 2. Production levels of IL-10 and IL-4 after intra-articular injection of the respective adenoviral constructs in the knee of normal mice. Values represent ELISA measurements in washouts of synovial tissue. Note the peculiar kinetics of IL-4.

When adenoviral IL-10 is injected in the knee joint of collagen type II-immunized mice, shortly before expected onset of arthritis, this treatment has some suppressive effect on the local arthritis, but the decrease is not impressive. This is probably owing to the fact that IL-10 has proinflammatory potential as well, like upregulation of adhesion molecules and Fc receptor expression, herein enhancing leucocyte infiltration at the local site (23,24). Moreover, IL-10 is a potent suppressor of TNF, but has limited effect on IL-1 production in vivo. Remarkably, the most pronounced effect of IL-10 overexpression in the knee joint is the complete suppression of arthritis in the ipsilateral paw (Fig. 3), without a consistent effect on other paws. This fits with the concept that TNF is an important mediator in spreading of arthritis to ipsilateral sites and that the local suppression of TNF and IL-1 is sufficient to prevent significant diffusion of these mediators to the nearby paw.

Additional studies of a number of investigators showed efficacy of systemic (iv) injection of an adenoviral construct of viral IL-10 in CIA. The effect was convincing before onset of arthritis, but virtually absent in established arthritis (25,26). Viral

Disease Incidence (%)ipsilateral paw

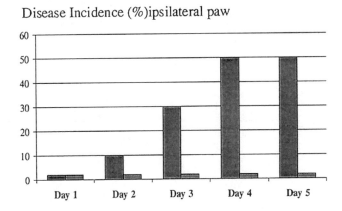

Fig. 3. Arthritis incidence in the ipsilateral paw after injection of Ad IL-10 in the knee joint of mice with CIA. First bars, control virus; second bars, Ad IL-10. Note the absence of arthritis spreading to the paw. IL-10 was marginally effective in the knee itself (*see* ref. *22*).

IL-10 lacks immunostimulatory properties and is predominantly immunosuppressive, making it more suitable for therapy. A recent study also examined local efficacy after periarticular injection in mouse paws *(27)*. Intra-articular injection in the ankle is technically hardly possible, and periarticular localization might explain the common finding of suppression of arthritis expression in the injected paw by this approach. It probably generates more of a local depot of IL-10, with sufficient leakage to the joint spaces and limited direct activation of the synovial tissue by viral antigens. The common observation of efficacy in noninjected paws is probably linked to the use of high dosages, causing a systemic suppressive effect on CIA, including manipulation of collagen type II immune responses in lymphoid organs.

With respect to cartilage damage, transfer studies in severe combined immunodeficient (SCID) mice identified that IL-10 reduces invasion of fibroblasts into the articular cartilage, a therapeutic activity not found with TNFR gene transfer *(28,29)*. However, perichondrocytic cartilage degradation was still ongoing after IL-10 gene transfer, whether from murine or viral origin, and effective suppression of this characteristic element of cartilage destruction is only found with IL-1Ra. These observations further underscore separate activities of IL-10, TNFR, and IL-1Ra and argue for combination therapies.

Adenoviral IL-4 and Arthritis

As a follow-up of the IL-10 studies, murine IL-4 was overexpressed in the knee joint, again using the murine CIA model. In contrast to IL-10, endogenous IL-4 levels are low in inflamed joints, making IL-4 an obvious therapeutic modality. When evaluating the levels of IL-4 produced in the knee joint after local gene transfer, it was evident that the kinetics of IL-4 expression are curious. Low expression in the first days and higher expression after a week (Fig. 2). So far this is the only adenoviral gene construct where this kinetic pattern was seen; all other gene constructs analyzed, including IL-1Ra, IL-12, IL-15 , IL-17, and TGFβ showed the highest expression in the first days. The reason for these peculiar kinetics is unclear. The high levels at later stages were not owing to substantial elicitation of endogenous IL-4 production, because similar kinetics were observed in IL-4 knockout mice.

Table 1
Reduced Cartilage Damage After Local Adv-IL-4 Treatment
in Murine Collagen Arthritis (*see also* ref. *30*)

Degree of cartilage damage	Chondrocyte death		Cartilage erosions	
	Ad control (10^7)	Ad IL-4 (10^7)	Ad control (10^7)	Ad IL-4 (10^7)
Arthritic mice	20/22	21/21	20/22	21/21
Non	0	3	0	7
Mild	0	10	0	14
Moderate	8[a]	8	15[a]	0
Severe	12	0	5	0

[a]Number of mice showing a particular degree of cartilage damage.

First observations in the CIA model were disappointing. No significant reduction of inflammation in the IL-4-injected knee joint was seen. In line with this, no significant suppression of spreading to ipsilateral paws was seen either. However, upon more careful analysis of joint histology of the treated knee, it was clear that IL-4 had markedly reduced the erosive changes. Although proteoglycan loss from the articular cartilage matrix as identified by loss of Safranin-O staining was not reduced, the degree of chondrocyte death was highly diminished at d 7 after injection of IL-4. Moreover, excessive proteoglycan-breakdown neoepitopes, indicative for irreversible breakdown and occurrence of collagenase-mediated loss of collagen type II, were seen in the control arthritic group, but hardly in the IL-4-treated mice. Follow-up till d 14 revealed that the control group proceeded to major erosive cartilage damage, including marked surface erosions and tissue loss (Table 1), whereas the IL-4 mice were highly protected *(30)*.

Adenoviral IL-4 and Bone Erosion

In addition to prevention of major cartilage erosion, IL-4 also abolished excessive bone erosion in murine CIA. Pronounced osteoclast activation was found in the control, arthritic group with impressive ingrowth of granulation tissue from the synovial membrane, whereas this aggressive phenotype was hardly seen in the IL-4 mice. Reverse transcriptase polymerase chain reaction (RT-PCR) analysis and immunolocalization on the synovial tissue suggested that IL-4 exerted its suppressive activity at multiple levels. TNF and IL-1 were suppressed, stromelysin was inhibited, but also IL-12 and IL-17 levels were markedly reduced, implying that both nonimmune inflammatory and destructive pathways as well as Th1-driven activation was inhibited.

With respect to characteristic elements of bone erosion, it became evident that osteoprotegerin ligand (OPGL) is reduced, with similar levels of the endogenous inhibitor OPG. OPGL is recently identified as the crucial mediator of osteoclast differentiation and activation. Because OPGL upregulation can be induced both by the cytokines TNF and IL-1 as well as by the Th1 T-cell pathway (IL-17), a dual hit of IL-4-mediated suppression is conceivable *(31)*. As yet it is unclear whether IL-4 can directly reduce OPGL.

A recent study in rat adjuvant arthritis demonstrated efficacy of retroviral IL-4 injected in the ankle. As discussed for IL-10 injections in the paw, it is unlikely that paw injections target the joint spaces and most of the expression probably occurs at periarticular sites, compatible with significant serum levels of IL-4 and enhanced systemic Th2 function *(32)*. In line with the murine studies, IL-4 reduced bone destruction in adjuvant arthritis. Comparative studies with Chinese hamster ovary (CHO) cells engineered to produce IL-4, IL-10, or IL-13, and engrafted at weekly intervals, showed efficacy in TNF transgenic mice only for IL-4 *(33)*.

In conclusion, local IL-4 treatment provides impressive control of cartilage and bone destruction. However, the limited effect on cell infiltration implies that IL-4 should be combined with an anti-inflammatory treatment, to provide acceptable symptomatic relief at the site. Recent studies with systemic IL-4, combined with low-dose steroids, demonstrated marked synergy of this mixture *(34,35)*. It remains to be seen whether low steroid dose can be combined with local IL-4 gene therapy. Other options are to combine IL-4 with FasL *(36)* or to engineer cassettes of gene constructs, for instance carrying FasL, an IL-1 inhibitor, a modulatory cytokine like IL-4, and a protease inhibitor.

OTHER TARGETS

Apart from the overproduction of inflammatory cytokines and chemokines in the inflamed synovial tissue, chronicity of the arthritis is owing to abnormal local proliferation of cells and prolonged cell survival, resembling tumor-like behavior. Gene targeting of cell activation and promotion of cell apoptosis is a promising therapeutic goal.

Apoptosis and Proliferation

Cells undergo apoptosis when their Fas receptors engage FasL (Fas ligand). Because many cells in the synovial tissue express Fas, whereas FasL itself is scant, antibodies against Fas or genetic overexpression of FasL in the synovial tissue may serve as a general ablative approach. In CIA transfer of FasL appeared feasible. Direct injection of an adenoviral gene construct with FasL in inflamed joints of DBA mice with CIA ameliorated the disease activity *(37)*. In addition, overexpression of FasL-induced apoptosis in cells of human RA synovium that was implanted in SCID mice *(38)*.

However, it is not known whether sufficient numbers of cells susceptible to Fas-mediated apoptosis are present in the rheumatoid synovium. An interesting development is the further understanding of the Fas pathway, with identification of Fas-associated death domain protein (FADD) as a key element. FADD gene transfer induced apoptosis of RA synoviocytes. Moreover, local injection of FADD adenovirus eliminated synoviocytes in vivo, by induction of apoptosis of proliferating human RA synovium engrafted in SCID mice *(39)*. Remarkably, the transfer did not affect chondrocytes.

Another way to enhance cell death is to deliver the herpes thymidine kinase, followed by administration of ganciclovir. This will be effective only when sufficient numbers of proliferating cells are present in the synovial tissue, which is debatable in established RA. An interesting variant to this is the induction of selective apoptosis of T cells. Galectin-1 (GAL-1) has been shown to induce in vitro apoptosis of activated T cells and immature thymocytes. A single injection of syngeneic DBA/1 fibroblasts, engineered to secrete GAL-1 at the day of disease onset, was able to abrogate CIA *(40)*. Intriguingly, a skewing towards a type 2-polarized immune reaction was noted.

Cell Activation, NF-κB

In addition to apoptosis, interference with cell activation might be a promising strategy. NF-κB is expressed ubiquitously and is involved in the regulation of a large variety of genes, some of which are responsible for cytokine production and inflammatory responses in RA. Activation of NFκB by molecules such as TNF-α involved the rapid degradation of IkBa, the natural inhibitor. Efficacy of overexpression of IKBa has been demonstrated in streptococcal cell wall (SCW) arthritis *(41)*.

An alternative approach is the transfection of a NF-κB decoy. Synthetic double-stranded DNA that shows a high affinity for the transcription factor NF-κB was constructed and treatment was done using the hemagglutinating virus of Japan (HVJ)-liposome method *(42)*. Injection in the ankle joints of rats with collagen arthritis decreased severity of swelling and reduced joint damage.

It is expected that further understanding of signaling pathways will provide novel targets for gene therapeutic approaches, in particular those elements in pathways that are associated with agressive and destructive behavior of cells.

EFFECTS ON IPSILATERAL AND CONTRALATERAL JOINTS

As mentioned at the various cytokine sections, additional protective effects of local gene therapy in the knee were noted in the ipsilateral paw and sometimes also in the contralateral joint *(32,41,43)*.

The restricted effect on ipsilateral paws is seen under conditions of limited local dosing in the knee, not exceeding 10×8 pfu of the adenoviral vector and injections given at onset of arthritis. Local control of inflammatory mediators, otherwise responsible for spreading of arthritis to the paw, as well as some diffusion of the inhibitory protein itself, are the most likely explanations. Traffic of genes or cells carrying the gene are less likely, because adenoviral infection mainly transduced the synovial-lining cells, which consist of fibroblasts and macrophage-like cells.

The efficacy of local gene therapy may include contralateral sites when high local dosages are applied, with obvious leakage of inhibitor to remote sites. In addition, when the gene is applied periarticularly as is the case in ankle-joint injection, or when gene therapy is applied to joints, which are already heavily inflamed and carrying a florid exudate in the joint space. Under those conditions the adenoviral vector may infect or affect numerous cell types, including leucocytes and probably also dendritic cells. The latter are obvious candidates for traveling to other sites, and may influence arthritis at remote sites, dependent on the local priming with transduced genes and soluble cytokines (Fig. 4). Impact is expected in particular in models where immunity and local priming of T cells are important elements of the arthritis. The observation of contralateral protection may argue that local events in inflamed joints not only destroy joints, but also drive the disease at remote sites. Identification of the cells involved in transfer of protection to remote sites deserves major attention at present.

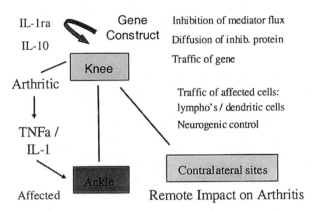

Fig. 4. Schematic view of linkage of arthritis at various sites and potential pathways of local gene therapy-mediated remote control.

On the other hand, one might argue that clinical application should be preferrably performed under controled conditions, which would imply that joints should be washed-out before adenoviral gene transfer, to deliberately target local synovial-lining cells.

IMPROVEMENT OF FOCAL THERAPY

Successful gene therapy depends on an effective gene-delivery system. Viruses are obvious vehicles, and three types of viruses are sufficiently cleaned and optimized to permit their use in clinical trials: retrovirus, adenovirus and adeno-associated virus (AAV). Retrovirus and AAV, unlike adenovirus, integrate their genetic material into the chromosal DNA, increasing the potential of long-term gene expression. Apart from retention of the gene, the targeting of cells, or selection of cells as a carrier to deliver the gene product at particular sites, is a crucial element of successful therapy.

Targeting of Synovial Cells with RGD Viruses

When adenoviral gene constructs are injected into the knee joint cavity of the mouse, the usual way to infect cells is through the Coxsackie adenovirus receptor (CAR) receptor on the fiber knob of the virus. It was noted that infection in normal mouse joints was high, but expression dropped dramatically (fivefold) in chronically inflamed joints, which is closer to the clinical situation in RA patients.

One way to enhance infection of cells under inflamed conditions is to make use of upregulated integrin expression of the synovial cells. Adenoviral vectors with a Arginine-glycine-aspargic acid RGD motif introduced in the fiber knob were constructed by the group of Curiel (44,45). This allowed this virus to enter cells through integrin interaction. Upon injection of these viruses, carrying GFP as a marker gene, it was found that infection was greatly enhanced (up to 70-fold) in chronically inflamed joints.

To get an impression of applicability in RA patients, ex vivo incubations of synovial-tissue specimens with RGD viruses were performed. Infection levels with normal viruses are highly variable in tissue specimens of various RA patients, probably linked to large differences in cellular infiltrates. However, a dramatic increase in transduction levels was consistently noted with the RGD viruses, ranging from 10–50-fold increments.

T Cells

Another way to express inhibitors or modulatory proteins at the site is to make use of the migratory capacity of T cells. It was found that pathogenic lymphoid cells, engineered to express TGF-β ameliorate CIA *(46)*. It is known that Th1 cells display good migratory characteristics (chemokine receptors) to enter joint tissues, whereas the protective Th2 cells have difficulty reaching this site. It will be technically possible to engineer T cells with the desired chemokine receptor make-up of a Th1 cells, yet additionally engineered to produce modulatory cytokines such as TGF-β and IL-4. By manipulation of the TCR on these cells, it is also possible to direct the antigen specificity, for instance, to the joint-specific, antigen collagen type II *(47)*, and to use such cells as gene carriers in anti-inflammatory gene therapy in autoimmune arthritis.

CONTROLLED EXPRESSION OF GENES

As mentioned earlier, it is expected that future therapies will make use of cassettes of genes, combining the targeting of multiple mediators as well as including growth factors to optimize recovery of the damaged joint. Apart from improved targeting to synovial tissue, a major challenge for the future will be the targeting of chondrocytes in the articular cartilage. Present adenoviral gene constructs are too large to allow for proper penetration of the dense cartilage matrix and further research is needed to design applicable carriers for this tissue. Lipid carriers might be an alternative *(48)*.

Apart from targeting, the controlled expression of the gene is an obvious goal. So far, most studies have been done with the constitutive cytomegalovirus (CMV) promotor. However, it makes more sense to create an intelligent promotor system, which can sense the need of expression of a particular inhibitor and only activates the gene, when needed. The group of Munford recently engineered a two-hybrid system, with a complement promotor activating the *Tat* gene, and Tat activating the HIV promotor in front of the gene of interest *(49)*. The complement promotor will be turned on under conditions of acute inflammation and will be silenced when inflammation is suppressed. Testing of such a hybrid system, with IL-1Ra as the gene of interest in the model of CIA, has been done (van den Berg and van de Loo, unpublished observation) and looks promising.

The recent observation of long term retention of AAV-IL-1Ra in the knee joint of rats and the reactivation of IL-1Ra production upon rechallenge with an inflammation-inducing agent such as lipopolysaccharide (LPS) *(16)*, provides a way to protect against exacerbations. This is important in arthritic diseases that undergo spontaneous flares and remissions.

SIDE EFFECTS AND PRECAUTIONS

Risks involved with gene therapy surround the use of the various vector systems and the traffic of genes to remote sites. Nonviral vectors holds the least concern, but show low efficacy of gene transfer. Viral vectors have been genetically disabled to minimize their ability to replicate and cause pathology. Engineering of viral vectors continues to improve, including removal of immunogenic components and further reduction of the risk of recombination events towards the impossible. An advantage of the ex vivo gene-therapy approach, with infection and selection of cells in vitro, is the opportunity to do safety screenings before transplantation of the cells.

The first clinical trials in RA patients have been done with the retroviral ex vivo approach, for safety reasons, but it is expected that further trials will focus on improved adenovirus or AAV as a carrier. If the focus of future therapy will be on local treatment in joints, the total amount of viral elements introduced is low and the risk negligible. Thousands of patients have participated in gene-therapy studies over the last decade and it is fair to say that the safety record is impressive so far.

REFERENCES

1. Evans, C.H., S.C. Ghivizzani, R. Kang, T. Muzzonigro, M.C. Wasko, J.H. Herndon, and P.D. Robbins. 1999. Gene therapy for rheumatic diseases. *Arthritis Rheum.* 42:1–16.

2. Evans, C.H., S.C. Ghivizzani, and P.D. Robbins. 1998. Blocking cytokines with genes. *J. Leukoc. Biol.* 64:55–61.

3. Evans, C.H. and P.D. Robbins. 1996. Pathways to gene therapy in rheumatoid arthritis. *Curr. Opin. Rheumatol.* 8:230–234.

4. Robbins, P.D. and S.C. Ghivizzani. 1998. Viral vectors for gene therapy. *Pharmacol Ther.* 80:35–47.

5. Robbins, P.D., C.H. Evans, and Y. Chernajovsky. 1998. Gene therapy for rheumatoid arthritis. *Springer Semin. Immunopathol.* 20:197–209.

6. Probert, L., D. Plows, G. Kontogeorgos, and G. Kollias. 1995. The type I IL-1 receptor acts in series with TNFI to induce arthritis in TNFI transgenic mice. *Eur. J. Immunol.* 25:1794–1797.

7. Van den Berg, W.B. and B. Bresnihan. 1999. Pathogenesis of joint damage in RA: evidence of a dominant role for IL-1. *Bailliere's Clin. Rheumatol.* 13:577–597.

8. Van den Berg, W.B., L.A.B. Joosten, G. Kollias, and F.A.J. van de Loo. 1999. Role of TNFI in experimental arthritis: separate activity of IL-1θ in chronicity and cartilage destruction. *Ann. Rheum. Dis.* 58(Suppl.I):S140–S148.

9. Van den Berg, W.B. 1998. Joint inflammation and cartilage destruction may occur uncoupled. *Springer Semin Immunopathol.* 20:149–164.

10. Van den Berg, W.B., L.A.B. Joosten, M.M.A. Helsen, and F.A.J. van de Loo. 1994. Amelioration of established murine collagen induced arthritis with anti-IL-1 treatment. *Clin. Exp. Immunol.* 95:237–243.

11. Joosten, L.A.B., M.M.A. Helsen, F.A.J. van de Loo, and W.B. van den Berg. 1996. Anticytokine treatment of established type II collagen-induced arthritis in DBA/1 mice: a comparative study using anti-TNF(, anti-IL-1I/θ, and IL-1ra. *Arthritis Rheum.* 39:797–809.

12. Bakker, A.C., L.A.B. Joosten, O.J. Arntz, M.M.A. Helsen, A. Bendele, F.A.J. van de Loo, and W.B. van den Berg. 1997. Prevention of murine collagen-induced arthritis in the knee and ipsilateral paw by local expression of human IL-1ra protein in the knee. *Arthritis Rheum.* 40:893–900.

13. Van den Berg, W.B. and L.A.B. Joosten. 1999. Murine collagen-induced arthritis. *In* In Vivo Models of Inflammation. D.W. Morgan and L.A. Marshall, editors. Birkhauser Verlag, Basel. 51–75.

14. Müller-Ladner, U., C.R. Roberts, B.N. Franklin, R.E. Gay, P.D. Robbins, C.H. Evans, and S. Gay. 1997. Human IL-1ra gene transfer into human synovial fibroblasts is chondroprotective. *J. Immunol.* 158:3492–3498.

15. Ghivizzani, S.C., E.R. Lechman, R. Kang, C. Tio, J. Kolls, C.H. Evans, and P.D. Robbins. 1998. Direct adenovirus-mediated gene transfer of IL-1 and TNF(soluble receptors to rabbit knees with experimental arthritis has local and distal anti-arthritic effects. *Proc. Natl. Acad. Sci. USA* 95:4613–4618.

16. Pan, R.Y., S.L. Chen, X. Xiao, D.W. Liu, H.J. Peng, and Y.P. Tsao. 2000. Therapy and prevention of arthritis by recombinant adeno-associated virus vector with delivery of IL-1ra. *Arthritis Rheum.* 43:289–297.

17. Bessis, N., L. Guery, A. Mantovani, A. Vecchi, J.E. Sims, D. Fradelizi, and M.C.Boissier. 2000. The type II decoy receptor of IL-1 inhibits murine collagen-induced arthritis. *Eur. J. Immunol.* 30:867–875.

18. Quattrocchi, E., M. Walmsley, K. Browne, R.O. Williams, L. Marinova-Mutafchieva, W. Buurman, et al. 1999. Paradoxical effects of adenovirus-mediated blockade of TNF activity in murine collagen-induced arthritis. *J. Immunol.* 163:1000–1009.

19. Le, C.H., G. Nicolson, A. Morales, and K.L. Sewell. 1997. Suppression of collagen-induced arthritis through adenovirus-mediated transfer of a modified TNFI receptor gene. *Arthritis Rheum.* 40:1662–1669.

20. Mageed, R.A., G. Adams, D. Woodrow, O.L. Podhajcer, and Y. Chernajovsky. 1998. Prevention of collagen-induced arthritis by gene delivery of soluble p75 TNF receptor. *Gene Ther.* 5:1584–1592.

21. Joosten, L.A.B., E. Lubberts, P. Durez, M.M.A. Helsen, M.J.M. Jacobs, M. Goldman, and W.B. van den Berg. 1997. Role of IL-4 and IL-10 in murine collagen-induced arthritis: protective effect of IL-4 and IL-10 treatment on cartilage destruction. *Arthritis Rheum.* 40:249–260.

22. Lubberts, E., L.A.B. Joosten, M.M.A. Helsen, and W.B. van den Berg. 1998. Regulatory role of IL-10 in joint inflammation and cartilage destruction in murine SCW arthritis. More therapeutic benefit with IL-4/IL-10 combination therapy than with IL-10 treatment alone. *Cytokine* 10:361–369.

23. Lubberts, E., L.A.B. Joosten, L. van den Bersselaar, M.M.A. Helsen, A.C. Bakker, Z. Xing, et al. 2000. Intra-articular IL-10 gene transfer regulates the expression of collagen-induced arthritis (CIA) in the knee and ipsilateral paw. *Clin. Exp. Immunol.* 120:375–383.

24. Ma, Y., S. Thornton, L.E. Duwel, G.P. Boivin, E.H. Giannini, J.M. Leiden, et al. 1998. Inhibition of collagen-induced arthritis in mice by viral IL-10 gene transfer. *J. Immunol.* 161:1516–1524.

25. Kim, K.N., S. Watanabe, Y. Ma, S. Thornton, E.H. Giannini, and R. Hirsch. 2000. Viral IL-10 and soluble TNF receptor act synergistically to collagen-induced arthritis following adenovirus-mediated gene transfer. *J. Immunol.* 164:1576–1581.

26. Apparailly, F., C. Verwaerde, C. Jacquet, C. Auriault, J. Sany, and C. Jorgensen. 1998. Adeno-virus-mediated transfer of viral IL-10 gene inhibits murine collagen-induced arthritis. *J. Immunol.* 160:5213–5220.

27. Whalen, J.D., E.L. Lechman, C.A. Carlos, K. Weiss, I. Kovesdi, J.C. Glorioso, et al. 1999. Adenoviral transfer of the viral IL-10 gene periarticularly to mouse paws suppresses development of collagen-induced arthritis in both injected and uninjected paws. *J. Immunol.* 162:3625–3632.

28. Jorgensen, C., F. Apparailly, F. Canovas, C. Verwaerde, C. Auriault, C. Jacquet, and J. Sany. 1999. Systemic viral IL-10 gene delivery prevents cartilage invasion by human rheumatoid synovial tissue engrafted in SCID mice. *Arthritis Rheum.* 42:678–685.

29. Müller-Ladner, U., C.H. Evans, B.N. Franklin, C.R. Roberts, R.E. Gay, P.D. Robbins, and S. Gay. 1999. Gene transfer of cytokine inhibitors into human synovial fibroblasts in the SCID mouse model. *Arthritis Rheum.* 42:490–497.

30. Lubberts, E., L.A.B. Joosten, L. van den Bersselaar, M.M. Helsen, A.C. Bakker, J.B. van Meurs, et al. 1999. Adenoviral vector-mediated overexpression of IL-4 in the knee joint of mice with collagen-induced arthritis prevents cartilage destruction. *J. Immunol.* 163:4546–4556.

31. Lubberts, E., L.A.B. Joosten, M. Chabaud, L. van den Berselaar, C.J.J. Coenen-de Roo, C.D. Richards, et al. 2000. Prevention of bone erosion in murine collagen arthritis by local IL-4 gene therapy. Implications in human rheumatoid arthritis. *J. Clin. Invest.* 105:1697–1710.

32. Boyle, D.L., K.H. Nguyen, S. Zhuang, Y. Shi, J.E. McCormack, S. Chada, and G.S. Firestein. 1999. Intra-articular IL-4 gene therapy in arthritis: anti-inflammatory effect and enhanced Th2 activity. *Gene Ther.* 6:1911–1918.

33. Bessis, N., G. Chicchia, G. Kollias, A. Minty, C. Fournier, D. Fradelizi, and M.C. Boissier. 1998. Modulation of proinflammatory cytokine production in TNF(-transgenic mice by treatment with cells engineered to secrete IL-4, IL-10 or IL-13. *Clin. Exp. Imunol. 111:*391–396.

34. Joosten, L.A.B., M.M.A. Helsen, T. Saxne, D. Heinegard, L.B.A. van de Putte, and W.B. van den Berg. 1999. Synergistic protection against cartilage destruction by low dose prednisolone and IL-10 in established murine collagen arthritis. *Inflamm. Res.* 48:48–55.

35. Joosten, L.A.B., E. Lubberts, M.M.A. Helsen, T. Saxne, C.J.J. Coenen-de Roo, D. Heinegard, and W.B. van den Berg. 1999. Protection against cartilage and bone destruction by systemic IL-4 treatment in established murine type II collagen-induced arthritis. *Arthritis Res.* 1:81–91.

36. Guery, L., F. Batteux, N. Bessis, M. Breban, M.C. Boissier, C. Fournier, and G. Chiocchia. 2000. Expression of Fas ligand improves the effect of IL-4 in collagen-induced arthritis. *Eur. J. Immunol.* 30:308–315.

37. Zhang, H., Y. Yang, J.L. Horton, E.B. Samoilova, T.A. Judge, L.A. Turka, et al. 1997. Amelioration of collagen-induced arthritis by CD95 (Apo-1/Fas)-ligand expressing APCs as a therapy for autoimmune disease. *J. Clin. Invest.* 100:1951–9157.

38. Okamoto, K., H. Asahara, T. Kobayashi, T. Matsuno, T. Kobata, T. Sumida, and K. Nishioka. 1998. Induction of apoptosis in the rheumatoid synovium by Fas ligand gene transfer. *Gene Ther.* 5:331–338.

39. Kobayashi, T., K. Okamoto, T. Kobata, T. Kato, H. Hamada, and K. Nishioka. 2000. Novel gene therapy for rheumatoid arthritis by FADD gene transfer: induction of apoptosis of rheumatoid synoviocytes but not chondrocytes. *Gene Ther.* 7:527–533.

40. Rabinovich, G.A., G. Daly, H. Tailor, C.M. Riera, J. Hirabayashi, and Y. Chernajovsky. 1999. Recombinant galectin-1 and its genetic delivery suppress collagen-induced arthritis via T cell apoptosis. *J. Exp. Med.* 190:385–398.

41. Miagkov, A.V., D.V. Kovalenko, C.E. Brown, J.R. Didsbury, J.P. Cogswell, S.A. Stimpson, et al. 1998. NF-kappaB activation provides the potential link between inflammation and hyperplasia in the arthritic joint. *Proc. Natl. Acad. Sci. USA* 95:13,859–13,864.

42. Tomita, T., E. Takeuchi, N. Tomita, R. Morishita, M. Kaneko, K. Yamamoto, et al. 1999. Suppressed severity of collagen-induced arthritis by in vivo transfection of nuclear factor kappaB decoy oligodeoxynucleotides as a gene therapy. *Arthritis Rheum.* 42:2532–2542.

43. Lechman, E.R., D. Jaffurs, S.C. Ghivizzani, A. Gambotto, A. Kovesdi, Z. Mi, et al. 1999. Direct adenoviral gene transfer of viral IL-10 to rabbit knees with experimental arthritis ameliorates disease in both injected and contralateral control knees. *J. Immunol.* 163:2202–2208.

44. Krasnykh, V.N., G.V. Mikheeva, J.T. Douglas, and D.T. Curiel. 1996. Generation of recombinant adenovirus vectors with modified fibers for altering viral tropism. *J. Virol.* 70:6839–6846.

45. Reynolds, P.N., I. Dmitriev, and D.T. Curiel. 1999. Insertion of an RGD motif into the HI loop of adenovirus fiber protein alters the distribution of transgene expression of the systemically administered vector. *Gene Ther.* 6:1336–1339.

46. Chernajovsky, Y., G. Adams, K. Triantaphyllopoulos, M.F. Ledda, and O.L. Podhajcer. 1997. Pathogenic lymphoid cells engineered to express TGFθ1 ameliorate disease in a collagen-induced arthritis model. *Gene Ther.* 4:553–559.

47. Annenkov, A. and Y. Chernajovsky. 2000. Engineering mouse T lymphocytes specific to type II collagen by transduction with a chimeric receptor consisting of a single chain Fc and TCR zeta. *Gene Ther.* 7:714–722.

48. Madry, H. and S.B. Trippel. 2000. Efficient lipid-mediated gene transfer to articular chondrocytes. *Gene Ther.* 7:286–291.

49. Varley, A.W., G. Coulthard, R.S. Meidell, R.D. Gerard, and R.S. Munford. 1995. Inflammation-induced recombinant protein expression in vivo using promoters from acute-phase protein genes. *Proc. Natl. Acad. Sci. USA* 92:5346–5350.

35

Modulation of the IκB Kinase/Nuclear Factor-κB Pathway by Gene Therapy

Paul P. Tak and Gary S. Firestein

CONTENTS

INTRODUCTION

In rheumatoid arthritis (RA), the synovium is hypertrophic and edematous, and villous projections of synovial tissue protrude into the joint cavity. Cartilage degradation primarily results from the action of extracellular proteolytic enzymes produced in the local microenvironment at the invasive front of the synovial tissue (pannus). Although the etiology of RA remains elusive, immune-mediated mechanisms are of crucial importance. It has become clear that macrophages and fibroblast-like synoviocytes play a critical role as effector cells in chronic synovial inflammation (1–3). T cells could contribute to the excessive production of proinflammatory cytokines by stimulation of these effector cells (4–6). Both macrophages and fibroblast-like synoviocytes are highly activated and secrete a variety of cytokines as well as matrix metalloproteinases.

Fibroblast-like synoviocytes are also able to produce other factors, such as proteoglycans and arachidonic acid metabolites. Relatively little is known about the factors that influence the specific retention of macrophages and the interaction between cells in the intimal lining layer. It has recently been suggested that the ligand pair CD55/CD97 could be involved (7). Of note, intimal macrophages exhibit stronger expression of the 7-span transmembrane receptor molecule CD97 than macrophages in the synovial sublining, illustrating their highly activated phenotype. In addition to proliferation, migration, and retention of cells, inhibition of apoptosis provides an important explanation for the increased cellularity in the synovium (8). Various mechanisms may be involved in causing inadequate apoptosis: the development of mutations of the *p53* suppressor gene

From: *Modern Therapeutics in Rheumatic Diseases*
Edited by: G. C. Tsokos, et al. © Humana Press, Inc., Totowa, NJ

as a result of chronic oxidative stress *(9)*, deficient functional Fas ligand expression *(10)*, overexpression of anti-apoptotic molecules, such as sentrin *(11)*, and activation of nuclear factor (NF)-κB *(12)*.

The significance of activated inflammatory cells in the synovium is supported by clinical observations. Local disease activity is particularly associated with the number of macrophages and the expression of proinflammatory cytokines *(3,13)*. There is also a significant positive correlation between macrophage infiltration and radiographic signs of joint destruction after follow-up *(14)*. The pivotal role of tumor necrosis factor-α (TNF-α)—at least in the majority of RA patients—has been confirmed by the impressive effects of specific therapeutic strategies targeting the TNF-α molecule *(15)*. The importance of pro-inflammatory cytokines, which are mainly derived from macrophages and fibroblast-like synoviocytes, is also illustrated by the effects of treatment aimed at blocking the effects of interleukin-1 (IL-1) and IL-6 *(17)*.

PATHOGENIC MECHANISMS THAT RATIONALIZE
THE THERAPEUTIC TARGET

NF-kB Activation in Synovial Inflammation

Synthesis of many cytokines, including TNF-α, IL-1β, IL-6, and IL-8, is mediated by the transcription factor NF-κB, which is able to induce transcription of proinflammatory gene arrays (Table 1) *(18–20)*. NF-κB is also involved in Th1-dependent, delayed-type hypersensitivity responses *(21)*. The induction of matrix metalloproteinses, cyclo-oxygenase-2 (COX-2), and inducible nitric oxide (iNOS) add to the detrimental effects of NF-κB activation in inflammatory disease *(20)*. Moreover, NF-κB activation leads to upregulation of adhesion molecules, such as E-selectin, vascular cell adhesion mlecule (VCAM-1), and intracellular cell adhesion molecule ICAM-1, whereas NF-κB inhibition reduces leukocyte adhesion and transmigration *(22)*. Thus, NF-κB activation may lead to accumulation and activation of inflammatory cells at sites of inflammation. As noted earlier, NF-κB activation also appears to be a pivotal factor in protecting specific cells against apoptosis, which may further enhance cell accumulation *(12)*.

NF-κB is highly activated in a variety of inflammatory diseases. In RA, NF-κB is overexpressed in the inflamed synovium *(23–25)*. The NF-κB family includes NF-κB1 (p50/p105), NF-κB2 (p52/p100), p65 (RelA), RelB, and c-Rel *(26)*. Except for RelB, which does not form homodimers, every member of this family can form heterodimers or homodimers with each other. The most prevalent activated form of NF-κB is a heterodimer consisting of a p50 or p52 subunit and p65, which contains transactivation domains necessary for gene induction. Both p50 and p65 have been localized to nuclei in the intimal lining layer cells and in mononuclear cells (MNCs) in the synovial sublining. Increased NF-κB activity in RA synovium compared with osteoarthritis (OA) controls has been shown by electrophoretic mobility shift assays *(25)*. Of importance, heterodimers of p50 and p65 are intimately involved in activation of inflammatory gene sets by IL-1 or TNF-α in human monocytes. Both p50 and p65 also play a role in constitutive IL-6 production by RA fibroblast-like synoviocytes *(27)*. Studies in rabbit synovial fibroblasts revealed a role for p50 homodimers in the induction of matrix metalloproteinase-1 (MMP-1), suggesting a mechanism of NF-κB mediated cartilage degradation in RA *(28)*.

Table 1
Deleterious Effects on Synovial Inflammation
and Joint Destruction Regulated by NF-κB

Production of proinflammatory cytokines and chemokines
Induction of matrix metalloproteinases
Induction of cyclooxygenase-2 (COX-2) and inducible nitric oxide (iNOS)
Upregulation of adhesion molecules
Protection against apoptosis

Previous studies have shown that asymptomatic synovitis precedes clinically manifest arthritis *(13)*. In line with this notion, NF-κB activation precedes the development of collagen-induced arthritis (CIA) in mice *(25)* and adjuvant arthritis in rats *(29)*. In addition, selective activation of NF-κB by in vivo gene transfer of adenoviral constructs encoding wild-type IKKβ to the joints of normal rats led to synovial inflammation and clinical signs of arthritis *(30)*. Hence, these studies confirm the pivotal role of NF-κB activation in the development of arthritis.

Regulation of NF-κB Activation

NF-κB exists in the cytoplasm in an inactive form associated with regulatory proteins called inhibitors of κB (IκB), including IκBα, IκBβ, and IκBε. Phosphorylation of IκB is an important step in NF-κB activation and is regulated by IκB kinase (IKK). The IKK complex comprises at least three subunits, including the kinases IKKα and IKKβ (also called IKK1 and IKK2) *(31)* and the regulatory subunit IKKγ *(32)*. In addition, a novel lipopolysaccharide-inducible kinase, termed IKKi, was recently described *(33)*. IKK activation initiates IκBα phosphorylation at specific N-terminal serine residues. Phosphorylated IκBα is then ubiquinated and degraded by proteasomes in the cytoplasm. This leads to release of NF-κB dimers from the cytoplasmic NF-κBIκB complex followed by nuclear translocation. NF-κB then binds to κB enhancer elements of target genes, inducing transcription of an array of proinflammatory genes.

IKK is a critical regulator of NF-κB activation in many cell types and serves as a conduit between multiple activation signals and nuclear translocation of NF-κB *(34)*. IKKβ is the primary pathway for proinflammatory stimuli, resulting in NF-κB activation, whereas the involvement of IKKα has not been shown *(35,36)*. To determine if IKK regulates NF-κB in primary cells isolated from rheumatoid synovial tissue, IKK was characterized in cultured fibroblast-like synoviocytes isolated from synovium of patients with RA and OA *(34)*. Immunoreactive IKK protein was abundantly expressed by fibroblast-like synoviocytes in both patient groups. IKKα and IKKβ genes were constitutively expressed and IKK activity was greatly increased by stimulation with proinflammatory cytokines. This was associated with degradation of endogenous IκBα and nuclear translocation of NF-κB. IKKβ activation resulted in increased expression of IL-6, IL-8, MMP-1, and ICAM-1 *(37)*. Inhibition of IKKβ activity by transfection with dominant-negative adenoviral constructs prevented TNF-α-mediated, NF-κB nuclear translocation and proinflammatory gene expression in these cells. However, a dominant-negative IKKα mutant had no effect *(34,37)*. Similarly, IKKβ specifically regulates NF-κB activation and inflammatory gene transcription in human monocytes

Table 2
Therapeutic Strategies Aimed at Blocking NF-κB Activity

Strategy	Reference
IKKβ-dominant-negative gene therapy	(30)
NF-κB decoy oligonucleotides	(12,49)
T cell-specific NF-κB inhibitor	(47)
Corticosteroids	(41)
Sulfasalazine	(42)
5-aminosalicylic acid	(43)
Aspirin	(44)
Tepoxalin	(45)
Leflunomide	(46)
Curcumin	(54)
Antioxidants	(55)
Proteasome inhibitors	(56)

(38) and in human CD4+ T lymphocytes (39), which are also likely to be involved in the pathogenesis of RA. Upstream of IKK, kinases such as NF-κB inducing kinase (NIK) and MEKK1, both members of the MAPKKK family, and an IKK-related kinase, named NAK (NF-κB activating kinase) (40) can activate IKK in response to proinflammatory stimuli.

REVIEW OF DATA

Various conventional drugs used to treat RA have effects on NF-κB activity (Table 2). For instance, the effects of corticosteroids are probably in part mediated through inhibition of NF-κB activation (41). Other examples include sulfasalazine (42), 5-aminosalicylic acid (43), aspirin (44), tepoxalin (45), and leflunomide (46). Several of these drugs appear to inhibit IKK or upstream signals. However, they are not specific and require relatively high concentrations to inhibit effectively NF-κB activity.

The effects of specific inhibition of NF-κB activity have been shown in various animal models of arthritis. Screening libraries for compounds that inhibit NF-κB activation identified a compound termed SP100030 as a potent inhibitor of NF-κB activation in a T-cell lymphoblastoid line (47). IL-2, IL-8, and TNF-α production by activated Jurkat cells and other T-cell lines were inhibited by SP100030. The effect of SP100030 was also evaluated in murine CIA. Joint swelling was significantly decreased in animals that were treated with SP100030 before the onset of joint swelling (47). Clinical efficacy was accompanied by diminished NF-κB activation in joint extracts, suggesting that the compound acted through this mechanism in vivo. In line with these observations inhibition of NF-κB in T cells in transgenic mice overexpressing IκBα resulted in decreased incidence and severity of CIA (48). Protection against disease was associated with reduced interferon-γ (IFN-γ) production, suggesting that the protective effects were mediated in part by decreased Th1 responses. Specific NF-κB inhibition, using intra-articular administration of NF-κB decoy oligonucleotides (12) or in vivo transfection of NF-κB decoy oligonucleotides (49), also resulted in clinical improvement

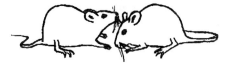

Intra-articular gene therapy with IkB kinase-β
• Synovial inflammation is induced by overexpression of wild type IKKβ
• Synovial inflammation is suppressed by overexpression of dominant negative IKKβ

Fig. 1. Use of intra-articular gene therapy to evaluate the role of key signal transduction pathways like IκB kinase.

in streptococcal cell wall-induced arthritis and in CIA in rats in association with suppressed IL-1 and TNF-α production. Of interest, histologic and radiographic studies revealed marked protection against joint destruction in the treated joints *(49)*. The inhibitory effects of NF-κB inhibition on production of proinflammatory cytokines and MMPs in animal models of arthritis were confirmed using human RA synovial tissue in culture. It is possible to reduce the production of TNF-α, IL-1, IL-6, IL-8, MMP-1, and MMP-3 by overexpression of IκBα by adenoviral gene transfer *(50)*.

NF-κB blockade can also lead to induction of apoptosis. This was shown using the proteasome-inhibitor peptide aldehyde MG132, which inhibits NF-κB activity by preventing Iκ-Bα degradation *(12)*. Treatment with MG132 induced apoptosis in the joints of rats with streptococcal cell wall arthritis. Likewise, adenoviral gene transfer of super-repressor IκBα enhanced apoptosis in joints of rats with streptococcal cell wall arthritis and similar results were obtained in pristane-induced arthritis *(12)*. TNF-α may be one of the important factors involved in the induction of apoptosis in fibroblast-like synoviocytes in response to inhibition of NF-κB translocation *(51)*.

Activation of IKKβ by forced overexpression of the gene using intra-articular gene therapy leads to NF-κB activation and histologic evidence of inflammation (*see* Fig. 1) *(30)*. Hence, activation of this kinase is sufficient to initiate the synovial inflammatory cascade. On the other hand, IKKβ can be selectively blocked by injecting a dominant-negative IKKβ adenoviral construct into the joints of rats with adjuvant arthritis. This treatment effectively suppressed local IKK functional activity and reduced NF-κB translocation. Moreover, intra-articular gene therapy using this construct significantly suppressed arthritis activity as measured by paw swelling.

Despite clinical improvement, however, there was no decrease in joint destruction. As noted earlier, inhibition of the production of MMP-1 and MMP-3 has been described after IκBα overexpression, but it is not clear what proportion of MMP expression can be inhibited by blocking NF-κB *(52)*. It is also possible that other transcription factors, especially AP-1, are more important than NF-κB in joint destruction. For instance, previous studies have demonstrated that AP-1 activation occurs very early in murine CIA, whereas NF-κB peaks later *(25)*. Early AP-1-driven MMP expression would be unaffected by NF-κB blockade in this model. Alternatively, the absence of a protective effect on joint destruction could be because the therapeutic protocol led to IKK inhibition too late to alter the irreversible damage that occurs early in disease. Nevertheless, the data suggest that blocking NF-κB activity by direct intra-articular gene therapy with a dominant-negative IKKβ mutant ameliorates rat adjuvant arthritis, whereas activation of NF-κB by wild-type IKKβ gene transfer induces arthritis in normal rats, identifying this pathway as a potential therapeutic target *(30)*.

SIDE EFFECTS AND PRECAUTIONS

The NF-κB/IKKβ pathway plays a key role in synovial inflammation. Intra-articular gene therapy aimed at interfering with this pathway could represent an attractive strategy for the treatment of RA. However, there should some precautions in light of the potential toxicity of NF-κB blockade, which might result in liver apoptosis. It has previously been shown that IKKβ knockout mice develop liver failure owing to hepatocyte apoptosis, especially in the presence of TNF-α *(36,53)*. This issue is clearly relevant in RA, where TNF-α overproduction is a hallmark of disease. Furthermore, NF-κB blockade could obviously compromise the normal host defense. Finally, it is conceivable that anti-inflammatory mediators might be inhibited as well, although the production of IL-10, IL-11, and IL-1RA appears to be unaffected *(50)*.

CONCLUSION

The eventual effects of blockade of the NF-κB/IKK pathway by gene therapy will depend on the delicate balance between suppressing inflammation and interfering with normal cellular functions. By selectively targeting specific NF-κB subunits, IκB proteins, or kinases that have some specificity for the synovial compartment as well as for arthritis activity, one might achieve therapeutic efficacy and minimize side effects.

REFERENCES

1. Firestein, G.S. 1996. Invasive fibroblast-like synoviocytes in rheumatoid arthritis. Passive responders or transformed agressors? *Arthritis Rheum.* 39:1781–1790.
2. Burmester, G.R., B. Stuhlmuller, G. Keyszer, and R.W. Kinne. 1997. Mononuclear phagocytes and rheumatoid synovitis. Mastermind or workhorse in arthritis? *Arthritis Rheum.* 40:5–18.
3. Tak, P.P., T.J.M. Smeets, M.R. Daha, P.M. Kluin, K.A.E. Meijers, R. Brand, et al. 1997. Analysis of the synovial cellular infiltrate in early rheumatoid synovial tissue in relation to local disease activity. *Arthritis Rheum.* 40:217–225.
4. Sebbag, M., S.L. Parry, F.M. Brennan, and M. Feldmann. 1997. Cytokine stimulation of T lymphocytes regulates their capacity to induce monocyte production of tumor necrosis factor alpha, but not interleukin-10: possible relevance to pathophysiology of rheumatoid arthritis. *Eur. J. Immunol.* 27:624–632.
5. McInnes, I.B., B.P. Leung, R.D. Sturrock, M. Field, and F.Y. Liew. 1997. Interleukin-15 mediates T cell-dependent regulation of tumor necrosis factor alpha production in rheumatoid arthritis. *Nature Med.* 3:189–195.
6. Vey, E., J.M. Dayer, and D. Burger. 1997. Direct contact with stimulated T cells induces the expression of IL-1 beta and IL-1 receptor antagonist in human monocytes. Involvement of serine/threonine phosphatases in differential regulation. *Cytokine* 9:480–487.
7. Hamann, J., J.O. Wishaupt, R.A.W. Van Lier, T.J.M. Smeets, F.C. Breedveld, and P.P. Tak. 1999. Expression of the activation antigen CD97 and its ligand CD55 in rheumatoid synovial tissue. *Arthritis Rheum.* 42:650–658.
8. Tak, P.P. and G.S. Firestein. 1999. Apoptosis in rheumatoid arthritis, in Apoptosis and Inflammation. J.D. Winkler, editor. Birkhauser Publishing Ltd., Basel, pp. 149–162.
9. Tak, P.P., N.J. Zvaifler, D.R. Green, and G.S. Firestein. 2000. Rheumatoid arthritis and p53: how oxidative stress might alter the course of inflammatory diseases. *Immunol. Today* 21:78–82.
10. Cantwell, M.J., T. Hua, N.J. Zvaifler, and T.J. Kipps. 1997. Deficient Fas ligand expression by synovial lymphocytes from patients with rheumatoid arthritis. *Arthritis Rheum.* 40:1644–1652.

11. Franz, J.K., T. Pap, K.M. Hummel, M. Nawrath, W.K. Aicher, Y. Shigeyama, et al. 2000. Expression of sentrin, a novel antiapoptotic molecule, at sites of synovial invasion in rheumatoid arthritis. *Arthritis Rheum.* 43:599–607.

12. Miagkov, A.V., D. V. Kovalenko, C.E. Brown, J.R. Didsbury, J.P. Cogswell, S.A. Stimpson, et al. 1998. NF-kappaB activation provides the potential link between inflammation and hyperplasia in the arthritic joint. *Proc. Natl. Acad. Sci. USA* 95:13,859–13,864.

13. Kraan, M.C., H. Versendaal, M. Jonker, B. Bresnihan, W. Post, B.A. 't Hart, et al. 1998. Asymptomatic synovitis precedes clinically manifest arthritis. *Arthritis Rheum.* 41:1481–1488.

14. Mulherin, D., O. FitzGerald, and B. Bresnihan. 1996. Synovial tissue macrophage populations and articular damage in rheumatoid arthritis. *Arthritis Rheum.* 39:115–124.

15. Elliott, M.J., R.N. Maini, M. Feldmann, J.R. Kalden, C. Antoni, J.S. Smolen, et al. 1994. Randomised double-blind comparison of chimeric monoclonal antibody to tumour necrosis factor alpha (cA2) versus placebo in rheumatoid arthritis. *Lancet* 344:1105–1110.

16. Bresnihan, B., J.M. Alvaro-Gracia, M. Cobby, M. Doherty, Z. Domljan, P. Emery, et al. 1998. Treatment of rheumatoid arthritis with recombinant human interleukin-1 receptor antagonist. *Arthritis Rheum.* 41:2196–2204.

17. Yoshizaki, K., N. Nishimoto, M. Mihara, and T. Kishimoto. 1998. Therapy of rheumatoid arthritis by blocking IL-6 signal transduction with a humanized anti-IL-6 receptor antibody. *Springer Semin. Immunopathol.* 20:247–259.

18. Baldwin, A.S., Jr. 1996. The NF-kappa B and I kappa B proteins: new discoveries and insights. *Annu. Rev. Immunol.* 14:649–83:649–683.

19. Firestein, G.S. and A.M. Manning. 1999. Signal transduction and transcription factors in rheumatic disease. *Arthritis Rheum.* 42:609–621.

20. Tak, P.P. and G.S. Firestein. 2000. Nuclear factor-κB: a key role in inflammatory diseases. *J. Clin. Invest.*

21. Aronica, M.A., A.L. Mora, D.B. Mitchell, P.W. Finn, J.E. Johnson, J.R. Sheller, and M.R. Boothby. 1999. Preferential role for NF-kappa B/Rel signaling in the type 1 but not type 2 T cell-dependent immune response in vivo. *J. Immunol.* 163:5116–5124.

22. Chen, C.C., C.L. Rosenbloom, D.C. Anderson, and A.M. Manning. 1995. Selective inhibition of E-selectin, vascular cell adhesion molecule-1, and intercellular adhesion molecule-1 expression by inhibitors of I kappa B-alpha phosphorylation. *J. Immunol.* 155:3538–3545.

23. Handel, M.L., L.B. Mcmorrow, and E.M. Gravallese. 1995. Nuclear factor-kappa B in rheumatoid synovium: Localization of p50 and p65. *Arthritis Rheum.* 38:1762–1770.

24. Marok, R., P.G. Winyard, A. Coumbe, M.L. Kus, K. Gaffney, S. Blades, et al. 1996. Activation of the transcription factor nuclear factor- kappa B in human inflamed synovial tissue. *Arthritis Rheum.* 39:583–591.

25. Han, Z.N., D.L. Boyle, A.M. Manning, and G.S. Firestein. 1998. AP-1 and NF-kappa B regulation in rheumatoid arthritis and murine collagen-induced arthritis. *Autoimmunity* 28:197–208.

26. Chen, F., V. Castranova, X. Shi, and L.M. Demers. 1999. New insights into the role of nuclear factor-kappaB, a ubiquitous transcription factor in the initiation of diseases. *Clin. Chem.* 45:7–17.

27. Miyazawa, K., A. Mori, K. Yamamoto, and H. Okudaira. 1998. Constitutive transcription of the human interleukin-6 gene by rheumatoid synoviocytes: Spontaneous activation of NF-kappa B and CBF1. *Am. J. Pathol.* 152:793–803.

28. Vincenti, M.P., C.I. Coon, and C.E. Brinckerhoff. 1998. Nuclear factor kappaB/p50 activates an element in the distal matrix metalloproteinase 1 promoter in interleukin-1beta-stimulated synovial fibroblasts. *Arthritis Rheum.* 41:1987–1994.

29. Tsao, P.W., T. Suzuki, R. Totsuka, T. Murata, T. Takagi, Y. Ohmachi, et al. 1997. The effect of dexamethasone on the expression of activated NF-kappa B in adjuvant arthritis. *Clin. Immunol. Immunopathol.* 83:173–178.

30. Tak, P.P., D.M. Gerlag, K.R. Aupperle, D.A. van de Geest, M. Overbeck, B.L. Bennett, et al. Role of IκB kinase-2 in synovial inflammation. *Arthritis Rheum,* in press.

31. Zandi, E., Y. Chen, and M. Karin. 1998. Direct phosphorylation of IkappaB by IKKalpha and IKKbeta: discrimination between free and NF-kappaB-bound substrate. *Science* 281:1360–1363.

32. Yamaoka, S., G. Courtois, C. Bessia, S.T. Whiteside, R. Weil, F. Agou, et al. 1998. Complementation cloning of NEMO, a component of the IkappaB kinase complex essential for NF-kappaB activation. *Cell* 93:1231–1240.

33. Shimada, T., T. Kawai, K. Takeda, M. Matsumoto, J. Inoue, Y. Tatsumi, et al. 1999. IKK-i, a novel lipopolysaccharide-inducible kinase that is related to IkappaB kinases. *Int. Immunol.* 11:1357–1362.

34. Aupperle, K.R., B.L. Bennett, D.L. Boyle, P.P. Tak, A.M. Manning, and G.S. Firestein. 1999. NF-kB regulation by IkB kinase in primary fibroblast-like synoviocytes. *J. Immunol.* 163:427–433.

35. Delhase, M., M. Hayakawa, Y. Chen, and M. Karin. 1999. Positive and negative regulation of IkappaB kinase activity through IKKbeta subunit phosphorylation. *Science* 284:309–313.

36. Li, Z.W., W. Chu, Y. Hu, M. Delhase, T. Deerinck, M. Ellisman, et al. 1999. The IKKbeta subunit of IkappaB Kinase (IKK) is essential for nuclear factor kappaB activation and prevention of apoptosis. *J. Exp. Med.* 189:1839–1845.

37. Aupperle, K.R., B.L. Bennett, A.M. Manning, D.L. Boyle, and G.S. Firestein. IκB kinase (IKK2), but not IKK1, is the convergent pathway for cytokine-induced NF-κB signaling in fibroblast-like synoviocytes. *Arthritis Rheum.* 42:S177. 1999.

38. O'Connell, M.A., B.L. Bennett, F. Mercurio, A.M. Manning, and N. Mackman. 1998. Role of IKK1 and IKK2 in lipopolysaccharide signaling in human monocytic cells. *J. Biol. Chem.* 273:30,410–30,414.

39. Khoshnan, A., S.J. Kempiak, B.L. Bennett, D. Bae, W. Xu, A.M. Manning, et al. 1999. Primary human CD4+ T cells contain heterogeneous IkappaB kinase complexes: role in activation of the IL-2 promoter. *J. Immunol.* 163:5444–5452.

40. Tojima, Y., A. Fujimoto, M. Delhase, Y. Chen, S. Hatakeyama, K. Nakayama, et al. 2000. NAK is an IkappaB kinase-activating kinase. *Nature* 404:778–782.

41. Marx, J. 1995. How the glucocorticoids suppress immunity. *Science* 270:232–233.

42. Wahl, C., S. Liptay, G. Adler, and R.M. Schmid. 1998. Sulfasalazine: a potent and specific inhibitor of nuclear factor kappa B. *J. Clin. Invest.* 101:1163–1174.

43. Nikolaus, S., U. Folscn, and S. Schreiber. 2000. Immunopharmacology of 5-aminosalicylic acid and of glucocorticoids in the therapy of inflammatory bowel disease. *Hepatogastroenterology* 47:71–82.

44. Kopp, E. and S. Ghosh. 1994. Inhibition of NF-kappa B by sodium salicylate and aspirin. *Science* 265:956–959.

45. Fiebich, B.L., T.J. Hofer, K. Lieb, M. Huell, R.D. Butcher, G. Schumann, et al. 1999. The non-steroidal anti-inflammatory drug tepoxalin inhibits interleukin-6 and alpha1-anti-chymotrypsin synthesis in astrocytes by preventing degradation of IkappaB-alpha. *Neuropharmacology* 38:1325–1333.

46. Manna, S.K. and B.B. Aggarwal. 1999. Immunosuppressive leflunomide metabolite (A77 1726) blocks TNF-dependent nuclear factor-kappa B activation and gene expression. *J. Immunol.* 162:2095–2102.

47. Gerlag, D.M., L.J. Ransone, D.L. Boyle, P.P. Tak, A.M. Manning, and G.S. Firestein. 2000. Effect of a T cell specific NF-κB inhibitor on in vitro cytokine production and collagen-induced arthritis. *J. Immunol.* 165:1652–1658.

48. Seetharaman, R., A.L. Mora, G. Nabozny, M. Boothby, and J. Chen. 1999. Essential role of T cell NF-kappa B activation in collagen-induced arthritis. *J. Immunol.* 163:1577–1583.

49. Tomita, T., E. Takeuchi, N. Tomita, R. Morishita, M. Kaneko, K. Yamamoto, et al. 1999. Suppressed severity of collagen-induced arthritis by in vivo transfection of nuclear factor kappa B decoy oligodeoxynucleotides as a gene therapy. *Arthritis Rheum.* 42:2532–2542.

50. Bondeson, J., B. Foxwell, F. Brennan, and M. Feldmann. 1999. Defining therapeutic targets by using adenovirus: Blocking NF-kappa B inhibits both inflammatory and destructive mechanisms in rheumatoid synovium but spares anti-inflammatory mediators. *Proc. Nat. Acad. Sci. USA* 96:5668–5673.

51. Zhang, H.G., N. Huang, D. Liu, L. Bilbao, X. Zhang, P. Yang, T. Zhou, D.T. Curiel, and J.D. Mountz. 2000. Gene therapy that inhibits nuclear translocation of nuclear factor kB results in tumor necrosis factor-a induced apoptosis of human fibroblasts. *Arthritis Rheum.* 43:1094–1105.

52. Nawrath, M., K.M. Hummel, T. Pap, U. Muller-Ladner, R.E. Gay, K. Molling, and S. Gay. 1998. Effect of dominant negative mutants of Raf-1 and c-myc on rheumatoid arthritis synovial fibroblasts in the SCID mouse model. *Arthritis Rheum.* 41:S95.

53. Tanaka, M., M.E. Fuentes, K. Yamaguchi, M.H. Durnin, S.A. Dalrymple, K.L. Hardy, and D.V. Goeddel. 1999. Embryonic lethality, liver degeneration, and impaired NF-kappa B activation in IKK-beta-deficient mice. *Immunity* 10:421–429.

54. Jobin, C., C.A. Bradham, M.P. Russo, B. Juma, A.S. Narula, D.A. Brenner, and R.B. Sartor. 1999. Curcumin blocks cytokine-mediated NF-kappa B activation and proinflammatory gene expression by inhibiting inhibitory factor I-kappa B kinase activity. *J. Immunol.* 163:3474–3483.

55. Blackwell, T.S., T.R. Blackwell, E.P. Holden, B.W. Christman, and J.W. Christman. 1996. In vivo antioxidant treatment suppresses nuclear factor-kappa B activation and neutrophilic lung inflammation. *J. Immunol.* 157:1630–1637.

56. Hellerbrand, C., C. Jobin, Y. Iimuro, L. Licato, R.B. Sartor, and D.A. Brenner. 1998. Inhibition of NFkappaB in activated rat hepatic stellate cells by proteasome inhibitors and an IkappaB super-repressor. *Hepatology* 27:1285–1295.

36 Regulation of Apoptosis in Rheumatoid Synoviocytes

Kusuki Nishioka and Tetsuya Kobayashi

CONTENTS

INTRODUCTION
FAS-SIGNALING PATHWAYS IN SYNOVIOCYTES
NOVEL THERAPEUTICS BY FAS/FAS L/FADD SYSTEM
ACKNOWLEDGMENTS
REFERENCES

INTRODUCTION

Rheumatoid arthritis (RA) is a systemic autoimmune disease characterized by early synovitis following synovial proliferation and infiltration of various inflammatory cells *(1,2)*. The process of disease progression, characterized by activation and hyperplasia of synoviocytes, mainly of synovial fibroblasts, results in cartilage and bone destruction *(1,2)*. Proliferation of synoviocytes is, however, not limitless, and spontaneous remission or arrest of synovial proliferation are occasionally observed *(3,4)*. First, our laboratories following by others have demonstrated that RA synoviocytes express functional Fas antigen (CD95/APO-1) and that these cells undergo Fas-mediated apoptosis both either in vivo and in vitro *(5–8)*. These findings suggest that Fas-mediated apoptosis may play a critical role in the regression of synovial hyperplasia in RA. It also implies that induction of intractable synovial hyperplasia in RA may occur when Fas-mediated apoptosis ceases to operate partially or completely leading to accumulation of Fas-positive proliferating synoviocytes. However, the regulatory mechanisms that control apoptosis are not well understood. Identification of the regulatory mechanisms in RA synoviocytes may provide important insights into not only understanding of the pathophysiology of RA but also the development of novel strategies for RA therapy. In this chapter, current of the study by our laboratory on the regulatory mechanisms of Fas-mediated apoptosis in RA was described. We also propose a novel gene therapy strategy in the treatment of RA based on induction of the apoptosis gene synovectomy in patients with RA.

From: *Modern Therapeutics in Rheumatic Diseases*
Edited by: G. C. Tsokos, et al. © Humana Press, Inc., Totowa, NJ

FAS-SIGNALING PATHWAYS IN SYNOVIOCYTES

JNK/AP-1 Pathway

Fas-mediated apoptosis is highly observed in synoviocytes of patients with RA and a few with osteoarthritis (OA) or normal subjects, despite the equal expression level of Fas molecules on their cell surface *(5)*. Therefore, the signaling pathway(s) downstream the Fas molecule is thought to be responsible for the regulation of Fas-mediated apoptosis in RA synoviocytes (Fig. 1).

We have found that Fas-ligation using its agonistic monoclonal antibody (MAb) termed CH-11, induces a rapid tyrosine phosphorylation of JNK (c-JUN amino-terminal kinase) and formation of AP-1 (activator protein-1) corresponding to apoptosis of RA synoviocytes but not OA synoviocytes *(9)*. JNK, a member of the mitogen-activated protein kinase (MAPK), is a protein serine/threonine kinase that activates *c-jun* and subsequent AP-1 transcriptional factor *(10–12)*. It has been reported that JNK is activated by Fas ligation in apoptosis of a human T-cell line (Jurkat cells) and peripheral blood lymphocytes *(13–16)*. In addition, overexpression of Daxx, a novel Fas death domain-associating protein, induces activation of JNK and protentiated Fas-mediated apoptosis *(17,18)*. Furthermore, FAP-1 (Fas-associated phosphatase 1), a protein tyrosine phosphatase, binds to the distal negative regulatory tail of Fas. FAP-1 functionally blocks Fas-mediated apoptosis in developmental stage in T-cell or colon cancer-cell lines *(19,20)*. In RA synoviocytes, we have also demonstrated that treatment with the protein tyrosine phosphatase inhibitor orthovanadate significantly enhances Fas-mediated apoptosis *(9)*. In a series of experiments, we also showed that RA synoviocytes express Daxx and FAP-1 mRNA (Okamoto et al., unpublished data). Based on these findings, it seems that the JNK/AP-1 signaling pathway is probably involving in Fas-mediated apoptosis of RA synoviocytes (Fig. 1).

FADD/Caspase-8/Caspase-3/PARP Pathway

More recently, several studies using the yeast two-hybrid system or biochemical techniques have identified Fas-interacting signal-transducing molecules, such as Fas-associated death-domain protein (FADD) *(21,22)*, FAP-1 *(19,20)*, and receptor-interacting protein *(23)*. In addition, caspase-family proteases have been implicated as key regulators of apoptosis in various cells *(24,25)*. It has been demonstrated that Fas ligation induces oligomerization of Fas molecules on the cell surface, leading to the recruitment of two key molecules and formation of the death-inducing signaling complex (DISC) *(26–28)*. FADD is recruited to bind the intracellular domain of Fas through each death domain *(21,22)*, and then Caspase-8 (FLICE) is also recruited to the Fas and FADD complex through the death-effector domains *(29,30)*. Activation of Caspase-8 promotes the caspases cascade, leading to the transmission of the apoptotic signal to the nucleus. We have also found that the same signaling pathway plays a critical role in Fas-mediated apoptosis of RA synoviocytes *(31)*. Fas-ligation induces activation of Caspase-3, with subsequent cleavage of PARP (poly [ADP-ribose] polymerase), a substrate of activated Caspase-3 *(31)*, corresponding to Fas-mediated apoptosis in RA synoviocytes. PARP is reported to be involved in DNA repair, genome surveillance, and integrity *(32–34)*. The Ca^{2+}/Mg^{2+}-dependent endonuclease implicated in internucleosomal DNA cleavage, the hallmark of apoptosis, is negatively regulated by poly(AP-ribos)ylation *(32–34)*. Thus, the loss of normal function of PARP may activate

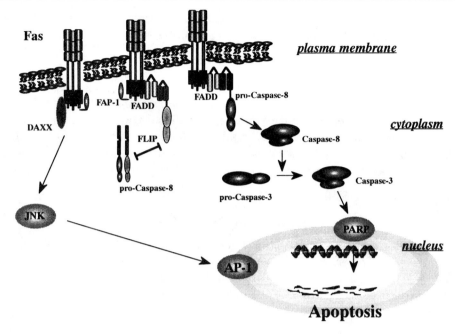

Fig. 1. Schematic diagram of the mechanisms involved in the regulation of Fas-mediated apoptosis in RA synovial cells.

this nuclease in dying cells. Caspase-8 is also activated following Fas ligation, and this occurs prior to the activation of Caspase-3 in RA synoviocytes. In addition, we found that a Caspase-8-specific inhibitor blocks the activation of Caspase-3, suggesting that Caspase-8 appears to operate upstream of Caspase-3 in Fas-mediated apoptosis of RA synoviocytes, in agreement with previous studies using other cells *(29,30)*. Importantly, we also demonstrated that the recruitment of FADD to the Fas death domain is augmented after Fas ligation in RA synoviocytes but not in OA synoviocytes. These findings strongly indicate that Fas-mediated apoptosis of RA synoviocytes may be regulated at the recruitment of FADD to Fas molecule, which initiates a sequential activation of the FADD/Caspase-8/Caspase-3/PARP signaling pathway (Fig. 1).

We demonstrated that Fas-mediated apoptosis might be regulated by at least two signaling pathways. Fas-mediated apoptosis in RA synoviocytes is almost completely blocked by specific Caspase-8 or Caspase-3 inhibitors. Therefore, FADD/Caspase-8/Caspase-3 /PARP pathway seems to be a key signal for Fas-mediated apoptosis in RA synoviocytes. It should be noted that neither signaling pathway could not be detected in OA synoviocytes after Fas-ligation, suggesting that Fas-mediated apoptosis in synoviocytes may be regulated by Fas signal transduction.

Actually, the FADD/Caspase-8/Caspase-3/PARP pathway is a main stream of Fas-mediated apoptosis in synoviocytes, and in particular the activation of Caspase-8. On the other hand, FLIP (also called I-FLICE, FLAME, CLARP, Casper, or CASH) *(45–51)* has been identified independently by several groups as an apoptosis-inhibitory molecule. FLIP has two death-effector domains, and it can interact with either FADD or Caspase-8 through each death-effector domain and can inhibit the activation of Caspase-8 *(45,46)*. Because RA and OA synoviocytes express both long and short forms of FLIP (FLIP$_L$ and FLIP$_S$) mRNA, as detected by reverse transcriptase polymerase chain reaction (RT-PCR) *(35)*, these proteins are probably involved in the induction of Fas-mediated apoptosis of synoviocytes (Fig. 1).

Interestingly, we investigated that TNF-α enhances the sensitivity of RA synoviocytes to Fas-mediated apoptosis, whereas basic fibroblast growth factor (bFGF) did not affect this process *(35)*. Both TNF-α and (bFGF) can equally induce proliferation of synoviocytes, suggesting that sensitivity to Fas-mediated apoptosis in synoviocytes of RA may be differentially regulated by cytokines, following the different sensitivity to Fas. The phenomenon may be closely associated with the disease progression.

NOVEL THERAPEUTICS BY FAS/FAS L/FADD SYSTEM

Anti-Fas MAb for RA Therapy

Synovial proliferation in RA joints may ultimately lead to cartilage and bone destruction *(3,4)*. This suggests the presence of an imbalance between the proliferative process and Fas/FasL system-mediated apoptosis, in favor of proliferation of the synovium. It is thus possible that active induction of apoptosis via the Fas/FasL system may produce effective control of RA (Fig. 2). In fact, we have reported that intra-articular injection of agonistic anti-mouse Fas MAb improved the arthritis in the several animal models. Histologic examination showed a clear disappearance of Fas-expressing cells, such as synovial cells, CD3+ T cells, and B220+ B cells from the synovium of arthritic mice after local injection of anti-Fas MAb owing to induction of apoptosis of these cells. Furthermore, to evaluate the effectiveness of anti-Fas MAb on human RA, we also investigated the effects of agonistic anti-human Fas MAb on proliferating rheumatoid synovium engrafted in mice with severe combined immunodeficiency (SCID), which show histologic features similar to RA synovium *(53)*. Apoptosis of Fas-expressing cells in the transplanted RA synovium occurred 36 h after intraperitoneal injection of anti-Fas MAb *(53)*. These results clearly suggest that active induction of apoptosis mediated via Fas/FasL system by administration of anti-Fas MAb may be useful as a new therapeutic intervention for RA (Fig. 2). Currently, several MAbs have been developed without serious cytotoxicity in bone or cartilage.

Ex Vivo Gene Transfer of hFasL for RA Therapy

Although anti-Fas MAb and soluble FasL might be useful against RA, they exhibit serious adverse effects, such as lethal hepatic injury *(54,55)*. In addition, it is difficult to prepare a chimeric anti-Fas MAb that avoids the host immune response. Thus, it is important to develop a safer therapeutic modality based on the Fas/FasL system when considering clinical application. For this purpose, we evaluated the usefulness of cells transfected with human FasL (hFasL) gene against proliferative RA synovium, acting through cell-to-cell interaction, because FasL-positive activated T cells and natural killer (NK) cells play an important role in the induction of apoptosis under physiologic conditions. We first examined the effect of the murine T lymphoma cell line, which does not express Fas antigen, transfected with hFasL gene on RA synoviocytes in vitro *(56)*. hFasL transfectants exhibited cytotoxicity against cultured RA synoviocyte in a dose-

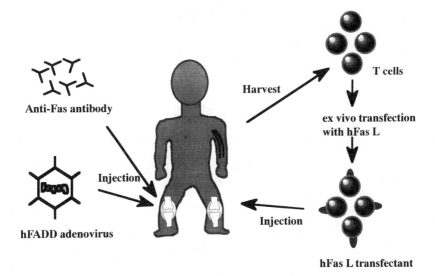

Fig. 2. Schematic diagram of novel strategies currently under investigation for the treatment of RA based on modulating the apoptotic process.

dependent manner. On the other hand, soluble FasL in the culture supernatant of hFasL transfectants did not induce cytotoxic activity against RA synoviocytes *(57)*. These findings suggest that cell-to-cell interaction via the cell membrane-bound FasL plays an important role in the apoptotic effect of hFasL transfectants on RA synoviocytes. In the next series of studies, we evaluated the effects of hFasL transfectants in vivo by injecting irradiated-hFasL transfectants into the joints of SCID-RA mice engrafted with RA synovium. Histologic examination demonstrated that synoviocytes and mononuclear cells (MNCs) disappeared in engrafted synovium treated with these transfectants 7 d after injection without accumulation of polymorphocytes, such as neutrophils, and subsequent neutrophil-mediated killing action. These results strongly suggest that FasL-transfectants can eliminate these cells by inducing apoptosis through cell-to-cell interaction. Thus, ex vivo gene transfer of FasL is an effective and safe therapeutic modality and might be a clinically useful therapy for RA.

As mentioned earlier, we have recently reported that FADD plays a key role in Fas-mediated apoptosis of synovial cells in patients with RA. In this study, we determined whether FADD gene transfer could induce apoptosis of RA synoviocytes in vitro and in vivo. Transfection of FADD gene by adenoviral vector into cultured RA synoviocytes induced upregulation of FADD expression and apoptosis. In addition, local injection of FADD adenovirus (Ad-FADD) eliminated synoviocytes in vivo by induction of apoptosis of proliferating human rheumatoid synovium engrafted in SCID mouse, which is the most suitable animal model of RA for the evaluation of treatment strategy in vivo. In addition, Ad-FADD-induced apoptosis was limited to cells of the synovium tissue and did not affect chondrocytes. Our results strongly suggest that FADD gene transfer can induce apoptosis of RA synoviocytes both in vitro and in vivo, suggesting that FADD gene transfer might be effective in the treatment of RA.

ACKNOWLEDGMENTS

This work was supported by grants from the Ministry of Education, Science, Sports and Culture of Japan, Santen Grant, and The Organization for Drug ADR Relief, R&D Promotion and Product Review.

REFERENCES

1. Harris, E.D. 1990. Rheumatoid arthritis. Pathophysiology and implications for therapy. *N. Engl. J. Med.* 322:1277–1289.

2. Stamenkovic, I., M. Stegagno, K.A. Wright, S.M. Krane, E.P. Amento, R.B. Colvin, et al. 1988. Clonal dominance among T-lymphocyte infiltrates in arthritis. *Proc. Natl. Acad. Sci. USA* 85: 1179–1183.

3. O'Sullivan, J.B. and E.S. Cathcart. 1972. The prevalence of rheumatoid arthritis. Follow-up evaluation of the effect of criteria on rates in Sudbury, Massachusetts. *Ann. Intern. Med.* 76:573–577.

4. Feigenbaum, S.L., A.T. Masi, and S.B. Kaplan. 1979. Prognosis in rheumatoid arthritis. A longitudinal study of newly diagnosed younger adult patients. *Am. J. Med.* 66:377–384.

5. Nakajima, T., H. Aono, T. Hasunuma, K. Yamamoto, T. Shirai, K. Hirohata, and K. Nishioka. 1995. Apoptosis and functional Fas antigen in rheumatoid arthritis synoviocytes. *Arthritis Rheum.* 38:485–491.

6. Firestein, G.S., M. Yeo, and N.J. Zvaifler. 1995. Apoptosis in rheumatoid arthritis synovium. *J. Clin. Invest. 96:1631–1638.*

7. Hasunuma, T., T.T.M. Hoa, H. Aono, H. Asahara, S. Yonehara, K. Yamamoto K, et al. 1996. Induction of Fas-dependent apoptosis in synovial infiltrating cells in rheumatoid arthritis. *Int. Immunol.* 8:1595–1602.

8. Asahara, H., T. Hasunuma, T. Kobata, H. Yagita, K. Okumura, H. Inoue, et al. 1996. Expression of Fas antigen and Fas ligand in the rheumatoid synovial tissue. *Clin. Immunol. Immunopathol.* 81:27–34.

9. Okamoto, K., K. Fujisawa, T. Hasunuma, T. Kobata, T. Sumida, and K. Nishioka. 1997. Selective activation of the JNK/AP-1 pathway in Fas-mediated apoptosis of rheumatoid arthritis synoviocytes. *Arthritis Rheum.* 40:919–926.

10. Déijard, B., M. Hibi, I.-H. Wu, T. Barrett, B. Su, T. Deng, et al. 1994. JNK1: a protein kinase stimulated by UV light and Ha-Ras that binds and phosphorylates the c-Jun activation domain. *Cell* 76:1025–1037.

11. Kyriakis, J.M., P. Banerjee, E. Nikolakaki, T. Dai, E.A. Rubie, M.F. Ahmad, et al. 1994. The stress-activated protein kinase subfamily of c-Jun kinases. *Nature* 369:156–160.

12. Davis, R.J. 1994. MAPKs: new JNK expands the group. *Trends Biochem. Sci.* 19:470–473.

13. Wilson, D.J., K.A. Fortner, D.H. Lynch, R.R. Mattingly, I.G. Macara, J.A., Posada, and R.C. Budd. 1996. JNK, but not MAPK, activation is associated with Fas-mediated apoptosis in human T cells. *Eur. J. Immunol.* 26:989–994.

14. Latinis, K.M. and G.A. Koretzky. 1996. Fas ligation induces apoptosis and Jun kinase activation independently of CD45 and Lck in human T cells. *Blood* 87:871–875.

15. Goillot, E., J. Raingeaud, A. Ranger, R.I. Tepper, R.J. Davis, E. Harlow, and I. Sanchez. 1997. Mitogen-activated protein kinase-mediated Fas apoptotic signaling pathway. *Proc. Natl. Acad. Sci. USA* 94:3302–3307.

16. Juo, P., C.J. Kuo, S.E. Reynolds, R.F. Konz, J. Raingeaud, R.J. Davis, et al. 1997. Fas activation of the p38 mitogen-activated protein kinase signaling pathway requires ICE/CED-3 family proteases. *Mol. Cell Biol.* 17:24–35.

17. Yang, X., R. Khosravi-Far, H.Y. Chang, and D. Baltimore. 1997. Daxx, a novel Fas-binding protein that activates JNK and apoptosis. *Cell* 89:1067–1076.

18. Chang, H.Y., H. Nishitoh, X. Yang, H. Ichijo, and D. Baltimore. 1998. Activation of apoptosis signal-regulating kinase 1 (ASK1) by the adapter protein Daxx. *Science* 281:1860–1863.

19. Sato, T., S. Irie, S. Kitada, and J.C. Reed. 1995. FAP-1: a protein tyrosine phosphatase that associates with Fas. *Science* 268:411–415.

20. Yanagisawa, J., M. Takahashi, H. Kanki, H. Yano-Yanagisawa, T. Tazunoki, E. Sawa, et al. 1997. The molecular interaction of Fas and FAP-1. A Tripeptide blocker of human Fas interaction with FAP-1 promotes Fas-induced apoptosis. *J. Biol. Chem.* 272:8539–8545.

21. Chinnaiyan, A.M., K. O'Rourke, M. Tewari, and V.M. Dixit. 1995. FADD, a novel death domain-containing protein, interacts with the death domain of Fas and initiates apoptosis. *Cell* 81:505–512.

22. Boldin, M.P., E.E. Varfolomeev, Z. Pancer, I.L. Mett, J.H. Camonis, and D. Wallach. 1995. A novel protein that interacts with the death domain of Fas/APO1 contains a sequence motif related to the death domain. *J. Biol. Chem.* 270:7795–7798.

23. Stanger, B.Z., P. Leder, T.-H. Lee, E. Kim, and B. Seed. 1995. RIP: a novel protein containing a death domain that interacts with Fas/APO-1 (CD95) in yeast and causes cell death. *Cell* 81:513–523.

24. Cohen, G.M. 1997. Caspases: the executioners of apoptosis. *Biochem. J.* 326:1–16.

25. Medema, J.P., C. Scaffidi, F.C. Kischkel, A. Shevchenko, M. Mann, P.H. Krammer, and M.E. Peter. 1997. FLICE is activated by association with the CD95 death-inducing signaling complex (DISC). *EMBO J.* 16:2794–2804.

26. Peter, M.E., F.C. Kischkel, S. Hellbardt, A.M. Chinnaiyan, P.H. Krammer, and V.M. Dixit. 1996. CD95 (APO-1/Fas)-associating signaling proteins. *Cell Death Differ.* 3:161–170.

27. Boldin, M.P., T.M. Goncharov, Y.V. Goltsev, and D. Wallach. 1996. Involvement of MACH, a novel MORT-1/FADD-interacting protease, in Fas/APO-1- and TNF receptor-induced cell death. *Cell* 85:803–815.

28. Muzio, M., A.M. Chinnaiyan, F.C. Kischkel, K. O'Rourke, A. Shevchenko, J. Ni, C. Scaffidi, et al. 1996. FLICE, a novel FADD-homologous ICE/CED-3-like protease, is recruited to the CD95 (Fas/APO-1) death-inducing signaling complex. *Cell* 85:817–827.

29. Nicholson, D.W., A. Ali, N.A. Thornberry, J.P. Vaillancourt, C.K. Ding, M. Gallant, et al. 1995. Identification and inhibition of the ICE/ CED-3 protease necessary for mammalian apoptosis. *Nature* 376:37–43.

30. Yoshihara, K., Y. Tanigawa, and S.S. Koide. 1974. Inhibition of rat liver Ca^{2+}, Mg^{2+}-dependent endonuclease activity by nicotinamide adenine dinucleotide and poly(adenosine diphosphate ribose) synthetase. *Biochem. Biophys. Res. Commun.* 59:658–665.

31. Yoshihara, K., Y. Tanigawa, L. Burzio, and S.S. Koide. 1975. Evidence for adenosine diphosphate ribosylation of Ca^{2+}, Mg^{2+}-dependent endonuclease. *Proc. Natl. Acad. Sci. USA* 72:289–293.

32. Tanaka, Y., K. Yoshihara, A. Itaya, T. Kamiya, and S.S. Koide. 1984. Mechanism of the inhibition of Ca^{2+}, Mg^{2+}-dependent endonuclease of bull seminal plasma induced by ADP-ribosylation. *J. Biol. Chem.* 259:6579–6585.

33. Raff, M.C. 1992. Social controls on cell survival and cell death. *Nature* 356:397–400.

34. Steller, H. 1995. Mechanisms and genes of cellular suicide. *Science* 267:1445–1449.

35. Kobayashi, T., K. Okamoto, T. Kobata, T. Hasunuma, T. Sumida, and K. Nishioka. 1999. TNF-α regulates Fas-mediated apoptosis signaling pathway in synovial cells. *Arthritis Rheum.* 42:519–526.

36. Chu, C.Q., M. Field, M. Feldmann, R.N. Maini. 1991. Localization of tumor necrosis factor α in synovial tissues and at the cartilage-pannus junction in patients with rheumatoid arthritis. *Arthritis Rheum.* 34:1125–1132.

37. Di Giovine, F.S., G. Nuki, and G.W. Duff. 1988. Tumor necrosis factor in synovial exudates. *Ann. Rheum. Dis.* 47:768–772.

38. Saxne, T., M.A. Palladino Jr., D. Heinegd, N. Talal, and F.A. Wollheim. 1998. Detection of tumor necrosis factor α but not tumor necrosis factor α in rheumatoid arthritis synovial fluid and serum. *Arthritis Rheum.* 31:1041–1045.

39. Alvaro-Gracia, J.M., N.J. Zvaifler, and G.S. Firestein. 1990. Cytokines in chronic inflammatory arthritis. V. Mutual antagonism between interferon-gamma and tumor necrosis factor-alpha on HLA-DR expression, proliferation, collagenase production, and granulocyte macrophage colony-stimulating factor production by rheumatoid arthritis synoviocytes. *J. Clin. Invest.* 86:1790–1798.

40. Butler, D.M., D.S. Piccoli, P.H. Hart, and J.A. Hamilton. 1988. Stimulation of human synovial fibroblast DNA synthesis by recombinant human cytokines. *J. Rheumatol.* 15:1463–1470.

41. Gitter, B.D., J.M. Labus, S.L. Lees, and M.E. Scheetz. 1989. Characteristics of human synovial fibroblast activation by IL-1α and TNFα. *Immunology* 66:196–200.

42. Fujisawa, K., H. Aono, T. Hasunuma, K. Yamamoto, S. Mita, and K. Nishioka. 1996. Activation of transcription factor NF-κB in human synovial cells in response to tumor necrosis factor α. *Arthritis Rheum.* 39:197–203.

43. Irmler, M., M. Thome, M. Hahne, P. Schneider, K. Hofmann, V. Steiner, et al. 1997. Inhibition of death receptor signals by cellular FLIP. *Nature* 388:190–195.

44. Meinl, E., H. Fickenscher, M. Thome, J. Tschopp, and B. Fleckenstein. 1998. Anti-apoptotic strategies of lymphotropic viruses. *Immunol. Today* 19:474–479.

45. Hu, S., C. Vincenz, J. Ni, R. Gentz, and V.M. Dixit. 1997. I-FLICE, a novel inhibitor of tumor necrosis factor receptor-1 - and CD-95-induced apoptosis. *J. Biol. Chem.* 272:17,255–17,257.

46. Srinivasulam, S.M., M. Ahmad, S. Ottilie, F. Bullrich, S. Banks, Y. Wang, et al. 1997. FLAME-1, a novel FADD-like anti-apoptotic molecule that regulates Fas/TNFR1-induced apoptosis. *J. Biol. Chem.* 272:18,542–18,545.

47. Inohara, N., T. Kosekim, Y. Hu, S. Chen, and Núñez, G. 1997. CLARP, a death effector domain-containing protein interacts with caspase-8 and regulates apoptosis. *Proc. Natl. Acad. Sci. USA* 94:10,717–10,722.

48. Shu, H.-B., D.R. Halpin, and D.V. Goeddel. 1997. Casper is a FADD- and caspase-related inducer of apoptosis. *Immunity* 6:751–763.

49. Goltsev, Y.V., A.V. Kovalenko, E. Arnold, E.E. Varfolomeev, V.M. Brodianskii, and D. Wallach. 1997. CASH, a novel caspase homologue with death effector domains. *J. Biol. Chem.* 272:19,641–19,644.

50. Fujisawa, K., H. Asahara, K. Okamoto, H Aono, T. Hasunuma, T. Kobata, et al. 1996. Therapeutic effect of the anti-Fas antibody on arthritis in HTLV-I tax transgenic mice. *J. Clin. Invest.* 98:271–278. This paper demonstrates improvement of arthritis in tax transgenic mice following local injection of anti-Fas antibody.

51. Sakai, K., H. Matsuno, I. Morita, T. Nezuka, H. Tsuji, T. Shirai, et al. 1998. Potential withdrawal of rheumatoid synovium by the induction of apoptosis using a novel in vivo model of rheumatoid arthritis. *Arthritis Rheum.* 41:1251–1257.

52. Ogasawara, J., R. Watanabe-Fukunaga, M. Adachi, A. Matsuzawa, T. Kasugai, Y. Kitamura, et al. 1993. Lethal effect of the anti-Fas antibody in mice. *Nature* 364:806–809.

53. Rensing-Ehl, A., K. Frei, R. Flury, B. Matiba, S.M. Mariani, M. Weller, et al. 1995. Local Fas/APO-1 (CD95) ligand-mediated tumor cell killing in vivo. *Eur. J. Immunol.* 25:2253–2258.

54. Kayagaki, N., A. Kawasaki, T. Ebata, H. Ohmoto, S. Ikeda, S. Inoue, et al. 1995. Metalloproteinase-mediated release of human Fas ligand. *J. Exp. Med.* 182:1777–1783.

55. Okamoto, K., H. Asahara, T. Kobayashi, H. Matsuno, T. Hasunuma, T. Kobata, et al. 1998. Induction of apoptosis in the rheumatoid synovium by Fas ligand gene transfer. *Gene Ther.* 5:331–338.

56. Nishioka, K., T. Hasunuma, T. Kato, T. Sumida, and T. Kobata. 1998. Apoptosis in rheumatoid arthritis: A novel pathway in the regulation of synovial tissue. *Arthritis Rheum.* 41:1–9.

57. Zhang, H., Y. Yang, J.L. Horton, E.B. Samoilova, T.A. Judge, L.A. Turka, et al. 1997. Amelioration of collagen-induced arthritis by CD95 (Apo-1/Fas)-ligand gene transfer. *J. Clin. Invest.* 100:1951–1957.

58. Kobayashim T,, K. Okamoto, T. Kobata, T. Hasunuma, T. Kato, H. Hamada, and K. Nishioka. 2000. Novel gene therapy for rheumatoid arthritis by FADD gene transfer: inducton of apoptosis of rheumatoid synoviocytes but not chondrocytes. *Gene Ther.* 7:527–533.

37 Gene Therapy for Arthritis

Conception, Consolidation, and Clinical Trial

Christopher H. Evans, Steven C. Ghivizzani, James H. Herndon, Mary C. Wasko, and Paul D. Robbins

CONTENTS

INTRODUCTION

More than 10 years have passed since we conceived the idea to use gene therapy in the treatment of arthritis. The original concept of delivering therapeutic genes to the synovial linings of arthritic joints (Fig. 1) *(1)* was quickly joined by additional strategies, including the systemic delivery of genes to extra-articular locations *(2)*. Subsequent evaluation of these possibilities in animal models of disease (reviewed in refs. *3* and *4*), confirmed that both approaches have merit. However, for a variety of technical and safety reasons, we decided to develop local gene delivery to the synovium for the first clinical trials *(5)*, while continuing to investigate other strategies at a preclinical level.

As a result of this decision, considerable effort was devoted to evaluating the abilities of different vectors to deliver genes to the synovial lining of rabbits' knee joints by in vivo and ex vivo means *(6)*. These studies confirmed the efficiency of adenovirus as a vector for in vivo synovial delivery, as first observed by Roessler et al. *(7)*, and a growing number of subsequent investigators are using this technique for preclinical studies *(8–14)*. However, although experimentally very useful, this means of gene transfer did not seem well-suited to early human application because of inflammatory

From: *Modern Therapeutics in Rheumatic Diseases*
Edited by: G. C. Tsokos, et al. © Humana Press, Inc., Totowa, NJ

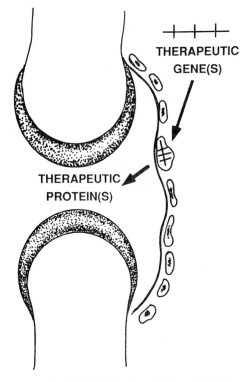

GENE TRANSFER TO THE JOINT

Fig. 1. Gene transfer to synoviocytes as a treatment for arthritis. (For details, *see* text.)

responses to adenoviral infection and the brevity of gene expression. Retroviral, ex vivo methods, although more tedious, gave longer gene expression, albeit at a lower level, and were not associated with inflammation. Moreover, ex vivo gene delivery brings advantages of safety, because no transducing agents are introduced directly into the body and all genetically modified cells can be thoroughly tested before reimplantation.

The remainder of this chapter describes the development of the ex vivo gene therapy protocol used in the first human clinical trial. Additional information can be found in refs. *5* and *15*.

PATHOGENIC MECHANISMS THAT RATIONALIZE THE THERAPEUTIC TARGET

In general terms, pathophysiological events in rheumatoid arthritis (RA) are driven by a series of interrelated processes involving inappropriate immune reactivity, and the excessive production of immunostimulatory, inflammatory, and destructive mediators *(3)*. Agents that restore immune homeostasis and interfere with the activities of arthritogenic mediators are of obvious potential utility in treating RA. In recent years, it has become clear that biology provides a number of such agents *(16)*. Many of them, however, are proteins and thus awkward drugs in chronic conditions such as RA. Gene therapy was primarily suggested as a means of solving the delivery problem *(1)*, but it may bring additional advantages. For example, there is growing evidence that molecules synthesized endogenously following gene transfer have greater biological potencies than the corresponding recombinant proteins *(17,18)*. Moreover, the anti-erosive potency of certain proteins may be enhanced by local, intra-articular synthesis.

In planning a clinical protocol based on the delivery of genes to the synovium, particular attention was paid to the selection of the transgene. The gene product needed to have therapeutic potential, yet be resoundingly safe. The latter requirement was a difficult one to satisfy, because many molecules that modulate immune reactivity and cytokine behavior are pleiotropic, and have complicated dose-response properties. Nevertheless, the interleukin-1 receptor antagonist (IL-1Ra) *(19)* appeared to satisfy these demanding criteria. IL-1Ra shows anti-arthritic activity in animal models of RA *(20–22)* and has recently shown efficacy as a recombinant protein in human clinical trials *(23)*. As a result of its use in phase III trials for septic shock, there is considerable information confirming the remarkable safety of IL-1Ra in humans *(24,25)*. IL-1Ra was also attractive because of experimental evidence that IL-1 antagonism might be particularly useful in preventing erosion of the articular surfaces, which is difficult to prevent by existing drugs *(22)*.

REVIEW OF THE DATA

Preclinical Efficacy Studies

Pre-clinical development of the local, retroviral, ex vivo delivery of a human IL-1Ra cDNA used the rabbit knee as a model. A cDNA containing the entire coding sequence of human IL-1Ra was cloned into a recombinant, Moloney-based retrovirus to produce the vector MFG-IRAP with expression of the transgene driven by the 5′ LTR of the virus *(26)*. This virus was used in an ex vivo gene delivery protocol.

As a prelude to gene delivery, synovial biopsies were recovered from the knee joints of rabbits by partial surgical synovectomy. Synovial cell cultures were established from each of the individual rabbits, and infected with MFG-IRAP. Autologous, transduced cells were then returned to the appropriate knee joints; gene expression was monitored by serial lavage of the knees and enzyme-linked immunosorbent assay (ELISA) measurement of human IL-1Ra in the lavage fluids.

Several nanograms of hIL-1Ra could typically be lavaged from the knee joints during the first week after gene transfer. This value fell progressively, reaching the limit of detection of the assay by 6 wk post-transfer *(26)*. The reasons why gene expression are lost remain to be identified, but they could include immune reactions by the rabbit to human IL-1Ra, death of the transduced synovial fibroblasts, and promoter extinction. Nevertheless, gene expression remained high enough for long enough to encourage further development of the technology, while the longevity of gene expression was addressed as a separate issue.

Expression of IL-1Ra was sufficient to protect genetically modified knee joints from an intraarticular challenge with IL-1 *(26,27)*. In antigen-induced arthritis (AIA), ex vivo IL-1Ra gene therapy protected the matrix of articular cartilage from degradation and maintained biosynthetic rates at normal levels *(18)*. As an anti-inflammatory modality, IL-1Ra gene therapy was less comprehensive; it reduced the influx of leukocytes into the joint space, but had little effect on synovitis or joint swelling. Later research suggested that it is necessary to block both IL-1 and tumor necrosis factor (TNF) in this model to reverse the latter two pathologies *(13,14)*.

For unknown reasons, intra-articular expression of hIL-1Ra was several-fold higher in knees with AIA than in normal knees *(18)*. Moreover, expression of hIL-1Ra reduced the concentrations of rabbit IL-1β in the lavage fluid, possibly by inhibiting autocrine-induction loops. This may help explain why the anti-arthritic effect of the IL-1Ra transgene was greater than predicted on a quantitative basis. Indeed, Lewthwaite et al. *(28)* found no effect of purified, human, recombinant IL-1Ra on early AIA in rabbits. The concentrations of hIL-1Ra in the lavage fluid were similar following gene *(18)* and protein *(28)* delivery, suggesting that gene delivery provides a more potent effect. Along these lines, Makarov et al. *(17)* have calculated that local delivery of the *hIL-1Ra* gene is four orders of magnitude more effective than systemic delivery of recombinant hIL-1Ra in treating streptococcal cell wall arthritis in rats.

Ex vivo intra-articular gene delivery using MFG-IRAP also showed efficacy in zymosan-induced arthritis and collagen-induced arthritis (CIA) in mice *(29)*. Thus, including Makarov's studies in rats *(17)*, ex vivo transfer of the *hIL-1Ra* gene has proved effective in four quite different experimental models of RA, a circumstance that encourages confidence in its possible utility in human disease.

Preclinical Studies with Human Tissues

Before entering clinical trials, it was necessary to determine, insofar as possible, whether human tissues would respond to the gene therapy procedures in the same manner as those of experimental animals. To do so, we entered into a collaboration with Professor Steffen Gay, then of the University of Alabama, who had developed a model in which human rheumatoid synovial tissue is coimplanted with human cartilage in severe combined immunodeficiency (SCID) mice *(30)*. Under these conditions, the synovial cells reform a pannus, which degrades the adjacent human cartilage by direct invasion and by stimulating chondrocytic chondrolysis. Transduction of the human rheumatoid synoviocytes with MFG-IRAP prior to implantation strongly inhibited chondrocytic chondrolysis *(31)*, thereby confirming the importance of IL-1 in this process and demonstrating the responsiveness of tissue from human rheumatoid joints to gene transfer and gene therapy. Of considerable additional interest, human synovial cells recovered from the SCID mice 60 d after implantation were still expressing the transgene. This supports the case for an important role of the immune system in curtailing *hIL-1Ra* gene expression in rabbits.

Preclinical Safety Testing

Because the human arthritis gene therapy protocol would be the first clinical use of gene transfer in a nonlethal disease, it was essential to examine the issue of safety in considerable detail. Several types of safety studies were performed.

In one series of experiments, MFG-IRAP was used to transduce the hematopoietic stem cells of mice *(32)*. Sera of mice with engineered stem cells contained several hundred ng/mL of hIL-1Ra for the life of the animals, yet no adverse sequelae were apparent. However, the mice were more resistant to endotoxin than control mice expressing the *Lac Z* gene. Mice expressing the *sTNFR* gene in an equivalent fashion

(33), unlike the hIL-1Ra$^+$ mice, had altered peripheral blood mononuclear-cell (MNC) profiles.

None of the rabbits used in the preclinical development of the arthritis protocol had shown adverse reactions to the gene transfer procedure. To examine this matter in greater detail, two additional sets of studies were performed. One was a cell tracking experiment, in which genetically and fluorescently labeled cells were injected intra-articularly into normal knee joints and joints with AIA. At intervals, groups of rabbits were euthanized and various organs, including the gonads, were examined for the presence of labeled cells or transgene sequences. These investigations failed to detect extraarticular cells or transgene sequences after injection of engineered cells into normal joints. A small number of labeled cells were recovered from the liver of one animal and the spleen of another 2 wk after injection into arthritic joints. However, there was no detectable pathology in these, or any other organs of any of the rabbits from either control or arthritic groups of animals *(34)*. In a complimentary series of experiments, labeled autologous synoviocytes were injected into rabbits intravenously. This mimicked the worst possible case in which all cells would exit the joint after intraarticular injection. Under these conditions, labeled cells could be recovered from the lungs, livers, and spleens of various animals but again, there were no associated pathologies. From the results of these types of experiments, we concluded that cells exit from the joint only rarely after intra-articular injection, and that even when they do, this is unlikely to have adverse sequelae.

CLINICAL PROTOCOL

Based on the foregoing considerations, we developed a clinical protocol for a phase I study, the basic aim of which was to determine whether it is possible to transfer genes to human rheumatoid joints, to express them within those joints, and to do everything in a manner that is safe and acceptable to the patients *(34)*.

Maximum emphasis was placed on safety. Because this is an ex vivo protocol, it enabled the cells to be extensively screened before injection into the patients. Furthermore, genetically modified cells were introduced into the target joints 1 wk before they were removed during a previously scheduled joint-replacement surgery. This tactic not only introduces a large safety cushion, but also provides ample tissue for post-procedure analysis.

To be eligible for the trial, patients needed to be post-menopausal females with end-stage RA, requiring, as part of its surgical management, the replacement of metacarpophalangeal (MCP) joints 2–5 on one hand, and additional surgery on one other joint. The latter procedure provided autologous synovium from which to establish cultures of autologous synovial fibroblast. These surgeries were already indicated as part of the surgical management of the patients and were not imposed as part of the protocol. Indeed, the entire study only required the participants to have a small number of intra-articular injections and venupunctures that they would not otherwise have undergone.

The study was explained to prospective participants by an informed clinician who also consented to the patients' participation, but played no other role in the trial. Once

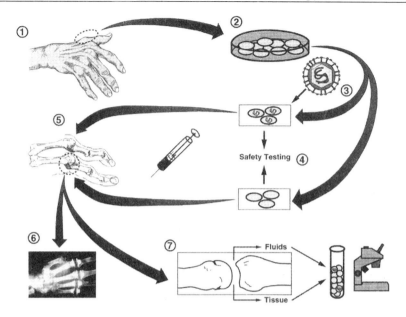

Fig. 2. Gene transfer to the human rheumatoid joint. The first patient to undergo gene transfer first underwent surgery to fuse the first metacarpophalangeal (MCP) joint of the right hand (1). Autologous synovium was recovered at this time. Cells were grown in culture (2). Half the cultures were transduced with a retrovirus carrying a human interleukin-1 receptor antagonist cDNA (3), and both transduced and untransduced cells were subjected to rigorous safety testing (4). Cells were returned to the second through fifth MCP joints of the same hand (5) 1 wk prior to surgical replacement of these joints (6). Tissues recovered at the time of total joint replacement are being analyzed for evidence of successful gene transfer and gene expression, as well as for indications that the transgene product was biologically active within the joint (7). Reproduced with permission from the University of Pittsburgh Medical Center, Pittsburgh, PA, 1996.

enrolled in the study, synovial biopsies were obtained from the patients during the first surgery; in eight of the nine patients this involved hand surgery, such as a thumb fusion (Fig. 2). Biopsies were used to established autologous cell cultures, which were split in two. One half was transduced with MFG-IRAP, whereas the other remained an untransduced control. Transduced cells were required to produce at least 30 ng IL-1Ra/10^6 cells/48 h. The bulk of each culture was then cryopreserved while aliquots were tested for endotoxin, mycoplasma, and bacterial and fungal contaminants; transduced cells were also tested for the presence of replication-competent retrovirus. Once given a clean bill of health, cells were thawed, recultured, and harvested. In a double-blinded fashion, two MCP joints were injected intra-articularly with control cells and the other two MCPs received genetically modified cells. One week later, all four MCPs were removed surgically.

Synovial material removed intraoperatively from the MCP joints was divided into several portions. One was analyzed by reverse transcriptase-polymerase chain reaction (RT-PCR) for expression of the transgene. Another was trypsinized, the cells placed into culture and the IL-1Ra content of the conditioned medium measured by ELISA. A third was sectioned and stained.

Permission to proceed with this protocol was given by the Recombinant DNA Advisory Committee of the National Institute of Health (NIH), the Director of NIH, the Food and Drug Administration (FDA), and an External Monitoring Board. All nine patients have completed the protocol, the first having received the genes over 5 yr ago. Data collection and analysis are in progress. The preliminary data suggest that the procedure is safe and results in successful gene transfer, with intra-articular gene expression. We are in the early stages of planning a phase II trial.

A similar phase I study is underway at the University of Dusseldorf in Germany, where three patients have been treated. The preliminary data from this study are similar to those from the American study (Wehling, Personal Communication). Another phase I protocol, based on the concept of a "genetic synovectomy" *(35)*, has recently begun at the University of Michigan under the direction of Dr. Blake Roessler.

CONCLUSIONS AND FUTURE DIRECTIONS

In shortly over 10 years, we have conceived the idea to use gene therapy to treat arthritis, consolidated the concept experimentally, and completed a phase I clinical trial. The concept has stood up well to intellectual scrutiny and there is now a critical mass of investigators that have collectively generated impressive proof of principle in animal models of RA. The early results from the first clinical trials are encouraging, and should lead to further interventionial studies in humans.

The ex vivo protocol reported here, while helping to maximize safety and thus facilitate use in humans, is cumbersome. Development of a useful method for in vivo delivery would help simplify the process and accelerate its clinical application. Further work is needed to identify the best gene or combination of genes to use in arthritis gene therapy, as well as to determine whether gene therapy could be used advantageously in conjunction with traditional anti-arthritic drugs. Our recent observation of a "contralateral effect" *(13,36,37)* suggests ways to improve the efficiency of local gene therapy.

The degree to which gene therapy will become a standard treatment for RA depends on a number of factors, including the performance of competing, nongenetic therapies *(38)*. There is preliminary evidence that gene therapy might have value for treating other forms of arthritis, such as osteoarthritis (OA) *(39–41)*, as well as for aiding the repair of cartilage, bone, ligament, tendon, and other connective tissues *(42,43)*.

Based on past progress, prospects for successful arthritis gene therapy in humans appear quite good. Before too long it may be possible to add to the title of a chapter such as this, a fourth alliterative noun: cure.

ACKNOWLEDGMENTS

We thank Elvire Gouze and Maria Delvecchio for critically reading an earlier version of this chapter and making many improving suggestions.

REFERENCES

1. Bandara, G., P.D. Robbins, H.I. Georgescu, G.M. Mueller, J.C. Glorioso, and C.H. Evans. 1992. Gene transfer to synoviocytes: prospects for gene treatment of arthritis. *DNA Cell Biol.* 11(3):227–231.

2. Evans, C.H. and P.D. Robbins. 1994. Gene therapy for arthritis. *J. Rheumatol.* 21:779–782.

3. Evans, C.H., S.C. Ghivizzani, R. Kang, T. Muzzonigro, M.C. Wasko, J.H. Herndon, et al. 1999. Gene therapy for rheumatic diseases. *Arthritis Rheum.* 42(1):1–16.

4. Evans, C.H., J.J. Rediske, S.B. Abramson, and P.D. Robbins. 1999. Joint efforts: tackling arthritis using gene therapy. First International Meeting on the Gene Therapy of Arthritis and Related Disorders. Bethesda, MD, 2–3 December 1998. *Mol. Med. Today* 5(4):148–151.

5. Evans, C.H., S.C. Ghivizzani, J.H. Herndon, M.C. Wasko, J. Reinecke, P. Wehling, et al. 2000. Clinical trials in the gene therapy of arthritis. *Clin. Orthop. Rel. Res.* 397S:300–307.

6. Nita, I., S.C. Ghivizzani, J. Galea-Lauri, G. Bandara, H.I. Georgescu, P.D. Robbins, et al. 1996. Direct gene delivery to synovium. An evaluation of potential vectors in vitro and in vivo. *Arthritis Rheum.* 39(5):820–828.

7. Roessler, B.J., E.D. Allen, J.M. Wilson, J.S. Hartman, and B.L. Davidson. 1993. Adenoviral-mediated gene transfer to rabbit synovium in vivo. *J. Clin. Invest.* 92(2):1085–1092.

8. Goossens, P.H., G.J. Schouten, B.A. t Hart, A. Bout, H.P. Brok, P.M. Kluin, et al. 1999. Feasibility of adenovirus-mediated nonsurgical synovectomy in collagen-induced arthritis-affected rhesus monkeys. *Human Gene Ther.* 10(7):1139–1149.

9. Ikeda, T., T. Kubo, Y. Arai, T. Nakanishi, K. Kobayashi, K. Takahashi, et al. 1998. Adenovirus mediated gene delivery to the joints of guinea pigs. *J. Rheumatol.* 25(9):1666–1673.

10. Lubberts, E., L.A. Joosten, L. van Den Bersselaar, M.M. Helsen, A.C. Bakker, J.B. van Meurs, et al. 1999. Adenoviral vector-mediated overexpression of IL-4 in the knee joint of mice with collagen-induced arthritis prevents cartilage destruction. *J. Immunol.* 163(8):4546–4556.

11. Taniguchi, K., H. Kohsaka, N. Inoue, Y. Terada, H. Ito, K. Hirokawa, et al. 1999. Induction of the p16INK4a senescence gene as a new therapeutic strategy for the treatment of rheumatoid arthritis [see comments]. *Nature Med.* 5(7):760–767.

12. Sawchuk, S.J., G.P. Boivin, L.E. Duwel, W. Ball, K. Bove, B. Trapnell, et al. 1996. Anti-T cell receptor monoclonal antibody prolongs transgene expression following adenovirus-mediated in vivo gene transfer to mouse synovium. *Human Gene Ther.* 7(4):499–506.

13. Ghivizzani, S.C., E.R. Lechman, R. Kang, C. Tio, J. Kolls, C.H. Evans, et al. 1998. Direct adenovirus-mediated gene transfer of interleukin 1 and tumor necrosis factor alpha soluble receptors to rabbit knees with experimental arthritis has local and distal anti-arthritic effects. *Proc. Natl. Acad. Sci. USA* 95(8):4613–4618.

14. Evans, C.H., S.C. Ghivizzani, E. Lechman, Z. Mi, D. Jaffurs, and P.D. Robbins. 1999. Lessons learned from gene transfer approaches. *Arthritis Res.* 1999;http://arthritis-research.com/08jul99/ar0101r01.

15. Muzzonigro, T.S., R. Kang, J. Reinecke, P. Wehling, M.C. Wasko, and J.H. Herndon. 2000. Gene therapy for rheumatoid arthritis: clincial studies, in Gene Therapy in Inflammatory Diseases. C.H. Evans and P.D. Robbins, editors. Birkhauser Verlag, Basel, Switzerland, pp. 53–63.

16. Moreland, L.W., L.W. Heck Jr., and W.J. Koopman. 1997. Biologic agents for treating rheumatoid arthritis. Concepts and progress. *Arthritis Rheum.* 40(3):397–409.

17. Makarov, S.S., J.C. Olsen, W.N. Johnston, S.K. Anderle, R.R. Brown, A.S. Baldwin, Jr., et al. 1996. Suppression of experimental arthritis by gene transfer of interleukin 1 receptor antagonist cDNA. *Proc. Natl. Acad. Sci. USA* 93(1):402–406.

18. Otani, K., I. Nita, W. Macaulay, H.I. Georgescu, P.D. Robbins, and C.H. Evans. 1996. Suppression of antigen-induced arthritis in rabbits by ex vivo gene therapy. *J. Immunol.* 156(9):3558–3562.

19. Arend, W.P. 1993. Interleukin-1 receptor antagonist. *Adv. Immunol.* 54:167–227.

20. Bendele, A., T. McAbee, M. Woodward, J. Scherrer, D. Collins, J. Frazier, et al. 1998. Effects of interleukin-1 receptor antagonist in a slow-release hylan vehicle on rat type II collagen arthritis. *Pharm. Res.* 15(10):1557–1561.

21. Schwab, J.H., S.K. Anderle, R.R. Brown, F.G. Dalldorf, and R.C. Thompson. 1991. Pro- and anti-inflammatory roles of interleukin-1 in recurrence of bacterial cell wall-induced arthritis in rats. *Infect. Immun.* 59(12):4436–4442.

22. Van Lent, P.L., F.A. Van De Loo, A.E. Holthuysen, L.A. Van Den Bersselaar, H. Vermeer, and W.B. Van Den Berg. 1995. Major role for interleukin 1 but not for tumor necrosis factor in early cartilage damage in immune complex arthritis in mice. *J. Rheumatol.* 22(12):2250–2258.

23. Bresnihan, B., J.M. Alvaro-Gracia, M. Cobby, M. Doherty, Z. Domljan, P. Emery, et al. 1998. Treatment of rheumatoid arthritis with recombinant human interleukin-1 receptor antagonist [see comments]. *Arthritis Rheum.* 41(12):2196–2204.

24. Granowitz, E.V., R. Porat, J.W. Mier, J.P. Pribble, D.M. Stiles, D.C. Bloedow, et al. 1992. Pharmacokinetics, safety and immunomodulatory effects of human recombinant interleukin-1 receptor antagonist in healthy humans. *Cytokine* 4(5):353–360.

25. Van Zee, K.J., S.M. Coyle, S.E. Calvano, H.S. Oldenburg, D.M. Stiles, J. Pribble, et al. 1995. Influence of IL-1 receptor blockade on the human response to endotoxemia. *J. Immunol.* 154(3):1499–1507.

26. Bandara, G., G.M. Mueller, J. Galea-Lauri, M.H. Tindal, H.I. Georgescu, M.K. Suchanek, et al. 1993. Intraarticular expression of biologically active interleukin 1-receptor-antagonist protein by ex vivo gene transfer. *Proc. Natl. Acad. Sci. USA* 90(22):10,764–10,768.

27. Hung, G.L., J. Galea-Lauri, G.M. Mueller, H.I. Georgescu, L.A. Larkin, M.K. Suchanek, et al. 1994. Suppression of intra-articular responses to interleukin-1 by transfer of the interleukin-1 receptor antagonist gene to synovium. *Gene Ther.* 1(1):64–69.

28. Lewthwaite, J., S.M. Blake, T.E. Hardingham, P.J. Warden, and B. Henderson. 1994. The effect of recombinant human interleukin 1 receptor antagonist on the induction phase of antigen induced arthritis in the rabbit. *J. Rheumatol.* 21(3):467–472.

29. Bakker, A.C., L.A. Joosten, O.J. Arntz, M.M. Helsen, A.M. Bendele, F.A. van de Loo, et al. 1997. Prevention of murine collagen-induced arthritis in the knee and ipsilateral paw by local expression of human interleukin-1 receptor antagonist protein in the knee. *Arthritis Rheum.* 40(5):893–900.

30. Geiler, T., J. Kriegsmann, G.M. Keyszer, R.E. Gay, and S. Gay. 1994. A new model for rheumatoid arthritis generated by engraftment of rheumatoid synovial tissue and normal human cartilage into SCID mice. *Arthritis Rheum.* 37(11):1664–1671.

31. Muller-Ladner, U., C.R. Roberts, B.N. Franklin, R.E. Gay, P.D. Robbins, C.H. Evans, et al. 1997. Human IL-1Ra gene transfer into human synovial fibroblasts is chondroprotective. *J. Immunol.* 158(7):3492–3498.

32. Boggs, S.S., K.D. Patrene, G.M. Mueller, C.H. Evans, L.A. Doughty, and P.D. Robbins. 1995. Prolonged systemic expression of human IL-1 receptor antagonist (hIL- 1ra) in mice reconstituted with hematopoietic cells transduced with a retrovirus carrying the hIL-1ra cDNA [see comments]. *Gene Ther.* 2(9):632–638.

33. Doughty, L.A., K.D. Patrene, C.H. Evans, S.S. Boggs, and P.D. Robbins. Constitutive systemic expression of IL-1Ra or soluble TNF receptor by genetically modified hematopoietic cells suppresses LPS induction of IL- 6 and IL-10. *Gene Ther.* 4(3):252–257.

34. Evans, C.H., P.D. Robbins, S.C. Ghivizzani, J.H. Herndon, R. Kang, A.B. Bahnson, et al. 1996. Clinical trial to assess the safety, feasibility, and efficacy of transferring a potentially anti-arthritic cytokine gene to human joints with rheumatoid arthritis. *Human Gene Ther.* 7(10):1261–1280.

35. Sant, S.M., T.M. Suarez, M.R. Moalli, B.Y. Wu, M. Blaivas, T.J. Laing, et al. 1998. Molecular lysis of synovial lining cells by in vivo herpes simplex virus-thymidine kinase gene transfer. *Human Gene Ther.* 9(18):2735–2743.

36. Lechman, E.R., D. Jaffurs, S.C. Ghivizzani, A. Gambotto, I. Kovesdi, Z. Mi, et al. 1999. Direct adenoviral gene transfer of viral IL-10 to rabbit knees with experimental arthritis ameliorates disease in both injected and contralateral control knees. *J. Immunol.* 163(4):2202–2208.

37. Whalen, J.D., E.L. Lechman, C.A. Carlos, K. Weiss, I. Kovesdi, J.C. Glorioso, et al. 1999. Adenoviral transfer of the viral IL-10 gene periarticularly to mouse paws suppresses development of collagen-induced arthritis in both injected and uninjected paws. *J. Immunol.* 162(6):3625–3632.

38. Evans, C.H. and P.D. Robbins. 1999. Will there be a role for gene therapy, in Challenges in Rheumatoid Arthritis. H.A. Bird and M.L. Snaith, editors. Blackwell Science Ltd. London, UK, pp. 245–257.

39. Pelletier, J.P., J.P. Caron, C. Evans, P.D. Robbins, H.I. Georgescu, D. Jovanovic, et al. 1997. In vivo suppression of early experimental osteoarthritis by interleukin-1 receptor antagonist using gene therapy. *Arthritis Rheum.* 40(6):1012–1019.

40. Frisbie, D., P.D. Robbins, C.H. Evans, and C.W. McIlwraith. 2000. In vivo gene therapy of an equine model of osteoarthritis, in press.

41. Fernandes, J., G. Tardif, J. Martel-Pelletier, V. Lascau-Coman, M. Dupuis, F. Moldovan, et al. 1999. In vivo transfer of interleukin-1 receptor antagonist gene in osteoarthritic rabbit knee joints: prevention of osteoarthritis progression. *Am. J. Pathol.* 154(4):1159–1169.

42. Evans, C.H. and P.D. Robbins. 1999. Genetically augmented tissue engineering of the musculoskeletal system. *Clin. Orthop.* (367 Suppl.):S410–S418.

43. Evans, C.H. and P.D. Robbins. 1995. Possible orthopaedic applications of gene therapy. *J. Bone Joint Surg. Am.* 77(7):1103–1114.

V   OTHER RHEUMATIC DISORDERS

38

Recent Advances in the Pharmacotherapy of Spondyloarthropathies

Jürgen Braun, Joachim Sieper, and Muhammad A. Khan

CONTENTS

INTRODUCTION AND OVERVIEW

Ankylosing spondylitis (AS) and related spondyloarthropathies (SpA) are relatively common *(1)* chronic inflammatory rheumatic diseases of uncertain etiopathogenesis *(2)*, frequently involving the axial skeleton, including sacroiliac joints *(3)*. The therapeutic options for the treatment of these diseases mostly involve physiotherapy and nonsteroidal, anti-inflammatory drugs (NSAIDs) as stated in recent overviews on the subject *(4–9)*. The newer cyclooxygenase (COX)-2 selective inhibitors celecoxib and rofecoxib provide significant symptomatic benefit, and cause less gastric ulcers, but are no more effective than established NSAIDs *(10)*. Up to 20% of AS patients are intolerant or show lack of adequate response to NSAIDs *(11)*. Corticosteroids are effective when injected locally or intra-articularly *(12)*, but oral dose, unlike in rheumatoid arthritis (RA), rarely provides systemic relief in AS, an interesting difference for which the underlying pathophysiologic basis is unclear.

From: *Modern Therapeutics in Rheumatic Diseases*
Edited by: G. C. Tsokos, et al. © Humana Press, Inc., Totowa, NJ

Sulfasalazine, a disease-modifying anti-rheumatic drug (DMARD), benefits SpA patients with peripheral arthritis and, possibly, those with gut inflammation and those in early and in active disease stages of the disease *(13–15)*. Of interest, quite a few rheumatologists use methotrexate (MTX) to treat AS when there is lack of response to NSAIDs and sulfasalazine *(16)*, despite the absence of randomized controlled clinical trials for this indication *(17–19)*. A very recent report on a few AS patients who received a high loading dose of azathioprin was promising *(20)*. Possible beneficial effects of thalidomide *(21)* and of pamidronate *(22)* for the treatment of AS were recently reported from two open studies. These two drugs work at least partly by blocking the proinflammatory cytokine tumor necrosis factor-α (TNF-α), that is mainly produced by monocytes and macrophages and to a lesser degree by T cells, and that mediates inflammatory and immunoregulatory activities *(23,24)*. This cytokine is also the target of recently introduced, newer therapies for the treatment of RA *(25)* and Crohn's disease *(26)*. Thus, there is a clear need for effective new drug therapies in the treatment of AS and related SpA.

TNF-α BLOCKADE

The efficacy of anti-TNF-α therapy in severe AS and related SpA has now been reported in open-label pilot-studies *(27–29)* and in a recently performed controlled clinical trial in Germany (unpublished results). There are two specific receptors for TNF-α—a 55 kD and a 75 kD size—that are present on many cell types. The biologic effects of TNF-α, that are discussed in this book (Chapters 1 and 6) and also reviewed elsewhere *(30)* are mostly proinflammatory, but it also has important physiologic functions in immune responses against pathogens, and in suppressing autoimmunity and malignancy *(31)*. Therefore, blocking of some of these functions might lead to undesired side effects.

BIOLOGICALS BLOCKING TNF-α

The antibody used for blocking TNF-α in the recently published German *(27)* and Belgian *(28)* studies on SpA patients was infliximab (Remicade®, Centocor)—the first such antibody approved for treating patients with severe RA and Crohn's disease. It is of interest that Crohn-like gut lesions have been detected in a significant percentage of SpA patients *(32)*.

There are other agents acting against TNF-α, such as the TNF-α-75kD-receptor-IgG1 fusion protein (Etanercept, Enbrel®, Lederle) that have also been proven effective in severe RA patients *(33)*. It is as yet unclear whether etanercept works in Crohn's disease.

ANTI-TNF-α THERAPY IN PATIENTS WITH ACTIVE AS

Several years after the description of TNF-α mRNA in sacroiliac biopsies of SpA patients *(34)* and the failure to detect bacterial DNA there *(35)*, the group from Germany has performed an open pilot study with an anti-TNF agent (infliximab) in AS *(27)*. In this study, 11 AS patients who had active disease for at least 3 mo (range 3–72 mo) were treated with infliximab at wk 0, 2, and 6 in a dosage of 5 mg/kg. Ten patients were male, one female, the mean age was 36 yr (range 27–56 yr), and the median disease

Table 1
Comparison of Outcome Parameters (Median) Before, After 2 and After 12 wk
of Treatment with Infliximab in Patients with Severe Ankylosing Spondylitis

	Wk 0	Wk 2	p =	Wk 12	p =
BASDAI (range)	6.5 (5.2–8.5)	1.9 (0.4–4.6)	0.001	2.4 (0.4–6.3)	0.004
BASFI (range)	5.3 (1.3–8.2)	2.3 (0.2–6.4)	0.002	2.4 (0.2–6.5)	0.008
BASMI	3.0	1.0	0.031	1.5	0.1
VAS for IBP (range)	7.8 (6.0–9.8)	2.0 (0.3–5.1)	0.002	2.5 (0.7–5.1)	0.004
CRP (SD; mg/L)	15.5 (±23.5)	<6.0[a]		<6.0[a]	0.008
ESR (SD; mm/1.h)	32.0 (±31.0)	<15[a]		<15[a]	0.008

BASDAI, Bath Ankylosing Spondylitis Disease Activity Index; BASFI, Bath Ankylosing Spondylitis Disease Functional Index; BASMI, Bath Ankylosing Spondylitis Metrology Index; VAS, Visual Analog Scale; CRP, C-Reactive Protein; ESR, Erytrocyte Sedimentation Rate; [a]normal range of CRP and ESR; p was calculated by the Wilcoxon-test concerning the difference between the median and mean values before treatment (wk 0) and wk 2 and 12.

duration was 5 yr (range 0.5–13 yr); 10/11 were HLA B27 positive. Five patients had AS-relevant radiologic changes of the spine with three or more syndesmophytes and/or fusions of vertebrae, and three of them had active spinal inflammation as detected by dynamic spinal magnetic resonance imaging (MRI). All patients except one had C-reactive protein (CRP) levels >6 mg/L before treatment, and in 3 of them it was documented several times over at least 1 yr. The Bath AS disease activity index (BASDAI), the functional index (BASFI), pain on a visual analog scale (VAS), and a metrology index (BASMI) were assessed. Quality of life was assessed using the SF-36 instrument. Laboratory markers of disease activity including interleukin-6 (IL-6) were determined. Dynamic MRI of the spine was performed in five patients, that showed evidence of spinal inflammation (spondylitis and spondylodiscitis) in three of them. One patient had a rash after the first infusion, and she was withdrawn from the study. The study found that anti-TNF-α therapy is very effective in AS. Table 1 lists the comparison of outcome parameters (median) before the initiation of therapy, and at 2 and 12 wk of treatment with infliximab. The subjective improvement started on the first day after the first infusion. The mean improvement of the BASDAI after 4 wk was 72 ± 17%. At wk 2 and 4, improvement ≥50% in activity, function, and pain scores was documented in all patients. In the direct comparison between wk 0 vs wk 2 and 12, the medians of all parameters had improved significantly (Table 1). The clear-cut benefit persisted until wk 12 in 8 of the 10 patients (6 wk after the third infusion). The CRP decreased from 15.5 ± 9.6 mg/L to normal and IL-6 from 12.4 ± 11.6 ng/L to normal (<5 ng/L). Quality-of-life assessments as regularly performed using the validated questionnaire SF-36 showed improvements in this global health assessment measure before and after 4 wk of treatment with infliximab, as shown in Table 2. The median values of 6 out of 9 concepts (physical functioning, role functioning physical, bodily pain, vitality, social functioning, and reported health transition) between wk 0 and 4 had improved; this was statistically significant. Three other concepts also improved, but not significantly: general health, role functioning emotional, and mental health. It remains to be shown whether this anti-inflammatory therapy is safe and effective over long period of time, and whether it will prevent ankylosis.

Table 2
**Improvement of Global Health Assessment Concepts (SF36) Before and After 4 wk
of Treatment with Infliximab in Patients in Severe Ankylosing Spondylitis**

SF 36	Wk 0	Wk 4	p =
Physical functioning (%)	44.4	72.0	0.01
Role functioning physical (%)	0.5	62.5	0.05
Bodily pain (%)	12.0	46.0	0.002
Vitality (%)	37.5	42.0	0.02
Social functioning (%)	37.5	68.8	0.03
Reported health transition[a] (range)	4.0 (5–3)	3.0 (4–2)	0.004
General health (%)	37.5	42.0	0.08
Role functioning emotional (%)	66.0	100	0.1
Mental health (%)	46.0	60.0	0.07

[a]Transformed scale scores are not calculated for this item, median values are shown.

p was calculated by the Wilcoxon-test concerning the difference between the mean values before treatment (wk 0) and wk 4.

In all, three patients were withdrawn from the study because of significant infusion reactions (all easy to handle). It has to be studied whether patients treated with infliximab should receive concomitant MTX or azathioprine to minimize such untoward effects.

ANTI-TNF-α THERAPY IN PATIENTS WITH ACTIVE SPONDYLOARTHROPATHY

In the Belgian study *(28)* spinal pain of 7/11 AS patients improved significantly at 2 and 6 wk after anti-TNF-α therapy given as an induction therapy at wk 0, 2, and 6. Clinical improvement was already noticed on the day after the first infusion; function also improved significantly, and most elevated CRP values became normal after therapy. In this study, they were also 18 SpA patients with peripheral arthritis who were treated with good result.

There is an ongoing study with Enbrel® for the treatment of AS in California (Davis, personal communication). Clinicians have used Enbrel for some patients with active AS relatively unresponsive to conventional therapy, and the patients seem to respond very well (R. Bluestone, personal communication).

ANTI-TNF-α THERAPY IN SEVERE PSORIATIC ARTHRITIS

In one study, eight patients with psoriasis were treated with infliximab *(35)*. Peripheral joint and skin symptoms ameliorated significantly after 7 and 14 d. In another open study *(36)*, ten patients with severe psoriatic arthritis under therapy with MTX (15–25 mg/wk) received additional therapy with infliximab. All patients developed quick and persistent improvement of joint and skin symptoms (C. Antoni, personal communication). A randomized controlled trial with Enbrel in addition to MTX has proven efficacy of this agent in patients with psoriatic arthritis (P. Mease, personal communication). Thus, blockade of TNF-α seems to be effective in patients with severe psoriatic arthritis.

THERAPY OF UNDIFFERENTIATED SPA

It is remarkable that no therapy study dealing with this condition has ever been performed to date. The two patients of the aforementioned Belgian study *(28)* improved, similar to the other SpA. This is in accordance with our present experience in six cases *(37)*. Of note, this included a patient with multilocular enthesitis who significantly improved after infliximab. The 5 mg/kg dose tended to be better than the 3 mg/kg dose in this small study.

EFFECTS OF ANTI-TNF THERAPY ON LABORATORY PARAMETERS

Some rather unexpected laboratory findings after infliximab therapy have been reported. Feldmann measured increased TNF-α serum levels, while both soluble TNF receptor levels remained unchanged and elevated. However, measuring serum TNF-α is difficult (only 50% of the RA patients treated had elevated levels), because the half-life is short and the TNF measured in that study was not in its bioactive state *(38)*. This might indicate that immune complexes of soluble TNF and infliximab were measured. In contrast, the TNF secretion capacity of peripheral blood (PB) T cells was found to be reduced in AS patients and in HLA B27-positive healthy controls as compared to HLA B27-negative normal persons *(39)*. This might indicate that the cytokine pattern of PB cells is the reverse of what is happening in the gut, the synovium, or in the joints. This might indicate active regulatory suppression in order to prevent damage at other sites or it might be from effector cells having left the previously inflamed sites. Of interest, in accordance with findings in RA patients after infliximab *(40)* we found a somewhat increased TNF-α secretion capacity after treatment in six patients *(41)*.

There is also a discrepancy regarding total lymphocyte counts after infliximab. Although Paleolog et al. *(42)* reported somewhat of an increase, similar to other RA patients *(43)*, we found lower lymphocyte counts and somewhat less circulating CD3+ T cells in AS patients 1 wk after infliximab *(40)*. This might depend on the timepoint when the measurement was performed.

SIDE EFFECTS OF ANTI-TNF-A THERAPY WITH INFLIXIMAB

Some undesired effects of infliximab therapy have been observed *(25,44,45)*: side effects directly associated with the infusion (2–5%); autoimmune phenomena (DNA antibodies in 10–16%); and somewhat more upper respiratory-tract infections, which were reported to have occurred in about 20–30% of the patients *(25)*. This was not statistically significant. However, in an ongoing study, a young AS patient with a negative tuberculin reaction developed systemic tuberculosis after three infusions of infliximab. Another female patient in the same study developed a lupus-like syndrome with polyarthralgia and fever.

The risk of developing malignancy has been discussed thoroughly, but there is no evidence of a significantly increased risk to date. Lymphoma were observed in a few anti-TNF treated patients with Crohn's disease *(46)*. However, all such reported increases were not significantly different from normal population prevalences. Thus, the concern of malignancy bases mainly on theoretical calculations and is not based on evidence to date *(47)*.

The murine and the human part of anti-TNF antibodies have significant immuno-genic potential. Human antichimeric antibodies (HACA), possibly associated with hypersensitivity infusion reactions and human antihuman antibodies (HAHAs) have been described *(25,44)*. However, it is not clear whether the production of HACA has influence on the efficacy and frequency of special side effects. Concomitant therapy with MTX or azathioprine might reduce the risk of antibody development but further study is clearly needed.

COURSE AND SEVERITY OF SPA: WHICH PATIENTS SHOULD BE TREATED?

Can there possibly be an indication for expensive biologic therapies in SpA at all? Are SpA courses of disease severe enough to justify such costly interventions? In a recent discussion with experienced rheumatologists, the argument was raised that one could just wait for ankylosis to occur in AS patients with inflammatory back pain and sacroiliitis; then the symptoms might improve by the natural course of disease. This statement is partly true, but seems also typical for doctors who have had no major therapy to offer for decades.

However, rheumatologists are well aware of rapidly progressing severe courses in AS *(48)* and it is well-known that the majority of the burden of disease develops in the first 10 yr *(49,50)*. This would argue for early therapy. However, there is limited knowledge on prognostic factors in SpA *(51)*. The recently raised hypothesis arguing for enthesitis as favorable prognostic sign in arthritic conditions *(52)* clearly needs confirmation.

The total burden of disease in AS is incompletely defined, but a significant percentage of young AS patients has a chronic recurrent course of disease resulting in significant disability *(53)*. Because there is still a significant diagnostic delay of 5 yr and more, there are almost no studies on AS patients with a disease duration of <10 yr. This was an important difference between the Belgian (mean disease duration 15–19 yr) and the German study (5 yr) on infliximab in AS.

Although the study of radiographic progression seems to be difficult *(54)*, we should aim for preventing widespread spinal ankylosis—an essential factor for disability in AS. Modern imaging techniques such as MRI are promising new tools as activity and outcome parameters *(55)*.

In summary, therapy directed against TNF-α seems to work in AS and other SpA. However, controlled trials need to be performed to compare the effects to standard treatment regimen. Infections and autoimmune phenomena seem to be a problem which, however, can be handled. Tuberculin skin test-positive patients might be safer when being prophylactically treated with a tuberculostatic drug such as INH. Because we do not yet have significant long-term experience, we do not know about long-term side effects.

Because of the high costs of therapy, we need to study minimal dosage requirements, but should also think about the possibility of high-dose induction therapy, which might be even more effective. Twenty mg/kg may be the highest dose ever tried, but no more than 10 mg/kg was used in the studies discussed earlier.

Do we have to treat regularly, and what is the optimal interval between each infusion? A randomized, controlled trial on AS is now being performed in Germany in which the drug infusion will be given every sixth week. The 6-wk-interval was chosen because at about 7 wk after the third treatment, beginning of symptomatic worsening was noted, and 4 out of 10 patients showed significant worsening of the BASDAI index at 8 wk. Thus, to suppress constantly disease activity, infliximab infusions every 6 wk seem appropriate. However, for individual patients, lower doses and longer intervals of infusions might work equally well. This is relevant because of the high costs of anti-TNF therapy.

Which patients should be treated? Initially, probably only those with very severe and active disease, and later, probably those patients in early stage of their disease, to investigate if early interruption of inflammation will prevent cartilage damage and prevent or delay progressive ankylosis.

If the present promising results can be confirmed in controlled prospective studies in a larger number of patients, one can hope that we have found, for the first time, a very effective therapeutic option in severe AS and related SpA. This could become a major breakthrough in the therapy of this group of diseases that, it is hoped, may even prevent progressive ankylosis so typical of AS.

REFERENCES

1. Braun, J., M. Bollow, G. Remlinger, et al. 1998. Prevalence of spondylarthropathies in HLA B27-positive and -negative blood donors. *Arthritis Rheum.* 41:58–67.

2. Sieper, J. and J. Braun. 1995. Pathogenesis of Spondylarthropathies. *Arthritis Rheum.* 38: 1547–1554.

3. Braun, J. and J. Sieper. 1996. The sacroiliac joint in the spondylarthropathies. *Curr. Opin. Rheumatol.* 7:275–283.

4. Dougados, M., A. Gueguen, J.P. Nakache, P. Velicitat, E.M. Veys, H. Zeidler, and A. Calin. 1999. Ankylosing spondylitis: what is the optimum duration of a clinical study? A one year versus a 6 weeks non-steroidal anti-inflammatory drug trial. *Rheumatology* 38:235–244.

5. Gran, J.T. and G. Husby. 1992. Ankylosing spondylitis. *Current drug treatment* 44:585–603.

6. Creemers, M.C.W., P.L.C.M. van Riel, M.J.A.M. Franssen, L.B.A. van de Putte, and F.W.J. Griibnau. 1994. Second line treatment in seronegative spondyloarthropathies. *Semin. Arthritis Rheum.* 24:71–81.

7. Toussirot, E. and D. Wendling. 1998. Current guidelines for the drug treatment of ankylosing spondylitis. *Drugs* 56:225–240.

8. Leirisalo-Repo, M. 1998. Prognosis, course of disease, and treatment of the spondyloarthropathies. *Rheum. Dis. Clin. North Am.* 24:737–751.

9. Koehler, L., J.G. Kuipers, and H. Zeidler. 2000. Managing seronegative spondarthritides. *Rheumatology* 39(4):360–368.

10. Langman, M.J., D.M. Jensen, D.J. Watson, S.E. Harper, P.L. Zhao, H. Quan, et al. 1999. Adverse upper gastrointestinal effects of rofecoxib compared with NSAIDs. *JAMA* 282:1929–1933.

11. Amor, B., M. Dougados, and M.A. Khan. 1995. Management of refractory ankylosing spondylitis and related spondyloarthropathies. *Rheum. Dis. Clin. North Am.* 21:117–128.

12. Braun, J., M. Bollow, S.F. Seyrekbasan, et al. 1996. Computed tomography corticosteroid injection of the sacroiliac joint in patients with spondylarthropathy with sacroiliitis: clinical outcome and followup by dynamic magnetic resonance imaging. *J. Rheumatol.* 23:659–664.

13. Nissila, M., K. Lehtinen, M. Leirisalo-Repo, R. Luukkainen, O. Mutru, and U. Yli-Kerttula. 1988. Sulfasalazine in the treatment of ankylosing spondylitis. *Arthritis Rheum.* 31:1111–1116.

14. Bosi-Ferraz, M., P. Tugwell, C.H. Goldsmith, and E. Atra. 1990. Meta-analyis of sulfasalazine in ankylosing spondylitis. *J. Rheumatol.* 17:11.

15. Clegg, D.O., D.J. Reda, M.H. Weisman, W.D. Blackburn, J.J. Cush, et al. 1996. Comparison of sulfasalazine and placebo in the treatment of ankylosing spondylitis. A Department of Veterans Affairs cooperative study. *Arthritis Rheum.* 39:2004–2012.

16. Creemers, M.C., M.J. Franssen, L.B. van de Putte, F.W. Gribnau, and P.L. van Riel. 1995. Methotrexate in severe ankylosing spondylitis: an open study. *J. Rheumatol.* 22(6):1104–1107.

17. Sampaio-Barros, P.D., L.T. Costallat, M.B. Bertolo, J.F. Neto, and A.M. Samara. 2000. Methotrexate in the treatment of ankylosing spondylitis. *Scand. J. Rheumatol.* 29(3):160–162.

18. Biasi, D., A. Carletto, P. Caramaschi, M.L. Pacor, T. Maleknia, and L.M. Bambara. 2000. Efficacy of methotrexate in the treatment of ankylosing spondylitis: a three-year open study. *Clin. Rheumatol.* 19(2):114–117.

19. Ward, M. and S. Kuzis. 1999. Treatment used by patients with ankylosing spondylitis. Comparison with the treatment preferences of rheumatologists. *J. Clin. Rheumatol.* 5:1–8.

20. Durez, P. and Y. Horsmans. 2000. Dramatic response after an intravenous loading dose of azathioprine in one case of severe and refractory ankylosing spondylitis. *Rheumatology* 39(2):182–184.

21. Breban, M., B. Gombert, B. Amor, and M. Dougados. 1999. Efficacy of thalidomide in the treatment of refractory ankylosing spondylitis. *Arthritis Rheum.* 42:580–581.

22. Maksymowych, W.P., G.S. Jhangri, S. Leclercq, K. Skeith, A. Yan, and A.S. Russell. 1998. An open study of pamidronate in the treatment of refractory ankylosing spondylitis. *J. Rheumatol.* 25(4):714–717.

23. Corral, L.G. and G. Kaplan. 1999. Immunomodulation by thalidomide and thalidomide analogues. *Ann. Rheum. Dis.* 58(Suppl.1):I107–I113.

24. Pennanen, N., S. Lapinjoki, A. Urtti, and J. Monkkonen. 1995. Effect of liposomal and free bisphosphonates on the IL-1 beta, IL-6 and TNF alpha secretion from RAW 264 cells in vitro. *Pharm. Res.* 12(6):916–922.

25. Maini, R., et al. 1999. Infliximab (chimeric anti-tumour necrosis factor alpha monoclonal antibody) versus placebo in rheumatoid arthritis patients receiving concomitant methotrexate: a randomised phase III trial. ATTRACT Study Group. *Lancet* 354(9194):1932–1939.

26. Present, D.H., P. Rutgeerts, S. Targan, et al. 1999. Infliximab for the treatment of fistulas in patients with Crohn's disease. *N. Engl. J. Med.* 340:1398–1405.

27. Brandt, J., H. Haibel, D. Cornely, W. Golder, J. Gonzalez, J. Reddig, et al. 2000. Successful treatment of active ankylosing spondylitis with the anti-tumor necrosis factor α monoclonal antibody infliximab. *Arthritis Rheum.* 43:1346–1353

28. Van den Bosch, F., E. Kruithof, D. Baeten, F. De Keyser, H. Mielants, and E. Veys. 2000. Effects of chimeric monoclonal antibody to tumor necrosis factor-a (infliximab) in spondyloarthropathy: an open pilot study. *Ann. Rheum. Dis.* 59(6):428–433.

29. Braun, J. and J. Sieper. 2000. Anti-TNFalpha: a new dimension in the pharmacotherapy of the spondyloarthropathies!? *Ann. Rheum. Dis.* 59(6):404–407.

30. Beutler, B.A. 1999. The role of TNF in health and disease. *J. Rheumatol.* 26 S57:16–21.

31. De Vos, M., C. Cuvelier, H. Mielants, E. Vexs, F. Barbier, and A. Elewaut. 1989. Ileocolonoscopy in seronegative spondyloarthropathy. *Gastroenterology* 96:339–344.

32. Weinblatt, M.E., J.M. Kremer, A.D. Bankhurst, K.J. Bulpitt, R.M. Fleischmann, R.I. Fox, et al. 1999. A trial of etanercept, a recombinant tumor necrosis factor receptor: Fc fusion protein, in patients with rheumatoid arthritis receiving methotrexate. *N. Engl. J. Med.* 28(4):253–259.

33. Braun, J., M. Bollow, L. Neure, et al. 1995. Use of immunohistologic and in situ hybridization techniques in the examination of sacroiliac joint biopsy specimens from patients with ankylosing spondylitis. *Arthritis Rheum.* 38:499–505.

34. Braun, J., M. Tuszewski, S. Ehlers, et al. 1997. Nested PCR strategy simultaneously targeting DNA sequences of multiple bacterial species in inflammatory joint diseases. II. Examination of sacroiliac and knee joint biopsies of patients with spondyloarthropathies and other arthritides. *J. Rheumatol.* 24:1101–1105.

35. Antoni, C., C. Dechant, H. Lorenz, A. Olgivie, D. Kalden-Nemeth, and J. Kalden. 1999. Successful treatment of severe psoriasis arthritis with infliximab. *Arthritis Rheum.* 42(Suppl):S371.

36. Mease, P., B. Goffe, J. Metz, and A. Vanderstoep. 1999. Enbrel® (Etanercept) in patients with psoriatic arthritis. *Arthritis Rheum.* 42:S377.

37. Brandt, J., H. Haibel, J. Reddig, J. Sieper, and J. Braun. 2001. Successful short-term treatment of severe undifferentiated spondyloarthropathy with the anti-tumor necrosis factor α monoclonal antibody infliximab. *J. Rhematol.*, in press.

38. Charles, P., M.J. Elliott, D. Davis, A. Potter, J.R. Kalden, C. Antoni, et al. 1999. Regulation of cytokines, cytokine inhibitors, and acute-phase proteins following anti-TNF-alpha therapy in rheumatoid arthritis. *J. Immunol.* 163(3):1521–1528.

39. Braun, J., J. Tsian, J. Brandt, H. Maetzel, H. Haibel, P. Wu, et al. 2000. Treatment of spondyloarthropathies with antibodies against tumor necrosis factor (TNF) α—first clinical and laboratory experiences. *Ann. Rheum. Dis.* in press

40. Rudwaleit, M., S. Siegert, A. Thiel, Z. Yin, A. Radbruch, J. Sieper, and J. Braun. 2000. Low T cell production of TNFλ and IFNγ in ankylosing spondylitis: ist relation to HLA B27 and influence of the TNF-308 gene polymorphism. *Ann. Rheum. Dis.* 59:1–6.

41. Paleolog, E.M., M. Hunt, M.J. Elliott, M. Feldmann, R.N. Maini, and J.N. Woody. 1996. Deactivation of vascular endothelium by monoclonal anti-tumor necrosis factor alpha antibody in rheumatoid arthritis. *Arthritis Rheum.* 39:1082–1091.

42. Ohsima, S., Y. Saeki, T. Mima, M. Sasai, K. Nishioka, H. Ishida, et al. 1999. Long-term follow up of the changes in circulating cytokines, soluble cytokine receptors, and white blood cell counts in patients with rheumatoid arthritis after monoclonal anti-TNF-α antibody therapy. *J. Clin. Immunol.* 19:305–313.

43. Maurice, M.M., W.L. van der Graaff, A. Leow, F.C. Breedveld, R.A. van Lier, and C.L. Verweij. 1999. Treatment with monoclonal anti-tumor necrosis factor alpha antibody results in an accumulation of Th1 CD4+T cells in the peripheral blood of patients with rheumatoid arthritis. *Arthritis Rheum.* 42(10):2166–2173.

44. Kavanaugh, A.F. 1998. Anti-tumor necrosis factor-alpha monoclonal antibody therapy for rheumatoid arthritis. *Rheum. Dis. Clin. North Am.* Aug; 24(3):593–614.

45. Moreland, L.W. 1999. Inhibitors of tumor necrosis factor for rheumatoid arthritis. *J. Rheumatol.* 26(Suppl.)57:7–15.

46. Sandborn, W.J. and S.B. Hanauer. 1999. Antitumor necrosis factor therapy for inflammatory bowel disease: a review of agents, pharmacology, clinical results, and safety. *Inflamm. Bowel Dis.* 5:119–133.

47. Cope, A.P. 1998. Regulation of autoimmunity by proinflammatory cytokines. *Curr. Opin. Immunol.* 10:669–676.

48. Ward, M. 1999. Health-related quality of life in ankylosing spondylitis: a survey of 175 patients. *Arthritis Care Res.* 12:247–255.

49. Carette, S., D. Graham, H. Little, J. Rubenstein, and P. Rosen. 1983. The natural disease course of ankylosing spondylitis. *Arthritis Rheum.* 26(2):186–190.

50. Gran, J.T. and J.F. Skomsvoll. 1997. The outcome of ankylosing spondylitis: a study of 100 patients. *Br. J. Rheumatol.* 36(7):766–771.

51. Amor, B., R.S. Santos, R. Nahal, V. Listrat, and M. Dougados. 1994. Predictive factors for the longterm outcome of spondyloarthropathies. *J. Rheumatol.* 21:1883–1887.

52. McGonagle, D., W. Gibbon, and P. Emery. 1998. Classification of inflammatory arthritis by enthesitis. *Lancet* 352:1137–1140.

53. Zink, A., J. Braun, A. Listing, J. Wollenhaupt, and the German Colloborative Research Centers. 2000. Disability and handicap in rheumatoid arthritis and ankylosing spondylitis—results from the German rheumatological database. German Collaborative Arthritis Centers. *J. Rheumatol.* 27:613–622.

54. Spoorenberg, A., K. de Vlam, D. van der Heijde, E. de Klerk, M. Dougados, H. Mielants, et al. 1999. Radiologic scoring methods in ankylosing spondylitis: reliability and sensitivity to change over one year. *J. Rheumatol.* 26:997–1002.

55. Braun, J., M. Bollow, and J. Sieper. 1998. Radiologic diagnosis and pathology of the spondyloarthropathies. *Rheum. Dis. Clin. North Am.* 24:697–735.

39 Modern Therapy of Crystal Arthropathies

Kanyakorn Jaovisidha and Ann K. Rosenthal

CONTENTS

INTRODUCTION

Crystal-induced arthritides include the common diseases of gout and calcium pyrophosphate (CPPD) deposition disease, as well are the less common forms of arthritis associated with basic calcium phosphate (BCP) (Table 1). Other crystals, including those listed in Table 2, can be seen in synovial fluid. However, most of these rarer crystals are of uncertain pathogenicity. Although the clinical syndrome associated with gout was described centuries ago, some treatment aspects of gouty arthritis remain poorly studied. Furthermore, patients often have significant comorbidities, which affect responses to and limit choices of therapy. To date, no specific treatment exists for CPPD deposition disease. Therefore, the management of patients with these common crystal arthropathies can be quite challenging. A better understanding of the pathogenesis of crystal-induced arthritis, including the identification of factors that turn on and off crystal formation and crystal-induced inflammation, may lead to better therapies for both gout and CPPD deposition disease. We discuss here standard therapies for gout, CPPD, and BCP arthritis and introduce some promising new therapies for patients refractory or intolerant to standard treatment regimens.

GOUT

Gouty arthritis usually presents as an acute monarthritis affecting the joints of lower extremities. The typical attack begins suddenly with severe pain, erythema, swelling, and tenderness of the involved joint. Common risk factors include advancing age, male gender, renal insufficiency, hypertension, alcohol use, obesity, and a family history of gout. Physical examination shows classic signs of inflammation of the joint itself and

From: *Modern Therapeutics in Rheumatic Diseases*
Edited by: G. C. Tsokos, et al. © Humana Press, Inc., Totowa, NJ

Table 1
Articular Crystals and Their Associated Clinical Syndromes

Crystals	Appearances	Associated clinical syndromes
Urate	Needle-shaped, negatively birefringent	Gout
CPPD	Rhomboid-shaped, positively birefringent	Pseudoosteoarthritis
		Pseudogout
		Pseudorheumatoid arthritis
BCP	Light microscopy is not useful	Calcific periarthritis
		Milwaukee shoulder syndrome
		Tumoral calcinosis

Table 2
Rare Crystals or Crystals of Uncertain Significance in Synovial Fluid

Charcot-Leyden crystals	Cryoglobulins
Cholesterol	Hemoglobin
Calcium oxalate	Xanthine-hypoxanthine
Amyloid	Cystine
Lipid liquid	Aluminum
Hematoidin	Corticosteroids

often in the skin overlying the involved joint. Although less common, early attacks can be polyarticular. Attacks are typically self-limited, lasting 5–15 d, and are followed by an intercritical phase in which crystals can be obtained from the joint, but no inflammation or symptoms exist. Recurrent attacks are common, although some patients may not have a second episode. Untreated, the intercritical phases become shorter, attacks more frequent and more often polyarticular, and eventually joint damage and soft-tissue deposits of urate known as tophi may occur.

Making a firm diagnosis is often the first challenge in treating the patient with suspected gout. The differential diagnosis of acute gout includes trauma, infection, CPPD deposition disease, palindromic rheumatism, calcific tendinitis or periarthritis, and degenerative joint disease. Gout is often overdiagnosed on clinical grounds. A definite diagnosis of gout can only be made by needle aspiration of the inflamed joint. The aspirated fluid should be examined with a compensated polarized light microscope. Urate crystals are needle-shaped negatively birefringent crystals. Serum uric acid levels are not helpful in the acute setting in either confirming or refuting the diagnosis. Unfortunately, the use of polarizing microscopy to identify synovial fluid crystals requires experienced observers, and test accuracy may vary considerably between laboratories. False-negative rates can be as high as 67% when crystals are rare [1]. An analysis of four studies on crystal identification showed that the odds of having gout in the presence of a positive test were 14 times higher than that of having gout before the test results were known. A negative likelihood ratio was 0.33 [2]. Although it is ideal to examine the synovial fluid, a presumptive diagnosis of gout can be made by the triad of monarthritis, hyperuricemia, and a response to colchicine. When a patient

Table 3
Treatment Options for Acute Gout

Colchicine PO or IV
NSAIDs PO or IM
Steroids IA, PO, IM, IV, or SC
Rest
Splinting
Cold application
Therapeutic arthrocentesis
Pain medications

presents during intercritical period, a study has shown that synovial fluid analysis of knees and the first metatarsophalangeal joint is helpful, because crystals have been seen months after the acute attack. *(3)*.

Treatment of Acute Gout

Acute gouty arthritis is self-limiting and if untreated, lasts for a few days to several weeks. Treatment goals are to relieve pain, decrease inflammation, and shorten the acute attack. Treatment options include non-steroidal, anti-inflammatory drugs (NSAIDs), colchicine, and intra-articular or systemic corticosteroids (Table 3).

NSAIDs are the most commonly used drugs for acute gout. Indomethacin has historically been used for gout, but probably is not significantly more effective than the newer NSAIDs. As one of the earliest available NSAIDs, it was well-studied initially and remains in common use. Doses of 150–200 mg/d given BID to TID are appropriate to control inflammation. Because indomethacin has central nervous system (CNS) side effects such as headache and mental status changes, as well as a high incidence of gastrointestinal (GI) side effects, other NSAIDs may be preferable in high-risk or elderly patients. Sulindac, piroxicam, ibuprofen, and ketoprofen were equally effective in clinical studies *(4)*. A single dose of 60 mg of intramuscular ketorolac was also equivalent to 50 mg of oral indomethacin for pain relief in the emergency room *(5)*. Traditional NSAIDs are contraindicated in patients with renal insufficiency, peptic ulcer disease, in patients who also take anticoagulants, and in some elderly patients. Sulindac may be preferable to other NSAIDs in the setting of mild renal insufficiency. In general, one should choose a drug with a rapid onset of action for acute pain. Unlike colchicine, NSAIDs remain effective after the attack is well established.

The cyclooxygenase (COX)-2 inhibitors, rofecoxib and celecoxib, have not been specifically studied in gouty arthritis. However, these drugs may be excellent options for treating gout in patients with a history of peptic ulcer disease or those on oral anti-coagulants. Fifty milligrams of rofecoxib is recommended for relief of acute pain and has an onset of action within 45 min.

Colchicine is also commonly used to treat acute gout. It can be given orally or intravenously. There are varieties of dosage schedules published. These vary from hourly administration to a twice-a-day basis for acute gout. If the hourly schedule is used, 0.5 mg of colchicine is given per hour until relief or side effects occur. Relief of pain occurs in 12–24 h if the drug is started within the first 24 h of the onset of the attack. Commonly, such frequent dosing results in diarrhea and crampy abdominal

Table 4
Proper Use of IV Colchicine

Maximum dose for single injection is 2–3 mg; for cumulative injection, 4–5 mg.
Do not use if a patient is already on oral colchicine.
Do not give more oral or IV colchicine for 7 d after a full IV therapeutic dose.
Adjust dose for renal or hepatic insufficiency and avoid in patients with
    creatinine clearance <10 mL/min or severe liver disease.
IV dose is 50% of the oral dose.
Give the dose slowly.

pain, thus limiting its use. Colchicine given 0.6 mg every 4–6 h causes less diarrhea and can be used alone or as an adjunctive treatment to NSAIDs or steroids. A study of rheumatologists suggests that combination therapy with colchicine and NSAIDs is the most commonly used regimen for acute gout *(6)*. Colchicine is metabolized in the liver and excreted in the urine. Because this drug interferes with cell division, it can cause bone marrow failure in patients unable to metabolize it efficiently. Close monitoring of blood counts is necessary when colchicine is used in patients with mild renal or hepatic insufficiency *(7)*. Those with oliguria, severe renal insufficiency (creatinine clearance <10 mL/min) and biliary obstruction should use alternative agents. Colchicine toxicity occurs in a dose-dependent fashion.

Intravenous (IV) colchicine can be useful in patients, such as preoperative patients, unable to take oral medication. GI toxicity is reduced with IV administration. The recommendations for IV use should be followed strictly and are shown in Table 4. Physicians prescribing IV colchicine should adhere strictly to the guidelines suggested by Wallace et al. *(8)*. A recent study suggested errors in the use of IV colchicine in hospitalized patients are not uncommon *(9)*. The most common errors include its use in patients with contraindications to IV colchicine and those exposed to oral colchicine prior to administration of IV colchicine *(9)*.

Intra-articular (IA) corticosteroids represent a third option for acute gout. They are an excellent choice for patients with monarthritis or oligoarthritis who are at risk for toxicity from NSAIDs or colchicine. Triamcinolone acetonide, a long-acting crystalline corticosteroid, is used most commonly. The dose is dependent on the size of the joint.

Systemic corticosteroid can also be used effectively in patients who cannot tolerate colchicine and NSAIDs or have joint involvement that is not amenable to intra-articular therapy. However, the serious side effects of systemic steroids cannot be underestimated and are widely appreciated. Recommended regimens and forms of steroids for acute gout vary widely. Prednisone can be given orally in doses of 30–50 mg/d initially with a taper over 7–10 d. Intravenous methylprednisolone (50–150 mg/d with a taper over 5 d) was used successfully in two patients *(10)*. Sixty milligrams of intramuscular (IM) triamcinolone acetonide was comparable to 50 mg of oral indomethacin TID and was safe and useful in patients with contraindications to NSAIDs *(11)*. In one study of 76 patients, parental adrenocorticotropic hormone (ACTH) was found to have a more rapid onset of action and to be associated with fewer side effects than oral indomethacin 50 mg QID *(12)*. ACTH doses range from 40–80 IU IM, IV, or SQ q 8 h with a 3-d taper for polyarticular attacks to 40 IU IM once for single joint involvement. ACTH probably

Table 5
Treatment Options for Prophylaxis

Prevention of acute attack
    Colchicine
    NSAIDs
Treatment of hyperuricemia
    Inhibition of uric acid synthesis
        Allopurinol
        Oxypurinol
    Promotion of urate secretion
        Probenecid
        Sulfinpyrazone
        Benzbromarone
        Urate oxidase

has no advantage over other more readily available steroid forms. Its use has been associated with an increase in rebound attacks, fluid retention, electrolyte imbalances, and anaphylaxis. For example, Siegel et al. compared 40 IU of intramuscular ACTH to 60 mg of intramuscular triamcinolone acetonide. They found that ACTH caused more rebound attacks demonstrated by a higher rate of retreatment for recurrent symptoms than triamcinolone. Resolution of all symptoms occurred at an average of 8 d for both groups *(13)*.

Lastly, for the rare patient intolerant to NSAIDs, colchicine, and steroids, simply treating the pain of acute gout may be the best and safest option. The short-term use of narcotics may be necessary to control pain during the acute attack. Analgesics, rest or splinting of the inflamed joint, therapeutic arthrocentesis, and cold application may be useful adjunctive measures in the treatment of acute gout.

Prophylaxis of Acute Attacks in Gout

Most patients with gout experience a second episode within 2 yr of the first attack. However, a small percentage of patients may not have a recurrent attack for a decade. Furthermore, in an otherwise healthy patient, acute attacks are easily treated, whereas in a patient with multiple comorbidities, treatment of an acute attack may be quite challenging. Thus, the issue of when and whom to prophylaxis with antihyperuricemic drugs is controversial and is often decided on an individual basis. Certainly, the presence of tophi, a history of frequent recurrences, or the existence of contraindications to standard therapy for acute attacks lowers the threshold for initiating prophylaxis. In a Canadian analysis of cost effectiveness using hypothetical cohorts of patients, prophylaxis was recommended if attacks occurred two or more times per year *(14)*. The goal of prophylaxis is to prevent attacks. This can be done by preventing inflammation or lowering serum uric acid levels. Options include antihyperuricemic drugs, colchicine, or combination regimens (Table 5). Antihyperuricemic drugs are most commonly used and include the uricostatic drug allopurinol and the uricosurics probenecid and sulfinpyrazone. In Europe, the drug benzbromarone is available.

Urate-lowering agents should not be started during an acute attack, although recommendations on the timing of initiating these drugs after an acute episode has resolved vary from days to months. Furthermore, because any flux in urate level can theoretically promote crystal formation or dissolution and initiate an attack, urate-lowering drugs should be started along with either colchicine or an NSAID. The length of time that an NSAID or colchicine should be coadministered after initiation of an antihyperuricemic drug has never been studied. One author recommends that anti-inflammatories be used for a period of 1–2 mo *(15)*. Emmerson suggests continuing prophylaxis at least a year after the serum urate concentration has normalized *(4)*. Kelly suggests to use an anti-inflammatory until the serum uric acid level is in the normal range and there has been no attack for 3–6 mo. Wortmann suggests continuing colchicine or NSAIDs for 1–3 mo after the serum uric acid is controlled *(16)*.

Allopurinol is the most commonly used prophylactic drug for gout. It is generally well-tolerated and very effective. Allopurinol is effective in both under and overexcretors of uric acid. It acts by blocking the conversion of hypoxanthine to xanthine and of xanthine to uric acid. The dose is adjusted from 100 mg/d to a maximum dose of 800 mg/d, with an average dose of 300 mg/d. The onset of action is quite rapid and serum urate levels can be checked several weeks after initiating therapy *(15)*. Contraindications to allopurinol include concomitant azathioprine therapy, severe liver or kidney dysfunction, or known hypersensitivity to allopurinol. Side effects of allopurinol are usually mild and include skin rash, headache, diarrhea, and abdominal discomfort. Concomitant use of allopurinol and ampicillin increases the frequency of skin rash. Rarer, but more serious side effects include fever, eosinophilia, bone marrow suppression, liver toxicity, renal failure, Stevens-Johnson syndrome, and hypersensitivity vasculitis. Renal insufficiency and concomitant use of thiazide diuretics are risk factors for side effects.

Patients who are allergic to allopurinol may be desensitized *(17)* or given a trial of oxypurinol. Those with serious reactions to allopurinol such as acute interstitial nephritis, toxic epidermal necrolysis, hepatitis, leukopenia, or vasculitis are not candidates for desensitization. Alternative drugs should be used in these patients. In the desensitization regimen most commonly used, initial doses of allopurinol were 0.05 mg/d and the dose was slowly escalated. Some patients developed a mild cutaneous reaction, but allopurinol was safely reintroduced again slowly *(18)*. Oxypurinol, the active metabolite of allopurinol, can be substituted for allopurinol in some patients with allopurinol allergy *(17)*. The drug is not approved by the Food and Drug Administration (FDA), but can be obtained on a compassionate-use basis. In a multicenter, randomized, double-blind crossover trial, uric acid levels fell by 3.0 mg/dL with 300 mg of allopurinol and 2.6 mg/dL with an equimolar dose of oxypurinol *(19)*. Hamanaka et al. studied lymphocyte stimulation in patients who had hypersensitivity to allopurinol and found that there were significant lymphoproliferative reactions to oxypurinol but not allopurinol *(20)*. Thus, some patients may be allergic to both drugs.

Uricosuric drugs are also used commonly to prevent gouty arthritis. They are probably used less commonly than allopurinol because of the need for a divided dose schedule, their lack of efficacy in patients with renal insufficiency, and their slower onset of action. Because underexcretion of uric acid is the most common abnormality in idiopathic gout, these drugs are useful in many gout patients. They are most effective in patients with normal or near-normal renal function and should be avoided in patients with a history of kidney stones. Probenecid is the most commonly used uricosuric drug in the United States. It is given in divided doses of 0.5–3 g/d. Because of concern that any flux in urate levels may precipitate an acute attack, like allopurinol, probenecid should be initiated after acute inflammation has resolved and given concomitantly with colchicine or an NSAID for several weeks. Adequate fluid intake may prevent nephrolithiasis. The initial dose of probenecid is typically 250 mg BID and is increased 0.5 g every 1–2 wk until urate levels are optimized. Side effects include dyspepsia, hypersensitivity, and skin rash.

Sulfinpyrazone is derived from phenylbutazone and is a more potent uricosuric drug than probenecid. It is well absorbed. The starting dose is 50 mg twice a day and is adjusted up to 300–400 mg/d until the serum uric acid is normalized. Sulfinpyrazone has antiplatelet activity and should be used with caution in anticoagulated patients. In case of tophaceous gout with renal disease and allopurinol allergy, sulfinpyrazone may be useful. Because of its potency, uric acid crystalluria can occur. GI disturbance occurs in 10% of patients and the drug should be avoided in patients with peptic ulcer disease.

Benzbromarone is a uricosuric drug that inhibits postsecretory tubular reabsorption of urate and is active in the presence of renal insufficiency. It is not available in the United States, but is widely used in Europe. It is given in doses of 50–100 mg/d. Benzbromarone can also precipitate xanthine lithiasis, but is generally well tolerated. Recurrent but self-limited liver toxicity has also been reported. Monitoring of liver function is recommended as subfulminant hepatitis owing to an analog of benzbromarone was also reported, especially when benzbromarone is used with other benzofurans such as amiodarone *(21)*.

In patients who cannot take allopurinol or uricosurics to prevent gout attacks, colchicine is a safe and effective alternative. It can be given at doses of 0.5–2 mg/d *(22)*. Colchicine does not prevent long-term complications associated with hyperuricemia such as urate nephropathy or tophi, because it does not have antihyperuricemic property. Therefore, antihyperuricemic drugs are preferable.

Patients on prophylactic therapy for gout should be regularly monitored clinically. Serum uric acid levels are useful for monitoring therapy in patients treated with antihyperuricemic agents. Serum and urinary uric acid are now measured by automated enzymatic method using urate oxidase. A recent study suggested that serum uric acid levels are mirrored in saliva and hair *(23)* and in the future blood drawing may not be necessary. The value of measuring 24-h urinary excretion of uric acid remains controversial, because most patients are underexcretors and most respond well to allopurinol. Yamanaka et al. recommends lowering serum uric acid levels to 4.6–6.6 mg/dL by the sixth month after the initiation of an antihyperuricemic drug. Patients who achieved these levels had the lowest relative risk for an acute gouty attack *(24)*.

Patients with Refractory Gout

In the patient who is refractory to usual therapy, a wide range of possibilities should be considered. Treatment failures can be owing to noncompliance, failure to treat or recognize underlying causes of hyperuricemia, and least commonly, a true lack of response to adequate doses of medications. Patient understanding of the recurrent nature of this disease and acceptance of the need for prolonged treatment is crucial.

Secondary or hereditary forms of gout should be considered in the patient who has premature, poorly controlled, or progressive disease despite adequate therapy. The onset of gout before age 30 should lead to thorough evaluation for likely enzymatic or metabolic defect or secondary causes of hyperuricemia. Familial juvenile hyperuricemic nephropathy is an autosomal dominant disorder with high penetrance, which causes gout and renal failure in young patients owing to low fractional uric acid clearance. A 6-yr follow-up study of 31 patients from 12 kindreds showed that allopurinol 50–300 mg/d reduced plasma uric acid in responders by 30%. Patients with good compliance and GFR> 50 mL/min maintained normal or relatively stable renal function *(25)*. Secondary hyperuricemia occurs in the setting of renal insufficiency, hematologic malignancies, chemotherapy, or diffuse psoriasis. Management of these conditions can significantly improve control of urate levels.

A careful history can reveal other reversible causes of resistance to therapy. The use of certain drugs in gout patients can precipitate or worsen attacks. Drugs such as alcohol, diuretics, ethambutol, pyrazinamide, levodopa, cyclosporine, theophylline *(26)*, and low-dose aspirin can exacerbate hyperuricemia. Capsi et al. *(27)* recently showed that aspirin at doses of 75–325 mg/d in elderly hospitalized patients decreased uric acid excretion by 15% and increased serum uric acid levels. The reduction in creatinine clearance and daily uric acid excretion were most prominent in patients with low albumin levels. Danaher et al. studied the effect of 325 mg of aspirin on urate excretion in patients on probenecid for gouty arthritis. They found significantly decreased urate excretion ($p < 0.05$) in those who took probenecid and aspirin concomitantly compared to those who took aspirin 6 h after ingesting probenecid. The investigators recommend taking these two medications at least 6 h apart *(28)*.

Once hereditary and secondary causes of gout are identified and urate-elevating factors are minimized, most patients should be controlled on standard therapy. A small group exists, however, who continue to have acute attacks and/or elevated serum urate levels with a single prophylactic drug. These patients may benefit from combination therapy. Colchicine is frequently used prophylactically along with allopurinol or probenecid in refractory patients. The combination of benzbromarone or probenecid and allopurinol has also been helpful in patients with a poor response to single agents. *(29)* For example, in patients with tophaceous gout, once serum urate levels were <6 mg/dL, combined therapy with allopurinol and benzbromarone significantly reduced the size of tophi when compared to allopurinol alone or benzbromarone alone *(30)*. In a case report of an allopurinol nonresponder who also had tophi and renal insufficiency, benzbromarone added to allopurinol helped to decrease serum uric acid level *(31)*. There is anecdotal evidence that the combination of probenecid and allopurinol may be helpful in patients whose gout is difficult to control *(29)*.

Urate oxidase is a nonmammalian enzyme that converts uric acid to allantoins. Allantoins are 10 times more soluble than uric acid and are easily eliminated by the kidneys. Small studies and case reports describe the use of urate oxidase to treat short-term hyperuricemia often in the setting of malignancy or during chemotherapy, where rapid cell turnover dramatically elevates urate loads. Urate oxidase has been used to prevent and treat hyperuricemia associated with lymphoid malignancy *(32,33)*. Its use is contraindicated in patients who are pregnant, have allergies, or with G6PD deficiency. Serious allergic reactions ranging from urticaria to anaphylaxis have developed in some patients. A recombinant urate oxidase, SR29142, is now being studied for patients with hyperuricemia associated with malignancies in Europe and the United States *(33)*.

Losartan is an angiotensin 2-receptor antagonist that was found to have uricosuric effect in a rat model of CRF *(34)*. It increased urate clearance and decreased plasma uric acid in rats, but has not been studied in humans. Finally, surgery, such as joint-replacement surgery or removal of tophi, can be useful in managing certain problems in patients with chronic gout.

Gout in Transplant Patients

Transplant recipients are at high risk for gout. This increased risk is largely owing to cyclosporine use, but may be compounded by the concomitant use of other drugs including diuretics, and by renal insufficiency. Cyclosporine decreases fractional excretion of uric acid and causes gout in 4–11% of patients. Although particularly common after renal transplants, patients with heart and liver transplants also experience gout. Burack reported hyperuricemia in 72% of male and 81% of female cyclosporine-treated heart or heart/lung transplant recipients. Of these patients, gout developed in 10% of the men *(35)*. Cyclosporine clearly accelerates the clinical course of gout. Gouty arthritis occurred after a mean of less than 15 yr of hyperuricemia and polyarticular tophaceous gout developed in half of patients within 3 yr of the first attack. In the pretransplant waiting period, preexisting gout should be treated aggressively.

Treatment of the transplant patient with gout is a challenge. They often have contraindications to NSAIDs, and are susceptible to bone marrow and neuromuscular toxicity of colchicine. An acute attack can be treated with systemic or local corticosteroids, although these patients are frequently already on these drugs. Colchicine can be used if necessary provided that renal function and neutrophil count are in an acceptable range *(36)*. Arthrocentesis and splinting can be helpful in the acute setting. Most of these patients require urate-lowering therapy. Typically, transplant patients cannot take full-dose allopurinol because of the interaction between allopurinol and azathioprine. In the absence of other alternatives, the dose of azathioprine can be reduced to 25% of the usual dose, and low-dose allopurinol can be initiated. Blood counts must be closely monitored on this regimen. This increases the risk of inadequate immunosuppression and an azathioprine substitute may be required. Mycophenolate mofetil (MMF) inhibits inosine monophosphate (IMP) dehydrogenase and blocks *de novo* purine synthesis. It was used in five kidney transplant patients instead of azathioprine so that allopurinol could be used for recurrent acute gouty arthritis *(37)*. After starting MMF, serum uric acid levels decreased within 10 wk and renal function improved. Allopurinol-related adverse reactions were not noted. Thioguanine may be another alternative immunosuppressant. Uricosuric drugs may be preferable to allopurinol in transplant recipients with adequate renal function *(38)*. Although it is experimental, the enzyme urate oxidase degrades uric acid to allantoins and may be used as a short-term, urate-lowering agent. A nonrecombinant form of urate oxidase, purified from cultures of *Aspergillus flavus*, has been used in transplant gout. No changes in azathioprine doses were needed in six heart transplant patients, on cyclosporine, azathioprine, and prednisone, treated with nonrecombinant urate oxidase (Uricozyme) 1000 U IM/d for 15 consecutive days *(39)*. A normal serum uric acid level was maintained for 20–30 d after the last dose.

CPPD DEPOSITION DISEASE

CPPD deposition disease is commonly found in elderly patients and is caused by articular calcium pyrophosphate (CPPD) crystals. Affected patients often present with an acute arthritis clinically indistinguishable from gout (pseudogout). Alternatively,

Table 6
Metabolic Abnormalities Associated with CPPD

Hypomagnesemia
Hypophosphatasia
Hemochromatosis
Gout
Hyperparathyroidism
Familial hypercalciuric hypercalcemia

they may develop severe, degenerative arthritis. Less commonly, CPPD deposition disease may imitate rheumatoid arthritis (RA) or neuropathic arthropathy. CPPD disease is rare under age of 55 yr in the absence of familial or metabolic predispositions. Evidence of hyperparathyroidism, hypothyroidism, hypomagnesemia, hemochromatosis, hemosiderosis, hypophosphatasia, and amyloidosis should be sought in the young patient with CPPD deposition disease (Table 6). Screening for underlying disease should include serum calcium, magnesium, alkaline phosphatase, ferritin, and thyroid-function tests. In pseudogout, patients complain of sudden onset of pain, swelling, and redness in a single joint. Attacks are self-limited, but typically last longer than gout. The knee joint is most commonly involved. In the polyarticular form of CPPD deposition disease, patients typically complain of chronic joint pain, which may involve the shoulders, wrists, MCPs and other joints not usually affected by osteoarthritis (OA). Some of these patients have clear attacks superimposed on their baseline disability, whereas others are otherwise clinically indistinguishable from osteoarthritis.

As in gout, an exam of the synovial fluid is the only way to make a definitive diagnosis of CPPD deposition disease. Under polarized light microscopy, CPPD crystals are weakly positively birefringent rhomboid-shaped crystals. These crystals may be more difficult to detect than MSU crystals. Consequently, even greater variability exists in the ability of different laboratories to accurately identify CPPD crystals. In the absence of a good synovial fluid exam, CPPD deposition disease is suggested by clinical and radiological findings. It is associated with radiologic chondrocalcinosis, defined as the presence of finely stippled calcifications in the articular hyaline and fibro-cartilage. Conventional radiographs of the pelvis, hand, and knee reveal chondrocalcinosis in only 35% of patients with radiographic, arthroscopic, and surgical chondrocalcinosis *(40)*. Magnetic resonance imaging (MRI) may be more sensitive than plain radiographs for detecting chondrocalcinosis. On MRI images, it appears as low signal intensity using gradient-recalled echo (GRE) techniques *(41)*.

Treatment of Acute Attacks of CPPD Deposition Disease

Unlike gout, our understanding of crystal formation in CPPD deposition disease is limited. We do know that intra-articular CPPD crystals are inflammatory and we can interfere with their effects using anti-inflammatory drugs. Because we do not understand the abnormalities that underlie the formation of CPPD crystals, we have no specific therapies to prevent CPPD deposition diseases (Table 7).

Acute attacks can be treated with colchicine, NSAIDs, and intra-articular or systemic corticosteroids. Intravenous colchicine is not as effective as in acute gouty arthritis

Table 7
Treatment Options for CPPD

Acute pseudogout
    Therapeutic arthrocentesis
    Colchicine PO or IV
    NSAIDs PO
    Steroid PO, IA, IV, IM, or SC
Chronic inflammatory arthritis
    Hydroxychloroquine
    Probenecid
    Methotrexate
    $MgCO_3$
    Colchicine
    Surgery

but has been used successfully in case reports. In one postoperative patient with a polyarticular attack, an initial dose of 2 mg was followed in 24 h by an additional 1 mg with an excellent response *(42)*. Oral colchicine is used clinically in acute pseudogout attacks but has not been well studied. Dose recommendations are similar to those used in gout. Similarly, NSAIDs are in common use with little data to support their efficacy. No single NSAID appears to be superior to any other in the treatment of pseudogout. Intra-articular corticosteroid injections are very useful when a single or several joints are involved, and these have been shown to shorten the duration of symptoms in acute pseudogout from 3.5 to 1.5 d *(43)*. Triamcinolone 60 mg IM was tested in a small uncontrolled study for acute pseudogout and was effective. Most patients responded in 3–4 d after receiving the triamcinolone, and no toxicity was observed *(44)*. This approach can be beneficial in patients with polyarticular involvement, contraindications to NSAIDs, and for physicians not skillful in joint injection. Methylprednisolone 125 mg IV *(4)* and parenteral ACTH have also been used in pseudogout with resolution of the symptoms within an average of 4.2 d. Because this is a self-limited disease and the attack varies in duration, controlled trials are necessary to document the efficacy of these treatments.

Prophylaxis of Acute Attacks in CPPD Deposition Disease

Detection and treatment of an underlying metabolic abnormality is crucial in managing premature CPPD deposition disease. Unfortunately, in hyperparathyroidism and hemochromatosis, treatment of the underlying condition may not improve the arthritis. In the typical elderly patient with idiopathic CPPD deposition disease, NSAIDs and colchicine *(45,46)* can be used to ameliorate chronic or recurrent joint symptomatology. Whether NSAIDs alter the frequency or severity of attacks if taken long-term is not known. Colchicine 0.6 mg BID was used in a prospective, controlled trial in 10 patients and found to decrease the number of attacks from 3.2 to 1 attack/patient/yr *(47)*.

Although not in common use, other drugs may prove useful in reducing symptoms and attack frequency in CPPD deposition disease. Hydroxychloroquine (HCQ), an anti-inflammatory agent and probenecid, which reduce levels of a crucial component of CPPD crystals, have been reported to be effective in small trials of CPPD deposition disease. In a 6-mo, parallel group, double-blind study of chronic active inflammatory CPPD disease followed by a 6-mo, open-label, crossover trial for nonresponding placebo patients, HCQ, started at 100 mg/d and increased to a maximum of 400 mg/d, reduced the number of affected joints, compared to placebo. HCQ response rate was 76% compared to placebo 32%. Although the authors concluded that HCQ was an effective and safe alternative to NSAIDs in chronic inflammatory CPPD disease, further study is warranted *(48)*. Probenecid was given *(49)* at 500 mg BID in an open study of patients with CPPD disease resistant to or intolerant of IA steroids, HCQ, MTX, colchicine or prednisone, and NSAIDs. Symptomatic relief was observed. Magnesium carbonate 30 mEq TID was studied in a small, double-blinded, placebo-controlled trial for 6 mo. A pronounced placebo effect was observed. Yet, patients reported the active treatments as better than the placebo. At the end of 6 mo, no change in the appearance of radiographic chondrocalcinosis was demonstrated *(50)*.

Several hyaluronan preparations have recently been introduced in the United States for the intra-articular treatment of osteoarthritis. Their use in CPPD deposition disease is controversial. Intra-articular hyaluronan was reported to precipitate acute attacks of pseudogout in several case reports within hours of injection *(51,52)*. In contrast, no local flares occurred in 30 knees with chondrocalcinosis treated with five weekly intra-articular injections of 20 mg sodium hyaluronate and followed for 6 mo *(53)*. Patients should be cautioned about the possibility of flare, and more experience with these drugs is needed.

Other potential drugs based on their effects in a laboratory model of CPPD deposition disease require further study. These include transglutaminase inhibitors *(54)*, phosphocitrate *(55)*, and taxol *(56)*.

Joint replacement has an important role in the treatment of chronic CPPD deposition disease in severe cases. Whether the presence of CPPD crystals in the joint at the time of surgery affects surgical outcome is unknown.

ARTICULAR SYNDROMES ASSOCIATED WITH BCP CRYSTALS

BCP crystals in or near joints cause calcific periarthritis and Milwaukee shoulder syndrome (MSS) (Table 8). Tumoral calcinosis is also produced by BCP crystals and usually occurs in the setting of renal disease.

Calcific periarthritis is probably the most common of the BCP-associated articular syndromes. In this form of periarthritis, a deposit of BCP crystals forms in a tendon or soft tissue near a joint. Often large joints such as the shoulder are involved. Many patients with such calcium deposits remain asymptomatic. However, for unknown reasons, some deposits can cause acute painful inflammation. These patients present with the sudden onset of severe joint pain. In the shoulder, the diagnosis is usually made on X-ray, where a radioopaque calcium deposit can be seen near the involved joint *(57)*. Hydroxyapatite pseudopodagra is a term used to describe acute inflammation of the first metatarsophalangeal joint owing to BCP deposits. It often occurs in young women, where it presents with acute pain and inflammation in the great toe. A similar syndrome occurring in the MCPs and proximal interphalangeal joints (PIPs) has also been reported in young women *(58)*. These attacks are often self-limited. Treatment of calcific periarthritis includes intra-lesional steroids, NSAIDs, or colchicine. In a

Table 8
Articular Syndromes Associated with BCP Crystals

Calcific periarthritis, tendinitis, and bursitis. Rotator cuff calcification, hydroxyapatite
    pseudopodagra
BCP arthropathies: Milwaukee shoulder syndrome
Tumoral calcinosis

---

double-blind, placebo-controlled, randomized trial of 100 patients with mixed causes
of shoulder pain including calcific tendinitis, either a lesional injection of 40 mg
triamcinolone or 500 mg BID of Naproxen was superior to placebo, but combined
treatment failed to add further benefit *(59)*. There are few other studies comparing
the efficacy of these treatments. Some patients may need surgical removal of large
or recurrent calcific deposits.

MSS is chronic destructive arthritis of the shoulders, which occurs in elderly patients
and is more common in women. Symptoms are variable but most patients present with
chronic shoulder pain and limited range of motion. Affected patients may have very
severe pain especially after use and at night. Physical examination often reveals bony
deformities and very large effusions (hydrops). On X-ray, there is degeneration of the
true shoulder joint with calcified soft tissues and loose bodies. Destruction of the rotator
cuff is suggested by upward subluxation of the humeral head. MSS may also involve
the knee joint, where it has a predilection for the lateral compartment. Joint fluid from
involved joints is typically noninflammatory. MSS may be a difficult diagnosis to
confirm. BCP crystals cannot be seen under ordinary polarizing light microscopy. An
alizarin red stain may be used to visualize BCP crystals, but may nonspecifically stain
other joint fluid particles *(57)*. A semi-quantitative assay for BCP crystals, based on
their ability to bind diphosphonates, is more specific than alizarin red staining, but is
not widely available *(57)*. Therefore, the diagnosis of MSS is often based on physical
exam and radiologic findings.

Treatment of MSS is usually unsatisfactory and many patients go on to have very
severe destructive arthritis. BCP crystals are less inflammatory than CPPD or urate
crystals *(57)*. They are, however, capable of eliciting destructive enzymes such as
proteases and prostaglandins from synovial and cartilage cells. Their presence in the
joint is well correlated with the severity of joint degeneration seen on radiographs
(60). Our best hope for effective therapies for MSS lies in better understanding the
mechanisms through which BCP crystals form and how they promote joint destruction.
Nonspecific therapies such as NSAIDs, repeated joint aspiration with or without steroid
injection, and decreased joint use sometimes satisfactorily control the symptoms of
MSS. In a report of one patient with bilateral shoulder involvement owing to MSS,
colchicine 0.6 mg BID and choline magnesium trisalicylate 1500 mg BID were used
successfully *(61)*. McCarthy et al. recently showed that BCP crystal-induced stimulation
of prostaglandin E2 was dependent on COX-2 induction. These data support further
study of the use of COX-2 inhibitors in BCP crystal-associated arthritis *(62)*. Tidal
irrigation and complete arthroplasty may decrease pain in patients refractory to other
measures. Physical therapy may a useful adjunct to other therapies.

SUMMARY

Effective treatment is available for the common forms of crystal arthropathies. The first challenge in treating these diseases is to make an accurate and firm diagnosis. This should be based on the presence of crystals in synovial fluid. Treatment of gout and CPPD deposition disease can be a challenge in elderly or ill patients. A thorough knowledge of the risks and toxicities of both NSAIDs and colchicine will prevent harm from their misuse. Intra-articular corticosteroids and pain medication are useful alternatives for patients unable to tolerate systemic therapy. The key to better treatment for crystal arthropathies lies in a deeper understanding of the pathophysiology of these diseases.

REFERENCES

1. Schlesinger, N., D.G. Baker, and H.R. Schumacher Jr. 1999. How well have diagnostic tests and therapies for gout been evaluated? *Curr. Opin. Rheumatol.* 11:441–445.

2. Segal, J.B. and D. Albert. 1999. Diagnosis of crystal-induced arthritis by synovial fluid examination for crystals:Lessons from an imperfect test. *Arthritis Care Res.* 12:376–380.

3. Pascual, E. , E. Batlle-Gualda, A. Martínez, J. Rosas, and P. Vela. 1999. Synovial fluid analysis for diagnosis of intercritical gout. *Ann. Intern. Med.* 131:756–759.

4. Emmerson, B.T. 1996. The management of gout. *N. Engl. J. Med.* 334:445–451.

5. Shrestha, M., D.L. Morgan, J.M. Moreden, R. Singh, M. Nelson, and J.E. Hayes. 1995. Randomized double-blind comparison of the analgesic efficacy of intramuscular ketorolac and oral indomethacin in the treatment of acute gouty arthritis. *Ann. Emerg. Med.* 26:682–686.

6. Schlesinger, N., W.G. Johanson, Jr., J. Rao, J. Rao, and H.R. Schumacher Jr. 1999. A survey of current evaluation and treatment of gout. *Arthritis Rheum.* 42(Suppl.):S160 (Abstract).

7. Ben-Chetrit, E. and M. Levy. 1998. Colchicine:1998 update. *Semin. Arthritis Rheum.* 28:48–59.

8. Wallace, S.L. and J.Z. Singer. 1988. Review: Systemic toxicity associated with the intravenous administration of colchicine-guidelines for use. *J. Rheumatol.* 15:495–499.

9. Maldonado, M.A., A. Salzman, and J. Varga. 1997. Intravenous colchicine use in crystal-induced arthropathies: a retrospective analysis of hospitalized patients. *Clin. Exp. Rheumatol.* 15:487–492.

10. Groff, G.D., W.A. Franck, and D.A. Raddatz. 1990. Systemic steroid therapy for acute gout: a clinical trial and review of the literature. *Semin. Arthritis Rheum.* 19:329–336.

11. Alloway, J.A., M.J. Moriarty, Y.T. Hoogland, and D.J. Nashel. 1993. Comparison of triamcinolone acetonide with indomethacin in the treatment of acute gouty arthritis. *J. Rheumatol.* 20:111–113.

12. Axelrod, D. and S. Preston. 1988. Comparison of parenteral adrenocorticotropic hormone with oral indomethacin in the treatment of acute gout. *Arthritis Rheum.* 31:803–805.

13. Siegel, L.B., J.A. Alloway, and D.J. Nashel. 1994. Comparison of adrenocorticotropic hormone and triamcinolone acetonide in the treatment of acute gouty arthritis. *J. Rheumatol.* 21:1325–1327.

14. Ferraz, M.B. and B. O'Brien. 1995. A cost effectiveness analysis of urate lowering drugs in nontophaceous recurrent gouty arthritis. *J. Rheumatol.* 22:908–914.

15. Anonymous. 1985. Treatment of gout. *Drug Ther. Bull.* 23:47–48.

16. Wortmann, R.L. 1998. Effective management of gout: an analogy. *Am. J. Med.* 105:513–514.

17. Fam, A.G., J. Lewtas, J. Stein, and T.W. Paton. 1992. Desensitization to allopurinol in patients with gout and cutaneous reactions. *Am. J. Med.* 93:299–302.

18. Gillott, T.J., A. Whallett, and G. Zaphiropoulos. 1998. Oral desensitization in patients with chronic tophaceous gout and allopurinol hypersensitivity. *Rheumatology* (Oxford). 38:85–86.

19. Walter-Sack, I., J. Xaver de Vries, B. Ernst, M. Frei, S. Kolb, J. Kosmowski, et al. 1996. Uric acid lowering effect of oxipurinol sodium in hyperurecemic patients-therapeutic equivalence to allopurinol. *J. Rheumatol.* 23:498–501.

20. Hamanaka, H., H. Mizutani, N. Nouchi, Y. Shimizu, and M. Shimizu. 1997. Allopurinol hypersensitivity syndrome: hypersensitivity to oxypurinol but not allopurinol. *Clin. Exp. Dermatol.* 23:32–34.

21. van der Klauw, M.M., P.M. Houtman, B.H.Ch. Stricker, and P. Spoelstra. 1994. Hepatic injury caused by benzbromarone. *J. Hepatol.* 20:376–379.

22. Yü, T.F. and A.B. Gutman. 1961. Efficacy of colchicine prophylaxis in gout. *Ann. Intern. Med.* 55:179–192.

23. Kobayashi, K., Y. Morioka, Y. Isaka, and T. Tozawa. 1998. Determination of uric acid in scalp hair for non-invasive evaluation of uricemic controls in hyperuricemia. *Biol. Pharm. Bull.* 21:398–400.

24. Yamanaka, H., R. Togashi, M. Hakoda, C. Terai, S. Kashiwazake, T. Dan, and N. Kamatani. 1998. Optimal range of serum urate concentrations to minimize risk of gouty attacks during anti-hyperuricemic treatment. *In* Purine and Pyrimidine Metabolism in Man IX. Griesmacher, A., et al., editors. Plenum Press, New York. 13–18.

25. Mc Bride, M.B., H.A. Simmonds, C.S. Ogg, J.S. Cameron, S. Rigden, L. Rees, et al. 1998. Efficacy of allopurinol in ameliorating the progressive renal disease in familial juvenile hyperuricaemic nephropathy (FJHN). A six-year update. *In* Purine and Pyrimidine Metabolism in Man IX. Griesmacher, A., et al. Plenum Press, New York. 7–11.

26. Toda, K., K. Goriki, M. Ochiai, H. Tokunou, S. Uehara, H. Takahashi, and K. Okusaki. 1997. Gout due to xanthine derivatives. *Br. J. Rheumatol.* 36:1131–1132.

27. Caspi, D., E. Lubart, E. Graff, B. Habot, M. Yaron, and R. Segal. 2000. The effect of mini-dose aspirin on renal function and uric acid handling in elderly patients. *Arthritis Rheum.* 43:103–108.

28. Danaher, P.J., L.R. Bryant, J.A. Alloway, and M.D. Harris. 1999. The effect of low dose aspirin on serum urate levels and urinary excretion in patients receiving probenecid for gouty arthritis. *Arthritis Rheum.* 42(Suppl.):S173. (Abstract).

29. McCarty, D.J. 1987. Intractable gouty arthritis. *Hosp. Pract.* (Office Ed.). 1999. 34:95–103.

30. Perez-Ruiz, F., M. Calabozo, A. Alonso-Ruiz, A. Herrero-Beites, and J. Duruelo. 1999. Influence of urate-lowering therapy on the rapidity of resolution of tophi in chronic gout. *Arthritis Rheum.* 42(Suppl.):S172. (Abstract).

31. Reiter, S., R. Engelleiter, H. Proske, A. Müller, F.J. van der Woude, J.A. Duley, and H.A. Simmonds. 1998. Severe debilitating polyarticular gout and terminal renal failure in an allopurinol 'non-responder'. *In* Purine and Pyrimidine Metabolism in Man IX. Griesmacher, A., et al. Plenum Press, New York. 51–55.

32. Pui, C-H., M.V. Relling, F. Lascombes, P.L. Harrison, A. Struxiano, J-M. Mondesir, et al. 1997. Urate oxidase in prevention and treatment of hyperuricemia associated with lymphoid malignancies. *Leukemia* 11:1813–1816.

33. Mahmoud, H.H., G. Leverger, C. Patte, E. Harvey, and F. Lascombes. 1998. Advances in the management of malignancy-associated hyperuricaemia. *Br. J. Cancer* 77(Suppl. 4):18–20.

34. Hatch, M., R.W. Freel, S. Shahinfar, and N.D. Vaziri. 1996. Effects of the specific angiotensin II receptor antagonist losartan on urate homeostasis and intestinal urate transport. *J. Pharmacol. Exp. Ther.* 276:187–193.

35. Burack, D.A., B.P. Griffith, M.E. Thompson, and L.E. Kahl. 1992. Hyperuricemia and gout among heart transplant recipients receiving cyclosporine. *Am. J. Med.* 92:141–146.

36. Jones, R.E. and E.V. Ball. 1999. Gout: beyond the stereotype. *Hosp. Pract.* (Office ed.). 34:95–103.

37. Jacobs, F., M.F. Mamzer-Bruneel, H. Skhiri, E. Thervet, Ch. Legendre, and H. Kreis. 1997. Safety of the mycophenolate mofetil-allopurinol combination in kidney transplant recipients with gout. *Transplantation* 64:1087–1088.

38. Perez-Ruiz, F., A. Alonso-Ruiz, M. Calabozo, and J. Duruelo. 1998. Treatment of gout after transplantation. *Br. J. Rheumatol.* 37:580.

39. Ippoliti, G., M. Negri, C. Campana, and M. Vigano. 1997. Urate oxidase in hyperuricemic heart transplant recipients treated with azathioprine. *Transplantation* 63:1370–1371.

40. Fisseler-Eckhoff, A. and K.M. Müller. 1992. Arthroscopy and chondrocalcinosis. *Arthroscopy* 8:98–104.

41. Beltran, J., E. Marty-Delfaut, J. Bencardino, Z.S. Rosenberg, G. Steiner, F. Aparisi, and M. Padrón. 1998. Chondrocalcinosis of the hyaline cartilage of the knee: MRI manifestations. *Skeletal Radiol.* 27:369–374.

42. Meed, S.D. and I. Spilberg. 1981. Successful use of colchicine in acute polyarticular pseudogout. *J. Rheumatol.* 8:689–691.

43. O'Duffy, J.D. 1976. Clinical studies of acute pseudogout attacks. Comments on prevalence, predispositions, and treatment. *Arthritis Rheum.* 19:349–352.

44. Roane, D.W., M.D. Harris, M.T. Carpenter, D.R. Finger, M.J. Jarek, J.A. Alloway, et al. 1997. Prospective use of intramuscular triamcinolone acetonide in pseudogout. *J. Rheumatol.* 24:1168–1170.

45. Spiliotis, T.E. 1981. Colchicine and chronic pseudogout. *Arthritis Rheum.* 24:862–863.

46. Gonzalez, T. and M. Gantes. 1987. Prophylaxis of acute attacks of pseudogout with oral colchicine. *J. Rheumatol.* 14:632–633.

47. Alvarellos, A. and I. Spilberg. 1986. Colchicine Prophylaxis in pseudogout. *J. Rheumatol.* 13:804–805.

48. Rothschild, B. and L.E. Yakubov. 1997. Prospective 6-month, double-blind trial of hydroxychloroquine treatment of CPPD. *Compr. Ther.* 23:327–331.

49. Trostle, D. and H.R. Schumacher Jr. 1999. Probenecid therapy of refractory CPPD deposition disease. *Arthritis Rheum.* 42(Suppl.):S160 (Abstract).

50. Doherty, M. and P.A. Dieppe. 1983. Double blind, placebo controlled trial of magnesium carbonate in chronic pyrophosphate arthropathy. *Ann. Rheum. Dis.* 42(Suppl.):106–107.

51. Luzar, M.J. and B. Altawil. 1998. Pseudogout following intraarticular injection of sodium hyaluronate. *Arthritis Rheum.* 41:939–941.

52. Maillefert, J.F. and C. Tavernier. 1999. Pyrophosphate arthritis after intraarticular injection of hyaluronan: comment on the article by Luzar and Altawil. *Arthritis Rheum.* 42:594.

53. Daumen-Legre, V., T. Pham, P.C. Acquaviva, and P. Lafforgue. 1999. Evaluation of safety and efficacy of viscosupplementation in knee osteoarthritis with chondrocalcinosis. *Arthritis Rheum.* 42(Suppl.):S158 (Abstract).

54. Rosenthal, A.K., B.A. Derfus, and L.A. Henry. Transglutaminase activity in aging articular chondrocytes and articular cartilage vesicles. *Arthritis Rheum.* 40:966–970.

55. Cheung, H.S., J.D. Sallis, and J.A. Struve. 1996. Specific inhibition of basic calcium phosphate and calcium pyrophosphate crystal-induction of metalloproteinase synthesis by phosphocitrate. *Biochim. Biophys. Acta.* 1315:105–111.

56. Rosenthal, A.K. 1998. Calcium crystal-associated arthritides. *Curr. Opin. Rheumatol.* 10: 273–277.

57. Halverson, P.B. and D.J. McCarty. 1997. Basic calcium phosphate (apatite, octacalcium phosphate, tricalcium phosphate) crystal deposition diseases; calcinosis. *In* Arthritis and Allied Condition. 13th ed. W.J. Koopman, editor. Williams & Wilkins, Baltimore. 2127–2167.

58. McCarthy, G.M., G.F. Carrera, and L.M. Ryan. 1993. Acute calcific periarthritis of the finger joints: a syndrome of women. *J. Rheumatol.* 20:1077–1080.

59. Petri, M., R. Dobrow, R. Neiman, Q. Whiting-O'Keefe, and W.E. Seaman. 1987. Randomized, double-blind, placebo-controlled study of the treatment of the painful shoulder. *Arthritis Rheum.* 30:1040–1045.

60. Halverson, P.B. and D.J. McCarty. 1986. Patterns of radiographic abnormalities associated with basic calcium phosphate and calcium pyrophosphate dihydrate crystal deposition in the knee. *Ann. Rheum. Dis.* 45:603–605.

61. Patel, K.J., D. Weidensaul, C. Palma, L.M. Ryan, and S.E. Walker. 1997. Milwaukee shoulder with massive bilateral cysts:effective therapy for hydrops of the shoulder. *J. Rheumatol.* 24:2479–2483.

62. Morgan, M.P., D.J. Fitzgerald, and G.M. McCarthy. 1999. Basic calcium phosphate crystals induce cyclooxygenase-2 and prostaglandin E2 production in human fibroblasts. *Arthritis Rheum.* 42 (Suppl.):S159 (Abstract).

40 Treatment of Musculoskeletal Infections

Arthur Weinstein

INTRODUCTION

Infection may occur in bone, joints, bursae, muscle, or tendon sheaths although osteomyelitis, infectious arthritis, and septic bursitis are by far the commonest musculoskeletal infections *(1,2)*. Varieties of microorganisms may infect joints and other musculoskeletal tissues including bacteria, viruses, fungi, and parasites. Most musculoskeletal infections result from hematogenous spread of the organism to the site. *Staphylococcal aureus* is the commonest cause of all types of musculoskeletal infection. The predispositions to musculoskeletal infections include penetrating trauma, joint-replacement surgery, joint damage from inflammatory disease, and systemic immunosuppression.

ACUTE BACTERIAL ARTHRITIS (SEPTIC ARTHRITIS)

Classification and Pathogenesis

Septic arthritis is a medical emergency and a cause of significant morbidity and mortality *(3)*. Acute infectious arthritis is usually classified by the type of infecting organism (Table 1). Not all cases of bacterial joint infection lead to a purulent synovitis; for instance, with gonoccocal arthritis, the synovial fluid may be inflammatory, not

From: *Modern Therapeutics in Rheumatic Diseases*
Edited by: G. C. Tsokos, et al. © Humana Press, Inc., Totowa, NJ

Table 1
Acute Infectious Arthritis: Infecting Bacteria

Gram positive cocci:
   Staphylococci - aureus, epidermidis
   Streptococci - pyogenes (beta-hemolytic group A),
   Other β-hemolytic groups (esp B, G), pneumoniae, viridans group
Gram negative cocci:
   Neisseria gonorrhoeae
   Neisseria meningitidis
   Other - *Moraxella, Kingella, Branhamella*
Gram positive bacilli:
   Listeria monocytogenes
   Corynebacterium pyogenes
Gram negative bacilli:
   Pseudomonas aeruginosa
   Serratia marcescens
   Salmonella species
   Hemophilus influenzae
   Pasteurella multocida
   Escherischia coli
   Proteus mirabilis
   Klebsiella pneumoniae
   Brucella species
Anaerobes:
   Propionobacterium acnes
   Bacteroides fragilis
   Fusobacterium necrophorum
   Peptococcus and Peptostreptococcus species
   Clostridium species
Spirochetes:
   Borrelia burgdorferi
   Treponema pallidum
Mycoplasma:
   Mycoplasma hominis
   Mycoplasma pneumoniae
   Ureaplasma urealyticum

purulent and with Lyme arthritis, inflammatory fluid is the rule. Bacteria commonly infect the synovium through hematogenous spread from a distant site or occasionally directly from penetrating trauma, iatrogenic joint needling, or an adjacent osteomyelitic focus. Microorganisms may also lead to arthritis by indirect means, such as immune complex formation, molecular mimicry, or unknown mechanisms. Predispositions to septic arthritis are given in Table 2. Rheumatoid arthritis (RA) patients are especially predisposed to septic arthritis because of the systemic illness, the use of immunosuppressive medications, including corticosteroids, and the inflammatory joint damage. Polyarticular septic arthritis occurs in approx 15% of cases of septic arthritis, and is seen with a high prevalence in patients with RA *(4)*. Polymicrobial infections occasionally occur with penetrating trauma and with joint prostheses. *S. aureus* is the

Table 2
Septic Arthritis: Predisposing Factors

- Old age
- Comorbidities: cancer, diabetes, chronic renal failure, chronic liver disease, RA
- Preexistent joint disease: RA, crystal disease, hemophiliac arthropathy
- Penetrating trauma
- Joint aspiration
- Prosthetic joint
- Intravenous drug use
- Immunosuppresssion
    congenital: hypogammaglobulinemia, complement deficiency
    acquired: AIDS, immunosuppressant medication

Table 3
Common Causes of Nongonococcal Acute Bacterial Arthritis

Organism	Approximate prevalence (%)
Staphylococcal aureus	60%
β-hemolytic streptococci	15%
Gram negative bacilli	15%
Streptococcus pneumoniae	5%
Other and polymicrobial	5%

most common cause of nongonococcal septic arthritis and generally occurs in joints that were abnormal prior to infection (arthritis, trauma, prosthesis, and surgery) (Table 3). In contrast, *Neisseria gonorrhoeae* is more likely to infect previously intact joints and otherwise healthy individuals or rarely those with inherited deficiency of the complement components of the membrane attack complex (MAC) (C5-C9) *(5)*. *S. aureus* causes the majority of joint infections in the elderly and in patients with RA.

Bacteria in the synovial membrane induce a cellular and humoral inflammatory reaction by a number of mechanisms including: release of bacterial products: lipopolysaccharide endotoxins (gram negative organisms) or exotoxins (gram positive organisms), cell wall fragments, or bacterial antigens with immune complex formation. This leads to early cartilage loss as a result of proteoglycan breakdown. In the joint-cavity bacterial products activate the complement system and phagocytosing neutrophils release lysosomal enzymes, further enhancing the inflammation and contributing to tissue destruction. With ongoing untreated infection, synovial pannus is formed with further erosion of cartilage and bone. An immune-mediated post-infectious synovitis may persist after eradication of the organism by antibiotics, probably related to the stimulatory effects of the intra-articular bacterial products and the release of neoantigens from cartilage. These infection-induced inflammatory processes in experimental *S. aureus* arthritis can be inhibited by the concomitant use of nonsteroidal, anti-inflammatory drugs (NSAIDs) with antibiotics and this treatment has been shown to lessen cartilage damage and reduce postinfectious synovitis *(6)*. These experimental observations await clinical studies to determine if concomitant use of NSAIDs or even corticosteroids with antibiotics in septic arthritis improves morbidity and prognosis.

Diagnosis

The stereotypical clinical picture of septic arthritis is an acutely painful monoarthritis with a red, hot swollen joint, mainly the knee, and with associated systemic symptoms of chills and fever and a high peripheral white blood cell count. However, atypical presentations are common and depend on the age (atypical in the very young and very old) and demographics of the patient population, the infecting organism, associated systemic illnesses, and coincident treatment such as immunosuppressive drugs, NSAIDs, or inadequate doses of antibiotics. The differential diagnosis includes crystal disease, trauma, and causes of acute inflammatory monoarthritis or oligoarthritis, including Reiter's syndrome and juvenile rheumatoid arthritis (JRA). Infectious arthritis with *Borrelia burgdorferi* (Lyme arthritis) typically presents with an acute or subacute arthritis of the knee. The clinical presentations of disseminated gonoccocal infection (DGI) and culture results are shown in Table 4 *(7)*. The bacteremic phase occurs in 65–70% of patients with DGI and is characterized by fever, migratory polyarthralgia, tenosynovitis of the wrists, hands, ankles, or feet, and a dermatitis with scattered, usually painless, pustular, vesicopustular, or hemorrhagic macular lesions. Septic monoarthritis occurs in 30–40% of patients, most commonly involving knees, wrists, and ankles. The definitive diagnostic test of septic arthritis is synovial fluid aspiration for gram stain and culture. Synovial fluid leukocytosis is a helpful but imperfect test. Counts of over 50,000 white blood cells/mm^3 occur in 70% of patients but "pseudoseptic" fluids may also occasionally be seen with crystal synovitis, RA, and spondyloarthropathies. On the other hand, 10% of patients with proven intra-articular infections may have initial synovial fluid white blood cell count less than 25,000/mm^3 *(8)*. Synovial fluid glucose levels may be depressed (relative to serum levels), but this is neither sensitive nor specific enough to have diagnostic utility. Synovial fluid lactic acid, produced by bacteria and synovial cells, is elevated in septic arthritis but also in other inflammatory arthropathies. However, a normal synovial fluid lactic acid level virtually excludes septic arthritis. In nongonococcal septic arthritis, organisms can be seen on gram stain in 50–70% of cases, more frequently with gram positive than gram negative infections. Synovial fluid cultures generally yield positive results in over 70% of patients and blood cultures are positive in 50%. The use of blood culture bottles (BCB) or isolator tubes (pediatric BCB) may increase the frequency of bacterial isolation *(9)*. Detection of specific bacterial DNA by polymerase chain reaction (PCR) is possible, especially for *N. gonorrhea* and *B. burgdorferi*, which are often synovial fluid culture-negative *(10–11)*. With gonococcal arthritis, the synovial fluid is often in the inflammatory range, with white blood cell counts less than 50,000, rather than frankly purulent fluid. Cultures of mucosal surfaces for *N. gonorrhoeae*—genitourinary, rectal, oropharynx—yield a higher positivity rate than blood or synovial fluid cultures. Thayer-Martin medium and chocolate agar are the culture media employed.

Imaging techniques play a limited diagnostic role in routine cases but may be helpful when infectious arthritis occurs in deep-seated sites such the hip, sacroiliac joints, and spine. Radionuclide scanning is very sensitive but not specific, however, three-phase technetium scanning can help to localize the process to the underlying bone when

Table 4
Disseminated Gonococcal Infection

Clinical picture	Phase	Culture (% positive)
Fever, polyarthralgia, tenosynovitis, dermatitis	Bacteremic	Blood (10%) Synovial fluid (0%)
Septic arthritis	Arthritic	Synovial fluid (<50%)
Asymptomatic mucosal	During either of above	Mucosal surfaces (80%)

Table 5
Infectious Arthritis: Principles of Treatment

- Treatment with parenteral antibiotics; initial choice dependent on clinical situation
- Daily aspiration of accessible joints
- Arthroscopic lavage or open surgical drainage when required
- Monitor clinical response and synovial fluid white blood cell count and culture
- Avoid NSAIDs until diagnosis is confirmed
- Splint extremity for pain relief but institute range of motion exercises in 2–3 d

there is overlying soft-tissue inflammation. Magnetic resonance imaging (MRI) may be especially helpful in the diagnosis of vertebral or sacral osteomyelitis.

Treatment and Outcome

The principles and specifics of treatment are summarized in Tables 5 and 6 *(2,12)*. The initial antibiotic regimen, prior to culture confirmation, will depend on the clinical setting and results of the gram stain. In general, hospitalization and parenteral (intravenous) antibiotics are indicated for suspected septic arthritis. Intra-articular antibiotics are not used because high concentrations are achieved in infected synovial fluid during intravenous administration. Furthermore, direct intra-articular administration may lead to a "chemical" synovitis.

Coverage for *S. aureus* with a β-lactamase-resistant penicillin (methicillin, oxacillin, nafcillin) or cefazolin, or vancomycin for suspected methicillin-resistant *S. aureus* or *S. epidermidis*, is generally indicated until definitive bacteriologic identification is made. Over 25% of *S. aureus* joint infections are methicillin-resistant (MRSA). Vancomycin-resistant organisms can be treated with linezolid (Zyvox), although there are no studies of effectiveness in septic arthritis. If a gram negative organism is suspected (including Neisserial), then a third-generation cephalosporin, such as ceftriaxone or cefotaxime, or in the case of *Pseudomonas aeruginosa*, ceftazidime and an aminoglycoside, should be used. Concurrent treatment for Chlamydial infection with oral doxycycline for 7 d is also recommended for patients with disseminated gonococcal infections. The treatment of Lyme arthritis will be discussed separately. When the bacteriological diagnosis has not been confirmed and empirical antibiotic therapy is being employed, NSAIDs should be avoided in the first week so the clinical response to the antibiotic treatment can be assessed. Pain relief can be effected by narcotic analgesia and by joint immobilization during the acute phase. When signs of inflammation abate, passive followed by active range of motion exercises should be instituted to help prevent joint contractures.

Table 6
Infectious Arthritis: Antibiotic Therapy[a]

Organism	Antibiotic	Alternative	Oral drug
S. aureus S. epidermidis	Nafcillin 2 g q4h iv	Cefazolin 1–2 g q8h iv	Dicloxacillin, cephalexin, Ciprofloxacin-Rifampin (implants)
MRSA	Vancomycin 1 g q12h iv	?Linezolid 600 mg q12h poor iv (Vancomycin resistant)	Clindamycin
Streptococcus sp.	Penicillin G 2 m units q6h iv	Cefazolin	Penicillin V, Cephalexin
N. gonorrhoeae	Ceftriaxone 1–2 g iv daily	Cefotaxime 1–2 g q6–8h iv	Ciprofloxacin, Cefuroxime axetil (+ doxycycline for Chlamydia)
Gram negative bacilli (depends upon susceptibility)	Ceftriaxone 1–2 g iv daily	Cefotaxime	Ciprofloxacin
Ps. aeruginosa	Ceftazidime 1–2 g q8h iv + Gentamicin 1 mg/kg q8h iv/im	Piperacillin 4–5 g q6h iv + Gentamicin	Ciprofloxacin
B. fragilis	Metronidazole Loading dose: 15 mg/kg iv Maintenance: 7.5 mg/kg q6h iv	Clindamycin	Metronidazole, Clindamycin
Other anaerobes	Clindamycin 600 mg q8h iv	Penicillin G	Clindamycin

[a]Adapted from refs. 2 and 12.

Recommendations for the optimal duration of therapy are empirical because there are no controlled studies to provide guidance. In general, for nongonococcal septic arthritis, intravenous therapy is continued for a minimum of 2 wk followed by 2–4 wk of oral treatment. Patients with disseminated gonococcal infection can be treated with parenteral antibiotics for 1 wk if started during the bacteremic phase, but generally 2 wk for infectious monoarthritis. Penicillins and cephalosporins can be safely used during pregnancy. Clinical response of infectious arthritis to antibiotic treatment with defervescence and reduction in joint pain and erythema is usually seen within 2–3 d. Within 5–7 d synovial fluid white blood cell counts should have decreased by 50% and sterility should have been achieved.

In clinically accessible joints, such as the knee, initial closed-needle aspiration followed by daily or alternate-day aspirations (to remove inflammatory products and monitor response to treatment) is preferable to open surgical drainage because of faster recovery of joint mobility. However, initial arthroscopic lavage may result in more complete removal of inflammatory products and yield a better outcome, but this has yet to be confirmed. Arthrotomy with surgical drainage is generally indicated in infections of the hip, especially in children, in those joints that demonstrate loculated pus on initial aspiration, and in patients who fail to demonstrate synovial fluid response (decreased white blood cell count and negative culture) after 5–7 d of appropriate antibiotic therapy. Sterile inflammation with joint effusion may persist for many weeks owing to a postinfectious synovitis.

The risk factors for a poorer prognosis include older age, the presence of comorbid conditions, the presence of a joint prosthesis, and a longer duration of symptoms prior to the institution of treatment. Delay in treatment beyond 7 d leads to incomplete joint recovery in the majority of patients. A recent prospective analysis demonstrated that 50% of patients had preexisting joint disease and 29% of the infected joints had synthetic material. Mortality was 10% and outcome was poor in 33%, especially in those patients who were older, or who had preexistent joint disease or joint prostheses *(13)*.

PROSTHETIC JOINT INFECTIONS

The overall infection rate in total joint replacement is approx 1%, slightly higher for the knee than for the hip *(14)*. However to put prosthetic infections in perspective, only 10% of all hip failures are owing to infection. Bacteria can adhere to the inert solid surface of the prosthetic joint, elaborate polysaccharides to form a glycocalyx, and coalesce to form a protective biofilm, which accounts for persistent infection despite antibiotic therapy and normal humoral and cellular immunity *(15)*. This pathophysiology accounts for the partially suppressive effects of long-term antibiotic therapy with the lack of a durable response and the necessity for removal of the prosthesis to effect a bacteriological cure in most cases.

Early-Onset Prosthetic Infections

Early-onset infections account for 70% of all prosthetic infections and occur within the first 3–6 mo of joint-replacement surgery. They are related to intraoperative and perioperative infection and are most commonly due to *S. epidermidis*, *S. aureus*, gram negative bacilli, or polymicrobial infection. Risk factors for early-onset infections include concomitant systemic illnesses such as RA, concomitant extra-articular infections, the duration of surgery and the operative procedures, and postoperative hematoma formation. These risks have been substantially reduced by giving prophylactic antibiotics just prior to surgery (e.g., cefazolin 1–2 g intravenously) and continued for 1–2 d postoperatively, using antibiotic-impregnated methylmethacrylate cement, and employing clean air systems in operating rooms. Intravenous vancomycin can be used as prophylaxis in hospitals with a high frequency of MRSA or for patients allergic to penicillins or cephalosporins. The clinical manifestations are often suggestive of infection with fever and joint pain and associated erythema, induration and drainage at the incision site. Wound cultures or joint aspiration may yield a microbiological diagnosis.

Late-Onset Prosthetic Infections

Late-onset infections are owing to bacterial seeding of the prosthesis during hematogenous spread. The commonest organisms are *S. aureus* (45%), streptococci (25%), gram negative bacilli (15%), coagulase-negative staphylococci (10%), and anaerobes (5%). Most patients with late-onset infections have a subacute or chronic course with joint pain as the predominant symptom. Radiographs may demonstrate prosthetic loosening, but it should be noted that this can occur without infection. More specific radiologic findings for infection are periosteal new bone formation and severe radiolucency at the prosthesis-bone interface. Radionuclide scanning lacks sensitivity and specificity. Joint-fluid aspiration and occasionally open synovial-tissue or bone biopsy may be needed for definitive microbiological diagnosis of late-onset infection.

Treatment of Prosthetic Joint Infections

Cure rates in patients with prosthetic infections using surgical debridement and antibiotics alone are only 20–30%, although they are higher in those with early-onset infection. Those with late-onset infections resulting in prosthetic loosening will require surgical removal in addition to antibiotics for cure. Thus, treatment of most patients will require removal of the prosthesis, debridement of the joint, a prolonged course of parenteral antibiotic therapy (6–8 wk) and subsequent reimplantation of a new prosthesis employing antibiotic-impregnated cement. This two-stage approach yields a higher success rate, but even under these conditions, the reinfection rate may be very high (10–30%). Initial parenteral antibiotic therapy followed by long-term, oral, suppressive antibiotic therapy with a cephalosporin (e.g., cefazolin) or fluoroquinolone (e.g., ciprofloxacin) may be needed for those unable or unwilling to undergo prosthesis removal. In a recent study, patients with relatively early-onset, implant-related infections (symptoms less than 1 yr) with *S. aureus* or coagulase-negative staphylococci were randomized to receive 3–6 mo of oral ciprofloxacin (750 mg every 12 h) with either oral rifampin (450 mg every 12 h) or placebo. Patients had neither clinical nor radiological signs of implant loosening and prior to oral therapy underwent thorough debridement and 2 wk of intravenous therapy with either nafcillin or vancomycin and oral placebo or rifampin. The implants were left in place. With a median follow up of 33 mo, the cure rate was about twice as high in the ciprofloxacin-rifampin compared to the ciprofloxacin-placebo group *(16)*. Thus, rifampin may be valuable adjunctive therapy in the treatment of early-onset prosthetic joint infections where preservation of the prosthesis is desirable if possible.

Although perioperative and operative preventive strategies as described previously have been shown to reduce infection rates, there is no scientific evidence that antibiotic prophylaxis is needed for patients with joint prostheses undergoing dental procedures. Oral infections however, should be treated promptly and appropriately. Arthrodesis may be necessary in those patients who are unable to have reimplantation because of mechanical factors in the joint.

BACTERIAL ARTHRITIS IN CHILDREN AND THE ELDERLY

The presentation of joint infection in very young children (neonates) is often subtle and therefore presents a diagnostic challenge, especially with septic arthritis of the hip, the commonest joint to be infected. Nonspecific tests such as a very elevated erythrocyte sedimentation rate (ESR) or C-reactive protein (CRP) provide clues to a serious underlying systemic problem, including infection. The coexistence of osteomyelitis and contiguous septic arthritis is not uncommon in children under 2 yr because of metaphyseal-epiphyseal interconnecting blood supply. The frequency of *Hemophilus influenza* arthritis has declined with the introduction of the conjugate vaccine in 1990. *H. influenza* infections can be treated with parenteral cefuroxime (75 mg/kg/d). Infections of the knee, hip, and ankle account for 80% of septic arthritis in children, with gram positive cocci the commonest organisms. Infections of the hip require primary surgical decompression and drainage. Penetrating wounds of the feet can cause infectious arthritis or osteomyelitis, occasionally with *Pseudomonas aeruginosa*. Almost 50% of all adults with nongonococcal septic arthritis are over the age of 60. This likely occurs because of a high frequency of comorbid illnesses, diminished immune function and preexisting joint disease, including joint prostheses. Furthermore, bacteremia in the postoperative period is a commoner cause of septic arthritis in older than younger patients. Like young children, the presence of fever and leukocytosis are insensitive markers of septic arthritis in the elderly, but acute-phase reactants (ESR, CRP) are usually significantly elevated. Antibiotic dose adjustments are needed in these groups. Morbidity with poor functional outcome and mortality is higher in older patients.

BACTERIAL ARTHRITIS WITH OTHER CONDITIONS

Patients with long-standing, erosive, seropositive RA on corticosteroid therapy are particularly prone to septic arthritis and account for a disproportionately high percentage of cases in many series *(3,13)*. Polyarticular involvement is common. The sources of infection include skin ulcers, ulcerated rheumatoid nodules, and wound infections. Patients may present with subacute worsening of joint complaints, mimicking active RA and delaying the diagnosis. Septic arthritis should be considered in any RA patient who develops acutely inflamed monoarthritis or oligoarthritis. Even adequately treated patients suffer a high recurrence rate of joint sepsis and mortality is significant (20–40%), especially with polyarticular infection. Prolonged treatment with oral antistaphylococcal antibiotics (dicloxacillin) may be required to prevent recurrences.

Intravenous drug abusers have many risk factors for septic arthritis or osteomyelitis including the development of soft-tissue infections and transient bacteremias, and the presence of serious cormorbid conditions such as hepatitis and bacterial endocarditis. Surprisingly, septic arthritis is relatively uncommon in patients with AIDS, whereas pyomyositis has been well documented. Septic arthritis and osteomyelitis in drug abusers may occur with atypical organisms such as pseudomonas and other gram negative bacteria and at unusual sites, especially fibrocartilagenous joints (sternoclavicular, costochondral, symphysis pubis) and the axial skeleton (vertebral osteomyelitis, sacroliitis). Systemic candidiasis with costochondral or sternoclavicular joint infection has been described in addicts using contaminated brown heroin. Simultaneous crystal arthropathy, gout or pseudogout, and septic arthritis is unusual but has been described *(17)*. To complicate matters, both gout and pseudogout can cause a pseudoseptic arthritis with fever, leukocytosis and synovial fluid white blood cell count greater than 50,000/mm^3.

LYME DISEASE

Lyme disease (LD) is the most common vector-borne (Ixodes tick) infection in the United States, with 15,000 new cases reported yearly *(18)*. It has focal endemicity with moderate to very high frequencies along the eastern seaboard and in parts of Wisconsin and Minnesota. This illness has protean manifestations including an early acute infection with dermatological, neurological, cardiac, and musculoskeletal features and a late or chronic phase with predominately arthritis in North America. There is also a Lyme-induced fibromyalgia-like syndrome, which may cause chronic musculoskeletal symptoms.

Clinical Features of LD

LD is caused by infection with the spirochete *Borrelia burgdorferi* (Bb). The clinical picture of LD can be classified in stages: early (localized or disseminated) and late. Early LD occurs most frequently from spring through early fall, when nymphal and adult ticks are abundant and feeding. Early localized disease is characterized by an expanding, often asymptomatic, erythematous rash (erythema migrans; EM) starting at the site of the tick bite. It is often accompanied by fever (usually less than 102°F) and a flu-like syndrome characterized by arthralgia and myalgia. These constitutional features may occur without EM but in highly endemic areas, EM is the most common presenting early feature of LD, approaching 80–90%. Early disseminated LD, related to hematogenous spread of Bb, is characterized predominately by involvement of any of three organ systems—skin, nervous system, heart—and includes disseminated EM lesions, facial palsy, meningitis, or radiculoneuropathy, and, rarely, heart block (of any degree). About 20% of patients who present with EM have a disseminated rash. Facial palsy may be isolated or accompanied by subtle or flagrant meningitis and may occasionally be bilateral. Early LD may remit spontaneously, but if untreated, over 50% of patients develop late features, mainly arthritis or neurological involvement (peripheral neuropathy, encephalopathy).

Coinfection with the agent of human granulocytic ehrlichiosis (HGE), a rickettsia-like organism, or with Babesia microti, an intraerythrocyte microorganism, may occur with LD because all three microorganisms use the Ixodes tick as vector *(19,20)*. HGE often presents with an acute illness with high fever, arthralgia, and myalgia. Leukopenia, thrombocytopenia, and high transaminases, which are not features of LD, occur quite commonly with HGE. HGE may be particularly severe and even fatal in the elderly. Thus the rare fatalities attributed to LD may have been related to coinfection. Diagnosis

Table 7
Lyme Disease: Rheumatic Features

Stage	Rheumatic feature
Early	Arthralgia/myalgia
Late infectious	Intermittent arthritis
	Chronic mono- or oligoarthritis
Late "autoimmune"- post-antibiotics	Chronic monoarthritis
Late somatic - post-antibiotics	Arthralgia/myalgia

of both HGE and Babesiosis is best performed by specific polymerase chain reaction (PCR) assays, although antibody testing and thick blood smear for the organisms in granulocytes or red cells, respectively, have also been utilized.

The rheumatic features of LD are shown in Table 7. With early LD, arthralgia and myalgia are common. Over 50% of patients with untreated or incompletely treated LD develop arthritis. Initially, this is an intermittent transient asymmetric mono- or oligoarthritis, appearing within weeks to months after infection. Recurrent joint inflammation may continue over many months, eventually settling into a persistent arthritis in 10% of patients, with large effusions and even Baker's cysts, usually in one or both knee joints. The differential diagnosis includes JRA (children and adolescents), spondyloarthropathy such as Reiter's syndrome, other causes of bacterial arthritis, and crystal arthritis. The synovial fluid is inflammatory and tests for LD are positive (*see* below), so the diagnosis is generally not difficult, especially if a patient lives in or has traveled to an endemic area. Chronic arthritis, which persists after antibiotic treatment, may be related to local autoimmunity *(21)* and chronic arthralgia and myalgia to a post-LD syndrome *(22)*.

Diagnosis of LD

The presence of an EM rash on a patient in an endemic area is characteristic enough that other tests are not needed and treatment may be instituted. Culture of Bb is impractical for routine diagnosis because the organism is slow-growing and it is relatively insensitive. The majority of synovial fluids in patients with Lyme arthritis are culture negative. However, the results of molecular tests for Borrelial DNA sequences by PCR have good sensitivity (>90%) in the synovial fluids of patients with untreated Lyme arthritis *(11)*. Testing for anti-Borrelial antibodies, although an indirect diagnostic technique, is the mainstay of laboratory diagnosis for early and late LD *(23)*. A two-step approach has been recommended: a screening enzyme-linked immunosorbent assay (ELISA) followed, in equivocal and positive cases, by a more specific Western blot test. IgM Western blot testing, which suffers from significant false-positivity rates, is recommended within the first 4 wk of infection when true-positive results are more likely to occur. IgG Western blot testing, which has a very high specificity, can be performed at any time during the course of illness but is much more likely to be positive with disseminated or late-stage LD. Virtually all patients with Lyme arthritis are IgG Western blot positive, making it an excellent diagnostic test for patients in a Lyme-endemic area who present with an oligoarthritis or monoarthritis. Effective treatment for early LD may abrogate an antibody response. Because of high variability from laboratory to laboratory and time to time, serial antibody testing is inadequate as a measure of response to treatment.

Treatment of LD

Evidence-based guidelines for the treatment of LD have recently been published *(24)*. Early localized LD (EM) is generally treated with 2–4 wk of doxycycline 100 mg bid or amoxicillin 500 mg tid (in children ≤8 yr). Doxycycline is also active against HGE. Patients with early disseminated or late disease are usually treated with oral or parenteral antibiotics depending on the severity of illness and the organ system involved. In general, neurological involvement is treated with intravenous ceftriaxone 2 g daily for 4 wk. Isolated facial palsy may be treated with oral antibiotics. Carditis with third-degree heart block may be treated with iv antibiotics initially followed by oral antibiotics when the heart block reverses. Lyme arthritis may be treated with oral antibiotics, followed, if there is no response, by another course of antibiotics, oral or iv. There is no scientific evidence that more prolonged courses of antibiotics alter the course of Lyme disease infection. A chronic inflammatory synovitis, which is PCR-negative, may persist after adequate antibiotic therapy for Lyme arthritis. This may have an autoimmune pathogenesis and thus is generally treated with anti-inflammatory therapy and occasionally synovectomy *(21)*. A small percentage of patients have persistent or recurrent arthralgia, myalgia, and fatigue following LD, despite adequate courses of antibiotics. This is often called post-LD syndrome or Lyme-induced fibromyalgia (FM) *(22)*. The symptoms wax and wane but the overall course is chronic. Objective findings of arthritis are lacking. The treatment of these patients is supportive and symptomatic and includes nighttime amitriptyline or cyclobenzaprine, antidepressant therapy when needed, exercise programs, and coping strategies. A recent controlled trial was unable to detect chronic infection in these patients or to support the use of aggressive antibiotic therapy in its treatment *(25)*.

Prevention of LD

Prevention of LD by the use of antibiotics for asymptomatic individuals with Ixodes tick bites is not recommended, except possibly if the tick is engorged, a sign of feeding for more than 24–48 h *(26)*. However, a recent trial showed that one dose (200 mg) of doxycycline was effective in preventing LD if given within 72 h of the tick bite *(27)*. Otherwise, the incidence of developing either symptomatic LD or asymptomatic seroconversion is very low, equaling the risk of developing a side effect from the antibiotic therapy. A LD vaccine, which utilizes a single recombinant protein—outer surface protein A (OspA)—has been proven to be safe and effective (70–80%) in clinical trials *(28)*. Protective antibody levels decrease quickly after the first two vaccine injections, 1 mo apart, and a booster injection after 1 yr is recommended. It is expected that more booster injections will be required to maintain a protective anti-OspA level.

ACUTE BACTERIAL INFECTIONS
OF OTHER MUSCULOSKELETAL STRUCTURES

Septic Bursitis and Tenosynovitis

Septic bursitis is a common soft-tissue infection *(29)*. The vast majority of cases are post-traumatic, with transcutaneous inoculation of microorganisms into the bursa.

Diabetes, alcoholism, and systemic corticosteroid therapy are risk factors. Involvement of the olecranon and prepatellar bursae account for the majority of the cases. An overlying tissue inflammation or cellulitis is common. In distinction from septic arthritis of the elbow or knee, passive extension is full and pain free. Bursal fluid white blood cell counts are elevated, although lower on average than synovial fluid counts in septic arthritis, and the bursal fluid is not usually purulent. Inoculation of bursal fluid into liquid media (blood culture bottles) may increase the yield of positive cultures *(30)*. *S. aureus* is the commonest cause of septic bursitis and with streptococci account for over 90% of cases. Uncomplicated olecranon bursitis, with little overlying cellulitis, in an otherwise healthy individual may be treated with a course of oral antibiotics (e.g., dicloxacillin or cephalexin) and close follow-up, including repeat bursal aspirations. Treatment should continue until the bursal fluid is sterile, usually 7–10 d. Indications for parenteral therapy include an older or immunocompromised patient, an accompanying cellulitis or systemic symptoms, and prepatellar septic bursitis. The duration of therapy should be about 2 wk. Occasionally septic bursitis may require surgical drainage. An occasional sequela of septic bursitis is a chronically inflamed aseptic bursa, which is cured by bursectomy.

Acute digital flexor tenosynovitis is a true emergency, because delay in treatment will result in tendon necrosis. Patients almost always have a history of a cut or puncture wound on the palmar side of a finger or a chronic hand condition with skin ulceration, such as scleroderma. *S. aureus* and *Streptococcus pyogenes* are the most likely causes. Patients with an acutely inflamed digital tendon sheath should be referred immediately to a hand surgeon for appropriate drainage and irrigation as well as antibiotic therapy. If there is some question about the diagnosis, ultrasonography may be a useful imaging technique *(31)*.

Pyomyositis

Pyomyositis is an acute bacterial infection of muscle, usually caused by *S. aureus*. Although common in the tropics, it was rarely described in temperate climates until the advent of HIV/AIDS *(32)*. The infection is seeded in muscle through hematogenous spread. Patients present with fever, constitutional symptoms, and localized muscle pain. The muscle is tender and indurated, not fluctuant. One or a few muscle groups may be involved, most commonly the quadriceps femoris. Blood cultures are rarely positive but cultures of the muscle aspirate usually reveal the infecting organism. The creatine phosphokinase levels may be normal or slightly elevated and local asymmetric muscle pain, not weakness, is the main clinical feature. Therefore, pyomyositis is easily distinguishable from inflammatory muscle diseases. The diagnosis is made by ultrasound which may show a fluid collection, or more definitively by computed tomography (CT) scan or magnetic resonance imaging (MRI), which show intramuscular inflammation and abscess formation. Treatment requires parenteral antibiotics and drainage of the abscess, if present.

Osteomyelitis

Osteomyelitis is an infection in bone characterized by progressive inflammatory destruction and relative resistance to medical therapy *(33,34)*. Bacteria gain access to bone either through hematogenous seeding, contiguous spread of infection, or direct trauma (compound fractures). Otherwise healthy children are more frequently affected than adults with osteomyelitis after bacteremia and it most commonly involves the metaphysis of the femur, tibia, and humerus. In adults, especially intravenous drug abusers and the elderly, hematogenous infection may involve the axial skeleton—vertebrae, sacrum and sacroiliac joints, symphysis pubis, clavicle and sternoclavicular joints. Diabetic patients with peripheral vascular insufficiency or foot ulcers are especially susceptible to osteomyelitis of the bones of the feet. Prosthetic joint infections as described earlier involve bone and joints. A microbiological diagnosis is critical for appropriate therapy and needle biopsy or open surgical biopsy is generally required. The predominate organism is *S. aureus*, but the clinical situation often dictates other likely organisms, such as *Pseudomonas* in intravenous drug abusers, streptococci or anerobic bacteria in the diabetic foot, *Salmonella sp.* or *Streptococcus pneumoniae* in sickle cell disease, and opportunistic infections and *M. tuberculosis* in immunocompromised patients. Imaging helps to both anatomically localize the infection and to aid in diagnosis. Plain radiographs may be normal, but may also show cortical destruction and periosteal new bone formation, a relatively specific finding. Technetium bone scanning is sensitive for an inflammatory process, but not specific for infection. CT scanning can identify the extent of bone edema, inflammation, and destruction, the presence of necrotic bone (sequestra), and the surrounding soft-tissue involvement. MRI is best for detection of spinal infection. Acute osteomyelitis, especially when caused by hematogenous spread and when treated early, may be cured with parenteral antibiotics alone. The principles of therapy are to employ the appropriate parenteral antibiotics in adults for 4–6 wk. For *S. aureus* infections, there is some evidence that a higher cure rate is obtained when rifampin is added to standard anti-staphylococccal regimens. Children may be treated with a shorter course of parenteral antibiotics followed by several weeks of oral therapy. Chronic osteomyelitis, by definition, is refractory to medical treatment and requires surgical debridement with removal of necrotic bone, in addition to appropriate antibiotic therapy. Therapy with fluoroquinolones, with or without rifampin, given for some months, has been used to suppress the symptoms and signs of chronic refractory osteomyelitis, as in the diabetic foot.

CHRONIC OSTEOARTICULAR INFECTIONS

Osteoarticular tuberculosis

With the advent of HIV, the incidence of tuberculosis (TB) and the frequency of extrapulmonary TB have risen dramatically. Skeletal TB occurs in approx 3–5% of cases *(35)*. Osseous infection with *M. tuberculosis* typically occurs during hematogenous spread, either with primary infection or after many years with late reactivation. Spinal osteomyelitis with seeding to the vertebral bodies is the commonest skeletal manifestation of TB. Joint involvement may occur secondary to hematogenous spread or from a contiguous focus of tuberculous osteomyelitis. The clinical syndromes associated with osteoarticular TB are shown in Table 8. Although pulmonary involvement (abnormal chest X-ray) is found in only 30% of patients with skeletal TB, the tuberculin skin test is positive in almost all immunocompetent patients. Tuberculous spondylitis (Pott's disease) accounts for 50% of all osteoarticular TB *(36)*. Soft-tissue extension from the anterior vertebral bodies with abscess formation may occur, resulting in pressure on neurological structures. If left untreated, cord compression with paraplegia can be the

Table 8
Osteoarticular Tuberculosis: Clinical Syndromes

- Spondylitis (Pott's disease)
- Tuberculous arthritis
- Extraspinal osteomyelitis
- Tenosynovitis
- Poncet's disease

outcome. However, most cold abscesses respond to chemotherapy and do not require surgical drainage. Tuberculous sacroiliitis can also occur.

Tuberculous arthritis usually presents as an indolent monoarthritis of a weight-bearing joint, especially the knee, occasionally with mild constitutional features *(37)*. Adjacent osteomyelitis may be present. While the synovial fluid is inflammatory and TB cultures may be positive, the diagnosis is best made by synovial biopsy where histology shows a granulomatous synovitis and acid-fast stains and culture are more likely to be positive. Prosthetic joint infections with *M. tuberculosis* can rarely occur *(38)*. Tuberculous osteomyelitis generally involves the long bones in adults and may be multifocal, especially in immunocompromised patients. Dactylitis of the metacarpals and phalanges owing to TB has been described mainly in children. Tenosynovitis of the wrists and hands can mimic other infectious as well as noninfectious causes of tendonitis. Poncet's disease is a "reactive" polyarthritis, mainly hands and feet, in the setting of active TB, which resolves with antituberculous therapy. Treatment of osteoarticular TB is by combination chemotherapy, usually for 12–18 mo: isoniazid 5 mg/kg/d po to a maximum of 300 mg/d, rifampin 10 mg/kg/d po to a maximum of 600 mg/d. Pyrazinamide 25 mg/kg/d po to a maximum of 2 g/d is also used in the first 2 mo *(2)*. Articular infections with atypical mycobacteria, especially *M. marinum*, *M. kansasii*, and *M. avium intracellulare*, may occur with a predominance of arthritis and tendonitis in the hands and wrists. Definitive diagnosis is often delayed and treatment usually requires combination chemotherapy and surgical debridement.

Fungal Arthritis

Fungal musculoskeletal infections, especially osteomyelitis and arthritis, often create diagnostic difficulties because of a lack of clinical suspicion *(38)*. Candidal organisms can cause arthritis by hematogenous spread in intravenous drug abusers or in seriously ill, immunosuppressed, hospitalized patients with indwelling vascular lines, by direct intra-articular inoculation and by infection of prosthetic joints. Acute monoarthritis, especially of the knee, can be seen with Candida, whereas most other fungal infections cause an indolent chronic monoarthritis. Treatment with parenteral fluconazole is as effective and less nephrotoxic than amphotericin B. The optimal dose and duration of therapy have not been the subject of randomized controlled trials. Systemic candidiasis in a non-neutropenic patient is usually treated with fluconazole 400 mg poor iv daily or amphotericin B 0.7 mg/kg iv daily for a minimum of 2 wk. General characteristics of arthritis caused by other fungi including coccidioidomycosis, sporotrichosis, blastomycosis, cryptococcosis, and histoplasmosis are: chronic monoarthritis, mainly

Table 9
Virus Infections Associated with Arthritis

Virus	Mechanism	Frequency of arthritis
Parvovirus B19	?IM	C
Rubella	DI	C
Alphaviruses (arboviruses)	?IM	C
Chikungunya		
O'nyong-nyong		
Ross River (epidemic polyarthritis)		
Other		
Hepatitis viruses		
Hepatitis A	?	U
Hepatitis B	IM	C
Hepatitis C	IM	U
Retroviruses		
HTLV-1	DI	U
HIV	?	C
Other		
Mumps	?	U
Echoviruses	?DI	U
Varicella-Zoster	?DI	U
Epstein-Barr	?DI	U
Adenovirus	?	U

DI, direct invasion-culture of virus from synovium or detection of viral DNA/RNA by PCR; IM, immune-mediated, viral antigen/antibody in serum and/or synovial fluid; C, common; U, uncommon.

of the knee; coexistent pulmonary and skin involvement; diagnosis best made by staining and culture of synovial tissue. Amphotericin B is the drug of choice for invasive fungal infections. It is generally given at a dose of 0.5–1.0 mg/kg/d iv. Duration of therapy is generally for 4–6 wk. Synovectomy may also be required. Amphotericin B frequently induces renal tubular injury, resulting in a lowered glomerular filtration rate with resulting azotemia and metabolic abnormalities, including hypokalemia, hypomagnesemia, and hyperchloremic acidosis. Other preparations—amphotericin B colloidal dispersion (ABCD) and liposomal amphotericin—appear to be effective antifungals with a lower risk of nephrotoxicity.

VIRAL ARTHRITIS

Although arthralgia commonly accompanies many viral infections, arthritis is a well-recognized feature of but a few viral illnesses *(39)*. Table 9 lists the viruses that may be associated with arthritis, some commonly and others rarely. The mechanism of the arthritis accompanying viral infections is direct invasion for a few, immune complex formation for many and unknown for some. The arthritis often occurs during the viral prodrome, at the time of the rash. Viral arthritis is generally characterized by the sudden onset of symmetrical small- and medium-joint pain and stiffness with or without joint swelling (RA-like), lymphocytic/monocytic joint fluids, and a self-limited, nondestructive course. Treatment is generally symptomatic with anti-inflammatory agents.

REFERENCES

1. Weinstein, A. 2000. Musculoskeletal infections, in Educational Review Manual in Rheumatology. R. Lahita, A Weinstein, editors. Castle Connolly Graduate Medical Publishing, New York, pp. 1–24.

2. Fung, M.F. and J.S. Louie. 1995. Infectious agent arthritis, in Treatment of the Rheumatic Diseases. M.H. Weisman, M.E. Weinblatt, editors. WB Saunders, Philadelphia, pp. 321–334.

3. Pioro, M.H. and B.F. Mandell. 1997. Septic arthritis. *Rheum. Dis. Clin. North Am.* 23:239–258.

4. Dubost, J.J., I. Fis, P. Denis, R. Lopitaux, M. Soubrier, J.M. Ristori, et al. 1993. Polyarticular septic arthritis. *Medicine* 72:296–310.

5. Wurzner, R., A. Orren, and P.J. Lachmann. 1992. Inherited deficiencies of the terminal components of human complement. *Immunol. Rev.* 3:123–147.

6. Smith, R.L., G. Kajiyama, and D.J. Schurman. 1997. Staphylococcal septic arthritis: antibiotic and nonsteroidal anti-inflammatory drug treatment in a rabbit model. *J. Orthop. Res.* 15:919–926.

7. Goldenberg, D.L. 1997. Bacterial arthritis. *Curr. Opin. Rheumatol.* 6:394–400.

8. Krey, P.R. and D.A. Bailen. 1979. Synovial fluid leukocytosis. *Am. J. Med.* 67:436–442.

9. Ike, R.W. 1998. Bacterial arthritis. *Curr. Opin. Rheumatol.* 10:330–334.

10. Liebling, M.R., D.G. Arkfield, G.A. Michelini, M.J. Nishio, B.J. Eng, T. Jin, and J.S. Louie. 1994. Identification of Neisseria gonorrheae in synovial fluid using the polymerase chain reaction *Arthritis Rheum.* 37:702–709.

11. Nocton, J.J., F. Dressler, B.J. Rutledge, P.N. Rys, D.H. Persing, and A.C. Steere. 1994. Detection of *Borrelia burgdorferi* DNA by polymerase chain reaction in synovial fluid from patients with Lyme arthritis. *N. Engl. J. Med.* 330:229–234.

12. The Medical Letter. 1999. The choice of antibacterial drugs. 41:95–104.

13. Kaandorp, C.J.E., P. Krijnen, H.J.B. Moens, J.D.F. Habbema, and D. Schaardenburg. 1997. The outcome of bacterial arthritis. A prospective community-based study. *Arthritis Rheum.* 40: 884–892.

14. Tsukayama, D.T., R. Estrada, and R.B. Gustillo. 1996. Infection after total hip arthroplasty. A study of the treatment of one hundred and six infections. *J. Bone Joint Surg. (Am).* 78:512–523.

15. Costerton, J.W., P.S. Stewart, and E.P. Greenberg. 1999. Bacterial biofilms: a common cause of persistent infections. *Science* 284:1318–1322.

16. Zemmerli, W., A.F. Widmer, M. Blatter, R. Frei, and P.E. Ochsner. 1998. Role of Rifampin for treatment of orthopedic implant-related staphylococcal infections. *JAMA* 279:1537–1541.

17. Baer, P.A., J. Tennenbaum, A.G. Fam, and H. Little. 1986. Coexistent septic and crystal arthritis. *J. Rheumatol.* 13:604–607.

18. Nadelman, R.B. and G.P. Wormser. 1998. Lyme borreliosis. *Lancet* 352:557–565.

19. Nadelman, R.B., H.W. Horowitz, T.-C. Hsieh, J.M. Wu, M.E. Aguero-Rossenfeld, I. Schwartz, et al. 1997. Simultaneous human granulocytic ehrlichiosis and Lyme borreliosis. *N. Engl. J. Med.* 337:27–30.

20. Krause, P.J., S.R. Telford, A. Spielman, V. Sikand, R. Ryan, D. Christianson, et al. 1996. Concurrent Lyme disease and babesiosis. *JAMA* 275:1657–1660.

21. Gross, D.M., T. Forsthuber, M. Tary-Lehmann, C. Etling, K. Ito, Z.A. Nagy, et al. 1998. Identification of LFA-1 as a candidate autoantigen in treatment-resistant Lyme arthritis. *Science* 281:703–706.

22. Bujak, D.I., A. Weinstein, and R.L. Dornbush. 1996. The clinical and neurocognitive features of the post Lyme syndrome. *J. Rheumatol.* 23:1392–1397.

23. Tugwell, P., D.T. Dennis, A. Weinstein, G. Wells, B. Shea, G. Nichol, et al. 1997. Laboratory evaluation in the diagnosis of Lyme disease. *Ann. Intern. Med.* 127:1109–1123.

24. Wormser, G.P., R.B. Nadelman, R.J. Dattwyler, D.T. Dennis, E.D. Shapiro, A.C. Steere, et al. 2000. Practice guidelines for the treatment of Lyme disease. *Clin. Infect. Dis.* 31(Suppl. 1):S1–S14.

25. Klempner, M.S., J. Evans, C.H. Schmid, G.M. Johnson, R.P. Trevino, D. Norton, et al. 2001. Two controlled trials of antibiotic treatment in patients with persistent symptoms and a history of Lyme disease. *N. Engl. J. Med.* 345:85–92.

26. Sood, S.K., M.B. Salzman, B.J.B. Johnson, C.M. Happ, K. Feig, L. Carmody, et al. 1997. Duration of tick attachment as a predictor of the risk of Lyme disease in an area in which Lyme disease is endemic. *J. Infect. Dis.* 175:996–999.

27. Nadelman, R.B., J. Nowakowski, D. Fish, R.P. Falco, K. Freeman, D. McKenna, et al. 2001. Prophylaxis with single-dosed doxycycline for the prevention of Lyme disease after an *Ixodes scapularis* tick bite. *N. Engl. J. Med.* 345:79–84.

28. Sigal, L.H. 1999. Lyme disease and the Lyme disease vaccines. *Bull. Rheum. Dis.* 48:1–4.

29. Canoso, J.J. and P.R. Sheckman. 1979. Septic subcutaneous bursitis: report of sixteen cases. *J. Rheumatol.* 6:96–102.

30. Stell, I.M. and W.R. Grandsen. 1998. Simple tests for septic bursitis: comparative study. *BMJ* 316:1877.

31. Jeffrey Jr., R.B., F.C. Laing, W.P. Schechter, R.E. Markison, and R.M. Barton. 1987. Acute suppurative tenosynovitis of the hand: diagnosis with US. *Radiology* 162:741–742.

32. Wildrow, C.A., S.M. Kellie, B.R. Saltzman, and U. Mathur-Wagh. 1991. Pyomyositis in patients with human immunodeficiency virus: an unusual form of disseminated bacterial infection. *Am. J. Med.* 91:129–136.

33. Haas, D.W. and M.P. McAndrew. 1996. Bacterial osteomyelitis in adults: evolving considerations in diagnosis and treatment. *Am. J. Med.* 101:550–561.

34. Lew, D.P. and F.A. Waldvogel. 1997. Osteomyelitis. *N. Engl. J. Med.* 336:999–1007 .

35. Evanchik, C.C., D.E. Davis, and T.M. Harrington. 1986. Tuberculous arthritis of peripheral joints: an often missed diagnosis. *J. Rheumatol.* 13:187–189.

36. Nussbaum, E.S., G.L. Rockswold, T.A. Bergman, D.L. Erickson, and E.L. Seljeskog. 1995. Spinal tuberculosis: a diagnostic and management challenge. *J. Neurosurg.* 83:243–247.

37. Garrido, G., J.J. Gomez-Reino, P. Fernandez-Dapica, E. Palenque, and S. Prieto. 1988. A review of peripheral tuberculous arthritis. *Semin. Arthritis Rheum.* 18:142–149.

38. Harrington, T.J. 1998. Mycobacterial and fungal arthritis. *Curr. Opin. Rheumatol.* 10:335–338.

39. Smith, C.A. 1990. Virus-related arthritis, excluding human immunodeficiency virus. *Curr. Opin. Rheumatol.* 2:635–641.

Index